BOSTON MARATHON

Year-by-Year Stories of the World's Premier Running Event

Tom Derderian

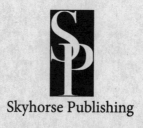

Skyhorse Publishing

Skyhorse Publishing books may be purchased in bulk at special discounts for sales promotion, corporate gifts, fund-raising, or educational purposes. Special editions can also be created to specifications. For details, contact the Special Sales Department, Skyhorse Publishing, 307 West 36th Street, 11th Floor, New York, NY 10018 or info@skyhorsepublishing.com.

Skyhorse® and Skyhorse Publishing® are registered trademarks of Skyhorse Publishing, Inc.®, a Delaware corporation.

Visit our website at www.skyhorsepublishing.com.

10 9 8 7 6 5 4 3 2 1

Library of Congress Cataloging-in-Publication Data is available on file.

Cover design by Tom Lau
Cover photo credit: Victah Sailer

Print ISBN: 978-1-5107-2428-0
Ebook ISBN: 978-1-5107-2429-7

Printed in the Canada

Dedicated to those who tried and tried again

A Boston Ballad
To get betimes in Boston town I rose this morning early,
Here's a good place at the corner, I must stand and see the show.

The Runner
On a flat road runs the well-train'd runner,
He is lean and sinewy with muscular legs,
He is thinly clothed, he leans forward as he runs,
With lightly closed fists and arms partially rais'd.

Walt Whitman, "By the Roadside 1854," from *Leaves of Grass*

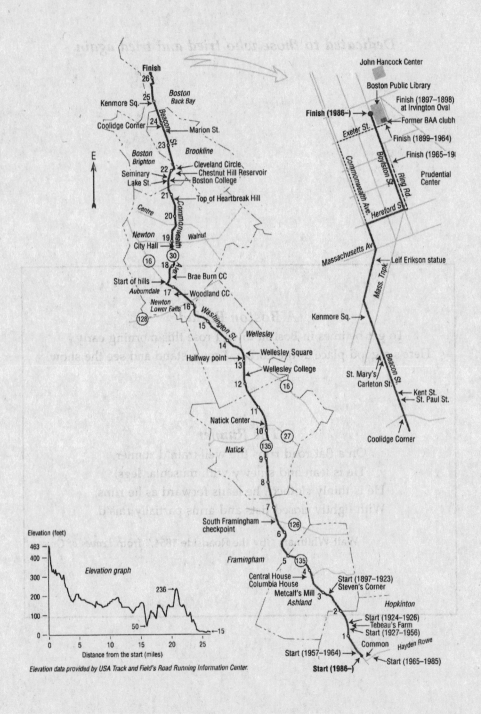

Finish
26
25 ← Kenmore Sq.
Boston
Back Bay
24
Coolidge Corner — Beacon St.
Marion St.
23
Boston
Brighton
Brookline
22 — Cleveland Circle
Seminary — Chestnut Hill Reservoir
Lake St. — Boston College
21
Top of Heartbreak Hill
20 — Commonwealth Ave.
Centre
Newton
City Hall 19 — Walnut
30
(16) 18
Start of hills — Brae Burn CC
Auburndale 17 — Woodland CC
Newton
Lower Falls 16 — Washington St.
(128) 15
Wellesley
14
Wellesley Square
13 — Wellesley College
Halfway point
12
(16)
11
Natick Center
10 — (27)
Natick (135)
9
8
7
South Framingham — (126)
checkpoint 6
5 — (135)
Framingham
Central House 4 — Start (1897–1923)
Columbia House Steven's Corner
Metcalf's Mill 3
Ashland Hopkinton
2 — Start (1924–1926)
Tebeau's Farm
Start (1927–1956)
1
Common
Start (1957–1964) Hayden Rowe
Start (1986–) — Start (1965–1985)

E ↑

John Hancock Center
Boston Public Library
Finish (1897–1898)
at Irvington Oval
Finish (1986–) — Former BAA clubh
Exeter St. — Finish (1899–1964)
Finish (1965–19
Commonwealth Ave. — Boylston St. — Ring Rd. — Prudential Center
Hereford S
Massachusetts Av — Leif Erikson statue
Mass. Tpk.
Kenmore Sq.
St. Mary's
Carleton St.
Kent St.
St. Paul St.
Coolidge Corner — Beacon St.

Elevation (feet)
463
400
300 — Elevation graph
236 →
200
100
50 →
← 15
0 5 10 15 20 25
Distance from the start (miles)

Elevation data provided by USA Track and Field's Road Running Information Center.

Contents

Forewords

I've enjoyed listening to Tom Derderian's running stories since our first meeting at a road race in the early 1970s. As a matter of fact, I think it was Tom's own story and his enthusiasm for running that in part motivated me to train for my first Boston Marathon in 1979.

It has always been a treat to run with Tom, because he can make long training runs fly by with his seemingly endless store of running and racing stories. Whether we are running, carbo-loading, or watching over our young children, Tom continues to share with me countless running tales, stories with a special emphasis on his favorite event, the Boston Marathon. His memories of runs, races, and running-related gatherings are always vivid and on the mark. Tom has truly given all of us a gift in writing *Boston Marathon: The First Century of the World's Premier Running Event*. He is a student of the sport and an authority and historian of the Boston Marathon.

Perhaps the most special memories of my first run and win at Boston in 1979 are those of having dinner at Tom's house the night before the race. As he prepared plates of pastas and sauces for his running friends, Tom recounted Boston Marathon lore from the early years right up to his current prerace strategy, which he hoped would make him competitive the next day among the elite athletes in the 83rd running of the marathon. Tom Derderian's knack for describing competitors' personalities, styles, and careers is extraordinary. In *Boston Marathon*, it is almost as if Tom gives each of us our own pair of running shoes to race beside the leaders from year to year, decade to decade. After reading Tom's book, everyone will want to head to Boston, to run or to cheer.

Joan Benoit Samuelson
*Two-time winner of the Boston Marathon and gold medalist
in the first Olympic women's marathon*

It is a special honor to be writing this foreword for *Boston Marathon: The First Century of the World's Premier Running Event*, not only because I know and respect Tom Derderian as a writer and runner, but especially because of his ability to focus on what is most important in the race—the human side. This book is no dry statistical tome; it is alive in the same way the Boston Marathon is.

If you have ever been to the Boston Marathon, you know the excitement, energy, and goodwill that surround this special event. Of course, what makes Boston a unique race, different from the marathons in New York City and London and Tokyo, is its old age—it has been run every year since 1897 over nearly the same course.

Being a marathoner himself, Tom Derderian is aware that the center stage must be for the athletes themselves, and rightly so! Tom details the lives of the men and women who have made Boston the best marathon in the world. They are a particularly hardworking group. What I enjoy most in the book is seeing the similarities of the athletes of 50 and more years ago to the present-day runners—how they all became obsessed with the Boston Marathon and kept coming back year after year.

To be honest, I believe there are few sweeter victories in sport than winning Boston. When you read Tom's book, you will see how hard these athletes tried to make that dream come true. There are some touching stories and some outrageous ones. Tom doesn't shy away from the real story of the Boston Marathon, noting political and social events of each decade and the trends that changed the race over time.

I have always felt that the marathon is the king of sports. And certainly Boston is the king of marathons. Tom's book is unique. There is nothing like it. He makes you feel as if you're at the race itself, running for victory.

Bill Rodgers
*Four-time winner of both the Boston Marathon
and New York City Marathon*

Foreword to the 2017 Edition

By Amby Burfoot, 1968 Boston Marathon winner, Writer-at-large, *Runner's World*

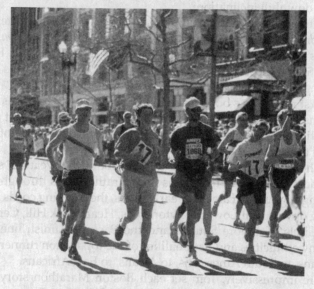

I can't prove that reading about the Boston Marathon will add some sizzle to your long runs and your marathon racing at Boston. But I think it's almost a guarantee. That's why I'm so excited about Tom Derderian's update of his classic Boston Marathon history book.

I've got one year to go before the 50th anniversary of my Boston win in 1968, and I want to be as fit as a creaky 71-year-old can be on that occasion. Which means I'll have to put in a regular dose of training miles—the kind of focused effort that takes a lot of motivation.

Since the beginning of my marathon-running career in the mid-1960s, I've used books and articles about the Boston Marathon to inspire that training. The strategy always worked well in the past, and I'm counting on it to keep me going in the future.

I must have almost a dozen Boston Marathon books on my office shelves. The first I remember reading was a little pamphlet-type thing put together by famed *Boston Globe* writer Jerry Nason. His obvious respect for the Boston Marathon and its participants literally thrilled me. We were so unappreciated by everyone else, particularly the newspaper types, in those early days.

I would say the same about Joe Falls's classic 1977 book, *The Boston Marathon*, the first to find itself behind the hard covers that denote a serious book (unless you're counting Clarence DeMar's autobiography, which is also in my office). Falls was a noted baseball writer, but enamored of both the super-talented and wonderfully zany marathoners who showed up every April in Hopkinton.

Three years later, a *Runner's World* editor, Ray Hosler, gathered a series of essays, reports, and fact sheets together to provide a deeper, more technical insider's view of Boston. I remember my wonderment at seeing a topographical map of the treacherous Boston course. Really? How could such a difficult route have such a downhill inclination?

Once my friend and longtime running rival Tom Derderian entered the Boston-Marathon-book field in 1994 with his 600-page *Boston Marathon: The History of the World's Premier Running Event*, the race was essentially over. His book became the definitive Boston story, a rank it has held ever since. This new edition will only lengthen Tom's lead over all other contenders.

When I first read Tom's book more than two decades ago, I was stunned. So was everyone else I talked to. Most road race histories are content to provide a list of race winners and their times, with just a few biographical notes about the champs and their staunchest rivals.

Tom reached so much higher. He told us about the weather, so critical in marathon races. And about the towns the marathon runs through, along with the course highlights: the careening early miles, the cheering coeds at Wellesley, the crushing downhill at Lower Newton Falls, Heartbreak Hill, Cemetery Mile, Cleveland Circle, Kenmore Square, and the Back Bay finish line. He delved into the many ethnicities and nationalities of the top Boston runners, Indians to Scandinavians, to South Americans, to Asians, to East Africans.

Even more impressively, Tom set each Boston Marathon story against the historical epoch in which it happened. The world changes. There are global and regional wars, the *Titanic* and other vessel sinkings, civil rights movements, feminist revolutions, moon landings, economic challenges, political trends, and much more. Somehow Tom managed to bring these into his narratives about every April's Boston Marathon. The overall effect is a telling of Boston Marathon history that leaps off the pages. It feels almost cinematic in its color and energy.

The last two decades have brought many highs and lows to the Boston Marathon, and in this new edition Tom continues to weave together the whole Boston story, and not just isolated anecdotes. Yes, top runners have apparently used drugs. Yes, the bombings of 2013 rocked the Boston Marathon to its (fortunately very strong) core.

Most importantly, more runners than ever before have found their way to Hopkinton, particularly more women. The modern Boston Marathon promotes women's running as actively as it fought to deny women in the 1960s and early 1970s when calcified regulations stood in the way.

And then you've got the 2014 Boston Marathon. We've all got the 2014 Boston Marathon, even those runners who weren't lucky enough to secure a race number.

For almost 20 years, I had been telling people that the 1996 Centennial Boston was the greatest single footrace in the history of humankind. Of course, the 2014 Marathon outstripped the Centennial and all other races by a wide margin. The day was gorgeous; the fans loud, supportive, and far greater in number than any other year; and we runners were fully aware that we were lucky to be on the roads from Hopkinton to Boston.

We also realized that we had a responsibility: to reclaim the Boston Marathon from the fear of terrorism. We understood that we had to run with courage and resilience. And so we did, all 35,000 of us.

The result, on April 21, 2014, was the greatest, most celebratory road race in history. There will never be another day to match it. I simply can't imagine it.

Similarly, there won't be another Boston Marathon book to match this fully updated treasure trove. Tom Derderian has set the standard by pouring his soul (and seemingly infinite research skills) into the book you are holding.

It's big, but you don't have to read it all at once. I find myself dipping back into it at many different times—wherever I want to learn more about a particular Boston Marathon or a historical running figure.

Read it year by year, or however you choose. And then enjoy the lightness and exuberance of your next training run. That's what I'll be doing.

Foreword to the 2017 Edition

By Shalane Flanagan

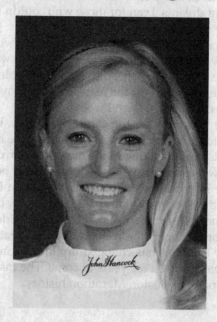

Obsession and heart break. The Boston Marathon is both to me.

I watched my first Boston marathon from the corner of Hereford and Boylston. Pressed up against a metal railing, waiting impatiently, counting hundreds of tired, but joyful, runners passing by . . . I was trying to spot my favorite runner: my dad. He was running in the 100th Boston Marathon.

On this day in 1996, at age 15, I decided that one day I too would run Boston. Growing up only 16 miles north of the city, the only thing New Englanders would talk about on Patriots Day was the Boston Marathon. This is where my obsession began. Watching my father in blissful agony run down Boylston Street towards the finish line made me so proud. I knew I wanted to become part of this thrilling historic event and part of the marathoning club.

In high school I met Tom Derderian through my father. Many times we would have dinner at his house with his amazing family. Tom was always a supportive mentor when it came to my running. Most poignantly, when he wrote an article defending and supporting my aggressive racing tactics in high school. At the time, some were critical of my kamikaze racing because it yielded some heartbreaking moments. His words of support at the time were critical, and just what a young girl needed. To not fear failure and to go all in when you have big dreams. Tom has never wavered in his support throughout my running career.

Since 1996, the sport of running has grown wildly. There have been many changes on the elite level, including the dominance of East Africans and, unfortunately, drugs. My goal of just running the marathon quickly changed over the years to trying to win the Boston Marathon. My best Boston race, and one I am most proud of, was in 2014, the year after the horrific bombings. I ran with the nation's hopes and dreams. I ran for those who couldn't. I ran with so much purpose and love for my city.

I ran the marathon in 2:22.02. The fastest an American woman has ever run it. Normally, this time would win all but a few Bostons and would have even won the men's race on occasion. But on this day, I was only able to attain 6th. After I crossed the finish line, wiped away the tears, collected myself, I told reporters, "I don't wish it were easier. I just wish I were better."

I believe everyone who runs Boston can relate to this. We are all constantly working to give Boston our best because it demands the best from us. My obsession with Boston is heartbreaking in the most wonderful way. I know that if I ever win Boston it will change my life. I would forever be a Boston Marathon champion. But more importantly, a Bostonian who won Boston. I relentlessly train, chasing down the opportunity to change my life by becoming part of history and bringing a nation of runners along the joyous ride with me.

Thank you Tom for capturing and celebrating the greatest road race. Thank you for going all in. This race has changed my life. Runners across the world will be reading *Boston Marathon* for years to come. The inspiration within fuels us to write our own piece of Boston Marathon history.

Why They Come Back to Boston

Many of the things most people spend their lives pursuing do not exist. So it is with the perfect painting, poem, man or woman, the perfect wave for surfers, the perfect ice for skaters, the perfect performance for musicians, the perfect erotic experience for lovers, the perfect wood for a cello, or the perfect marathon for runners. Marathon winners want to run faster, and record setters fear someone might break their record; they want to come back to try again. Perfection? Not yet. The possibility exists to do it better; let me try it just one more time. Male, and later female, winners and near-winners of the Boston Marathon came back time and again. This was their artistic pursuit. They came in pursuit of the unicorn, the beast that does not exist.

The unicorn is the symbol of the Boston Athletic Association (BAA), the originator and current manager of the Boston Marathon. The unicorn appears on all uniforms of the BAA running club and on the medal given to the winner of the marathon. The unicorn is a creature of myths that say it has the legs of a buck, the tail of a lion, the head and body of a horse, and a single horn—white at the base, black in the middle, and red at the tip—in the middle of its forehead. The body of the unicorn is white, the head red, the eyes blue. The unicorn symbolized the power of things good. The unicorn was a common symbol in Scotland. The Scottish brought track and field to America in the 19th century with their Caledonian games. Perhaps they brought the unicorn symbol as well.

There is an element of whimsy to the unicorn. A popular Irish song has it that the reason there are no unicorns in the world today is that as the rains began to fall and Noah loaded his ark, the two silly unicorns frolicked and forgot to get on board. Marathon runners are like that—frolicking and forgetting in a perpetual youth to get on board with the burdens of life. Some of the men and women we will meet in this story are like frolickers who never grow up and will not anticipate rain. They are hopeful people, some of whom meet tragic ends while others defy aging in their pursuit of the unicorn.

According to the legends of the Middle Ages, one could catch the unicorn only by placing a virgin in its haunts; upon seeing the virgin, the creature would lose its fierceness and lie quiet at her feet. But it could be that the unicorn, like permanent victory, can never be possessed, and if captured, never held. Like virginity, the very value in it is the losing of it.

Gerard Cote, four-time winner and dozen-time loser of the Boston Marathon said, "If I am beaten the next time I run, I do not mind. If you have a salad that is all one thing, all lettuce, it is not good. It has no flavor. So victory, always, would be flat. You must mix it with defeat to gain the flavor.'' This book is a history of the men and women who time and again tasted victory and defeat in the Boston Marathon.

I believe that there is something inherently good and noble about the Boston Marathon. It has given extraordinary purpose to people whose lives might otherwise have been tedious. There is a religious purity, as well as piety, to the pursuit. A pagan rite of spring is manifest in the outstretched hope of small children who lift their hands to touch the passing marathoners. The Boston Marathon has opened the wealth of the world to some and a wealth of worldliness to others. The Boston Marathon continues to symbolize what Bostonians, and Americans generally, think is important beyond the necessities of everyday life. The style of life of participants comprises all of America's instincts, from puritanism to the work ethic to fanaticism to the recent hedonistic get-fit-stay-young-live-forever cult of those who exercise to look pretty.

We can see in the Boston Marathons over the past century a reflection of the changes in the average person's hopes, heroes, and dreams. The marathon filled different needs in the minds of the public. The ways the Boston Marathon has been important to the public have changed as well. When the public needed heroes, the Boston Marathon provided them, and when the public needed empowerment—the delicious notion that anyone can overcome time and distance to finish a marathon, the New Age idea that there is a god within—the Boston Marathon was there. During World War I a military relay from Hopkinton to Boston replaced the marathon. The relay stupidly and vaingloriously mixed patriotism and propaganda with athletics. It failed at both. When the public needed a feminist statement, there in 1967 was Jock Semple, dead-center in the viewfinders of press cameras shoving Kathrine Switzer. Reconciliation came 5 years later when Jock, welcoming women to the marathon, gave Switzer a notorious kiss in clear view of more press cameras.

Changes in politics, the arts, demographics, economy, technology, and the temper of the times influenced the competitors and can be seen here in this history of the Boston Marathon. If there is a political attitude throughout this book, it is that the pursuit of something unattainable is an object of art—and a world full of such dreamers is the way the world should be. The runners who tried and tried again are the artists in this particular sense, who in their pursuit of the Boston Marathon have affirmed that there is something wholly different between human beings and all the other animals of Earth. Perhaps humans are the only animals who know that they will die and so while living do more than sustain themselves; they live with a rush and a fury.

Each April a new hero rushes out to greet and celebrate life and its consequences as the flowers rush out to welcome spring. I have done that rushing and furious greeting. I have never emerged the hero, but I have touched those hopeful, outstretched hands of children. I started with the marathon at the youngest age and it has shaped me.

I came to glimpse the unicorn, according to my parents, 6 weeks after my birth and in every following year of childhood as our family went to watch the start of the marathon each Patriots' Day on the Hopkinton town common. When you lived in the next town you did that. As a child on my father's shoulders all I cared about was getting a balloon, which I held tightly. The runners waited behind a snow fence. I saw numbers pinned to their chests, motion, music, bright colors. The runners walked out of their cage to the starting line. Once or twice the starting gun startled me and I lost my balloon. All the bright-colored runners ran away. I could see their backs going down the hill. I did not know where they were going, if they were chasing something or being chased. My balloon floated up into the sky. Everything moved out of reach, quieted and disappeared. I was little. I cried.

'Rejoice. We conquer!'

What was running like in America before the Boston Marathon? To understand Boston we must be able to hold in our minds at least a snapshot understanding of America itself, its view of itself in the world, and then of running in America before the first Boston race in 1897. The first major running events in America were professional and highly promoted. In 1844 four English runners challenged a field of 32 Americans over 10 miles for a prize of $1,000. Between 25,000 and 30,000 people turned out to watch an unheralded American Indian named John Gildersleeve upset the favorite, John Barlow. These runners were fast even by today's standards. Later that year Barlow ran 54:21 for 10 miles to win $1,400 in a rematch.

The Scottish seemed to have brought organized running competition to the New World. The Boston Caledonian Club held their first games, a tradition carried to Boston by Scottish immigrants, in 1853 in Boston. The games included a 3-mile running race and other track and field–type events like caber tossing.

Certain writers in the decade of the 1850s waged the literary campaign known as the Muscular Christianity Movement; its most famous book, *Tom Brown's School Days*, by Thomas Hughes (1857) documented the athletic phenomena of the day. Until the 1870s organized running competitions had not been common except among the ancient Greeks, but elite schools such as Harvard, Yale, and Amherst quickly picked up the Caledonian types of competitions. These became track and field.

"The Caledonians were actually preceded by other professional runners in the United States, and their foot races and walking contests had been common during the first half of the nineteenth century. Participants in this activity that became known as pedestrianism, like John Barlow of England, Thomas Jackson (alias the

American Deer), George Seward of New Haven, and Louis Bennett (a Seneca Indian known everywhere as 'Deerfoot') provided goodly wages in their time for crowds of thousands."

These pedestrians were professional runners who came from classes lower than the low classes who paid to watch them and bet for their favorites. "In America the runners, who were (not surprisingly) usually poorer than the spectators, were very often blacks and American Indians." The pedestrians of the late 1800s followed a "go-as-you-please" rule that allowed them to run, walk, rest, eat, drink, skip, or crawl over the distance. Edward Payson Weston went as he pleased over the 1,326 miles from Portland, Maine, to Chicago in 25 days to earn $10,000.

Six-day indoor track races established a benchmark for brutality in the 1880s when runners struggled to the exhortations of spectators who had bets riding on them to continue day after day and lap after lap for nearly a week. The 6-day record for 1888 was 623.75 miles in New York's Madison Square Garden.

Show biz, hype, and a lack of standards marked early pedestrianism and long-distance racing. Ultimately those aspects, public boredom, and the eternal suspicion of a "fix" by the bettors who lost money killed the sport/business of long-distance racing. What replaced it?

Amateur (no wagering) collegiate track and field began in America in 1876. It arose in part because of an industrial-age desire for precision in measuring and comparing performances. Colleges like Harvard, Yale, Amherst, Wesleyan, and Bowdoin took part. These were upper class institutions whose members had the leisure to participate in sports while the mass of the population worked from sunup to sundown in factories or on farms. So it should come as no surprise that a Harvard track man was the first to take the lead in the Boston Marathon—the first to go in pursuit of the unicorn.

The BAA started in 1887, wealthy, opulent, and big. It had a five-story clubhouse on Exeter Street in Boston's newly created, land-filled, prestigious Back Bay. The Back Bay used to be a salt marsh—a stinking fen of mudflats at low tide—until it was filled in with soil carved from the top of Beacon Hill. The club had tennis courts, racquet courts, Turkish baths, a bowling alley, and a running track. Its members included the Adamses, Saltonstalls, Cabots, and Lodges—as the old saying goes, "Boston: the home of the bean and the cod, where the Lowells talked to the Cabots and the Cabots talked to God."

The Amateur Athletic Union (AAU) of the United States established itself the following year, on January 21, 1888. The AAU and the BAA would determine the form of the Boston Marathon.

In the early years of the marathon, only a very few strong and durable young men contested the BAA's marathon. There were few other marathons, and none of equal notoriety. In those days the movers and shakers, Boston's wealthy, the scions of the codfish aristocracy, returned from their African

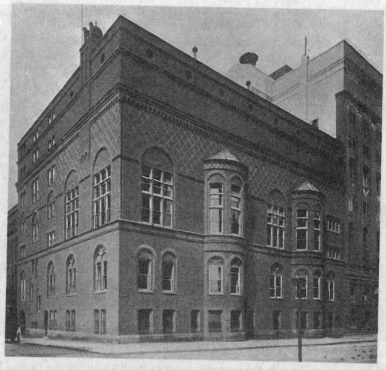

The BAA clubhouse, completed in 1888, was an opulent palace for athletics, complete with swimming pool, indoor track, Turkish baths, bowling alley, boxing room, tennis courts, barbershop, and a wine and cigar department. Courtesy of the Boston Athletic Association.

safaris to smoke and talk about the hunt in dark-paneled rooms with stuffed animal heads poking out of the walls. It was into just such a room that Jack Caffery, a Canadian laborer and teamster, wandered looking for the BAA officials after he finished the marathon of 1900. Those old founders never dreamed that Africans would come to Boston almost 100 years later to win their marathon.

The old money came from the Yankee traders dealing in rum, sugar, and slaves. Some money came from the profits of whaling—creating the oil barons of the day—and Yankee trading in clipper ships. The Boston aristocracy did not directly govern, but through their wealth they set the tone, pace, and style of Boston. Their sons and the sons of their friends were most of the U.S. team for the first Olympics in Athens in 1896. No Olympic committee paid their way. Thomas E. Burke of the BAA won the 100- and 400-meter races. Teammate Ellery H. Clark won the broad jump and the high jump. James B. Connolly of South Boston won the hop, step, and jump. In 1896 Boston was Olympic track and field in America, and the BAA team was the most powerful on earth.

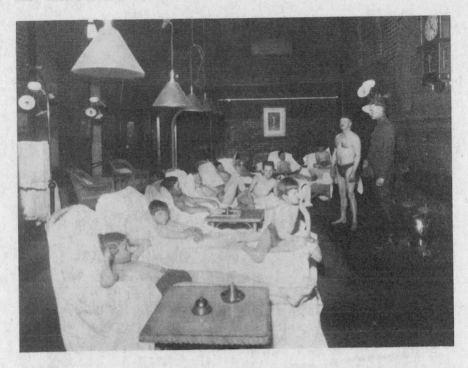

A soldier instructs boys in the lounging room of the BAA clubhouse during World War I. Courtesy of the Boston Public Library, Print Department.

The old Boston Yankees—the Brahmins on Beacon Hill, Protestant descendants from Puritans—watched as wave after wave of Catholic Irish, up to 1,000 a month, flooded Boston. The guard would change forever—the Kelleys were coming! The old guard founded the AAU in 1888. In part they attempted to keep working people out of athletics by eliminating any way of making a living through the sport. For clear reasons, athletics, and principally footraces, corrupted easily. Footraces, like horse races, attracted flimflam men and crooks. People bet on races, and some of the runners, out of necessity or greed, "fixed" their races. Enforced amateurism—regulated sport for the love of the sport—was intended to prevent those abuses. But amateurism also worked to keep sport aristocratic against the growing forces of popularism. It kept women out. The opposing ideas of professional running and amateur running have remained in conflict for the entire history of the Boston Marathon.

In the late 1800s people planned public relations events worldwide for the first time. The communications technology had never existed before. These new events planned for the public and media came without precedent in traditional religious or cultural rituals and customs. The village market day had given way to the county fair and then quickly to world's fairs and expositions. The first modern Olympic Games really had no precedent. The ancient Greeks could only attend local events; the fresh idea of a worldwide Olympic Games appealed to the world of 1896. The elite and 10-year-old BAA set out in imitation of the Olympics with a marathon of its own.

Where did that marathon idea come from? The Greeks had no race in their ancient Olympics longer than about 3 miles. They raced in the stadium between two poles. They ran barefoot over soft sand. At the turns they could push, pull, and trip each other or kick sand in the face of the following runner.

The Greeks, however, did employ intercity messengers who ran long distances splendidly. These were skinny, tough, wiry professionals. The Greeks did not see road-running messengers as athletes. They toiled anonymously. They had no nobility and did not possess the classic mesomorphic features that the ancient Greeks saw as athletic. There may have been hundreds of runners with the ability to run sub-3:00 marathons, but they were no more athletic heroes than are letter carriers today. Pheidippides was such a toiler.

Supposedly Pheidippides ran 24 hilly miles from the Battle on the Plains of Marathon on a summer's day in BC 490 to announce that the Athenian

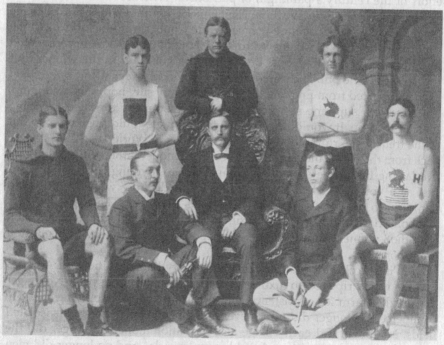

Most of the first USA Olympic team were BAA athletes: standing (from left), Thomas E. Burke, T.P. Curtis (trainer/manager), Ellery Clark; seated, W.W. Hoyt, S. Paine, John Graham, J.B. Paine, Arthur Blake. Courtesy of the Boston Public Library, Print Department.

army, outnumbered six to one, had killed 6,400 invading Persians and driven the rest into the sea. Pheidippides staggered into the ruling chamber and shouted, "Rejoice. We conquer!" then dropped dead.

As researched by Sandy Treadwell in *The World of Marathoners*, Richard D. Mandell in *Sport, A Cultural History*, and others, the historian Herodotus recorded everything else about the battle, but no dying messenger, no "Rejoice. We conquer!" Herodotus was too good a reporter to miss such a story. He did write about a Pheidippides who ran 150 miles in 48 hours to Sparta to recruit their help. But it is unlikely that Pheidippides made the marathon, then died. He was, however, a great runner, a great patriot, but not, in the Greek sense, a noble athlete.

The confusing story comes from the melding of the Battle of Marathon to an event reported by Plutarch a half century later. Plutarch wrote of a messenger named Eucles who ran to Athens to announce victory and then died. Eucles, not Pheidippides, proclaimed, "Rejoice. We conquer!" Time compresses and neatens history when necessary to generate an essential myth.

In the 19th century every cultured European student knew the neat, compressed story of Pheidippides's sacrifice. The idea of the supreme glorious effort fit the century's paradigm of patriotism. When Frenchman Baron de Coubertin decided to revive the ancient Greek Olympic Games, his colleague Michel Breal at the Sorbonne persuaded de Coubertin to include a 24-mile run from Marathon to Athens. At first the thought of such an unprecedented long race seemed outrageous. Breal offered a gold cup to the winner. But the press and the public cheered the idea of a local Greek event rather than events imported from England like the apparently silly hop, step, and jump. The idea of a supreme sacrifice for God and Country appealed to young men at the time. It would be this same feeling that would push men up out of the trenches to run into death by the millions in World War I. To stagger back from the battle and shout, "Rejoice. We conquer!" then die would grant everlasting life in the eyes of his compatriots to a young Christian soldier. Just as a young Moslem soldier killed in Jihad—holy war—would go to paradise, to die for God and Country was the ideal. The marathon race symbolized that 19th-century ideal. In 1914 that ideal killed one Boston Marathon winner just a few days after he would have defended his Boston Marathon title.

Only in the closing years of the 19th century had conditions in America and the world ripened so luxuries like marathons could appear. No longer did families farm for subsistence with occasional barter supplying the only commerce. No longer did nearly every man bend over a hoe in his isolated fields. No longer did each village face starvation alone. No longer did the only power come from animal and human muscle. And no longer did men regard physical warfare—life-and-death fighting with an ax, spear, sword, lance, or bow, man against man—as the only worthwhile athletic competition.

The growing industrialization yielded an agricultural surplus. In America the frontier closed. Rails ran from sea to sea. Steam power replaced sailing ships, powered by a hundred athletic men climbing up and down the rigging. The volume and value of international trade increased. The rifle and cannon equalized men in warfare. As the trigger finger replaced the muscled body of the trained warrior, a soldier could be killed by a man he never saw.

For more people than ever, life became less harsh and more healthy at the end of the 19th century. Personal hygiene became popular. People bathed. The marathon began in 1897 during a time of transition, when personal hygiene hadn't been a widespread American habit. In fact, through much of U.S. history cleanliness was inconvenient or religiously proscribed. Colonial America leaders deemed bathing impure, since it promoted nudity, which could only lead to promiscuity. Laws in Pennsylvania and Virginia either banned or limited bathing, and for a time in Philadelphia, anyone who bathed more than once a month faced jail. Americans lived in wretched filth and many died of associated diseases.

In such an environment no one would be inclined to train for running or be able to do so. In 1700 in a society fearful that any exposure of leg would promote promiscuity, you could not run far down the public road in short pants. The sensually iconoclastic poetry of Walt Whitman heralds the transition to a respect for the human body as a source of joy and wonder from a condemnation of it as a repository of original sin. Not since the early Christians closed the ancient Roman baths—which the BAA clubhouse of the late 1800s came to resemble—had people cared enough about their bodies to keep them clean.

In addition to hygiene, economic progress granted just enough convivial leisure time for the masses to pursue sport—a prerogative for centuries taken only by royalty and the landed aristocracy. High society granted high status to sport, but only for those already of high status. In the 1870s as machines freed more common men from lives of backbreaking labor, the notion of sport for the masses boomed.

By the closing years of the 19th century, people developed great optimism that reason, science, and technology could make life physically better than it had been in all of humanity's time on earth. No longer did most men and women have to accept the lot they felt God gave them, to toil on earth, then rest only in the afterlife. As technology allowed the novel notion that life on earth could be improved, strange things began to happen. Clipper ships sold ice cut from New England ponds to India and China. Captains brought back wonderful artifacts from the East and later raw materials like molasses and rubber from distant colonies. Only by virtue of higher living standards could an activity as nonessential as long-distance running begin. A sporting event, no matter how recreational or entertaining, is not divorced from the larger society around it but instead is shaped by the same forces of change that act on the surrounding society. Those changes are reflected in the Boston Marathon and are in turn reflected by it. Those years shortly before the first

Boston Marathon in 1897 seemed like a pivot around which the world turned forever into a different economic, environmental, and political future.

The Boston Marathons run in 1897, 1898, and 1899 were not little, humble affairs but big sporting news in Boston. The newspapers reported their results on the front page. In the first decade of the 20th century, marathoners became major sports heroes in the world. They were the explorers, test-pilots, and astronauts of their era, boldly running where none had run before, and, in their perceptions and the public's, risking their lives and future health to do it. One cigarette company offered cards picturing marathon runners in every pack. The public lined the course to bet large sums on the outcome of the race and to watch whether any of the participants would actually drop dead from exhaustion.

The ideal of sacrifice would change with the decades. The reasons for running changed as the times and the men changed. "Rejoice. We conquer!" followed by death sounds a bit extreme to those of us who now run for fun. But it did not sound extreme to marathoners in the first decades of this century, who believed that a marathon "used a man up" and that any more than one marathon would permanently damage health.

The BAA and the city of Boston changed as the world changed. The first decade of the 20th century saw a sharp increase in marathon participants in what we could call the first running boom, only to drop off in the second decade. The first World War had caused the replacement of the marathon with an odd military relay. The Great Depression of the '30s wiped out the opulence of the club; throughout those years a few diehard old men held it together with shoestrings and athletic tape. The World War II years saw a record low in participants but high public interest; the race offered a contrast to the gruesomeness of war. And unlike during World War I, the race was not cancelled. Slowly it grew again. Numbers reached 200 and more again in the 1950s, at last matching some years in the 1920s. All these changes became apparent in the fortunes of Boston marathoners; they will be visible through the human narrative of this book.

From a not-so-humble beginning in a city that has the audacity to think itself the hub of the universe, the Boston Marathon rose and kept step with a country that became an industrial giant, survived two global wars to become the dominant nation on earth, and then twisted in the turmoil of two undeclared wars. As the relative international power of the United States declined, the Boston Marathon reflected that decline and stultified under the double burdens of neglect and the principle of amateurism. Suddenly in the mid-1980s it sank from an event of worldwide importance to a mere local road race. Their marathon was a small part of the BAA's original activities in 1897, but by 1985 the marathon granted the only glory that remained, and many observers predicted a quick death for the BAA and its race. Ownership of the marathon nearly passed into the hands of a man many claimed to be a crook. In 1986 the marathon rallied under the recognition of its marketing power and the worldwide dominance of American culture.

Bigger and bigger sponsors lined up to support the race, and by 1990 the marathon had money to give away. Ten thousand runners came, and the BAA found a $10-million sponsor. The Boston Marathon changed in nearly 100 years from an elite oddity to an elaborate, perhaps monstrous celebration of the industrial age's achievement principle. Now the Boston Marathon moves toward its 100th running to drive the public relations image of a financial giant, John Hancock Financial Services.

The Boston Marathon has traditionally been run every year on Patriots' Day, April 19, but since the 1960s it has been on the third Monday in April. Patriots' Day is a Massachusetts holiday that celebrates the 18th-century rides of Paul Revere and William Dawes through Lexington and Concord. Longfellow and Emerson wrote fanciful poems about those beginning days of the Revolutionary War. It would be neat if the marathon followed the route of Revere and Dawes, but it never did. By the late 1800s, Patriots' Day had become a day of spring celebration, parades, and sporting events. Principal among sporting events were footraces.

Each year the Boston Marathon has filled the minds of Bostonians and touched people in the rest of the country and the world. It is the biggest one-day press event in the world, yet little more has been recorded than the compiled summations of a few odd newspaper reports in one old book and bits and pieces in several others. Because the marathon happens in the flicker of one day, the public cannot see how the personalities and motivations of the individual athletes change during the year. Each marathon has a season, but the season and the dreams and tribulations of its contestants are mostly hidden. The story of the Boston Marathon, from its patrician beginnings to its pluralistic present, is a saga that spans the last century of American history. Until I collected it, most of the human stuff of the Boston Marathon was locked in the minds and attics of a few moribund men. Each contestant wanted something. The pursuit of the Boston Marathon provided the most exciting parts of the lives of dozens of men, men and later women who without the race would have led more ordinary lives. My intention in this book is to tell the stories I have found about what each wanted and how badly he or she wanted it.

I wanted to set this information down in a durable context before the memories die with the men and their attic memorabilia is lost to estate sales. The offices of the Boston Athletic Association had no complete records or files. Photographs of old Boston Marathons are rare and becoming rarer. There was no curator of the collective Boston Marathon memory. I hope this book will be that curator. As I have found it, here is the whole story.

Research Notes

The Boston Athletic Association itself had no archives and no complete race results from earlier than the 1980s, so old Boston newspapers supplied most factual information for this book. Because of the urgency with which they are produced, newspapers are often inaccurate or inconsistent in details, like the spelling of names and assignments of affiliation. From year to year they did not always report the things I wanted to know, such as the number of entrants or checkpoint times. Some years they reported runners' affiliations, other years just cities or states. (See Appendix B for a list of runners' affiliations. There affiliations are listed as acronyms and appear in italics in each year's results.) The more important errors are corrected in subsequent newspaper editions, but details like checkpoint times are not; I read all the Boston newspapers for several weeks before and after each year's marathon. Often biographical details surfaced in prerace or follow-up stories. Before the 1950s Boston had half a dozen daily papers, and most of them had both morning and evening editions. The spellings of runners' names, diminutives, initials, club affiliations, and residences often varied from year to year. I have attempted to be accurate and consistent, but sometimes I had to just choose what I hoped was correct.

Books proved to be more dependable, but until DeMar wrote his in 1937 there were none. Magazine articles provided a level of detail and accuracy not available in newspapers, but very little appeared in magazines before the 1970s. The *Long Distance Log* and *Distance Running News* in the 1960s offered only short articles. Later running magazines became a rich source.

Personal interviews with old runners produced a great deal of material, much of which conflicted with the details produced by another old runner's personal recollections. I found runners to be utterly unreliable when it comes to facts about races in their distant past unless they have newspaper clippings or their training logs in hand. Interviews were, however, a splendid way to capture anecdotes, attitudes, and relationships.

After becoming a runner in high school I ran the first of my 14 Boston Marathons in 1967, and I can testify personally to many of the events over the last 25 years. Throughout the 1970s I got to know most of the contenders as friends, teammates, training partners, or fellow competitors. I draw heavily on those memories and relationships.

In the race results I have included the top finishers along with other regulars, former winners, consistent contenders, interesting characters, and a few finishers from far back in the pack to indicate just how many runners ran under a certain standard in a given year. Winners (past and future) always appear in bold in the results.

I wish I had the time and the resources to discover the livelihoods and longevity of many of the earlier winners. Where I learned these facts I have included them. What ultimately happened to the winners from 1897, 1902, 1903, 1904, 1906, 1908, 1909, 1910, 1912, 1913, 1916, 1919, 1920, 1949, 1952, and 1958? Do you know? Perhaps I can find out by the next edition.

Introduction

Death in the Eye

Defiance of death gave birth to the first Boston Marathon in 1897, but as the decades passed, the reasons morphed to mirror the needs of the times. We may have come full circle to return to the original reason why we run—to look death in the eye. This update edition brings the story of the marathon full circle, back to its beginnings after an orbit of 120 years.

In the beginning, Baron de Coubertin seized on the idea of the marathon footrace as a culmination of the first modern Olympics, not because the ancient Greeks ran marathons (they did not) but because of the idea of a race in tribute to Pheidippides. After fighting in the battle on the Plains of Marathon, Pheidippides ran to the city of Athens to shout, "Rejoice, we conquer" (over the invading Persians), then dropped dead. The act, or the myth, crystalized the ideal of every young man at the end of the 19th-century sacrificing to the ultimate for country. Big countries needed young men to fill their armies, so the marathon acted as recruitment in a 19th-century world where battles could be won by charging the enemy line on foot or horseback.

The marathon served to symbolize that privilege of sacrifice for a concept larger than oneself or one's family, farm, or village.

The world had lingered on the fate of Dorando Pietri as he had staggered into the 1908 Olympic marathon stadium in London clearly in the lead. But he could not run on his own to the finish line. Officials carried him. Other officials later disqualified Pietri for being carried. He languished for days in the hospital with telegraphed reports tapping worldwide worrying about whether he would live or die. (He lived.)

The Great War, as WWI was called, was an industrialized war. At its start, military commanders expected battles to be won by long marches followed by running assaults by men on foot or horseback to engage the enemy in hand-to-hand combat. Winning sent the losers running for safety. By the end of the war, muscles and human endurance did not matter because war had become mechanized. Muscles mattered little against machines and, in fact, killed one Boston Marathon winner.

After the 1914 Boston Marathon, the symbolism became real. Jimmy Duffy, a jovial Canadian born in Ireland who moved to Canada to work as a stonecutter in Toronto, won the marathon over Eduard Fabre, a champion snowshoe racer, also from Canada. But the next June, when war broke out in Europe, Canada allied with England and joined the fight. So on April 22, 1915, Jimmy Duffy received orders and with his unit sprinted out of the trenches. A German flare lit up the night sky as German machine-gun emplacements fired and killed Jimmy Duffy in full sprint. He died running.

The war canceled the 1918 Boston Marathon, replacing it with a relay among teams from various American military units. As years passed, men older than military age ran the marathon year after year with vigor. People watched the marathon and wagered on it. Military attachments faded in favor of sports entertainment.

After all the death suffered by WWI the world moved away from sacrifice, and the marathon, although still looked upon as a risky business, took more of its risk from the business of gambling. The roaring 1920s with a rampant increase in wealth looked at the marathon as a big and increasingly popular game. After the stock market crash, the marathon became a vehicle in the 1930s for young men to demonstrate their ability to work hard and get a job. Marathons still had a death-defying ring, but mostly because young men running them had not trained very well and looked quite sickly after running for several hours. Running couldn't be good for you, was the thinking. That began to change through the fifties when such people as cardiologist Dr. Paul Dudley White, who was President Dwight Eisenhower's physician, advocated exercise to prevent heart attacks. Gradually the public accepted the notion that a person could run not only to train for competition but also to achieve good health. The meaning of "death defying" changed to maybe premature "death postponing." The marathon became a race for older men, but men only.

Women got the right to vote in 1920, Gertrude Ederle swam the English Channel in 1926, and Amelia Earhart flew an airplane solo across the Atlantic in 1932, but no women tried to run the Boston Marathon until 1966, in concert with the movement against the Vietnamese War. You could say she came in peace. Her running may have been the pivot away from the marathon as a celebration of a mass muscle warfare.

In 1973, conscientious objector Jon Anderson won the Boston Marathon. In 1980, Bill Rodgers, another conscientious objector, spoke out against Jimmy Carter's insistence that the U.S. not go to the Moscow Olympics because the Russians had invaded Afghanistan. A phone call made to the Bill Rodgers Running Center from an American terrorist said that Rodgers would not make it alive past Coolidge Corner. There it was: world politics comes to the Boston Marathon.

Then the numbers of runners began to grow. The marathon changed as people ran in a personal affirmation regardless of their placing in the race. Every finisher became a winner. The epitome seemed to be when people wore their names on the shirts as if they were their own cheer leaders—or branded products. In following years it changed again, but still kept bits of all its previous incarnations. People began to run for something outside of competition and self-aggrandizement: to bring recognition to something greater than themselves and to raise money to fund research to cure diseases. Then came the terrorist bombings of 2013.

Small groups could not build mechanized armies so they made bombs at home out of cookware. They could be deployed anywhere and for any reasons the makers could image. They did not follow a national agenda but a personal one, with effects just as deadly to its victims.

The bombings brought the marathon full circle back to its origins as something symbolic in the face of an enemy. Marathon runners and spectators became vulnerable to attack. This new warfare no longer targeted young men, but by its indiscriminate nature terrorism made everyone a soldier. Thus the essence of Boston Strong made everyone a foot soldier in the tradition of Pheidippides risking death to fulfill a duty.

Now the point is made, the circle is complete. The Boston Marathon is not a fragile line serving a few. Boston is now strong pulling all together, united. Pheidippides would rejoice in the closing of the circle. Yet of course young men came to Boston to race. To compete. To be the best. For that, they had to feel they deserved to win.

Only in the 1950s did the notion that running and exercise were good for health come into play. The sixties and seventies saw the marathon become a means to express the political importance of women and older runners and running as artistic pursuit of self-expression. The notion of the expansion of the self continued throughout the 1980s as the marathon became more popular, and the concept of sacrifice for a larger idea than one's self-improvement nearly vanished.

The advent of running to raise money by getting friends and family to donate to a specific charity in the 1990s and beyond took the idea of running to a different purpose. Some degree of selflessness tried to manifest itself but lost to a coming self-indulgence of Facebook-style self-aggrandizement. But the bombings have changed all that. The marathon has again become dangerous. In two flashes we saw that we must bind together to be strong. The marathon has again become an event that defies death. The marathon has come back to its origins as a symbol to unite people in a struggle for their identity. It may no longer be the emerging national state powered by industrial corporations, but perhaps memorialized in the words of eight-year-old Boston Marathon bombing victim Martin Richards: "No more hurting people."

Do we really want to call attention to the crimes that occurred on Marathon day? We want to wish away the bombings and all the ways they made us feel. We don't want to feel angry, afraid, vengeful, violated, or depressed. Do we have a choice? When death stares at you, don't you have to stare right back and run forward?

We may want our marathon to be fun and a celebration of springtime and not defined by a defiance of death provoked by the bombing. We are bolstered by over 120 years of running in the defiance of death.

Chapter 1

1897-1909
The First Marathon Runners

Presidents: *William McKinley, Theodore Roosevelt, William H. Taft*

Massachusetts Governors: *Roger Wolcott, Winthrop Murray Crane, William L. Douglas, Curtis Guild, Jr., Eben S. Draper*

Boston Mayors: *Joshia Quincy, Thomas Norton Hart, Patrick Andrew Collins, Daniel A. Welton, John Francis Fitzgerald, George Albee Hibbard*

1890 Populations: *United States, 62,979,766; Massachusetts, 2,238,947; Boston, 450,000*

1900 Populations: *United States, 76,212,168; Massachusetts, 2,805,346; Boston, 560,892*

Between 1897 and 1909 the U.S. and the world saw an American president shot and killed; work start on the Panama Canal; the suppression of the "Boxer" rebellion in Peking, China; Jack London write *Call of the Wild*; and the Wright Brothers fly the first airplanes (though the idea of flight for anything except entertainment did not ignite until the Great War in 1914). The changing world was still making its changes slowly.

Horses were everywhere in 1900. There was even a ubiquitous species of bird that flourished on the grain spilled around stables. Few of these birds can be found today. Horses pulled surreys, farm wagons, buggies, cabs, and delivery wagons. Paved surfaces were rare. Country roads had three tracks in them instead of two, the middle track made by the horse. In the whole of the United States were 8,000 registered automobiles. Many people had never even seen a car. Some who came to run the Boston Marathon saw more automobiles during the course of the race than they had during the course of their entire lives. Automobiles were the playthings of the sporting and adventurous rich, including those who liked to cruise alongside the marathon runners.

Without the automobile, radio, television, or airplanes, the world loomed a gigantic but largely irrelevant place—the lives of most Americans remained unaffected by events more than a few miles from their homes. News from Russia or Japan disturbed no one. Any insecurities remained local rather than global. Considerable financial and health problems faced the average person, but they were local problems, understandable if not solvable. There had never been a world war. No intercontinental ballistic missiles waited docile but omnipotent in submarines and silos, and no one had heard of the ozone layer.

Frederick Lewis Allen, in his book *The Big Change: America Transforms Itself 1900-1950*, noted that women of the era carried yards and yards of cloth in their daily garments. Their athletic talent lay concealed beneath layer upon layer of underpinnings—chemise, drawers, whalebone corset, and petticoat. The ideal woman, swathed not only in silk and muslin but in innocence and propriety, stayed sheltered, and the ideal man, whether a pillar of rectitude or a gay dog, virtuously protected the person and reputation of such tender creatures as were entrusted to his care. The men wore shirts with high stiff collars, and runners' shorts came down to their knees.

There were no hot showers for runners in winter, no refrigerators to keep drinks cold in summer. From autumn to spring there were no fresh fruits or vegetables. There was no orange juice in 1900. Baths were customarily taken once a week. There were no bathrooms, only outhouses. Imagine the runner's life in 1900—freezing in the privy before your winter morning run, then cold and clammy, afterward, knowing you'd have to wait until Saturday night to take a bath! Runners often ran in bicycling shorts and shoes, unyielding cowhide that had to be broken in with saddle soap and sweat until, if a runner was lucky, it conformed itself to the lumps and bumps of his foot. The shoes had no heels, and the soles gave no traction. (Women, of course, ran very rarely. We won't see women running in the Boston Marathon for another 70 years.)

In 1900 Andrew Carnegie's income from owning his steel company was $23 million—with no income tax to pay. Anyone with an income of $10,000 could live in a house full of servants, but the average wage of the American worker was only $400 or $500 a year.

Health care, even for the very rich, lacked technology. Doctors could do little more than demonstrate good bedside manners while their patients either recovered or didn't. By 1990s standards, private life for most in America at the turn of the century was quiet, simple, and harsh. It was believed that a man had the capacity in his body to run but one marathon, and that at peril to his longevity. Yet marathon running became hugely popular in this decade, as men like Jack Caffery, Tom Longboat, Tom Hicks, John Hayes, Alf Shrubb, and Dorando Pietri became household names. More people participated in marathon running in the 15 years before the Great War than in the 15 years after. One could consider 1900 to 1909 as the first running boom.

Boxing bouts at the Boston Athletic Association ring at the Exeter Street clubhouse attracted 200 members, most of whom placed bets on their favorites. The first marathon, scheduled to finish outside, would attract 25,000 spectators and more bets. Wagering drove the sport of marathon racing.

THE START AT METCALF'S MILL

MONDAY, APRIL 19, 1897

18 Men to Race Today in 'Marathon'

Monday, April 19, 1897, 12:15 p.m. Tom Burke dug his heel into one side of the hard and narrow dirt road in front of Metcalf's Mill in Ashland, Massachusetts. He dragged his heel to the other side of the road and stood there, about 25 miles west of the Boston Athletic Association track on Irvington Street in the Back Bay. As the double gold medalist sprinter from the first modern Olympic Games held in Athens the previous year, Burke was the most celebrated member of the association. Thus came to him the distinction of starting the runners in a new kind of race in America, a marathon. There had been only one other in the country. Burke drew the line without ceremony; the race needed a starting line and he had his boots on. Burke called out numbers for 18 men, 15 answered and stood next to the scuffed line. Burke had no gun. At exactly 12:19 he shouted "Go!" to start the BAA marathon.

Officials of the BAA observed the race with pride, knowing they had created something important. Reporters from all the Boston newspapers had come to watch. Burke and the BAA's John Graham had arrived with the reporters by the 9:12 train from the B & A Railway station on Boston's Kneeland Street. That Monday morning Patriots' Day train from Boston to Ashland bulged with the wheels and equipment of the Company B, Second Regiment and the ambulance corps, both of whom would accompany the "peds" along their route by bicycle to see to their needs.

Graham had represented the Boston Athletic Association when he attended the Olympic marathon, the world's first, in Athens in 1896. The appeal of long-distance racing centered on its danger. The ancient Greeks had no marathon or any such long race in their Olympic Games, but every American and European schoolboy had heard of the sacrifice of Pheidippides, the Greek soldier who, it was told, ran from the Plains of Marathon to Athens to announce the Greek victory over the invading Persians, and then dropped dead. The lesson was obvious: Someday you too may be called to sacrifice for your country. So the Olympic Games had to have a long race.

That first modern Olympic marathon was won by a Greek water carrier named Spiridon Louis. It ran from the Plains of Marathon through the flat village of Nea Makri past Rafina along the Pendeli hills up a 7-mile climb into the Hymettus hills then down 6 miles and into the new 50,000-capacity marble Panathinaikon Stadium near the Acropolis. Louis won the world's first marathon in 2 hours 58 minutes, 50 seconds. He was Greek, just like Pheidippides. It was perfect: The man matched the myth. The victory thrilled the men from Boston. How would BAA officials find a course like that near their city, the one they considered the Athens of the New World?

The officials from the BAA set out to design a course to match the original in Greece. They picked for the start a spot in Ashland, 25 miles west of the nearest thing they had to a stadium, the 220-yard Irvington Street Oval that served as their running track. The oval did not have 50,000 seats or even a chip of marble, the Newton hills weren't a very close match for the Hymettus hills—and Ashland, unlike Marathon, was not a plain, but the railroad did run in that direction.

The night before the first Boston Marathon, the six runners from New York, including Hamilton Gray and John J. McDermott, took their evening meal together in the dining room of the Central House in Ashland at a table apart from the Boston runners. Long before the days of carbohydrate loading, the meal of a marathoner on the night before the race, like that of a soldier on the eve of battle, took on the importance of the biblical Last Supper. McDermott and Gray, gaunt and lean, looked like they had trained well for distance running. One Boston observer noted that neither carried "an ounce of superfluous flesh." Clearly a rivalry had quickly developed between the host Bostonians and the invading New Yorkers.

Moments after the start Dick Grant seized the lead. He was the only man in the field without a handler to give him water and attend to his needs. Bostonians had their hopes and money on Grant, a Harvard man with a background in track racing. He felt the bright sun on his right shoulder and a cool west wind on his back. He felt the stiff leather soles of his black leather shoes slap the hard dirt road. Cross-country runner Hamilton Gray, running for the St. George AC (athletic club) of New York, followed him and matched strides. They made little puffs of dust with each unified footfall. The *Boston Globe* reporter's postrace story, in the lurid prose of the day, noted that "the sleepy old town rang with the cheers of her lusty sons."

As Grant and Gray ran, Gray's handler rode up and handed him a water canteen. He took a drink, then handed the rest to Grant. The two certainly felt a competition, one against the other, but they also held a common cause against the enormous distance. Fear of 25 miles bound them. What would happen to the human body while trying to race that distance was unknown. A man could drop dead, use himself up, shorten his life—or, most likely, break down and never reach Boston.

So great was their respect for the distance that J.J. Kiernan, representing the St. Bartholomew AC of New York, and John J. McDermott, a lithographer by trade, of the Pastime AC of New York, ran softly 30 yards behind hard-running Grant and Gray at South Framingham. McDermott at 123-1/2 pounds was the only man in the field who had won a marathon, the only other one yet held in America. The Knickerbocker AC sponsored the first-in-America race from Stamford, Connecticut, to New York City in 1896. That race had been a muddy slog—only a third of the field had finished, and it had taken McDermott 3:25:55. He traveled at a much faster rate now, but he did not know if he could keep up his pace. The newspapers considered McDermott the man who would reach Boston first, but no one knew much about what would happen in the race.

After leaving South Framingham the cyclists fell into a line as each spun up a cyclone of dust. People on horseback and in wagons followed. The loose road dirt rose on the spokes of each wagon wheel, then spilled off in cascades of dust. The papers described that, "the houses all along the line were filled with people and many handkerchiefs and good wishes were wafted upon the beautiful April day as the men with faces set, kept on."

The papers further reported that as Grant passed Wellesley College, the girls lining the streets cheered, "'Rah,' for Harvard" as if they were at a football game. Behind Grant, McDermott ran with beautiful form. McDermott caught the leaders on the hills between Wellesley and Newton. He took the heart out of Gray, who stopped to walk. As McDermott charged past on a downhill, Grant gave chase: "Although nearly played out he clung to the heels of the NY flyer." Grant grabbed a tiger by the tail. He had the speed to match McDermott, but McDermott's cautious early pace, his experience with a previous marathon, and probably greater conditioning allowed him to continue without slowing. Grant did not dare drop back; he wanted to win, so he clung for a mile to his relentless tiger on a downhill until the base of the next hill.

There, Grant staggered a few steps and quit running. McDermott continued. Grant walked to the top of the hill, arriving just in time to see McDermott turn the corner and disappear. Seeing a street-watering cart (used to keep dust down on town roads), Grant signaled the driver to stop. Grant lay in the street and asked the driver to run water over him. Once refreshed he tried to run again, but his feet were too badly blistered. He hobbled. Dick Grant, trained to race on the track, the man with the greatest speed in the field, was forced to leave the race. But the race would not leave him. The idea of winning the Boston Marathon would not leave him.

At Auburndale McDermott commanded nearly a mile lead. The churning and mobile bicycling, buckboard, horseback, electric-car crowd gathered around him so closely that his attendants had to work to keep the path open. McDermott plodded on in a pandemonium of dust. He asked attendant Eddie Heinlein to tell him when he had passed 20 miles. At the Evergreen Cemetery, a quarter mile from the Chestnut Hill reservoir, McDermott stopped to walk for the first time. He walked 220 yards, then suddenly sprinted for 200 more until a violent cramp seized his left leg. He stopped, and Heinlein pummeled his leg vigorously to exorcise the cramp amid the applause of the spectators.

Many thought he was gone, finished, and regardless of his position in the lead would have to retire from the race, but he held his leg stiff and yelled to Heinlein, "Rub!" Heinlein tore at the cramp with his fingers and held the quivering muscle fibers apart until they relaxed.

The cured McDermott jumped back into the race and ran on Beacon Street to Coolidge Corner and to St. Paul Street, where he walked to Carleton Street. Blisters filled his shoes, and the skin had begun to peel off the soles of his feet. When he heard that a runner had just come over the hill, he "shut his teeth and set his face and leaning well forward dug his shoes into the hard Beacon Street." Spectators said that he ran up the hill like a half-miler and down the other side to Commonwealth Avenue and across Massachusetts Avenue. There, sweaty and dusty, he plunged into the dignity of a funeral procession as it moved along Massachusetts Avenue. He so startled the drivers of two electric cars that they stalled their vehicles.

At the Irvington Oval spectators filled every available foot of standing room. "The fences were black with boys, young men and women." They had watched the BAA Open Handicap games, a track-and-field meet where slower runners started sooner so that often the races became great catch-up dramas (and better fodder for wagers, as the last starter, called the scratch man, tried to catch the runner who started with the gun and all those in between), where A.W. Foote of Yale had won the mile time prize in 4:48. McDermott, now weighing 114-1/2 pounds, ran onto the track and completed the 220-yard lap in exactly 40 seconds. The crowd pressed forward, "wishing to grasp the hand of the winner of the first marathon run in Massachusetts." The police "forgot their duty." The crowd hoisted McDermott onto their shoulders. "It was by the hardest kind of reasoning [Did he punch someone?] that he escaped and ran to the B.A.A. Clubhouse."

Newspapers proclaimed McDermott's time of 2:55:10—10 seconds faster than Spiridon Louis had run in Greece and faster than he himself had run 6 months earlier—was a new world's record and that McDermott was the marathon champion of America and the world.

"Grant is the hardest man I ever beat," McDermott told the *Globe* reporter. "He held me for a mile, although he was all pumped out. If he had trained for the race he would have given me a hard race. As it was it was hard enough to shake him. He ran the pluckiest race I ever saw." McDermott examined his feet. "This will probably be my last long race. I hate to be called a quitter and a coward, but look at my feet." They were bloody and blistered, with the skin peeling off.

But Grant and McDermott would both be back. And so would Lawrence Brignolia, a 20-year-old Cambridge oarsman finishing over an hour behind the winner. The *Globe* reporter described Brignolia as a "modest genial fellow [who] has a wonderful physique and confidence." He had been apprenticed to a horseshoer until age 15. Before the race Brignolia had been persuaded to take a big breakfast to prepare him for the ordeal, but he had gotten cramps while running. The 160-pound Brignolia finished in 4:06, but would train, eat carefully, and be back, too.

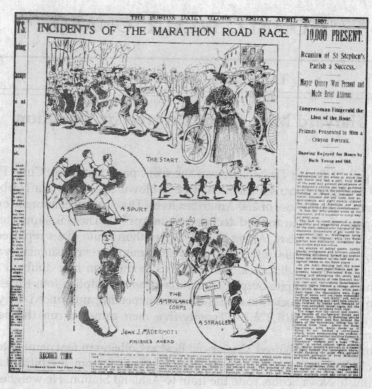

Before the advent of photojournalism, artists' renderings provided snapshots of newsworthy events, like this first running of the Boston Marathon (*Boston Daily Globe*, April 20, 1897).

1897 Results

1.	J. McDermott, *PAC*, NY	2:55:10[CR,WR]*	6.	J. Mason		3:31:00
2.	J. Kiernan, *SBAC*, NY	3:02:02	7.	W. Ryan		3:41:25
3.	E.P. Rhell	3:06:02	8.	**L. Brignolia**		**4:06:12**
4.	H. Gray, *SGAC*, NY	3:11:37	9.	H. Leonard		4:08:00
5.	H.D. Eggleston	3:17:50	10.	A.T. Howe		4:10:00

18 entrants, 15 starters, 10 finishers.
[CR] denotes course record. [WR]denotes world record. *Past and future winners always appear in bold in the results.

RONALD MACDONALD

TUESDAY, APRIL 19, 1898

Harvard Man Grant Favored in Marathon

The April 19 *Boston Daily Globe* ran the front page headline "Cuba Free." The U.S. armored cruiser *Maine* had been blown up in Havana Harbor in February, with the loss of 260 American lives. The country clamored for war with Spain over Cuba and did declare war on April 25. The U.S. supported the Cuban insurrectionists. Along the 1898 marathon route, flags replaced the waving handkerchiefs of the previous year. American expansionists wanted Hawaii and the Philippines, too. The U.S. population had doubled since 1820, and the per capita output of manufacturers multiplied four times. The Boston Athletic Association at its 10th annual meeting announced the year's gross income at $101,926.30. Twenty-five men came to run the second BAA marathon.

A curly and light-haired 22-year-old Boston College student named Ronald J. MacDonald, who had come to Boston at age 9 from his birthplace in Antigonish, Nova Scotia, rode the train to Ashland Station. He weighed 142 pounds, stood 5'7", and wore a pair of common bicycle shoes. A noble, nearly haughty look shot from his eyes as he posed for a newspaperman's sketch. He had never run a marathon before, but he had been running for the Cambridgeport Gym for 3 years and had won the July 4 mile handicap race in Newton. He had also won the New England 3-mile championship and 3 weeks earlier had won an 11-mile cross-country race. The pundits and predictors favored the 1897 winner, John J. McDermott, who had said he wouldn't run another marathon race, but there he was.

Most of the runners took the 8:30 train from Boston. The *Globe* reporter saw them: "Sauntering through the station came eight or ten healthy rugged looking men clad in sweaters, small caps and carrying small grips." At the start Tom Burke took a stout piece of pine instead of his heel (although some accounts say that he had dragged his toe) to scratch the starting line on the dirt road, but starter "Doc" Moran had to wait because some men were missing. They arrived on the next train to join the leaders in a start that took them through the mile in 5 minutes flat.

McDermott ran in a pack of five with elbows touching down the dusty road to Framingham. Hamilton Gray followed. Spectators and interested parties tagged along. "Carriages and a few motor wagons and equestrians followed as far as Natick where they dropped but others took up the chase." It was a dry day, and frequent collisions added to the din and dust. "Dust rose in a thick cloud until the runners and bicycle riders resembled [flour] millers." The use of noisemakers annoyed at least one observer: "The clanging of gongs and the constant ringing of bells was hideous." Young boys and men rode their bicycles alongside their favorite run-

Young boys and men rode their bicycles alongside their favorite runners and whispered words of encouragement or advice.

ners and whispered words of encouragement or advice. Members of Company B, First Regiment, had their hands full trying to keep a clear path through the ever-forward-leaning crowds.

Boys on bikes raced out of Natick to see who led, then raced back to town competing to be the first to announce the leaders. Eugene Estoppey of New York looked relaxed running into Natick. A runner named O'Conner whom the *Globe* reporter called "as fresh as a daisy" actually led the race, but he was doomed to drop out. But Estoppey, who had his own ideas about everything, including training for marathon running, was actually better prepared. Each year he readied himself for the rigors of the marathon by walking to Ashland from his home in New York. This habit of traveling from his native New York to Ashland, not by train, horseback, or carriage, but on foot to prepare himself for the race, would lead the press in subsequent years to label him eccentric. He arrived a week early and then practiced running.

Dick Grant had left Harvard and now represented the Cambridgeport Gym. He and R.A. McLean, a 21-year-old who had been born in Scotland, led a field of eight by 75 yards. Grant ran conservatively, so he thought. He controlled his speed and he had trained more this year. He waited like the clever McDermott for time to wear everyone else out. But MacDonald ran so conservatively that he was nowhere in sight of the leaders. Wearing a white shirt with the emblem of the Cambridgeport Boat Club and black trunks with a bright blue braid, he waited for the leaders to play themselves out so he could dash for the lead. "Ham" Gray tried to take the lead at Wellesley. He got it after a little spurt past O'Conner, who had been running on the sidewalk, and the eccentric Estoppey. McLean came up to the leaders. Leads shifted frequently. The day, the sun, and the dust wore on.

Somewhere between Wellesley and Newton Lower Falls, O'Conner disappeared from the course and MacDonald showed himself. He had been running 2 to 3 miles behind the leaders. There may have been method in his tactic, as was tentatively observed by the astute *Globe* writer: "He was noticed to apparently awake out of a stupor, throw his head back and start running in an altogether different style." The pursuit was on. MacDonald wanted the lead. Gray led at Auburn Circle but could not shake Estoppey. The runners dueled up the hill. The attending cyclists had to dismount their bikes and walk up. The reporter found it "painful to watch [the runners'] expressions of agony." Still MacDonald came on.

A shout from McLean's attendants told him that MacDonald was gaining. He appeared to be trying a desperate strategy, and many thought he would sizzle himself in the process. He sprinted downhill. His attendant whispered that he may have gone daft. Gray had passed McLean to take the lead again at Coolidge Corner. Gray had only 50 yards. He saw MacDonald. The *Globe* reporter tried to sort out what was happening: "MacDonald saw victory but Gray was determined not to be beaten . . . . [but perhaps] Gray [by letting MacDonald gain] was playing the Fox." By St. Paul Street MacDonald burst again, and now Gray could hear his footsteps. At Kent Street MacDonald caught Gray. With all their bursting spent, they moved like menacing fighters circling in molasses. Ever so slowly MacDonald pulled away. Gray could do nothing but persevere, alternating walking and running. MacDonald never stopped running and took no liquid during the entire race.

According to the *Globe* reporter, MacDonald did not enter the Irvington Oval lightly. "With a mighty bound he landed in the center of the cinder path." Boys gathered to run to the finish line with him like a bodyguard. Past the line the crowd hauled MacDonald to their shoulders and carried him. They set him down in time for Gray's finish. The two shook hands. Ten minutes later "Larry" Brignolia, the oarsman and apprentice to a horse-shoer, the man with the rippling physique, finished, over an hour and 10 minutes faster than the year before.

1898 Results

1. **R. MacDonald**, *CG*	2:42:00^{CR}	
2. H. Gray, *SGAC*, NY	2:45:00	
3. R.A. McLean	2:48:02	
4. **J. McDermott**, *PAC*, **NY**	**2:54:17**	
5. **L. Brignolia**, *BBC*	**2:55:49**	

6. E. Estoppey, Jr., *PAC*, NY	2:58:49
7. D. Grant, *CG*	3:08:55
8. J. Mason *SAC*, NY	3:09:30
9. D. Harrington, *BC*	3:09:30
10. J.E. Enwright, *PAC*, NY	3:16:20

25 entrants, 15 finishers at least.

LARRY THE BLACKSMITH

WEDNESDAY, APRIL 19, 1899

Grant's Third Attempt for Victory

"Pale, thin people suffer from want of nourishment," read the advertisement on page 3 of the *Boston Daily Globe* on April 20, 1899. That pitch for John Hoff's malt extract explained that their product "makes flesh and blood." Another advertisement extolled the wonders of Dr. T. Sanden's Electric Belt, nature's strengthener of ailing men and women that cured nervous debility, rheumatism, lumbago, lame back, kidney, liver, and stomach disorders, poor circulation, and sleeplessness. Accompanying the advertisement was a drawing of shirtless men wearing Electric Belts and basking in the little wiggly lines that emanated from them. Lydia E. Pinkham's Vegetable Compound or its competitor, Paine's Celery Compound, might have had more appeal for the electrically squeamish. But the idea of marathon running had reached advertisers: They offered running shoes at $2 a pair.

Before the Ashland start a doctor examined the 17 starters and pronounced each one fit. John Graham fired a pistol to start the race. Twenty-nine minutes later four leaders, a hound dog named Prince, and their attendants detailed from Battery B, First Heavy Artillery under the command of Captain Walter Lombard, reached South Framingham. (Prince had no attendant.) According to the *Globe* reporter, sensitive to the necessary nautical terminology of the day, against their faces pressed "half a gale of wind." The curious sailing terminology used in describing the early races—"beating," "quartering wind," "overhauled," "heave to," "fetch," "reach"—disappeared in later years. The big man at 161 pounds, blacksmith Larry Brignolia ran with Dick Grant and two others. Following at a respectable distance ran three members of the Highland Club, two named Sullivan and one named Harrigan.

Between Natick and Wellesley Brignolia and the dog Prince seemed to allow Grant to lead. Grant, ever the Harvard man, entered Wellesley with a 25-yard lead to greet a "bevy of pretty girls all gowned in fashionable and varicolored gowns, but with crimson predominating, shout[ing] for the Harvard man." Men nearby realized that the women cheered only for the Harvard runner, so out of a sense of fair play and balance they instead gave their cheers to the blacksmith. As may be expected, the blacksmith was more than a mere horseshoer. He was an oarsman who rowed front for the Bradford Boat Club and was an expert with single sculls. One day he won a novice singles regatta on the Charles River and 15 minutes later entered the intermediate race and placed second by only 1-1/2 lengths. He planned to race in the national intermediate rowing championships on the Charles in July.

The "Brig vs. Dick" battle waged in earnest on the long hill up Commonwealth Avenue. On that hill foot trouble struck one Sullivan, who had to stop to remove his shoe. Brignolia wore special shoes, with light leather uppers that laced nearly to the toes, rubber heels, and leather soles. By the top of the hill Brignolia had 200 yards on Grant. By Coolidge Corner Brig had 11 minutes on Dick and ran 5 minutes faster than MacDonald's course record from 1898. When Grant reached Coolidge Corner he fell in exhaustion to the street.

Grant's handlers rushed to rub and bathe him with water, then help him to his feet. John Bowles, who "coached" (handled) MacDonald in 1898, performed the same function now for Brignolia. Brignolia had said he could not spare time or money to train more than a month for this race. He had a lead, but his limited conditioning would not allow extravagances. Bowles told his charge to rest until a competitor came into sight. He slowed to consolidate his energy.

All ran well for Brignolia until near St. Mary's. He had conserved, but he didn't see a stone in the road. He turned his ankle and, lacking the quickness he might ordinarily have had to balance himself, fell to the ground. He tried to rise, but his trainers seized him and carried him to the grass, where he rested for 5 minutes while they vigorously rubbed him all over. He walked and ran the remaining distance to Exeter Street. There he lightly sprinted. Dick Grant finished 3 minutes later.

1899 Results

1.	L. Brignolia, CG/BBC	2:54:38	7.	D.J. Sullivan, HC	3:21:30
2.	D. Grant, Cambridgeport, MA	2:57:46	8.	J.O. Lynch, PAC	3:23:51
3.	B. Sullivan, HC, Roxbury, MA	3:02:01	9.	J.H. Kelley, PAC	3:30:12
4.	J. Maguire, Cambridgeport, MA	3:02:29	10.	J.E. Enwright, PAC	3:39:15
5.	R.F. Hallen	3:04:59	11.	D.P. Harrigan, HC	3:44:45
6.	E. Estoppey, Jr., PAC	3:13:34			

17 starters, 11 finishers.

JACK CAFFERY AND BILLY SHERRING

THURSDAY, APRIL 19, 1900

Mysterious Canadians Invade Boston

"No weaklings will be permitted to start in the marathon tomorrow," reported the Boston Herald on Wednesday, April 18, 1900. The next day physicians examined each of the 29 participants to see if any might be judged unfit for the ordeal of the fourth running of the Boston Marathon. None was.

The 19th dawned overcast, but a late-morning sun dried the dirt roads except for 5 or 6 miles of thick mud ruts along South Framingham. Spectators in bowler hats collapsed their umbrellas, used them as canes, and waited for the start. Canadian businessmen wearing overcoats, pockets stuffed with cash, hoped to make back their money and more in their bets on a mysterious group of Canadians. On the train to the start the businessmen milled about placing their bets, as did similarly well-heeled Bostonians. Canadian money went to a couple of runners from Ontario named Caffery and Sherring. Boston bettors had never heard of this pair. Temperatures went past 70 °F. The overcoats came off.

America was young, brash, rural, and big-shouldered. So was Lawrence Brignolia, the Cambridge, Massachusetts, blacksmith and defending champion who shined with supreme confidence as he accepted the attention of the crowds at the start. Most American money rested on those big shoulders. Last year's early leader and second-place finisher, Dick Grant, wrapped in a big quilt, looked nervous. The rest of the American money hovered over him.

The arrival of a Canadian team cracked the isolation of the all-U.S. race. America had begun to turn around to face the rest of the world. The U.S. balance of trade leaped in this decade from $100 million to $500 million, and Bostonians received more than their share. They had money to wager. Boston had grown throughout the previous century to be a world center of commerce and culture. With the new foreign contact Bostonians had with trading partners, there is no surprise that some came to run the marathon. No surprise either then that the United States' biggest and closest trading partner, Canada, sent the first racers. It was not, however, the entire country of Canada that sent them. Wealthy men like Webber Bessey, the manager of the Star Theatre in Hamilton, Ontario, paid the expenses of the marathoners, intending to bet heavily on them and pocket a profit. This was adventure capitalism. The runners left Hamilton, not the commercial or cultural hub of anywhere, for Boston with considerable fanfare. The loyal fans of the Hamilton runners waited outside city newspaper offices for postings of telegraphed results as the marathon developed.

> *The arrival of a Canadian team cracked the isolation of the all-U.S. race.*

John Peter Caffery, a dark and hardy 21-year-old standing 5'8-1/2" and weighing 127-1/2 pounds, and a boyish William Sherring held the most impressive credentials of the five-man Canadian team. Jack and Billy, as their teammates called them, ran for St. Patrick's AC in Hamilton and wore its single shamrock on their chests. They intended to challenge the Americans, champion Brignolia and Grant, the popular and swift former Harvard man now running for the Cambridgeport Gym. Caffery made his living driving a team of horses and had trained for 2 months especially for this race. He spoke modestly when he spoke at all about himself. Caffery had won a big 1898 race in Hamilton by going 19 miles, 168 yards in 1:54:00 and had run a 10-mile race in 58:48, but he had placed second to Sherring in the Hamilton *Herald* Thanksgiving Day 20-mile race. John N. Barnard and Fred Hughson, also of Hamilton, waited eagerly in Ashland to run along with the braggadocio Brignolia and the trembling Grant.

The runners waited in three rows on an iron railroad bridge in Ashland. Runners, handlers, and spectators had taken the 9:15 train to Ashland, where they arrived at 10:10 and then loaded onto barges pulled by a motor car for the last mile (and the first mile of the race). The large party from the city included many older cigar-smoking men with pockets bulging with cash; they accompanied the young runners to the start, from where they planned to take the electrics to watch at the South Framingham checkpoint.

At 11:30 the motor carriage of official starter John Graham arrived at the Ashland station. He drove the one mile west to the railroad bridge, where he presided over 29 men packed into three close-ordered ranks. The Canadians huddled together, but officials placed them in separate positions on the line. Something chittered in the nerves of John Barnard, the Canadian man the *Boston Globe* called "a fleet little sprinter." Before Graham's invocation to race, Barnard, with his Canadian teammates in tow, bolted from the line. The entire field followed and had to be called back to begin again in a true start. But to the runners and handlers the Canadians had showed their intentions to race aggressively from the gun.

In the true start, the Canadians again took a quick lead, followed by an array of bicycles, carriages, and motor machines. They intended to burn off their competition. John Bowles, who was Grant's and Brignolia's handler, told his charges to "hold on to the leaders at all hazards." Captain Lombard of the bicycle corps, having given each of his men a number that corresponded with that of a runner, instructed them to spread themselves over the first half mile of the course. To avoid confusion each cyclist picked out his man as he came by, then followed alongside.

Experienced judges of the 4-year-old race said that the Canadians could not hold that pace beyond 10 miles. Shocked American bettors watched with emptiness in their stomachs and fear for their wallets. They pulled alongside their picks and swore at them to run faster. After a mile Caffery held a 25-yard lead while Grant kept up with the tail end of the Canadians. At 4 miles the once-confident Brignolia took a stitch. Those on the inside knew that he had "shot his bolt and that it would be only a matter of time until he would have to withdraw from the race."

The pack of five Canadians set what locals called a "wicked pace" with Sherring "beating," as the local reporter wrote, past Caffery—who himself took a stitch—to a 100-yard lead at 10 miles in West Natick at 57 minutes. Grant sat in 6th place in 58 minutes and Brignolia languished in 15th. Sherring continued leading into Newton but looked in distress. With a 2-minute lead over Caffery, Sherring flopped down by the roadside in "a helpless manner." Attendants rubbed restoratives into his legs for several minutes. Caffery came into Sherring's view, then passed; the supine Sherring gave recognition with only a faint sigh. His assistants lifted him to his feet and helped him hobble, walk freely, then break into a slow run.

Fourteen miles from home Brignolia fell out and took a car to the finish. The heat had begun to wilt the strongest of men. Lawrence Brignolia continued to live in Cambridge for the rest of his life. He continued shoeing horses until there were none to shoe. He died in an automobile accident on February 13, 1958, at the age of 82 and weighing about 300 pounds.

Dick Grant had learned the lessons of restraint in marathon racing. He had trained more and was a year stronger. He picked his way one by one past the fagged Canadians and closed to within 100 yards of Caffery. Caffery turned to see Grant stalking him. Grant had finished second to Brignolia in 1899, and this year he wanted an improved place. Winning the race would do the trick. But all traces of Caffery's earlier stitch had vanished, leaving him with plenty of fight. He burst away from the pursuing Grant, who continued to try to overtake the accelerating Canadian. Slowly at first and then more quickly, Grant went to pieces. Sherring, seemingly refreshed, caught Grant.

A royal battle broke out between the two as Grant refused to surrender his second-place position. Grant used himself up in the struggle. He suffered severe cramps, took a warm drink, and walked. Another Canadian passed but there was nothing Grant could do. Teammates and local runners paraded past as Grant kept one foot traveling past the other. After this race Grant's name no longer appears in Boston Marathon results, but he is mentioned in 1918 by *Boston Herald* columnist Duffy as being an athletic director in Havana, Cuba.

The spectators cheered wildly as Caffery, running with ease, approached the new finish line. The crowd in its exuberance closed on Caffery as he closed on the finish line. Through their thickness he had trouble finding the line. Once he crossed what he believed to be the official finish line he slipped away from the crowd and through the doors of the BAA clubhouse. Caffery wandered through the building until he located the officials on the third floor, sequestered as they organized the results of the concurrent BAA track meet. Men of wealth and position in the city of Boston, they were not used to being accosted by a sweating, exhausted man who made his living driving a team of horses. They asked him a surprising question. Had he broken the finishing tape? Had he run through it? Caffery was astounded. He stood dumbfounded. He had not even seen it. The officials refused to declare him the winner and waved him off. They had work to do. They kept the official clock running. As they saw it, the winner had not yet appeared.

Caffery dutifully, manfully, turned and made his way back down the three stories while the clock still ticked. He waded through the crowd to the official finish line for the second time, then returned to the clubhouse. No one else had yet finished. Caffery had to go back into the building, find the officials and their clock, then persuade them to stop it. Through crowds and fatigue Caffery wandered back through the BAA clubhouse. Which way was it to the third floor? Hamilton, Ontario, had nothing like this magnificent clubhouse. Caffery had never been in a building like it.

Ground for this splendid place had been broken on May 1, 1887, and it opened on December 29, 1888. Caffery left the basement mezzanine and ascended the front staircase, which consisted of four short flights to reach the main, or social, floor, 12 feet above the sidewalk. Over the entrance of the building was a room for nonmembers, designated the Strangers' Room. Caffery passed the dining hall, finished in cherry. Its walls hung with buff cartridge paper on which a simple green and cream pattern was stenciled to harmonize with the light finish of the cherry. Architect J.H. Sturgis fitted the ceiling with heavy beams finished in bronze. The dining room was worked up as light as possible because it was on the dark side of the building.

Caffery had yet to report to the officials, who waited somewhere in the building. The wine room was to the rear of the coatroom, both finished in ash. To the rear of the wine room was the billiard makers room. The morning room had big bay windows that looked onto Blagden Street. The drawing room was done in white painted pine. Dust stuck to the dried sweat on Caffery's legs. A rich Brussels carpet in a red pattern covered the floor, and at night heavy red tapestry curtains could be drawn to keep out the gloom of night. The BAA's board of governors spared no expense to create an elaborate structure—bowling alleys, bicycling room, running track, tennis courts, boxing rooms, a fencing room, a barbershop, a restaurant, a wine and cigar department. This was a palace to athletics.

Caffery had no interest in the running track in the balcony. He had done his running for the day. But such an indoor track would be a godsend in their Canadian winters. A 3-1/2-foot balustrade separated it from the gymnasium below. The fastest and best-covered running track in America, it cost $1,000—23 laps to a mile, with 8-foot wide banked corners. The felt-and-rubber covering was patented by a Dr. Sargent of Harvard. The heated swimming tank measured 37 by 29 feet. Complicated brassworks conducted hot water through pipes to heat the pool water.

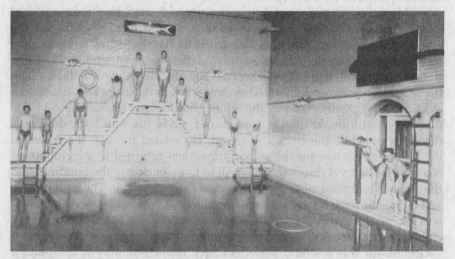

A complex brassworks heated the pool in the BAA clubhouse. The golden fish on the wall alludes to the moniker of the old elite of Boston, the "codfish aristocracy." Courtesy of the Boston Public Library, Print Department.

The first room of the Turkish bath had walls of glazed brick in white, green, and buff. Caffery needed a bath but had no time for one, he must find his way to the officials' room. The clock ticked on. Four horseshoe arches topped with voussoirs of the same stone celebrated the entrances to the second room of the baths. The rough plaster above the brick held decorations in Persian patterns of green and blue. The main dome featured a series of medallions; above and between them were circular stained glass windows, lighted from the room above. A Moorish pendant hung from the center to light the room. But the officials were not in the Turkish bath—they were in a third-floor office. At last Caffery found the right room.

The BAA officials finally accepted Caffery as the winner and at last stopped the clock. A minute later the boyish and bedraggled Sherring arrived at the finish line. The officials believed that now the real finishers were coming in, finishing in what were reasonable times. Caffery's trainers complained that he had lost 5 minutes wandering in the building and protested that his time be adjusted. The stubborn officials refused.

Caffery had a pulse of only 108 at the finish line after his 25 miles averaging 6:22 per mile, but perhaps he ran faster if the disputed 5 minutes were subtracted. Ironically, Caffery's prize for first place was a marble clock. Newspapers reported that the Boston ladies admired the handsome Sherring. Both men cheered wildly as a third Canadian and fellow Hamiltonian, Fred Hughson, ran into view through the 1-yard wide corridor of cheering crowds to complete the Canadian sweep. Police and officials struggled to keep a line open to the finish as each straining spectator leaned past another's shoulder to catch sight of the next finisher.

Sherring called for something to eat. He was weary at first but within an hour regained his energy. Canadians Dennis Carroll and the false-starting Barnard failed to finish. Carroll had vowed that if he did not win the Boston Marathon he would never return to his native Hamilton. The next day he sent for his trunk and settled in Boston for the rest of his life.

But back in Hamilton the breaking news that not one but three of their sons swept to victory in the sophisticated city in the prosperous country to the south set Hamiltonians dancing in the streets. Or at least those Hamiltonians who had backed their boys and won a load of money were dancing. The next day's *Hamilton Spectator* gleefully and snidely gloated,

Hamilton's runners won glory for themselves and brought honor to their native city by their grand performance in the marathon race, the greatest event of its kind on the continent, competed for as it was by the crack American amateur long distance runners. They swept everything before them and opened the eyes of the Americans who thought it was presumptuous of runners from Canada to imagine that they could carry off such a trophy. But gallant runners from the northern zone showed they could bring as much glory to their country as the brave Canadians in the battlefield of South Africa. Even the most sanguine did not imagine that they would make such a sweep as they did, and leave nothing for the Americans to console themselves with. They captured all the honors in sight to the amazement of cultured Boston. Nothing was left to the Bostonians but the credit of being able to cook pork and beans to perfection, and the culture they prize so highly. The critics did not like the style and training of the Canadians but after this they will probably adopt it. The result of the race was a cruel disappointment to them.

A band, the mayor, and townspeople met the marathoners at the train station on their return. Roman candles shot into the air. The mayor made a speech. Jack Caffery, with typical marathoner introversion and reticence, said only thank you. The crowd cheered anyway and along with the band escorted their hero to his door.

After only 4 years the Boston Marathon was already an international event that was beginning to draw a fierce and fanatical following of men who would live and breathe for it. Dick Grant was one, as was the 1898 winner, Ronald MacDonald. At the finish of the 1900 race MacDonald said, "I never expected to see either Caffery or Sherring finish as they went away at a mile clip; they run very differently from the way we do here. I noticed that they were running flat footed, while we always run with the heel off the ground." MacDonald said that he only wished that he had "fitted" (trained himself to get fit) for this race. Complaining that during his victory run he had had a sore knee and the wind in his face, he proclaimed he could beat Caffery's new world record time next year.

1900 Results

1. J. Caffery, Hamilton, ON   2:39:44[CR]
2. W. Sherring, Hamilton, ON   2:41:31
3. F. Hughson, Hamilton, ON   2:49:08
4. J. Maguire, Cambridgeport, MA 2:51:36
29 starters, 26 finishers.

5. J. Fay, Roxbury, MA   2:55:07
6. T.J. Hicks, Cambridge, MA   3:07:19
7. B. Sullivan, Roxbury, MA   3:13:20
8. D. Grant, Cambridgeport, MA   3:13:57

RONALD MACDONALD'S RETURN

FRIDAY, APRIL 19, 1901

Boston College Student Plans to Top Canadians

Ronald MacDonald came to Ashland to win, as he said he would. He had done it before and he thought he could do it again. He predicted that he would break Caffery's record. Quiet Caffery returned with a larger entourage of Canadian runners and partisans, arriving with the calm confidence of a man who had run a 25-mile time trial in 2:25 flat when his own course record for Boston stood at 2:39. Both Caffery and MacDonald passed the prerace medical examination, which deemed 38 men physically perfect. Four judged to be imperfect were not allowed to start. Readers of the newspaper that day found predictions of rain with fresh to brisk easterly winds. Headlines read that fighting continued in the Philippines. Contrary to predictions, in Ashland, Massachusetts, the fighting began an hour after the sun came out. The 38 perfect ones faced a battery of cameras as well as starter John Graham's gun at the stroke of noon. Some of those cameras would make the photographs that for the first time replaced the line drawings of the previous years' newspapers.

Betting at the Columbia House before the race rested chiefly on Caffery against the field, even money, or Caffery against MacDonald, 2 to 1. "Thousands of dollars changed hands on bets," which were not illegal.

With the light lunch from Ashland's Columbia House in their bellies and the bicycled soldiers from Battery D&E of the First Regiment in attendance, the runners bounced off to a downhill 4:40 first mile. The favorites soon overhauled the wild enthusiasts on a soft, sandy road halfway to South Framingham. A gallery of spectators—passengers in automobiles, motor carriages, and stylish equipages, equestrians, and youngsters who tried to keep pace with the runners—watched.

Money rode on this race; it was the reason for most cheering. A public used to betting on boxing and horse racing practiced the same sort of support for marathon runners. A large contingent of Canadians, many of whom wore "buttons with the picture of Caffery on them and a rosette of ribbons with the green and red of the St. Patricks AC" came to support their runners. If a Canadian won they would be "comfortably provided as to pockets, and will go home none the poorer." Money was poised, about to change hands. The Canadians waited eagerly for it. "They made what appeared to be a prodigal gift of offering to back Caffery's chances of beating 2h 32m." The record stood at 2:39. The weather seemed right for a record, and the runners wanted it.

Caffery running in his slouchy style and MacDonald looking pretty up on his toes ran with William Davis, a Mohawk Indian from Canada. Fred Hughson, (the 1900 third-place finisher, also from Canada), Crimmins of Cambridge, and a rank outsider, Sammy Mellor of Yonkers, New York, ran together for the early miles. A Greek runner, the first-ever race entrant not from North America, John Vrazanis, kept up in the early miles, but blisters forced him to drop out—though another account holds that he ran in last place from the start but finished the race out and succeeded in beating one man. But as the Greek dropped out or finished out, another creature dropped in.

Between Natick and Wellesley a horse joined the race. The *Boston Daily Globe* and the *Boston Herald* ran conflicting accounts. The *Globe* reported that applause frightened a horse, causing a dangerous situation, and that only an act of heroism by an unknown cyclist prevented injury. The *Herald*, however, reported that "a horse ran away soon after [the runners were] passing Natick and was having some fun all to himself when a clever wheelman swept along side him and brought him to a stop so skillfully that even the runners applauded."

Going into Wellesley Hughson led Caffery, but there Caffery "waked up" and caught Hughson. Word passed back to MacDonald that Caffery had started on to the finish. MacDonald dug in. He caught Hughson at the top of a hill. They raced each other. MacDonald prevailed. Hughson developed problems with his knee. Later he fell to the road a couple of times from cramps. At the reservoir he stopped for help from his attendants.

Near this point in the race, a bizarre series of events instigated by MacDonald began to unfold. MacDonald would go on to graduate from Boston College and become a physician who would set up practice in his native Antigonish, Nova Scotia, and there spend his days. But if you believe his version of the story, you'll see that he was lucky to live through this marathon.

MacDonald accepted a soaked sponge from a stranger in the crowd and, curiously, held on to it even as he was seized by what appeared to observers to be cramps. He stopped to walk, and while he did Hughson, walking himself, passed. Both men, spent and discouraged, retired from the race. Here the story of what happened to MacDonald splits into two versions. Dr. Thompson, a physician in attendance to MacDonald, says MacDonald retired to a cart that took him and the sponge to MacDonald's home. There the physician examined the sponge and detected chloroform on it. A reporter asked Dr. Thompson whether he thought that, if MacDonald was really chloroformed, was it intentional or an accident? Thompson replied, "It couldn't have been an accident when there was so much money up on the race." MacDonald claimed that had it not been for the doctor's quick work the chloroform might have proved fatal. Trainer John Bowles had another version: Bowles accused Dr. Thompson of having given MacDonald some pills when he appeared exhausted; but instead of stimulating him they had the opposite effect. Bowles cited the case of a Brown University runner, Dave Hall, in the marathon from Stamford to New York City who practically collapsed after accepting pills from an outsider. The controversy raged without conclusion for days after the race.

Caffery ran unimpeded and uncontroversially to the finish, "jogging much as [one] would in slippers that were on the point of falling off—just skimming the ground with an even monotony of movement." Those who came south to bet on Caffery returned to Canada happy and richer. The *Herald* reporter noted, that "as Caffery actually beat the crazy mark [2:32, set by the odds makers] by three minutes the result from a financial point of view may be imagined." The rest of the racers were nearly a mile behind and had running to do.

The bony Canadian Mohawk, William Davis, ran with a loping, deceiving gait, knees wide apart and head erect. The *Boston Post* reporter saw Davis run "utterly devoid of style . . . in a squat fashion." Next to him ran a light, 111-pound, 20-year-old Sammy Mellor, who represented the Hollywood Inn AC. A raw east wind struck both men at the top of the Newton hills. They fought the wind and each other. The *Herald* reporter saw that Davis "came home like a wild man, finishing as fresh as many athletes finish runs of a mile." Ten minutes later Mellor struggled to the finish. Cambridge runner John C. Lorden, a smooth-running, muscular man, followed in 5th place about 7 minutes later, but no one bothered to record the 10th-place time of J.J. Kennedy of Roxbury. Both men would play important parts in the 1902 race.

1901 Results

1.	J. Caffery, Hamilton, ON	2:29:23^{CR}	6.	T. Hicks, YMCA, Cambridge, MA	2:52:32
2.	W. Davis, Hamilton, ON	2:34:45	7.	P. Lorden, CG, MA	2:55:40
3.	S. Mellor, *HIAC*	2:44:34	8.	J. McAuliffe, CG, MA	2:56:44
4.	C. Crimmins, CG, MA	2:47:15	9.	E. Grussel, Jr., NY	3:02:20
5.	J. Lorden, CG, Cambridge, MA	2:51:29	10.	J.J. Kennedy, Roxbury, MA	*NT

38 starters.
*NT: no time available.

THE STRENUOUS LIFE

SATURDAY, APRIL 19, 1902

Medical Student Favored in Marathon

A bullet from the gun of the anarchist Leon Czolgosz killed President McKinley and propelled 42-year-old Theodore Roosevelt to the presidency. In a country governed by a young, vigorous military man, a former roughrider, a big-game hunter, the Boston Athletic Association's activities, including the marathon, epitomized upper-class American values. In a speech in Chicago in April of 1899 Roosevelt had said, "I wish to preach, not the doctrine of ignoble ease, but the doctrine of the strenuous life." Ronald MacDonald, with his supercilious gaze, curls, and principled frown, epitomized the men of the BAA, the ruling elite of Boston and America, and of course the strenuous life. He was well educated, noble, a sportsman who did not have to work with his hands or sweat for anything but the fun of it. MacDonald came back to Ashland in the bright sun to win again. He had been at Boston College but had now moved on, his eyes on life as a doctor. This time he would drink from no chloroformed sponge. He was confident that his pretty running form would carry him to victory as it had in 1898.

In contrast, little and scrappy Sammy Mellor traveled north from Yonkers to improve on his third-place finish of the previous year. He worked with his hands, so he typified all that was not genteel in class-conscious America. In the previous year's Thanksgiving Day 20-mile race in Hamilton, Ontario, Mellor defeated MacDonald by 10 seconds. Two-time Boston Marathon winner and record holder Jack Caffery came south from Canada intending to win again—and in record time again. J.J. Kennedy, a man with an angelic face, had won the 3-mile members' run at the Apollo Garden in Roxbury, Massachusetts, the summer before and so had sharpened his speed. John C. Lorden of Cambridge had started in an 8-mile handicap cross-country race on the previous Saturday but failed to finish. Eugene Estoppey had again walked from his home in New York to the marathon start in Ashland. Thomas J. Hicks, who had finished sixth in each of the past 2 years, came to improve on that by the maximum. Except for Estoppey, each man thought winning was a reasonable achievement for himself.

The odds makers picked Caffery. While smart money weighed on him, however, dysentery festered within his bowels and catalyzed cramps during his final rubdown at Scott's Hotel in Ashland. With so much money riding

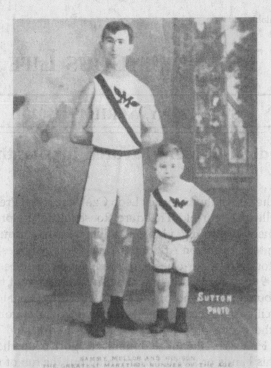

Marathons and marathoners were so popular at the turn of the century that Sammy Mellor and his son were pictured on a promotional postcard for a New York luncheonette. Courtesy of the Boston Public Library, Print Department.

on him Caffery decided, there on the starting line, to take the safe route and not run at all, leaving the road clear for MacDonald and Mellor. With Caffery gone, the odds makers had to make new odds.

MacDonald and Mellor ran side by side for 12 miles. Mellor wore #11 on a white shirt with white knee-length pants. Hair parted in the middle topped his head, which looked small on his little body. The *Globe* reporter, riding in his flagged Crestmobile, wrote that Mellor "was continually gazing far across the fields and woods and appeared to be all absorbed in the scenery of the country side as if he were engaging in a morning constitutional rather than a race." MacDonald, a head taller and 30 pounds heavier, wore blue. Charles Moody, a high schooler from Natick, was taller but thinner than MacDonald and moved with what the *Globe* reporter saw as a "businesslike stride." As the racing grew more serious the leaders seemed to be fencing with each other without consideration for time or distance or any of the other racers. First Mellor would worry MacDonald with little stabs of speed, then MacDonald would respond with a thrust of his own that Mellor would parry by slipping behind the bigger man, then following with a burst and a surge. This man-on-man duel had to continue until one man broke the other or both men broke.

At Wellesley hills MacDonald slowed. A carriage load of his supporters urged him on, administering restoratives and sponging his head. MacDonald could not respond to their ministrations and did not speak to their exhortations. Instead he rubbed his hand in a circular motion on his stomach. Then he began to walk. Word reached John Lorden by way of his elated handlers that up ahead MacDonald was walking. Lorden caught MacDonald, but MacDonald started running again with that pretty stride of his. Lorden fell in behind and waited. As they ran downhill into Newton Lower Falls, Lorden tossed in a burst and MacDonald tottered to the sidewalk. Or so the *Globe* reporter wrote—maybe that reporter had previously covered boxing—but Lorden never laid a glove on MacDonald. MacDonald waited there until his brother arrived in a wagon to collect him and drive him home. Quickly Hicks passed MacDonald, but his name did not appear in the top 12 in the final results.

By then Mellor had left the dusty country roads behind and skimmed the macadam on Washington Street at Auburndale. The *Globe* reporter, pressing his bowler hat to his head as the Crestmobile zipped along, wrote,

> Every foot of the course from the reservoir to Coolidge Corner, both sides of the boulevard, were black with shrieking spectators and Brookline's aristocracy leaned out of windows and waved lace handkerchiefs in the April breeze as the "white shadow" wended his way, acknowledging the salutations with a smile and nod.

One of the saluters at Coolidge Corner was no other than Jack Caffery himself. His dysentery had taken furlough long enough for him to run several steps with Mellor, shake his hand, and wish him well. Within a year the two would not be on speaking terms.

Mellor was free to win as he pleased, but pains in his ankles threatened his victory more than did Kennedy. By Chestnut Hill, Mellor had 4 minutes on Kennedy. But Mellor won in a time much slower than Caffery's record, saying, "If it hadn't been for [painful ankles] I would have broken the record." Mellor wanted that record; he resolved to get it some day, at any cost.

Kennedy, the runner no one bothered to time last year, finished 2 minutes and 9 seconds later. Looking distressed, Lorden finished alone, over 10 minutes behind the winner, but he had improved from his previous year's fifth place and was now a man who had made up his mind to win the Boston Marathon. At 27 years old, Lorden had been running since he was 16, but mostly as a sprinter. He went back to his job working 10 hours a day in the shipping department of the Pump Manufacturing Company in East Cambridge. He trained mostly at night, under gaslights when he could find them.

1902 Results

1.	S. Mellor, Jr., *HIAC*, NY	2:43:12	7.	E.F. O'Brien, Jr., Dorchester, MA	3:09:15
2.	J.J. Kennedy, *SPAC*, Boston, MA	2:45:21	8.	W.H. Hunter, New Haven, CT	3:09:50
3.	**J.C. Lorden**, *CG*	**2:54:49**	9.	J. Flynn, Dorchester, MA	3:13:15
4.	C. Moody, *BHS*	3:03:47	10.	A. Ziegler, *PAC*	3:20:20
5.	W.A. Schlobohm, *HIAC*	3:05:49	11.	F.L. LeMonier, Boston, MA	3:22:53
6.	E. Poole, Cambridge, MA	3:07:14	12.	E. Estoppey, *Polo AC*, NY	3:23:20

42 starters.

IN DEFIANCE OF THE DOCTOR

MONDAY, APRIL 20, 1903

Mellor Determined to Break Caffery's Record

On the night before the Boston Marathon of 1903, Irish immigrant John C. Lorden visited the offices of Dr. J.F. Fair in East Cambridge. The doctor examined Lorden, then wrote the following letter: *This is to certify that I have advised Mr. John Lorden not to participate in the race to be held Monday, April 20, 1903, owing to trouble with his bowels, which are not in a healthy condition at the present time.* (The race ran on Monday the 20th that year because the Patriots' Day holiday of the 19th fell on a Sunday, the Lord's day of rest.)

Lorden took the doctor's letter, carefully folded it, tucked it into his pocket, and left for home.

In the morning Lorden presented himself for registration in the marathon. The registration official asked Lorden if he had been examined by a physician. Lorden replied that yes, he had. Dr. Fair's letter remained safely tucked in his pocket. The official gave Lorden his race number and he made for the starting line, but whatever condition Dr. Fair had diagnosed lingered in Lorden's intestines.

Sammy Mellor headed for the starting line, too. He was a small man full of fight. As the previous year's winner he was a heavy favorite, but many bettors had put their money on Jack Caffery, the course record holder from 1901. Mellor made for the starting line with vengeance on his mind. He still seethed from the treatment he had received in Jack Caffery's hometown of Hamilton, Ontario, during the annual Around the Bay 20-miler the previous November. Mellor explained the reasons for his rage in an interview in the *Boston Daily Globe.*

In the introduction to that interview, published on April 20, the writer compared Mellor with Caffery: "There are those who maintain that if Mellor had been pushed he would have broken Caffery's record." Mellor felt the same way. But there was more at work than athletic rivalry to fuel Mellor's desire for revenge. Mellor explained what had happened in the past year to destroy the cordial relationship the two had when Caffery congratulated Mellor at Coolidge Corner. The incident that incensed Mellor in the Hamilton 20-miler occurred as he led the field with 4 miles to go. Caffery, hometown favorite and holder of that course record, had dropped out.

> I saw the chance [of a course record] in my grasp [2 minutes ahead of the record], when suddenly, one of the most prominent of the promoters and a well known newspaper man in Hamilton suddenly reined in his horse, for he had followed the race in a carriage, and applying the whip, swerved the animal toward me. The horse was a spirited one and the sudden lashing infuriated him. It was a deliberate attempt to run me down and disable me. . . . I jumped out of the horse's path, but the driver again turned its head toward me and made another attempt. This time I caught at the bridle and was dragged a considerable distance. . . . I am afraid that I lost some of my form. . . . When I finished the timers told me that I had broken the record by over a minute. Immediately I went into the newspaperman's private office and as small as I am expressed my feelings. After the mix-up in the private office I was told that I had failed to lower the record by 39 seconds. Now what puzzled me was the fact that if the incident was an accident, such a prominent individual should allow my assault on him to go unheeded. I believe there is a police court in Hamilton.

With such seething ferocity Mellor took his place on the Ashland starting line. John Lorden, the 1902 third-place finisher, slipped, intestinal distress and all, quietly into the starting array wearing #62, white shorts, and a dark shirt displaying the emblem of his Cambridgeport club. Below his bulging sprinter's calf muscles he wore dark socks. He stood in the front line looking relaxed and feeling no internal rumbles. Mellor, dressed again all in white, with his shirt displaying a dark diagonal stripe and the *M* with crossed arrows of his new club, the Mohawk Athletic Club of Yonkers, waited to thrash Caffery. As the race settled through the first few miles, it was Caffery who took the pace, with Mellor back in the field waiting to pounce. Lorden languished in seventh place after 2 miles as the doctor's prediction of bowel trouble unraveled. In the next day's *Globe* Lorden described his distress: "The cramps seem to have gotten hold of my skin, and I felt as though the skin across my abdomen was pulling all up in knots. I grabbed at it, pulled with both hands and soon the cramps seemed to be letting go." Meanwhile Mellor moved through the pack.

Midway to South Framingham Mellor caught Caffery. Both men began to hammer themselves thin as they distanced themselves from the pack.

In Natick J.J. Kennedy ran 600 yards behind the leaders along with boyish but swarthy Mike Spring from Brooklyn, wearing the blue Maltese Cross of the Pastime AC. Lorden, innards under control, was pursued by a crowd-pleasing, childlike 16-year-old named Arthur Ziegler, and at last the mischievous Fred Lorz of New York followed. About 300 bicycles, the *Herald*'s photo automobile, a St. Louis gasoline runabout, and the *Globe*'s flag-flying white steamer Crestmobile paralleled the leaders. The *Herald* reporter was so impressed with his conveyance in an automobile that he dedicated six paragraphs of his marathon story to describing his ride.

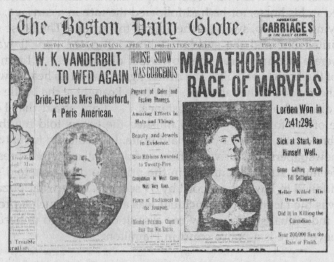

John C. Lorden (*Boston Daily Globe*, April 21, 1903) defied doctor's orders not to run and won the marathon.

At Wellesley, Mellor "trotted over to Caffery and eyed him from head to heel. After a few sarcastic remarks . . . Mellor jumped in front." Both men played to the crowd in Newton Lower Falls. Caffery doffed his cap, and Mellor waved. Mellor ran away up Auburndale Hill, but Caffery caught him at the Washington Street and Commonwealth Avenue corner. "As the leaders swung around from the Auburndale Hotel into the boulevard both squared away for the hill." There Mellor crossed over to the concrete gutter that ran beside the trolley tracks. Here Caffery encountered difficulty. His running form deteriorated as he seemed to be experiencing stomach problems. Lorden, meanwhile, had overcome his own intestinal trouble and felt stronger and stronger. "I kept coming, getting stronger, you know," he would say after the race. Kennedy ran in third but dropped out at Auburndale. Lorden passed man after man until ahead of him remained the death duel between Caffery and Mellor. Caffery looking "used up" fell onto the grass with leg cramps. Lorden approached as Caffery's handlers rubbed his legs to banish the cramping. Caffery saw him coming and rose to his feet, but he could not run. He tried to hail a watering wagon, but the driver did not understand and did not stop. Caffery, the fastest man ever over the Boston Marathon course, was helpless. He accepted further aid from his handlers but at last had to retire from the race. He was driven to the finish in a carriage, inconsolable.

That July Caffery married Miss Jane Campbell. He never returned to race the Boston Marathon. Thereafter he worked as a laborer, hardware store clerk, chauffeur, carpenter, and shoe merchant. He tried to make a comeback for the 1908 Olympic Games in London and in fact traveled with the unlimited Canadian team of 12 marathoners, finishing in 11th place, in his career-slowest time of 3:12:46. In 1918 at age 38, John Peter Caffery contracted "Spanish" influenza in the worldwide epidemic and died at home on February 2, 1919, leaving six children. He is buried on Plains Road on the far side of Hamilton Bay, in sight of his longest training loop.

Lorden continued his pursuit of Mellor. He had a 6-minute lead, nearly a mile at their pace. At Walnut Street in Waban, Mellor showed signs of distress. He stopped at Hammond Street in Newton Center, where he managed to persuade the driver of a water cart to sprinkle water on his legs and ankles. The treatment gave him new life, and he dashed down the hill into Brighton. Slowly the refreshment wore off and Mellor's fighting spirit began to slip away, but Lorden felt stronger by the mile. He ran with the inner fortitude of a man whose troublesome bowels were quiet. Mellor had done in Caffery but perhaps had also done in himself. By St. Paul Street Mellor could hear Lorden's footsteps. Mellor tried to hold Lorden off, but it was like fighting the tide. Lorden swept past, leaving Mellor with a wobbling gait. Lorden ran steadily on to the finish and the cheers of his new countrymen.

In fourth place, flourishing Fred Lorz, the joking bricklayer, made what one observer called a "grand finish." Lorz brought some showmanship to running; others brought something else. Dr. J.B. Blake examined many of the finishers after the race and concluded that "the use of stimulants during the race was not conducive to the best condition of the men who used them," though no official accusations were made that specific marathoners had used stimulants. At the time there were no rules against their use nor against any kind of drugs, stimulants, or narcotics. But drugs could not replace training, so most runners thrived on a spartan life of simple living and training. The year's third-place finisher was one of those.

Michael Spring from Brooklyn finished third. He had won two races, a quarter-mile and a 3-mile, on the same day a year earlier, but little distinguished him from others in the field. He was 20 years old, 5'6" and 118 pounds, Jewish, and a graduate of a technical institute who was employed by the Edison Company designing powerhouses. He spent his nights after work running from his home 2 miles over the newly constructed Brooklyn Bridge over the East River and back. Then he'd take a bath and go to bed, day after day until the next year's Boston Marathon.

1903 Results

1. J. Lorden, Cambridgeport, MA	2:41:29	6. A.B. Ziegler, PAC, NY	3:01:53
2. S. Mellor, MAC, NY	2:47:13	7. E. Fay, Cambridge, MA	3:04:50
3. M. Spring, PAC, NY	2:53:01	8. J.S. Hunt, South Boston, MA	3:06:40
4. F. Lorz, MAC, NY	2:53:42	9. J. Leadbetter, NewYMCA	3:08:14
5. J.J. Donovan, MAC, NY	3:01:37	10. J.B. Coakley, Roxbury, MA	3:10:47

56 starters.

THE STREAK OF YELLOW

TUESDAY, APRIL 19, 1904

Lorden, Mellor, Cream of the Marathon Field

On the other side of the world from Boston in 1904, the Japanese fought the Russians, and by April shocked the Western world because it was they who controlled the seas with a navy superior in size and technology to the neglected czarist force. Ships themselves had become bigger and faster. The emperor's men were winning. The Boston newspapers reported on the Russo-Japanese War on most of their April front pages, but on April 20 replaced the world news with that of the local conflict in the marathon. Marathoners had become faster, too, and competition denser and the fields bigger. The old world order was changing. The old marathon order was changing along with the world; a record number of runners turned out to race the Boston Marathon in 1904. Technical details changed for the marathon, too. Automobiles, a superior technological conveyance in the opinion of the *Herald* reporter who had written so profusely in 1903 about the thrills of riding in one, replaced bicycles as the transportation used by the runners' handlers.

In Ashland, 118-pound, 21-year-old former half-miler Mike Spring, designer of powerhouses for the Edison Company, pulled on his racing shoes. They were old shoes but had new soles. The cobbler, though, had left big stitches inside without hammering them down. But there was nothing Spring could do about the poor cobbling—the race was about to begin. He did not expect to win. He had not won anything in 2 years. He thought that winning did not really suit him. He felt he lacked the courage. He had tried boxing but had given that up, blaming his previous year's third-place finish on weakness caused by his attempts to make weight for the 115-pound class for boxing. Sammy Mellor stood in Ashland too; he had won in 1902 and intended to win again. Mellor had plenty of courage, perhaps too much. Fred Lorz, the fourth-place man in 1903 when John Lorden won, came back. He didn't seem to have a great deal of emotional involvement in this or any race. Lorz crowned himself with a devil-may-care attitude. Running was fun and he was having it. It was better than his job laying bricks.

Lorden himself returned to defend. He reasoned that Caffery had won twice, why shouldn't John Lorden? He had no medical problems. But perhaps because he had no problems to distract him, he thought too much. Maybe the thinking weighed him down. Tom Hicks, running for the Cambridge YMCA, had come in from Minneapolis for some serious running; he had not run at Boston the year before, but this was his fourth attempt to win there. He had run 3:07 back in 1900, and 2:52 in 1901, each for sixth place, and did not finish in 1902. Perhaps Hicks had not done enough thinking about race tactics. Later in the year Hicks would win the Olympic gold medal in St. Louis under dreadful conditions of heat and dust. But in Ashland skies were overcast. The day blew chilly. The prizes offered by the BAA were large gold and silver loving cups.

Mellor took the early lead. He ran erect; his little body was a perfect machine. He slipped over the miles oblivious of the receding competition, but oblivious as well of the invisible deterioration of his own body. Winning was not enough for Mellor—he had to win big. Driven by the grudge he still held against Caffery because of the incident at Hamilton in 1902, he wanted Caffery's course record. Lorz, Spring, Tom Cook, and Bill Schlobohm waited. They were either fearful or not hungry enough to challenge Mellor. Hicks ran leisurely in eighth place as the field filed through South Framingham.

By Wellesley hills it was Spring who tried but could not close on Mellor. Mellor seemed slightly bent forward, refusing to stop slamming himself after the record. The bending continued and Mellor slowed in proportion. Or perhaps he slowed and bent. It was not clear to Mellor or anyone which was cause and which was effect. Spring could not help but gain on Mellor. For Lorden, the burden of having run the race over and over in his mind in the nights before proved too heavy to carry. It forced him to retire from the race in Wellesley. By Auburndale, Spring pulled even with Mellor and pushed ahead into the lead over the Commonwealth Avenue hills. Spring ran up the first hill but walked up the others. Still he maintained his lead. He ate three oranges. He kept his moistened handkerchief in his mouth. Mellor was not out of sight. At Coolidge Corner Mellor, totally bent over and slowed to shuffling, capitulated to a walk. Four more men marched past, the last of them was affable Fred Lorz. Later Hicks charged by, looking full of energy.

Meanwhile, on another part of Commonwealth Avenue—the steep hill in Brighton—another race unfolded. Gasoline cars defeated steamers and electrics in a one-fifth-mile hill climb. The 2-1/2-horsepower electrics took a minute and 15 seconds to climb the hill, the steamer took 21-3/5 seconds, but the 60-horsepower Mercedes took only 15-2/5 seconds (a top speed of 48 mph).

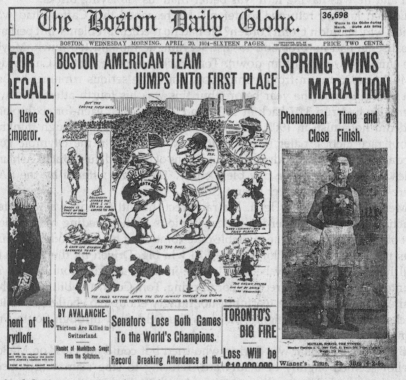

Michael Spring, wearing the Maltese cross of New York's Pastime Athletic Club (*Boston Daily Globe*, April 20, 1904), surprised himself and everyone else by winning.

After his finish in the marathon, Spring found himself at last down to fighting weight at 112-1/2 pounds. He said, "I am sort of surprised at winning, as I always thought there was a streak of yellow in me. . . . I can't say that I will go to St. Louis [the Olympics] to compete." Spring had made up his mind that he would not run another big race. Hicks came sprinting onto the Irvington Oval for second place; he had miscalculated, starting his charge too late. Both Hicks and Lorz would go to St. Louis, and what happened there would change both forever.

1904 Results

1. **M. Spring**, *PAC*, NY	**2:38:04**	6. S.A. Mellor, *MAC*	2:44:43
2. T.J. Hicks, *CbYMCA*	2:39:34	7. J. Easley, Cambridge, MA	2:46:30
3. T.E. Cook, *SBG*	2:42:35	8. D. Bennett, Hamilton, ON	2:50:35
4. W.A. Schlobohm, *MAC*	2:43:48	9. F. Perreault, *CRC*, Malden, MA	2:52:45
5. **F. Lorz**, *MAC*	**2:44:00**	10. J.S. Hunt, South Boston, MA	2:53:15

96 entrants, 67 starters, at least 40 finishers.

THE JOKER GOES WILD

WEDNESDAY, APRIL 19, 1905

'Cheater' to Run Marathon

A shadow of controversy had been following Fred Lorz since the previous summer. He could run well. He knew it. He enjoyed running and had not taken it seriously until now. He had placed fourth and fifth in Boston in the last 2 years, but his antic at the St. Louis Olympic Games haunted him. No one would let him forget it. On a mad dog, midsummer, midwest day, running on churned-up dusty roads, Lorz had dropped out of the Olympic marathon. To race on a day like that stretched beyond his own craziness. As he rode in a car to the finish, he waved to the runners still on the course; then as a whim seized him, he jumped out of the car and ran into the stadium, accepted the cheers of the crowd, and took a victory lap—still no other runner had appeared. It was grand comedy, no doubt propelled by endorphins, and Lorz stood, about to take the gold medal from Alice Roosevelt, the daughter of president Teddy, when hot, tired, dusty officials who had followed Tom Hicks as he ran, walked, and coughed along every step of the route drove into the stadium and accused Lorz of cheating. He didn't deny it. He laughed. He was joking! The temperature reached over 100 °F on the course. Nobody could have run that fast. Didn't they get it? The judges did not share Lorz's sense of humor.

Now Lorz wanted to exorcise the demon that said he was a cheat. He trained nights after his day job as a bricklayer. At age 26, he carefully planned his redemption.

At the Ashland starting line Lorz had more to worry about than his own reputation: past winners—Sammy Mellor, 1902; John Lorden, 1903; Michael Spring, 1904. Each intended to win again. Tom Hicks had an Olympic gold medal but only a second place at Boston. Mellor, the man who charged to the front last year hell-bent for record pace, said,

> Because I failed last year many think I have gone back and cannot repeat my performance of 1902. You have to feel right to win such a race as this is going to be, and I can safely say that this year I feel right. Of course the field is a big one and a good one, but my hopes are high and I believe I will reach the finish first again.

Spring had said in 1904 that he would not go to the Olympic Games, which he didn't, but he had also said that he would not run another big race. He had been surprised to win the year before, in spite of his self-admitted "streak of yellow." Just before the 1905 race he told the *Boston Post*, "I am out for a new record in this run. I weigh 119 pounds and feel fine. This will be my last long distance race and I mean to make a name for myself." But a month before Spring had said he was not ready for a record run. He thought he was not running as well so he took a 2-week layoff. But he felt he had come back rapidly. The *Post* reported on April 14, "Spring's entry assures the management of the great run, that it will be the greatest of the annual runs from Ashland into the Exeter Street clubhouse."

Lorden had long since solved the stomach problems that plagued him before his 1903 win. He told the *Post*, "You can count on my being well up at the finish. I have not been training for the past four months for nothing. Spring, Hicks and the rest of the bunch will have to do some tall hustling to defeat me." Tom Hicks, the champion of the St. Louis Olympic marathon, appeared in Ashland. Joseph Martell appeared in Ashland ready to run, too, but upon examination by doctors he was ordered out of the race as unfit. He sneaked in regardless. Forty-nine-year-old Peter Foley was allowed to run and became a sentimental favorite of the crowd because of his age.

No one pinned any doubts on the fitness of Louis Marks of the Pastime AC. He had come to Boston a week earlier from New York to prepare for the race with trainer Clarence Powers. Powers had been Spring's handler the year before and would be with Spring again on race day, but for the week before the marathon he helped Marks through his training. Powers and other friends accompanied Marks on a 2-hour run from Grove Hall in Boston out Blue Hill Avenue to the Blue Hills south of Boston and back to the city. They saw no fatigue in him.

The Boston Athletic Association offered a gold-lined punch bowl with 12 matching goblets for first prize. Second place got the bowl alone.

Many in Boston rested their hopes and bets on 10-mile cross-country champion, miler, and 2-miler F.H. Haarer. Others predicted good things from Harvard man H.F. Miller. Some said the marathon favors small men like Mellor and Spring, both under 120 pounds. Others felt that big men such as the blacksmith Brignolia, 163 pounds, or moderately sized men like Marks, 143 pounds, or Lorz at 132 pounds could run well but that the big men like Brignolia or Haarer, a head and a half taller than Mellor or Spring, did have a disadvantage. The theory was that the ankles on such men could not carry their weight for a fast, full marathon.

On race day a mild quartering wind blew over most of the course. A tall, thin high school boy named Charles "Chuck" Neary from Natick took the early lead as he had the year before. He hoped to hold the lead into his hometown, but just after South Framingham the pack of Mellor, Spring, Haarer, Lorz, and Marks absorbed him. The group, accompanied by their ever-present handlers, presented an aerodynamic wedge, with the little men (Mellor and Spring) in front, the medium-sized men (Marks and Lorz) next, and the large Haarer following. Against such a juggernaut a high school boy had no rally. He wilted.

In Natick Mellor spurted. Spring and Haarer responded. Lorz and Marks waited. They conversed. Sometimes in long-distance racing what you don't do is more important than what your aggression leads you to do. Lorz and Marks did not chase the leaders. Mellor and Spring carried with them the great weight of past victories. Nothing but first would be good enough for either. Suddenly Spring stumbled and fell. He got up, limped, but the "kinky tendon in his knee" would allow no headway.

In Wellesley Mellor responded to the cheers of the college girls by boldly bursting away from Haarer. Marks and Lorz ran together in an easy and restful stride; Marks gave Lorz a drink of the special tonic that he had prepared in New York. Lorz used the experience he had gained in his two previous Boston Marathons, and because Marks had dropped out of Boston 2 years before with stomach problems he ran a cautious pace. They waited, planned, and shared the tonic. They had been carefully preparing for this race for months.

By Auburndale the aggressive running of "plucky Sammy," as the papers of the day called him, brought him 1 minute behind Caffery's record. Haarer struggled. Mellor was too much for him. By Brighton Seminary Haarer failed. He gave up. He let himself fall heavily to the ground and out of the race. Mellor had a mile on Marks and Lorz. The wind from the side whipped up annoying eddies of dust.

A thousand people watched from the electrics (streetcars) that followed the race along Commonwealth Avenue; Mellor looked sure to win again. He crested the hill but began to falter on the descent toward the reservoir at Chestnut Hill. He wanted the record and the win. But cramps in his quadriceps made it impossible to take advantage of the downhill. He could not run. His body did not work, yet he kept forcing it forward. Depression set in when his body told him that a record was skittling out of reach. By 22 miles all enthusiasm had drained from Mellor's body. He yielded to fatigue. He surrendered. He walked. Mellor now traveled at half Lorz's speed. Lorz had separated himself slightly from Marks, and on Beacon Street when he saw Mellor walking, he ran humorlessly past. Mellor had no fight left. Marks followed. Mellor quit the race.

Difficulties caught up with Lorz by Coolidge Corner. His handlers implored him to win: "Keep at it, Fred. Keep at it, only a little more. For heaven's sake keep it up. Marks is coming." They poured water on his head and swabbed him with sponges as he ran. They begged him to win; their fortunes depended on it.

The undisciplined crowds left a zigzag maze behind Lorz. It confused Marks. He could no longer see the leader.

At Massachusetts Avenue a jumble of bicycles and automobiles clotted into a tangle directly in front of Lorz. One of his handlers on a bike fell in front of him. He "leaped like a bird over the fallen rider and kept on amid cheers," running freely to the BAA clubhouse. There, in sight of the finish

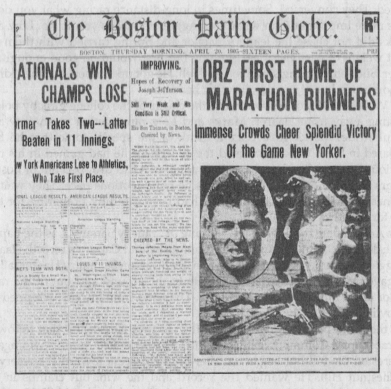

Winner Frederick Lorz—accused of cheating to win the Olympic marathon—fell over a bicycle at the finish line of the 1905 race (*Boston Daily Globe*, April 20, 1905).

line tape, Lorz encountered his biggest obstacle. Steps before the tape a bicycle swerved and tangled up Lorz, who fell forward, tumbled, and smashed the tape on his way to the ground.

Lorz chatted gaily in the victory circle. In the rush of the win, his humor restored, Lorz forgot his difficulties: "It's a cinch to run 25 miles. I never walked from the start." Lorz predicted he would come back the next year and break the record. Marks claimed he felt fresh as a daisy and would have won if only he could see through the crowds how close he ran. Robert Fowler, who finished third, said, "I lost the race by holding back too long." He blamed his handler, none other than the 1898 winner, Ronald MacDonald. "When I asked for a chance to go faster I was refused." MacDonald said that the race would be won in 2:40 because of the crosswind and dust and so ordered his charge to run with the Olympic champion, Hicks. Hicks had a bad day and never saw the leaders.

Lorz won his redemption. He said, "I guess those people who said I tried to steal the St. Louis race will now do a little thinking. I want to get myself right with the sporting people. I never claimed to have won the Olympic race and after I finished I told secretary James E. Sullivan of the Amateur Athletic Union that I rode in that automobile."

Joseph Martell, the entrant declared medically unfit, finished 31st, one place ahead of the "ancient" 49-year-old Peter Foley, in 3:25. Foley's "progress from start to finish was a continuous ovation."

Seventeen-year-old Timmy Ford of Cambridge, a plumber's assistant, plodded through the day to finish 15th with a 3:01. He resolved to come back.

1905 Results

1.	F. Lorz, MAC, NY	2:38:25	7.	T.J. Sullivan, SPAA	2:52:47
2.	L. Marks, PAC, NY	2:39:50	8.	J.F. Kennedy, Tileston	2:53:17
3.	R. Fowler, CG	2:41:07	9.	M.J. O'Neil, Cambridge, MA	2:53:56
4.	H.F. Miller, Jr., HAA	2:42:44	10.	J.S. Hunt, South Boston, MA	2:54:51
5.	E.S. Farnsworth, CG	2:43:01	11.	B. Jacobs, Boston, MA	2:56:00
6.	D.J. Kneeland, SPAA	2:48:32	12.	J. Lorden, Cambridgeport, MA	2:57:51

78 starters, 38 under 3:30.

RATHER SLOW PLUMBER'S HELPER

THURSDAY, APRIL 19, 1906

Hopeful Mellor Bound for Record Run

San Francisco still burned from the earthquake that on April 18 shook the city "like a terrier shaking a rat." San Francisco would burn building by

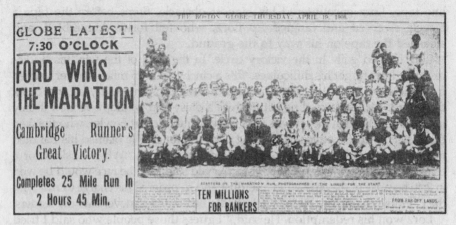

GLOBE LATEST!
7:30 O'CLOCK

FORD WINS
THE MARATHON

Cambridge   Runner's
    Great Victory.

Completes 25 Mile Run In
    2 Hours 45 Min.

TEN MILLIONS
FOR BANKERS

FROM FAR-OFF LANDS.

The 1906 field of runners waited at the start on the railroad bridge in Ashland; some feared their chances would be hurt by the noxious mixture of dust and automobile exhaust fumes they were forced to inhale (*Boston Globe*, April 19, 1906).

building for the rest of the week. News of the earthquake pushed all news of the marathon from its customary first-page spot in the Boston newspapers. Americans lined up to donate money. Bostonians pledged generously. The inside pages of the papers reported that in France a team of horses had knocked Pierre Curie, husband of Madame Curie and codiscoverer of radium, to the street. The horses' hooves missed him, but the wagon wheel crushed his skull. Susan Brownell Anthony had sickened and died weeks before. Women in America could not yet vote.

For the marathon in Boston only one previous winner returned, the lately omnipresent and furiously hopeful Sammy Mellor. The 1905 winner, Fred Lorz, had promised to return and break the course record, but he did not enter. The 105 runners entered included Tom Hicks and J.J. Kennedy. East Cambridge boy Timmy Ford—18 years old, blue-eyed, sandy-complexioned, a plumber's apprentice—entered at the last minute. He had finished a nondescript 15th the year before. Five feet tall and weighing 113-1/2 pounds, he raced in an odd cap that looked squashed onto his head and a Hampshire Athletic Association light green singlet with a single bandolier strip brandishing the monogram "AHA." He had begun training in December with long walks under the direction of his trainer, Frank Gormly. He took his first run on February 3. On the week before the race he ran a timed trial from South Framingham to Cleveland Circle in a time faster than Caffery's record-setting pace. He ran in 10th place at Natick, chewing a piece of straw and smiling to the crowds. His father waited in Boston behind a stretch of red yarn.

Meanwhile Mellor battled against a chilly headwind. David Kneeland of Roxbury ran with Mellor. Kneeland had placed sixth in the St. Louis Olympics and at Boston the year before and was the reigning New England 5-mile champion. For a living he hustled coal. He weighed 123 pounds. He boasted of having never taken a day off work because of his running. In Wellesley Hicks began to walk. He walked all the way to the finish. Mellor quit the race in Wellesley. With no effort on Ford's part his place improved. He ate two oranges.

Kneeland, alone and in the lead, faced a dilemma as well as a headwind. How much should he conserve himself and defend his lead? Might he burn himself up in an attempt at a big victory? His handlers advised him. A hundred bicycles churned up dust around him. Most of it blew back in his face. Kneeland ran up the first long hill in Newton. His graceful stride served him well. He walked up the next hill. Then he ran. While Ford was chewing his straw, Kneeland had bashed out the miles with Mellor. Now that fight began to show its bruises. "Elevated eyebrows proclaimed internal distress." Ford chewed, ran, and closed. "Kneeland's sleek legs were stretched for greater activity." Kneeland could hear the people cheering for Ford. "[Kneeland] bent his body forward, straining every fiber, and there was a look of agony on his face."

Crossing the bridge just before Commonwealth Avenue, a wagon broke down in front of Kneeland. Again he walked. "His discouraged coaches applied sponges and epithets of cheer." Ford was nearer now. Kneeland "saw with eyes that blinked with fatigue and despair a diminutive figure in green trunks shoot past him." Later Ford said, "After I trailed him some distance I knew I had him. I could see his knees were wobbly."

But the race was not over for Ford. A cyclist fell directly in front of him. He had to sidestep quickly. The crowd pressed so close that Ford had to slow down to penetrate it. He had to shepherd his own way. Kneeland followed the parted path, where he gained on Ford because he could move more easily. Even on Exeter Street's final straightaway Ford had to slow while the official vehicles made a path through the crowd for him. Kneeland gained. Ford smiled on Exeter Street as he saw the red yarn stretched and waiting. He gave a little sprint, then "threw himself across the line and against the barrier of human flesh pressed close against it." A giant policeman tried to catch Ford but an elderly man twirling his hat quickstepped around him. "Ford's blue eyes closed for an instant as he rested in the arms of his father."

Six seconds later Kneeland finished. It was the closest finish of all 10 Boston Marathons. It was also 16 minutes slower than Caffery's record. "Rather slow," read the *Daily Globe*'s headline.

1906 Results

1. **T. Ford**, *HamAA*, MA	**2:45:45**	6. M.J. O'Neil, *RAA* — 2:56:55
2. D. Kneeland, *RAA*	2:45:51	7. T.J. Sullivan, *SPAA* — 3:02:06
3. **T. Morrissey**, *MercAC*, NY	**2:53:41**	8. B. Mann, *NHAC*, NY — 3:02:06
4. P. Laffargue, *SBAC*, NY	2:53:56	9. W.R. Prouty, Hyde Park, MA — 3:07:11
5. J. Hayes, *SBAC*, NY	2:55:38	10. H. Brawley, *SAAA* — 3:08:11

105 entrants.

THE MOST FAVORED FAVORITE

FRIDAY, APRIL 19, 1907

Canadian Indian Longboat Unbeatable

H.H. Potter, a half-Sioux Indian living in Roxbury and running for the local athletic association, trained for the BAA marathon and entered for the 8th year. His hope, as he expressed it to a reporter, was to have the pleasure of meeting Mr. Thomas Longboat. Longboat was an Onondaga Indian from Canada who had become an instant legend as a long-distance runner. Potter was not a mere fan but also a serious contender for the Boston Marathon; he had always finished better than 14th. Potter, however, never mentioned racing and defeating Longboat or even dreaming to do so; he wanted only to shake his hand. When Tim Ford won the marathon in 1906 Tom Longboat was quite unknown, but a year later he was such a favorite to win "The Boston" that his backers could find few people willing to take their bets at any odds. The Longboat legend grew quickly but had its origins in the 1901 Boston Marathon.

In 1901 Canadian Mohawk Indian Bill Davis finished second to the Canadian Jack Caffery. Both had broken Caffery's year-old course record. In subsequent years, as Davis suffered a series of setbacks and languished in semiretirement, he heard a story about a teenage Indian on the reservation near Caledonia, 15 miles from his home in Hamilton, Ontario. He heard that the boy could run. He heard tall stories. As the story was reported in the Sunday edition of the *Boston Post*, young Longboat had accompanied his family on a wagon drawn by a couple of grays for a rare visit to Hamilton.

The boy was told that the team would leave at 3:00 p.m., with or without him. At the appointed hour the city still held the boy in its spell and did not release him until 5:00. His strict family had indeed left without him. The boy ran home; taking a slightly different but equally long road, he arrived at the family home before the wagon. Davis sought Tom Longboat and urged him to train seriously. Longboat had been born on June 4, 1887, in a log cabin on the Six Nations Reserve south of Brantford, Ontario. He carried the Onondaga name of Cogwagee, which means "everything." Tom Longboat's father died when he was a boy, leaving his mother to raise the family of two sons and two daughters in rural poverty.

Longboat had in fact already been training for racing. He happily covered miles and miles of rolling farm country on the west bank of the Grand River in the Six Nations Reserve. On April 24, 1907, the *Toronto Telegram* printed this, quoting an Indian guide:

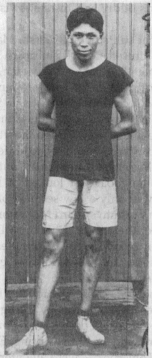

The 1907 winner, Tom Longboat, an Onondaga Indian, came to Boston from the Six Nations Reserve in Canada as the most heavily favored runner in the marathon to date. Courtesy of the Boston Public Library, Print Department.

> Tommy practice running two years. He run every morning and every night. He run down at the council on 24th May and get beaten. Then he come home and run more. He run round this block. It five miles and a half around and Tommy get so he run it in twenty-three and a half minutes. Next 24th of May Tommy go down to the council and run again. It a mile race and Tommy win by near a quarter of a mile.

For his first big race Davis coaxed Longboat to Hamilton for the big Thanksgiving Day 20-mile race. Davis had trained him for the 4 previous weeks. On race day Longboat showed up in a wildly striped bathing suit and old bicycle shoes. Some odds went 100 to 1 against him. "One such bet between an unnamed bookmaker and a citizen named J. Yaldon was penciled into the sheet at one thousand dollars to two dollars.

Davis instructed Longboat to shadow the Englishman John Marsh or whoever held the lead and to sprint at the very end. Longboat stuck like glue to the leader. When the leader sprinted, Longboat sprinted. When the lead slowed, Longboat slowed. Crowds laughed at Longboat in the early miles. "He held his hands oddly and his feet swished sideways in a peculiar manner."

After 15 miles Longboat still stuck to Marsh. Marsh put in a burst to do in Longboat but did in himself. Marsh sat down on the side of the road. Longboat sat on the other side, looked at Marsh, and grinned. Longboat was a man with a big toothy smile. He enjoyed himself at whatever he did. He was a young man, and according to the *Toronto Star* journalist Lou Marsh (no relation), "His head is full of ideas and he is one of the greatest kidders who ever came down the line to fame." Soon the sitting runner, John Marsh, heard the other runners coming. He jumped to his feet and resumed running. Longboat followed. But Marsh had run himself out. He "fell in a heap," the newspapers explained. Longboat just looked at him, then jogged to the finish. Longboat's time was only a few seconds off the course record. Ten days later Longboat won Toronto's Ward Marathon, a 15-mile road race, by 3 minutes. His next race, the annual Christmas Day 10-miler, he won in 54:50, setting a Canadian record by 2-1/2 minutes. Newspapers all called him "the greatest distance runner the world has ever seen." With that fanfare he arrived in Boston in April of 1907.

The 1906 winner, Tim Ford, chose not to run. He said he believed that other runners had injured their chances by trying to win the second time. He was in good condition and had been training but would wait until 1908. Other previous marathon winners—Mike Spring, Fred Lorz, Sammy Mellor, Olympic gold medalist Tom Hicks—were all entered. Race director George V. Brown got a letter from Caffery backing Longboat. Longboat's trainer said, "There is many a slip 'twixt the cup and the lip."

Harry Rosenthal, a Toronto businessman, was Longboat's first manager, but questions about the amounts of expense money changing hands cast doubt on Longboat's amateur status. The association with Rosenthal lasted only a few months. "At the direction of the Canadian Amateur Athletic Association Longboat joined and took up residence at the West End YMCA in Toronto." The Y entered him in the BAA Marathon, but controversies and allegations followed Longboat down from Canada.

Convoluted press reports dogged Longboat in Boston. The *Post* on April 15 gave this twisted account of what Rosenthal said that the YMCA manager, C.H. Ashly, did not say: "Ashly did not say that Longboat is a bad boy and required care to keep him away from liquor and other excesses but he makes it plain that the runner requires very careful handling." Innuendo of a drunken Indian followed Longboat all during his Boston stay.

The Ashland start had problems. Repairs closed the railroad bridge at Metcalf's Mill, so runners could not line up on it. George Billings of the BAA changed the course so the race could start at Steven's Corner on the Hopkinton road. The change made the start wider to accommodate a record 124 racers and to avoid forcing the runners to cross the railroad track after only a short distance. Billings also arranged for a watering trolley to wet the road to keep down the dust.

Longboat himself was in need of repairs. Reports floated about that he had fallen in training, injuring his knee. Dr. Frank Burt examined Longboat on April 17, reporting "temporary indigestion of the stomach which has affected his throat, and a cough which bothers him considerably." Longboat had a cold, but he had prepared thoroughly.

His training consisted of systematic increases in distances run on the measured concession roads on the reserve, then running into neighboring towns. Once after returning from running and walking, he told his mother he had gone to Dunnville and back, a total of 50 miles. She told him she'd throw him out of the house if he ever lied to her again. But more than merely chalking up brutal mileage, Longboat allowed himself a full recovery from hard efforts so his body had time to strengthen itself before the next on-slaught. These training principles would remain sound for the next century and serve Longboat well in Boston.

The Boston papers gave viewing instructions to marathon spectators: Take a street car to Ashland, then board one of the special cars leaving Ashland Square and follow beside the runners the whole distance from Ashland to Lake Street in Brookline. The practice, started in 1905, was so successful that the streetcar company decided to use some of its largest cars to accommodate the growing interest.

Flaxen-haired Jimmy Lee from Roxbury led from the start. Fred Lorz, the 1905 winner, followed him. Into South Framingham Lee and Lorz led, pursued 30 yards back by four men, including Canadian Charlie Petch. Ten yards behind them Longboat ran flat-footed, followed by the cagey crew of John "Chuck" Neary, the fast-starting youth from Natick who seemed to have mended his ways; Mike Spring, the 1904 winner; and Sammy Mellor, the 1902 winner.

Longboat held his hands at hip level, contrary to the recommended chest-high pumping style of 1900s trainers. Robert Fowler, John Hayes, and Tom Hicks planned a catch-up race with a slow start to allow the leaders to destroy themselves. The herd of following cars and bicycles and their attendant dust annoyed Longboat. The promised wetting cart never arrived to wet. He worried that a car might knock him down. He never knew there were so many bicycles and automobiles in the world. On the reservation roads he rarely saw one. He did however enjoy the cheers of their occupants.

Slowly a freight-laden train cut across the road in Framingham after the lead group of 10 passed. It blocked the road for its duration. Longboat said later, "I heard it behind me and had to chuckle when I thought of the others getting shut off."

As the train continued to trundle by, it dammed the course. Runners flooded the road behind it, their reservoir growing deeper and angrier with the arrival of each frustrated runner. The best of them had to wait the longest. Fowler, the fittest he had ever been in his life, waited. Hayes waited. The train had no mercy for royalty—Olympic gold medalist Hicks waited too. The day blew blustery and squally. Spits of sleet began to keep the dust down. It was a cold day, good for fast running. It was not a good day to start slowly. The dam held for a minute and 15 seconds.

Through Wellesley leader Lee ran a minute inside Caffery's record. Just before the junction of Washington Street and Commonwealth Avenue Longboat passed Lee, but to the surprise of the streetcar riders and other watchers, Petch ran stride for stride with Longboat. A snowsquall struck on the hills. The *Boston Post* wrote under the subhead "Hills had no terror for Redskin," that "these [hills] killed off Petch and caused him to drop back, but the noble son of the Onondagas did not seem to notice them." From there Longboat ran on alone, swiftly and easily smashing Caffery's record with each stride.

On the last part of the course a pretty girl handed a Canadian flag to Longboat. He made a bow and a big grin and waved the silk. Fowler, Hayes, and teenager James O'Mara charged past Petch over the final miles, making up the train delay, but Petch, weary Petch, flushed with high spirits and patriotism, wrapped a Canadian flag around his waist and proudly finished.

Longboat returned to Canada a hero because of his Boston victory. He was taken in a torchlight parade to city hall in Toronto where the mayor read a congratulatory address. "Young women gazed at Longboat in rapture as bands played and fireworks exploded around him." But in the end Longboat was an Indian—a member of a recently conquered race, tolerated as a performer in the conqueror's nation but credited not on having the qualities of a winner but on manageableness. The *Toronto Star* wrote,

> His trainers are to be congratulated, not only for having such a docile pupil, but on being able to show such excellent results from their regimen. It is to be hoped that Longboat's success will not develop obstinacy on his part, and that he will continue to be manageable.

Longboat never returned to defend his Boston title. The following year the New England Athletic Union banned him from Boston for taking money for running. He was reinstated. In the 1908 Olympic Games in London, Longboat collapsed at the 19-mile mark while running in second place. John Hayes won after officials disqualified Italy's Dorando Pietri because enthusiastic spectators helped him across the finish line. So discouraged was Longboat that he almost announced his retirement. Instead, at the persuasion of his manager, he turned professional. He raced indoor match race marathons on 10-laps-to-the-mile board tracks to capacity crowds of bettors. He won $17,000 in prize money alone as a professional. He was wealthy and became world famous.

One such professional race was against Dorando Pietri, who had in the previous month defeated Johnny Hayes in a match race marathon. The match with Longboat packed New York's Madison Square Garden with total gate receipts of $15,000. Pietri and Longboat each were guaranteed 25%, or shares of $3,750. Longboat won in 2:45:05.

In 1916 Longboat volunteered to serve in the Great War and joined the 180th Sportsmen's Battalion.

> Longboat competed in military races and was once assigned the dangerous job of carrying messages from one battlefield post to another in France. He was wounded and reported dead, leading to a jolting personal experience on his return to Canada in 1919. His wife Lauretta had remarried. The development was wrenching for both of them but, happy as she was to see Longboat alive, Lauretta decided to remain in her new marriage.

Longboat accepted his loss and later remarried and had four children. Thomas Longboat, Cogwagee of the Onondaga, died on January 9, 1949, at age 61 of pneumonia on the Six Nations Reserve.

> Although he had been baptized so he could marry in a church, he had kept to the longhouse religion all his life. His god was still the Great Spirit, and he was buried according to the traditional faith. He was dressed in new cotton and wool, which had been hand-stitched by the women in his family. . . . On his feet were new buckskin moccasins. A friend whittled a V in the top of the coffin to permit his spirit to escape. The entire service was spoken in Onondaga, the chants led by his two sons.

1907 Results

1. T. Longboat, *WEYMCA*, ON	2:24:24^{CR}	
2. R. Fowler, *CG*	2:27:54*	
3. J.J. Hayes, *SBC*, NY	2:30:38	
4. J. O'Mara, Cambridgeport, MA	2:35:37	
5. J.J. Lee, *SAAA*, Roxbury, MA	2:36:04	
6. C. Petch, *NEAC*, Toronto, ON	2:36:47	
7. S. Hatch, Chicago, IL	2:37:11	
8. J.H. Neary, Natick, MA	2:37:59	
9. J. Lindquist, *SAGC*	2:38:58	
10. C. Schlobohm, *MAA*, NY	2:42:02	
12. D. Kneeland, *SPAA*	2:45:54	
13. T. Hicks, Cambridge, MA	2:46:05	
15. M. Ryan, *MercAC*, NY	2:47:54	
17. T. Morrissey, *MercAC*, NY	2:49:23	

124 entrants, 102 starters, 53 finishers.
*Also broke John Caffery's record set in 1901.

No Favorite at All

MONDAY, APRIL 20, 1908

Sticking to Schedule Brings Victory

No newspapers picked a favorite this year. Last year everyone had picked Longboat as unbeatable, and everyone was right. The 1908 field, by contrast, was the most unpredictable yet in the BAA marathon. The wagering became a true lottery. To be sure, there was no shortage of quality—previous winners Sammy Mellor (1902), Mike Spring (1904), and Fred Lorz (1905) were all as fit as ever. The 1907 second-place finisher, Bob Fowler, who had been held back by the train in South Framingham for 1:15, was ready to run and hungry after that frustration on top of his second place of 1907 and third place in 1905. No one but Longboat had run faster in 1907. David Kneeland, the second-place runner from 1906, came to run, as did 1906's fifth place John Hayes, who had improved to third in 1907. Except for Longboat, most of last year's top 10 were back. Olympic gold medalist Tom Hicks came to improve on his second place at Boston in 1904. Chuck Neary, the tall, thin runner from Natick whom the newspapers called "elongated," came to race. Any of them could take it. It promised to be a mystery marathon.

On April 16 Bob Fowler told the newspapers, "Marathons are hard things to make predictions about. Everything is against any one man winning out. . . . what an uncertain proposition a marathon is." He listed cramps, climate, stones, and ankle sprains as dangers that add to the uncertainty.

Fowler did not include A. Roy Welton in his recitation of hazards. Welton, of the Lawrence, Massachusetts, YMCA, wearing a dark diagonal stripe on his singlet and a dark, wrinkled cap pulled onto his head, snatched an early lead and stretched it out to break all of Longboat's records up to 16 miles. It was a day for records. No dust blew on the roads because cooling snow-flakes and drizzle kept the day perfect for rapid, sweatless running.

During all this speeding John Hayes sat back in 32nd place in South Framing-ham, and behind him waited Mike Ryan in 38th. Ryan carried with him an enormous well of self-confidence, self-assertion, and pride. He knew he could finish far ahead of his present place. Even the rambunctious Sammy Mellor waited calmly in 13th place. But Fowler, Jimmy Lee (the fine-featured fifth-place runner of the previous year), and a gang of others hovered moments behind the brazen Welton. Lee wore the unicorn symbol of the BAA. The hosts' hopes weighed on him. Wouldn't it be nice if a golden-haired boy of the BAA could win their road race? This dream would haunt the BAA for the next half century. Fowler swung between his restlessness to win quickly and the temperance that experience had taught him. But in the middle stages he ran abreast of Lee as grim, cold cyclists followed, waiting to see who would crack.

Welton cracked in Wellesley. As the *Boston Herald* put it, "a sickly smile to his rivals told of Welton's disappointment at his physical inability to reach his goal." Fowler and Lee raced each other up the Newton hills on to the boulevard now called Beacon Street. They knew nothing of what and who waited behind them. A not quite 20-year-old electrician's assistant from Yonkers lurked behind them. Thomas P. Morrissey, running for the Mercury AC, ran with a lock of his black hair swinging on his forehead. He had a workman's muscular arms and wore ankle-high tennis shoes. He weighed 133-1/2 pounds. Unnoticed, he had been unconsidered before the race but was not unaccomplished.

Morrissey had been third in Boston in the slow year of 1906 with a 2:53 for the 25 miles, but in 1907 he finished a dismal 17th. But to redeem himself he had won the national indoor 25-mile championship in New York and shortly thereafter placed 10th in the Yonkers Marathon. He had trained running 10 to 15 miles three nights a week and walking on three other nights. He ran a 20-miler once every 3 weeks. The *Boston Post* reported that on Sundays he went to vespers. He didn't expect to win, but he did expect to place in the top three in under 2:30. Though Morrissey could not see the Fowler–Lee battle ahead of him, he could tell their position from the cluster of cars. That cluster had grown closer with each of the Newton hills.

Fowler and Lee fought each other and traded minor victories spurt for spurt, which of course means that each lost precious energy spurt for spurt. The urgings of the partisans, spectators, and fans in the automobiles and on the streetcars took on the character of a crowd at a prizefight. They wanted a knockout—now. Fowler and Lee could not help but be infected by their screaming for immediate resolution. In their spurts and surges, their Pyrrhic victories before the mobile cheering section spelled mutual doom for Fowler and Lee. On April 22 *Post* writer J.D. Delaney would write, "American runners have always had too much slash and bang in their running." Delaney favored those whose racing adhered to a schedule. Fowler and Lee fell off-schedule.

Morrissey stuck to a schedule that led him to a rendezvous with the first-place runner at St. Paul Street. (The record does not show whether it was Fowler or Lee who clung to the lead longest.) The *Globe* reported that "on came [Morrissey] as relentlessly as an Indian seeking vengeance." Nothing seemed in Morrissey's way once he took the lead, except an insistent young man wearing a cap. That was 1906 Boston winner Tim Ford wearing the cap, riding in an automobile next to Morrissey. Morrissey feared disqualification for accepting aid and coaching from someone other than the BAA assigned handler. Though he told Ford to go away, Ford would not quit coaching. Morrissey snatched Ford's cap off his head and tossed it into the crowd, forcing Ford to choose between continuing to kibitz and his lucky hat. Ford ran for the hat, and Morrissey ran for the finish, unaided to a solo victory as he broke the red woolen string across Exeter Street.

Behind Morrissey, Hayes had stuck to his own schedule, which had him pass through South Framingham in 32nd place, 30th by Natick, 25th at Wellesley, a relentless 13th just before the hills, and 5th at Coolidge Corner; he passed Fowler and Lee to come on to the finish. The *Herald* described him "fresh as a daisy in a meadow." His only regret was that he had not started his real running sooner. Fowler finished third again; in acute despair at his continual almost-winning, he vowed to quit running this marathon.

The first six finishers ran faster than Caffery had in his 1901 record race. Sammy Mellor, who ran every race since 1901 and won in 1902, ran the fastest marathon of his life but finished eighth. Fred Lorz's seventh place was his last appearance—by 1922 he was dead of pneumonia at 42.

1908 Results

1.	T.P. Morrissey, *MercAC*, NY	2:25:43	6.	J.J. Lee, *BAA*		2:28:34
2.	J.J. Hayes, *IAAC*	2:26:04	7.	F. Lorz, *MAC*		2:32:20
3.	R.A. Fowler, *CG*	2:26:42	8.	S. Mellor, *MercAC*		2:41:17
4.	M.J. Ryan, *IAAC*	2:27:08	9.	A.R. Welton, Lawrence, MA		2:43:25
5.	W. Wood, Somerville, MA	2:27:48	10.	J.J. Goff, CG		2:43:54

120 entrants.

THE INFERNO

MONDAY, APRIL 19, 1909

Marathon Mania Grips Boston

Since 1897 the Boston Marathon field had increased more than 10-fold, and the numbers of spectators rose to an estimated 300,000. A marathon mania gripped Boston in 1909. The catalyst for this craziness was the Olympic marathon of the previous summer. It grabbed the public attention as nothing but death can.

Headlines in American newspapers ran variations of "Dying Man Wins Olympic Marathon." That dying man was Dorando Pietri of Italy—but he didn't win and, further, he didn't die. He merely almost won and almost died. Dorando entered the Olympic stadium in London clearly the leader and about to become the winner when he began to stagger. To the horror of the crowd he fell. He got up, ran, staggered, and fell again. The shocked crowd could only watch. At last officials could take no more and helped Dorando across the finish line. Later that day other officials had to consider that Dorando did not run unaided to the finish; they disqualified him and crowned the next-place finisher, American Johnny Hayes, Olympic champion. Hayes had finished second in Boston in 1908. Another American, Joe Forshaw of St. Louis, earned the bronze in those Olympic Games. A. Roy Welton, who had broken Longboat's checkpoint records for most of the 1908 Boston race, finished fourth. These men became celebrities. In fact, by 1911 the Mecca Cigarette

> *By 1911 the Mecca Cigarette Company issued "runner" cards, featuring 150 different athletes, that were distributed in packages of cigarettes.*

Company of New York issued "runner" cards, featuring 150 different athletes, that were distributed in packages of cigarettes. The public thirsted after stories of marathoners. Hundreds of marathon races were scheduled in the United States that year. In Massachusetts alone there were Patriots' Day running races in nearly every town.

The April 18 issue of the *Boston Daily Globe* carried an 11-stanza poem about marathon racing. Each stanza sang praise to a different ethnic group of competitors: Irishmen, Indians, Italians, Canadians, French, and others.

People worldwide had waited during Pietri's hospitalization to see if he would live or die. Day by day newspapers reported his recovery. A cry went up that the marathon was a more savage and dangerous event than boxing. An editorial in *The New York Times* on February 24, 1909, instructed,

> It is only the exceptional man who can safely undertake the running of 26 miles, and even for them the safety is comparative rather than absolute. The chances are that every one of them weakens his heart and shortens his life, not only by the terrible strain of the race itself, but by the preliminary training which produces muscular and vascular developments that become perilous instead of advantageous the moment a return to ordinary pursuits and habits puts an end to the need for them. For the great majority of adults particularly in an urban population, to take part in a Marathon race is to risk serious and permanent injury to health, with immediate death a danger not very remote, and it is little better than criminal to let growing boys make any such demands upon their powers of endurance. For boys, indeed, even the shorter races are of very questionable desirability, since at any distance the expenditure of energy under the stimulus of competition is excessive. . . . The truth is that exercise should always be purely subordinate to the business and pleasure of life. To make it or the bodily changes it produces ends instead of incidents is a dangerous as well as an absurd mistake.

The lewd lure of death—the titillating possibility that they might see someone die—held unprecedented numbers of people along the streets of Boston to watch the 1909 marathon. Those in the crowd of 300,000 who came to see someone die were nearly not disappointed.

On April 19 a warm southwesterly flow of air brought what was then a record high temperature of 83.4 °F to Boston with high humidity. Worse still, the ill wind blew more or less at the runners' backs, more or less at the same speed they ran. Stale air followed them. Sweat pooled on their skin and dripped off rather than evaporating. In even, still air runners generated enough wind by their own motion so that sweat evaporated to carry away excess heat, but on this day the racers stewed in their own juices. There were none of the snowflakes and drizzle of the previous 2 years to cool their hot skin. With no recent experience running in heat, runners expected fast times and planned to run to get them. Disaster awaited.

The field in 1909 could not include the marathon heroes of the day. Hayes had turned professional and raced the recovered Pietri and Tom Longboat in a much-publicized series of prize-money indoor match marathons. They packed venues like New York's Madison Square Garden with overflow crowds of cigar-smoking gamblers. They raced each other on board tracks, 10 or 11 laps to the mile, while bettors screamed encouragement or dismay. The amateur Boston Athletic Association, through its membership in the Amateur Athletic Union, the governing body of the sport, would not allow Hayes, Pietri, Longboat, or other professionals to run in their marathon. The amateur Boston Marathon field did, however, have its own stars.

Tom Morrissey had won the year before and intended to win again. Sammy Mellor, the 1902 winner, had run his best time of 2:41 for eighth place the year before. Mellor had developed a mystical love for the Boston Marathon: "I have run in every race since 1901, and when I come along on race day every rock on the course seems to jump up and shake hands with me." Bob Fowler, third the previous year, hoped to fix himself on the apparent tradition of third-place succession that had seen Mellor, Lorden, Spring, and Morrissey crowned with first place after their thirds of previous years. But the press favored a young man from the Carlisle Indian School, a Hopi named Lewis Tewanina who had placed ninth in the 1908 London Olympic Games but had never run in Boston. He was pictured in newspaper cartoons racing wearing a feather, deerskin pants, and moccasins. Hayes arrived in town to advise his pupil, Mike Ryan of New York City, who had finished fourth the year before. Hayes planned to follow Ryan on a bicycle.

A. Roy Welton and Jimmy Lee of Yonkers, ninth and sixth in 1908, respectively, came to race. Carl Schlobohm took an early lead but relinquished it shortly. Tewanina took the lead with Louis Fine of Providence, Rhode Island. Harry Jensen of New York hung close, as did Jimmy Lee and Sammy Mellor. At South Framingham Pat Grant of Brooklyn ran easily in 62nd place. Henri Renaud of Nashua, New Hampshire, ran in 53rd place and held no notion of winning the race. But Renaud would be the man of the day.

Renaud's father had persuaded his son to enter the marathon. The father, who had come to New Hampshire from his native Trois-Rivieres, Quebec, had been a noted ultra-long distance racer in his youth. Nineteen-year-old Henri ran with his pants held up by a black leather belt and his socks rolled down his ankles to his polished black leather running shoes. His grin displayed a gap left by a departed upper front tooth, which together with his sweat-plastered hair made him look a bit goofy. He did not know it at the time, but he had reason to grin. He gained places in the race without passing anyone. His job in a cotton mill in Manchester, New Hampshire, required him to work from 6:30 a.m. to 6:00 p.m. in a hot and humid room operating a weaving loom. The heat and humidity were required to prevent a buildup of static electricity and cotton fibers in the air. Unlike other racers that day at Boston, Renaud had already been in summer weather for 12 hours a day.

Renaud had started racing the previous September and had placed 14th in the New England AAU cross-country championships and 13th and 16th in other local races. He was neither fast nor strong, nor was he well regarded as a runner, but he alone was heat-acclimated. He weighed 158 pounds and stood 5'11" (though another report has him at 5'9", which seems more likely from photographs). He claimed a diet that included little meat.

Mellor and Lee took the lead. Mellor had been there many times before. He had tried to win the marathon every year since 1901. But it was too hot, and Mellor had to surrender the lead. As the sun pressed down on Mellor perhaps he did begin to see the stones reaching up to shake his hand. Fine and Tewanina took the lead back again.

Fine suffered. He drove himself until the machinery of his body stopped. The heat seized him, and the sun put him in the Newton hospital. Welton dropped out at 18 miles. Tewanina stopped and asked for something to eat. His coach from the Indian school collected him and drove him to the finish line. Morrissey had given up and walked by the Wellesley hills. John Goff of Cambridge took a turn leading before himself dropping out. Fowler suffered, but stubbornness kept him in the race. Every runner sponged himself frequently. *Globe* writer Lawrence J. Sweeney was amazed at the retreat of dyestuffs from the fabrics of the runner's uniforms: "The colors from their suits outlined fantastic designs on their weary legs."

Up the long hill Mellor and Lee did not attempt to push themselves. They had made a peace treaty of sorts to prevent what had happened to Lee and Fowler the previous year, when both raced themselves out in an attempt to beat Morrissey but ended up only defeating each other. All hopes for good times died. Mellor and Lee made peace not to save themselves for victory but from the weather. No longer was racing paramount; mere survival became the goal. Just keep going and get it over and done. The *Globe* reported that Ryan in his desperation resorted to stimulants.

Renaud had eaten nothing and taken only two drinks of water. Only in Auburndale, after he had broken into the top 20, did he think of winning. His co-workers back at the mill had laughed at him and told him to give up running because he would never win anything. During the hills Renaud passed runner after runner. After the Newton hills he ran in third place.

Pat Grant held the lead for a short time, until he himself had to walk. He broke into a run as Harry Jensen passed him but could not prevent the passing. At St. Paul Street, less than 3 miles from the finish, Renaud caught and passed Jensen. Once Renaud got the lead he swore that no one would pass him even if it cost him his life. Renaud said later, "I am American for speed and French for gameness."

Perhaps Howard A. Pearce of New Bedford was too game, or perhaps it was the heat or marathon mania, but after he dropped out of the race at 8 miles and rode with other dropouts to near the finish, he jumped out of the car and burst through the crowd and began to run on the course. The people who saw him break into the race took no note, but those who saw him running quickly and freshly behind the BAA official lead vehicle took him to be the winner. They gave him their full cheers. He accepted them. Officials such as John Graham and George V. Brown doubted that he had run the whole way, so they pulled their car up to him to ask. Pearce ignored them as he ran down Commonwealth Avenue and on toward the Exeter Street finish line. Pearce the imposter headed for the tape. The officials decided that he must not reach it. They implored him to stop, but he refused. The officials asked to police to stop him and remove him from the course. Only with the finish line in sight did the police catch up and nab Pearce and physically force him from the course.

Henri Renaud, the legitimate winner, plugged along nearly a mile ahead of Jensen and Grant. Renaud accepted his deserved ovation from a crowd that had been waiting a long time in what for them was quite pleasant weather. His time was the slowest-winning Boston Marathon time of the century. He crossed the finish line with road dust caked on to his sweat. Little rivers from the spongings eroded those fantastic designs of mud and dye on his legs. He lifted his arms in victory and gave his goofy missing-tooth grin as he broke the red worsted wool finish line.

"Survivors of the Inferno of 1909" shows the positions of the top eight finishers at each checkpoint. As the day wore on, more and more runners dropped out because of the excessive heat. For some of these finishers, it wasn't so much their speed but their ability to withstand the heat that won them their places.

	South Framingham	Natick	Wellesley	Commonwealth Avenue	Coolidge Corner	Final place
Henri Renaud	53	38	28	19	3	1
Harry Jensen	3	5	9	4	1	2
Patrick Grant	62	26	22	7	2	3
James Crowley	6	10	10	6	6	4
Samuel Mellor	8	1	3	8	5	5
Joseph McHugh	21	13	7	5	7	6
Edward Ryder	28	24	19	10	4	7
Carl Schlobohm	39	30	24	22	10	8

Survivors of the Inferno of 1909

Bob Fowler finished 10th and swore again that this race would be his last marathon. Mike Ryan, with or despite Hayes's help, slogged along to finish 35th in 3:35. Sammy Mellor, at 5th, took his best place in years.

Later in the year two resolutions concerning the safety of marathons passed at the AAU annual convention. The first barred all competitors under 16 from marathons, and the second required a medical examination for all marathon competitors.

1909 Results

1. **H. Renaud, Nashua, NH**   **2:53:36**
2. H. Jensen, *PAC*, NY   2:57:13
3. P.J. Grant, *TAC*, Brooklyn, NY 2:57:17
4. J.F. Crowley, *IAAC*, NY   2:59:42
5. **S.A. Mellor, Jr., *MercAC*** **3:00:53**

6. J.P. McHugh, South Boston, MA 3:01:52
7. E.G. Ryder, *OAA*, MA   3:02:48
8. C. Schlobohm, *MercAC*, NY   3:06:10
9. E. McTiernan, Worcester, MA   3:08:08
10. R. Fowler, Cambridge, MA   3:09:31

182 entrants, 164 starters.

Chapter 2

1910-1919
The Great War Decade

Presidents: *William H. Taft, Woodrow Wilson*

Massachusetts Governors: *Eben S. Draper, Eugene Foss, David I. Walsh, Samuel W. McCall, Calvin Coolidge*

Boston Mayors: *John F. Fitzgerald, James Michael Curley, Andrew J. Peters*

1910 Populations: *United States, 92,228,496; Massachusetts, 3,366,416; Boston, 686,092*

As the second decade of the century opened, the English and the Germans conducted a high-stakes competition of battleship construction. The Germans thought if they could build enough dreadnoughts they would drive the English from the seas; the German army was already the best in Europe. But if the English could add to their fleet, they could maintain naval superiority. All that plus the growing international trade of the U.S. in industrial (rather than agricultural) products woke up the giant country and linked the fates of America and Europe.

In 1916 Americans reelected Woodrow Wilson with the slogan "He kept us out of war." In 1914 Joe Kennedy of Boston married Rose Fitzgerald of Dorchester, the daughter of Boston mayor John F. (Honey Fitz) Fitzgerald; their child, John Fitzgerald Kennedy, was born along the Boston Marathon course in Brookline in 1917. By then the Great War in Europe had sucked the United States into involvement. It touched nearly everyone in the civilized world. Millions of young men, off to fight in the glorious war, ran out of their trenches with the glee of the mythic Pheidippides, eager to shout, "Rejoice. We conquer!" The war touched the Boston Marathon and changed its history. It killed one winner.

By the close of the decade the international awakening of America had come full circle; Americans wanted the world to go away and leave them alone on their continent.

MEN WITH SCHEDULES

TUESDAY, APRIL 19, 1910

Fowler: Victory This Year for Sure?

In 1910 cities had many daily newspapers, some with morning, evening, and "extra" editions. They were the only media. From time to time readers saw photos documenting the travels of former President Theodore Roosevelt. The week of the Boston Marathon readers saw Roosevelt in the Middle East riding a camel. They read that Mark Twain lay on his deathbed and that a vociferous band of suffragettes were demanding that women get the right to vote. In the second week of April readers of Boston newspapers read about the frustrations of marathoner Bob Fowler.

Fowler, from Cambridge, Massachusetts, had his heart set on winning this year's Boston Marathon. The year before he had finished 10th in "the inferno." He finished third in 1908; was stopped by a freight train and so he finished second to Longboat in 1907, but also under the course record; placed third in 1905. Wasn't it finally his turn? Fowler, now with a receding hairline, said that if he won this year it would be his last marathon. He felt he deserved to win, that this was his year. On New Year's Day of 1909, Fowler had run the fastest time ever in the world, 2:52:45.4, for the full 26-mile, 385-yard marathon in Yonkers, New York. Natural succession meant that Fowler, who had paid his dues, should win. But neither the world nor the marathon worked in predictable patterns; events conspired against those with even the best of intentions.

Fowler loved runners as well as running, so he encouraged a Canadian named Fred Cameron to come to Boston this year. Fowler had met Cameron, an apprentice machinist, at a race in Halifax, Nova Scotia, a year earlier. A boyish 23-year-old, Cameron stood at 5'3-1/2" and 127 pounds with a high forehead and deep-set blue eyes. Anyone who met him found him likable, well mannered, and articulate. But he had never run 25 miles in his life, though he had gone 5 miles in 26:01 to better Tom Longboat's Canadian record by 3 seconds. He saw himself as a 10-mile runner and had the credentials to back that up. He won the 1909 Halifax 10-miler in 54:46, a Canadian record, beating Bob Fowler. But friendly Fowler brought Cameron to Boston and trained with him for the week before the race.

Why, to Fowler's dismay, did Patriots' Day have to be warm, upward of 70 °F? That was just the worst kind of weather for Fowler's body. Why did a different train have to block his way this year?

By race day 193 men had entered. Sammy Mellor came back, as did old-timer Peter Foley, a diamond cutter from Winchester, Massachusetts. Foley,

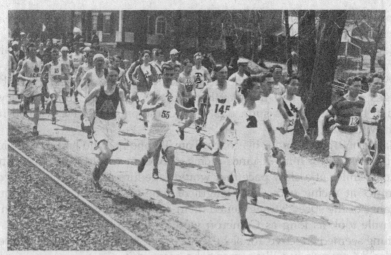

The 1910 field started their race, running along the rail line in Ashland. Prerace favorites Harry Jensen, #13, and Daniel Sheridan, #55, did not finish. Courtesy of the Boston Public Library, Print Department.

now 52 with a face full of gray whiskers, had become a celebrity for running marathons at such advanced ages. People marveled that he could still run a marathon. But the BAA officials didn't marvel; they banned him. They said he was too old and had no chance to win. But old Foley fooled them. He shaved off his whiskers, slipped into the starting throng at Ashland, and ran away to Boston, a hoary old bandit.

Mike Ryan, the high-strung red-headed Irishman of New York, came to race alongside his bicycle-mounted handler and advisor, 1908 Olympic gold medal marathoner and now professional, Johnny Hayes. Ryan had been fourth in Boston in 1908, just behind Fowler. Three times during the 1910 race Hayes's bicycle would break down, and each time he would have to commandeer a new one.

The fashion of training this year dictated that to run his best race a man should decide what time he expected to run, then construct a timetable for the checkpoints based on that even pace. The old-style tactic had been to burst away from your opponent at precisely the correct moment, much like a boxer might erupt in a flurry of punches at a critical match moment. But it seemed that in recent years the men who had stuck to even pacing and did not run in spurts had done best. So this year each contender appeared to have his own schedule in hand.

Newcomer Cameron zipped out to an early lead. Fowler ran conservatively and according to his schedule. Ryan stuck to his schedule, and newcomer Clarence DeMar stuck to his. DeMar kept a vision of the distance before him. He thought this was the way to run: Imagine the course before you, and imagine yourself running it as you plot your position on your mental map. Overall conditions seemed moderately fast, the heat not severe. But just what schedule did young Cameron intend to keep?

Cameron wore a cap with a visor to protect his eyes, which were said to be rather weak. No runner went with him, but bicycles and cars did. The BAA tried but failed to keep unofficial machines off the course. Automobiles, badges of prestige and the playthings of the rich, and common bicycles ridden by excited boys spun dust into Cameron's face. He washed it off with witch hazel.

Cameron trained under his coach, Tom Trenholm, who had definite ideas about training for long-distance racing. Cameron would train with runs of 16 to 18 miles at a slow pace that would take him as much time as would 25 miles at racing pace. That length of time on his feet, rather than the distance or the speed, strengthened them. Eighteen miles at about 8 minutes per mile took as long as Cameron would take to run the marathon. The training seemed effective, for as he led the race, he showed no strain. Spectators said Cameron ran like a man who enjoyed it.

In South Framingham a freight train again crossed the route after 25 runners had passed. Fowler went right on schedule, in 29th place, running an even pace on a warm day. Every year since 1907 a freight train had blocked the path of some marathoners. BAA officials had spoken to the superintendent of the railway division each year since the first incident, and each year he agreed that no trains would run on the spur from 12:15 to 12:45 on race day. Yet each year someone forgot to tell the engineer. Fowler lost 1:16 this year to the train, and it destroyed his schedule. Fowler may have the distinction of being the most unlucky runner in Boston Marathon history. In cooler weather he might have made up the time, but the railway and the weather had seemingly conspired against him. Fowler gamely continued to Lake Street, then, overcome with frustration, disappeared from the course.

Cameron ran according to his own scheduled, even pace. In a story written by Cameron himself in the *Boston Post* on April 20, 1910, he said, "I had the whole race doped out." He never faltered or lost his lead. Boston mayor John Fitzgerald's car followed Cameron over the last parts of the course. No one passed him. The mayor invited the victor to lunch the next day. Lunch, too, fit into Cameron's schedule.

Clarence DeMar's schedule put him in 23rd place in South Framingham— ahead of the train. DeMar is perhaps thus the luckiest racer in Boston Marathon history. Gradually his schedule worked to merge with Cameron's. DeMar passed runner after runner. Had the race been only a few miles longer . . .

DeMar caught sight of the leader for the first time at Exeter Street, where Cameron turned, saw the finish line, and took victory. As DeMar had a minute to run he could hear the cheers for Cameron. The tantalizing closeness of his finish, his continual gain on the leader, and the ease of the entire run captivated Clarence DeMar. It was in that forgiving minute that he contracted the marathon syndrome. Victory had become palpable; he had tasted victory like a shark tasted blood in the water but could not feed. He watched another man devour the spoils. This near victory changed DeMar's life and, perhaps more so than an easy win, infected him with marathon fever for the next four decades. Mike Ryan moved from eighth at South Framingham to fifth at the finish. He too got a whiff of victory. Yet Ryan's marathon fever raised symptoms that would in following years provoke conflict with DeMar, making each the other man's harshest critic.

Others criticized DeMar this year, telling him that a man is never the same after running a marathon, so he must expect to finish way back in any subsequent races. Common sense told those who volunteered their advice to DeMar that one or two marathons should do for a lifetime. But DeMar thought too much, liked running, and resented unsolicited advice. As a compositor for a printing firm, he worked meticulously. He minded if his p's appeared where his q's should be. And he trained meticulously. After the race the 21-year-old said, "I feel that I have lots of time in which to develop as a runner."

1910 Results

1.	F. Cameron, *RAC*, Amherst, NS	2:28:52	9.	E.P. Devlin, *MHAC*, NY	2:41:34
2.	C. DeMar, *NDAA*	2:29:52	10.	J. Cleary, Cherry Valley, MA	2:44:58
3.	J.J. Corkery, *CanAC*	2:34:25	11.	C. McCarthy, *YMCA*	2:47:54
4.	J.R. Roe, *WEAC*, Toronto, ON	2:38:06	12.	G.F. McInerney, *ShanAC*, PA	2:49:45
5.	M.J. Ryan, *IAAC*, NY	2:38:24	13.	R.F. Piggott, *CG*	2:50:59
6.	J.J. Reynolds, *NJAC*	2:40:03	24.	H. Renaud, Nashua, NH	3:03:24
7.	R.E. MacCormack, *TecAC*, ON	2:40:25	35.	S. Mellor, Yonkers, NY	3:08:42
8.	E.A. White, *HCL*, NY	2:40:50			

169 starters.

CLARENCE, FESTUS, FABRE, AND FOWLER

WEDNESDAY, APRIL 19, 1911

Snowshoe Racer Heads Field for Patriots' Day Marathon

Before he ever ran his first marathon, young Clarence DeMar carefully studied a 10-cent Spaulding book about distance running, wanting to be sure that he understood the theory before putting it into practice. He would rather read and study than be coached; coaches rattled him. When he had absorbed the lessons of the little book and added his own experience of

cross-country running at the University of Vermont and his second place in
the Boston Marathon of 1910, he really began to train. He trained nearly 100
miles a week for a couple of months, including several 20-mile jaunts in
addition to his regular runs to and from work. There is no record of anyone
before DeMar training that much for a marathon. But Clarence DeMar
wanted to be thorough. He believed that only with hard work would God
grant success in any venture. A few nights before this year's Boston Marathon, he dreamed that he had won. But he knew the dream was only a
dream, and he discounted any prediction of victory.

Bob Fowler also dreamed that he would win. He predicted he would do
it, and he believed his dreams. Fowler hoped for a drizzly day. This would
be his 25th marathon. It was now or never.

Old Sammy Mellor would not be running. Over the years Mellor had
placed in six of the top eight trophy positions. Perhaps he had at long last
given up the pursuit.

Andrew Sockalexis, a Penobscot Indian from Old Town, Maine, had run
well in the past year and might be a factor. He was the cousin of Louis, a
professional baseball player for Cleveland. Joe Lorden seemed to be even
faster than his older brother, 1903 winner John Lorden. The press also favored
Mike Thomas, an Indian from Lenox Island, off Prince Edward Island in
the Canadian Maritimes.

The prerace press paid attention to another Canadian, 6-footer Edouard
Fabre, a champion snowshoe racer. Some said that Fabre had Indian blood,
and the common opinion of the day insisted that Indian heritage conferred
special powers of endurance and the ability to withstand pain. Some even
considered it unfair for pure-blood Indians and white men to run in the
same races.

Festus J. Madden, a bulky and muscular Irishman and South Boston freight
handler, had attracted press attention when he ran extraordinarily well in
the Cathedral 10-mile handicap that spring. Madden's blood flowed pure
Irish. His people had endured the threat of starvation in 1845 after a blight
killed Ireland's potato crop. Many younger sons emigrated to America,
where they became laborers, sportsmen, boxers, runners, sharing with native
Americans low social status. Madden had arrived in America with this wave.

Madden had his own notions about training. He tried to mix endurance
and speed training. One day he would run 18 miles, then take a day off and
come back on the third day to run a fast 8 or 9 miles with his North Dorchester
AA clubmate Israel Saklad or Joe Marino. The press favored Madden, Fowler,
and DeMar—but they favored many runners. Marathoners were big heroes
in Boston that year. The *Boston Post* of April 19 had head shots of 21 favorites
bordering their first page.

These 21 lined up with about 100 others for an uneventful start. After 6
miles DeMar tempered himself in 15th place; Fabre ran in 33rd, Fowler in
12th, and Madden in 3rd. DeMar ran with a slight limp because of a sore
knee. He told the *Boston Post* reporter that, "At the start of the race I held

myself in check somewhat. That is, I don't mean I ran slowly, but I kept what you might call a reserve force in me. . . . I did not let my eagerness to pass them get the better of me."

DeMar had his schedule in hand. The limp remained, but the knee gave him no problem. The weather blew in a few cooling drops of rain, making conditions ideal.

Madden took the lead by Wellesley and held it to the beginning of Commonwealth Avenue and the hills. DeMar took the lead from Madden at 19 miles. By Coolidge Corner DeMar ran 3:26 slower than Caffery's 1901 checkpoint record of 2:04:00. From there to the finish a remarkable thing happened. Where Longboat had run his last 3 miles in 17:58 to set his course record of 2:24:24, DeMar ran 14:13 for the same distance to smash Longboat's record.

Could DeMar really have run 4:45 per mile for the last 3 miles of a marathon? That pace seems too fast, and in his autobiography DeMar made no mention of running the closing miles a minute per mile faster than his average. The newspapers reported these relative times, but the distances may not be precise. This sort of imprecision haunted the race until the 1980s, but it did nothing to diminish the wild enthusiasm and respect for marathon running.

The *Boston Daily Globe* marathon writer, Lawrence Sweeney, started his story about the 1911 marathon with the exclamation, "Let the Eagle scream!" and proceeded to hail DeMar and his new world record. Subsequent announcements in the *Globe* and other papers proclaimed that DeMar would be at Boston Arena with Governor Foss and Mayor Fitzgerald and would speak briefly. DeMar had become an instant celebrity. In an era with few other sports personalities, DeMar became a media star. At first he enjoyed the attention, the glory, the fame, and the appreciation, but later the attention of sports fans and sport itself would sound hollow to DeMar.

In an era with few other sports personalities, DeMar became a media star.

Bob Fowler again did not gain the glory he so much wanted. He ran the best that he knew how to run to take fourth place. He said he was deeply disappointed that he did not win, that he had lost the spring in his muscles.

Fabre ran a clever race, moving steadily through the field from checkpoint to checkpoint. He had plans for future Boston Marathons. DeMar, on the other hand, appeared to retire for the rest of the decade from the Boston race; he disappeared. He would be back, a mature and changed man, a man who had undergone a spiritual awakening, rebirth, and return to his roots (but that would not be for a long time). Mike Ryan had more immediate plans.

1911 Results

1.	C. DeMar, *NDAA*	2:21:39^{CR}	10.	J. Lorden, *SMAC*, MA	2:36:33
2.	F.J. Madden, *SouthBAC*	2:24:31	11.	J. Cleary, *WAC*	2:37:07
3.	E. Fabre, *NAC*, Montreal, PQ	2:29:22	12.	A.K. Sturgis, Boston, MA	2:38:46
4.	R. Fowler, Cambridge, MA	2:29:31	13.	E.W. McTiernan, *AAA*	2:38:56
5.	R.F. Piggott, Medford, MA	2:30:45	14.	C. Horne, *YMCA*, MA	2:42:00
6.	D. Sheridan, *VAC*	2:31:44	15.	C. McCarthy, *LYMCA*	2:42:15
7.	A. Harrop, Fall River, MA	2:32:31	16.	C. Appleyard, *MAA*	2:42:41
8.	W. Galvin, *MercAC*	2:33:10	17.	A. Sockalexis, Old Town, ME	2:43:45
9.	M.J. Ryan, *IAAC*, NY	2:36:15			

141 entrants, 127 starters.

MUD, RAIN, AND RYAN

FRIDAY, APRIL 19, 1912

The Ancient Marathoner Returns

The marathon again promised to be the big news story for Boston in early April of 1912. Nearly every day articles described the entrants. Heroes were nominated and endorsed, and marathon stories spilled off the sports pages. The many daily papers used stories about potential winners to scoop their competition. The marathon was the lottery of the day; much money waited to change hands because of well-placed or poorly placed bets. The April editions of the *Boston Post* read like a racing form dedicated to the marathon— almost an official daily program.

So it appeared until April 15, the day the Titanic sank. Suddenly room for endless marathon stories evaporated. The unsinkable ocean liner sank on its maiden voyage with 1,500 people on board. The papers reeled with the stories of the survivors and the heroism of the dead. Nasty accusations flew. Who to blame? Men who survived while women and children drowned had their manhood questioned. The press celebrated the heroism of the man who took out his pistol to hold other men off life rafts while women and children boarded them. The pistol wielder as well as the cowards went down with the ship. He was an old-fashioned man, as was marathon runner Mike Ryan.

Red-headed, clear-skinned, imperious Mike Ryan of the Irish-American AC of New York City was a principled, uncompromising man of his time. He held there was a right way to do things, and usually it was his. Ryan would have gone down with the ship and taken the cowards with him.

Ryan had raced Boston before, with a 15th place to Longboat in 1907, 4th in 1908 to Morrissey, DNF in 1909 (he was recovering from a bout of blood poisoning), 5th in 1910, and 9th in 1911. He had broken all world records in the East vs. West Marathon in Pittsburgh in 1909, but because of controversy about the course those records were not accepted. He had set a course record in the Hamilton, Ontario, *Spectator* Marathon and finished second in the British championship. Ryan came to race this year in a white running suit with emerald trim. Soon the resplendent suit would be splattered with muck.

A northeast storm dumped rain all the night before and through three quarters of the marathon, rendering the roads inches deep in mud. Some runners took to the sidewalks, while others picked their way around puddles. Checkers had problems recording the numbers of all the competitors because some passed behind them on the sidewalk.

Cool, moist air, perfectly brewed for runners to inhale, filled New England. Not a particle of dust hovered anywhere. The air was especially suited for Bob Fowler, whom the newspapers called the "ancient marathoner." The day was made for him, and no trains got in his way. Loyal money rode on him.

Festus Madden's training partner, Israel Saklad of the North Dorchester AA, took the lead through Framingham in 22:18, only 18 seconds slower than Caffery's checkpoint record from 1901. The North Dorchester club had its own mobile cheering section in a big touring car with a sign on the back listing the names of its racing members. Saklad ran along reading his own name.

From Natick, Yale man Johnny Gallagher took over. He looked unstoppable and uncatchable, but he was given chase by South Boston Irishman Madden, now of the aggressive and growing North Dorchester club, and Penobscot Indian Andrew Sockalexis, raised in Maine but recruited by the same club along with three Indians of the Carlisle school with the wonderful names of Arquette, Telyumptewa, and Hermequatewa. Ryan ran in eighth place through the Newtons, full of confidence. There is no record that his advisor, Johnny Hayes, tried this year to wallow through the mud on a bike. Fowler and Olympian Joe Forshaw seemed unable to get moving and trailed.

Gallagher ran 4 minutes ahead of DeMar's record at Lake Street, but he turned his ankle on a stone in the mud and slowed. (More likely fatigue allowed him to twist the ankle.) Sockalexis and Madden passed him near Cleveland Circle. As Ryan came up on Gallagher, he tried to hold Ryan off, but the bad ankle was too much for him. Really Gallagher had simply run too fast in the early stages, and the ankle was a good excuse. Sockalexis led through Coolidge Corner, where Gallagher quit. Mud stuck to Sockalexis's skin and clothes, but all he needed to do was persevere and the race would be his. But fatigue weighed on him as on a deer chased by wolves in deep snow. Relentlessly Ryan drew closer to Madden, who seemed stuck in his own pace. Madden had no power to resist Ryan. Sockalexis remained in the lead. But nothing could stop Ryan's run. Full of energy and covered with muck, Ryan charged past Sockalexis and on to a powerful sprint for new

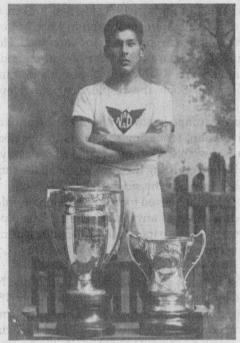

Andrew Sockalexis of Old Town, Maine, a Penobscot Indian, placed second in Boston in 1912 and 1913 in heartbreakingly close and dramatic races. Courtesy of the David Kayser collection.

course and world records. Sockalexis finished 34 seconds later, and Madden kept third.

In an article in the *Globe* under his own byline, Ryan pronounced, "Well, I told you I would win."

1912 Results

1. **M.J. Ryan**, *IAAC*, NY	2:21:18^{CR,WR}	10. H.J. Smith, *PAC*, NY	2:27:46
2. A. Sockalexis, *NDAA*	2:21:52	11. A.K. Sturgis, *AcAA*	2:27:59
3. F. Madden, *NDAA*	2:23:24	12. S.W. Root, *MercAC*, PA	2:28:47
4. T. Lilley, *NDAA*	2:23:50	13. W. Rozett, *PAC*, NY	2:28:55
5. **F. Carlson, Minneapolis, MN**	**2:25:38**	14. S. Hatch, Chicago, IL	2:30:29
6. H. Jensen, *PAC*, NY	2:25:50	15. A. Hermequatewa, *CIS*	2:31:46
7. R.F. Piggott, Medford, MA	2:26:07	16. J. Silver, *BAA*	2:32:34
8. **E. Fabre, *NAA*, Montreal, PQ**	**2:26:23**	30. J. Forshaw, St. Louis, MO	2:36:52
9. W. Galvin, Yonkers, NY	2:26:50	32. R. Fowler, Cambridge, MA	2:37:38

123 starters.

SWEDISH REVENGE

SATURDAY, APRIL 19, 1913

Sockalexis Runs to Win Hand in Marriage

Before the Boston Marathon in 1912, newspapers had reported selections for that year's U.S. Olympic team, which included the top runners of the day. Festus Madden was not on the list because he had neglected to take out citizenship papers. But Swedish immigrant Fritz Carlson had done all the right things to become an official U.S. citizen, and he made the list.

U.S. Olympic marathon runners for the Games in Stockholm, 1912

Clarence DeMar, North Dorchester AA, Boston

Mike Ryan, Irish-American AC, New York

Andrew Sockalexis, North Dorchester AA, Boston

Thomas Lilley, North Dorchester AA, Boston

Fritz Carlson, Cook's Gymnasium, Minneapolis

Harry Jensen, Pastime AC, New York

Richard Piggott, Medford, Massachusetts

John J. Gallagher, Yale

Lewis Tewanina, Carlisle Indian School

Sidney Hatch, Chicago

L. Pillivant, Chicago

After finishing fifth in the 1912 American Marathon Run, as the Boston Marathon was alternately billed, and after seeing his name in lists in newspapers, Carlson believed that he had been selected for the U.S. Olympic team. He left the next day on a train for New York, where at his own expense he boarded a boat for Stockholm to visit his family. Carlson had emigrated from Sweden 10 years earlier and moved to Minneapolis, where he worked in a sawmill and trained under Tom Cook, who had moved to Minneapolis from Boston. Cook had placed third in the Boston Marathon in 1904. (Tom Hicks, who had placed second in Boston in 1904 and won the St. Louis Olympic marathon that year, had also moved to Minneapolis.) Carlson was joyous at the prospect of representing his new country in the Olympic Games in his birth country.

Carlson had learned little English and was not a confident speaker. He did not know how to write English and consequently communicated through his friend and traveling companion, John C. Karlson.

Carlson stayed with his parents, who lived about 50 miles from Stockholm; he trained diligently for the Olympics and practiced on the Olympic course itself. What finer way could there be to pay respect to your new country than to win for her an Olympic gold medal? When the U.S. delegation arrived, Carlson presented himself. But U.S. official and head of the Amateur Athletic Union, James E. Sullivan, refused Carlson a place on the team. He said the U.S. already had enough men and did not need Carlson. Carlson was shocked and angry. He had neither the money nor the clout to sort it out.

In the 1912 Stockholm marathon, the 1911 Boston winner DeMar finished 12th in 2:50:46. Ryan dropped out, and Sockalexis finished 4th after a duel with Canadian Jimmy Duffy, who ran 5th in 2:42:18.8. Sockalexis prevailed by 11 seconds at 2:42:07.9. Edouard Fabre finished 11th in 2:50:36.2. Kenneth McArthur of South Africa was the winner in 2:36:54.8, on a hot day when Portuguese runner Francisco Lazaro suffered apparent sunstroke and collapsed at 19 miles. He thrashed about in delirium through the night and died in the morning. The death revived the debate on the humaneness of marathon running.

Three days later in cooler weather Carlson ran the same course and cruised in at 3 minutes faster than McArthur's winning time. He should have been in that Olympic race. But for the AAU, Carlson might have been the gold medalist. But he was the only man who felt that way. At Boston he planned to beat all the runners who had run in Sweden. He came to Boston in 1913 looking to prove himself and to seek revenge.

Sockalexis came looking for something entirely different—love. Or so the Boston Evening Transcript reporters would have us believe. Their April 19 headline read "Win, or Lose Her Hand." The paper described the would-be Sockalexis bride, Pauline Shay, as a "pretty little Indian maid of the Penobscot tribe." They maintained that she imposed on the Indian athlete the task of winning the famous BAA race before she would consent to marry him. "Her suitor must dangle the scalps of the finest athletic warriors in America at his belt or she will have none of him." Neither revenge nor love would fuel last year's winner, Mike Ryan. Recovery from an appendectomy kept him from the race.

A sultry gray day greeted the runners, who could run on firm roads this year. Harry Smith took the lead at South Framingham. Twenty-nine-year-old Carlson sat back in 12th at the advice of Tom Cook. Bob Fowler had given up running and advised Sockalexis, who ran alone behind the lead pack. Fabre led Madden, Cliff Horne, and Al Harrop. Smith ran almost as fast as Gallagher had the year before. By Wellesley, Carlson saw Madden in distress. He thought it might be the Irishman's heart, but the problem was lower, in Madden's stomach, and Madden dropped out of the race at 17 miles. Carlson plowed through the pack. He stared at the runners he chased.

Carlson watched Fabre and Smith leave the hard oiled roadway for the grass. He knew they experienced troubles with their feet. Carlson

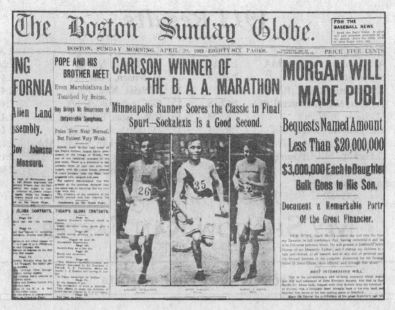

The top three of the 1913 race appeared dead center on page 1 of Sunday's *Boston Daily Globe* (April 20)—from left, Andrew Sockalexis, Fritz Carlson (the winner), and Harry J. Smith.

passed them and easily took the lead. Still Sockalexis stayed behind, letting time and distance wear on Carlson. The year before he had run out too hard and had done himself in. He did not want to make that mistake again. But now he ran too far behind, and as the miles passed he did not gain on the Swede. Fowler advised him to speed up. The newspapers reported that Pauline pleaded with him. "Miss Shay called upon her lover to hurry. 'Faster, Andrew,' was her appeal." Sockalexis sprinted up to and past the runners ahead of him. But Carlson sprinted too. Sockalexis had given away too much time at the start. Although Sockalexis ran the last miles faster than Carlson, Carlson had enough in him to respond. Sockalexis simply ran out of race.

Sockalexis gambled and lost—second again. He still did get his bride, though, and Carlson got his revenge, soundly defeating the fourth-place Olympian by 2 minutes. But in Stockholm Sockalexis had run 6 minutes behind the winner. Of course this did not prove that Carlson would have won the Olympic gold, but he made people think about such a might-have-been. He satisfied himself that he had indeed belonged in the Stockholm Olympic marathon running for the U.S.

Finishing fifth was the French-Canadian Edouard Fabre, who spent his winters on snowshoes and intended to use his experience to win the 1914 Boston Marathon. But there would be one tiny complication.

1913 Results

1.	F. Carlson, *CkG*, MN	2:25:14	11. T. Dwyer, *MAC*, NY	2:36:09
2.	A. Sockalexis, *NDAA*, MA	2:27:12	12. S.C. Pavitt, *NDAA*	2:36:13
3.	H.J. Smith, *BCH*, NY	2:28:23	13. H. Jensen, *BCH*, NY	2:41:00
4.	G. McInerney, *SCC*, PA	2:31:51	14. J. Weiss, *NBC*, PA	2:42:48
5.	E. Fabre, *NAA*, Montreal, PQ	2:32:18	15. G. Crosby, *BCH*, NY	2:44:05
6.	J.J. Stack, *BCH*, NY	2:32:38	16. C.B. Lucas, Fall River, MA	2:45:07
7.	J.M. Lorden, *SMAC*, MA	2:33:04	17. J.C. Karlson, *MinnAC*	2:46:01
8.	W. Brown, *NDAA*, MA	2:33:46	18. J.J. Monaghan, *SMAC*, MA	2:47:10
9.	G. Gaskill, *NDAA*, Boston, MA	2:34:00	19. T.M. Lilley, *NDAA*	2:49:22
10.	A.K. Sturgis, *NDAA*	2:35:42	20. W.J. Fallon, *NDAA*	2:50:20

83 entrants, 60 starters.

MY SHADOW RAN FASTER

MONDAY, APRIL 20, 1914

Lorden to Battle Canadian Invasion

Edouard Fabre knew the course. Jimmy Duffy knew Fabre knew, but Duffy knew he could sprint faster than Fabre. Duffy planned to follow Fabre and run away at the end. Fabre knew all this too. But what could he do except run as fast as he dared? Fabre had placed third at Boston in 1911, eighth in 1912, and fifth in 1913. He hungered to win. He could taste it. Fabre stood 6 feet tall, strong and silent; Duffy stood shorter (5'8") and chattered.

Jimmy Duffy hungered for cigarettes and beer. He drank and roistered, thrusting himself through life. He loved action and was in turn loved by those who knew him. A good singer, Duffy often led his pals in drinking songs. His rollicking lifestyle contrasted with that of many top marathoners of the day. Most seemed introverted, taciturn, disciplined, often righteous. DeMar, the perspicacious printer, may have been in his meticulousness the antipode of Duffy. Whereas DeMar, Caffery, and Ryan all liked to make their own way, Duffy went along, got along, and had a great time. Trainers wrung their hands at his tendency toward reckless abandon, but they could not stay angry with him. His charm evoked in his friends the urge to protect him from his faults. Duffy was born in Sligo County, Ireland, on May Day 1890. He grew up with his parents in Edinburgh, Scotland, until he emigrated to Canada in 1911, where he worked as a stonecutter in Toronto. Duffy shattered Sammy Mellor's course record for the Hamilton Bay 19-mile race in 1912 by over 2 minutes. Like Fabre, Duffy came to Boston to win. He had more fun trying to win.

Joe Lorden, younger brother of the 1903 winner, John Lorden, took the early lead through South Framingham in 22:23, much slower than Caffery's 1901 checkpoint record of 20:00. A Finn, Villir "Willie" Kyronen took the lead at Natick and held it into the hills. Early on Fabre ran in eighth place and Duffy, his shadow, in ninth. Together they moved up into third and fourth behind Kyronen and, for a time, Arthur Roth.

Roth, of the north Dorchester Club, moved into second place on the hills. The *Post* reporter observed, "Roth is a mere slip of a youth who runs as though he was about to drop with his head wobbling from one side to the other and apparently exerting himself to the limit at all times." Joe Lorden fell back to fifth. Duffy had tacked onto Fabre at the start and did not ever let him get more than a foot away. From time to time Duffy ran up to Fabre's elbow and made him spurt. Duffy wore a white shirt with a maple leaf and the word "Canada" front and center. Fabre's white shirt bore the name of his Montreal club, Richmond. It was perhaps a cruel exercise for Duffy to harry Fabre. Like a wanton boy plucking legs off flies, Duffy tortured Fabre, keeping him agitated and racing while constantly probing him for weakness. Duffy figured that weakness would eventually show itself in Fabre's lack of response to one of his surges. The *Post* reported the day after the race that Duffy tried to break away from Fabre 16 times; but runners in marathons cannot make 16 serious attempts to break another runner. Three perhaps, but really only one is necessary. Such pseudobreaks as the *Post* reporter observed were not full anaerobic stabs at escape but feints in advance of the one mighty run-through. When the other man reaches a state of unresponsiveness to a false surge it is time for a real one. Fabre tried to run the sprint out of Duffy on the hills, imagining that if he just tried a little harder the shadow of Duffy would drift away. But Duffy lingered like a leech searching for the soft spot.

Duffy felt Fabre go soft after 22 miles at Coolidge Corner. There Duffy blasted away, leaving the all-but-helpless Fabre to struggle for second place a mere 15 seconds later.

Duffy's first words after crossing the finish line were "Give me a cigarette." After his physical he had a beer. Later that night he went to see "The Queen of the Movies" with, among others, Bob Fowler.

The rambunctious Duffy reported that "the BAA marathon is a great race and I hope to win it again." It had been the race of his life and the last amateur race of his life.

James Duffy: Runner, Soldier

On June 28, 1914, in the Bosnian town of Sarajevo, a chauffeur misunderstood his instructions, made the wrong turn, tried to correct his blunder, and delivered Archduke Francis

Ferdinand to a waiting assassin. On September 23 James Duffy enlisted in the Canadian army to fight in the Great War that followed the events of June. The following April 19 Duffy was not in Boston, as he had thought he would be a year earlier, defending his Boston Marathon crown. Duffy huddled that day with the men of the 16th Battalion in a dank trench dug into the rolling countryside outside Ypres, a small town in west Belgium. Ypres was the place where poisonous gas was first used in human combat, catching Allied troops unaware. The soldiers of the 16th had been outside Ypres for several days, shoring up positions held by French soldiers they had been called in to relieve. The task was a messy one of reinforcing parapets, constructing latrines, and removing the putrid flesh of the dead. Duffy looked forward to the following day, when the Canadians were due to be relieved themselves and would retire to billets for a welcome rest.

Relief came on schedule, but the break was short-lived. Two days later the Canadians were back at the front, fighting alongside other Allied troops to hold a 3-mile front that was the only remaining barrier between advancing German armies and the strategic channel port of Calais. The fateful moment occurred at 5:00 on the afternoon of April 22. Suddenly and silently, after what had been an almost beautiful day of warmth and spring sunshine, clouds of gas billowed up from the facing German lines and drifted on prevailing breezes toward the Allied trenches. French soldiers, to the left of the Canadians, took the brunt of the attack, floundering in defenseless bewilderment. Choking and gagging, they stumbled in retreat, allowing the Germans to surge forward into the vacuum.

The charge gave the Germans control of the French trenches and command of a small wood containing four British machine guns. But the Canadians managed to regroup to form a new line that held the advance from going further. Then, as darkness fell, and with it a tense silence, Canadian soldiers received orders to counterattack under cover of night and retake the captured wood. The task, little short of suicidal, fell to the 10th and 16th Battalions, a direct charge into the face of concentrated German troop fire. A few minutes before midnight, the wood no more than a blur before them in the starlight, the Canadians moved out of their trenches, almost certainly knowing the fate that awaited them. They advanced in eight lines, overcoats and packs removed, bayonets fixed in place. The faint sound of bayonet scabbards clinking on a wire hedge gave them away. The Germans sent a flare aloft. When the light exposed the Canadian advance, the German guns erupted.

> The battlefield became as bright as day. The ranks wavered and swayed for an instant; they got their balance: they merged one into the other; the charge recovered momentum, and the mass went lunging ahead. The crash of rifle fire bewildered the senses. The bullets made resounding cracks on either side and hit the eardrums like blows of a hammer.

The light caught Jimmy Duffy in full sprint up the hill, running top speed into the bullets. Carried to a field hospital in a nearby farmhouse, he died within hours. Of 300 soldiers and 5 officers in the 16th Battalion, only 27 survived the night.

1914 Results

1. J. Duffy, *RBC*, ON	2:25:01	9. T. Lilley, Dorchester, MA	2:38:53
2. E. Fabre, *RichAC*, PQ	2:25:16	10. F. Madden, South Boston, MA	2:38:57
3. J. Lorden, *SMAC*, MA	2:28:42	11. H. Honohan, Worcester, MA	2:41:17
4. W. Bell, *ShamAA*, PQ	2:30:37	12. J. Anthony, *GAAA*, NY	2:42:55
5. A. Roth, *DC*, Roxbury, MA	2:31:08	13. J. Weiss, Philadelphia, PA	2:44:53
6. W. Kyronen, *KAC*, NY	2:34:38	14. C. de Steffano, *OzAC*	2:46:28
7. G. McInerney, *ShanAC*, PA	2:35:56	15. A.R. Hollis, Cambridge, MA	2:46:28
8. F. Carlson, *MinnAC*, MN	2:37:19		

SNOWSHOE

MONDAY, APRIL 19, 1915

Strong Canadian Comes to Boston

Edouard Fabre did not feel at his best on April 19, 1915. He had the great ambition to win the Boston Marathon, but he also had a chest cold, and it looked like a hot day. Canadian snowshoe racers do not like hot days. And his knee hurt. He did not think he had a chance. Jimmy Duffy was hunkered down in trenches in France with only 3 days to live; no other runner waited in Fabre's way. Newspapers that week reported German sinkings of American ships and that Jimmy Henigan had won the Cathedral 10-Mile Handicap in 52:14 running as scratch man. Henigan did not yet think of himself as a marathoner but rather as 5- to 10-miler and cross-country runner.

Fabre was born to French-Canadian parents at Ste. Genevieve, Quebec, on August 21, 1885. Orphaned at an early age, Fabre grew up in a home for abandoned children in the St. Henri district of Montreal. He ran away from the orphanage one night and after crossing the Victoria Bridge to the south shore of the St. Lawrence crawled exhausted into a clump of bushes on the Indian Reserve of the Caughawaga Iroquois. In the morning an Iroquois family discovered him and took him in. He caught their passion for endurance running, and like so many young men from the reservation he became an iron worker.

Although the facts are not known, some speculated that Fabre paid his own way to the 1906 Olympic Games and also participated in the Olympic Games of 1908. In the 1912 Olympics he placed 11th in 2:50:36. Since 1911 at Boston Fabre had run third, eighth, fifth, and the previous year's second to Jimmy Duffy. It was in a race against Duffy before the outbreak of war that Fabre had almost lost his amateur standing. Duffy had turned professional, and Fabre tainted himself by running against him. The rules were strict, but no evidence was found that Fabre had received money, and he received only a temporary suspension.

In preparation for Boston Fabre trained as no one had for a marathon. He ran a thousand miles in the first three months of 1915, meanwhile developing a kidney infection and a sore leg. Perhaps he had overtrained, but still the press picked him as their favorite.

At Natick, Hugh Honohan of New York, with his handler, the famous track man Mel Sheppard, led with Sidney Hatch of Chicago and Dorchester's Cliff Horne nearby. Fabre trotted along in 15th place. Dust and exhaust fumes plagued them again. Year after year BAA officials said they would do something about the cars on the course, but year after year the cars came back. In 1914 Lieutenant Governor Edward P. Barry had suggested legislation to make the marathon a state institution in order to wrest authority for traffic control from the cities and towns on the route, but the legislation never passed.

In the heat of that day checkpoint times did not approach those of 1901, 1908, or 1912. All the way up to Coolidge Corner Honohan looked like the winner. His 1:29:34 to the earlier Commonwealth Avenue (the "Boulevard") checkpoint was much slower than Welton's 1908 record of 1:23:55. Honohan's strategy did not seem to be reckless. Horne, a half mile in arrears, did not expect Honohan to slow to a walk. Horne surprised himself as he ran past the utterly spent Honohan and into the lead. The Boston crowds loved the idea of a Dorchester boy in the lead and cheered wildly. Meanwhile, back in the pack, Fabre had moved relentlessly from 15th to 11th at Wellesley, then 3rd by Coolidge Corner. Here Fabre's high mileage paid off. He picked up a minute per mile on Horne and sailed past him so quickly that Horne could not respond. Fabre arrived alone on Exeter Street.

Fabre lost 7-1/2 pounds during the race; according to the *Boston Post* reporter, after his victory Fabre called for beer after beer until a half dozen bottles surrounded him on the bench. By the time he was ready to go into the street he had regained much of the lost weight. He felt quite happy about himself and his victory.

Sydney Hatch of Chicago placed third. He wanted to come back and improve on that.

1915 Results

1.	E. Fabre, *RichAC*, PQ	2:31:41	9.	J. Mullen, *DC*, MA	2:50:02
2.	C. Horne, *DC*, MA	2:33:01	10.	A. Horne, *WinAC*, Everett, MA	2:51:36
3.	S. Hatch, *IAC*, Chicago, IL	2:35:47	11.	A. Merchant, *WinAC*, MA	2:55:00
4.	H. Honohan, *NYAC*, NY	2:37:02	12.	J. Costello, *BCH*, NY	2:56:04
5.	E.L. Byrne, *BCH*, NY	2:37:15	13.	H. Garvin, *SCC*, NY	2:56:28
6.	G. McInerney, *SCC*, NY	2:38:14	14.	W. Bell, *ShamAA*, Montreal, PQ	2:58:30
7.	P. Wyer, *MonAC*, ON	2:45:16	15.	B. Kennedy, *IAC*, IL	3:01:24
8.	F. Travalena, *MAC*, NY	2:46:58			

73 entrants, 58 starters.

FINNISH CATCH-UP

WEDNESDAY, APRIL 19, 1916

Fast Finn Comes to Boston

The talents of most runners hide deep within their bodies. Even close inspection cannot separate the talented from the merely thin. Jimmy Henigan had run third this year in the St. Alphonsus 8-miler from a 4:45 handicap while Arthur Roth ran from 3:15 to seventh place. The next week Henigan won the Cathedral 10-Mile Handicap run from 5:45 to win in 52:24. Henigan clearly was talented. Roth looked merely thin, not the least bit talented. He rested for the next week's Boston race, glad that Henigan did not run marathons. Roth was surprisingly fast for a marathoner, especially one who looked so frail and ungainly when he ran. He was far from the Greek ideal of an athlete—in running clothes he looked starved and awkward, more like a man running away from something than toward it. But Roth had done his training.

Bricklayer Bill Kennedy ("Bricklayer" seemed to be Kennedy's handle; it preceded his name whenever he was mentioned), who the year before rode a freight train from Chicago to Boston and finished 15th, used a passenger train this time. No previous winners entered. But the previous year's third-place finisher, Sydney Hatch, came to run his 40th marathon. Last year's fourth-place runner, Hugh Honohan, also came to race. Twenty-three-year-old Finnish Willie Kyronen of New York's Millrose AA looked like the speed man in the field.

The BAA would not let Peter Foley run officially because he was deemed too old. But he planned to celebrate his 60th birthday by defying them and following the runners.

Governor McCall came to the start in ideal running weather to pose for photos with the runners. The course from Ashland to Framingham alternated from soft sand and dust to mud. Perhaps that is why leader Michael J. Lynch's time at the South Framingham checkpoint was the slowest in the history of the race, 24:18 compared to Caffery's 1901 record of 20:00.

The hopes and fortunes of marathoners do not often follow neat progressions. The name of Honohan disappears from the race records. He was running 12th when he turned his ankle. Pores moved from 17th to 5th at one point, then developed cramps; he too disappeared. Jepson finished 27th, about an hour behind the winner. James J. Corkery does not appear on any checkpoint lists, yet he provided great drama in the 1916 race. At Newton Lower Falls Corkery, in the words of a *Post* reporter the next day, "unloosed in a fashion that many believed would carry him to victory." He caught up to a pack including Arthur Jamieson, Pores, Honohan, John Mullen, William Brown, and James McCurnin and ran into them like a bowling ball into

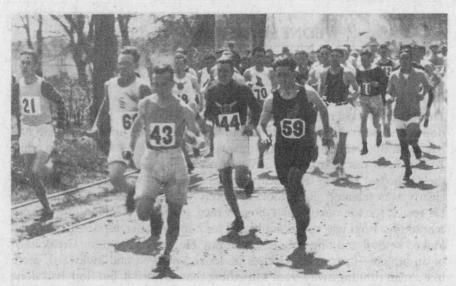

John H. Brady (#43), who finished 32nd, led early by the rails out of Ashland on the dusty dirt road, accompanied by Herbert Robinson (#59), Robert Briggs (#44), and Frank Liffert (#21). Courtesy of the Boston Public Library, Print Department.

tenpins. The whole pack burst at his approach. They sprinted away with their eyes on the back of Roth's head. Mullen was the first to break.

As the pack crumbled, Hatch ran up into the rubble. Kyronen burst past Jamieson, Corkery, John Phillips, and Hatch. He alone gave chase to Roth. Roth, frail and wobbling, looked vulnerable, running as if on his last legs. The spectators saw him, and they saw Kyronen fit and flying after him. It looked like only a matter of time before the fresh runner caught the gasping and spent one. But the spectators did not know a vital something about frail, 116-pound Arthur Roth.

Roth, who made his living as a tracer in an architect's firm, ran with a short stride, his head tilted to one side and his arms swinging about as he sucked in great gasps of air. The crowds assumed he was at his limit, but a runner's degree of fatigue is only ascertainable from his stride and appearance in a relative way. Only those who knew Roth understood that he always looked moribund. He never ran with a serene face, a classic arm swing, or a high back-kick. He tilted. Roth always looked like death, even in his quickest running. He looked bad even when he looked good.

Kyronen did have superior speed. And given more running room he would have cut down Roth. Kyronen cut Roth's lead from 600 yards in the last couple of miles to 75 yards on Exeter Street. But the Finn ran out of time. He made the same mistake as Sockalexis had in 1913 and others would again. Kyronen watched Roth break the finish line tape. The winner's clock stopped. Eleven seconds later the second-place watch clicked.

After the finish Governor McCall told Roth that it was not only Roth's body that won the race, but his head as well. The governor's comment echoed the common myth of victory being the result of willpower. Roth disagreed, saying his victory was thanks to Jimmy Fallon, his trainer and handler who kept him on schedule. It was the training, governor, the training that brought out the talent from deep within Roth's body.

Hatch found himself in third place again, and Kennedy, representing the Bricklayers' AC from Chicago, heard his time read off as he finished sixth. Kennedy enjoyed his sport and the company of marathon runners more than anything. He found laying brick harder work than running marathons.

1916 Results

1. **A.V. Roth**, *DC*, MA	2:27:16	9. M. Lynch, *CI*, Washington, DC	2:41:22
2. W. Kyronen, *MillAA*, NY	2:27:27	10. G.B. Moss, *HCL*, NY	2:43:39
3. S. Hatch, *IAC*, Chicago	2:28:30	11. L. Davis, *BunAA*, Lowell, MA	2:45:24
4. J.J. Corkery, *SPA*, Toronto	2:30:34	12. H.C. Schuster, *SAAC*, NY	2:45:41
5. W.D. Brown, *DC*, MA	2:34:18	13. F. Travalena, *MAC*, NY	2:51:16
6. **B. Kennedy, *BAC*, Chicago**	**2:35:17**	14. J. Mullen, *DC*	2:53:34
7. J.P. Phillips, *BCH*, NY	2:39:39	15. G. Kirkwood, *PaulAC*, NY	2:53:34
8. A.L. Jamieson, *SPA*, ON	2:41:09		

58 starters.

WAR CLOUDS AND WAR FLAGS

THURSDAY, APRIL 19, 1917

DeMar and Roth Return

Chuck Mellor so desperately wanted to race in Boston that he decided to jump a freight train in Chicago. But Mellor, with wire-rimmed glasses and wiry, wavy hair, was not a jumper, and he did not have enough spring to land securely on the train. He got a grip and dangled as the train approached a bridge. He banged and bruised his thigh on a steel girder, but with a marathoner's mindless tenacity, he held on tightly to keep from tumbling off the train. When Mellor got to Boston he found accommodations in the South End—on a pool table.

The rest of the world tumbled topsy-turvy in war, and the U.S. had joined in on April 6 with a Congressional Declaration of War against Germany. But all Chuck and his pal Bill Kennedy wanted to do was race marathons. American flags popped out again all along the marathon course, the most since 1902, during the Spanish-American War. The *Boston Daily Globe's* car sported a flag on its front bumper in addition to its white triangular *Globe* pennant.

Wandering 35-year-old bricklayer Bill Kennedy, representing the new Morningside Athletic Club in New York City, took a temporary job laying bricks in Boston to pay his expenses there. A few years earlier Mellor and Kennedy had journeyed from Chicago on an adventure. "We beat it to New York on a Pullman to get jobs," Kennedy reported. Kennedy got one but Mellor could not find work until Kennedy hired him as his helper. After a few days Mellor quit, saying that hod-carrying and mortar-mixing were too much like work. This year in Boston Kennedy had a room with a single bed. When he found Mellor sleeping on a pool table he offered to share his lodgings. They paid 15¢ for their meals and sustained themselves in between on a large loaf of stale bread.

Kennedy continued his work with mortar and brick the week, and the day, before the race. Before the race he knotted the corners of a plain white handkerchief and stitched on a small American flag for inspiration; reluctant or not Kennedy would soon be in the army along with many of his countrymen. He laid his makeshift covering over his graying hair as protection from the sun. The week before the marathon Kennedy had run the Cathedral 10-miler in 52:58, so he was in shape and fairly fast. Kennedy, who had run 23 marathons, feared Sydney Hatch, a fellow Chicagoan, because he figured that it would take an old-timer to win. Hatch had run more than 40 marathons.

Kennedy gambled that the favored pair of "Flying Finns," Willie Kyronen and Hannes Kolehmainen, would race each other out. Kennedy felt it was important in this time of war for American runners to repel the foreigners. Hannes, of the illustrious brothers Kolehmainen, was Johannes Petter Kolehmainen, who had run a third-place 3:06:19 marathon at age 17 in Helsinki in 1907 behind his second-place older brother, Taavetti Heikki, known as Tatu. A third brother, August William ("Willie") held the world's fastest professional time in 1912.

Hannes had won the 5,000 meters and 10,000 meters in the 1912 Stockholm Olympics and would go on in 1920 to win the Olympic marathon gold medal for Finland in Antwerp, Belgium. But for now he had his compatriot and the Boston course to challenge him.

Kyronen had finished a flying, closing second to Roth in Boston the year before. Roth, wiry, frail, and relentless as ever, wanted to win again. The Boston crowds would like their Boston boy to win again. Hans Schuster, the Swede who had won the Brockton (Massachusetts) Marathon in the fall of 1916 wanted Boston too. Clarence DeMar had won the race in 1911 and was back, but he hadn't done much racing since his 1911 victory. Most people thought it was not likely that he would run well. Where had he been for the last 6 years? DeMar had come to a personal understanding about his motivations for running and how he would react to fame, something he simultaneously sought and abhorred, so he had started training again.

But Hatch was the man who had really trained. He had recently run and won a 100-mile race. He relied not on talent but on training mileage for the strength necessary not to slow down. The old-timers had learned that the winner of a marathon is the man who slows down least in the final miles, that victory is seldom a matter of a glorious kick at the end of the race, as is often true in a track race. Some quick runners, like Kyronen, nourished the hope that a marathon could be a kicker's race, but kicks wouldn't win marathons for another 60 years.

A strong east wind blew on April 19, but DeMar remembered it as a fairly warm day. Hannes Kolehmainen took the pack out to a reasonable 22:44 at the South Framingham checkpoint. A.F. Merchant, running with the BAA unicorn on his shirt, hung on to Kolehmainen. The marathon had bewitched Merchant and held him under its spell, instilling in him a fanatical and crazed desire to win at any cost. His handler, H.H. Potter, fell victim to the same incantation. Equipped only with urgings, sponges, and water, Potter pedaled alongside.

Kyronen did not want to settle back in the pack either, but he did not feel well. Kennedy felt perfectly relaxed. He ran fifth through Natick in pursuit of the pack of Schuester, Hatch, Merchant, and Kolehmainen. Going into Wellesley Kennedy caught them and took the lead. As Kennedy, closely pursued by the pack, passed the college a Wellesley girl dashed out to place

As Bill Kennedy passed the college, a Wellesley girl dashed out to place an American flag in his hand.

an American flag in his hand. He took it with a smile and a bow and ran waving the flag for a quarter of a mile before giving it to his handler.

By Newton Lower Falls Kennedy led Schuster, Kolehmainen, and Merchant by 5 yards. Kyronen and Hatch followed. On the hill Kyronen gripped his stomach in pain and halted. The physician accompanying him ordered him inside the physician's automobile. DeMar, who had been in 25th place in Framingham, passed runner after runner on the hills. Kennedy cruised comfortably but Merchant began to fall back, a cramp seizing his leg muscle. He punched at it to relax the tension and relieve the pain. He did not want to settle for finishing back in the pack. He had come too far. This cramp was an aberration, an unreal thing that was supposed to happen to someone else. It should not be happening to him, not when he ran so close to first place. It must be some kind of mistake. Merchant could not accept his own demise. He felt he deserved another chance. He sought escape.

A Boy Scout assigned as an extra bicycle attendant saw Merchant get into a car. Merchant did not appear at the Coolidge Corner checkpoint. Chuck Mellor had passed Merchant, then miles later he saw Merchant ahead of him climb under the ropes and get back onto the course. For Merchant everything was right again. He was back running where he should be. The cramp was not supposed to have happened, and Merchant convinced himself that it never really did. It was OK—he hadn't really needed the ride, therefore he hadn't really taken it.

DeMar, with his brother Bob following on a bicycle, moved up and passed Kolehmainen with a half mile to go. Or, more accurately, Kolehmainen slowed and DeMar did not. Hatch did not slow. Kennedy did not slow. The lesson here stuck with DeMar. High mileage works and age is not a handicap. Kennedy was 35, Hatch 34, and DeMar himself only 29. DeMar said, "If those two old fellows improve with age why isn't there a chance of a young fellow like myself emulating their example?"

Few people would like to emulate Merchant, who crossed the finish line fifth. Immediately upon finishing Mellor protested Merchant's finish. Potter corroborated Merchant's insistence that he had run the whole course, but the preponderance of evidence told BAA officials that Merchant had not run the entire way. They disqualified Merchant, and the AAU considered banning him for life. Merchant was bewildered. No, no, he really did run, fifth was where he was supposed to finish. In Merchant's mind the illusion was complete.

In victory Kennedy said that America should endeavor to prove itself superior in all branches of effort. Kennedy and Hatch soon enlisted—Kennedy joined the 23rd Engineers and Hatch won the Croix de Guerre. DeMar joined the army. The men were used to training; the army would be a different sort of training, but nevertheless their duty. They wanted to do whatever was necessary to win the war. It was what a man must do, reluctant or not, and it was, so they thought, where the glory waited. They all served in France.

1917 Results

1.	B. Kennedy, NY	2:28:37	9.	P.M. Dean, Rochester, NY	2:44:28
2.	S. Hatch, Chicago, IL	2:30:19	10.	L. Davis, Dorchester, MA	2:44:28
3.	C. DeMar, Melrose, MA	2:31:05	11.	A.V. Roth, Roxbury, MA	2:45:29
4.	H. Kolehmainen, NY	2:31:58	12.	J. Mullen, Dorchester, MA	2:49:23
5.	C. Mellor, Chicago, IL	2:36:20	13.	W. Brown, Dorchester, MA	2:51:11
6.	H. Schuster, NY	2:37:28	14.	G. Costarkis, Boston, MA	2:52:59
7.	C. Linder, Quincy, MA	2:38:38	15.	C. Leventhal, Brooklyn, NY	2:53:32
8.	M.J. Lynch, Washington, DC	2:40:06			

70 entrants, 48 starters.
Unofficial: Peter Foley (age 61) 4:11.

THE KHAKI-WHITE RELAY

FRIDAY, APRIL 19, 1918

Marathon Cancelled

When Congress declared war against Germany, the Boston Athletic Association went on record saying that they would do everything possible for men in the service. What they ultimately did was to cancel their marathon. To support the boys who were about to go "over there" they replaced the two-decade-old marathon with a special event. You may wonder after you read this account how much the BAA did for the participating servicemen, the sport of long-distance racing, or itself with this unprecedented relay. This perfervid display of patriotism perhaps assuaged a guilt rising because an athletic association could do little to help the war effort. However, in all areas, athletic and propagandistic, the effort proved feckless. But it was not the BAA that made the silly rule that turned the entire idea from an athletic event to a publicity stunt. It was the military itself that required the racing men to wear their full service uniforms and carry batons with messages inside for 25 miles. These rules made the race a mockery, but it was still a very difficult thing to do athletically.

Navy men wore their whites, with their spit-polished, high-laced boots and spats. They wore their big collar with the thin blue stripes and a blue—navy blue—kerchief. They wore long pants and long sleeves. The army men wore regulation khaki—shirts with epaulets, buttons, collars, and cuffs; pants with belts, flap pockets, and cuffs. They too wore regulation spit-polished, high-laced leather boots and spats. Mercifully they did not have to wear hats and coats.

The rules for this novelty marathon, as the *Boston Evening Transcript* called it on April 19, required 10 men to a team, with each running about 2-1/2 miles. Red and blue shields marked the exchange zones, red for Army and blue for Navy. Sixty automobiles would transport the runners. The *Herald* expected no end of confusion for BAA officials. Few of the men were in serious running shape. All had undergone military training that consisted of fields of men doing calisthenics in unison. One photo in the Boston papers showed such a workout. While a band played, all of the men stood in perfect rows, each with his expedition hat at his feet as he followed the leader's instruction. The caption said that the battalion acted as one man—exactly what an infantry battalion would do in the European war as they rose from their trenches with bayonets fixed to go over the top. A relay would be like that. The teams would run as one man.

Only one man of the 140 in the race had run the marathon. Al Harrop of Fall River, Massachusetts, had finished seventh in 1911 in 2:32. He ran for the 302nd Infantry team from Camp Devens in Ayer, Massachusetts. Several others on the military teams had been good runners. Mike Devaney, who as a civilian had run middle distances for the Millrose AC, now ran anchor leg for the navy. James Sullivan, who ran anchor leg for the Camp Devens Divisional team, had run cross-country for the Irish-American AC of New York. Harold Weeks had been the New England 3-mile and 5-mile champ. The naval cadet team had a host of excollegiate runners in Colbarth of Bowdoin, Bent of Massachusetts Institute of Technology, Cummings and Eaton of Harvard, and Havener of Yale.

In all white, Henry Pain of the Boston Navy Yard, took the early lead out of Ashland. He handed off 10 yards ahead of Paul Defazio. Charley Phillips, formerly of Exeter and Dartmouth, ran against Abbot of Camp Devens Divisional. With his racing experience Phillips stayed on Abbot's shoulder. The college runner had a big kick in the last half mile that took him to a 60-yard lead. After a half mile Charley Lewis of Army caught Murphy of Navy. Lewis gave a quarter-mile lead to teammate Griffin, and the navy never came close to the lead again. That was the end of the racing. The last 16 miles was a procession of fatigued men in dress uniforms, each running alone carrying a baton down the middle of the road. It wasn't a race and it wasn't a parade.

Few spectators lined the course, and for the first time in years automobile traffic was no problem. No one had favorites to bet on. The race simply did not generate spontaneous public interest. Official interest, however, was high—as high as the secretary of the navy, Josephus Daniels. At the postrace ceremony in the BAA gymnasium, intraservice politics showed up as the secretary got big applause, especially from naval petty officers.

The teams ran so slowly that Harrop, in running regalia without the other nine members of his team, would have placed seventh overall based on his 1911 marathon time. DeMar, Ryan, Sockalexis, or Madden would have beaten *all* the military relay teams. The soldiers looked silly trying to do something for which they

The clumsiness of the military relay effort echoed the clumsiness of the Great War.

were not dressed and not trained. The whole event proved to be neither good athletics nor good public relations. The clumsiness of the military relay effort echoed the clumsiness of the Great War, where millions of men, poorly trained and ill equipped, sprinted out of trenches to be mowed down by machine gun fire.

Oh yes. The message inside the baton? Pure propaganda. It was an appeal to buy Liberty Bonds: "We will fight to the limit; we expect you to buy to the limit."

1918 Results

1.	Camp Devens Divisional team	2:24:53		4.	301st Signal Battalion	2:29:14
	(Defazio, Horton, Abbot,			5.	Naval Cadet School	2:29:23
	Lewis, Griffin, Brooks, Moore,			6.	304th Infantry Devens	2:32:20
	Palmeter, Paulson, Sullivan)			7.	Bumkin Island	2:37:20
2.	302nd Infantry	2:28:10		8.	Radio School	2:44:26
3.	Boston Navy Yard	2:28:45				

14 teams started, all finished.

WHY CARL SMILED AT FRANK

SATURDAY, APRIL 19, 1919

Henigan Hub Hope

Once Jimmy Henigan announced himself a starter in the 1919 Boston Marathon, the headlines read, "Henigan Hub Hope." The press admired his ability with good reason: He had won every race around. Henigan was strong, fast, and he smiled when he ran. They called him "Smilin' Jimmy Henigan." Others called him "Hinky Henigan." The establishment picked popular and talented Henigan to win . . . so the local pressure sat on him. But not all runners react to pressure the same way.

Willie Wick, in his first marathon, happily plugged along the hills of the 1919 race with his short, stocky pal Carl Linder. Spectators in Newton found amusement in Wick, who stood at 4'10-1/2", displayed a bald head, and ran on bowed legs. The leaders and favorites in the race ran a palpable distance ahead of Wick and Linder, who shuffled comfortably and contentedly with his pal. The day felt warm, but not oppressively so, and a crosswind blew. The leaders were the fast favorites—the Flying Finn Willie Kyronen, the Flying Swedes Runar Ohman and Hans Schuester, and the Flying Boston

10-miler Jimmy Henigan were all the press picks. Nobody picked the shuffling Finns, Carl or Willie.

Linder and Wick lived in Quincy, Massachusetts. Linder, 29, was born in the village of Rauma on the western coast of Finland and had emigrated to America 17 years earlier. He was a short man of bulk and muscle, and his head seemed massive and cubistic on his wide shoulders. Linder had been an all-round champion athlete and had won New England championships in decathlon and javelin. He could hurdle, sprint, throw, and high-jump. He supported his wife and two children as a pattern maker in the Fore River shipyard in Quincy.

During the Great War Linder tried to enlist in the U.S. Army to fight for his adopted country. Twice they turned him down because he had flat feet, despite his pleas to the recruiting officer that if he could run marathons and cross-country races he could shoulder a gun and march for his country. The press of 1919 knew that Linder had run marathons before. They well knew that he had placed 17th in Boston in 1916 and 7th in 1917. What they didn't know was that Linder was tired of being an also-ran and had decided to do something about it. He solicited the help of Finnish champion runner Hannes Kolehmainen, who was then living in West Virginia. He coached Linder by mail, and Carl dutifully followed Hannes's instructions.

Wick dutifully followed Linder. Wick had started his life in the interior of Finland, the land of cold lakes and long summer days. He made his living in Quincy baking bread. Newspapers cartooned him wearing a baker's hat with the caption "He did not loaf." But ahead of both favorites and Finns and not picked as a contender ran long, lean, high-stepping Frank Gillespie of Chicago.

Gillespie had run conservatively in 12th place in a field that ran conservatively through the first checkpoint. The time of 24:15 at South Framingham was nearly the slowest ever. The runners just looked around, each waiting for the other to take the lead and make the race. No one would. At last Gillespie could take the suspense no longer. He bolted into the lead at Natick. Ohman followed but did not pass Gillespie or dominate the race as had been predicted. He did not dare. Snowstorms in Sweden, a long boat ride, and a new city had prevented him from training effectively. Otto Laakso, another Finn, ran up into 4th place, and Arron Morris ran into 3rd. *Globe* reporter Lawrence J. Sweeney noted on April 20 that Morris was "the first colored boy to ever attain prominence in the running of the classic." The favorites, however, did not look favorable.

Hub Hope Henigan cracked first. He quit on the hills. Kyronen dropped out. Ohman dropped back. Schuster dropped out. Gillespie ran well up the hills, but on the downhills his feet jammed into the lumpy stitches and raw leather of his new shoes. Blood and fluid filled his shoes and oozed out the lace holes. Meanwhile Carl and Willie ran merrily along, passing runner after runner. The inevitable happened and Carl drifted ahead of his pal Willie. When Linder looked ahead he saw Gillespie coming back to him. As

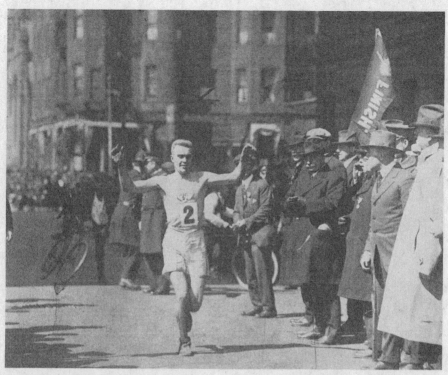

Carl W.A. Linder won in 1919, followed by countrymen Willie Wick and Otto Laakso; thus began a long tradition of Finnish influence in the Boston Marathon. Courtesy of the Boston Public Library, Print Department.

Linder passed Gillespie with 2-1/2 miles to go and moved into the lead, Gillespie looked at him. Linder smiled. Gillespie knew he could not race a man who smiled. He especially could not race a smiling man who ran quickly but with control and grace. Linder felt strong, with plenty of power in reserve. Kolehmainen's training methods had worked. Gillespie's feet screamed in pain. He walked. He had to walk. Wick passed him too. By the time Laakso came up on Gillespie, his feet had numbed. He ran slowly to the finish.

1919 Results

1.	**C. Linder**, *HAC*, **Quincy, MA**	**2:29:13**	6. A. Morris, *STCC*, NY	2:37:31
2.	W. Wick, Quincy, MA	2:30:15	7. **P. Trivoulidas**, *MornAC*, **NY**	**2:38:10**
3.	O.J. Laakso, *KAC*, NY	2:31:31	8. R. Ohman, Sweden	2:41:38
4.	F. Gillespie, Chicago, IL	2:36:44	9. A.K. Sturgis, Natick, MA	2:51:15
5.	M.J. Lynch, Washington, DC	2:36:58	10. H. Kanto, *HAC*, Quincy, MA	2:51:53

37 starters, 25 finishers.
Unofficial: Peter Foley (age 63) 4:08.

Chapter 3

1920-1929
The Running Twenties

Presidents: *Woodrow Wilson, Warren G. Harding, Calvin Coolidge, Herbert Hoover*

Massachusetts Governors: *Calvin Coolidge, Channing H. Cox, Alvan T. Fuller, Frank G. Allen*

Boston Mayors: *Andrew J. Peters, James M. Curley, Malcolm E. Nichols*

1920 Populations: *United States, 106,021,537; Massachusetts, 3,852,356; Boston, 748,060*

This fast, furious, xenophobic, jazz decade began with the election and short presidency of Warren G. Harding, a return to normalcy after war, the hypocritical Prohibition, and the revival of the Ku Klux Klan. It ended with the stock market crash in the fall of 1929 that signaled the economic depression of the 1930s. In the intervening years the country bathed in prosperity. Nearly everyone grew richer. Americans had never had it so good.

The U.S. reigned supreme in the Boston Marathon throughout the '20s with the domination of the event by Clarence DeMar of Melrose, Massachusetts. The press named him Mister DeMarathon. Was there any connection between DeMar's victories and America's xenophobia and prosperity? Foreign entries did remain at an all-time low during the decade.

On August 23, 1927, the U.S. government executed Nicola Sacco and Bartolomeo Vanzetti for murders committed in April 1920, ending a celebrated contest between the old Massachusetts Protestants and the new immigrants. The immigrants brought prosperity, or at least indicated its existence, but fear of them and the changing order they heralded produced a resistance in the more settled Americans—the Mayflower immigrants, the Yankees. The Massachusetts Supreme Court ruled against Sacco and Vanzetti's appeals for a new trial, but ultimately their execution came to mark the end of Yankee domination of the politics of Massachusetts and Boston.

Control of the Boston Marathon also fell from Yankee power, and with it prestige of the BAA. The lack of international competition allowed the local runner, DeMar, to win many races when he was well below top form. At his peak he had finished third in the world in the 1924 Paris Olympic Games.

DeMar emphasized quality and accomplishment over personality. He exemplified the last of the ascetic, frugal, tight-lipped, close-mouthed, intolerant Yankees, those from the same mold as Calvin Coolidge. These kinds of men would never dominate America or the Boston Marathon again.

This era changed the women too. The 1920s saw a liberation of women with the passage of the universal suffrage amendment. "Flappers" with "bobbed" hair swilling bootlegged liquor from pocket flasks forever submerged the ideal, demure Victorian lady, and conservatives warned of a breakdown in moral standards. By 1920 the cost of living had doubled in just 7 years, but there was money to be made and to go around; this decade marked the beginning of America's change to urban industrialism. In his 1931 book *Only Yesterday*, Fredrick Lewis Allen characterized the decade with neologisms that the Great War decade had never heard and subsequent generations would not forget, new terms and phenomena like racketeers, Teapot Dome, Coral Gables, radio, Al Capone, automatic traffic lights, confession magazines, the Wall Street explosion, and Charles A. Lindbergh. America turned its back on the League of Nations in its postwar return to—Harding's neologism—normalcy.

In a time when hard news traveled slowly but rumors spread in a flash, millions of Americans expected news of a Red Revolution to reach them the next week or next month. They heard of bombings, riots, strikes, and feared chaos. The Boston police strike of 1919 had sent a shiver through Americans and sent the governor of Massachusetts to the White House, where he declared, "There is no right to strike against the public safety by anybody, anywhere, at any time." By the end of the decade it became clear that there was no coordinated conspiracy (Bolshevism did not sweep across Europe), strikes did not stop prosperity, and bombings were only the work of a few fanatics. Despite the fear, the xenophobia, nothing bad happened in the '20s until the crash of '29.

The first radio station began broadcasting on November 2, 1920, and by the end of the decade the Boston Marathon could be followed live. Allen wrote that the tabloids boomed, presenting life not as a political and economic struggle but as a three-ring circus of sport, crime, and sex. A lively competition among the many Boston dailies busied the reporters and editors in covering track, long-distance running, the Olympic Games, and, the first 3 weeks of every April, the Boston Marathon. They chronicled endless details of the lives and times of the Boston runners.

F. Scott Fitzgerald wrote stories about the country's wealthy, and H.L. Mencken made vicious fun of the wealthy and everyone else. William Jennings Bryan gave his last gasp against Clarence Darrow in the Scopes monkey trial that in the public mind established the separation of science and religion. In the previous decade Clarence DeMar had quit racing; as a serious Baptist he had begun to feel "that the whole game of running was a selfish vainglorious search for praise and honor." But he had no such qualms in the '20s.

Even such a temperamental, stubborn, principled man as DeMar could not run against the temper of his times; he yielded and got back into the vainglorious game of running down the middle of the street in front of cheering crowds in his short pants. The temper of the '20s became freer. Hemlines rose above the knee, and young people flocked to petting parties—unthinkable 10 years earlier. They sang the popular songs—"Yes, We Have No Bananas," "The Sidewalks of New York," "It Ain't Gonna Rain No More." As much as he resisted the tide, it swept DeMar up with it.

Prohibition of alcohol in the form of the Eighteenth Amendment passed into law January 16, 1920. Its passage led to blatant and legendary lawlessness, when a man like Al Capone could become the virtual dictator of Chicago. The popularity and declining cost of the automobile helped make Capone's bootlegging possible, and it also helped runners get to odd little races in odd little places. Now towns off the railroad could have their own festival races and attract fields from afar.

The Coolidge prosperity crashed in the fall of 1929 to become Hoover's burden, and the weight of economic depression fell hard on the Boston Marathon and the Boston Athletic Association, making the '30s a decade of utterly different character. But until then, the '20s roared.

A new population of men began to run marathons in the 1920s and the public watched them with awe. Marathoners became heroes in a way that hadn't been true since the beginning of the century. (They were faster too.) The war was over and it was time to play.

PETER THE GREEK

MONDAY, APRIL 19, 1920

Linder, Roth, 73 Others Enter Patriots' Day Grind

The war had made mockery of Olympic principles in 1916, so no games could be contested, but now the world had returned to normal and American long-distance runners wanted more than anything else to represent their country in the August Games in Antwerp, Belgium. On April 6 the press reported the BAA officials' desire that their race would be the trials; 4 days later the Olympic Committee announced that the Boston Marathon would indeed host the Olympic marathon trials. By race day the "classiest field ever" boasted 75 names. It was not the biggest field ever, nor the fastest, but it attracted three previous winners: Finnish Carl Linder, "Bricklayer" Bill Kennedy, and frail Arthur Roth.

Other glorious pursuers came to ripen the field and perhaps change their luck: Linder's little pal Willie Wick, smiling Jimmy Henigan, train-jumping Chuck Mellor, and the flying Finn Willie Kyronen. Everyone had to have a handle; a mere name wasn't enough. The Olympic Committee's selectors would pick six Americans for the traveling team, but the marathon coach, 1912 Boston winner and record holder Mike Ryan, would pick only four to start and two to watch from the bench.

The pressure to win weighed heavily on Kyronen, who had tried time and again to win at Boston and had come close in 1916. Arthur Duffey said in his *Boston Post* column, that "if Willie Kyronen does not win, New Yorkers are off him for life." The *Post* picked Chuck Mellor to win based on his recent 2:30:30 marathon on a 26-mile course in the Auto City Marathon in Detroit. Frank Zuna, a plumber from Newark, New Jersey, who had won the Brooklyn–Seagate Marathon, seemed to be rapidly improving. The third-place runner from last year, Otto Laakso, came back to race. The 1919 seventh-place finisher, Peter Trivoulidas, a Greek national and a busboy in John Wanamaker's store in New York City, traveled north again. They all shuffled and milled around until starter George V. Brown raised his gun.

While Henigan again bounded away in the lead, Trivoulidas, a little, dark, deep-chested man with round eyes, a round head, and a big nose, ran in 23rd place, just behind squared-headed Linder and his pal, little bald-headed Wick. Trivoulidas's sturdy legs flicked up each step with a high back-kick. A satin binding accented his shorts, but his socks would not stay up; they bunched around his ankles. During the war Trivoulidas had served in the Greek navy. Born in 1891 in the village of Vateca, near Sparta, which was not far from the eponymous Marathon, he had run his first marathon on that original course in 1911. Trivoulidas weighed 131 pounds. Soon he would get his American citizenship.

A few places behind Trivoulidas, representing the 74th regiment, ran battle-scarred Robert Conboy. As he ran spectators could see on his body the ugly marks of the Great War. Kennedy still wore the flag on a hat; the armistice had come, but patriotism still raged. Peace with Germany had not been formally adopted. America for Americans, believed these proud veterans.

Clifton Mitchell ran nearby; the *Globe* described him as a "diminutive colored boy." But it was frail-looking Arthur Roth who harbored the dearest hopes of winning. He wanted to be the first American double winner of the Boston Marathon. Canadian Caffery was the only double winner so far (1900 and 1901). The little Trivoulidas harbored only hopes of pacing himself intelligently and of finishing well.

Trivoulidas came up on Kennedy. "Are you Bill Kennedy?"

"I am."

"Then I'm going to stay with you."

Kennedy thought about how his feet hurt. "You better get going; you'll never win if you stay with me." Though by Natick Henigan held a 300-yard lead, Roth did not take the lead seriously. Optimism carried Henigan only so far. Although a splendid, speedy, and powerful 5- and 10-mile racer, he had not prepared for marathons. By Wellesley wiry and light Roth settled into the #2 slot. Trivoulidas left Kennedy and eased along into 14th. Henigan suffered until the 17-mile mark, when Roth caught him. Roth's attendants sponged his face, "blackened with dust, gasoline fumes and perspiration," reported Lawrence J. Sweeney in the *Globe* the next day. Henigan, Kyronen, Mellor, Laakso, and others disappeared from the course as if snatched by goblins.

They each had seriously intended to win. When winning became obviously impossible, depression set in. Emotion can modify fatigue. A hopeful runner does not tire as fast as a despairing one. Each man who dropped out thought no one felt as bad as he did. Had any one of those men about to stop running known of Roth's condition he might have brightened and toughed it out.

Trivoulidas had no expectations of winning, so as he moved up through the field his mood brightened to dazzling, as without passing runners he suddenly found himself in second place. The leader, Roth, had no energy left. His death-rattle running style, at its best unsightly, now deteriorated. He staggered. He swung from side to side. He kept his lead until only 5/8 of a mile—3 minutes of running—remained.

Elated Trivoulidas caught Roth between the Hotel Puritan and the Harvard Club just after the statue of Leif Eriksson, or about halfway between Kenmore Square and Exeter Street. Roth dropped his arms at the approach of Trivoulidas, "that high-stepping, heavy treading little Greek born near the plain of Marathon," wrote Sweeney in the *Globe*. He unconditionally surrendered. Trivoulidas after his victory said in his broken English, "Sure, me pretty tired, but my how light I feel when I see only one man ahead of me! Happy too, I can make a gain. I know I win. No tired any more." Or at least that's how the *Herald* reporter took down the victor's words.

Linder and Wick ran consecutively again and finished third and fourth. The plumber from Newark, Frank Zuna, stopped on Exeter Street to remove his shoes and ran to the finish in his stockings, for seventh place. Trivoulidas and Wick were not American citizens so could not represent the U.S. in the Olympics. The Committee's preliminary picks were Roth, Linder, White, Conboy, Zuna, and Mitchell for the Olympic team. But Coach Ryan would reject at least one man as not fit enough to compete in the Olympic Games.

1920 Results

1. P. Trivoulidas, NY	2:29:31	8. C. Mitchell, *SCAC*, NY	2:41:43
2. A. Roth, *SAAA*, Roxbury, MA	2:30:31	9. J. Tuomikoski, Quincy, MA	2:43:06
		10. R. Ohman, *DC*, MA	2:43:41
3. C. Linder, *HAC*, Quincy, MA	2:33:22	11. S. Hatch, IAC	2:45:43
4. W. Wick, *HAC*, Quincy, MA	2:34:37	12. W. Carlson, *SAAC*, Chicago, IL	2:48:38
5. E.H. White, *HCL*, NY	2:36:10	13. H. Kauppinen, Brooklyn, NY	2:50:32
6. R. Conboy, 74th Reg., NY	2:37:34	14. J. Rossi, *CAC*, NY	2:52:44
7. F. Zuna, *WPAL*, Newark, NJ	2:39:34	15. B. Kennedy, *MornAC*	2:53:13

75 entrants, 60 starters.

A CELEBRATION OF PALS

TUESDAY, APRIL 19, 1921

Zuna and Mellor to Challenge Records

In the summer of 1920 Coach Mike Ryan had not let Frank Zuna run in the Olympic marathon. Zuna traveled with the team to Antwerp, but Ryan, the Boston Marathon course record holder at 2:21:18, said Zuna had not been able to demonstrate his fitness to his satisfaction. Zuna did not give demonstrations on demand. He went his own way. At the Olympic Games he did not go to the stadium to see the events because he preferred to not fall victim to "spectatoritis"—watching someone else rather than performing himself.

Zuna came from Bohemian ancestry in Czechoslovakia and made his living as a plumber. During the war he had run with Clarence DeMar in the Interallied Games, an informal Olympics among allied servicemen. As DeMar later remembered it, in order to be on the Interallied mile squad one had to go the distance in under 5 minutes. Because Zuna could easily break 5 minutes for a mile, he didn't bother to try 10 miles. And as he needed only his running clothes and shoes to run in the Boston Marathon, he wore his running outfit as underwear, dressed in shabby street clothes, and, run-

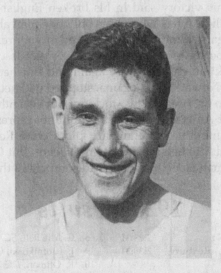

Olympian Frank Zuna was one of the few runners Clarence DeMar actually approved of, but 1912 winner Mike Ryan did not appreciate Zuna's carefree and independent streak. Photo courtesy of the *Boston Herald*.

ning shoes in his hip pocket and carrying nothing else, rode the train from Newark to Boston.

Frank Zuna, born in 1894, grew to 5'9" and 151 pounds. He wore straight dark hair and an impish grin and represented the Paulist AC of New York. Zuna looked like a happy workman. He did his work in a big Newark plumbing shop from 8:00 to 5:00. He trained every other day. He had first caught the marathon craze from reading back in 1908 about Johnny Hayes and Dorando Pietri. Hayes's declaration that no man with a yellow streak wins a marathon stuck with Zuna and motivated his desire to become a marathoner. He won the Brooklyn–Seagate 20-miler and the Brockton Marathon in 1914. In 1916 he served with General Pershing in the Mexican border dispute with Pancho Villa. During World War I he fought with the 27th Pioneer Division in France. In Boston in 1921 Zuna joined his great pal and Olympic teammate Chuck Mellor, to race all comers. Mellor wore a shirt blatantly announcing as he went his Chicago club: Logan Square AC. He looked as fit as could be and had made a habit of winning marathons.

April 19 gave runners cold and raw air. Tom Burke, who had shouted "Go!" to start the very first marathon back in 1897, remembered that it was such a day as this that John J. McDermott had set the first course record. Burke predicted a new record on this day. Zuna had company in pursuit of records. Mellor, for one, was game. On April 2, Mellor had won the Detroit Auto City Marathon over the full 26 miles, 385 yards by 8 seconds over Zuna. The old-timers said a man could not run two very good marathons in the same month. But here raced two very good men. Great pal or not Zuna wanted to beat Mellor to teach Ryan a lesson; Ryan had let Mellor run in Antwerp where he placed 12th, while he prevented Zuna's participation. Zuna wanted to break Ryan's Boston course record to rub Ryan's face in his own error.

Edouard Fabre, the 1915 winner from Canada, had taken a job with the United States Tire Company and had come to live in Boston. Fabre had run third in Detroit. He could spoil Zuna's plan.

The 1920 winner, Peter Trivoulidas, had run for Greece in the recent Olympic Games but now represented the Millrose AA. Carl Linder, the pattern maker from the Fore River Shipyards in Quincy and 1919 Boston winner, came back representing the BAA. Finnish Willie Kyronen and Otto Laakso completed the formidable Millrose team.

Zuna and Mellor ran together at record course pace until the 17-mile mark. Neither Fabre nor Trivoulidas could challenge either of them, nor could any human. Avoiding automobiles became their challenge. Once the thing to do was to follow the race on the train, but now the thing to do on Patriots' Day in Boston was to drive your new automobile alongside the marathon runners. So many cars occupied the course that the *Herald* reporter wrote of the worsening problem, "Every Henry Ford purchased since Christmas was out." Zuna and Mellor managed to avoid the cars, but the hills tired Mellor.

He had to leave his teammate and friend on his own. Too bad for Mellor—he was having so much fun.

Zuna ran on alone, continuing his record-setting pace. No one came near him. Zuna ran like a sprinter. He did not shuffle like Arthur Roth or run with Longboat's free and easy stride or move with Fabre's forward-thrusting snowshoe gait. In the eyes of former world-great sprinter Arthur Duffey, who had become a columnist for the *Boston Post*, Zuna did not prance like Trivoulidas but bounded along, shrugging his shoulders with every stride like a sprinter does in that moment before breaking the tape—except Zuna shrugged a thousand times each mile. He shrugged himself along under Mike Ryan's course record pace.

No one came close to catching Zuna that day. A second after he broke his record victory tape, Zuna turned to *Globe* reporter Lawrence Sweeney to resist his questions: "Wait 'till I see Chuck finish." Zuna and the reporter waited, but the raw wind quickly sent Zuna indoors. Mellor trotted in 3 minutes later. In the BAA clubhouse, to the amusement of reporters, the friends shared the same hot bath. The reporters and officials implored Zuna to stay the evening for celebrations and to be introduced to the public in a big Boston theater. But Zuna refused at first, saying he had to be back for work in the morning. "I have never allowed my running to interfere with my work as a plumber."

Officials persisted, pressing Zuna to be a good fellow and stay. "'Like to very much,'" he said as reported the next day by Tom McCabe of the *Herald*, "'but you know . . .' and he raised his hands in that inimitable way certain classes of people use to express their feelings." The officials and other "good fellows" secured a place for him on the overnight train back to New York, but he agreed to stay only when they included Mellor in the celebrations. Zuna smiled a lot. Mellor broke training and had himself a good smoke. The pals celebrated each other.

Zuna's victory and dismantling of Ryan's course record delighted Clarence DeMar. In his autobiography he wrote,

> Zuna always interested me . . . For Zuna now to break the cherished record of the one who had considered him mediocre seemed to me like a reasonable athletic revenge. The marathon record had passed from an Irishman to a Bohemian, from one who capitalized on its possession to one who thought no more of it than he did of a good meal.

1921 Results

1. F.T. Zuna, *PaulAC*, NY	2:18:57[CR]	4. C. Linder, *BAA* 2:28:02
2. C. Mellor, *LSAC*, Chicago, IL	2:22:12	5. A.R. Michelson, Stamford, CT 2:30:35
3. P. Trivoulidas, *MillAA*, NY	2:27:41	6. E. Fabre, *SAAA* 2:31:34

7. W. Kyronen, *MillAA*	2:32:36	12. A. Rodgers, *ImpAC*, NS	2:38:51
8. O.J. Laakso, *MillAA*	2:33:39	13. C. Mitchell, *STCC*, NY	2:40:12
9. J. Goff, *STCC*, NY	2:37:35	**14. B. Kennedy, *MornAC*, NY**	**2:40:40**
10. R. Conboy, 74th Reg., NY	2:38:18	15. W. Carlson, *SAAC*, IL	2:42:37
11. M.J. Lynch, *AC*, DC	2:38:38		

THE HENIGANS

WEDNESDAY, APRIL 19, 1922

Can DeMar Show Old-Time Speed?

A sleetstorm in November of 1921 broke many trees, which fell and blocked the streets. Clarence DeMar, the old marathon winner from 1911, could not ride his bicycle to work. The trolley from Melrose to Medford would have taken hours, so he tried running to work, for the first time in years. He felt so good doing it that he continued, long after crews had cleared the streets. Before New Year's Day he had decided to run the marathon again. He weighed only 6 pounds more than in 1911. He had been born 33 years earlier in Ohio and moved to Massachusetts with his mother when he was 10 years old. Who did DeMar think would win the BAA Marathon? DeMar thought Chuck Mellor would win.

Mellor had won the three previous Detroit Auto City marathons. Other Boston Marathon winners—Zuna, Kennedy, Linder, and Fabre—had come to repeat, but all except Zuna had lately performed far from their best. The old-timers said that a man never comes back from running a good marathon, that a marathon uses him up. Jack Caffery, with his wins in 1900 and 1901, had been an exception. The *Globe* intoned on race day, "Whether DeMar can cope with the present day marathoners after a gap of eleven years is something to be doubted." The writer generously continued, "He was a great runner in his prime and today will tell whether he can show anything like his old time speed. No matter what he does, his running will offer an interesting lesson for the students of athletics."

In other places the newspaper held up other hopes. One headline put impossible pressure again on the top local 5- and 10-miler, Smilin' Jimmy "Hinky" Henigan. "Henigan Has Great Hopes" declared the *Globe*. Jimmy had a brother, Tommy, who was quite fast; he entered as well.

An Indian racer with the acquired name of Smoke drifted down from Canada. Albert Smoke, a trapper and fisherman of the Missausuggi tribe from Petersboro, Ontario, did indeed often smoke big black cigars. He held them in his teeth, grinning as he talked through the tobacco.

The weather blew gloriously cool under a cloudy sky. The light rain of the night firmed the roads and left neither mud nor dust. Jimmy Henigan took the lead and held it easily at Framingham's Union Station. Zuna, under siege as defender, felt obligated to follow. DeMar had observed at the start that Zuna did not look himself. He looked too content. His cheeks had no hollow, and the backs of his hands lacked road map relief. In the year since his victory a patina of fat had grown over Zuna's lean body—not enough to make him look jolly, but enough that a keen competitor and observer such as DeMar, who knew Zuna well, would know that he had not been training with the vengeance of the previous year. Willie Ritola, a nearly translucent-skinned, blond 26-year-old carpenter and Finnish immigrant, followed. Tommy Henigan followed Ritola.

At Natick Jimmy Henigan led by 80 seconds. Zuna ran at record pace in second place. By Wellesley Jimmy Henigan led by 300 yards. Zuna seemed to have disappeared. At Newton Lower Falls the idea of winning dawned on DeMar.

At Auburndale Jimmy Henigan dropped back, and brother Tommy joined him. DeMar had moved steadily through the pack. He had to do battle with the Indian, Smoke. The Henigans fought hard. Jimmy, running with hunched shoulders, was the last to give up family glory. His shoulders hunched more and more, fatigue contracting his body as he lashed himself up and over each of the Newton hills.

Mellor and Trivoulidas dropped out. DeMar ran on through what the *Globe's* Sweeney called a "blue-black smoke of petrol and oil," and Henigan raced him for every inch. Henigan could run much faster than DeMar over 5 or 10 miles so could easily respond to DeMar with surges, but after 17 miles Henigan's quick leg muscles would not follow orders. He could not hold a steady pace. At last DeMar passed Henigan at Boston College and shook him on the downhill to Lake Street. Henigan stopped. A helper gave Henigan a yardstick, and he struck his calves to make them quit their clenching. But they would not relax, so Henigan could not finish. His incandescence had evaporated like luminescent carbon from the filament of a light bulb only to be deposited as soot trapped inside the glass. Smilin' Jimmy Henigan had burned out, but he would not be able to escape his obsession with the marathon—the guiding light of his life— for many more years.

At the Coolidge Corner checkpoint DeMar ran over a minute faster than had Zuna, with a time only 4 seconds slower than Caffery's checkpoint record. A course record by the old man seemed possible. Willie Ritola of Finland ran right on schedule. He had no cramps and no problems except that he was too far back for even his superior speed to catch up. He caught Smoke and whipped past him, but DeMar ran too far ahead. Ritola went on to win Olympic gold medals in both the 10,000 meters (30:23.2) and the steeplechase (9:33.6) and finished second to Paavo Nurmi in the 5,000 meters in 1924 in Paris. In 1928 Ritola would win a gold medal in the 5,000 meters (14:38) in the Amsterdam Olympics. His Olympic 10,000 record of 30:23 put together more sub-5-minute miles in one race than DeMar ran singly in his life. What would have happened had Ritola decided to lead from the start? Timing is the thing, and Willie Ritola had consulted the wrong schedule and missed his train.

Clarence DeMar astounded all observers as he steamed on alone to victory and a new course record. Eleven years after his first victory, the press wrote as if confronted by a miracle. Sweeney of the *Globe* said, "The superman of marathon runners is Clarence H. DeMar of Melrose." The headline read "Defying Father Time." Neal O'Hara of the *Post* wrote, "Eleven years ago Jack Dempsey couldn't swing a fist. . . . Babe Ruth was a bushleaguer." Superlative piled upon superlative as the press told the story of the great DeMar. But not everyone had superlatives for him.

Mike Ryan criticized DeMar in an article for the April 20 *Boston Herald*: "He carries his chin high and did not have sufficient swing in his leg action to give him a smooth working appearance. He insisted on running down the hills instead of loosening out and letting his stride carry him down." Ryan continued on to say that if only DeMar would pay attention to these details he would chop a minute off his time.

DeMar wrote a first-person story for the *Boston Post* that appeared the day after the race: "I must confess that I expected to win the race. I do not say this with any conceitedness. . . . I never feel so well as when I have a canter. . . . I do not know whether or not I will ever do any more marathon running. If I find time I certainly will, but it is business for me first, and marathon running afterwards." With that DeMar went back to work at his job in a print shop.

1922 Results

1.	C.H. DeMar, *DC*, MA	2:18:10^CR*	9.	H. Frick, *GAC*, NY	2:28:16
2.	W. Ritola, *FAAC*, NY	2:21:44	10.	E. Fabre, *NAA*, Montreal, PQ	2:29:00
3.	A. Smoke, *PAA*, ON	2:22:49	11.	C. Mitchell, *STCC*, NY	2:30:24
4.	V. MacAuley, *DC*	2:24:02	12.	J. Tuomikoski, *BAA*	2:32:06
5.	W. Kyronen, *MillAA*, NY	2:24:42	13.	B. Kennedy, *CAC*, NY	2:32:50
6.	O.J. Laakso, *MillAA*, NY	2:24:45	14.	C. Morton, *WLAC*, Detroit, MI	2:38:23
7.	C. Linder, *BAA*	2:25:29	15.	A.K. Sturgis, *DC*	2:40:29
8.	F.T. Zuna, *PaulAC*, NY	2:26:26	16.	S. Hatch, *IAC*, Chicago, IL	2:43:42

78 starters.

Unofficial: Peter Foley 3:48.

*Permanent course record for 24.5 miles.

SAVED BY A SAFETY PIN

THURSDAY, APRIL 19, 1923

Can Old DeMar Make It 2 in a Row?

"I intend to lead all the way," said Jimmy Henigan, his brightness in full glow. "I do not see why I should not win." And why not? He was the fastest man around. He should win the Boston Marathon. He had been running for 14 years. "He stated positively that he would run his last race in the Ashland to Boston grind this coming Patriots' Day." And why not win? DeMar was sick in bed—he might not run!

In early February Clarence DeMar ran down Fulton Street in Medford between high banks of snow. A big dog obstructed his path and made a lunge for him. With his sneakers DeMar kicked the dog and tried to run past. Instantly a man charged DeMar and punched him in the face. "Kick my dog, will you? He was barking a welcome to me." Blood rushed from a gash on his upper lip. The rupture made way for erysipelas, or Saint Anthony's fire. Redness and pain followed an infection that spread over DeMar's entire face and ignited a systemic fever that confined him to bed for 10 days. Sickness distressed DeMar, who kept careful track of his illnesses. He had been ill a total of 13 days since 1903. His lifetime sick-day total had nearly doubled. Smilin' Jimmy Henigan never felt better in his life.

Frank Zuna had not been ill, either. In early April he won the Detroit Marathon in 2:34. On April 19 DeMar crawled out of bed; he would run regardless. He saw Zuna at the start, a bright-eyed man with hollow in his cheeks and trim in his every motion. DeMar figured that Zuna would be the toughest, but what had Detroit cost him? At noon in Ashland sharp shadows rushed over the ground in answer to the starter's gun. A warm sun tapped the runners' right shoulders as they ran east to Boston. The pressure of the tapping sunshine grew with the miles. The sun beat down on DeMar's head, but he ran in his characteristic way: chin up, no counterbalancing arm action, rolling from the waist and pounding with the balls of his feet. Zuna ran like a sprinter, but like one who knew the marathon and knew that runners often wilt on hot days. Zuna held back, waiting for DeMar to wilt first. Henigan waited for no one.

But it was Tommy Henigan who led the race at South Framingham, not the faster Jimmy, despite his bragging. This day Jimmy mysteriously never contended. DeMar, however, remained behind Tommy as did yet another in the ever-growing list of blond Finns in Boston Marathon history, Albert T. "Whitey" Michelson of Stamford, Connecticut.

Bill Kennedy had adopted Whitey Michelson as his protégé and Cygnet AC teammate. Kennedy, now 41, had won the race in 1917 and had since settled in Port Chester, New York. He had become a spokesman/philosopher for the marathon sport. He said that every marathoner he ever met was more or less a dreamer. In a letter to *Globe* reporter Sweeney, who had been present at every Boston Marathon since 1897, published in the *Globe* on April 18, Kennedy wrote, "Why else would a man spend three months of hard training three or four times a week from five to twenty miles, cutting out the smokes and chews and going to bed at nine or ten o'clock?" Kennedy loved his sport and the people in it. He said he would "lend every nickel he had to a marathoner because he knew he would pay him back." On the day before the race, marathoners elected Kennedy president of the International Association of Marathoners. They elected taciturn Clarence DeMar secretary. If there was anything critical to be said, the often acerbic DeMar would say it.

But DeMar felt far from happy on that hot marathon course. Having patched the hole, he wore the same shoes he had won in the previous year. In a last-minute notion he stuck a safety pin through his socks and into the shoe leather to keep his socks from descending into his shoes and bunching up to raise blisters. That idea turned out to be fortuitous.

After Tommy Henigan quit, DeMar let Michelson lead. At 13 miles DeMar had crossed over to the sidewalk and Michelson to the middle of the car track in order to use the softer footing. Michelson cast curious glances at DeMar from the corner of his eye to assess his condition, as if wondering when the old man might make his move. In Newton Lower Falls DeMar gave the youngster an example: He burst away on the downhill. Michelson responded and took the lead back; DeMar did not retaliate. The hills stood ahead. On the last one Michelson, still leading, walked. He walked past Boston College, then ran slowly down the hill toward Lake Street. DeMar ran quickly down the hill to pass Michelson, who had no fight left. Zuna did have fight, and he zeroed in on DeMar.

DeMar had serious problems with fatigue and with the wheeled spectators who rolled alongside him. Just before Cleveland Circle an automobile hit a bicycle, which in turn ran over DeMar's shoe. But because a pin held the shoe to the sock, only the heel came off DeMar's foot and folded underneath it. DeMar had a dilemma: The folded shoe hurt and required him to pay inordinate attention to every other step; it would not fall off, but if he stopped to correct the problem Zuna might close. What should he do? The errant shoe only hurt him, it did not slow him. Zuna was resourceful and not about to surrender. DeMar had his shoe and relentless Zuna on his mind.

When Zuna was a boy the police caught him and friends in the Essex County park in New Jersey. They were shooting illegal craps. A policeman grabbed young Zuna by the coat. He slipped out of the coat, leaving the officer holding it, and ran away. The police gave chase in their cars, but they had governors on the cars limiting them to only 6 mph. Zuna could run much faster. He toyed with them for 4 miles; the police thought he would get tired and stop. But he did not tire, and he did not surrender.

DeMar worried. Zuna might not be tired now. DeMar ran scared, with no way of knowing how much zip Zuna had left. The rolling spectators shouted conflicting advice to DeMar, ranging from "Stop and fix it" to "Take the shoe off and run barefoot." DeMar resented the suggestions, as he did most advice. As the miles passed, the shoe did not fall off. Zuna could not catch DeMar. The great Zuna got tired. Saved by a safety pin, DeMar won again.

The biggest crowd ever yet on hand to watch a Boston Marathon gave DeMar universal applause, but the press had used up all its superlatives the year before. Tom McCabe of the *Herald* said, "Last year we were dumbfounded; now we are lost in amazement."

Wallie Carlson, brother of 1913 winner Fritz Carlson, finished third. Carl Linder, the 1919 winner, took seventh and Kennedy eighth.

The 1915 Boston winner, Edouard Fabre, now age 38, plowed into 11th place. He had left the Boston area and the tire business to move back to Canada. As he headed for a bowl of pea soup, he brushed past the medical examiners, barbarous in his fatigue: "By God . . . don't bother me now for those things." He had his soup; he loved his beer, but the Volstead Act, the enforcement law for Prohibition, was now in force, so unlike in 1915, the press reported only his soup drinking.

But DeMar was the man with the fierce concentration that allowed him to overcome difficulties to win his third and most painful victory.

Waiting at the finish of this year's marathon were three curious scientists named Gordon, Levine, and Wilmaers. They had an X-ray unit installed on the second floor of the BAA building on Exeter Street, and they immediately ushered each finisher upstairs so they could take an X ray of his chest. They took a second X ray an hour later. In addition to taking X rays (a new medical diagnostic tool), the three scientists had taken measurements of each runner's "vital capacity"—the volume of air that can move in and out of the lungs with each maximal breath—before and after the race and again several days later. They were hoping to determine if marathon runners had larger hearts and

Waiting at the finish line were three curious scientists, hoping to determine with their X-ray machine if marathon runners had larger hearts and lungs than average people.

lungs than average people and whether the stress of the race temporarily enlarged either the heart or the lungs. Earlier researchers had observed by palpation and percussion (feeling and thumping) that a runner's heart was indeed larger.

But rather than clarify the issue, the new research muddled it. Their pictures showed no cardiac enlargement, and the measurements of lung capacity showed no differences from normal. Immediately after the race runners appeared to have less lung volume, but several days later it was the same as before the race. Postrace fatigue would account for the discrepancy. Gordon et al. concluded that "on considering the entire picture that a marathon runner presents . . . given a normal heart, the most important point in summary training is that of the legs rather than the heart." It was a good try, but subsequent findings would show that there was more to it. Although not elucidative by contemporary standards, scientists had at least begun to measure runners' physiology. And the next year they would attempt to measure the course according to Olympic standards.

1923 Results

1. C. DeMar, *MALP90*	2:23:47	9. J. Conto, *PAC*, NY	2:38:20
2. F. Zuna, *MillAA*, NY	2:25:30	10. A. Flanders, *BAA*	2:40:41
3. W. Carlson, *SAA*, Chicago, IL	2:27:10	11. E. Fabre, *NAA*, Montreal, PQ	2:41:09
4. A.T. Michelson, *CAC*, CT	2:28:27	12. S. Mirageas, *GAAC*, MA	2:44:01
5. G. Nilson, *FAAC*, NY	2:29:40	13. M.J. Lynch, *AC*, DC	2:45:19
6. N. Erickson, *FAAC*, NY	2:29:46	14. P. Porfolio, Cambridge, MA	2:46:47
7. C. Linder, *BAA*	2:30:03	15. H. Kanto, *CVC*, NH	2:47:15
8. B. Kennedy, *CAC*, NY	2:33:47		

70 entrants, 67 starters.

26 MILES, 385 YARDS?

SATURDAY, APRIL 19, 1924

Boston Selection Site for Paris Olympics

Clarence DeMar fiercely wanted to be on the U.S. Olympic team, as he had been in 1912. He wanted another crack at the gold. He was 35 years old, so no one, not even he thought another chance was likely. But in addition to his Boston victories, which had become commonplace, he wanted an Olympic gold medal. The Olympic Committee again picked the Boston Marathon to be the basis for team selection. DeMar knew the course and had won there three times, so Boston was a good place for him to race for an Olympic spot. A mediocre finish by DeMar, however, would place his selection in the hands of the committee. A runaway victory would keep his fate where he always wanted it—in his own hands. So DeMar had to do more than win; he had to win masterfully.

Because 1924 was an Olympic year and the official Olympic or full marathon distance had been arbitrarily set during the 1908 games as the distance from a starting line near Windsor Castle to the Olympic Stadium in London, the Boston Marathon officials decided to break tradition and lengthen their race to 26 miles, 385 yards. They measured the roads as best they could and pushed the start west out of Ashland into Hopkinton at the fork in the road near the Tebeau farm. From Ashland it was mostly uphill to that point.

The weather on April 19 at the new Hopkinton start promised a fast race. Gentle rain the night before weighed down the road dust, and a chill wind cut from the north to cool the runners. The newspapers expected an Alphonse-Gaston routine ("After you." "No, no, after you.") between DeMar and Zuna. Both had won the race before, DeMar three times, but Zuna had won two races this spring at the full marathon distance. DeMar thought the races had taken too much out of the big Bohemian. Zuna stood half a head taller than DeMar. Which would dare lead and show his hand to the other? Would Zuna bound off into the lead or would DeMar shuffle into one?

Though Zuna had beaten DeMar and Michelson in the Laurel-to-Baltimore Marathon, DeMar declared that he, DeMar, would win nevertheless in Boston. DeMar referred more to his own evolving fitness than to their apparent rivalry. The newspapers, used to boxing, pitted man against man, but these marathoners saw the challenge as a matter of training the body to be ready on race day to contend with time and distance; only incidentally, once they achieved fitness, could they race each other.

Moments after the start, careful observers noticed that DeMar, the great shuffler, no longer shuffled. He had had a shuffle-ectomy. During the winter he had jumped over a snowbank and wrenched his back. He visited an osteopath, who poked at him to correct a limb length discrepancy. All those years he shuffled because one leg was longer than the other, and the doctor's poking put Clarence together again. Or so DeMar said. His newfound boldness and uplifting running style were obvious as he took the lead at Natick. He left Louis Tikkanen, Chuck Mellor, and Billy Churchill. A fan yelled at DeMar to hurry up, and DeMar told him to shut up. Shuffling or bounding, DeMar did not like to be told what to do.

DeMar had met Churchill in California during an American Legion convention, where they ran a 5-mile race together, with DeMar winning. DeMar represented the Melrose American Legion Post 90, which paid his expenses on that California trip. He liked Churchill and invited him to Boston to run the marathon. Churchill stayed at DeMar's house for the weekend.

Churchill made a game attempt to stay with his high-stepping host. He led Mellor by 60 yards and Zuna by 300. Frank Wendling followed with

Victor MacAuley, who survived a queasy passage from Halifax and who Nova Scotians said would be the next Freddy Cameron. The big Zuna did not look good.

DeMar sailed along. His attendant, Bob Campbell, the foreman in the print shop where he worked, rode along to see to his needs, but he had few. DeMar hooked his sight on the bend in the road and pushed. He squeezed every second from the road. His body seemed electric. He had never felt like this before. His physiology sang down the streets. He felt big and above the road, and the road seemed little to him. Nothing bothered DeMar.

For Zuna the road seemed too big and too close. He developed stomach problems; nothing could be done, so he dropped out. Churchill came back on DeMar going into Wellesley and took the lead. DeMar ripped it back. At Wellesley College DeMar passed 12 college girls in a row, each wearing a full-length fur coat. They cheered him and he waved. He could be cavalier and undauntable because he ran his finest 2-1/2 hours.

DeMar ran with no socks in a pair of custom-made Arnold Glove-Grip shoes with pneumatic inner soles. They sold for $10 a pair. DeMar's photo frequently appeared in ads for Arnold's Glove-Grips placed next to the news stories about that year's marathon. Part of the ad text read thus:

> In his many spectacular endurance feats, Clarence DeMar always wears a running shoe constructed on the Arnold Glove-Grip arch-fitting last. There are few things that Clarence worries about before his races, but he always insists upon Glove-Grips for shoes.

DeMar's inner soles twisted and bunched up, raising blisters, but he blamed the inner soles and lack of socks as the irritants, not his Glove-Grips.

Regardless of foot problems, DeMar flew down the roads and up the Newton hills past the checkpoints on the new course, establishing new records. By the time he reached Exeter Street, second-place Mellor ran a mile behind. DeMar apparently smashed Hannes Kolehmainen's world record of 2:32:35, set when he won the gold medal in the 1920 Olympics.

The press dug deeper for superlatives to describe DeMar. Having exhausted their thesauruses, they resorted to punning: Mister DeMarvelous, Mister DeMarathon. Now DeMar shined a true star. The papers speculated on whether and when and who he would marry. Back in the Melrose mayor's office, DeMar shook hands with 2,000 people. Photographers came to the print shop to photograph his bare feet. And no doubt Arnold sold lots of Glove-Grips.

DeMar made the Olympic team, as did Frank Wendling, Churchill, Zuna, Mellor, and Ralph Williams. On to Paris!

THE BOSTON GLOBE—FRIDAY, APRIL 20, 1928

DeMar wins again with

ARNOLD GLOVE-GRIP SHOES

$10

The CONTINENTAL

Boylston Street Store

Open Saturday Evenings

HENIGAN BEING CONGRATULATED BY C. F. GORMAN OF DORCHESTER CLUB

ELIGIBLE FOR THE OLYMPIC TEAM ON THEIR SHOWING IN THE MARATHON

DE MAR ON JOB TODAY, BUT DIDN'T RUN TO WORK

Marathon Victor Plans to Compete in Several Races —Sure to Be on Olympic Team

TWO ARRESTED IN WATERTOWN RAID

Revere and Boston Men at Garage

FILES WRIT AGAINST MAYOR McGRATH

Seeks Removal of Mrs Dunn as Quincy Auditor

MILLIONAIRES MADE BY STOCK MARKET MEET

Matthew C. Brush Among Those at Dinner to W. C. Durant, About to Sail For Europe

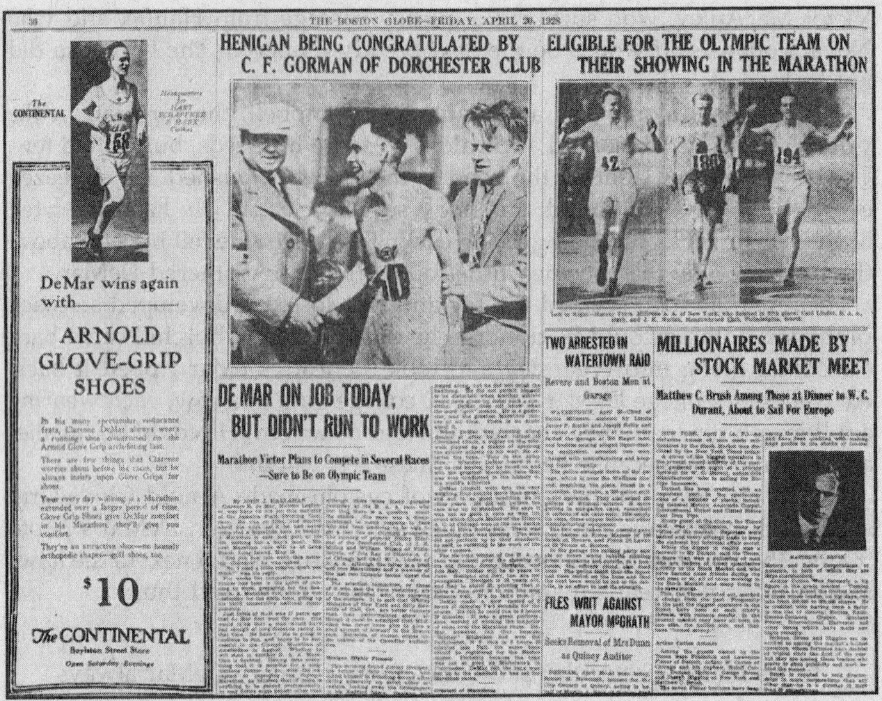

Clarence DeMar frequently appeared in advertisements for Arnold Glove-Grip shoes (shown here in the *Boston Globe*, April 20, 1928). It is not clear what, if anything, DeMar received for the endorsement or how the era's strict amateur rules allowed such a commercial relationship. Reprinted courtesy of the *Boston Globe*.

Checkpoint Splits

S. Framingham	31:25
Natick	52:56
Wellesley	1:10:08
Newton Lower Falls	1:25:47
Woodland Park	1:34:58
Lake Street	2:00:08
Coolidge Corner	2:10:05
Finish	2:29:40

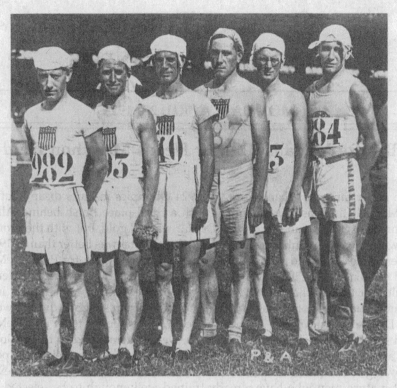

The "hats" (handkerchiefs knotted at the corners) were probably not official USA team regalia, but they signaled how hot the 1924 Paris Olympic marathon was expected to be. The team included (from left) Frank F. Wendling, William J. Churchill, Clarence DeMar, Frank Zuna, Charles Mellor, and Ralph Williams. Courtesy of the Boston Public Library, Print Department.

1924 Results

1.	**C. DeMar, *MALP90***	**2:29:40**[CR]	9.	L. Tikkanen, *FAAC*, NY	2:46:31
2.	**C. Mellor, *IAC*, Chicago, IL**	**2:35:04**	10.	S. Mirageas, *MillAA*	2:50:49
3.	F.F. Wendling, *WidAC*, NY	2:37:40	11.	M.J. Dwyer, *MAC*, NY	2:50:51
4.	W.J. Churchill, *OC*, CA	2:37:52	12.	M.J. Lynch, *AC*, DC	2:52:50
5.	**C. Linder, *BAA***	**2:40:12**	13.	N. Erickson, *FAAC*, NY	2:53:18
6.	V. MacAuley, *WAA*, NS	2:40:36	14.	G. O'Neil, *DC*	2:55:22
7.	R. Williams, *HAC*, MA	2:41:58	15.	J. Rossi, *CAC*, NY	2:56:05
8.	**B. Kennedy, *CAC*, NY**	**2:43:03**			

Chewing Tobacco
and the Daily News

MONDAY, APRIL 20, 1925

Bronze Medalist DeMar Heads Marathon Field

The Americans came back from the 1924 Olympics in Paris disappointed. DeMar felt the least disappointed, with a third-place finish behind Albin Stenroos of Finland and an Italian. DeMar wanted gold, but with the bronze he was at least not unhappy. His experience in total was better than in 1912, when Mike Ryan had bossed him around. Before leaving for Paris, DeMar had stipulated that if he were to be on the Olympic team, his experience could not be like that in 1912. In Stockholm DeMar had had to train in a manner that was not of his own determination. Ryan's regime did not work for DeMar or for anyone else on the team, so the entire team and DeMar had finished dismally. In 1924, in Paris, DeMar demanded to be let alone. He and Ryan avoided each other, but DeMar attributed the relatively poor showing of the rest of the Americans to forced team coaching. He believed that mature men who have already trained well enough to be selected for an Olympic team need no additional coaching. In the humid continental summer heat a bronze medal was, indeed, honorable, but DeMar was unfulfilled. In his official report Mike Ryan said that the team had done poorly because of their own fear of the heat. He said DeMar should have won but was too yellow and afraid. Frank Wendling finished in 16th, Frank Zuna, at last on the Olympic team, in 18th, and Billy Churchill in 23rd. They all were disappointed. Chuck Mellor in 25th felt the worst of the American bunch.

But disappointment did not seem to drive Mellor to train harder. He spent January ice skating with Mrs. Mellor and began training in February with 5-mile runs, lengthening them to 15 miles twice a week. On Sundays he took long walks. Such a genteel approach did not match the DeMar style, but Mellor, like nearly every other top marathoner, had more natural talent than DeMar.

Mellor's Illinois Athletic Club teammate Schous Christianson led the 1925 Boston race early on. He often performed this "rabbit" role. Dutifully Victor MacAuley of Nova Scotia, Mellor, DeMar, and Whitey Michelson followed in a bunch. Tommy Henigan and Willie Kyronen chased them. The runners ran into a winter gale of snow flurries, and bare arms reddened in the cold. Mellor, ever resourceful from his days of train-hopping and pool table–sleeping, stuffed the day's newspaper in his shirt to shield his belly from

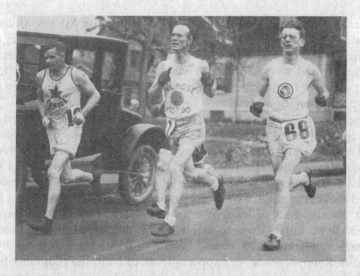

Canadian Victor MacAuley (left) Clarence DeMar (middle) with Chuck Mellor, who has the day's newspaper stuffed into his shirt to protect him from the cold. Photo courtesy of the *Boston Herald*.

the chill. He wore gloves but no hat. He fortified himself with a cheekful of chewing tobacco.

At Natick the call rang out: Christianson, DeMar, MacAuley, Michelson. Along the route 300,000 people watched. They hunkered down with their backs to the east wind to watch the runners come squinting and grimacing into the squall.

Into Wellesley Kyronen caught a stitch. He gripped his side as if shot. Mellor lagged into Newton Lower Falls. MacAuley led after Christianson dropped back as a prelude to dropping out. Ralph Williams of Quincy chased MacAuley. Much to the dismay of DeMar and the other U.S. Olympic marathoners, the Committee had selected Williams for the 1924 team over 1919 BAA winner Carl Linder, who had finished ahead of Williams in the trials at Boston. Williams was the only member of the Olympic team to drop out in the Paris heat. This year at Boston Williams dropped out because of the cold. Bill Kennedy, the bricklayer who won in 1917, stopped in a garage to use the toilet (New England bushes have no leaves in mid-April). Henigan dropped out at Woodland, leaving Mellor with the lead and DeMar 10 yards behind.

DeMar ran close to the curb and into the wind. Most of the runners wore long-sleeved shirts, but Mellor and DeMar bared their shoulders to the wind and now occasional snowflakes. Did old DeMar have a plan he was playing close to his vest? Both seemed to have something in reserve. So did Frank Zuna, who ran in third place. On Beacon Street DeMar gained. Victory this year would bring a special honor. The Amateur Athletic Union had designated this year's Boston Marathon the first national marathon championship. DeMar would like that. He liked winning. He took his every advantage. It had worked in 1923, when he waited for Michelson to wilt, but that was a hot day. Runners don't wilt in snowflakes. They may stiffen and stop, but they don't wilt.

Mellor stiffened nothing but his resolve. Mellor and DeMar raced down Beacon Street with an unclosable, unwavering gap, as if a tether connected them. Those two and Zuna ran this section of the race faster than ever. All three ran at a relative sprint. As much as DeMar glared at Mellor's back and tried to haul in that tether, Mellor let out more line. DeMar, powerless, watched Mellor turn onto Exeter Street. As he did so DeMar could see Mellor spit his 26-mile wad of tobacco onto the street. Then DeMar ran as he watched Mellor finish. Zuna took third in his last appearance in Boston. In 1971 Frank Zuna, at age 79, visited Boston to watch the marathon. By then he lived in Reno, Nevada, in happy retirement from the plumbing trade.

As Mellor, the new National AAU and Boston Marathon champion, waited for his pal, Zuna, to finish he said simply "I'm happy."

1925 Results

1. C. Mellor, *IAC*, Chicago, IL	2:33:00		9. W.J. Kennedy, *CAC*, NY	2:43:46
2. C.H. DeMar, *MALP90*	2:33:37		10. F. Wendling, Buffalo, NY	2:48:59
3. F. Zuna, Newark, NJ	2:35:35		11. S. McLellan, Noel, NS	2:49:57
4. A. Michelson, *CAC*, NY	2:37:22		12. C.W.A. Linder, *BAA*	2:50:33
5. K. Koski, *FAAC*, NY	2:39:26		13. J. Rossi, *CAC*, NY	2:51:28
6. W. Kyronen, *FAAC*, NY	2:40:36		14. J. Carleton, E. Sandwich, MA	2:52:21
7. V. MacAuley, Windsor, NS	2:42:14		15. G. Duncan, *DC*	2:54:49
8. N. Erickson, *FAAC*, NY	2:43:08			

110 starters.

DeMar

MONDAY, APRIL 19, 1926

Gold Medalist Comes to Smash Record

Clarence DeMar did not have a happy childhood. He was born in 1888, and before he reached 10 years old his father died. His mother could not support the household in rural Warwick, Massachusetts, so she sent young Clarence off to the Boston Farm School on Thompson's Island in Boston Harbor. The Farm School had merged with the Boston Asylum for Indigent Boys in 1885.

The Deer Island House of Correction stood nearby, as did a rendering factory on Spectacle Island for the disposal of dead horses. Boston Harbor Islands since the 1700s held quarantine hospitals for smallpox victims, garbage dumps, and sewage outlets.

Even at such a young age Clarence did not want anyone acting for him in loco parentis. He tried to escape the island with several other boys by swimming and pushing a rowboat through the cold, murky waters of Boston Harbor to Savin Hill, over a mile away. Clarence and his accomplices were caught and humiliated. The superintendent made particular fun of Clarence, calling his peculiar swimming kick a "twin screw propeller on a Chinese Junk." The ridicule and shame pushed Clarence deeper into the shell of himself, deeper into a hunger to be left alone, deeper into an obsession with self-reliance. The only thing that made Clarence's isolation humane to him was books. Clarence did learn one thing at the Farm School: Eschew indigence and any of the trappings thereof.

Finally, in 1904, when Clarence was 16, they let him go to work on a real farm in South Hero, Vermont. Between bouts of hard labor he found his way to the Maple Lawn Academy, where his inclination to bookish retreat gave him escape from adolescent socializing. He lived by himself until he entered the University of Vermont. DeMar kept to himself and spoke little. *Post* columnist Arthur Duffey wrote this line after a visit to DeMar's print shop the day after one of his victories: "He seldom speaks to anyone and if anyone wants to really offend him all they have to do is talk about his victory."

Adolescent Clarence DeMar only daydreamed of being an athletic hero. Every attempt at sport proved him inept; he was found either too slight, too weak, or too slow. A fortuitous event occurred for DeMar in the winter of 1908. It was an event that, on the face of it, is unimportant, yet for DeMar it proved catalytic. He attended a college smoker where the speaker, Professor Stetson of the German department, related his theory that there was some sport in which every man could become a champion. There were lots of kinds of men and lots of sports. If each one would look around, he could find something in which to excel. Right then DeMar decided to try out for cross-country. The trials were the next day. DeMar tried. Everything that made Clarence DeMar famous followed from that singularity. Where would he be if the German professor had come to speak on the day after the cross-country trials?

On the cross-country team the captain took it upon himself to tell DeMar how to run. "Run on your toes, on your toes!" DeMar ran on his heels, on his heels. He never pranced. But he did work hard. He escaped indigence by running 100-mile weeks in 1910 and 1911. He probably ran more consistent mileage than any of his competitors. What he lacked in talent, he made up for in work.

Finnish Albin Oscar Stenroos promised to be DeMar's competition for the Boston Marathon title this year. On the day of the race the *Herald*'s front

page ran the bold headline "Stenroos Out to Make New Marathon Record."
Stenroos stood a stocky 5'8" and 150 pounds. His Finnish head sported the
requisite blond hair. Modest and bashful, he made his living as a machinist.
He came to the U.S. in 1925, according to Hugo Quist, the guardian of
Finnish athletes. Stenroos the Olympic champion had already beaten DeMar
in the heat of Paris, but in Boston DeMar held the hometown advantage, so
the press and the bookmakers gave him a slight edge. Stenroos was older
than DeMar's 37 years. These were the men of wisdom and marathon understanding. Everyone predicted a battle of titans. On the day before the race the
Globe's John J. Halloran wrote, "Chances of an unknown winning are small."

They also thought highly of Whitey Michelson, who came up from Stamford, Connecticut, in an automobile and stayed at the "Marathon Inn" at
the Tebeaus' farm in Hopkinton. He was fast, groomed by his Cygnet teammate Bill Kennedy, who said prophetically before the 1926 race, "There is
one thing certain—no runner can hold back in the Boston race and hope to
win." Kennedy thought that pacing could get one into the prizes, but the
days of coming from way back to take first place were over.

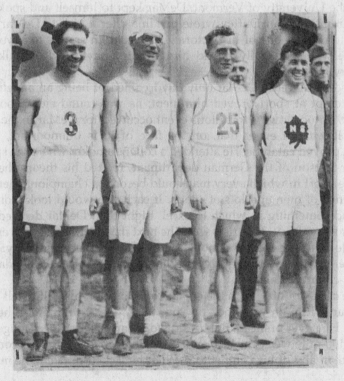

Runners (from left) Jimmy Henigan, Clarence DeMar, Albin Stenroos, and Johnny
Miles after the 1926 upset race. Photo courtesy of the *Boston Herald*.

Meanwhile, back at the Tebeaus' farm, just before the start Whitey Michelson heard an unknown, cocky youngster yipping about how he would win the race. The curly-haired, freckle-faced kid talked in a porridge-thick brogue to anyone who would listen. The BAA served coffee and sandwiches to anyone who wanted them. The kid drank the coffee and ate the sandwiches. This kid, a 20-year-old Canadian from the very tip of Nova Scotia in a place called Sydney Mines, had actually gone into the BAA headquarters at the clubhouse the Tuesday before the race and said straight-faced to manager Tom Kanaly, "You won't be disappointed if I win this race." On April 2 this kid had run 27 miles in 2:40. On Thursday before the race he walked the entire marathon course. He persuaded his parents to come watch him win. He had done little other running. He had run and won a few 3- and 5-mile road races in 1922, 1923, and 1924, but the year before in an obscure 10-mile track race in Amherst, Nova Scotia, he ran 53:48. He chattered as if he were God's chosen runner, so unshakable was his faith that he would win. In October Michelson had run a marathon in 2:29:01.8 on an accurate course in Port Chester, New York. He beat DeMar by 2 minutes. It was the first sub-2:30 marathon in the world, except for DeMar's short Boston in 1924. Michelson was the fastest marathon runner in the world. He said to the cocky kid, "What's that you say, you . . . win? What's your name?"

"Jack Miles."

"You have a fine chance to win," said Michelson sarcastically.

"Well, you just watch me. I'll be in the shower before the second-place runner comes in. You wait and see."

"You're crazy." Michelson said. "You're another one of those marathon nuts they talk about."

Michelson didn't know about the 10-mile track time, but he did know that Miles had never run a marathon before, so he dismissed him. The kid wore a pair of 98¢ sneakers, not $10 Arnold Glove-Grips.

Michelson and others were also in the habit of dismissing both of the Henigans. Tommy grabbed an early lead in this year's race and delivered the field to Ashland 10 seconds faster than the record. Pepino Porfilo of Harvard followed him along with Silas McLellan of Nova Scotia, DeMar, Stenroos, Wallie Carlson, Michelson, Kennedy, and of course The Kid, named Johnny, Jack, or Jackie Miles. They hit 31:14 in South Framingham.

DeMar looked stiff. Jimmy Henigan looked powerful as ever along with Louis Gregory. Miles stuck with DeMar, but when Stenroos got too far ahead Miles shot after him. By Natick, which they reached in 51:46, Miles ran 50 yards behind Stenroos. At Wellesley Gregory ran third with DeMar, Carlson, Karl Koski, Michelson, and the Henigans. Stenroos and Miles continued as before with the kid tailing, seeming afraid to pass or come up on the older man's shoulder, through Wellesley in 1:08:07. Jimmy Henigan quit in Newton Lower Falls and Tommy 3 miles later.

Gregory collapsed near the Brae Burn Country Club. What had been heralded as a DeMar–Stenroos duel had turned into a Stenroos–Miles duel.

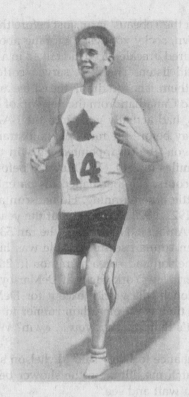

Brash young Johnny Miles of Nova Scotia carried a crumbled photo of Olympic marathon winner Albin Stenroos in his pocket as they raced Boston in 1926. Photo courtesy of the *Boston Herald*.

Miles's face flushed ruddy in the cold wind, but Stenroos looked sallow and pale. Miles followed Stenroos by only 10 yards up the hills. At the top of the hills Miles moved to within arm's length of Stenroos, looked him over, then dropped back. Miles continued his little tests until he felt no response from the old man. Then after the hills, in the manner of a disinterested spider that had sucked its victim dry, he passed him by, unmolested and unchallenged.

But in truth Miles ran far from disinterested. He had carried a faded, crumbled photo of the Olympic champion in his pocket for months. Now he had gone and passed his idol. Was it a crazy thing to do? Doubts filled him. Was Stenroos just playing with him? A hundred yards later Miles got his answer as he looked back to see Stenroos grab his side. The Olympic champion was beaten. From this point Miles unhinged himself and ran away down the hills and onto the broad boulevards and through the geometry of Boston's Back Bay to Exeter Street. Everything worked for Johnny Miles that day, manifesting itself true to his prophecy. After the race he humbly said, "I could never have won the race on my own strength alone. There was a supreme power behind it which aided me." The *Post*'s front page headline read "Unknown Kid Smashes Record."

DeMar said, "If, at his age, he can better my record by four minutes, I don't know what he'll do when he's my age." That day began a long friendship for Miles with DeMar and Michelson. Nobody likes a cocky kid—unless he's right.

1926 Results

1.	J. Miles, Sydney Mines, NS	2:25:40[CR]*	9.	J. Carleton, E. Sandwich, MA	2:44:20
2.	A. Stenroos, *FAAC*, NY	2:29:40	10.	A.R. Scholes, *GladAC*, ON	2:48:14
3.	C. DeMar, *MALP90*	2:32:15	11.	T.E. Quinlan, *MALP45*	2:53:32
4.	A. Michelson, *CAC*, NY	2:34:03	12.	C. Bolekis, *OstAA*, MA	2:54:49
5.	W. Carlson, Dorchester, MA	2:40:35	13.	J.A. Dellow, *GladAC*, ON	2:54:52
6.	K. Koski, *FAAC*	2:41:22	14.	F.T. O'Donnell, *MAAA*, PQ	2:55:29
7.	N. Erickson, *FAAC*	2:42:35	15.	M.J. Lynch, *AC*, DC	2:56:46
8.	B. Kennedy, *CAC*, NY	2:44:01	16.	H. Frick, *MillAA*, NY	2:57:26

*Permanent course record for 26 miles, 209 yards.

MILES

TUESDAY, APRIL 19, 1927

Coal Miner's Son Comes Back to Boston

By 1927 a public that thirsted for a new hero celebrated returning winner Johnny C. Miles, the kid with confidence and a quick smile. They welcomed smiling Johnny. Coolidge prosperity bloomed. Incomes had caught up with the cost of living. The relative price of automobiles dropped; a new Ford could be had for several hundred dollars. People made fortunes on the stock market. Goodness and riches looked to have no end in America. Americans and Bostonians wanted to put the distasteful war and troubles of Europe and the rest of the world behind them.

Yet in the spring of 1927 Nicola Sacco and Bartolomeo Vanzetti waited for their gruesome execution. Riots flared protesting their innocence while patriots and defenders of the American way against the imagined worldwide Red-Bolshevik-Socialist-menace wanted them dead. The newspapers hovered over this moribund pair like vultures. But too much of the grisly on the front page depressed the public. They welcomed news that would make them feel that their human race was not debased, vengeful, cruel, sinister, or conspiratorial. Johnny Miles, the Sunday school teacher, coal mine worker and marathon winner, planned to bestow that kind of relief on Boston. In another month a stunt flyer named Charles A. Lindbergh would sit alone in his airplane for a long time and grant the nation an excuse for happiness. Miles wanted to break 2:20 for an accurate Boston Marathon course, thereby winning the race and setting a new world record. He wanted to show that man could go faster, longer than anyone ever thought possible. The spirit of the day was to do what had never been done. If Paavo Nurmi and Joie Ray could break records over a mile, why not Jackie Miles over a marathon?

Before Johnny Miles came to Boston the year before he had kept that picture of Albin Stenroos crumpled in his pocket. Perhaps that hero worship was why Johnny was reluctant to pass Stenroos, and perhaps that's why Johnny ran so fast afterward. Once an iconoclast succeeds, the idol is left behind and the original drive is gone. Then what? What drove Johnny Miles? It was more than adulation for DeMar and Stenroos. Ultimately it was faith in what made his Nova Scotian heart to fear, an amazing grace. And like the settlers sung about in the hymn, "Amazing Grace," Johnny had come "through many dangers, toils and snares."

The Miles family emigrated to Canada from Cardiff, Wales, where Johnny's father, a streetcar operator, fell under the spell of an advertisement for pleasant living and high-paying work in the coal mines of Nova Scotia. Mr. Miles left his family for Nova Scotia. The illusion of a wonderful new life soon gave way to hard work, low pay, and a tough life. Eliza (Kendall) Miles joined her husband in Canada with their eldest son, John C. Miles, who had been born on October 30, 1905. The family settled in Sydney Mines on Cape Breton in 1907. Mining presented constant danger underground, and the number of pleasant days on the surface of Cape Breton numbered only two sunny ones in October. The senior Miles went to work in the No. 1 Princess Mine, dug far beneath the bottom of the Atlantic Ocean. Mrs. Miles made the money stretch to support them.

In 1916 Johnny's father, a veteran of the Boer War, announced that he would go to do his share to help the Canadian war effort. After the mines, a war seemed like pleasant work. When his father went to war, Johnny, the oldest son, went into the mines to earn the money necessary for the family's survival. Johnny turned 11 that year.

They called Johnny's underground job in the mine trapping. He spent his time sitting alone in the dark, listening for the rumble of the coal trains so he could open the trap doors that isolated portions of the mine shaft to prevent the accumulation of explosive gas at the mine face. Between trains he listened to the drips of water—water from the ocean above—and the rustle of hungry rats. He liked the rats. Their presence indicated that there was no accumulation of poisonous gas. He tossed the last bits of his sandwich, the dirty parts propped up by his continually coal-soiled thumbs, to them. He worked after school on the 3-to-11 shift for 3 years until his father returned from the war in 1919.

Upon the return his father, who came back with only slight shrapnel wounds and returned to work, Johnny faced a giant chunk of leisure time.

He decided to become a boxer like his father had been. He skipped rope, lifted weights, punched the bag, and did push-ups. He trained hard but showed no promise. So, as it is with many runners, there came a singular moment when Johnny decided to become a runner to the exclusion of all else. A friend who was a middle-distance runner dropped off a book about training for running by Alf Shrubb, a renowned runner in his day and then a coach.

Johnny paid no attention to the book until one day he passed a display in a shop window showing the prizes offered to the first 16 finishers in the 3-mile Victoria Day race in Sydney. He saw an all-purpose jackknife, a fishing rod, and other luxuries. Johnny went home, dug out the Shrubb book, read a little, and zipped outside to do sprints in the road. In the race he placed 17th, just out of the prizes he coveted.

Of course, being so close meant that he had to try again the next year. In the 1922 Dominion Day race in North Sydney he placed third overall and won a 98-pound bag of Robin Hood flour for being the first runner to pass the shop of a particular nearby merchant. He also won a small table lamp for third place. The win and the prizes captured the attention of his parents. Thus his father became his coach.

The senior Miles, an elder in the Presbyterian-United Church, did not drink and rarely smoked. He also held the stopwatch. Mr. Miles dedicated himself to his son's training to the point of clearing a 1/8-mile track behind their home and elevating Shrubb's little book to the status of second Bible in the Miles's household. By the spring of 1925 Johnny had run 3 miles in 15:18 to win the Victoria Day race. By the spring of 1926 he worked as a delivery man driving a team of horses who pulled a grocery wagon for the cooperative store. On his way home with an empty wagon, he lengthened the reins and ran along behind the wagon. During the snowy winter he trained by running out and back along the only plowed surface in town—the tram track. He trained and improved. In 1926 he won nearly every race he entered. His best time for the year was a 54:14 track 10-mile in Halifax, Nova Scotia, in July. But Johnny Miles had won a Boston Marathon; his life had changed irrevocably. People expected greater things than usually emerged from a mere miner's son.

Johnny Miles quickly became a big hero in Boston at a time when the public ached for one. Johnny was perfect—young, handsome, friendly, talkative, and best of all the darkest of dark horses, the lowest of underdogs ever to sweep into Boston Marathon history. No Boston Marathon had ever been won by an unknown, unfavored, unconsidered runner. Henri Renaud's win in the 1909 inferno had come as a surprise, but he did not forge his own victory; rather the weather fried the favored runners. Renaud survived but broke no records; he did not outrun an Olympic champion, and he had not announced at the start that he would win. Miles smashed records and defeated two legends, DeMar and Stenroos, with one blow. A fairy tale had come true.

But with victory a burden descended. Could Johnny carry it and defend his title, or would success spoil him? He proved that he could be a runner, but could he be a hero and a runner? Immediately after his Boston victory the Canadian Club took the Miles family from the boardinghouse they had found for themselves and placed them in a suite of rooms at the Hotel Bellevue. Johnny set out on a 2-day itinerary of appearances and speaking engagements about the city arranged by the enthralled *Boston Post*. Governor Fuller and the Mayor Nichols came to pose with Johnny. He was a good hero: He spoke to schoolchildren, answered questions on radio, even preached a sermon. He held 3,000 people in rapt attention at the Tremont Temple as he preached his Gospel message.

> There is no secret to this marathon game. You must think clean, live clean, obey the laws of nature and God. You may fool the people for a time if you don't obey these rules, but you won't fool God, and if you don't live clean you will ultimately have to pay, both here and in the life hereafter.

Post reporter Bill Cunningham followed Johnny home to Sydney Mines to report on his welcome there. Throngs mobbed Johnny at railway stations along the route. The mayor of Moncton, New Brunswick, presented roses to Johnny's mother. In Nova Scotia crowds carried him shoulder-high to the hotel where the family stayed for the night. A crowd gathered, and Johnny addressed them from the balcony as though he were the Pope. When things quieted down and Johnny returned to his delivery route, people along the way invited him into their homes. "They'd make me drink these eggnogs until they'd be coming out of my ears. Well, gee, you know I couldn't insult them. I had to try and drink it." Success had come so progressively that it seemed destined to continue right into Boston, 1927. To insure that the Cinderella tale continued, Mr. Miles made special fairy slippers for Johnny.

Coach, trainer, dietitian, masseur, and father John Miles took out Johnny's 98¢ sneakers and weighed them. Nine ounces each. He picked up a straight razor and carefully flensed all excess rubber. Four ounces each—featherweight and paper-thin. The elder Miles calculated that the reduced weight would cut several minutes off Johnny's time. In training he had never gone longer than 15 miles so as to be well rested for a supreme effort to shatter the world's record by running under 2:20 for the full and corrected (+176

Johnny Miles's father picked up a straight razor and carefully flensed all excess rubber from his son's shoes. Four ounces each—featherweight and paper-thin.

yards) course in Boston. He was up every morning at 6:00 for a bath and a rubdown. He would walk 10 to 20 miles, then in the midafternoon run 10 to 15 miles. Johnny, full of confidence, gathered his parents, packed up the magic shoes, and departed for Boston. "Winning would be a cinch," Miles recalled. "Nothing to it, just a walkaway. That was the way it was figured out. I never wore the shoes until the day of the race."

In Boston the Mileses stayed at the luxurious Somerset Hotel. Johnny again declared, "I will win." But Boston bet on DeMar. Detractors said Miles had gone soft, that fame had changed his lifestyle and would be his undoing. In those days newspapers carried adages recycled by President Coolidge: "Do the task that lies nearest you." DeMar faced up to the task at hand. And it would be formidable.

No wind stirred at the start. Miles wore a bathrobe and a cap as his father escorted him to the line. DeMar wore a handkerchief knotted at the corners and sitting on his head; it could be wetted and reflect the sun but still be light. Time and sunlight had faded his running suit, and the trunks were so large he had to make a tuck in the waist with a safety pin. He pinned his socks to the counters of his old tried-and-tested shoes so they would not slip under his feet and bunch up.

The temperature passed 76 °F and would rise to 84 °F by midafternoon. The roads had been freshly tarred. Dust would not be a problem, but bituminous ooze would—the science of paving was in its infancy. Arthur Duffey of the *Post* wrote, "At frequent intervals yesterday the erstwhile macadam was a sea of live sticky tar. . . . [The] sun boiled this pitch from the road." In the heat and gunk 35 men dropped out in the first mile or two. DeMar, Miles, and a man named Bricker ran in a pack of five. By 6 miles DeMar had 25 yards on the field. Miles, who had spent his winter training through snow, ice, and wind, suffered from the heat. He could feel it creeping through the thin soles of his shoes. Before he got to 3 miles the blood soaked through his sneakers, those little fairy slippers. He lost the toenails on both feet; big blisters came up under each one. He tried to pull his toes up because the sock pulled on his toenails. Then the top of the toes skinned off and blistered.

At 7 miles he popped into a car. "Too hot," he said cheerfully to mask his disappointment. "There are other races." He rode to the finish. Johnny Miles did not by nature complain, so he did not mention or display his bloody feet. This cheeriness proved to be a public relations error.

When told that Miles had quit, Jimmy Henigan said, "Oh, gee." A reporter riding nearby said not to let that fact put ideas into his head. "I'd like to take a header in that lake," said Henigan, looking at the lake in Natick. Henigan ran through the tar. At 11 miles he caught up with DeMar.

DeMar had crossed the road to avoid the tar, which reeked acrid fumes. He ran on the dirt walkways and in the lumpy gutters. He greeted Henigan, " 'Lo, Jim," smiled DeMar, "glad to have you around."

"Come on and run," said Jim as he shot ahead by 3 yards. DeMar took him up on it and pulled even on the crest of the hill going into Wellesley.

Side by side they swung past the cheering Wellesley girls. This year none wore fur coats. True to his history, Henigan soon dropped out, and DeMar had to run on alone. But lots of people dropped out in that heat. As they dropped the old-timers looked better and better. Edouard Fabre, the 1915 winner, moved from 31st to 6th, Carl Linder from 14th to 5th, and Karl Koski moved into 2nd by Woodland Park as Bill Kennedy, age 49, moved from 16th to 3rd. Positions did not change from there to the finish. Only DeMar, Koski, and Kennedy broke 3 hours, whereas at least 17 had in the cool year before, even with the lengthened course.

The press, having no record to boast of, no new hero, and a top three of running veterans who had between them barely a full head of hair and that gray, turned their attention on the loser of the day—Johnny Miles. His biggest fan, reporter Bill Cunningham, took furious offense at Miles's DNF. He wrote,

> Johnny Miles—the great Johnny Miles the crowd was all waiting for—let go without even a fight. That isn't the way champions perform. That isn't the way championships pass. Miles should have finished the race if he had to crawl across the line on his hands and knees after the hour of midnight with his bleeding feet wrapped in newspapers. Good losing is as much a part of the code as good winning. The loser who walks off the field is some part of a thief. He robs his opponent of legitimate victory and the full measure of glory that goes with one.

Johnny returned to Cape Breton, having learned a bitter lesson. One by one his toenails fell off, and he healed inside and out. He wanted to return to Boston to show people like Bill Cunningham that he could win again.

This race did not prove, as Miles had hoped, that a marathon could be run under 2:20, but it did show a hungry public that balding, gray-haired old men have some running left in them. For an America that wanted desperately to believe in something, geriatric running had to suffice for now.

1927 Results

1. C. DeMar, *MALP90*, MA	2:40:22[CR*]	
2. K. Koski, *FAAC*, NY	2:44:41	
3. B. Kennedy, *CAC*, NY	2:51:58	
4. C. Bricker, *YMCA*, Galt, ON	3:00:54	
5. C. Linder, *BAA*	3:02:21	
6. E. Fabre, *NBYMCA*, PQ	3:06:12	
7. H. Frick, *MillAA*, NY	3:07:10	
8. T. Bury, West Lynn, MA	3:12:33	
9. G. Duncan, *DC*	3:17:46	
10. B. Reynolds, *YMCA*, ON	3:21:20	
11. A. Michelson, *CAC*, NY	3:26:30	
12. W. Agee, Hamilton, MA	3:26:30	
13. F.E. McCone, Medford, MA	3:33:07	
14. G. Bird, *NBYMCA*	3:35:40	
15. E.W. Ferson, Needham, MA	3:36:02	

195 entrants, 186 starters, 34 finished under 4 hours.

*Course record for 26 miles, 385 yards, adjusted by 176 yards from Miles's victory in 1926.

JOIE RAY

THURSDAY, APRIL 19, 1928

Track Star Enters Marathon

For his own reasons, the most celebrated and popular American miler of his era (1917-1925) decided to move up to the marathon. No other world-caliber miler had ever done it. On February 10, 1923, Joie "Chesty" Ray ran a world record for the 2-mile in 9:08.4 on a flat (not banked) indoor track—without spikes—in the Brooklyn Armory. In 1919 he had won the 800 and 1,500 in the Amateur Athletic Union national championship. He had run a mile in 4:12. He had run more sub-4:20 miles than anyone. He was the U.S. national mile champ eight times.

Joie Ray was fast, successful, and apparently at the end of an athletic career. He could have retired. For a living he drove a taxi in Chicago. Of course Chesty Ray had a barrel chest, and in addition he played the clown. In the Antwerp Olympic Games Ray got a laugh from the crowd by running behind the famous and peculiar Finnish runner Paavo Nurmi. Nurmi, also a barrel-chested man, usually ran holding a stopwatch. Following Nurmi, Ray stuck out his chest and parodied Nurmi by frequently consulting his own imaginary watch. Spectators chuckled. Ray grinned.

Ray had had his fun in a dazzling career as a miler, but he turned now to the marathon attempting to join another U.S. Olympic team by running 26 times his best distance. Joie Ray came to the 1928 Boston Marathon, again the U.S. Olympic trials, with his speed bottled up and ready to pop. Would he be another Johnny Miles, winning in his first attempt, or another Jimmy Henigan, a morning glory out fast and early to fade?

In contrast to men like Henigan and Ray, Clarence DeMar could not run fast. Nothing popped with Clarence. He metered his efforts meticulously. He could not generate the emotional outbursts necessary to race a mile. He did not joke. He had run a mile in less than 5 minutes only a few times in his life. Once he ran 4:48 and was quite proud of that. Is there something limiting about a human body that excels in racing marathons, or are speed and talent ultimately everything? Does endurance preclude speed and vice versa? Are the volatility and spontaneity of speed antithetical to the guts necessary for the long run? Can men who joke and smile not run marathons? Must marathoners be dull and dour to endure?

Smilin' Jimmy Henigan had speed and talent but seemed to lack the stick-to-it-iveness necessary to win a marathon. Like Ray, he won nearly everything in his specialty—5 to 15 miles—yet he could not translate that ability to a marathon. How could Ray expect to do better when his specialties, the middle distances, were even farther removed from the marathon? For 7 years Henigan had jumped into the marathon, looked like a winner for better than half the race, then dropped out. Henigan entered again this year. He could not stay away. He was a veteran of 480 races and had won 270 prizes during his 20 years of racing. At 36 years old, he had been on the Olympic team and placed 10th in the Olympic cross-country run. This, 1928, was an Olympic year. The Olympic Committee would use Boston to select six men to go to the Amsterdam Games. The committee could make some exceptions. But more candidates than ever before came to race; 285 in all showed up in Hopkinton to start.

The press went with experience and picked DeMar. They thought Henigan would drop out again, but they didn't know what to make of Ray. Why wouldn't he just retire gracefully?

On March 17 DeMar won the Providence-to-Boston 44-mile race with ease. He claimed that these long races didn't take as much out of him as shorter, faster marathons. He felt it much easier to go the 7-1/2 miles per hour than the 10 required in a classic marathon race. At the slow pace he could eat as he went. On that same St. Patrick's Day, Henigan ran second to Whitey Michelson in the Pawtucket, Rhode Island, marathon. Michelson also threatened to make the Olympic team.

The weather settled in to be average for April in Massachusetts—a shady sky after a blustery morning covered the biggest Boston Marathon field ever. And with radio coverage of the race, you could follow the marathon in progress without leaving your home, with bulletins every hour and continuous coverage after 2:15. The newspapermen still followed the race, each in an automobile provided in exchange for a photo in the next day's paper of the car full of the reporting staff and a caption establishing the make and model of the car. Police controlled unofficial traffic better than ever before.

The field slipped through South Framingham in 31:23, a good but unremarkable time. DeMar carried malted milk tablets in his hip pocket and wore shoes so old that the soles had separated in places. William Taylor of Sydney Mines, Nova Scotia, ran alongside. Johnny Miles didn't come to Boston, but Taylor, a runner from the same tiny town, filled himself with hope and made the trip. Perhaps he would be the unknown kid this year. Unfortunately all he had was optimism, and at nearly 30 he wasn't a kid.

William Wilson from Philadelphia, a mesomorphic man of broad shoulders with a bald spot on the top of his head, led the field. Joe Mullen knew him. "He won't go the distance; we'll catch him and maybe DeMar," he said to Jimmy Henigan as they ran side by side. "Jimmy, I picked you to win; that's why I've been following you." Mullen's faith in him pleased Henigan. At least someone other than his wife, who had made him good chicken sandwiches and a bottle of hot tea that he consumed an hour before the race, believed in him. Maybe he'd finish this year.

To Henigan, Ray up ahead looked beautiful, like he could easily sprint past DeMar at any time. In contrast, DeMar ran with with a constant unorthodox wiggling of his hands and elbows. Natick passed in 53:01 and Wellesley in 1:10. Wilson hung on DeMar. He softened on the hills. DeMar threw in a little burst. Wilson walked at Walnut Street. Ray ran 300 yards behind. Was he preparing for the *Big Kick*?

No, in fact, he was trying to survive. A big blister ate away at his right big toe. At 15 miles he tried the shift his weight off the afflicted foot, but he could not fool Mother Nature or deny the fact that he was suddenly more tired than he'd ever been in his life. He had blistered badly, and his leg muscles twitched.

In the last 3 miles the sun came out, making it clear that no one would catch DeMar. But things weren't right for Clarence. Tireless in victory, he was irritated by little things that weren't quite right. His paper number felt too big and too heavy; it bothered him. It bothered him so much that after his finish he complained about it in a very un-Sunday-school-teacher way: He said "darn" twice. "The number tired me, it was too darned large and too darned heavy."

Henigan ate an orange that made him sick for a stretch, but the sickness did not stay. Inch by inch Henigan gained on Ray. He caught Joie after Coolidge Corner at St. Mary's. Jimmy didn't want Ray to get discouraged because he knew that Ray's feet were bleeding. Jimmy said later, "He is as game as any runner that lived. He was running on heart and that must have been bleeding too." Jimmy Henigan ran second. He said,

> It took me 17 years [beginning in 1911] of trying. I first got the idea while watching Longboat win in 1907—I heard the cheers of the crowd and determined then and there to become a marathon runner and win the BAA race, if possible. I was determined to finish this year so that the Dorchester team might win the team prize. But, it must have been my wife's chicken sandwiches—in all the other races I ran on an empty stomach. This is my eighth BAA and it will be my last.

Every year for each of those eight races, Henigan had said never again, but seven times he had gone back to line up on the BAA starting line.

When Ray crossed the finish line he let go of all effort. He had been trying so hard for so long to keep moving. How could it hurt so much to go so slowly? At the tape he ceased running, walking, even standing. He collapsed. They carried him into the BAA clubhouse. They had to cut the socks off his bloody feet. But game to the end, he said, "I'll be back next year."

Edouard Fabre finished 20th. He never came back to Boston again, though he continued running for many years and ran professionally into his 40s. Fabre won the professional Usher Green Stripe Snowshoe Marathon. His best year had been 1915, when he won nearly everything he entered, including the

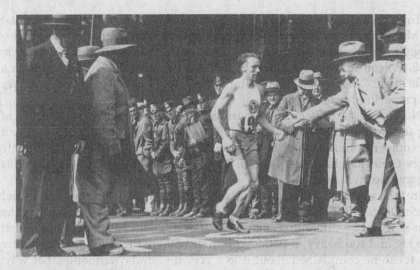

Celebrated miler Joie Ray, his feet run to a bloody pulp, just before his collapse into a politician's finish line handshake. Courtesy of the Boston Public Library, Print Department.

Boston Marathon. In 1937, at age 52, Fabre had a stroke that left him paralyzed on one side. He died July 1, 1939, of another stroke.

Whitey Michelson and Jack Lamb of Biddeford, Maine, both had bad days. When Whitey came upon walking Jimmy afflicted with leg cramps, he stopped, put his arm around Lamb, and walked. They walked in together in about 3:10. There would be next year for them. Excusing Michelson's poor Boston performance, the Olympic selection committee put him on the team for Amsterdam. Michelson went on to hold the best marathon time in the world for 1925, 1927, and 1931.

Later that year Ray won the Los Angeles Marathon by a large margin over DeMar. In the Olympic Games he placed 5th in 2:36:04, Michelson 9th in 2:38:56, DeMar 27th in 2:50:42, and Henigan 39th in 2:56:50. El Ouafi of Algeria won in 2:32:52. Karl Koski (under his Finnish name, Yrjo Korholin-Koski), representing Finland, finished 7th. Johnny Miles, running for Canada, finished 17th in 2:43:32. On his return from Amsterdam he began training for redemption at Boston.

1928 Results

1.	C. DeMar, *MALP90*	2:37:07[CR]	6.	C. Linder, *BAA*	2:50:13
2.	J.P. Henigan, *DC*	2:41:01	7.	W. Wilson, *MdC*, PA	2:51:02
3.	J.W. Ray, *IAC*, Chicago, IL	2:41:56	8.	L. Giard, Brockton, MA	2:51:11
4.	J. Mullen, *MdC*, PA	2:46:54	9.	C. Cahill, Dorchester, MA	2:52:02
5.	H. Frick, *MillAA*, NY	2:48:28	10.	S. McLellan, *NoAC*, Noel, NS	2:52:56

11. T. Bury, *DC*	2:54:55	20. **E. Fabre, *NBYMCA*, PQ**	**2:58:46**
12. O.T. Wood, *UV*	2:55:37	21. B. Bern, *DC*	2:59:36
13. B. Reynolds, Galt, ON	2:56:24	22. J.M. Harvey, *MdC*	2:59:52
14. L.G. Yeuell, *GCA*	2:57:04	35. A. Michelson, *MillAA*	NT
15. J.E. Holmy, Quincy, MA	2:57:40	36. J. Lamb, Biddeford, ME	NT
16. M. Lamp, *MillAA*	2:57:47	43. M. Lynch, *AC*, DC	NT
17. C. Soloman, *SJC*, NY	2:58:10	52. W. Taylor, *SyMAC*, NS	NT
18. H. Stanton, *ItAC*, RI	2:58:33	**John A. Kelley, DNF**	
19. G. Nyman, *FAAC*, NY	2:58:36		

285 starters.

REDEMPTION

FRIDAY, APRIL 19, 1929

Can Mister DeMar-athon Do It Again?

Billy Taylor of Sydney Mines, Nova Scotia, wanted to beat Johnny Miles, formerly of the same town but now living in Hamilton, Ontario. Taylor was older than Miles, but like him had emigrated from Great Britain with his father, who had accepted work in the mines. As a teenager Taylor signed on with the merchant marine and sailed around the world. The proprietor of the Strand Theatre had raised a collection in 1929 to pay Taylor's way to Boston. He was now 30 years old. This was his year to win Boston. But last year he had crumbled and finished dismally. Cape Breton's hopes, however, stayed with him, not Miles.

Miles had moved west in 1928 at the urging of the Canadian Olympic coach to take advantage of the training facilities in Hamilton. Miles had moved to the big time; he inspected twine for the International Harvester Company. He had learned to dance since the Olympic Games and courted Bess Connon, a friend of his sister. He lived in a house with his parents directly across the street from the Hamilton Civic Stadium track. On Sundays he taught Sunday school. Sometimes after a day of twine inspecting he would use a 2 by 4 to climb over the fence and run laps on the track in the moonlight while his father sat in their attic room and timed him. At the end of March, after weeks of 100 training miles, 15 and 20 miles at a time, Miles felt ready for Boston. In the spring of 1929 he took the lead in a Hamilton 15-miler at the gun and no one caught him. The week before Boston, Miles ran a 20-mile training run that left his legs tired. He brought several pairs of running sneakers to the start, wanting to leave nothing to chance. In case of a hot day one pair was constructed with extra-heavy soles. In short, Miles had become more careful and thorough in his preparations, like DeMar. He was not a coward or a quitter. He would prove that those with opinions like the reporter Bill Cunningham, who had hounded him for dropping out in 1927, were wrong.

Out of Hopkinton on a cool day, Max Lamp, a man with the perfect name for the leader of a race, took the quick lead. He ran through South Framingham half a minute slower than the course record. Miles thought this pace was too fast so he held to the back of a tight pack, but he did not dare let the pack go. They ran 23 seconds behind record pace at Natick, then brought the times down, 17 seconds at Wellesley. With each man cautious and wary while watching the others but like a snowball gathering momentum, the bunch rolled along. Koski, the bald Finnish carpenter, had won the Shepard Stores 44-mile Providence-to-Boston race, beating DeMar; he ran easily but cleverly behind the pack near another Finn, Willie Kyronen. Yet another Finn, Whitey Michelson, won the Port Chester, Buffalo, Pawtucket, and Baltimore marathons, but he tucked into the pack and looked good too. So it continued with no man yielding. At 20 miles the group still ran close, including Lamp, Miles, Michelson, Jack Lamb, Taylor, and Art Gavrin. DeMar, his face pinched and drawn, ran well behind.

Marathon wisdom says the race is only half over at 20 miles, but for Jimmy Henigan it was all over as he dropped out at Woodland Park. Lamp tired and his lightness left him. Then the hills began. Miles moved on Michelson, who took off his gloves, moved on Miles, took the lead back, and asked for water. By that request Miles knew Michelson had trouble. The two had become friends since Whitey mocked the unknown Johnny at the start of the 1926 race. But friendship or not, Miles wanted the win and had prepared for it.

A sudden burst at Boston College let Miles skim over the top of the last hill and race down to a 30-yard lead over Michelson by Lake Street and a half-minute lead on the record. Michelson struggled and Koski and Kyronen caught him while Miles got his redemption as he ran alone down the last glorious miles over Beacon Street to sweep to victory.

Michelson, Lamb, and Taylor finished upright and racing, unlike the previous year's stooped death march to Exeter Street.

Massachusetts governor Frank Allen congratulated Miles. Jubilant Johnny wore a bulky white cardigan with the word "Canada" and a maple leaf on his left breast. "Having led a clean life all the time, with no fear of diverting from God's ways, one cannot help but have success," said Miles. Again he had God's gift and Boston toasted him. Even the *Post* reporter, Bill Cunningham, took back the nasty words he had printed in 1927 about Miles not having the courage to fight. Redemption brought sweet pleasure for Johnny and his parents.

Miles returned to Hamilton a Boston winner. Like Jack Caffery in 1900 and 1901 and Olympic winner Billy Sherring in 1906, Miles gave the town a marathon hero. At a reception in City Hall, Bill Worth, the general manager of the Fiber and Twine Division of International Harvester, said, "If Miles puts as much time and energy into the interests of the International Harvester Company as he puts into this running, he could have a future." Miles couldn't sleep that night; he kept turning the general manager's words over and over. He had attained his goal. True, there were Olympics and other Bostons, but perhaps it was time to get on with the reality of working life and give up the fantasy. Why come back? This may be the top. If it is, then there is no place to go but down.

1929 Results

1. J. Miles, *OC*, Hamilton, ON	2:33:08[CR]	16. A.I. Gavrin, *MillAA*	2:49:59
2. K. Koski, *FAAC*, NY	2:35:26	17. J.E. Holmy, Quincy, MA	2:50:12
3. W. Kyronen, *FAAC*, NY	2:35:44	18. T. Gaul, Roxbury, MA	2:50:28
4. A. Michelson, *MillAA*, NY	2:37:22	19. B. Bern, *DC*	2:50:56
5. J. Lamb, *DC*, MA	2:39:25	20. L.G. Yeuell, *DC*	2:51:45
6. W. Taylor, Sydney Mines, NS	2:40:05	21. W.C. Zepp, Worcester, MA	2:51:47
7. G. Ruotsalaines, *NBYMCA*, PQ	2:41:06	**22. B. Kennedy, *CAC*, NY**	**2:52:51**
8. R. O'Toole, Newfoundland	2:43:07	23. A. Havey, South Boston, MA	2:54:46
9. C.H. DeMar, *MALP90*	**2:43:47**	24. A. Rodgers, *DAAA*, NS	2:55:17
10. F. Ward, Jr., *MillAA*, NY	2:44:13	25. J. Carleton, *CHP*, MA	2:56:04
11. H. Kauppinen, *KAC*, NY	2:44:13	26. T. Bury, *GEAA*, MA	2:56:32
12. F.T. O'Donnell, *ShanAC*, PA	2:45:39	27. L.S. Reed, *TWWC*, MA	2:57:45
13. M. Lamp, *MillAA*, NY	2:46:21	28. C.E. Cahill, Dorchester, MA	2:58:14
14. L. Giard, *DC*	2:47:06	29. J.D. Semple, West Lynn, MA	2:58:54
15. C. Linder, *BAA*	**2:49:11**	30. J.M. Harvey, *MdC*, PA	2:59:59

188 starters.

Chapter 4

1930-1939
The Depression Years

Presidents: *Herbert Hoover, Franklin Delano Roosevelt*

Massachusetts Governors: *Frank G. Allen, Joseph B. Ely, James Michael Curley, Charles F. Hurley*

Boston Mayors: *James Michael Curley, Frederick W. Mansfield, Maurice J. Tobin*

1930 Populations—*United States, 123,202,624; Massachusetts, 4,249,614; Boston, 781,188*

Frederick Lewis Allen, a prolific writer about American life in the 1920s and '30s, brackets the decade of the 1930s with two events. The first is the day the big bull market in the U.S. stock exchange reached its peak. On September 3, 1929, the prices of shares of American corporations reached their highest value. No one knew at the time that they would go no higher. Fortunes existed on paper. The prices of securities exceeded their values, and prices fell in the stock market panic and crash of October 1929. That event and its consequences characterized the following decade. America would stagnate until war broke out in Europe on September 3, 1939, the second of Lewis's brackets. The story of the Boston Marathon during this decade is a story of depression.

The Great Depression dominated American life; it touched everything and everyone in America. It shaped the values of the men who would later direct, manage, and report the Boston Marathon. An understanding of runners and running in the depression years will help explain the values men held as they directed policy through the '60s, '70s, and '80s—men like Will Cloney, Jock Semple, and reporter Jerry Nason. (By choosing what to report, Nason directed public attention and shaped attitudes to which the marathon managers reacted.) Attitudes toward women, prize money, and sponsors formed during the depression years in the minds and hearts of BAA directors, sponsors, and future race managers. Those who were young men in the 1930s emerged with the mark of those years.

For some young runners, the hard economic times did not depress their enthusiasm for the marathon. Men out of work had more time to train than men with jobs. The first thing a runner would do when unemployed was to train more. If nothing else was under his control, at least his running was. For other men, especially those with families dependent on them, unemployment brought only terror. Massachusetts high schools graduated record numbers of students, mainly because there were no jobs to be had, so students stayed to graduate. More interest accumulated in the marathon. Working, or in this case nonworking, class men began to participate. According to the *World Almanac*, by 1935 Boston had its greatest-ever population—817,713, or nearly 250,000 more than in 1990, 55 years later. The newspapers reported that a million people watched the Boston Marathon.

Unemployment reached its peak in 1933, with a quarter of the work force without jobs. Several unemployed Boston Marathon winners hoped that the publicity generated by their winning would land them jobs; for some it did and some it didn't, depending on the runner's skin color. Government stepped into the situation with the Works Progress Administration founded by Roosevelt in 1935 and run by Harry Hopkins, an eccentric but brilliant and dedicated social worker. By the time the WPA was disbanded in 1943 it had spent $11 billion dollars and employed 8.5 million persons.

In 1930 a radio set cost the relatively enormous sum of $135. On it could be heard Amos 'n' Andy, "Happy Days Are Here Again," and "Singing in the Rain." Paavo Nurmi's world record for the mile stood at 4:10.4, and in 1934 Glenn Cunningham ran 4:06.8. Miniature golf became a craze, as did flagpole sitting, backgammon, and marathon dancing. Erich Maria Remarque's *All Quiet on the Western Front* and Pearl Buck's *The Good Earth* were best sellers. Lou Gehrig matched Babe Ruth swat for swat. The kidnapping of the Lindbergh baby occurred in March of 1932. Juan Zabala of Argentina won the 1932 Los Angeles Olympic marathon in 2:31:36.

The winter of 1933-34 froze the ocean from Nantucket to the mainland, and Katharine Hepburn appeared in the movie "Little Women." Walter Pitkins's book *Life Begins at Forty* led the nonfiction bestseller list in 1933; Prohibition ended in December of that year. In 1936 Charlie Chaplin made the movie "Modern Times," Hitler's armies marched unopposed into the Rhineland, and Edward abdicated the throne of England for love of Mrs. Simpson. Ki Chung Sohn, a Korean forced to run under the colors of occupying Japan and under the yoke of a Japanese name, Kitei Son, won the Berlin Olympic marathon in 1936 (2:29:19) in front of Hitler. Dale Carnegie's book *How to Win Friends and Influence People* came out in 1937. On May 6 of that year the Hindenberg blew up, and in July Amelia Earhart disappeared in the Pacific. Clarence DeMar published his book *Marathon* in 1937.

Boston Marathon starting fields in the 1930s remained at a constant couple hundred men, but spectators swelled to the greatest numbers yet. The men who raced the marathon attracted the label *plodder*. They were considered neither fast nor athletic, but merely relentless. They were working men (or seeking, if not actually working) who adhered to a strict amateur code. They were not wealthy, nor were they generally well educated. They shared a resourcefulness and camaraderie as they picked their way to get to races as cheaply as possible—hitchhiking, riding trains or buses, or jamming their narrow bodies into cars. There were few races nationally, but nearly all of the runners traveled to nearly all of the races. On the night before a race they could be found sleeping on benches under newspapers or in churches or YMCAs for no particular consideration in career, money, or fame—except when they got to Boston. There, for a few hours, they got fame.

THE MASTER'S VICTORY

SATURDAY, APRIL 19, 1930

Miles to Run for Third Victory

On April 17, 1930, the front page of the *Boston Daily Globe* announced that a raid in Grove Hall, Roxbury, had uncovered a huge distillery and 3,000 gallons of beer in an abandoned car barn. The next day Stella Walsh, the great "girl" sprinter, arrived at Boston's South Station to run in the national indoor track championships at Boston Garden. She would win the 220 yards in her usual 26 seconds. Her picture appeared on the *Globe*'s front page. Buried back in the April 19 issue ran excerpts from a letter by Ronald J. MacDonald, the Boston Marathon winner from 1898, who wrote from his home in Antigonish, Nova Scotia, where he worked as a physician. He was now in his 50s and weighed over 200 pounds. He wrote, "A marathon victory should be a great tonic to a boy, a tonic to urge him on to greater things in life—to get there. I am very much afraid few of the Boston Marathon winners accomplished much through their victory." MacDonald had graduated from the Tufts Medical School in 1907. "This I am sure would never have been accomplished had I not won the marathon race." MacDonald now had a wife and five children. "I am giving you this [advice for marathoners' future lives] as perhaps you might use some of the dope [information] to spur on other marathon aspirants to greater things in their future life."

Johnny Miles had been thinking for a year about his future life. He traveled down from Hamilton, Ontario, with his father intent on winning Boston again. If Clarence DeMar could win six times, then Johnny, younger and faster, could win more than twice. His victory the year before had proved that his 1927 failure was not because of a lack of talent or willpower but because of hot weather. But Johnny had also been thinking about his future with the International Harvester Fiber and Twine division, and MacDonald's admonition planted doubt in Johnny's mind about a single-minded pursuit of the Boston Marathon. Economic times were not good this year, but everyone thought the business cycle would soon turn around to prosperity again, so maybe one more year, then Johnny could let the dream slide. Even MacDonald after all these years could not let go of the dream: He closed his letter with the hope that his son would one day win the Boston Marathon.

The papers picked Miles as the favorite for the 1930 marathon. He had set the course record twice, in 1926 and 1929, and his corrected time from 1926 was about 2:26—no one had run faster. Yet if it were to be a hot day, Johnny strongly suspected that his hard training through the Canadian winter in long pants, hats, and gloves would leave him helpless in the heat. Often Canadian runners would not have been able to venture out without winter gear before April 19, so their bodies would not have adapted to running in heat and humidity. A summer's worth of running allows a runner's body time to learn how to cool itself as it goes, but on a hot day in April, the body cannot go *and* cool itself—it has to slow down. A day that one might consider a fine day for running in August would be a killer in April.

This Patriots' Day proved to be a subtle killer. Southern Mississippi Valley air heavy with humidity had spread northward into New England during the night. A blanket of clouds waited to release a spit-warm drizzle into still air. At the race headquarters in the Lucky Rock Manor Inn Karl Koski, the Finnish carpenter from New York and recent AAU champ with a time of 2:35:21, decided to skip his usual hot weather protection of a knotted handkerchief stretched over his bald head. Koski ran smoothly, with the precision of a machine. He had run a 2:25:21.2 over a hilly course on New York's Staten Island a month earlier, but many doubted the accuracy of that course. Could he really have run 10 minutes faster than his best? Most marathoners of the time would find it easier to believe that officials had mismeasured or mismarked the course. But such uncertainties were common in those days—if a man suddenly ran a fast time, had he improved or was the course short?

How to respond as a competitor to such a report was a problem. Was DeMar to assume Koski was really that fast or to believe the more likely reason, that the course was short? If Koski went out fast, should DeMar follow or assume that Koski was merely full of himself and would soon pay for his foolishness? Or might the Staten Island course have indeed been accurate but left Koski coming to Boston tired from the effort? Only a wise old marathoner like DeMar at age 41 could sort out those complexities.

Koski's teammate Willie Kyronen, an emaciated wisp and also a member of the Finnish-American Club, waited with him. He was in relentless pursuit of a victory, having finished second in 1916, seventh in 1921, fifth in 1922, sixth in 1925, and third in 1929. Jimmy Henigan, another relentless pursuer, said that this might be his last race, but the press commented that he had been singing his swan song for so long that nobody took it seriously—he loved to run and that was all there is to it. One report speculated that it was his chief aim in life. These men and Clarence DeMar, the old soldier, printer, and now teacher, were this year's battery of "big guns." DeMar had moved from Melrose to Keene, New Hampshire, where he taught industrial history to a class of 28 girls in the Normal School.

DeMar had recently married, so people joked about what that would take out of a 41-year-old. He married Margaret Ilslley who had first suggested that he teach Sunday school. As she watched she wore a helmetlike hat in the style of the day; it fit closely around her head all the way down to the nape of her neck, allowing only an eye to be visible in profile. Her dress, also typical of the day, had a *V* neck and a waist, if it could be called that, at the hips (the ideal women's figure then was straight, with no breasts, no waist, and no hips). Her hair was shingled in back, pulled over the ears and held in place by the helmet. She was also pregnant.

Clarence ran in rubber-soled shoes for the first time. He had preferred leather soles, feeling they allowed him to slide along. But he ran in second place going into Ashland and found that the rubber soles offered him a bounce he had never before felt. A clean-striding Finnish runner from Buffalo, New York, named Hans Oldag insisted on leading, so the old horse DeMar let him. DeMar once had trained about 100 miles a week but now did only 70. He did not worry about young Hans, but he did worry about Koski, Billy Taylor, and Kyronen. Johnny Miles seemed unable to energize himself and languished behind. He had difficulty breathing the thick air.

The air posed DeMar no problem as Oldag led him into South Framingham in 31:28, 28 seconds under the record. The split time relieved DeMar, because only then was he sure that the pace that felt fast to him was indeed fast. While cruising through Natick DeMar developed a thirst. His parched lips wanted a sip of water or a tart drink. Then he saw a kid sucking on an orange. He wanted that orange, but racing rules forbade the acceptance of aid from anyone but the race officials. Clarence refused to break the rules and did not ask for even a wedge.

The time of 1:09 at Wellesley Square seemed fine to DeMar, but not to Oldag. DeMar ran up to the younger man's shoulder. Oldag turned to look at his rival; he did not speak but perplexed DeMar with a half smile. DeMar decided on a tactic that would wipe the smile off. He burst past at a speed he knew he could not maintain but would throw a scare into the youngster. From that spot 3 weeks earlier DeMar had run an easy time trial to the finish; if he could duplicate that time he would come in under the record. He thought of his wife during the race and believed that if the Lord wanted him to win he would. The Lord must have wanted his Sunday school teacher as the winner, because Oldag began a long slow stagger to the finish while more than 50 men ran past him.

DeMar ran alone. Koski and Kyronen moved steadily through the pack. Massachusetts Governor Frank G. Allen rode alongside in his car as honorary referee. At the finish he gave the gold medal to DeMar. Amid the excitement and the flurry of photographers at the awards ceremony, DeMar handed his medal back to the governor, who out of habit slid the gold into his pocket. It took some searching for DeMar to get his medal back.

Gambling on the Marathon

Since the establishment of the Boston Marathon in 1897, gambling had focused public attention on the race. With few professional sports available to bet on, the marathon provided plenty of opportunities to pick winners. At first bettors knew little about which marathoners might be faster, so the race seemed more like a lottery. But once Caffery and his backers came down from Canada in 1900 and won money at the expense of the Bostonians, bettors began to study the sport. With the rise of numerous national professional sports, horse and dog tracks, and state-run lotteries, betting on Boston has subsided to its present status as a mere curiosity. But in the '30s the methods for betting on the marathon had become baroque and corrupt.

In 1930 many of the half-million spectators along the way paid inordinate attention to numbers the runners wore on their chests. To many of them it was the digits, not the men, that mattered, for digits made winners out of spectators. Operators had illegally printed and sold 100,000 lottery tickets at a gross take of half a million dollars. The players in the pool had to pick three numbers between 1 and 200, the range that corresponded to the runners' numbers; for example, this year DeMar wore 157. In a complex scheme, points were awarded and added up to determine the winner. What did not add up was the winnings. First prize was $15,000, but the total of the prizes equaled just half the take, at only $250,000. The rules were unclear, but the rest of the money disappeared, the operators disappeared, and the attorney general of Massachusetts said he was surprised.

People could not believe that such an old man could win a world-class athletic event—especially a man whom doctors told two decades earlier that he had a heart murmur and should take it easy. The myth that marathon running shortens your life died hard, and it annoyed DeMar. He frequently told a reworked joke of a marathoner who died when he was 117—people said that it was the running that killed him. But in church the next day DeMar was all the Lord's business. When people asked him about the marathon he maintained that it was dead and gone; that was yesterday. But DeMar wasn't dead and gone, and he would be back the next year as the favorite.

The 1930 favorite, Johnny Miles, gave up fighting the muggy air. On Exeter Street he stopped to wait for popular "Bricklayer" Bill Kennedy; he offered Kennedy his hand and they ran in together, holding hands, to the finish. At the finish Miles saw his father in a red sweater and ran to him to smother his disappointment in his arms. Soon Johnny Miles had to be back at work in the Fiber and Twine Division.

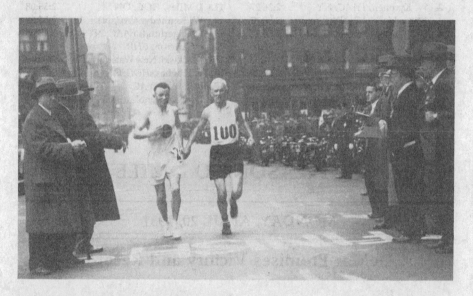

In mutual respect, Johnny Miles, (1926 and 1929 winner), and "Bricklayer" Bill Kennedy (1917 winner) finish the 1930 marathon together in a hand-holding tie for 11th and 12th. Courtesy of the Boston Public Library, Print Department.

Sixth-place finisher Ronald B. O'Toole from Newfoundland had shoe troubles at 17 miles, so he ran from there to the finish in his stocking feet.

John Duncan Semple, a Scottish 27-year-old finishing seventh, felt no disappointment at all. His friends called him Jack, but soon everyone would call him Jock. Semple had hitchhiked from Philadelphia, leaving there at 7:00 a.m. and arriving in Boston at 9:00 the next morning. Two days after hitchhiking back to Philadelphia he was fired from his job, so he moved to Lynn, Massachusetts. Tom McCabe of the *Herald* described Semple on April 20 as "one of those typical marathoners who ride in side door Pullmans [railroad cars] to get to the contest and do not know how they will get enough [money] to get home." But it was worth it. In the last 2 miles of the Boston Marathon Semple kicked past the famous Jimmy Henigan.

This time Henigan did not announce his retirement from running. How could he announce retirement at age 38 when the winner was almost 42 and planned to come back? Perhaps Henigan had resigned himself to the fact that the Boston Marathon was a permanent addiction for him. At least these days he was finishing them.

1930 Results

1.	C.H. DeMar, *MALP90*	2:34:48	10.	G.A. Norman, Malden, MA	2:53:17
2.	W. Kyronen, *FAAC*, NY	2:36:27	**11.**	**J. Miles, *HOC*, ON**	**2:55:08**
3.	K. Koski, *FAAC*, NY	2:38:21	**12.**	**W. Kennedy, *CAC*, NY**	**2:55:08**
4.	H. Webster, *HOC*, ON	2:39:27	13.	D. Fagerlund, *FAAC*, NY	2:58:08
5.	G. Routsalines, *NBYMCA*, PQ	2:41:05	14.	J. Carleton, *CHP*	2:58:32
6.	R.B. O'Toole, St. John's, NF	2:41:55	15.	J. McLeod, New Waterford, NS	2:58:40
7.	J. Semple, W. Philadelphia, PA	2:44:29	16.	F. Hughes, *HOC*, ON	2:59:05
8.	**J. Henigan, Medford, MA**	**2:46:38**	17.	R. Jekel, *NYAC*	2:59:38
9.	S. McLellan, *NHC*, NS	2:50:49	57.	H. Oldag, Orioles, Buffalo, NY	NT

216 entrants.

A Reason to Smile

MONDAY, APRIL 20, 1931

DeMar Promises Victory and Record

On Tuesdays and Thursdays, after his day's work as a foreman in the shipping department of a corrugated box company in Medford, Jimmy Henigan, whom they called Smilin' Jimmy, joined a couple of other top runners from his area for some hard training. On the other days he put in 10 to 15 miles alone. He had never trained this hard in his two decades of running. One day he took the train out to Lowell and ran the 20 miles back to Medford as fast as he could.

Henigan had had his secret training plan in the works for months. He was tired of winning almost everything but the Boston Marathon. He had tried to win 12 times, but the best he had done was second to DeMar in 1928. Henigan had 529 race prizes. He had medals and he had trophies, but if you live near Boston and run, you must run the marathon. If you win races you must win Boston or be forever unfulfilled. A job may give you money to fill your belly, but a Boston Marathon victory is glory far beyond corrugated boxes. Henigan had a wife, Florence, and five children, 12-year-old Jimmy Jr., Pauline, Rita, Florence, and baby Jackie. In a nutshell, that, and an occasional beer, was Henigan's life.

In a newspaper story a journalist had written that Henigan trained on beer. Henigan took offense to that characterization: He did not train on beer, he trained on training; he did not smoke, he ate sparingly, and he drank an *occasional* beer. The writer may have wanted, in the ever-more-common attempt to refute Prohibition, to flaunt the notion that beer drinking was harmless, and Jimmy quite agreed, but beer was not the cause of his success.

An oddball, Jimmy "Cigars" Connors of Roxbury, claimed that he owed his marathon success to smoking cigars. He said he could not do the marathon without a puff. Connors was a balding, burly man with hairy arms and a cigar constantly in his mouth. He said he would smoke 25 during the race—one puff per stride—and he claimed the world record for cigar smoking, 250 cigars in 24 hours. Connors wasn't particular about what kind of cigar he smoked—a Smoky City Stogie, Carolina Perfecto, Havana, or some guttersnipe variety. He admitted to being one of those marathon freaks of the BAA.

Why not Jimmy "Cigars"? The public had acquired a taste for stunts ever since they embraced Charles Lindbergh as the uncrowned prince of America for flying an airplane by himself a long way and landing where he said he would. Even now the stunt competition continued. On April 8, Amelia Earhart flew an airplane up to 19,000 feet for a new altitude record, but on April 10 Miss Elinor Smith flew up to 32,000 feet. There is no record of any woman requesting to enter the Boston Marathon, perhaps because marathon running was seemingly too hard? But stunts like the popular tree- and flagpole-sitting attracted public attention along with airplane flying. At least Cigars really did run a marathon, while most of these other stunts were merely a matter of sitting down for a long time, with occasional steering.

Johnny Miles intended to steer his career as well as his running and his personal life. He managed his International Harvester job as well as night school and the courtship of a young woman named Bess. He arrived late for this year's marathon because he did not want to miss any work. He hoped for a cool day.

Miles did not get his cool day, but neither did anyone else. By one o'clock the temperature reached 77 °F under a cloudless sky. Clarence DeMar, the defending champion and seven-time winner, had a plan for heat. He always ran well in hot weather relative to the rest of the field. They said his good results in adverse conditions came out of his head as much as his body—he thought as well as raced. This year DeMar had taken a room with a view in the Lenox Hotel looking down Exeter Street to the finish so his wife and 7-month-old baby could watch him win for the eighth time. "I will win the Boston Marathon this year and will break Johnny Miles's record for the distance," said DeMar. The *Boston Post* placed baby Dorothy DeMar's photo on the front page beneath the headline "DeMar, Koski to Fight Out Race."

Another photo identified DeMar in the pulpit of the Dudley Street Baptist Church in Roxbury on Sunday, the day before the race, addressing 1,000 parishioners. The *Post* picked DeMar, Karl Koski, and Willie Kyronen to finish, in that order.

The Boston newspapers all reported that a million people were expected to watch and that the BAA for the first time would award the winner with a traditional wreath fashioned of laurel leaves picked from the plain of Marathon in Greece. The winner's medal waited with the Greek inscription *NENIKHKAMEN* (Rejoice. We conquer!)—Pheidippides's alleged last words.

The night before the race Henigan couldn't sleep. For the first time before a Boston Marathon he felt nervous. He read until 4:00, then was up at 7:00 for a breakfast of two eggs, two cups of tea, and raisin bread. He kissed his wife, then rushed out to grab the train to Ashland. His last words to Florence were "I'll bring home the bacon this time sure."

The race headquarters at the Lucky Manor Inn, a 30-room hostelry in Hopkinton, reeked of wintergreen and arnica used as rubbing liniment. John Tebeau owned the vintage Revolutionary War–era inn. One of his daughters, Elenor, a physician with a Radcliffe degree, took the pulse of each runner. Another doctor measured blood pressure and a third checked weight. Bill Kennedy, the president of the International Marathoner's Association, helped by reading out the weights in a booming voice to be recorded.

At last the 203 runners all checked in, and George V. Brown raised his ancient starting gun. A nervous Canadian Finn named Komonen, whose name had been anglicized from Taavi to Dave, leaped into the lead. DeMar, Leslie Pawson, and Henigan along with Johnny Miles, Kennedy, and Carl Linder ran 25 yards behind to South Framingham. As Henigan passed DeMar he said, "Come on Clarence, step on it. We're going to leave you!" DeMar did not respond; he had his own ideas, "There goes Jimmy again . . . wonder where he'll drop out?"

By Natick Komonen, who had trained in Finland with the great Paavo Nurmi, had 20 yards on Henigan. Obviously Komonen planned to win, though he had not been picked as a contender. Another Finn, David Fagerlund, closely followed Henigan. DeMar waited in fifth, Koski in sixth.

DeMar moved up to fourth and put his plan to work. Koski followed into fifth in Wellesley, where Tommy Henigan gave his brother an orange. Jimmy, not such a stickler for rules as DeMar, sucked the orange and broke away from Komonen on the long downhill into Newton Lower Falls, where the course crosses the Charles River. Henigan had the lead and liked it. Komonen dropped rapidly back. DeMar moved into third by Woodland Park while Fagerlund remained behind Henigan, but Henigan pulled away. DeMar thought Henigan would tire—didn't he usually? For 10 years Henigan had never run well in the Boston Marathon. DeMar reassured himself. But it was DeMar who tired under the insistent sun. Fred Ward, who had been in 26th place in South Framingham, passed DeMar. This was especially demoralizing for DeMar to see, because Ward had defeated DeMar in a 20-

miler in Houston the year before by a mere foot. DeMar could not hold Ward off. He could not stay ahead of Koski. And he could not catch Henigan. The great Clarence DeMar just could not get going; his victory plan had fallen to pieces.

Henigan dumped water on his head and rubbed his wet palm up his high forehead. His hair stood straight up. He worried. He looked worried. His eyebrows arched. He squinted. The heat of the day and the pressure of the lead weighed on him. He thought of Dorando Pietri and his collapse in the Olympic stadium. That could happen to him. . . . or the Canadian Finn could come back. . . . or DeMar. . . . or Koski. Henigan said later that every stride felt like a tooth pulled. His toes hurt. His socks wrinkled and raised blisters. Smilin' Jimmy's smile became a grimace. But no one caught him. He had a half-mile lead, but only in the last yards would his grimace turn to a grin.

Percy Wyer, 96 pounds, 48 years old, caught lots of runners as he ran from 72nd place to 6th. German Paul deBruyn plowed through heat-defeated runners to move from 15th place to 8th. But Leslie Pawson dropped from the lead pack way back to 23rd place. Johnny Miles improved on his 11th place of 1930, but he ran about a half hour slower than he had in 1926. This was his last Boston Marathon. He would run in the Los Angeles Olympic marathon and place 14th, but thereafter he placed his full attention on his career with International Harvester. Miles married Bess in 1935. He earned a master's degree in business administration and stayed with IH for 43 years, including a lengthy stay in France, and eventually became division manager in charge of his former place of employment, the Fiber and Twine Division. He and Bess retired in 1968 to an apartment in Hamilton, Ontario. Miles last attended the Boston Marathon in 1991 at age 85.

Henigan turned onto Exeter Street. . . . he had finally done it. No one ran between him and the worsted yarn. At last he won the Boston Marathon, and a million people had seen him do it. Back home Florence and the kids listened on the radio, rejoicing. Jimmy celebrated. Medford was jubilant. Motorcycle police and fire trucks escorted him home. He rode on an open car waving to the people of Medford; the mayor came to shake his hand. First thing the next morning Henigan arrived back at work. The press came to visit him. They took his photograph, and for once he did not swear that he'd run his last marathon. He said instead that he'd be back next year to try to make the Olympic team for Los Angeles. Then the press left and Jimmy went back to work. Work was good. It was good to have work. It defined a man.

1931 Results

1.	J.P. Henigan, Medford, MA	2:46:45	5.	C. DeMar, Keene, NH	2:55:46
2.	F. Ward, Jr., *MillAA*, NY	2:49:03	6.	P. Wyer, *MonAC*, Toronto, ON	2:56:01
3.	K. Koski, *FAAC*, NY	2:53:41	7.	D. Komonen, Toronto, ON	2:58:31
4.	D. Fagerlund, *FAAC*	2:53:41	8.	P. deBruyn, NY	2:59:09

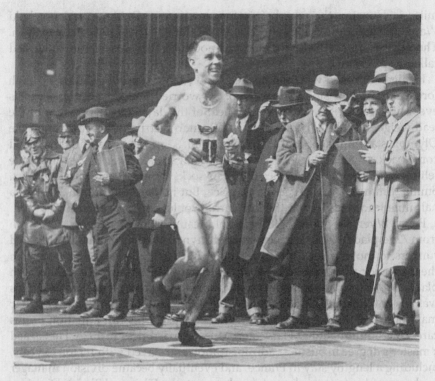

After trying to win the Boston Marathon for more than a decade, Smilin' Jimmy Henigan finally did it in 1931 (this photo shows his 1928 second-place finish). Courtesy of the Boston Public Library, Print Department.

9. G.A. Norman, Malden, MA	3:03:33
10. J.C. Miles, *HOC*, ON	3:04:56
11. J. Jakela, *CYMCA*, Toronto, ON	3:04:58
12. C. Linder, *BAA*	3:06:17
13. A.J. Brunelle, Revere, MA	3:06:57
14. E. White, *TP*, Staten Island, NY	3:07:52
15. G. Mulvaney, Providence, RI	3:08:58
16. T. Bury, *Lynn YMCA*, MA	3:09:43
17. A. Burnside, *MonAC*, ON	3:10:58
18. A. Moutsis, *GAAC*	3:11:19
19. C. Olson, *BucAA*, NS	3:13:53
20. B. Kennedy, *CAC*, NY	3:16:35
21. J. Peck, *KC*, Washington, DC	3:20:13
22. G. McCaffrey, Portland, ME	3:24:33
23. L. Pawson, *YMCA*, RI	3:24:41
24. F. Bleckinger, *MdC*, PA	3:25:37
25. P.R. Cassano, *MedAA*	3:27:37
26. J. Pearson, *MonAC*, ON	3:27:55
27. A. Rodgers, *DAAA*, NS	3:28:54
28. J. Semple, *Lynn YMCA*, MA	3:30:09

203 entrants.

WHAT DO YOU DO WITH A DRUNKEN SAILOR?

TUESDAY, APRIL 19, 1932

Olympic Trials for Finland

Jimmy Henigan said this would be his last marathon—win, lose, or draw—because this was an Olympic year; Boston was the trial, then he would go back to his favorite distance, 10 miles. He wanted to make his third Olympic team. He also wanted to win the Boston Marathon again.

Willie Ritola wanted a place on the Finnish Olympic team. He had three Olympic gold medals, from the 1924 steeplechase (9:33.6) and 10K (30:23.2) and the 1928 5K (14:38), but he hadn't run a marathon since he placed second to DeMar in 1922. He wanted to run the marathon in the Los Angeles Olympics on his third Olympic team. Winning Boston would assure Ritola a place on the Finnish team. The Finns held the Boston Marathon in such high regard that they made it their Olympic trials.

Paul deBruyn had already made Germany's Olympic team by winning the German national championship in Berlin. A week earlier he had run a time trial marathon in 2:30. He prepared himself to run with Teutonic thoroughness. He was experienced at Boston after his eighth place of the previous year.

DeBruyn had seen the world as a sailor for the North German Lloyd Steamships line, but now for a living he shoveled coal in the cellar of the Wellington Hotel in New York City, where he had lived for the past 2 years. Times were hard, and any job was a good job. When he was called on to make emergency repairs in the upper floors of the building, he would impress his superiors and the tenants by running full speed up as many as 26 flights of stairs. To him it was training, but to them it was obedience and loyalty to the job.

DeBruyn took his 5-mile morning runs in Central Park. He was a brawny 24-year-old, 163 pounds and fond of beer. And why not, said the newspapers, there is no Prohibition where he comes from. DeBruyn had been a swimmer in his youth in Oldenberg, South Germany. *Boston Post* reporter Ruth Bodwell described deBruyn in her prerace story on April 19: "A golden red-head with tiny freckles specking his smooth fair skin and blue eyes twinkling with fun and energy." DeBruyn's teeth shone like a toothpaste advertisement, and

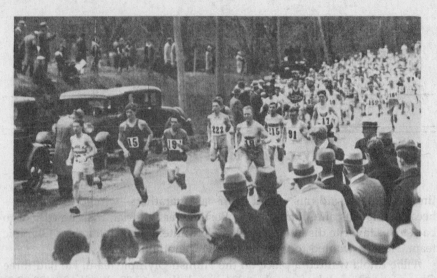

The start of the 1932 race shows German-born Paul deBruyn, #18, who made his living shoveling coal in the basement of a New York hotel. Courtesy of the Boston Public Library, Print Department.

on race day he wore a cream-colored shirt with the German eagle on his chest and green shorts. The only flaw in this seemingly perfect specimen was a bald spot on the back of the head. DeBruyn could run with abandon at Boston because he knew that, regardless of his showing, the Olympic spot for Germany was his.

"I used to be a sailor," deBruyn told Bodwell, "and spent a bad four years that way because two out of the four I was drunk." Since coming to the U.S. he had applied for citizenship.

Charles E. Bradford of Lowell, on the other hand, was already a U.S. citizen, subject to the laws of the state of Massachusetts. He had no job and no money, but he had a wife and child. He was supposed to support them but could not. Bradford hatched a scheme: What if he ran well in the Boston Marathon and got his name in the papers; would some sports-minded employer give him a job? He borrowed running togs and entered the race. Unfortunately he didn't tell his wife about his plan—in fact, he had not seen her in some time. She saw his name in the papers and notified the police, who waited for him at the finish line. He ran at 3:30 into the arms of a police officer, who gently arrested him for nonsupport. Bradford said that he would like to support his wife and child, but that he had no job and no money.

Bill Kennedy, who for years had had no trouble finding work wherever he went, hit upon hard times. He wrote a letter to John Halloran at the *Boston Globe* published a few days before the race:

I am well, but broke. . . . I've been out of work so much this winter that I've had much time to train. . . . I've run an average of 1000 miles a year for the past 25 years . . . about 130 hours alone with your mind wandering here and there—building air castles—tragedy and comedy. [A runner] thinks and pictures so many things. . . . To win the Boston Marathon, that is the dream of every runner. Sometimes I hardly believe I realized that hope fifteen years ago; I am still dreaming, still building castles, and actually believe I am going to win again. All marathon runners are dreamers; we are not practical. The hours we spend everyday every year! The strength we expend over long, lonesome roads and the pot of gold we aspire to receive for it all! The end of the rainbow, Johnnie, is a survivor's medal. Do you know that I always loved the old way best when they had the bicycle riders with us? It seemed more colorful and seemed to make you feel you had a protector at your side. I will be giving them all that's in me too and I look forward to that little thin string in front of the BAA clubhouse, a cot to lie on, and get those damn shoes off my feet! So long, old pal, I shall be in the prize winners.

Long lanky Johnny McLeod of Nova Scotia, aged 24, deeply tanned under his red shorts and white singlet, ripped away at the start to set a record-breaking pace for mile after mile. He zipped through Natick, on a day made for quick running, 48 seconds faster than anyone (52:13) and through Wellesley in 1:09:09, 106 seconds faster than anyone ever. He got to Lake Street in 2:00:40, 152 seconds faster than ever. Meanwhile deBruyn shadowed Ritola in 9th through South Framingham, where Ritola tossed away his canvas gloves. Henigan ran in 13th, Johnny Semple in 20th. McLeod had 300 yards on everyone by Wellesley Square.

On the downhill to Newton City Hall, Henigan caught Kyronen. On the next hill Henigan caught Ritola, suffering from a stitch in his side. Ritola called to the spectators for tea. Fifteen of them ran to get it. Ritola dropped back to fifth place, then dropped out.

DeBruyn took hot tea and Henigan took a water shower from a milk bottle. They ran in touching distance past Lake Street. They gained on McLeod, who ran in distress. DeBruyn held Henigan by 3 yards. Henigan, the 5- and 10-miler, was faster than deBruyn, so if it came down to a finishing sprint, it would be Henigan's race again. McLeod, ever the more slender, ran helplessly ahead; he dangled as bait. The Irishman and the German riveted their eyes on McLeod's back and closed. They caught McLeod. Offering no resistance, he waved them on. McLeod alternated walking, rubbing his legs, and running for the next 6 miles to place 27th. He said later it was the downhills, not the uphills, that did him in.

On Commonwealth Avenue Tommy Henigan came out with a water-soaked sponge for his brother. Jimmy took it and wiped it over his head

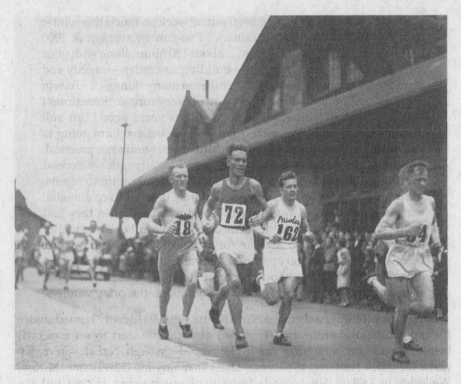

Paul deBruyn follows triple Olympic gold medalist Willie Ritola of Finland (#72, right) through Framingham. Courtesy of the Boston Public Library, Print Department.

and followed deBruyn. Suddenly a cramp seized his thigh. Slowing to nurse it and knead it into relaxation, he lost his hold on the German.

DeBruyn carried a watch in his hand like Paavo Nurmi, consulting it at every checkpoint. He was serious. He had done his homework. He kept to his schedule. But deBruyn was not the first runner seen by spectators in Kenmore Square a mile from the finish. Instead they saw someone who was not serious and possibly crazy: It was Jimmy "Cigars" Connors.

In the April 1 edition of the *Boston Post* Bill Cunningham wrote of his doubts about runners' sanity: "Psychologists have long since quit wondering about these boys. There are certain problems of human behavior that defy rational analysis." That especially applied to Jimmy "Cigars" Connors—the running clown—who claimed a record for running up and down the Boston Custom House Tower in 8:30. In the 1932 race he led the runners through Kenmore Square, a mile from the finish, puffing on a cigar. He had gotten to first place by riding on a car's running board. He had his laugh, the fans had their laugh. No one accused him of cheating, but such a joke infuriated a man like Semple, who closed on the leaders by benefit of his hard work and intense racing from 20th place to 10th. He saw the marathon as a serious athletic contest, not a parade or a circus freakshow. Semple hated what Connors did.

Semple had moved to Lynn, Massachusetts, from Philadelphia and found work as a locker room attendant in the YMCA. He slept on the daybed in his brother's house; although he couldn't afford to pay any rent, he bought an occasional ton of coal and gave his brother some of the merchandise prizes, including a gold watch, that he won in New England road races. He lived for running and runners. He had no patience with cigar-smoking clowns or jokers or fools or anyone who did not respect the sacrifices of marathon runners. His intolerance of any who disrespected the marathon or its runners would surface again and again in the coming decades, sometimes with embarrassing results.

DeBruyn paid no attention to the cigar smoke as he won by less than a minute over Henigan. Kyronen finished with a furious but futile stretch drive that brought him within half a minute of Henigan. Such a drive had taken Kyronen to within 11 seconds of victory in 1916 when he ran out of running room in the pursuit of winner Arthur Roth. The stretch drive did not work this time, either, because deBruyn was the man who had calculated correctly.

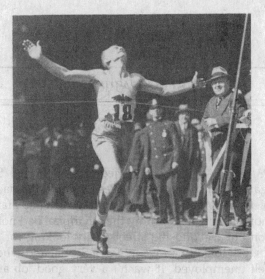

Paul deBruyn wins the 1932 Boston Marathon. Photo courtesy of the *Boston Herald*.

DeBruyn asked the BAA officials for a beer, but because of Prohibition the closest they could come was ginger ale. The newspapers reported that deBruyn wanted beer and left the Lenox Hotel to go where he could get some. Paul deBruyn went on to run for Germany in the Olympics in 1932 and 1936. He became a U.S. citizen and volunteered for the American Navy during World War II. Injuries he received in 1945 ended his running career. As of 1993, deBruyn lived in Holly Hill, Florida, and acted as the official starter and presenter of prizes in the annual Paul deBruyn 30 Kilometer in Ormand Beach, Florida.

Henigan went home to Medford, Florence and the kids, and another big celebration.

1932 Results

1.	P. deBruyn, *GermAAC*, NY	**2:33:36**	13.	K. Koski, *FAAC*, NY	2:44:20
2.	J.P. Henigan, *NMC*	**2:34:32**	14.	V. Callard, *MonAC*, ON	2:44:58
3.	W. Kyronen, *FAAC*, NY	2:34:55	15.	H. Oldag, Buffalo, NY	2:44:59
4.	A.R. Michelson, *MillAA*, NY	2:36:23	16.	F. Ward, *MillAA*, NY	2:45:38
5.	W. Steiner, NY	2:38:46	17.	W. Wilson, PA	2:45:38
6.	A. Burnside, *MonAC*, ON	2:39:42	18.	**C. DeMar, Keene, NH**	**2:46:15**
7.	E. Collins, North Medford, MA	2:40:59	19.	W. Malley, North Medford, MA	2:47:07
8.	**L.S. Pawson, Pawtucket, RI**	**2:41:36**	20.	E.H. White, Staten Island, NY	2:47:09
9.	E. Cudworth, *MonAC*, ON	2:42:32	21.	J. Shaw, Toronto, ON	2:47:45
10.	J.D. Semple, *Lynn YMCA*, MA	2:43:07	22.	**B. Kennedy, *CAC*, NY**	**2:49:58**
11.	H. Kauppinen, *FAAC*, NY	2:43:14	27.	J. McLeod, *DC*	2:51:31
12.	A.J. Brunelle, *Lynn YMCA*, MA	2:44:17		**John A. Kelley, DNF**	

A JOB FOR JIMMY

WEDNESDAY, APRIL 19, 1933

Olympians Come to Boston

In April of 1931 and April of 1932 Medford celebrated Smilin' Jimmy "Hinky" Henigan. In the 1932 Los Angeles Olympics he had dropped out with a leg problem, but Whitey Michelson placed 7th and Hans Oldag 11th. For the last 2 months, however, Jimmy the Olympian had not been training for the marathon but walking the streets daily looking for work. He had taken a day off work to go to a race in Nova Scotia, and when he returned he found himself unemployed. It wasn't a very good job anyway, but he now had eight mouths to feed, and his savings quickly disappeared. He walked and worried. The glory in striding through Los Angeles with Olympian stature vanished. Millions of other men throughout the country walked and worried as well. They walked to save carfare and worried because they were almost desperate. When a company in one city gave out apples on credit, suddenly every street corner had its apple salesman. President Hoover was gone, but Hoovervilles remained. Homeless men filled these shanty towns. Roosevelt had just taken office, but the prosperity of the Coolidge era was a distant memory. The United States was off the gold standard and you could buy 3.2 (low-alcohol) beer, but neither of those events cheered anyone. There was doubt that the BAA could sponsor the marathon beyond this year. A helpless hopelessness was the general mood of the country. Without a job, Jimmy Henigan was left without definition.

In Henigan's hopelessness the excitement to train disappeared. He had been loyal to his employer and he had worked hard. He never let running interfere with his work, except for once, but there was no work for him to do. What could he do? The demand for corrugated boxes was set by the production of what needed to be shipped in them. Those products needed customers. Those customers needed jobs to get the money to buy the products that had to be shipped in corrugated boxes. Nobody bought enough of the corrugated boxes made by Henigan's employer. Millions of men in America were out of work. Henigan had been transferred to piecework from his job as foreman in the shipping room, but the new job offered so little pay that he said he could not

In a plea for work Jimmy Henigan allowed his picture to appear on the front page of the **Boston Post.** *The BAA laurel wreath adorned his head.*

make carfare. Soldiers' relief in Medford helped some, but he had to grasp at anything to get work. In a plea for work Henigan allowed his picture to appear on the front page of the *Boston Post*. He wore a jacket and tie, the BAA laurel wreath adorned his head, and his marathon medals decorated his lapels. He smiled gamely. The details beneath the picture told of his need for work. He ran gamely but poorly in the marathon, finishing 18th in 2:49. DeBruyn dropped out at Boston College. A couple of men found Henigan at the finish to tell him they had a job for him. Hope returned. He forgot about his poor race; his smile came back. He rushed home to tell Florence.

Les Pawson, a millhand from Pawtucket, Rhode Island, raced against a monster headwind to break John Miles's 1929 course record. His arms turned lobster red from the raw ocean wind. Clouds covered the cold, stormy day and brought occasional showers. John DeGloria of the Mercury Club of Albany, New York, snatched the early lead, but he tired and slowed. The Canadian Finn, Komonen, picked up 2 minutes on Pawson over the last few miles, but Pawson still finished with the biggest lead in history. A young florist's assistant from Arlington, Massachusetts, named John A. Kelley tried to stay with the leaders. He lacked stamina and faded badly to 37th place in 3:03:56.

Dave Komonen, unemployed and nearly destitute, ran in a pair of shoes he had made himself of buckskin with spongy heels. After the race he sold them to someone in the crowd for $4.

1933 Results

1. **L. Pawson, Pawtucket, RI**	**2:31:01**^{CR}	13. J. Semple, Lynn, MA	2:46:59
2. **D. Komonen**, *MonAC*, ON	**2:36:27**	14. F. Dengis, *SDC*, Baltimore, MD	2:47:09
3. D. Wilding, *SilAC*, ON	2:38:00	15. W.K. Frick, Colebrook, NH	2:47:44
4. H. Webster, *HOC*, ON	2:38:31	16. F. Haupal, *ISC*, Glenville, CT	2:47:52
5. W. Kyronen, *FAAC*, NY	2:39:50	17. B. Spencer, *MonAC*, ON	2:48:03
6. A.R. Michelson, *MillAA*, NY	2:40:27	18. **J.P. Henigan, *NMC*, MA**	**2:49:01**
7. W.F. Hornby, *HOC*, ON	2:41:32	19. A. Burnside, *MonAC*, ON	2:50:21
8. **C. DeMar, *KNS*, NH**	**2:43:18**	22. A. Brunelle, *Lynn YMCA*, MA	2:51:48
9. J. DeGloria, *MerC*, NY	2:43:20	27. K. Koski, *FAAC*, NY	2:54:09
10. H. Kauppinen, *FAAC*, NY	2:46:01	32. **T. Brown, Westerly, RI**	**2:59:46**
11. F. Ward, *MillAA*, NY	2:46:08	37. **J.A. Kelley, *NMC*, MA**	**3:03:56**
12. N. Dack, *HOC*	2:46:12		

THE FROOD FINN

THURSDAY, APRIL 19, 1934

Henigan, Pawson Head Marathon Bill

On New Year's Day in 1934 Dave Komonen, facing poverty, made a desperate decision. In Boston after the 1933 race he had sold the shoes off his feet. But shoe making did not make him any money because he could barely sell the shoes for more than the cost of the materials. His real money-making skill was carpentry, but during these depression years he could find no work in Toronto. So, carrying all he owned, Komonen walked into the Toronto railway station and used most of the money he had to buy an $8 one-way ticket to Sudbury, Ontario. He stood a lithe, willowy 5'5", 125 pounds. One saw first Komonen's high forehead under blond hair, then how his eyes set deeply, and at last how his smile creased his face. America was supposed to be the land of opportunity, but none had surfaced for him. How did Dave Komonen fall to such desperation?

He was given the name Taavi when he was born in 1898 in Kakisalmi, Finland, where he became a farmer and carpenter. Though a frail and somewhat sickly youth, Taavi developed into a good middle-distance runner while serving in the military. He sometimes trained with his idol, Paavo Nurmi, who won six Olympic gold medals in the 1920s. Leaving a farm, wife, and two sons, Komonen emigrated to Canada, arriving on April 19, 1929, the day Johnny Miles set the course record at Boston. He looked for work as a carpenter but found little. So impoverished that at times he subsisted on soup and crackers, Komonen found the poor diet hurt his running.

Komonen joined the Monarch Athletic Club in Toronto and quickly became its star performer. Appeals through the club and through the newspapers for work failed to get him a job. Even the honor of having been elected Canadian Athlete of the Year in 1933 did not help. Komonen barely spoke English. He was not connected. He was indeed willing and able to work, but he had arrived in North America just in time for the Great Depression and was now only one of millions of ready, able, and redundant men. He moved to Sudbury because he had won a 10-mile race there and the people had treated him well. Running was the only connection he had. He thought perhaps something could be done for him in Sudbury; there was a large Finnish community there, so at least he would have people to talk to.

The leader of the local running club took Komonen to a Lions Club meeting and introduced him to members. The introductions worked; connections formed. Soon Komonen had work as a carpenter in the Frood nickel mine, and he found lodging with a local running chiropractor. He worked until 8:00 every night, then trained. When he couldn't run, he skied. Training through the northern Ontario winter was tough—snowdrifts in dead winter, mud and standing water in the spring. He often ran 8 miles before work and another 15 after. But at least now he had a regular income and would not have to sell his home-cobbled shoes.

But with a regular income came the ability to overcompensate for his starvation diet of the previous year. Komonen began to overeat, especially before races. In the winter of 1934 he fell ill. Whether it was from overeating, undereating, overtraining, or breathing the air in the nickel mine is not known, but he ran a temperature of 102 °F. But he recovered in time to come to Boston, ready to race and with plans to improve on his second place of the year before.

Komonen's marathoning had improved since his last Boston race, with his victory in the American Championship Marathon in June of 1933 (from Mt. Vernon to the steps of the White House) in 2:53:43 and the Canadian title in Toronto in August in 2:40:58. The *Boston Post* picked Komonen to win the 1934 Boston Marathon.

At the start Komonen knotted a handkerchief and pulled it over his head. He wore a dark singlet with "Frood Mines" printed on a diagonal, though only "Fro" appeared over his pinned-on race number. Leslie Pawson, the 1933 winner and record holder, Jimmy Henigan, Clarence DeMar, Willie Kyronen, Karl Koski, Albert Michelson, and who knows what dark horses came to race.

Dark horse, dark-haired, Jewish Bill Steiner, a 22-year-old New Yorker who won the Metropolitan AAU Championship Marathon in an astonishing 2:23:40, took the early lead. Those behind him wondered about the Metropolitan AAU race: Could that time have been right? It was a short course, wasn't it? Yes, but how short? Steiner led by 100 yards at South Framingham under a sunny sky, with Les Pawson and Bill Molloy of the North Medford Club running and wondering behind him. Kyronen and Paul deBruyn followed.

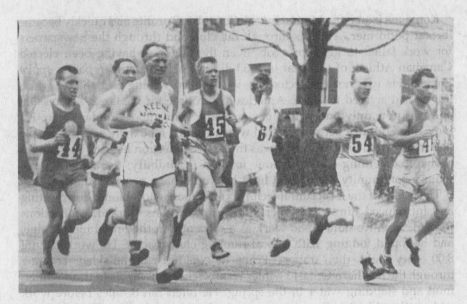

In the early going of the 1934 race a group surrounded seven-time winner, old man Clarence DeMar (#1), figuring he knew the right pace. Whitey Michelson is #45. Courtesy of the Boston Public Library, Print Department.

DeBruyn still worked nights shoveling coal into the furnaces of the Wellington Hotel in New York. He held onto his job despite the Depression and a desire to do something other than shovel coal. Next ran Komonen and a young man from Arlington, Massachusetts, Johnny Kelley. When a well-credentialed runner like Steiner jets out to an early lead, he cannot be considered a morning glory that will never survive the afternoon. But that doesn't mean you must follow. But if you don't follow he might steal the race. What do you do? The runners behind Steiner had this puzzle to ponder. By Natick Komonen and Kelley ran second and third behind Steiner. They let him go, gambling that he could not hold the pace. Kelley, a little man with a smooth running style, carried a supply of glucose tablets in a sack at his waist.

Kelley shared water with Komonen and together they caught Steiner before Woodland Park just as the sea breeze and clouds kicked in. Steiner did not look like a wilting flower, but neither did he look like a sturdy oak. There was a lot of uncertainty with a third of the course remaining. Pawson dropped out with cramps at Newton Lower Falls, and Henigan dropped out at 17 miles. Steiner did not respond to being passed by Komonen and Kelley but stoically maintained his pace. The road belonged to Kelley and Komonen if they stayed strong. Kelley ran out of glucose tablets on the last hill. He began breathing hard, developed what observers called a "pallor of the face," and weakened. Kelley let Komonen slip away on the downhill toward Lake Street. Komonen again wore his homemade crepe-and-buckskin shoes. In his belly rested a steak from the night before, and on top of that his oatmeal breakfast. Neither gave him any trouble.

Michelson dropped out. He and Henigan rode together to the finish line in a rumble seat. Alone, Komonen rumbled along the road with no difficulty. He ran away from Kelley from the Boston College crest to Lake Street. After that, Kelley posed no threat. Kelley ran remarkably well for one who had finished only 37th the year before. He cracked on the hills but had not broken. Komonen ran to the finish unhindered. The press punsters called it a "Finnish line." Others quipped that Mae West said, "Komonen see me some time."

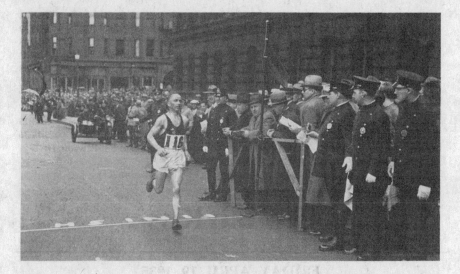

A miner from Sudbury, Ontario, Finnish immigrant Dave Komonen beat John A. Kelley to win the 1934 race. The previous year Komonen had been so poor he had to sell his homemade shoes. Courtesy of the Boston Public Library, Print Department.

Alex Burnside, a little man with a delicate moustache and an instrument maker in the weather bureau of the Dominion Government of Canada, placed fourth. His teammate, nearly 50 years old and less than 100 pounds, Percy Wyer, placed eighth. Both ran for Komonen's old Monarch AC. That other Finn, Karl Koski, who worked for a sandpaper manufacturer in New York, placed fifth. When asked how long he would stay in Boston, Komonen said he must get back to his job because a man was lucky to have work these days. Had Komonen remained with the Monarch AC in Toronto instead of moving to Sudbury, he along with Burnside and Wyer would have won the team prize; instead it went to Kelley's North Medford Club.

In the clubhouse Kelley ducked behind a curtain to be sick for several minutes. He came out smiling.

Fred Faller, who coached Kelley, said that all Kelley needed was stamina, because with his speed and judgment he'd be a wonder. Faller, a wonder himself, was born in 1895 in Germany. He won the AAU 10-mile and cross-country championships in 1919 and 1920 and ran 10,000 meters in 32:15. He lived to be over 90. He coached Kelley in these early days, although Kelley later disavowed his influence.

1934 Results

1.	D. Komonen, *FMAA*, ON	2:32:53	13.	P. deBruyn, *GermAAC*	2:52:44
2.	J.A. Kelley, *NMC*, MA	2:36:50	14.	A. Johnson, Lansing, KS	2:55:39
3.	W. Steiner, *GermAAC*, NY	2:40:29	15.	C. Welch, *NMC*	2:56:33
4.	A. Burnside, *MonAC*, ON	2:44:32	16.	C. DeMar *KNS*, NH	2:56:52
5.	K. Koski, *FAAC*	2:44:52	17.	W. Kennedy, *ISC*, NY	2:59:58
6.	G.A. Norman, *USMAA*, MA	2:45:00	18.	H.T. Sherman, *CALP14*, RI	3:02:50
7.	W.F. McMahon, *FAC*, RI	2:45:19	19.	P.R. Cassano, *NMC*	3:03:27
8.	P. Wyer, *MonAC*	2:46:06	20.	A. Jaaskela, *FAAC*, ON	3:03:47
9.	D. Fagerlund, *FAAC*	2:48:08	32.	T. Brown, Westerly, RI	3:13:15
10.	W.P. Molloy, *NMC*	2:48:56	33.	W. Young, *SWMC*, PQ	3:14:36
11.	M. Porter, *GermAAC*	2:49:56		James Henigan, Les Pawson, DNF	
12.	J.D. Semple, *USMAA*, MA	2:51:04			

THE BIG KISS

FRIDAY, APRIL 19, 1935

Komonen, Kelley, and Pawson Top Entrants

This was a year of weird weather in the U.S., a year of duststorms that blew away farms on the high prairie. The world's political climate also blew ill. Stories deep in the papers mentioned the dangers facing Polish Jews and referred to a rising politician in Germany named Adolf Hitler, who complained of the treatment of Germany's people under the Treaty of Versailles. Kelley and most potential marathon winners would soon be off to be soldiers, but now, in the midst of what came to be known as the Great Depression, few people had much to do. Kelley, however, had running.

Johnny Kelley was born on September 6 in the Boston victory year of Tom Longboat, 1907. He watched his first Boston Marathon in 1921, when Frank Zuna, the Bohemian plumber from New Jersey, won. A big policeman held up the crowd control rope for little Johnny so he could step forward to see Zuna finish. To Kelley, Zuna didn't even look tired. For decades Kelley would remember the look on Zuna's face. Marathon worship was sparked that day. Kelley was the eldest of a family of five boys and five girls raised in West Medford, Massachusetts. His father, William, delivered mail. Sometimes the Kelley children would walk the route with him. Kelley's mother, Bertha, cooked and cooked. Young Johnny tried football, but he was too small. He tried baseball, but gave it up after one time at bat. As all young ball players are instructed, Kelley kept his eye on the ball. He expected it to break and curve into the strike zone so he could swat it, but it kept straight on. He didn't flinch until the ball hit him in the head. So Kelley gave up baseball and tried footracing. In his first race he placed second. His prize was a baseball bat!

Kelley ran track at Medford High and then at Arlington High after his family moved. He ran 1-mile times around 4:38 to 4:45. At age 20 he tried his first marathon, an out-and-back course between Pawtucket and Woonsocket, Rhode Island. He ran 3:17. A month later, in his first Boston Marathon, he dropped out on the downhill after Lake Street. He tried again in 1932 and managed to stay with the leaders until Wellesley, then dropped out. Kelley worked as an assistant in the G.O. Anderson florist shop on Massachusetts Avenue in Arlington and shared a room with his brother in his father's house. He was 27 years old and lucky to have a job during this depression. In the last 2 years he had progressed from 37th to second, so he figured that this was his year to win.

But Dave Komonen figured this was his year to win again, and the *Post* agreed, projecting Leslie Pawson third after Kelley. But the *Post* did not know that Pawson had suffered a stress fracture in the past year and was not fit. The *Post* also did not know that Komonen drove down from Canada in a blizzard that delayed him near Rochester, New York. Komonen was tired from the night of sleep he had missed while stuck in the blizzard.

Kelley tried to leave nothing to chance. Under the guidance of his coach, Fred Faller, he planned to hang with Komonen until Wellesley, then break him with a sustained acceleration through Woodland Park. To prepare himself for this ordeal Kelley applied the best science the 1930s had to offer. Faller had said Kelley had to build up his stamina. Two years earlier Jimmy Henigan had introduced Kelley to Angus MacDonald, who was associated with the MacLean Hospital in Belmont, Massachusetts. Under MacDonald's supervision Johnny underwent a system of special baths and diets. He took salt glow baths, cabinet treatments, and various types of hydrotherapeutic treatments under the advice of Dr. Kenneth J. Tilotson. Kelley said he was put on a high-protein diet, rich in carbohydrates and fats. One must assume that he simply ate a lot.

Kelley had special shoes, too. A 70-year-old Englishman living north of Boston in Peabody named Samuel T. A. ("S.T.A.R.") Ritchins custom-made shoes for runners. These shoes were magic in a shoe-making world that focused on durability. New England made the best shoes in the world, but they were dress shoes, work shoes, boots, slippers, and sneakers—not running shoes. Jock Semple talked his employer, the United Shoe Machinery Company in Beverly, into sponsoring a running team, but the company did not

> *Runners ran in stiff, heavy, leather-soled "athletic" shoes. These monsters had to be carefully broken in before races.*

make their shoes. Runners ran in stiff, heavy, leather-soled "athletic" shoes. These monsters had to be carefully broken in before races.

Everyone knew you could run faster in light shoes, but no one until S.T.A.R. made them. Heavy shoes and the blisters caused by their unyielding materials caused marathon runners as much trouble as the distance itself. Semple paid extraordinary attention to his runners' feet. He inquired about their blisters, bunions, bruises, and cuts. He examined the blisters and treated them, sometimes lancing them himself. Semple could often be seen kneeling before a runner, tenderly caring for his foot. There was a touch of the Christ about it. A runner's worst enemy was his shoes. A joke about marathoners' shoes and the forces generated by their feet against the leather circulated at the time: A runner once put a dollar bill in his shoe before the marathon; when he finished, he found ten dimes there.

To toughen runners' feet, Semple used to take his United Shoe team out on Sunday mornings in the icy winter to Nahant Beach, where he would make them walk barefoot in the surf. He hoped the sun, the sand, the cold, and the salt would tan the soles of their feet in a process not unlike the one nearby tanneries used to change cowhide to shoe leather. Feet as tough as leather might protect a runner from his own shoes.

Shoe failure ending in bloody blisters caused more marathoners to drop out than illness, injury, or fatigue. Most runners wore canvas sneakers with dense rubber soles and heavy stitching. Folds, stitches, and seams chafed against the skin, and runners complained that the laces pinched the top of their feet. S.T.A.R. alone worked to solve those problems. He wore a black cape and worked at night, joked Semple. S.T.A.R. made white shoes instead of the standard black ones because white reflected heat and black, he calculated, absorbed 38% more heat. S.T.A.R. built in a metatarsal pad and made perforations in the side for ventilation.

Ritchins moved the laces to the outside of the shoe attached to an elastic that smoothly covered the top of the foot. He made the uppers of light kidskin, the strongest leather for its weight. The inner soles were of soft tanned calfskin and the outer soles of crepe rubber. They weighed 5-1/2 ounces. New England was a world center of shoe making, so all the best materials, art, and craftsmanship were available. These shoes, like most running shoes of the time, had a distinct heel and sole; there was no midsole. The rubber of the sole extended on the outside closer to the heel than on the inside for outside landing. Between the rubber sole and heel was only calfskin with stitching down the middle. Kelley believed shoes were important, a marathoner's tools. One year 8 of the top 10 Boston runners were in S.T.A.R.'s shoes. "S.T.A.R. Streamlines" took Ritchins 16 hours to make, for which he charged $7.50. Ritchins died in 1937.

For the 1935 race, S.T.A.R. shoes, a handkerchief given by a favorite aunt for good luck, and a pouch of 15 chocolate glucose tablets were Kelley's equipment. A runner by the name of Pat Dengis rode up from Maryland to spoil Kelley's carefully crafted plan. Dengis's real name was Frank, but for his own reasons he called himself Pat. He was born in Swansea, Wales, a pretty resort town on the coast. Dengis spoke often and without equivocation. He spit out his words. He would tell you exactly what he thought of you. Dengis was voluble but lovable. He was a toolmaker and designer in an aircraft factory and had worked on the clipper airship that had recently set aviation records in a trip from the West Coast to Hawaii. He had a belt buckle he had made for himself; into bronze he set his National Marathon Championship medals, worth about $300. In the Boston Marathon on this ideal day he wore not the usual singlet but a snappy blue silk shirt with sleeves, collar buttons, tails, and an equal amount of untucked fabric in the front. His intention was to capture Kelley.

Kelley kept to his plan. Weather was ideal for running, but because this was Good Friday only 300,000 of the usual 500,000 people turned out to watch. Kelley ran in 3rd place through the early miles and took the lead in Wellesley. By Woodland Komonen ran with difficulty and dropped out while in 4th place. Kelley kept popping his chocolate glucose tablets into his mouth until they were gone. Meanwhile Dengis and Dick Wilding ran conservatively in 13th and 17th places at South Framingham. They moved relentlessly through the pack. Paul deBruyn had trained hard for this race—perhaps too hard—and had leg trouble in the Newton hills. Dengis could not see Kelley but set his sights on the point where Kelley would come into view. He scanned over the crowds for Kelley's bobbing head. At last he saw it, and he pulled for it. He wanted that head on his plate. Dengis caught Kelley just beyond Wellesley and passed him. Dengis had no one between himself and victory. Suddenly, in his moment of success, Dengis caught a stitch. He said it felt like a knife slipping in under the heart. Kelley surged past the foundering Dengis and took a runaway lead down the hill into Newton Lower Falls. But as suddenly as it had come, Dengis's stitch disappeared. The dagger withdrew, and Dengis again held Kelley in his sights. Up over the Newton hills Dengis kept a steady pace, waiting for Kelley to falter. Dengis was used to calculating to catch whom he wanted.

Kelley looked like he would not be caught, but at Kenmore Square he suddenly stopped and bent over like a jackknife. The crowd in the packed square hushed. Kelley violently vomited up the 15 chocolate glucose tablets. They cost him the course record. Immediately he straightened, blessed himself, and ran on to the finish line. The officials were late, and there was no tape, and he lost the talisman handkerchief from his aunt, but regardless Kelley was delirious with joy.

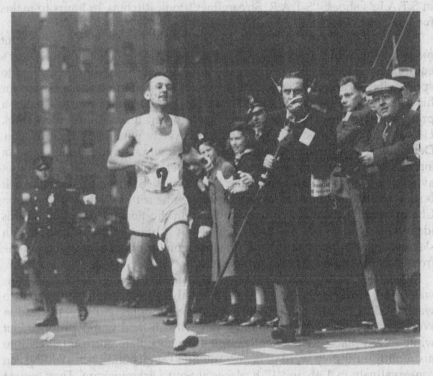

After stopping to vomit in Kenmore Square, John A. Kelley beat slow-starting Pat Dengis to win the 1935 Boston Marathon. Courtesy of the Boston Public Library, Print Department.

Dengis was too far behind to see Kelley vomit. He finished strongly. The officials had a tape ready for him to break. When they asked if he needed medical attention, he said, "Hell no, let's run this thing all over again." "Pat Dengis hopped around like a schoolboy," wrote a *Post* reporter in the April 20 edition. Dengis got a big kiss from Eva, his bride of 8 months. She, a beautiful long-haired blond, attracted considerable attention from the press photographers, who recorded the kiss for the pages of most of the local papers. Dengis was the surprise of the race. He lost 6 pounds, called for a beer, then shouted, "Where's Johnny, I've got to see Johnny! Would you imagine this: a *florist* runs 26 miles—for a laurel wreath! Where's Kelley?

I've got to see Kelley." Johnny Kelley told the *Post*, "I know this marathon glory will be over in a few days, so I've got to make the best of it."

1935 Results

1.	J.A. Kelley, Arlington, MA	2:32:07	13.	E. Brown, *NarrAC*, RI	**2:53:35**
2.	P. Dengis, *SDC*	2:34:11	14.	F. Bristow, *YAC*, ON	2:54:51
3.	R. Wilding, *YAC*, ON	2:39:50	15.	J. Shaw, *MonAC*, Toronto, ON	2:56:44
4.	G.A. Norman, *USMAA*, MA	2:40:57	16.	J.M. Clarke, *MdC*, PA	2:57:29
5.	H. Kauppinen, *FAAC*, NY	2:44:33	17.	G. Rolland, Long Island, NY	2:57:51
6.	E. Collins, *NMC*	2:44:39	18.	**C. DeMar, *KNS*, NH**	**2:58:27**
7.	J. Plouffe, *FAC*, RI	2:44:57	19.	C. Brederson, *FAC*, RI	2:59:12
8.	F. Ward, *MillAA*, NY	2:46:06	20.	W. Ray, *USMAA*, MA	3:00:13
9.	V. Callard, *MonAC*, ON	2:46:56	21.	K. Koski, *FAAC*, NY	3:04:21
10.	A. Brunelle, *USMAA*	2:47:23	23.	**W. Kennedy, NY**	**3:05:49**
11.	**J. Henigan, *NMC***	**2:48:43**	28.	**L. Pawson, *FAC*, RI**	**3:09:59**
12.	C. Hill, *USMAA*	2:50:52			

DEERFOOT OF THE NARRAGANSETT

MONDAY, APRIL 20, 1936

Who Can Catch Kelley?

The economy in these depression times provided little for most Americans and nothing for Indians. They were a conquered people living on the margin, living on the meager scraps tossed out from an impoverished marketplace. Ellison Myers Brown, born on the margin, saw running as his only way out of poverty.

In 1935's Boston race Brown's shoes had failed him with 5 miles to go. It had been 2 days after his mother's death. Wearing a shirt made from the fabric of her dress, he had run those last 5 miles barefoot and still finished 13th. This year he had new shoes—S.T.A.R.'s Streamlines. Though Brown had no money for shoes, he hustled and found support for himself and his training. But attracting such support in these depression years was difficult, and it did not come easily to Brown.

After finishing third in the North Medford Club's mid-March 20-miler, Brown won training support from William Waugh of the Tercentenary Committee of Providence, Rhode Island. The committee paid for Brown's keep in Middleboro, Massachusetts, near Lake Assawampsett. Jack Farrington, the Rhode Island AAU commissioner, coached Brown. He ran and ran and ate eggs and steak and drank vanilla sodas. From Middleboro he wrote to his sisters Gracie and Nina to say he would win. He stood 5'9" and weighed 139 pounds. Drawing had been Brown's favorite subject in school, and he drew quite well. He was bright and could be very funny.

Brown was one of six children of Bryan Otis Brown and a Spanish-Mexican mother. Born in Potter's Hill, Rhode Island, 22 years earlier on September 22, 1914, he was one of 300 surviving descendents of the Narragansett Indians who joined King Philip, the Wampanoag chief who united three tribes and forced white men to abandon the frontier and retreat in 1675-76. But the white men killed King Philip the next year and neutralized the Narragansetts. Ellison was named after his father's boss, Ellison Tinkham, and for Myers, the Indian baseball catcher for the New York Giants. His Narragansett tribal name was Deerfoot. Ellison, or Deerfoot, showed tremendous running talent at quite a young age.

Jock Semple told a story about the day when Ellison was 11 years old and saw a fine Indian runner called Chief (Horatio) Stanton out on the roads during a 15-mile run. His coach Tippy (Thomas) Salimeno waited at the end of the loop for his runner. An 11-year-old kid appeared suddenly from behind a bush and silently ran on the chief's heels. For 10 miles the kid followed silently. In the last 2 miles the chief pulled away. He was too tired to talk as the coach complimented him on his fast time. The chief finally caught his breath and said, "You think I ran fast?" He pointed behind him down the road. "There's a 10-year-old boy right behind me!" Well, there wasn't. Young Ellison had slipped into the woods to climb trees and continue his play. The coach thought the chief was crazy, so he made him go back and hunt for the boy. They found him playing in the trees. That began a long relationship of Salimeno helping keep Ellison Brown on track.

His contemporaries labeled Brown as a bit of a wild man. They say he felt at home in the trees, and for that as well as for his remarkable physique they called him Tarzan, after Edgar Rice Burroughs's character from 1914. "Muscled as the best of the ancient Roman gladiators must have been muscled, and yet with the soft and sinuous curves of a Greek god." The Boston newspapers gave colorful descriptions of Brown on the day of the race: "Tarzan Brown, a penniless, mahogany-hued and full-blooded Indian . . . dark-skinned warrior" (Jack Barnwell, *Post*); "brown-skinned and as smooth-cheeked as a girl" (Ruth C. Bodwell, *Post*); "silken muscled boy who speaks with the gravity of an ancestral chief" (Gerry Hern, *Post*); "penniless redskin," (Will Cloney, *Boston Herald*); "His schooling was sketchy. Tarzan would much rather learn to keep a good line of traps than to explore the alphabet" (Jerry Nason, *Boston Daily Globe*).

Brown was regarded as a freak—undisciplined, uncontrollable, unintelligent, a child of nature, an awesome natural talent—and if he won or lost it was because of his unalterable nature. In a way no different from Tom Longboat, the Onondaga Indian winner of the Boston Marathon in 1907, Brown was an Indian with special physical talents, but he would never get personal credit for what he accomplished. It was expected that he could run—he was an Indian, after all—so he got no credit for character, courage, or hard work for his success as a runner. If he succeeded it was because he did what his handlers prepared him to do, like a thoroughbred stallion. But if he failed at anything, he received all the blame.

Johnny Kelley thought nothing of all this. To him Tarzan Brown was a colorful character who never had a bad word to say about anyone. About Kelley, Brown said he'd lick that guy if nobody else.

Brown blasted away from the start and dismantled Johnny McLeod's checkpoint records from 1932:

Checkpoint Splits

Framingham	Ellison Brown	30:23
Natick	Ellison Brown	50:43
Wellesley	Ellison Brown	1:07:31
Woodland	Ellison Brown	1:31:49
Lake Street	Ellison Brown	1:59:43
Coolidge Corner	Ellison Brown	2:16:17

Kelley waited, a clever predator, for Brown to burn himself out on the hills. Indians in tribal dress, including Brown's father in a headdress, beat on tom-toms and cheered for their favorite son. Kelley lost his patience and exploded up the hills, intent on catching and dominating the prodigal Indian. He would teach that youngster the perils of going out too fast. It appeared that Kelley was right. Between the Woodland and Lake Street checkpoints Brown failed to increase the difference between his times and McLeod's old records. He appeared tired. He must be paying for his earlier speed. In a 3-mile acceleration Kelley made up Brown's entire half-mile lead. But it was Kelley who suffered from oxygen debt and a buildup of metabolic waste products in his leg muscles—a buildup that, although it started in the middle of the race, produced the same effects as he expected Brown's fast starting to have caused. Kelley caught Brown and cavalierly patted him on the back as if to say, "Nice running, boy, now let a real man take over." There was no malice in Kelley's gesture; he simply regarded Brown as a joker, a clown who didn't have what it takes to win big races. Kelley looked pink and pale. He didn't notice that Brown ran sweatless because he had been cruising over the hills. Brown thought, I'll get you later.

Later came fairly soon. Kelley led, and Brown cleverly skimmed the tangents from the peak of one curve to the other. He caught Kelley and surged past. This was the year and the race when Globe writer Jerry Nason named the last of the three Newton hills "Heartbreak Hill," a name that stuck. By Marion Street Kelley walked. His father had water and oranges for him, but they did not help. Kelley wanted to win Boston again, but his body would not let him. The next day Will Cloney of the *Herald* wrote that "Johnny was walking like an intoxicated man, his legs pushing crazily out to the sides." He walked six more times, while the runners from arrears marched past him. The best of these was William "Biddie" McMahon of Worcester. He ran on his way to a place on the Olympic team bound for Hitler's Germany. Jack Barnwell of the *Herald* wrote, "McMahon was the man who took up the white man's burden of catching the Indian."

Heartbreak Hill: Volcano or Molehill?

Many runners come to Boston fearing the legendary Heartbreak Hill. In their mind's eye they see a winding road up a windblown, snowcapped peak. They run through Natick and Wellesley in dread approach. Many runners on its slope feel as if they have altitude sickness as lactic acid freezes their leg muscles. Many a runner has approached the slope sure of sealing victory, but Heartbreak Hill changes the incipient winner into a loser looking for a place to drop out. Conversely, other runners settle for merely placing only to look up and see that the leader has surrendered to a walk. Still others run in fear but never even notice the hill.

Many runners have said they come to Boston anticipating a big, steep hill, but finding only reasonable slopes finally ask spectators how far it is to Heartbreak Hill, only to be told they have already passed it. For some it is nothing, for others a mountain, and for still others a wall. What is Heartbreak Hill exactly?

Economically it is an upper class neighborhood in Newton, Massachusetts, built on rolling hills and covered with big houses and big yards. Geologically, Heartbreak Hill is silt, sand, and clay, deposited by one or a series of glaciers 10,000 to 15,000 years ago. Topographically, its peak is 236 feet above sea level, but only 186 feet above the lowest previous place on the course. The start in Hopkinton is 227 feet higher than the top of Heartbreak Hill. So the hill is not technically formidable. But emotionally it can be a mountain.

Heartbreak Hill comes in the marathon when a runner is physically far from the start, 18 or 19 miles, and still physiologically far from the finish. It is the place where on a flat course a runner would hit the breaking point known as "the wall." It is the place where poorly prepared or poorly paced runners run out of energy stored as glycogen in the muscles and slow as if hitting a brick wall. Such fatigue evaporates hopes of a good place or time. What breaks hearts is the realization that willpower cannot overcome physiology, that desire cannot fool Mother Nature, that guts are not enough.

No one caught the Indian. He did run into difficulties of his own, saying he ran himself blind. Dengis ran into difficulties, too. He suffered a ruptured blood vessel in either his kidney or his bladder at 7 miles and continued to 10, but the pain was too great. By nightfall he was still in Massachusetts General Hospital for observation. Pawson dropped out at 12 miles.

After the race Ellison Myers "Tarzan" Brown, Deerfoot of the Narragansett, said, "I guess you white people can't say after this that the only good Indian is a dead Indian." King Philip would have been proud.

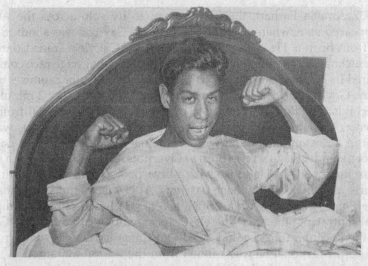

On the morning after his 1936 victory, Ellison Brown clowns for the cameras. Courtesy of the Boston Public Library, Print Department.

1936 Results

1. **E. Brown, Westerly, RI**	2:33:40	7. E. Collins, North Medford, MA	2:39:49
2. W. McMahon, Worcester, MA	2:35:27	8. A. Paskell, West Lynn, MA	2:40:07
3. M. Porter, New York, NY	2:36:48	9. V. Callard, Toronto, ON	2:40:25
4. L. Giard, Brockton, MA	2:37:16	10. J.M. Shaw, Montreal, PQ	2:42:38
5. **J.A. Kelley, Arlington, MA**	2:38:49	11. A. Johnson, Port Chester, NY	2:43:13
6. A. Burnside, Toronto, ON	2:39:05	12. C. Hill, Beverly, MA	2:44:24

13.	J. Paul, St. John, NB	2:45:30		22.	W.K. Ray, Beverly, MA	2:54:11
14.	L. Young, Beverly, MA	2:46:11		23.	**G. Cote, St. Hyacinthe, PQ**	**2:54:22**
15.	J. Lewis, *NMC*	2:46:34		24.	F. Worthington, PA	2:54:34
16.	**C.H. DeMar, Keene, NH**	**2:48:08**		25.	M. Bardsley, Pawtucket, RI	2:54:55
17.	W. Wicklund, Passaic, NJ	2:50:23		26.	**W. Young, Verdun, PQ**	**2:55:06**
18.	**J. Henigan, *NMC*, MA**	**2:50:37**		27.	D. Fagerlund, NY	2:55:11
19.	**B. Kennedy, Port Chester, NY**	**2:51:52**		28.	R. Kimball, Beverly, MA	2:55:32
20.	R. Hamilton, Florence, NS	2:52:08		29.	T. Bury, Lynn, MA	2:56:03
21.	F. Ward, NY	2:52:40		30.	J. Semple, Beverly, MA	2:57:02

UNEMPLOYED AND PENNILESS

MONDAY, APRIL 19, 1937

Kelley Expects a Win

In 1937 Amelia Earhart, the first woman to fly solo across the Atlantic, disappeared somewhere over the Pacific. Pete Gavuzzi was about to disappear from Boston. He used to be a runner in C.C. Pyle's Trans-Continental Race, nicknamed the Bunion Derby. That professional stage race commonly required its competitors to race 50 miles, day after day, for promises of prize money. Gavuzzi placed second in 1929 after 3,000 miles—by 2 minutes and 48 seconds. For that he received a promissory note for $9,250 from Pyle, known as Cash and Carry Pyle. Gavuzzi still had that note in his wallet as he sat in a Boston hotel room with no money to pay for the next day.

Short, slender Gavuzzi was born in Liverpool, England, of a French mother and an Italian father. He spoke with a Liverpool accent, moved with Italian gestures, and lived with French passions. After he emigrated to Canada, he spoke Quebec French with a British accent. He never retired from professional footracing; the sport merely evaporated beneath him. Pete Gavuzzi was the spiritual force behind nearly all Canadian long-distance runners, but as a professional he was banned from the Boston Marathon.

Now Gavuzzi coached. He sat in a cheap hotel room in Boston with a 24-year-old unemployed carpenter from Verdun, Quebec, who had finished third in the North Medford Club 20-miler in mid-March and wanted to remain in Boston to race in the marathon. But between the two of them they had but $2 to sustain themselves until race day, a month later, and still make their way home. The room cost a dollar a day. The Castor Athletic Club of Montreal had promised to wire money, but none had come. The two faced the fact that they would have to go home without his protégé's having run the Boston Marathon. They sat and calculated their finances and recalculated. Nope. They would have to go home.

Then the unemployed carpenter, Walter Young, remembered the precious Waltham watch he had won in the 20-miler. He could pawn it for money to go back to Quebec, where he might be able to get more money to come back and stay for the race. Gavuzzi urged him to do it. Young's wife, Muriel, and 3-year-old son waited back in Verdun, living on welfare.

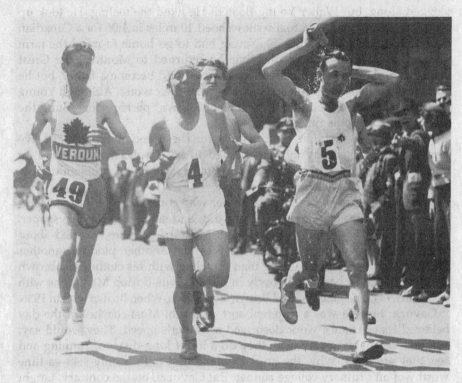

Unemployed Walter Young (#49 from Verdun, Quebec) had a job waiting for him, but only if he won at Boston. Johnny Kelley dumps water on his head as they pass the train station in Framingham. Courtesy of the Boston Public Library, Print Department.

Walter Young had been largely unemployed for several years. The Boston reporters said that he was a modest man, unassuming, who nonetheless commanded respect. He was born on March 14, 1913, to English-speaking parents in a tiny Quebec hamlet. He was raised on a farm in Greenlay and walked to school 3 miles away in Windsor Mills. Young did all those rugged and strenuous fetch-and-carry farm chores. By the eighth grade he struck out on his own for Montreal. He was nearly 6 feet tall and lanky. In the prosperous '20s he quickly got a job as a laborer in the steel mills. Later he became a carpenter's apprentice and made the acquaintance of boxers in a local gym. He boxed competitively as a welterweight and middleweight and won most of the 40 bouts he fought.

Young thought he was going to become a professional boxer until he was knocked out in two out of his first three professional fights. The knockouts turned him toward running to improve his boxing, and he found he could run quite far quite easily. Other boxers complained about running and slogged along, but Walter Young floated. He liked the feeling. He took up snowshoe racing and eventually snowshoed 10 miles in 1:06 for a Canadian record. When his father took ill, Young had to go home to mind the farm and he forfeited his job. By the time he returned to Montreal the Great Depression flared. Young had gotten married and become a father, but he seemed to run his best while his finances were their worst. Although Young knew that it had done nothing for Ellison Brown, perhaps for Young the racing could help his finances.

Young thought that if he could win Boston the attendant fame might give him a crack at a steady job. He wanted to be a policeman and had an application in with the city of Verdun. But first he had a problem of how to survive until the start of the race.

Gavuzzi believed in Walter as a runner who could win the Boston Marathon; Muriel did not; Clarence DeMar did, and said so in the newspaper. Johnny Kelley, who had won the North Medford 20-miler, worried about Young. Otherwise no one cared. He was just another plodder, another dreamer, another hopeful young man traveling with his clothes in a brown paper bag. Young had done poorly in his previous Boston Marathons with a 33rd in 1934, one place behind Brown, and a 26th, when Brown won in 1936.

Gavuzzi himself was a different sort of coach. Most coaches of the day believed that distance work destroyed a runner's speed. They would say, Witness the marathon runners; they do a lot of long-distance running and see, they are slow. Why, the great DeMar's best mile is only 4:48—a time worthy of an ordinary college runner. But Gavuzzi, on the contrary, taught that long, slow runs were best. He believed that a man could train slow and race fast. He thought that 3 hours done slowly would be more helpful than 2 done quickly. Gavuzzi would run for hours with the runner he trained. They would go slowly for 20 or even 40 miles. Gavuzzi said to save the hard running for the race.

Young pawned the watch, traveled back to Verdun, and begged the city mayor for help. Fortunately for Young, the mayor had troubles of his own and needed to convince people that the newly formed athletic commission was not a boondoggle. The mayor gave Young $50 and promised him a job on the police force should he win the Boston Marathon.

The magnificent Tarzan Brown had dropped out of the Olympic marathon in Berlin, as had Billy McMahon, leaving only Kelley to finish, 20 minutes behind the winner, Kitei Son, the Korean-born Ki Chung Sohn forced to run under a Japanese name and under the colors of occupying Japan. Son's time of 2:29:19 was the unofficial world record, or world's best time. Kelley finished 18th in 2:49:32. Brown had dropped out because of a hernia and was not willing or able to train for many months. He had started running again only 15 days earlier and entered because he felt he should defend his title, even if he could do so only nominally. Will Cloney of the *Herald* wrote that Kelley was more or less shunned by supporters because he demanded too much expense money (Brown and sometimes Kelley would ask for as much as $20 under the table for expenses to a race). Of past winners only Paul deBruyn, Les Pawson, Dave Komonen, and Kelley were thought by Young and the press to be serious threats. Pawson's running had been only ordinary lately and showed nothing of the course record-setting talent that he had demonstrated in 1933. His life had changed; he had a new career, a wife, and a baby. Perhaps he no longer had the passion to train for racing. Slow-starting Pat Dengis came back, full of bluster and fight. Another Quebec Canadian, Gerard Cote, looked good, but Young had recently defeated him in a 10-mile snowshoe race. The newspaper reporters almost unanimously predicted Kelley would win.

Kelley thought so, too. He said that he never felt better, that he had all his guns going. With his 1:52:59 in the North Medford Club 20-miler, he finished 3 minutes ahead of Young. Kelley cut back his training for a well-rested approach to the Boston Marathon.

Young traveled back to Boston from Verdun and bought his watch back from the pawnbroker. Young was not well rested. He searched for Gavuzzi in the cheap hotel but could not find him. Gavuzzi did not appear until he popped up in Hopkinton at the Lucky Rock Manor, the race headquarters on the Tebeau Farm, where about 200 runners performed their prerace rituals. Bricklayer Bill Kennedy sported a new moustache. Young had eaten a steak, salad, and tea 5 hours before the race. He did not eat starchy foods like bread, potatoes, or pasta because Gavuzzi told him that they slow a runner during a race. Young wore a singlet with the Canadian maple leaf and the word "Verdun" to show his appreciation of his sponsoring town, where he had lived for 10 years. The temperature was 60 °F and the sky was clear. George V. Brown started the race for his 39th time.

So confident was Kelley that he decided to run against no man but rather against time itself. He believed that he alone could maintain the pace he set. He doodled along in fourth place at South Framingham while Young ran in third. By Natick Kelley had the lead, but Young ran with him. From there until Coolidge Corner they exchanged leads 16 times. They ran together, cordially accommodating each other like training partners as they wove through the sometimes congested traffic. Every reporter, race official, and spectator who could commandeer a vehicle or bicycle followed along in a madding parade. Kelley cascaded himself with water while Young did not. Kelley drank water while Young did not.

On the hill by the Brae Burn Country Club Kelley stopped and vomited water. He said the vomiting actually helped, that when it stopped he felt much better. Kelley made up the 100 yards he lost and pulled even with

Young by the Boston College crest. He tried to run away from Young on the hills, but his constant bursting against gravity fatigued him. He hurled himself up the hills in an attempt to escape Young. He had won before and he should win again and he should do it now. His hubris did him in. By Coolidge Corner it was all over for Kelley. By Kenmore Square he alternated walking and running. Young ran alone from Coolidge Corner to win by 6 minutes.

Les Pawson came up from 8th place in Framingham to hold 3rd from Natick on. On this warm day the old-timers did well, with Fred Ward coming up from 20th place to 4th at the finish. Dengis dropped out with bladder problems again. DeBruyn dropped out. Lou Gregory, a 31-year-old math teacher in Earlsville, New York, finished in 12th place, with his feet beaten into a bloody mess. Old Clarence DeMar, now the father of twins and author of the newly published *Marathon*, placed 14th. DeMar offered Young a copy of his book.

At the start poor Jock Semple lost his number, and along the way after asking for a drink of water he got a bucketful thrown in his face. It drained into his shoes, and at the finish in the BAA clubhouse officials let a "girl" reporter into the locker room so Semple could not get dressed.

Walter Young's fame from winning the Boston Marathon did get him a place on the Verdun police force for a cadet's salary of $26.50 a week, and he had a regular paycheck for the next 41 years. Pawson had not run badly today. He couldn't call this race a comeback, but it was far better than he had been doing of late. Maybe he should train a little harder in the next year. Fame had worked for Pawson in 1933. It got him out of the mills and into a pleasant outside job. Too bad his running had not gone as well as it had before he was so favorably employed.

1937 Results

1.	W. Young, Verdun, PQ	2:33:20	14.	C. DeMar, Keene, NH	2:53:00
2.	J.A. Kelley, Arlington, MA	2:39:02	15.	C.R. Hill, *USMAA*	2:53:09
3.	L. Pawson, Pawtucket, RI	2:41:46	16.	M. Porter, Newark, NJ	2:54:00
4.	F. Ward, New York, NY	2:42:59	17.	W. Hornby, Hamilton, ON	2:55:35
5.	D. McCallum, Toronto, ON	2:43:16	18.	A.J. Brunelle, Medford, MA	2:55:38
6.	H. Kauppinen, Brooklyn, NY	2:46:06	19.	G.A. Norman, *USMAA*	3:00:02
7.	G. Cote, St. Hyacinthe, PQ	2:46:46	20.	P. Donato, *BClub*, MA	3:01:15
8.	J.W. Plouffe, Worcester, MA	2:46:53	21.	D. Komonen, Sudbury, ON	3:01:56
9.	J.D. Semple, *USMAA*	2:48:13	27.	B. Kennedy	3:04:44
10.	L. Giard, Brockton, MA	2:48:31	31.	E. Brown, RI	3:07:04
11.	G.L. Durgin, Beverly, MA	2:49:19	51.	F.W. Brown, *NMC*	3:23:15
12.	L. Gregory, *MillAA*	2:49:49	74.	W.H. Childs, Springfield, MA	NT
13.	A. Johnson, Port Chester, NY	2:50:02			

210 entrants.

NO FINER KING

TUESDAY, APRIL 19, 1938

Kelley and Dengis to Fight for Title

There was a joke afoot in 1938 that FDR's New Deal Works Progress Administration would put on the marathon. The country was still in the Great Depression and within that a recession that idled 20% of the work force. The Boston Athletic Association, once a pillar of fiscal strength, faced hard times, too, but they plowed on through to keep their marathon.

On the morning of the 1938 race, Les and Betty (Brooks) Pawson left their 13-month-old daughter, Joan, with the people downstairs and drove north from Pawtucket, Rhode Island, to Hopkinton. Les had eaten a steak breakfast at 9:00; on the drive he felt hungry, so he ate a hamburger. The last 5 years, since he had won Boston in course record time in 1933, had been an athletic disappointment for Pawson. He had suffered a stress fracture of the foot in that race, but recovered. He had not won anything significant since, yet he had not run so poorly as to think about quitting. He loved to run and really didn't want to give it up, but he was married and had a job and a daughter now. He wondered if this would be the last shot for him. To insure that if it were his parting shot it would be a good one, he had intensified his training. He usually ran hard when he ran, under 6 minutes per mile, but he often ran every other day. He had logged 450 miles of training since February, including a week with three 20-mile runs, and he weighed now what he weighed in 1933. Pawson's new job as foreman of People's Park in Pawtucket kept him outdoors and out of the stale air of the textile mill where he had been working before his 1933 win. The newspapers picked him along with five others as favorites for the marathon.

Pat Dengis came from Baltimore to race. His usual tactic was to start slowly and eat up the opposition to win. The story goes that he liked to warm up thoroughly and sometimes ran from Hopkinton to Framingham and back—at least 8 miles—just to warm up for a 26-mile race. He had taken Walter Young's coach, Pete Gavuzzi, as his own. Young himself could not get time off from his job on the Verdun, Quebec, police force, so he would not be racing this year to defend the title that got him the job. In the past year Dengis had won the Pan-Am Marathon in Dallas, the Yonkers Marathon, and the Port Chester Marathon, and in another marathon had finished second to Mel Porter, a 33-year-old civil engineer, in Washington, DC. Dengis was widely known for the sharply written barbs he aimed at other runners or races. Other runners, being members of a typically reticent breed, called Dengis flamboyant. He worked in an airplane factory and liked flying airplanes, which he did whenever he got the chance. His wife, Eva, blond and beautiful, attracted the press, who delighted in photos of her finish line embrace with Pat.

Johnny Kelley had outsprinted Gerard Cote, seventh in the Boston Marathon in 1937, in the North Medford Club 20-miler. Cote was staying in Arlington, not far from the Kelley residence. Kelley had left his job as a florist's assistant, spent many months unemployed, and now worked for the Boston Edison Company as a guard. His job was the envy of callous-handed marathoners because he could sit down at work and rest for his workout. Kelley no longer represented the North Medford Club but had dutifully transferred his loyalties to the Boston Edison Employees' Club. Canadian Duncan McCallum had run fifth last year. Pawson, Dengis, Kelley, Cote, McCallum, and the goodwill ambassador from Greece, 11th place (2:43:20) 1936 Olympian Stylianos Kyriakides, who would wear race #1 this year at Boston, waited with a couple hundred compatriots in Hopkinton. The prerace edition of the *Boston Post* put odds of 100 to 1 on DeMar, 15 to 1 on Semple, 4 to 1 on Dengis, Cote, and Kelley, and 6 to 1 on Pawson.

The day brought unexpected heat. (Weather prediction was not good in 1938—September 21 brought an unexpected hurricane that killed 682 people in New England. This was also the year of Wrong Way Corrigan's solo flight to Ireland instead of California and Hitler's consumption of Czechoslovakia.) The temperature in Boston reached an enervating 74 °F. The Boston papers agreed that 600,000 people came out to watch.

At Framingham Pawson and Kelley ran in 3rd and 4th while Dengis ran way back in 32nd. Kelley and Pawson shared water, sponges, and fruit provided by spectators and members of the large Kelley family. Walter Hornby, McCallum, Lou Gregory, Russell George, and Kyriakides bloomed early while old man DeMar, who would be 50 in June, ran 19th. Just before Natick, Pawson and Kelley took the lead. That hamburger churned in Pawson's stomach. As the minutes wore on, Kelley tired and faded, and by 18 miles Pawson ran alone. Kelley cast weary glances over his shoulder, knowing the relentless Dengis pursued him and would soon catch up.

Dengis figured that Pawson always fell back in the last 5 miles. But on this hot day, water stops were few. There was plenty of water from the officials for the leader and the next two, but after that there was little to be had. Cote had to beg for water from spectators. Pawson was glad he was out front, because he knew otherwise you didn't get any water.

Kelley stopped three times on Beacon Street and dumped water on his head. As Dengis passed him Kelley could not race, but the two exchanged pats on the back. At the start Kelley thought he could do no better than fourth, yet back on the Newton hills he had delusions of winning; but, in

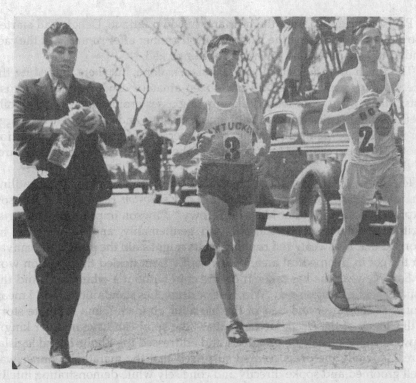

Les Pawson (#3) and Johnny Kelley (#2) are supplied a wet sponge by a well-dressed handler in the 1938 race. Courtesy of the Boston Public Library, Print Department.

his own words, "I got tired." Far ahead Dengis could see Pawson's red shorts bobbing as he ran down Beacon Street.

In the evening edition of the *Boston Daily Globe*, Jerry Nason, who was riding along in a Studebaker, described Pawson as "bronzed winged and free striding," running ahead of "grim pursuit by pulsating Pat Dengis." At Coolidge Corner Pawson almost stopped. He wore a white shirt with "Pawtucket" in a curve across his chest. His body begged for that internal quiet that comes after long, sustained effort. As he relaxed to yield to his craving, Betty was there. She yelled to him sharply. He straightened up and ran on.

Kyriakides dropped out at 21 miles with blisters. He said he could not run with blisters. He paid $1.25 for a taxi ride to the finish. He would come back to Boston in what would seem another lifetime to collect on that investment. While still running in the top five at 23 miles, McCallum collapsed into unconsciousness. He had to be carried from the course by two strong men. Later he had no recollection of the episode.

Pawson struggled with the heat and his own fatigue. Dengis had started too slowly. Like a sniper he had picked off runner after runner, but the race ended too soon for him. Pawson went unpicked.

The finish and the victory were Pawson's alone, but there, impeding the press photographers, were several dozen amateur candid camera enthusiasts. Many wore what looked like opera glasses around their necks, really German-made Leica cameras. With quick shutters and lenses relatively large for the postage-stamp-sized film, the cameras could snap excellent action shots. The press cameras took pictures of the candid cameras taking pictures of the runners.

The press, the runners, and the public loved Les Pawson. The headline for John W. English's story in the next day's *Boston Herald* read "Pawson Explodes Notion Plodder Must Be Screwy." Pawson impressed the sportswriters as intelligent, personable, and gentlemanly, and so neat that he worried that his sweaty red running pants might stain the pure white canvas on the cot in the medical area. Kelley said, "I am tickled that Pawson won it. For five years he has taken it on the chin without a whimper." And the usually acidic Dengis said, "Win, lose or draw, Les stands alone (and I mean alone) as the finest and best of the 'no alibi' runners." In a separate story Will Cloney of the *Herald* declared that "the sport can have no finer king." Pawson spoke on a radio broadcast and addressed the Rhode Island legislature. Generally the press seemed surprised that the marathon winner was well groomed and spoke directly and concisely while demonstrating intelligence in the handling of his personal affairs. They apparently believed that most marathoners were not clean, neat, or very bright.

The former great Tarzan Brown finished the race in a pathetic 3:38—more than an hour slower than he had run to win in 1936. Was he, in the stereotype of the day, a broken-down shiftless Indian, still penniless living in a tar paper shack with a wife and child and having done nothing useful with his fame? Some mocked Brown and called him worthless, but Ellison Myers Brown did not consider himself so. He possessed a degree of courage not generally acknowledged by the largely prejudiced American public to exist in native Americans.

1938 Results

1.	L. Pawson, Pawtucket, RI	2:35:34	13.	D. Komonen, Sudbury, ON	2:49:33
2.	P. Dengis, Baltimore, MD	2:36:41	14.	B. Steiner, New York, NY	2:50:53
3.	J.A. Kelley, Arlington, MA	2:37:34	15.	L. Giard, Beverly, MA	2:51:47
4.	M. Porter, New York, NY	2:39:55	16.	L. Evans, Montreal, PQ	2:52:21
5.	P. Donato, Roxbury, MA	2:42:05	17.	A. Brunelle, Medford, MA	2:52:37
6.	M. Mansulla, Brockton, MA	2:42:30	18.	G. Johnson, Port Chester, NY	2:56:43
7.	C. DeMar, Keene, NH	2:43:30	19.	B. Tilson, Hamilton, ON	2:58:57
8.	G. Cote, St. Hyacinthe, PQ	2:44:01	20.	C. Hill, Beverly, MA	2:59:06
9.	W. Hornby, Hamilton, ON	2:44:39	21.	J. Semple, Beverly, MA	3:00:26
10.	F. Ward, New York, NY	2:47:14	26.	B. Kennedy, NY	3:06:02
11.	A. Paskell, Cambridge, MA	2:47:34	29.	F. Brown, NMC	3:07:18
12.	H. Kauppinen, New York, NY	2:49:05	54.	E. Brown, Alton, RI	3:38:59

209 entrants, 180 starters.

JUST TARZAN IN THE RAIN

WEDNESDAY, APRIL 19, 1939

Dengis and Pawson to Battle for 26 Miles

During the 1936 Olympics Ellison Myers "Tarzan" Brown had gone into a bar in Berlin to drink some of the beer for which he had developed a fondness. There he met some Nazi blackshirts. He did not like them. They, no doubt, did not like him or his mahogany-hued skin. Brown fought them. He started it. He picked on them and rapped together a couple of their heads. Of course he was outnumbered, so he ultimately got the worst of it. The American team had to get him out of jail so he could run the Olympic marathon. And run he did. He looked like he would win the gold medal at 16 miles. Mysteriously he dropped out. He found out that he had a hernia. He did not tell anyone but went home to let it heal. There resided in Brown a quiet strength and a clear sense of moral indignation at what the Germans had become. Years before the American government mobilized to fight the racism of the Nazis, Tarzan Brown had fought them.

On April 19 a northeast storm darkened the skies in Hopkinton, a darkening that was compounded by a partial eclipse of the sun. The eagles who gathered to run and dallied around the Lucky Rock Manor before the start included the *Boston Post* favorite, Walter Young, who had at last achieved enough seniority on his police force to get the day off. He usually worked 15 hours a day with one day off in 15. Young felt fit because he had had no problems in a 32-mile run in the weeks before. His wife, Muriel, the one who doubted he would ever win the Boston Marathon, came to watch. She had become a believer.

Les Pawson, now an alderman in Pawtucket, seemed fit after his 56-minute 10-miler in Brighton, although Tarzan Brown had run a few seconds faster. Pawson had even been practicing. He had run a long one from Pawtucket to Attleboro and back, two 17-milers, and many 10-milers. Brown had won a 16.4-mile race in Syracuse and broke the course record. He seemed ready, but Kelley was not. Boston would be his first race of the season, and it showed in the extra 5 pounds he carried. But it was Gerard Cote, Young's teammate on the Verdun team, who had the best record going into this year's race. He had won the North Medford Club 20-miler, where Pawson ran third and Young fourth.

To a trained eye, Pat Dengis might be the man to watch. Dengis showed up in Boston with his pretty wife, Eva, and his strategist, old Bill Schlobohm. Bill had taken fifth place in the 1902 marathon. It was a surprise to see Dengis wearing suspenders. He said he was too skinny for his pants to stay up, and if he used a belt he had to tighten it so much that it hurt his back. He weighed 136 pounds and had a 27-inch waist. The prerace story by Will

Cloney of the *Boston Herald* called Dengis the "bellicose Baltimorean . . . with the roar of a lion and the heart of a lamb." That day another writer called him a spluttering Welshman, who had won 10 of his last 12 marathons. He wore a red sweatshirt to the start with his surname printed on it. The *Herald* reported that a man asked him, "May I shake your hand for luck?" Dengis replied, "You may kiss me if it will help."

George V. Brown, who usually fired an ancient gun to start the race, had died since the 1938 race. His son, Walter, fired the gun this year. By Framingham Pawson and Russell George, an Onondaga Indian, led with Cote in 3rd, Brown in 4th, and Young in 5th. Dengis stuck to his habit of starting slowly and ran in 15th place. In Framingham the leaders' time was a conservative 31:55 compared to Brown's blazing 30:23 in 1936. By Natick Brown had taken the lead. He was surprised that Young and Pawson let him do so. He passed Natick in 53:04 compared to his 50:43 in 1936. Young, Pawson, Cote, and Dengis had no recollection of how fast Brown had run before. They did recall that he had slowed considerably over the last several miles, so they paced themselves in expectation of a collapse. He passed Wellesley in 1:09:54, but he had gotten there in 1:07:31 in 1936. Brown ran easily. He had trained under Thomas Salimeno, who had seen to a regimen of plenty of long-distance running, steaks, and sleep. Rain came down in plastering sheets by Newton Lower Falls.

Brown hit the hills and accelerated. In the cool, wet air, uninhibited by heat, he could use his speed to the fullest. By the time he reached the other side, his Lake Street split was faster than in 1936, 1:57:47 compared to 1:59:43.

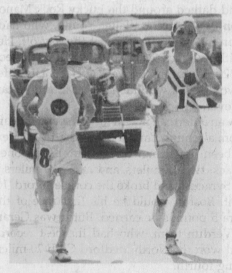

Johnny Kelley (#8) and Pat Dengis (#1) match strides. Within months Dengis would be dead. Photo courtesy of the *Boston Herald*.

It was faster yet by Coolidge Corner, as he flickered past in 2:12:39 compared to 2:16:17. Brown fooled them all. He did not slow. He did not tire. He did not drop back. Young, Pawson, Dengis, and especially Cote learned their lesson. On Exeter Street Brown saw the finish line ahead, slowed a little, and, in a compliment to his distant and invisible pursuers, looked back. He took a long look through the rain. He expected that someone would be there. But all he saw was the wind and the rain.

Tarzan Brown had just run a clever and an evenly paced marathon to victory, in a world best for the year at 2:28:51. The only accurate marathons ever run faster had been by Japanese runners: Kitei Son (Korean Ki Chung Sohn), 2:26:42; Yasuo Ikenaka, 2:26:44; and Fusashige Suzuki, 2:27:49, all in separate races in Tokyo in 1935. Ki Chung Sohn would run a 2:28:32 in 1940 in Tokyo, but had only run 2:29:19 in the Berlin Olympics. Brown, despite being the best marathon runner in the world, went home to his wife and 18-month-old child as he had left them that morning: an unemployed stonemason who would have preferred a job. Not only did he win, but he proved that he could come back from his poor performances and a virtual internal breakdown and win the Boston Marathon again. Still, the thrill for Brown had to remain in the pure sport of it. The prospects of a job for this Indian were low. He said he couldn't see any future in marathon racing, that he had earned a rest and would not run for the next couple of months.

A surprise was the 2nd-place finisher, Don Heinicke of Baltimore. He was a handsome man with clear blue eyes, who had come under the influence of Pat Dengis. Like Dengis, Heinicke started slowly, in 39th place at Framingham, and moved steadily through the pack. Dengis was 15th in Framingham and moved to 4th. He had expected to catch his protégé, but Heinicke kept just a bit ahead as both plowed ahead. Dengis expected Heinicke would one day win Boston. Dengis had been second twice, but he knew Heinicke had more natural speed to enable him to run a fast-enough time to win. Dengis had paid Heinicke's expenses to Boston from Baltimore, so jokingly, yet full of pride, he said young Don had bitten the hand that fed him.

Heinicke had taken up running after an accident with an old printing press in a tuberculosis sanatorium chewed four fingers off his right hand and ended his baseball career. He had been confined to the sanatorium with his stricken father and brother. They had died, but he survived. Heinicke worked in an industrial alcohol plant, where he held the unsavory job of extracting glycerin from molasses slops. It was dangerous work. Once a vat of boiling oil spilled, splashed, and burned both of Heinicke's arms. He bandaged them and ran anyway. Another accident gassed him and burned the insides of his already tuberculosis-scarred lungs, leaving him gasping with bloodshot eyes and flat on his back for a month. But Heinicke would be back to Boston again and again in pursuit of the gold medal with the unicorn on it.

1939 Results

1.	E. Brown, Westerly, RI	2:28:51^{CR}	12.	A. Mederios, *NMC*		2:41:24
2.	D. Heinicke, Baltimore, MD	2:31:24	13.	**J.A. Kelley, *BEEC***		**2:41:39**
3.	W. Young, Verdun, PQ	2:32:41	14.	G. Durgin, *BAA*		2:42:14
4.	P. Dengis, *MillAA*	2:33:22	15.	L. Evans, *MarAC*, Verdun, PQ		2:43:03
5.	L. Pawson, Pawtucket, RI	2:33:57	16.	J. Kleinerman, *STAC*, NY		2:44:25
6.	P. Donato, Roxbury, MA	2:34:25	17.	L. Young, *NMC*		2:45:24
7.	W. Hornby, *OC*	2:37:11	18.	J. Semple, *BAA*		2:45:45
8.	G. Cote, *MarAC*, Verdun, PQ	2:37:43	19.	A. Paskell, Cambridge, MA		2:46:15
9.	F. Bristow, *GladAC*, ON	2:38:44	20.	G. Dickson, Bronx, NY		2:46:24
10.	A. Brunelle, *NMC*, MA	2:39:09	30.	C. DeMar, Keene, NH		2:51:27
11.	F. McClose, *NYMCA*, MA	2:39:51	49.	F. Brown, *NMC*		3:08:54

Chapter 5

1940-1949
More War Years

Presidents: *Franklin Delano Roosevelt, Harry S. Truman*

Massachusetts Governors: *Leverett Saltonstall, Maurice J. Tobin, Robert Bradford*

Boston Mayors: *Maurice J. Tobin, John E. Kerrigan, James Michael Curley, John B. Hynes*

1940 Populations: *United States, 132,164,569; Massachusetts, 4,316,721; Boston, 770,816*

The 1940s featured big bands, blackouts, Rosie the Riveter, blitzkrieg, and Nazis. The names of Hitler, Himmler, Goebbels, Goering, Guderian's Panzers, and Rommel the Desert Fox countered those of Blood-and-Guts Patton, Ike Eisenhower, Monty Montgomery, and Douglas MacArthur in the newspapers. America went on rations, and propaganda flowed on all sides. The American public saw Humphrey Bogart in "Casablanca" and fell in love. Yet movies were only an escape from the ubiquitous war effort. America recycled, reused, and conserved anything that might be used as war material. The public feared a German or Japanese invasion. Automobile plants made tanks. Everybody worked. The economic depression lifted. Americans moved around the country to new cities for military and industrial purposes.

World War II depleted the numbers of Canadians who could come south to Boston to run. Canada had entered the war early with England. By the war's height any man in North America not in the military was suspect. Why did he not wear a uniform? Was he a draft-dodger? A coward? A German sympathizer? Of Japanese ancestry? In the mid-'40s it seemed that every other marathon entrant was a private, a sergeant, or an ensign. Some of these were the very men who had been chronically unemployed during the Great Depression.

Any innocence in the world died with the liberation of the concentration camps. The industrial killing of human beings horrified idealistic Americans, yet America itself remained a racially segregated society. The government forced Japanese-Americans into internment camps. And literally within sight of a future Boston Marathon winner, America used the most horrible weapon of all, the atomic bomb, in Hiroshima, Japan.

World War II ended in August of 1945, but immediately the Cold War began against a new enemy. Suspicion and fear of communism crept in. America emerged from the war with an economy as strong and powerful as the rest of the world's combined. Wealth and the good life, if either hadn't arrived for every American, seemed about to. Europe, Japan, and China lay in ruins. Africa still reeled from a dismemberment by colonial powers that themselves had been dismembered by the war. The American factories that had been converted to produce tanks now in their expanded form churned out automobiles. The U.S. population increased. The motion picture industry boomed. New highways ran everywhere. Suburbs sprang up. People in a postwar world began to dream again. Americans considered themselves the invincible, chosen people of Earth. As the world reordered before, during, and after the war, so did the sport of marathon racing.

The lowest turnout of entrants in the Boston Marathon had come during the height of the war in 1945. From that low, the numbers steadily rose.

By the end of the decade many American marathoners who had been in uniform took advantage of the GI bill and went to college. During the depths of the depression, they had never dreamed of this chance. In college they met the young speedy collegiate milers and 2-milers. The old vets planted the marathon bug in these youngsters' ears. The war provoked a change in the quality of men who would be attracted to the marathon. Younger, faster runners came. The aftermath of the war also drew in overseas runners, ending North American exclusivity forever.

Marathoners worldwide began to train as they had never trained before and to dream dreams of the Boston Marathon.

GERARD'S BIG CIGAR

FRIDAY, APRIL 19, 1940

Top Marathoner Dies in Plane Crash

On December 17, 1939, the single engine on a two-seater airplane flying 200 feet above the Maryland countryside sputtered, then quit entirely. The pilot, 21-year-old Richard Henry Sohn, banked sharply in the silence to avoid a clump of trees. The plane nosed over and slammed into a field. The impact killed the men in both seats, who worked for the Glen L. Martin airplane manufacturing company. Officials arriving on the scene found for identification only a note in the pocket of the passenger, an older, thinner man. The note held the name and address of marathon runner Don Heinicke. Officials investigated, but Don Heinicke answered at home, alive. The note had been carried by his mentor, his coach, marathoner Pat Dengis.

That morning Pat Dengis had forgotten to kiss his wife, Eva, goodbye. It was an oversight that could have been made up for later. He had kissed her in front of all the press at the finish of the Boston Marathon in 1935—photographs to prove it remained. A kiss is just a kiss. He was late; the kiss could wait.

He had been flight-testing the airplane that December day. Something went wrong. He could do nothing about it from his seat behind the pilot.

Dengis had been on the 1936 Olympic team, had won the prestigious Yonkers Marathon three times, and had won nearly every other marathon in the country except Boston. He planned that if he couldn't win Boston, his protégé would.

In the spring of 1940 Heinicke won the Pat Dengis Memorial Marathon in Baltimore. Running it severely compromised his chances at Boston, but he had to run for Pat. And wouldn't it be perfect if he could win "The Boston" for Pat too? The sudden death of Pat Dengis moved the entire running community as it did Fred Griffin and the sports editors of the *Boston Daily Globe*, who made room to print a poem to a dead marathon runner:

Pat Dengis

Ah, little we thought as he hurried past
That the die of Fate was already cast
And that he was running his final race
Though the hue of health was upon his face:
As he swept in view with a gallant zeal
And answered the challenger at his heel
It was plain to see by his twisted grin
He was claimed by all though he might not win.

How he liked to run in the wind and rain
With a boundless vim he could not restrain
Though never the laurel of brief renown
Might his brow adorn with a victor's crown
And his heart was seared with a mighty thirst
That could not be stayed till he entered first
But the Fates stepped in and they flogged his pride
Till he lost his pace and he stood denied.

O, the shot shall herald a braver start
But it shall not liven that stiffened heart

For the span of life is a thinning thread
And the conquered and conqueror soon are read:
But to those who dream in the haunts of yore
And to those whose senses are quick to score
He'll come sweeping down like a hurricane
With the gods that were in his swirling train.

—*Fred Griffin*

Eva would go with Pat's friend, old Bill Schlobohm, to the marathon start this year at the Lucky Rock Manor. It would be difficult for her to be there, but it might have been more difficult not to be. Running was Pat's life, and she was his.

Headlines on April 19 in the Boston newspapers told that Canadians would go to Norway to fight the Nazi invasion. Canadians stood with England against the Nazis as the battle for Trondheim neared. Gerard Cote of St. Hyacinthe, Quebec, intended to join them by way of the Royal Air Force as soon as they accepted his application. But for now he came to Boston to race the marathon again and improve on his eighth place of 1939. Jerry Nason of the *Globe* picked Cote to finish seventh and Tarzan Brown to win again. Jock Semple picked Les Pawson to win. Johnny A. Kelley thought that Canadian Scotty Rankine had built himself up to a marathon. Kelley said, "He doesn't look like a runner at all. . . . He fools you because he is so little. He has worlds of speed. He can run like a mad man at short distances." Rankine had won the Berwick modified marathon 5 years in a row at a distance of 12 miles, but he still ran a 2:34 marathon to win the Canadian championships. Paul Donato didn't look like a runner either, but many picked him to win. He was a little man with a big body and a bigger head. He was, in Nason's words, "squat, broad-chested, short legged. . . . [Donato,] with the hide of a leopard draping his powerful torso, . . . might easily pass as the strong man in the circus. Paul is power conveniently carried." And power, according to Nason, destined to closely follow Brown. Donato ran for the General Electric Athletic Association. He wore their big "GE" logo on his big chest.

Old Clarence DeMar at age 51 came to Boston looking for a job. The course he taught at the Keene Normal School had been dropped, and another temporary post had folded. He came to the *Boston Herald* offering to work as a compositor on the night of the marathon to pick up a night's pay. They took him up on it. After running 26 miles as hard as he could, he stood on those same feet setting type from dark until well after midnight.

Cote had prepared himself well. In 1935 he came under the wing of a refugee of the vanishing world of professional racing, Pete Gavuzzi. Gavuzzi's training philosophy of long, long, slow, slow distance had not changed since the days of Walter Young. He commonly advised 35- and 40-mile runs. In 1935 Cote ran a 50-mile time trial in 6:59.

Pete Gavuzzi trained and trained Cote. He ran along beside his athletes, talked and ran. Gavuzzi had trained Young and Dengis. Cote placed second to Dengis for 3 frustrating years at Yonkers—1937, 1938, 1939. One time Dengis, who usually started more slowly than anyone, caught up to Cote. Dengis paused as he passed. He leaned over and flamboyantly kissed Cote goodbye and ran away. Cote wanted to do that. Maybe not the kissing, but definitely the running away. Cote had been obsessed with Boston ever since Walter Young had won in 1937. In his preparation for Boston, Cote lowered Young's 10-mile snowshoe record from 1:06 to 1:03.

Cote stayed with his cousin, Charley Goulet, in Central Falls, Rhode Island. For the 2 weeks before the race Cote followed Gavuzzi's rule that 3 hours of slow running is better than 2 hours fast. He ran with heavy running shoes and a sweatsuit that stuck to him in the thick Rhode Island air. Cote was used to crisp Quebec air, so the weather in south Rhode Island felt like the humidity of midsummer. In the 2 weeks before the race, he ran a marathon in 3:50 and another in 2:50 over a course with a hill per mile.

Gerard Armand Cote passed his boyhood in a farmhouse in St. Barnabe, in the Quebec countryside east of Montreal. The Cotes had 26 cows and 7 horses. Summers were hot and rich, while winters were snowy and sparse. St. Hyacinthe was 10 miles away. The Roman Catholic church governed the actions of people as much as did the Canadian government. Quebec was nearly a country separate from English-speaking Canada. Will Cloney of the *Herald* wrote that Cote said this in his French-Canadian accent: "Eeef I talk In-gleesh at home in St. Hyacinthe I am a sissy. We have a popilation of twentee tousand, and only about five peeple are In-gleesh. French only is teached in school."

The Cote family had about 15 children; Gerard did not know exactly how many because some died in infancy. He was somewhere in the middle, born on July 28, 1913. As a child he ran errands for the family. He would be the one to go fetch: "From age five to eleven I was always on the go. . . . They say, 'Go over there and get me something,' you get rolling. You try to come back fast and prove that you're good."

For sports, boxing was everywhere, so Cote tried it. Like Walter Young he found that he was much better at the roadwork than the ringwork. When he heard of a professional race he showed up to run. A gruff, leathery-faced old man who was touted to win pulled young Cote away. Professional racing was dying, and the old man knew that. He said, "I'm an old man and I don't care if you beat me, but you're young. If I were you I wouldn't run this race." Had he run he would have sacrificed the amateur status necessary to run in the Boston Marathon. Cote did not run. The old man was Edouard Fabre, the 1915 Boston Marathon winner.

Cote led a bunched pack through Framingham in a time a little faster (31:39) than Brown's in 1939 (31:55) but much slower than Brown's in 1936 (30:23). Kelley, Pawson, Rankine, and Brown followed. By Natick Pawson took the lead, with Rankine, Cote, Kelley, and Heinicke moving up the way

Dengis had liked to move. Cote ran comfortably in third. Pawson had won in 1933 and 1938 but felt unfit. He was now a 32-year-old Pawtucket alderman and a parent who held down a full-time job. Those responsibilities cut into his training time. But he had no alibis. His endurance preparation had generally been 350 miles for the Boston race, but this year it was only 200. Pawson resolved to prepare himself thoroughly next time. He settled into survival pace. Next time he thought, next time.

Heinicke felt sick to his stomach. He had had too much endurance preparation. He knew the effort to win the Dengis Memorial Marathon hurt him, but perhaps the runners ahead would come back to him. Through Wellesley Kelley waved at the girls. They waved back. Brown burst into the lead. Few could read him. He did not wave. In 1936 he had been 2 minutes faster in Wellesley. This year his pace seemed reasonable. In Wellesley Square Kelley felt a grabbing sensation in his left leg. On the downhills it sent exquisite pains through him. He thought he would die. Brown looked like a winner again.

Nason described his pick: "The hunch players are putting their wampum on the flying feet of Ellison Brown." Brown indeed had feet that flew, but his face revealed nothing. When he ran he showed no expression—he did not smile, wave, or grimace. His face looked serene and his stride butter-smooth. Not Kelley, not his coach Tippy Salimeno, not Nason, perhaps not even Brown himself, could tell what he would do.

Through Wellesley Rankine, Pawson, Kelley, Heinicke, and Cote followed Brown. Six men essentially ran together. By Auburndale (1:32:55; Brown's 1936 record was 1:31:49), Cote had passed Pawson, feeling not the slightest bit tired. A brisk tailwind helped everyone. Cote ran in white shorts and a white shirt with a rich red Canadian mapleleaf. As Cote ran, the red dye ran from the leaf onto his shorts. At a quick glance he looked gruesome, as if his heart had burst.

Brown slowed on the uphill out of Newton Lower Falls, hungry. Someone offered him an ice cream bar. He ate it; it tasted good; he ate another. He slowed while his digestion worked. Kelley and Rankine battled for the lead up the hills. Cote ran in third, 200 yards behind their dueling. Brown saw that Cote was smart to let Kelley and Rankine wear themselves out fighting. But he could not take advantage of the situation. Ice cream bars filled him with complacency. He drifted back and away. Runner after runner passed him. Cote thought that Brown's good races happened mostly by grace or good luck. At Lake Street Kelley thought he had the race won as he burst away from Rankine, but out of nowhere came Cote. He jumped Kelley at the juncture of Beacon Street and Dean Road—4 miles from Exeter Street. Cote ran away from Kelley, whose glee in leading fled. He stumbled down the road as Cote ran smoothly and smugly down Beacon Street. Pat Dengis had said of Kelley, "Kelley's the greatest marathon runner in the world for 20 miles. He runs the next three miles on his guts and damned if I know how he ever manages to finish from there, but he does."

At Coolidge Corner Kelley reached for a piece of maple sugar candy. It came from the hand of 1919 Boston Marathon winner Carl Linder. Kelley said the candy saved his life. Good thing. Heinicke closed quickly. But Cote had already run too far away and felt too strong. Cote, with two gold teeth. Cote, the archetypal Quebec Frenchman. Cote, the man with vim and a wardrobe to match. Cote, the man who smoked a couple of cigars a day and sometimes a pipe. That zesty Cote won by almost 4 minutes. But there was more to this Cote than zest.

Two days before the race Jerry Nason of the *Globe* had written, to explode the myth of the exhausted marathon winner, that he "is supposed to flop at the tape in a dying swan act, his feet torn to ribbons, his sides heaving like a pair of bellows, and his thoughts as scattered as those of the recipient of a belt from an axe-helve." Nason rightly explained that the well-trained marathon runner does not flop at the tape as the myth seems to require. Cote ran to detonate that myth. At the finish he said, "I could have kept running for ten more miles." Indeed, he looked as if he could as he ran to the finish line on Exeter Street, waving and blowing kisses to the crowd.

Cote held court for the press in his Lenox Hotel room. His long-time

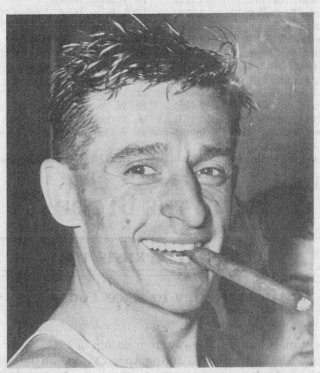

Gerard Cote knew how to win the marathons and enjoy life, but in a few years both pastimes would get him in trouble with the Canadian army. Courtesy of the Boston Public Library, Print Department.

dream of winning Boston had come true. It was time to celebrate. He ordered scotch and port wine from room service for himself and the reporters. He had a deal going with the manager of the hotel, so he got a free room every year. He lit a big cigar, put his feet up, and took all questions. They called him a dapper-dandy. Cote worked as a newspaper distributor, but it was a job that did not occupy much of his time. His father had become a building contractor in Montreal, but Gerard waited as the economy switched from depression to wartime. What the future would bring he did not know. He had been in the military reserves for years. That night Cote danced at the Hotel Statler until 2 o'clock.

Cote wanted to come back to defend his title at Boston, but he feared his military obligations would prevent a return: "I don't know what the war will do to us Canadians."

1940 Results

1. G. Cote, *MarAC*, PQ	2:28:28CR*	14. L. Young, *NMC*	2:44:57
2. J.A. Kelley, *BEEC*, MA	2:32:03	15. A. Mederios, *NMC*	2:48:14
3. D. Heinicke, *SDC*, MD	2:32:21	16. J. Smith, *NMC*	2:48:52
4. L. Pawson, Pawtucket, RI	2:33:09	17. L. Evans, *MarAC*, Verdun, PQ	2:48:55
5. P. Donato, *GEAA*	2:34:54	18. W. Smallcombe, *RRAC*, PQ	2:50:26
6. A. Brunelle, *NMC*	2:35:20	19. I. Amicangioli, *BAA*	2:51:02
7. R. Rankine, *SWH*, Preston, ON	2:37:44	20. A. Paskell, *NMC*	2:51:05
8. F. McGlone, *NYMA*	2:37:49	27. C. DeMar, Keene, NH	2:55:32
9. G. Durgin, *BAA*	2:38:21	29. J. Semple, *BAA*	2:58:10
10. F. Darrah, *NYMA*	2:43:38	33. J. Kleinerman, *GAC*, NY	3:04:37
11. A. Johnson, *ISC*, NY	2:44:01	40. W. Young, *MarAC*, PQ	3:14:57
12. J. Blaggie, Cambridge, MA	2:44:31	48. P. Polletta, Amesbury, MA	3:26:55
13. E. Brown, Westerly, RI	2:44:45	69. B. Chapinski, *PYMC*, MA	NT

193 entrants, 165 starters.
*Second fastest in the world that year. Ellison Brown ran 2:27:29.6 in Salisbury, Massachusetts.

IT'S IN THE BLOOD

SATURDAY, APRIL 19, 1941

Cote, Kelley to Race Today

The war kept most Canadians away from Boston in 1941. Hitler's Panzers swept down the Balkan peninsula during April. On the 18th the Greek prime minister, Alexander Koryzis, committed suicide. By the end of the month the British would again evacuate Europe, with the Germans on their heels. The United States still exported 400,000 to 600,000 barrels of oil a week to

Japan. Only Canadians Gerard Cote and Scotty Rankine came to race, Rankine by grace of a furlough from the Canadian army. Marathon defender Cote would become Sergeant Cote by November 15.

Les Pawson arrived at his best and could prove it. He had won the time prize a few weeks earlier in the Cathedral Handicap 10-miler in 51:38, and that race was a good predictor. It looked as if Pawson had re-earned his winning 1933 shape, when he set a Boston course record.

Johnny Kelley looked to be in good shape, too, but he had bad dreams of second places to banish. He was often nervous and sleepless. Kelley was unpopular with fellow runners because he was so anxious and disjointed before a race that he never talked to them. After a race, if he won he was so happy that he talked only to reporters. If he lost, he sulked in private. In bed the night before a race, and especially Boston, Kelley would run the race over and over in his mind. Jerry Nason of the *Boston Globe* wrote, "Kelley's lost at least a couple of marathons the night before." But Kelley had married Mary Knowles, a stenographer for the Bird's Eye frozen foods company, and perhaps marriage would calm him. He had moved in with Mary and her mother. He had met her at his Massachusetts Avenue streetcar stop in Arlington, asking her the time of day. Soon she made sandwiches for him and accompanied the Kelley clan to road races.

Fred McGlone, a railroad brakeman in Roxbury and born in Natick, had run 52 minutes in the Cathedral race. He looked dangerous. Lou Gregory, a schoolteacher from Batavia, New York, might finally put together a marathon as effectively as he put together races at the shorter distances.

U.S. Army Private Anthony "Hawk" Zamparelli took an immediate lead in the 45th running of the Boston Marathon. He had to. He knew he was not his fittest, but the boys back in 211th Coast Artillery, Battery B, at Camp Hulen, Texas, had each chipped in a dime or a dollar so "Hawk" could travel back to his hometown and race again. His falconine face gave rise to his nickname, but the name stuck because of his racing speed. He told his comrades that he had a game leg and would not be at his best, but they insisted. So Hawk, once in the battle, made his presence felt. Because of the bad leg he had to show himself sooner than later. With a bandage on his knee Zamparelli took the lead and held it as long as he could. But at 74 °F, he did not last long. Mother Nature could not to be fooled by bravery, and Zamparelli dropped back into the pack.

At the first checkpoint Pawson ran in sixth place with Rankine just behind him and Kelley, Cote, Gregory, long-jawed Joe Kleinerman of New York, and Don Heinicke ahead of him, in that order. After 1940's poor fourth-place performance Pawson wanted badly to win this race. Unlike the year before he had trained effectively and in quantity. He always trained at a 6-minute per mile pace or better, and this year he completed his self-required 400 miles of pre-Boston training. But he was 36 years old, not 28 as he had been in 1933. Pawson planned a sneak attack. He turned to Rankine and said, "When we go by these fellows we are going to go by for keeps." He wanted a psychological advantage. Each runner he passed allowed him to proceed unencumbered. But when Pawson tried to pass Kelley, Kelley hung on like a terrier. Pawson felt content to run side by side with Kelley. Pawson had eaten his breakfast of a bowl of meal with figs in it, then traveled in the family car with his wife, Betty, driving. She expected another child in July. Their 4-year-old daughter, Joan, rode along too. The family lived on the third floor of a three-family house in Pawtucket. Pawson still served as alderman in his town. They stopped on the way from Pawtucket to Hopkinton, in Milford, where Pawson ate two eggs.

Pawson—eggs, figs, and all—took the lead by Wellesley, with Kelley at his side. The hot sun sucked the energy out of both men. Pawson dumped water on his head at every chance. The *Globe* reporter wrote, ''His raven's wing hair was plastered in strings over his weather beaten face.'' The dye of his red shirt stained his white shorts. The burning daylight broiled Pawson's shoulders lobster-red. In 1933 it was cold wind that had reddened his skin.

Pawson ran as cars with water traveled alongside. A hundred times during the course of the race he took water from attendants in the vehicles and passed it across his chest from one hand into the other hand to offer the cup to Kelley. Over and over Pawson expended his own energy to hand water to his competitor. A small muscle in Pawson's left thigh bothered him. He knew he could press the pace as long as that sore muscle did not get worse. Pawson knew that the best place on this course to make up time was from Natick to the foot of the hills. He pressed. On one hand he tried to kill the enemy who ran next to him with a fast pace, and with the other hand he gave the enemy aid and comfort in the form of cool water and orange slices.

Don Heinicke watched this exchange. One of these years Boston would be his to win. Second place in 1939 was not enough; he wanted it all. But not this year; Heinicke's socks rolled up under his feet at Wellesley. He stopped to remove them. He got his body rolling again in the last few miles, but he rolled too little too late. It seemed too late as well for Brown and Gregory. They vanished from the course somewhere around Wellesley.

Pawson and Kelley ran away. They ran away from Heinicke, Cote, Joe Smith, Fred McGlone, and a neat little man with an efficient running style named Andre Brunelle. The thorough preparation began to pay for Pawson. At Lake Street he ran away from Kelley.

With a mile to go the pain in Pawson's thigh became intense. He stopped and walked a few steps. Kelley ran 250 yards behind. Pawson's pain settled back to a tolerable dullness, and he resumed running without interruption. He turned onto Exeter Street and won the Boston Marathon for the third time, in 2:30:38. Only DeMar had won more.

Defeat crushed Kelley—he had placed second for the fourth time in 8 years. "Kelley finished into the arms of his father and then his wife, upon whose shoulders he leaned heavily," wrote Will Cloney of the *Herald*.

After his victory Pawson sat on a cot and paused before answering reporters' questions. He said it was hot like in 1931 when Henigan had won. That year Leslie Pawson had finished in 23rd place in 3:24. He paused again. "Kinda warm," Pawson said.

Defeat crushed Johnny A. Kelley—he had placed second for the fourth time in 8 years. He finished into the arms of his father and then his wife.

Nason reported that a small man with a big smile approached the cot. "I've always wanted to meet you, Pawson. My name is Miles, Johnny Miles. I won this race back in the twenties." Pawson brightened, "Gee, I'm glad to meet you, Johnny. You ran a real marathon race."

To another question Pawson answered, "I will keep on marathoning. I suppose it's in the blood." Leslie Samuel Pawson did run for many more years and remained a close friend to Kelley. He served as best man at Kelley's third wedding. Pawson died at age 87 on October 13, 1992, in Pawtucket, Rhode Island.

Marathoning is definitely in the blood of Bricklayer Bill Kennedy, who finished his 28th Boston Marathon. He said he got more tired laying bricks than running marathons. Gerard Cote, effervescent even in defeat, said, "I lose so many races, I don't mind losing another one." Marathoning is in the blood of these men. It was in their heads too. In a literal, circulatory sense, it takes so much blood and heart to run a marathon. To run marathons may have been why these men had blood, veins, hearts, and minds in the first place.

The heat must have gotten Clarence DeMar's blood boiling, because he hit two spectators. One came up to him while he was running and asked for his autograph. DeMar socked him. The other dumped an unsolicited pail of water on DeMar's legs. DeMar socked him too. Again DeMar worked the night shift in the *Herald* compositing room.

O. Gardner Spooner, who was 53 and minus a right hand, finished 53rd. Three decades later he would die while out on a training run.

The captain of the BAA team, 37-year-old Jock Semple, made a big sprint for the finish to get the last of the prizes. He was now listed as an unemployed ship joiner. He proclaimed in his Scots brogue, "Mon, o, mon it's gude ta be in the mooney ageen!" His eighth-place finish made Semple the highest finishing member of the sponsoring club since Jimmy Lee's sixth place in 1908.

Milkman Joe Smith of the North Medford Club sprinted down Exeter Street to beat "Bud" McGlone of the Norfolk YMA. The month before the two of them had tied in the North Medford Club 20-miler. That lighthearted display brought down the wrath of Smith's teammates. They thought runners should not tie in races, and should *absolutely* not tie with members of other clubs. To runners of the North Medford Club, racing was serious business.

But the serious business of world war would soon smash into the lives of these men.

1941 Results

1. L. Pawson, Pawtucket, RI	2:30:38*	13. J. Anderson, *NYMA*	2:54:57
2. J.A. Kelley, *BEEC*	2:31:26	14. F. Kelley, Philadelphia, PA	2:56:42
3. D. Heinicke, Baltimore, MD	2:35:40	15. J. Riley, *NYMA*	2:58:26
4. G. Cote, St. Hyacinthe, PQ	2:37:59	16. W. Simons, *BAA*	2:58:52
5. J. Smith, *NMC*	2:40:32	17. G. Petrakos, Lowell, MA	2:59:56
6. F. McGlone, *NYMA*	2:40:44	18. L. Young, *NMC*	3:02:09
7. A. Brunelle, NMC	2:43:28	19. R. Eland, *BAA*	3:03:18
8. J. Semple, *BAA*	2:47:26	20. C. DeMar, *BT*	3:05:37
9. P. Donato, *GEAA*	2:49:02	21. A. Mederios, *NMC*	3:06:25
10. J. Kleinerman, *MillAA*	2:50:48	23. A. Zamparelli, Texas	3:10:30
11. M.J. O'Hara, *MillAA*	2:52:16	24. W. Kennedy, NY	3:11:29
12. L. Giard, North Randolph, MA	2:54:10	27. W. Childs, Springfield, MA	3:25:38

124 starters.
*Fastest marathon time in the world in 1941; Kelley's was second.

WAR!

SUNDAY, APRIL 19, 1942

McGlone Expected to Win Marathon

By April of 1942 the United States had been at war with Germany and Japan for 4 months, but MacArthur had abandoned the Philippines and Americans marched to death on Bataan. Corregidor would next fall to the Japanese. In Europe Hitler's armies ruined Stalin's armies.

A tradition had developed in the Boston Marathon to crown the winner with a wreath of laurel leaves picked in Greece, where the marathon originated. Greek-American George Demeter had for years gone to considerable expense to procure wreaths of real Greek laurel. He would wait at the finish line, and as the winner approached would ready himself. He would run the last few steps alongside the winner and place the wreath on the victor's head. Photos of Demeter chasing the winner, the laurel wreath hovering like a halo, appeared often in the papers. But this year the Greek laurel bushes belonged to the Nazis. No expense on Demeter's part could get real Greek laurel to Boston. The refugee mayor of Athens, Costas Kotsias, came to Boston to award the winner an olive branch grown in California and a wreath of American laurel.

The war brought other changes to the marathon. Traditionally, when Patriots' Day fell on Sunday, the race was held the following day. This year, Governor Leverett Saltonstall requested that the race be run on Sunday instead so defense workers could watch. Along the course air raid wardens stood on duty with badges and clubs. Gerry Hern wrote in the *Boston Post* that "the corner-of-the-mouth crack from insipid, lounging spectators won't seem half as funny this year, because a nation needs men of stamina and physical endurance."

In the fall of 1941 during the Salem-to-Lawrence (Massachusetts) road race an automobile slammed into Les Pawson, severely injuring him. He would not recover until 1943. Joe Smith, who had insouciantly tied the previous year's North Medford 20-miler with a runner from another club and then finished fifth in the Boston Marathon had recently recovered from a nervous ailment, but he suffered now from another mysterious malady. Smith's North Medford teammates knew that he had a gift for running but refused to ever make himself suffer any discomfort. They knew that if he'd ever push himself to the limit, he could run a very fast marathon.

Marathon day in eastern Massachusetts stayed 40 °F, chilly, gray, and windless. Fred McGlone, the runner Smith had tied with, originally of Natick and now of Roxbury, looked like a winner. He took the early lead. His hometown supporters stretched a banner across the road wishing "Bud" victory. Smith sat on marathon morning complaining about how rotten he felt. His wife, Isabell, told him he had moaned and groaned the same way on the morning before he won last year's National Championship at Yonkers. She told him to quit his bellyaching because he would win Boston too. Joe didn't think so. Joe felt that he would be lucky to make 13 miles. He told John W. English of the *Boston Herald*, "I was sick last winter. I only had six two-hour workouts, but I did get some speed work." He ran in eighth place through Framingham while McGlone held the lead. McGlone seemed a reasonable favorite. Last year he ran laughing into sixth place. That race had been a lark. What if he really tried? He had really tried in the Cathedral 10-mile handicap a few weeks earlier and posted the day's fastest time, 49:36 on the course. (How short was it?) But perhaps the pressure of being prerace favorite was too much for McGlone. Smith had looked at him at the start and saw a mirthless, ashen-white face. Johnny Kelley and Johnny Coleman wore the same bloodless mask. But Joe Smith felt lighthearted and just a bit cajoled by the missus.

Mayor Maurice Tobin rode in a car following favorite son McGlone, supplying him with water. In one attempt Hizzonner jammed his own hand into the the car door and required medical attention. McGlone did not look good himself. In Newton Coleman, a big, strong 20-year-old insurance clerk from Worcester, broke past McGlone and into the lead. Coleman wore the unicorn on his chest. Johnny Semple trained him. Coleman wanted to be the first BAA runner to win the marathon. Semple wanted someone he coached to win it if he himself could not do it. Semple had gotten the team captaining/coaching/training bug in the depression days when he organized a running team of the United Shoe Company in Beverly. That team had won the Boston Marathon team prize. Semple and his BAA team would love to beat the North Medford Club. To win the individual race seemed reasonable to Coleman. He had beaten Kelley, McGlone, Heinicke, Joe Smith, and the rest in the North Medford Club 20-miler in March. He had won the time prize in the Brighton Presentation Handicap a short time later. The marathon was the next step in his progression.

Kelley raced after Coleman, with McGlone racing after the two of them. They exchanged positions as they surged past each other on the hills. They had all run through a fast 10 miles and now brutalized each other on the hills. Kelley cracked first. He walked on the long hill by the Brae Burn Country Club. McGlone passed Coleman at Center Street. Coleman's mood changed from youthful aggression to despair. A mile later Coleman dropped out of the race. Ellison Brown dropped out of the race in Wellesley. His manager/trainer, Tippy Salimeno, picked him up in a car; he changed his clothes there and was in Rhode Island before the winner finished. Joe Smith ran comfortably through the hills in fifth place. He adapted his pace to his own feelings and not the surges of his overzealous competitors. It pleased him that he had made it past 13 miles. He never looked back. He kept a line on those in front and figured his own race.

McGlone wobbled and, notwithstanding the mayor's attentions, slowed. Lou Gregory caught McGlone at Boston College. Gregory had been training in the snows of upstate New York, where he taught school. He had been trying to win "The Boston" for years. He didn't want to let himself think that he had won it with 6 miles to go, but at the same time, he wanted to believe he had it won. With all the hills behind him at Lake Street Gregory looked like the winner. But McGlone had looked as invincible only a few miles earlier. Smith cruised past the early surgers. He still felt rotten, but not any more so than he had at the beginning. Every additional mile gave him a boost until only Gregory ran ahead of him. But Smith closed.

Smith ran because he liked to run when running felt good. He had told himself that he would train in order to win Boston and if he were lucky enough to win he would then retire from racing. Smith did not see himself as a fanatic. His fellow runners considered him rather lazy. And even as he was about to take the lead in the Boston Marathon, he had no intention of inflicting himself with pain. When Smith caught Gregory somewhere along Beacon Street, they looked in each others' eyes. Gregory did not want to believe Smith had arrived. Gregory's eyes had sunken and his eyebrows crumpled together. Gregory had dropped out last year. He had trained more this year. He had redoubled his efforts. But was it enough? He ran with tension in his face. Smith's face showed serenity; he may have felt queasy, but his face showed control. He was well past 13 miles and feeling no worse. That made him feel better. Gregory's training had not been enough. That made him feel worse. And finally, in the lead of the Boston Marathon, running did feel good for Smith, very good. Smith ran away to victory, feeling no pain.

An odd thing about Smith's race was that he did not break any checkpoint records. He did not arrive at Coolidge Corner as fast as Brown had in 1939 or even as fast as Cote the next year. But from Coolidge Corner to the finish

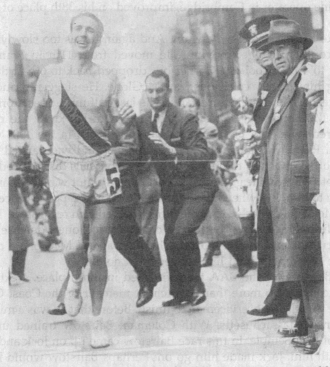

Milkman Joe Smith wins in 1942. Shortly after his victory a woman told him that he should be carrying a gun in the war, not running marathons. Photo courtesy of the *Boston Herald*.

Joe Smith ran faster than anyone. One reporter wrote that he "ran with fetching gayety." He smiled and waved to friends along the way. He was a milkman, a family man, president of the North Medford Club, a Medford resident, lanky, talkative and really named *Bernard* Joseph Smith. President Smith led his club to the team title. He was 6'2" and in winning broke Cote's course record by 1:37. Smith said, "When I don't train, I always do well. . . . I didn't train for Yonkers and look what happened. [He won.] I didn't think I had a chance today. I hadn't trained the way I wanted to." He told Arthur Duffey of the *Post*, "I run because I like to."

Costas Kotsias rushed up to Smith with his wreath of American laurel. As he presented it he said,

> The battle of Marathon marked the defeat of the barbarians. In historic Boston, the Athens of America, this event, symbolic of victory, promises that in the near future a triumphant soldier will arrive announcing to the American people and the world once again a victory over the barbarians."

Lou Gregory also broke the course record, and Carl Maroney, a 27-year-old machine operator in Cambridge, improved on his 38th place of last year with 3rd.

Heinicke had started slowly again. And again it was too slowly. Cote, it seemed, could never get moving. He moved from 11th in Framingham gradually to 4th at Coolidge Corner but dropped back to 6th at the finish. Following him, barely conscious, ran McGlone. He staggered and fell on Exeter Street. That was his third fall in the last half mile. Spectators offered help, but McGlone wanted to finish on his own. He knew the rules. He remembered what had happened to Dorando Pietri in the 1908 Olympic marathon. Pietri had fallen just before finishing and was carried by well-meaning officials across the finish line. Other officials disqualified him, so he was not awarded the gold medal. McGlone did not want the same thing to happen to him. But when he fell for the third time, a police officer helped him up. McGlone protested, but the officer helped him regardless. The BAA officials disqualified him. The mayor came to McGlone's defense, but the BAA officials would not be moved. They did award McGlone a duplicate prize, but everyone behind him moved up a notch.

Lloyd Bairstow of the BAA team finished in ninth place. Next year he planned to move up more than a notch. A member of the Coast Guard in Maine, he was the first serviceman to finish. Before that he was a millworker in Lawrence, Massachusetts. With Coleman, Bairstow trained under the tutelage of Jock Semple. In this race Bairstow came up on Jock and wanted to run with him. Jock made him go on. Perhaps Bairstow would be Jock's BAA Boston winner? But others had other priorities.

Kelley said that after the race a woman came up to Joe Smith to say, "You should be off carrying a gun in the war." The comment angered Smith.

1942 Results

1. J. Smith, *NMC*	2:26:51^{CR*}	
2. L. Gregory, *MillAA*, NY	2:28:03	
3. C. Maroney, *NMC*	2:36:13	
4. D. Heinicke, *WHC*, MD	2:37:24	
5. J.A. Kelley, *BEEC*	2:37:55	
6. G. Cote, *TC*, Montreal, PQ	2:39:59	
DSQ F. McGlone, *NYMA*, MA	2:40:07**	
7. W. Steiner, *MillAA*, NY	2:40:42	
8. M. O'Hara, *MillAA*, NY	2:41:08	
9. L. Bairstow, *BAA*	2:41:55	
10. J. Kleinerman, *MillAA*, NY	2:45:51	
11. A. Mederios, *NMC*	2:46:14	

12. B. Mazzeo, Portland, ME	2:47:19
13. R. Eland, *BAA*	2:48:32
14. J. Semple, *BAA*	2:49:03
15. A. Brunelle, *NMC*	2:49:45
16. F.L. Brown, *NMC*	2:50:31
17. P. Donato, *GEAA*	2:51:35
18. C. Robbins, Jr., CT	2:51:55
19. L. Giard, Randolph, MA	2:52:30
20. W. Wicklund, *PatAC*, NJ	2:53:45
24. C. DeMar, *BT*	2:58:14
33. F.W. Brown, *NMC*, MA	3:06:53

145 entrants.

*Fastest time in the world in 1942. Gregory's was second.

**Aided at the finish line.

MILITARY MARATHONERS

SUNDAY, APRIL 18, 1943

War Won't Stop Runners in Boston

Coxswain Lloyd Bairstow of the United States Coast Guard traveled down from his base on Cape Porpoise, Maine, to run the 1943 Boston Marathon. For fear of German U-boat attacks, a blackout order held for the coastline. A coat of opaque paint covered the top halves of automobile headlights to hide them from attacking Luftwaffe airplanes or bombarding battleships. Bairstow's coach, Specialist 1st Class of the United States Navy John Duncan Semple, entered too. No more locker room attending in Lynn at $11 a week for Semple. Lieutenant Lou Gregory entered—no upstate New York school-teaching for him for a while. Private Johnny Coleman traveled to Boston from camp—no insurance company for him.

Private Johnny Kelley came up from Fort McClellan in Alabama. In June of 1942 Kelley's wife of 3 years, Mary, died of cancer. Her death left Kelley at age 34 open to the draft and drove him to seek solace in his running.

Sergeant Alfred Libby entered the Boston race. Sergeant Gerard Cote of the Canadian army entered. He trained with a commando unit for special wartime deployment. When he could, he trained for the marathon. Les Pawson worked as a rigger operating a crane on the graveyard shift in the Walsh Kaiser shipyard in Providence, Rhode Island. Tony Mederios put down his welding torch in the South Boston Navy Yard to run the marathon.

Ellison Brown worked in a defense plant. Charley Robbins worked for United Aircraft. Soon Fred McGlone, the national marathon champion, and Charley Robbins would be drafted. Even Major Walter Brown was on duty; he passed the marathon starting job on to his brother, George Brown, Jr. Columnists reminded their readers that the marathon itself had its origins in war. Pheidippides was a courageous soldier who carried a message of victory in war.

Kelley wrote home from Fort McClellan, "Army life has given me a little more nerve and that is what I need for a marathon." The army made Kelley go for an 18-mile hike wearing a full pack. While the other recruits struggled, Kelley worried that he was getting out of shape. But he found ways to run enough to feel secure in his fitness for the marathon race. "Whoever beats me will have to run like the wind." Well, this year there was a wind, a sunny, brisk headwind. They all had to run into it.

Cote had gotten special permission from his commanding officer for a 21-day leave to go to his cousin's house in Rhode Island to train. Cote trained as a commando at Valleyfield, Quebec. He brought his young, attractive, raven-haired wife, Lucille, to Boston with him. He propped a picture of their 1-year-old daughter, Arlette, on the dresser of their room at the Lenox Hotel. The camp had a big send-off for him and expected him to win. But on the Wednesday before the race he stepped in a Boston pothole and severely strained the attachment of his Achilles tendon. A lump appeared. He worried. He could not refuse to start, not after getting special leave from the army. He walked with Lucille to the start. They did not talk. He did not want to talk.

Ancient Tom Burke, the double gold medalist from the 1896 Olympic Games, the man who fired the gun to start the first Boston Marathon in 1897, hustled the boys along to the line. Marathoner George Waterhouse of Roxbury said, "That guy has enough wind to beat us all."

During the race Lucille rode in the *Boston Herald*'s car. Boatswain's mate, former milkman, and last year's marathon winner, Joe Smith, rode in the *Boston Post*'s beach wagon. He did not want to race. "I said if I was lucky enough to win, I'd quit. I won, so I quit." Apparently he stayed quit. But Cote would not quit.

After the *Post* heard of Cote's tendon problem they abandoned him and picked Pawson to win. He had recovered from his automobile accident and won the North Medford Club 20-miler in 1:56, beating Lou Gregory in the last 3 miles. McGlone, as the national marathon champion, had to be considered a threat.

Lucille gave tea to her husband and to Kelley. For miles they ran side by side. Cote's shirt had "Army" printed beneath the Canadian mapleleaf and Kelley's singlet read "U.S. Army." Pawson stuck with Kelley and Cote until the Wellesley hills. At Wellesley no girls cheered; they had left for Easter vacation. The wind bothered McGlone. He let Kelley and Cote get too far ahead. He could not catch Kelley. Heinicke tried a reverse of his slow-start tactic. He started quickly, but faded and wound up sixth. Cote suffered from the pothole-afflicted Achilles. It hurt with every footstrike. He had never been in such pain in a marathon. So he tried to get the race over as quickly as possible. Kelley ran his fastest time at Boston. (He had run a lifetime best of 2:28:18 in Salisbury, Massachusetts, in May of 1940.) But his Boston Marathon personal record was not fast enough. Cote was too strong. Kelley lost him on the downhill to Lake Street. Cote's years of Pete Gavuzzi training helped him. Cote won Boston a second time. Kelley finished second again.

In his Lenox Hotel room Cote again held court, providing room service port and scotch for the reporters. He sat with his feet up, thumbs in his khaki suspenders and a big cigar in his mouth. Joe Smith celebrated with him. "Ah, Smeeth, my fran, don't I tell you t'at reck'ord of your's come down some day soon eh?" Smith grinned. Cote continued, "Joe, you are luckee today t'at there is a big wind out there. Right in the face. Otherwise your reck-ord is gone eh?" But Cote had not expected to win because of his injured heel. He thought he would crack at 20, and he worried not about Kelley but about McGlone and Heinicke. Cote had no certainty about his future plans. He could find himself at the front in France. He could find himself buried there not far from the graves of his ancestors or the grave of 1914 Boston Marathon winner Jimmy Duffy.

1943 Results

1. G. Cote, *CAN Army*	2:28:25*	11. B. Mazzeo, South Portland, ME	2:46:59
2. J.A. Kelley, *U.S. Army*	2:30:00*	12. F.L. Brown, *NMC*	2:48:55
3. F. McGlone, *NYMA*, MA	2:30:41*	13. J. Semple, *U.S. Navy, BAA*	2:52:10
4. L. Bairstow, *USCG, BAA*	2:33:47*	14. C. Robbins, Jr., *AirC*, CT	2:52:17
5. L. Pawson, Pawtucket, RI	2:35:58*	15. F. Bruhm, *CAN Army*	2:52:23
6. D. Heinicke, *WHC*, MD	2:38:52*	17. C. DeMar, *BT*	2:57:58
7. W. Wicklund, Clifton, NJ	2:41:46	21. E. Brown, Westerly, RI	3:01:52
8. A. Mederios, *NMC*	2:44:17	30. F.W. Brown, Sr., *NMC*	3:13:44
9. L. Young, *NMC*	2:44:44	38. F. Brown, Jr., *NMC*	NT
10. M. O'Hara, *U.S. Navy, MillAA*	2:46:14	41. O. Spooner, New Bedford, MA	NT

113 entrants.
*Fastest six marathon times in the world in 1943.

Boot Camp

WEDNESDAY, APRIL 19, 1944

Kelley Tired of Bridesmaid Role

For the past 4 years the North Medford Club had won the team prize in the Boston Marathon. Jock Semple, of the BAA, did not like that. Fred Brown,

Sr., an engineer at WHDH radio, organized the North Medford Club team. Jock captained the BAA team. The two men were fiercely and sometimes uproariously competitive, especially with each other. Fred said Jock wouldn't live long enough for his team to beat North Medford. Jock said, "Brown, I'll piss on your grave." (In fact both lived to the same ripe old age of 84: Jock Semple died in 1988 and Fred Brown in 1992.) Jock would tell potential recruits for his team that Fred Brown was a nuisance, that he was dictatorial and would try to steal an athlete for North Medford. Fred would tell potential recruits that Jock Semple had no control over his temper, that *he* was dictatorial. Fred said Semple had a hobby, making other people mad. A deep, dark, off-the-record rumor had it that the two men actually liked and respected each other. Each denied it.

This year, Semple vowed, things would be different. Semple was in the navy. He didn't have his BAA team. He had something better. He had access to what essentially was an all-star Navy team. Semple was a specialist first class stationed at Sampson Naval Base in Geneva, New York, which really was a monstrously large boot camp. The navy assigned Semple to drill the raw recruits in that camp. Semple had first crack at all the runners who came through. A couple of the best came through.

Ted Vogel from Watertown, Massachusetts, was a 17-year-old BAA runner when he popped a good race to win the 1943 Cathedral Handicap in 53:40 from a 4:30 lead over scratch runners like Cote and Kelley. By 1944 the navy had stationed Vogel at Sampson to be drilled by none other than Semple. The winner of the Cathedral time prize that day in 1943 (50:34) was Charley Robbins, an aircraft factory worker. In 1944 they drafted him. At the recruitment office Robbins bluffed and refused to take the oath or sign on the grounds that he was supposed to have a choice of service branches. He knew the invasion of Europe was near and figured the navy would be safer. The navy sent Robbins to Sampson—right into the waiting arms of Chief Petty Officer Jock Semple.

The navy enforced discipline so strict at Sampson that the recruits, or "boots," saluted even third-class petty officers. Officers beat the boots down until they feared them as much as the enemy. Rules and regulations left Robbins no place near his bunk to put his running shoes. The government had not issued running shoes. Regardless, he had no time to run. Boots had to march in step to meals, but they could walk back. Robbins's only training time was to run back to the barracks on a full stomach—until Semple came to the rescue. Semple had helped set up the camp and had a genius for slipping in, out, and around the system to get done what he wanted. Robbins said about Semple, "It was like a visit from God himself." Suddenly Robbins had a shelf to stow his running shoes. Semple got Robbins out for 2-hour runs on Sundays.

Robbins felt like royalty when he ran around the camp with Semple. Boots saluted them. One wiseguy made a crack as the two passed. Semple heard,

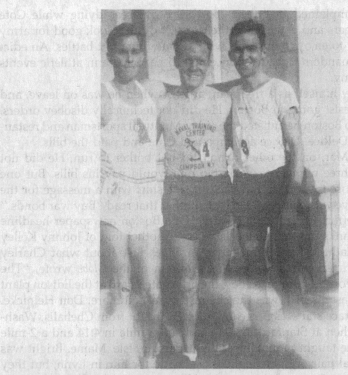

Jock Semple (#4 in the middle) rescued his Sampson Naval Training Center recruits (from left) Ted Vogel and Charley Robbins from the tedium of boot camp to race marathons. Photo courtesy of John D. Semple family.

turned, and speared the kid with a killing look: "Do you know whom you are talking to? I might be the captain!" The kid trembled, begged for forgiveness, saluted a dozen times. Semple and Robbins ran off. Semple knew the captain and persuaded him that a team from the camp could win the Boston Marathon team prize. Semple parted the military red tape like Moses parted the Red Sea. Semple got the captain to let his people go. He got them some flashy gold shirts for their Sampson Naval Training Station team uniform. It may have been the first time a couple of boots got off the station before completing basic training.

The Canadian army stationed Sergeant Cote in St. Jerome, Quebec. He took personal leave to go to Boston for the marathon. The year before he had gone under the auspices of the Canadian army to Boston and Yonkers. He won both races, and the army commanders basked in his success. But an army is both a military and a political entity, so when those same commanders received complaints that the dashing, dapper, debonair Cote traveled on army time and at army expense running races during wartime, putting his feet up and drinking port, they soured on him. Families of other servicemen complained that their sons were overseas dying while Cote smoked big cigars and entertained the press. It did not look good for army men to appear to enjoy themselves winning anything but battles. An edict from the commanders forbade servicemen to participate in athletic events outside the army.

But Cote saw himself as a free man, at least when he was on leave, and he could not resist going to Boston. He did not technically disobey orders. For expenses to Boston he enlisted the aid of Montreal sportsman and restauranteur Frank DeRice. DeRice accompanied Cote and paid the bills.

Clarence DeMar, on the other hand, did not bother to run. He did not want to take three nights off work. No one would pay his bills. But one Artin Black chose to run. He ran wearing a T-shirt with a message for the war effort: "Save waste paper." He had another that read "Buy war bonds."

Allied war effort turned for the better. One Boston newspaper headline announced "Yanks Capture 10 Jap Islands." Another told of Johnny Kelley winning the Cathedral race time prize in 50:39, just about what Charley Robbins had run the year before. Jerry Nason of the *Globe* wrote, "The sentimental favorite is Johnny Kelley, the little gate guard at the Edison plant in Southie." Nason's pick was the chemist from Baltimore, Don Heinicke.

Another prerace star was Sergeant Norman Bright from Chehalis, Washington, who when at Stanford in 1937 had run a mile in 4:14 and a 2-mile in 9:01. Now he taught mountaineering at Presque Isle, Maine. Bright was having a special pair of lightweight shoes made for him in Lynn, but they weren't ready yet. Cote gave him a pair of his own special lightweight shoes to wear in the race. Clayton Farrar had performed the hat trick of winning the Cathedral, Reddish, and North Medford Club 20-mile premarathon road races around Boston in the weeks before the Boston race. He had to be considered a threat, too.

This year in Boston Kelley ran in 12th place in Framingham, 10th in Natick, and 4th in Wellesley. Cote and Bright had the lead then. Cote ran hard and alone from 6 to 18 miles. He kept thinking about Kelley. Where's Kelley? By Lake Street Kelley ran only 35 yards behind Cote. With 3 miles to go Kelley caught Cote. Nothing happened. Kelley expected Cote would stop after being passed. Cote kept on. Kelley tried to break away. Cote responded defensively. He would not quit. He would not yield. He played a static defense like the tactic in arm wrestling: Rather than exhaust your arm in going for an immediate pin, you hold your position while the other guy exhausts himself going for the pin. Then, after the opponent's arm is exhausted, you go for the kill and crush him. Kelley, ever impatient, surged, going for an immediate pin. Cote waited. Kelley pushed and pushed. Through Kenmore Square he pushed, but Cote ran at his side, matching stride for stride, unyielding. Kelley trembled. Kelley cracked. Kelley broke. But he didn't break much. Little of the race remained. The men ran on Exeter Street in sight of each other. For the sixth time Kelley finished 2nd, this time by only 13 seconds. Cote flashed his big Quebec grin.

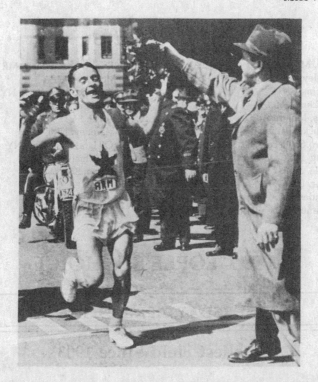

Gerard Cote wins the 1943 Boston Marathon, but all the attention would soon bring the wrath and revenge of the Canadian army down on him. Photo courtesy of the *Boston Herald*.

Semple and his Sampson team of Pharmacist's Mate 3rd Class Charley Robbins in 3rd, Semple in 9th, and Ted Vogel in 15th won the team prize. They celebrated their victory in their flashy gold Sampson uniforms. The North Medford Club took 8th with Louis Young, 16th with Carl Maroney, and 23rd with Fred Brown, Sr. himself. Willie Wicklund, a superintendent at the Wright Aircraft plant in Paterson, New Jersey, finished 4th.

Victorious Cote invited DeMar up to his hotel room for a celebratory postrace beer. DeMar declined, saying that he had other work to do. But he thought that Cote might be the man to equal his own record of seven wins.

When Cote returned to his post with the army at St. Jerome they did not greet him with cheers and congratulations. They did not grin. Commandos going off to run footraces did not make a wartime army look good. Cote's victory angered a particular general in Ottawa. For violating regulations against athletics outside the army, the general had to insure that Cote would not make sports page headlines again. Cote was in trouble, and it could cost him his life. D-day for the Normandy invasion approached. The Canadian army sent Gerard Cote overseas.

1944 Results

1.	G. Cote, Montreal, PQ	2:31:50*	11.	N. Bright, Presque Isle, ME	2:59:38
2.	J.A. Kelley, West Acton, MA	2:32:03*	12.	B. McCormick, PA	3:00:21
3.	C. Robbins, *SNTS*	2:38:31*	13.	J. Kernason, New York, NY	3:00:37
4.	W. Wicklund, *MillAA*	2:41:45*	14.	J. McKlissock, PA	3:00:54
5.	L. Evans, Montreal, PQ	2:43:20*	15.	T. Vogel, *SNTS*	3:03:36
6.	D. Heinicke, Baltimore, MD	2:47:52	16.	C. Maroney, *NMC*	3:08:09
7.	B. Mazzeo, South Portland, ME	2:49:06	17.	M. O'Hara, *U.S. Navy*, NY	3:09:49
8.	L. Young, *NMC*, MA	2:49:18	18.	J. Kashishian, PA	3:10:42
9.	J. Semple, *SNTS*	2:51:34	23.	F. Brown, Sr., *NMC*	3:20:14
10.	C. Farrar, *USCG*, NY	2:54:40			

33 finished under 3:48.
*Fastest five times in the world in 1944.

THE PEOPLE'S CHOICE

THURSDAY, APRIL 19, 1945

Smallest Field Since 1903

The Canadian army put Gerard Cote in England, away from Johnny Kelley, but closer to the Germans. The invasion of Europe had come, but Cote stayed in England. Canadian generals figured that if he was overseas they would not be criticized. They did not volunteer Cote for a Normandy landing.

With Cote out of the picture Kelley instantly became, as the newspapers called him, "the people's choice": the class of the field. But it was a small field. Ninety men entered and 67 started. Most young men who might run a marathon were fighting in the war. The Russians besieged Berlin, and the Allied air force swarmed over Germany. In the Pacific, Japanese soldiers chained themselves to their conquered archipelago to die rather than surrender.

This year marked a low point both for participation in the marathon and for spectators. The Boston Marathon had been bigger every other year since 1903, when only 56 runners showed up, than it was in 1945. The biggest field to date, 285 runners, was in 1928. This year marked a low for the world as well as for the Boston Marathon.

Much had changed since 1944. Walter Brown was now Lieutenant Colonel Brown, but he fired his same old family gun to start the race. A week earlier President Roosevelt had died. Charley Robbins, benefiting from more of Jock Semple's "arrangements," had become a pharmacist's mate 2nd class. Robbins had married Doris Stevens of Manchester, Connecticut, and had a

2-month-old daughter named Chris. Kelley became a civilian, remarried, and lived in West Acton, Massachusetts. Robbins had won the Reddish 10-mile handicap with a good lead over Kelley, who won the time prize by running 16 seconds faster than Robbins. Lloyd Bairstow had just come off 9 months of sea duty with the Coast Guard. Clarence DeMar planned not to run but to write about the race for the *Boston Daily Globe*.

Kelley did not work at his job in the electrical maintenance department at the Edison Plant in South Boston the day before the race. That night he entertained his Canadian houseguests, AB (Albert) Morton and Scotty Rankine. They showed up at Kelley's little white duplex on Massachusetts Avenue in West Acton with two huge pieces of Canadian tenderloin. (They didn't want to impose on Kelley and his new wife and use up their food ration points.) Kelley had married Barbara Raymond, a tall, blond war worker and forewoman in the Acton machine company. On April 12, the day Roosevelt died, she handed Kelley a telegram from the War Department telling the family that his youngest brother, Eddie, was missing in action over the Pacific. His parachute had been spotted as it left a disabled B-29 to splash into a stormy sea. He was never recovered.

Clayton Farrar, now of the Coast Guard Academy in New London, Connecticut, took the early lead. Don Heinicke wore a new shirt with a simple white horse to show his new affiliation as he bunched with Bairstow and Robbins. Robbins considered Heinicke remarkably bright and witty. The White Horse Social Club was a wonderful old fellows' tavern whose owner sponsored Heinicke and several other runners. Kelley and Canadian Lloyd Evans ran not far behind. At times Farrar's lead reached 500 yards. Semple's protégé, Bairstow, ran gracefully and reminded DeMar of the way Leslie Pawson ran, with power and bounding fluidity. The pace was slow until Auburndale. There DeMar, who now had a farm in Reading, Massachusetts, said he observed Farrar's head shake like a sick chicken's. When Farrar stopped on the third and steepest hill, Bairstow took over. Kelley ran a half mile behind. The pace was slow compared to that set by Pawson, Ellison Brown, Johnny Miles, and Joe Smith in their victory years. It was a brisk, bright, cool day, one made for fast running. DeMar speculated that the slow pace may have been because the men were relatively old. Kelley was 37.

When Kelley caught Bairstow at 23 miles, he did not fight back the way Cote had. DeMar defended Bairstow's passivity:

> As Kelley stepped into the lead, right at Coolidge Corner, Bairstow didn't even put up a struggle! And I am one to say that no struggle, when one is not in condition to fight, is sane and sensible. Windy *friends* may urge you to die rather than to yield, but there are hundreds more marathons coming. Why not yield gracefully to a better conditioned man and fit yourself so he will have to yield to you in the future?

Charley Robbins said that in his racing experience his biggest struggles had been losses while his best races, his wins, were easy.

Kelley looked easy. He ran waving to the crowd and blowing kisses. He looked fresher than when he started. He saw he was going to win and all the weight of worry lifted, so he had the energy to play to the spectators. Robbins made an observation about Kelley: "He runs on exhilaration. He is a great little running machine, but beatable as long as you could stay with him and keep him worried. Once he got a lead and became exhilarated, he was unbeatable." He was finally going to beat that second place jinx. Six second places! Kelley said, "I could have busted right out crying when I turned into Exeter Street." He clasped his hands together over his head and waved them around the way victorious boxers do. After he broke the finish line he asked to see his wife, Barbara. DeMar wrote, "Kelley's attractive wife and chic sister were bubbling over."

Victorious Johnny Kelley sat on a cot in the locker room after the marathon with Governor Maurice J. Tobin and the former mayor, John F. ("Honey Fitz") Fitzgerald. In front of the assembled all-male press they together sang "Sweet Adeline," the former mayor's theme song. The room filled with echoes and close harmony. For Kelley it was sweet victory. He proved himself a match for the politicians as he credibly crooned. The gentlemen of the press loved it, and Johnny loved them. He loved the whole world that day, he was so happy. He said "I knew they had to come back to me; I timed myself and knew what I had to make up. . . . You can't run the early part fast. I know; I tried it for years. It's the biggest thrill of my life. Ten years is a long time to wait."

The next day's *Globe* reported, "His face wreathed in a monster smile . . . [he] repeatedly blessed himself over the final miles." When asked how he did it, he replied, "How'd I do it? . . . I ran with patience." The newspapers reported that Barbara gave him a lump of sugar along the way. Kelley won by 400 yards. Happiness bubbled out of him. Yet in his time of joy he tried to do the right thing and considered sending his laurel wreath to the newly widowed Mrs. Roosevelt. Later Kelley told *Globe* reporter Cliff Keene, "But heck—I want to keep it. It certainly would be of more sentimental value to me than to Mrs. Roosevelt."

Reporters called Kelley to ask if he had any thoughts about going to Hollywood to be in pictures. To keep them guessing and perpetuate the joke, Kelley said yes. "I'm thirty-seven now and maybe the thrill won't come again. Sure, I'll keep running, but this is the race I really wanted." The ex-soldier and electrical maintenance man told Jerry Nason of the *Globe*, "Life merely begins at forty and I have three years to go. . . . let me at 'em."

DeMar noted that the crowds watching the marathon this year were the smallest he'd ever seen. Many doubted that the marathon, after surviving all these years, including through the Great Depression, would survive if the war continued any longer. DeMar wondered if it might bring more to the Patriots' Day holiday fun if he dropped a couple of typesetting jobs to run next year. The marathon needed something to survive. It was more than a sporting event, it was

> *Many doubted that the Boston Marathon, after surviving all these years, including the Great Depression, would survive if the war continued.*

a celebration of spring, a lifting of public spirit after another dreary New England winter. But it would need a new hero and a new story, one that would touch the pathos of the public in a postwar world.

1945 Results

1.	J.A. Kelley, West Acton, MA	2:30:40*	9. J. Semple, *U.S. Navy*	2:47:36
2.	L. Bairstow, *USCG*	2:32:50*	10. A. Morton, Toronto, ON	2:49:55
3.	D. Heinicke, *WHC*, MD	2:36:28*	11. G. Daniels, NYMA	2:50:50
4.	R. Rankine, ON	2:38:03	12. G. Dickson, *MillAA*	2:50:58
5.	L. Evans, Montreal, PQ	2:39:43	13. C. Maroney, NMC	2:55:26
6.	C. Robbins, *U.S. Navy*, MA	2:39:51	14. L. Jolin, Montreal, PQ	2:55:43
7.	L. Young, *NMC*	2:40:22	15. M. O'Hara, *U.S. Navy*	2:56:57
8.	T. Mederios, N. Medford, MA	2:41:04		

90 entrants, 67 starters.
*Fastest three times in the world in 1945.

STARVING GREEKS

SATURDAY, APRIL 20, 1946

50th Running of Classic Race

At last the war was over. But the suffering did not end. A *Boston Daily Globe* headline on April 17 proclaimed, "Truman [says] Eat Less Two Days a Week for Starving People of the World." In Greece 7 million people left destitute by the war faced starvation. Communist guerillas in the country's north resolved in February to continue the civil war. This new war raged at a cruel cost to the rural population, who saw many of their children captured to be raised as future guerilla fighters in border states under Communist control. Refugees numbering 700,000 fled to the cities under government control. The cities could not handle the influx. There was not enough food. Stylianos Kyriakides came to Boston to tell the world about the plight of the people of his country. But first he had to win the marathon.

Before he left Athens, Kyriakides told his family and friends that he would win the Boston Marathon or die trying. Echoing the Greek adage, "with this or on this," by which mothers would admonish their sons to return victorious from battle either carrying their shield or being carried upon it, he reminded Americans of the warring origins of the marathon.

Kyriakides had been to Boston to run the marathon in 1938. A dark, wiry, craggy-faced man, he had arrived in 1938 with the credentials of his 2:43:20 marathon in the 1936 Berlin Olympics, where he placed 11th. But in Boston he had developed horrible blisters, so he had to drop out at 21 miles and take an expensive taxi to the finish. But 1938 was a world and a lifetime ago. In 1938 Kyriakides was a young man, well fed and fearless. But in April of 1941, as Leslie Pawson won his last Boston Marathon, Hitler's Twelfth Army and Mussolini's Ninth Army fought a whirlwind blitzkrieg down the Balkans to conquer and occupy Greece. Kyriakides found himself a prisoner in his own ruined country. There was little to eat and nothing to do but what you were told.

One night during the occupation a Nazi patrol caught Kyriakides out of the bounds set by the Nazis. The Germans usually took no chances with their non-German subjects. They responded to partisan activity with pitiless cruelty. Usually after a quick court-martial a Greek caught out of bounds would be shot. The commanding officer ordered Kyriakides to empty his pockets. The officer saw a card.

"What is this?"

"It is my Olympic pass for the 1936 Games at Berlin."

"Were you there?"

"Yes."

"What did you do?"

"Marathon."

"Ah, marathon. An athlete. Why didn't you tell me that? Here, take your clothes. Go."

On another day a different group of German soldiers, bent on looting, visited the Kyriakides household. They saw a display case, which they ordered the family to empty. They saw a picture of Stylianos in his Olympic uniform. So great was the German respect for athletes that they replaced everything in the case, issued profuse apologies, and left the family alone. On these occasions Stylianos Kyriakides's athletic prowess had saved his life and his property. Now he would use his athletic ability to help save all of Greece. The electricity company paid his way to Boston. They got him extra food rations so he could train. They asked him to thank America for defeating the Nazis. Kyriakides wanted to win the Boston Marathon so he could beg for shiploads of food to be sent to his homeland. His was an act of desperation driven by an utter lack of material resources. A lot of things had to go right for it to succeed.

George Demeter, owner of the Hotel Minerva, performed as the marathon host of the Boston Greek community. It was in Boston that Kyriakides had his first steak in 8 years. Demeter was the man who chased Boston Marathon winners over the finish line to crown them with a wreath of laurel leaves picked in Greece. Before the race he gave Kyriakides a note with a message written in Greek to inspire him. In rough translation the message said, "Win or Die."

The Boston Marathon had survived the war years. This was the 50th marathon. As former runners and potential runners got out of the service, the ranks of men competing in long-distance running increased. A lot of things had changed this year for the Boston Marathon. For one thing the number of entrants was up—112 runners entered, and 102 started. And the old Tebeau farm would no longer be the prerace headquarters. A hundred marathoners were too many for the family with four children who now lived in the Lucky Rock Manor farmhouse. The headquarters moved to the Hopkinton Community Center. And no longer would police escorts ride the course on motorcycles. They rode instead in brand-new squad cars, equipped with two-way radios and amplifiers, to manage the crowds and especially the herds of young bicyclists.

Another new feature greeted runners at the start. Race officials herded them into a fenced enclosure—a slat-and-wire snow fence kept the official, numbered runners separate from spectators and riff-raff. An official checked them in and out of the corral. The thinly clad runners, coated with liniment and reeking of its wintergreen scent, milled about, resting or chatting with each other.

Gerard Cote survived the war and said he was in the best shape of his life. He was afraid only of Don Heinicke. Cote did not know that Heinicke had become a father on Tuesday. DeMar at 58 had fatherhood well behind him, but he came to run. Narragansett Indian Ellison Brown came back too. He and his wife, and four children lived in a tarpaper shack by Narragansett Bay. No more defense plant job. Typifying the racist views about Indians, Jerry Nason of the *Globe* wrote that Brown lived as if the white man had never come to this country. He hunted and fished as well as did an odd job or two to make a living.

Lou Gregory, the second-place finisher to Joe Smith in 1942, took the early lead. He had run the second fastest of the only four sub-2:30 marathons in BAA history; Cote had run one of the others. Gregory had 50 yards on the field by Framingham. A brisk and cold tailwind helped the runners, but the time in Framingham was 2 minutes slower than the record. It was an odd thing for this field to go out so slowly on such a good running day. Were they all watching each other like cats and mice?

By Natick Gregory had drifted back into a big pack while John Kernason of the Millrose Athletic Association played a solo lead by 75 yards. A tall skinny man who wore thick glasses, Kernason worked as a stenographer for the postmaster of New York City. He had a penchant for extremely fast starts. The big pack contained a population including Charley Robbins, Cote, Heinicke, AB Morton, Lloyd Bairstow, Kyriakides, and Johnny Kelley. By Wellesley the stenographer had 150 yards on Gregory and 350 yards on Kelley, Cote, Kyriakides, Robbins, and Bairstow.

A terrific traffic jam followed the runners. The war effort had forced gasoline rationing, so people did not drive frivolously. Traffic had annoyed marathon runners during the war years, but now it menaced them. It seemed that everyone from the mayor to the governor to each reporter had to have a car and had to drive next to the leaders. The officials had cars. VIPs all had their own cars. People lined the streets. The politicians saw a parade and had to get in on it. The autos vied for position, and spectators leaned out of car windows and shouted at their favorites. Pedestrian spectators had trouble seeing the runners, and the little racers seemed secondary to the big machines. But the men ran with deadly seriousness. Lou Gregory had passed Kernason and led until the Newton hills, where Kyriakides and Kelley caught and passed him. Both looked fresh and full of running.

Kelley feared the jinx of second place would grab him again. He expected to win, of course, but worried nonetheless. But for Kyriakides, grimmer terms framed the race. For he had to do or die, as George Demeter had written on that little scrap of paper. His sponsors, his employers, his cause for the starving people of Greece insisted on his victory. He had taken extra food in a country of underfed people. For them he could do nothing less than win. This race was not recreation for Kyriakides. With the food he took the responsibility to come home like an ancient Greek warrior—either victorious with his shield or carried upon it, dead. The Americans thought marathon running was a sport. But for Kyriakides the race was life itself.

When the pursuers had disappeared, Kyriakides and Kelley settled down to a death sprint. Kyriakides's best marathon was his Olympic 2:43. Kelley had run 10 minutes faster, but in Berlin he had only run 2:49. Every race is a new race. The past may predict, but it doesn't dictate. Kyriakides had more to lose and more to win than Kelley.

Kelley and Kyriakides slammed themselves into the hills. Kyriakides wore a shirt with "Greece" in a semicircle across his chest. Below it was a flag

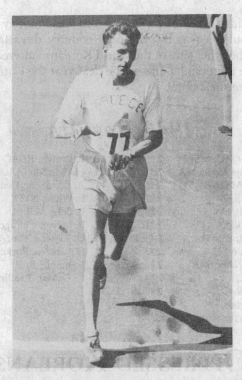

Stylianos Kyriakides came from war-ravaged Greece to carry a message; to deliver it he had to win the 1946 Boston Marathon. He did. Photo courtesy of the *Boston Herald*.

with a blue cross and the Greek initials of his home club. Kelley wore his Edison Employees' Club shirt. Kelley tried to run away, but Kyriakides stuck. For his country he had to crucify himself on Kelley and the course. From Lake Street to St. Mary's, Kelley and Kyriakides ran together.

In the last stages of the race Kyriakides broke from Kelley. As he did he thought of torches burning on the Acropolis. He thought of his two young children and his wife, Eugenia. Meals for them were often reduced to a few peas. Kyriakides drove his emaciated body to speeds and distances it had never reached. But Kelley found himself in a place he had been before— second place, now for the seventh time. Kyriakides felt the relief of a Christian let down off his cross.

After his glorious finish Kyriakides wept with joy as he talked to reporters. He said he planned to stay in the United States for a month and beg for Greece. He wanted a boatload of food, milk, and medicine for his country. Even Kelley, who was pushed back to second place again, gave up his disappointment as he was caught up in the Greek's emotions. He congratu- lated Kyriakides heartily: "It's great that you won, Stylianos. It's great for your country." Greece had indeed suffered under occupation during the war, and Kyriakides's victory in Boston did raise money to send relief to his homeland. But his was not the only country devastated by war and occupation. On the other side of the world Koreans suffered under the cruel occupation of the imperial Japanese. The next year the Koreans would come to Boston to make their point.

1946 Results

1.	S. Kyriakides, *OAC*, Athens	2:29:27*	12.	E. Brown, *RDAC*		2:48:47
2.	J.A. Kelley, West Acton, MA	2:31:27*	13.	J. Anderson, *AAC*		2:49:33
3.	G. Cote, *NAC*, Montreal, PQ	2:36:34	14.	A. Lundberg, Dedham, MA		2:52:09
4.	L. Gregory, *MillAA*	2:37:23	15.	L. White, *NYPC*		2:52:29
5.	A. Morton, Galt, ON	2:38:53	16.	L. Bolg, *MillAA*		2:55:09
6.	J. Kernason, *MillAA*	2:41:20	17.	R. Meyer, Chicago, IL		2:55:54
7.	L. Evans, Montreal, PQ	2:43:02	18.	O. Kissoon, *GoodAC*, ON		2:56:18
8.	C. Robbins, Jr., *NYMA*	2:43:59	19.	D. Mazzeo, Rockland, ME		2:57:07
9.	T. Vogel, *U.S. Navy*, BAA	2:44:24	20.	J. Semple, *BAA*		2:57:51
10.	L. Young, *NMC*	2:44:38	32.	C. DeMar, Reading, MA		3:09:55
11.	T. Mederios, *NMC*	2:47:25				

112 entrants, 102 starters.
*Fastest two times in the world in 1946.

OPPRESSED KOREANS

SATURDAY, APRIL 19, 1947

Olympic Champion Comes to Boston

Results of the 1936 Olympic marathon list the winner as Kitei Son, a young Japanese student. But the man's name was not really Kitei Son, and he was not Japanese. He was rather a Korean named Ki Chung Sohn, forced by the Japanese administration that had ruled Korea since 1905 to take a Japanese name and run under the colors of Japan. After all, the Japanese reasoned, the nation of Korea did not exist. But patriotic Koreans thought they still had a country and would again as soon as they got rid of the Japanese. When photos of Kitei Son, born Ki Chung Sohn, had arrived in Korea, the local newspaper editors painted over the rising sun on his Japanese uniform with Korean colors and printed his Korean name in the caption. When the occupying Japanese authorities saw the newspaper, they exploded. They closed down the paper, jailed the editors, and banned Koreans from all competitive running from that day on. The imperial Japanese were harsh masters, racists who regarded Koreans as garlic- and cabbage-reeking sub-humans.

But in the summer of 1945 American troops had pushed north into Korea, driving the Japanese before them. The Russian army blitzkrieged the Japanese holdings in Manchuria and drove the Japanese army across the Yalu into northern Korea. The Japanese military collapsed in mid-August. The empire surrendered. American occupiers came, but they were reluctant conquerors, benign and soon to leave. Korea could be a nation again; Korean marathoners could run for her; Ki Chung Sohn could reclaim his name. He had survived the war by moving from job to job to dodge the Japanese draft. He did manage to stay alive and in shape.

At service track meets in Korea, Korean runners impressed the American occupation soldiers, so they raised the money to send three Korean marathon runners to Boston. This would be the first time since 1910 that a Korean athlete had raced under the Korean flag.

With the American victory in World War II and with the American economy unscathed, everyone wanted to come to the U.S. The country's economy loomed as large itself as that of the rest of the world combined. For any marathoners anywhere in the world, the Boston Marathon was the race to run. For each of the previous 8 years, the world's fastest marathon time had been run in Boston. (To be fair, however, there had been few marathons anywhere during those war-ripped years. The war forced the cancellation of both the 1940 and the 1944 Olympic Games.) With Ki Chung Sohn, the most recent Olympic gold medalist, entered, the Boston Marathon became virtually the world championship.

Two Finns came, a Turk, two Greeks, three Guatemalans, many Canadians, as usual, and the three Koreans. No longer would the race be a New England/Canadian affair where the winner could be picked from local premarathon road races. The year before in a warring world the Boston Marathon's future had looked bleak, but Allied victory changed all that.

In other years men who were not citizens of America had won the race (German Paul deBruyn, Greek Peter Trivoulidas, Finnish-born Dave Komonen), but they were all immigrants who later became citizens. The new marathoners were all proud citizens of their own countries.

Ki Chung Sohn, Seung Yong Nam, and Yun Bok Suh made up the Korean team. Suh had been 13 at the time of the Japanese ban on long-distance racing. The gold medalist and the team coach, Sohn, saw in Suh his successor. Suh's family owned a profitable produce business in Seoul, but his father had died in 1938 and his mother in 1942. Suh was now 24, a sophomore at the University of Korea. He was 5'1" and weighed 115 pounds. Suh's marathon heroes were his teammate/teacher/coach Sohn and Johnny Kelley, whom he had read about. On April 10 the *Boston Post* printed a prediction: Kelley picked Suh to win Boston.

Ki Chung Sohn picked Suh to win, too. In order for the younger man to win, the teacher had to withdraw, because the student would never be so disrespectful as to overtake the teacher. Or perhaps Sohn was merely old, hadn't been training, or was injured. He never explained his withdrawal.

A sad-faced, bespectacled Turkish man named Sevki Koru took the early lead, wearing "Turkey" in a crescent on his plain white singlet. Clouds covered the day at 45 °F. Bill Steiner led through Framingham with Fred Brown in 3rd, and Kyriakides (well-fed at 6 pounds heavier than last year), behind him. Suh ran in 11th place. By Wellesley AB Morton led, with Suh on his heels. Lloyd Bairstow, now employed nights in a Lawrence, Massachusetts, bakery, moved into 3rd. In 4th ran Mikko Hietanen, a 35-year-old stockroom clerk from an ammunition plant in Jyvaskyla, Finland. He wore a kerchief knotted at the corners over his head, a blue-striped shirt under his jersey, and white gloves. In the tradition of Albin Stenroos, a formidable Finn had again come to Boston. Kyriakides moved into 10th. Johnny Kelley ran nowhere in sight. Charley Robbins, now a chemist at Pratt and Whitney aircraft in Connecticut, wasn't in sight either. Suh and Hietanen pulled away from the field. All the foreigners ran up at the front—you don't travel across half a world to jog. Excitement built at the new international character of the event.

At Newton Center a fox terrier created even more excitement—he darted under Suh's feet and tripped him. The fall cut Suh's hand and ripped the skin over his knee. He had carried a kerchief to wipe away sweat, but now he wrapped the kerchief around his bleeding hand. The ripped knee he let drip. The fall untied his shoelaces; he let them flap. On his shirt beneath the word "Korea" were a Korean flag and next to it an American stars-and-stripes shield. Hietanen came up on his shoulder. One last long hill remained. Suh flew up the hill like a wind-blown leaf and put 70 yards on Hietanen. For nourishment Suh had arranged for six boys to meet him with bread soaked in sugar water.

Bairstow ran in third position at Boston College when a bicyclist swerved into his path. The collision severely injured Bairstow. The roads had been cleared of extra cars but not bicyclists. The newspaper reporters were no longer allowed to ride in separate cars with flags advertising their papers. They all had to take the same press bus. A truck carried all the photographers. Only Governor Tobin and Mayor Curley rode in private cars. The BAA did not want a repeat of the previous year's race—the one nobody saw because of the traffic jam. But they could not shoo all the bicycles off the course. Bairstow tried to run after the accident with the bike, but he could not continue. Other runners had other difficulties.

The newspaper reporters were no longer allowed to ride along the course in separate cars with flags advertising their papers.

Ted Vogel had followed Kyriakides for the early miles because he thought the previous year's winner would be the man to beat. When Kyriakides failed to move up, Vogel took off along after the leaders. Out of the navy and running for Semple's BAA team while a student at Tufts University, Vogel moved into third by Lake Street.

At Lake Street the sun broke through the clouds, Suh ran 12 seconds slower than Joe Smith's 1942 record to that point. If there had been any doubt in the public mind about the relationship of size or ethnicity to endurance running, Suh's performance should have erased it. Yet many Americans still believed that native Americans held a natural advantage in endurance contests, and many Japanese and Koreans believed themselves unable to compete athletically against bigger ethnics, except in gymnastics and marathons. By the end Suh broke the 1942 record with a world record time, 1:12 better than Smith's.

"I won the race on that final long hill when the Finnish champion was at my shoulder," said Suh. "I'm glad I could win this race for my home country instead of having Japan take credit for the victory."

Jock Semple got his wish that year—the BAA finally won the team prize, with Ted Vogel, Ollie Manninen, and Semple. Clarence H. DeMar ran his 25th Boston Marathon at age 59. Cote had gotten a cramp and Kelley just looked very tired. The Finn in 9th place was 48 years old.

Vogel's coach at Tufts, Dinger Dessault, greeted his charge at the finish. He said, "Don't rush into the clubhouse. Enjoy the cheers. You've just run 26 miles." "And lost," Vogel contradicted. Ted Vogel was not happy. He thought he should be the best marathoner in the world.

Checkpoint Splits

Framingham	Bill Steiner	33:04
Natick	John Kernason	54:33
Wellesley	AB Morton	1:11:47
Woodland	Yun Bok Suh	1:35:25
Lake Street	Yun Bok Suh	1:58:12
Coolidge Corner	Yun Bok Suh	2:12:17

1947 Results

1.	Y. Suh, Korea	2:25:39$^{CR, WR*}$	9. V. Muinonen, Finland	2:38:59
2.	M. Hietanen, Finland	2:29:39	10. S. Kyriakides, Greece	2:39:13
3.	T. Vogel, BAA	2:30:10	11. L. Evans, Canada	2:39:41
4.	G. Cote, Canada	2:32:11	12. S. Nam, Korea	2:40:10
5.	A. Morton, Canada	2:33:08	13. J.A. Kelley, W. Acton, MA	2:40:55
6.	A. Ragazos, Greece	2:35:34	14. O. Manninen, BAA	2:43:26
7.	S. Koru, Turkey	2:37:50	15. C. Robbins, NYMA	2:43:33
8.	D. Mazzeo, Rockland, ME	2:38:03	16. D. Heinicke, Baltimore, MD	2:44:41

17.	J. Semple, *BAA*	2:45:09	21. W. Dupree, *BAA*	2:48:01
18.	R. Rankine, Canada	2:45:29	22. G. Waterhouse, *NMC*	2:49:59
19.	A. Mederios, *NMC*	2:45:34	**C. DeMar**	**NT**
20.	B. Steiner, NY	2:46:35		

184 entrants, 157 starters.

*Yun Bok Suh's winning time of 2:25:39 is considered a permanent record for 26 miles, 385 yards (1927-1950).

VOGEL VS. COTE

MONDAY, APRIL 19, 1948

Young BAA Runner Set to Win Big Race

Ted Vogel won the National Marathon Championship at Yonkers, New York, in the late spring of 1947. Running from scratch in the Cathedral 10-miler, he won the time prize within 11 seconds of the record with a 49:21. Vogel was the shining star of New England distance running, a nova among an aging elite, the blue-eyed boy of Boston. And on his uniform he wore the unicorn of the Boston Athletic Association. The experts picked Ted Vogel or Tom Crane, a 25-year-old from Springfield, Massachusetts, to win this 52nd Boston Marathon. Crane had run 22 seconds faster than Kelley's record in the North Medford 20-miler (1:53:21). Crane was second to Vogel at Yonkers. This Boston race would be a mostly American contest. No Finns, Turks, Greeks, or Koreans were coming. Yun Bok Suh cabled the Boston Athletic Association for traveling expenses to defend his title, but they were not forthcoming. But a bigger reason kept the foreigners away. This was an Olympic year. And it would be a big Olympic year, too, because war had quashed the previous two.

Other things changed too. College students began to adopt what had been a working man's race. Vogel attended Tufts University in Medford; Joe Smith delivered milk to his dormitory. Others had finished their wartime obligations and went to college on the GI bill. Charley Robbins had started at New York Medical School; he skipped an exam in embryology to keep his string of six BAA marathons intact. Paul Collins came to run. He studied violin at the Juilliard school. Guatemalans Luis Velasquez and Enrique Castilio came up to avenge their poor previous showings. Vogel and Jock Semple, now 43, met them at the East Boston Airport and as tour guides of the host BAA showed them around. Jock himself had given up marathon running and taken up race-walking.

Jock had arranged for 15 podiatrists to staff the Soden Building at the finish line and care for runners' blisters. The Soden Building, formerly the

BAA clubhouse, now housed the Boston University School of Physiotherapy, from which Semple had recently graduated. Now he owned certification for a higher paying form of locker room attendance.

The day looked good for running. A slight crosswind blew at 60 °F and the sun was shining. Young Ted Vogel ran next to old Gerard Cote. Vogel ran tall and fair with sandy hair flapping. He had height, a square jaw, square shoulders, and the crisp all-American good looks that would serve a salesman well. He looked bobbing, bright, and alert as he ran. He wore his BAA team jersey with the golden unicorn on a blue field. Cote, by contrast, was short and dark; he looked unwashed and unctuous, wearing the kind of strapped undershirt an auto mechanic might wear on a hot day. His shorts, of a garish scarlet satin, glared against his workmanlike looks. Next to Vogel, Cote looked like a carnival worker. There seemed to be a cocky strut to his jaunty stride. His hair did not flap. He was quite unflappable, but he decided on a tactic to rattle Vogel. Cote would push the issue. He used to be a boxer. Early in the race Cote stepped on Vogel's heel. It may have been accidental. It may have been arrogant. Cote kept wondering, "Where's Kelley? Where's Crane?"

Cote ran on, or at, Vogel's heels through Framingham in ninth and eighth place, then seventh and sixth at Natick. At Wellesley Dan Van Dorp of Seton Hall and the violinist Collins relinquished the lead to Vogel and Cote. Jesse Van Zant, another talented and smooth-running young man, moved steadily up through the pack. Cote took the lead by a stride and Vogel settled in to tag him. Cote began weaving and roving over the road. His repeated crossing in front of the long-legged and long-striding Vogel annoyed Vogel. Perhaps it was meant to annoy him. Cote said he searched for the springy spots in the macadam. At the water stops Cote grabbed his cup and threw its contents onto and over his head. A few drops fell on Vogel's legs. Vogel feared the cold water would trigger leg cramps. Cote's actions angered him. In his fatigue Vogel became waspish. Perhaps Cote initiated this war of nerves, or perhaps the older man was indeed oblivious to his own actions, or perhaps the younger man was too nervous, too high-strung.

Cote turned to Vogel at the bottom of the long hill and said, "You are going to win, but be careful. Tom Crane is coming." Was this an attempt to further rattle Vogel? Did Cote want to give the burden of victory to Vogel along with the burden of fear of runners who weren't even at the front? Was this cleverness, oblivion, or hypersensitivity? Cote kept at it. Elbows connected.

Finally Vogel had had enough. He said to Cote, "If you try any more of that stuff I'll slug you." Vogel was ready to square off with Cote right there in the middle of the street. Cote stopped jostling.

Cote worked as a corporal of a hospital security force in St. Hyacinthe, Quebec. He also trained a great deal. Cote pulled away from Vogel at Lake Street, but Vogel thought perhaps Cote was bluffing. Vogel had to find out.

He scurried to make up the 70 yards and caught Cote by Cleveland Circle. Cote shrugged. Cote did not bluff. At 22 miles Cote began to pour it on. Vogel could not respond.

Heinicke dropped out at 16. Lou Gregory dropped out at Newton Lower Falls. He intended to run this race as a memorial for his son, who had died a month earlier. Bairstow did not finish.

Cote flew down Exeter Street in complete control of himself to win the Boston Marathon for the fourth time. As the crowds cheered wildly he saw his cousin, Charley Goulet, in the window of the Lenox Hotel. Charley had lost an arm and fingers from the other hand in Germany during the war. Cote yelled, "Charley, come down and bring me a beer!" In postrace celebration Cote consumed a glass of milk and then a beer and finally smoked a cigar.

Before reporters Cote minimized Vogel's narrative of abuses and his threat. The *Post* reported, "I did not hear him say, 'If you do that again, I will slug you.' I do not believe he said that. What would we do? Stop in the middle of the street and fight? That's so much nonsense. It was nothing."

Van Zant finished third. Ollie Manninen of the BAA lived in Fitchberg, Massachusetts, and for a living made stoves in Gardner. Vogel, Van Zant, Kelley, and Manninen made the U.S. Olympic team based on their Boston Marathon finish in a point system that accounted for other races. Kelley said he wanted to be the U.S. flag bearer at the London Olympic Games.

Cote said he was hoping Vogel would win, that Vogel was young and fast and it would be good for the sport if he did win. Had Vogel won, it is interesting for us to speculate, would more quick college runners have entered the game of marathon running to push out the plodders? So important were the coming Olympic Games for Cote that he used the Boston as a training run. He still had to run in the Canadian Olympic trials to qualify for the team. Cote already had Boston gold, but he was not satisfied; he wanted Olympic gold. Cote told Joe McKenney of the Boston *Post*, "I won a race I had no intention of winning. As a matter of fact. I did not want to win." That comment cut Vogel to the marrow.

Cote continued to run the Boston Marathon through the mid-1950s and attended the Boston Marathon into the 1980s. He died suddenly at his home in St. Hycinthe at age 79 on June 12, 1993.

1948 Results

1.	G. Cote, St. Hyacinthe, PQ	2:31:02*	9.	D. Mazzeo, Rockland, ME	2:43:15
2.	T. Vogel, *BAA*, Watertown, MA	2:31:46	10.	W. Dupree, *TYC*	2:43:42
3.	J. Van Zant, *BAA*	2:36:53	11.	E. Castilio, Guatemala	2:44:38
4.	J.A. Kelley, *BEEC*	2:37:52	12.	T. Mederios, *NMC*	2:45:33
5.	O. Manninen, *BAA*	2:39:59	13.	P. Collins, *MillAA*, NY	2:47:00
6.	L. Evans, *TFC*, Montreal, PQ	2:41:05	14.	C. Robbins, Jr., *ANC*, CT	2:48:44
7.	W. Fedorick, *HOC*, ON	2:41:23	15.	L. White, *NYPC*	2:49:07
8.	L. Velasquez, Guatemala	2:41:27	16.	W. Steiner, *MacAC*, NY	2:50:52

17.	L. Bolg, *MillAA*	2:53:35	30.	D. Van Dorp, Seton Hall, NJ	3:01:03
18.	T. Horne, *NYMA*	2:54:30	31.	P. Donato, *GEAA*	3:01:45
19.	L. Young, *NMC*	2:55:46	39.	T. Wood, *BAA*	3:20:30
20.	D. Hudson, *BAA*	2:56:01	42.	T. Crane, Springfield, MA	3:22:30
21.	W. Grube, *OWU*	2:56:07	43.	F. Brown, *NMC*	3:22:45
22.	R. Sawyer, Jamaica Plain, MA	2:56:18	50.	A. Scandurra, *MillAA*, NY	3:33:20
24.	M. O'Hara, Ozone Park, NY	2:56:56	**51.**	**C. DeMar, Reading, MA**	**3:37:25**
27.	F. Ward, Dover, NJ	2:59:45			

*Fastest time in the world in 1948.

UNDONE BY A TIME TRIAL?

TUESDAY, APRIL 19, 1949

Swedish Champ Comes to Race

Ted Vogel had graduated from Tufts to employment with a greeting card company. He attended sales training in Kansas and did not have time enough to train for the marathon. He came home to watch this year's race, not to return for victory.

But Joe Smith decided to make a comeback. He had said in 1942 after his victory that he would not run the Boston marathon again, but he could not stay away. He had tried, riding the press car, but there is no glory in delivering milk. The only time he got his picture in the paper delivering milk instead of running a marathon was when he delivered milk to Ted Vogel's dormitory.

The Koreans, Suh and his teammates, wanted to come back to Boston but could not make airplane connections in Tokyo in time, so they returned to Seoul. Vic Dyrgall of New York's Millrose AA looked like a serious contender. He was the national champion at 15 and 20 kilometers. At 28, he was an accountant for a company that owned a chain of stores. While at the University of Idaho Dyrgall had met Mike Ryan, the 1912 Boston Marathon winner. It was Ryan, a trainer at the university, who filled Dyrgall with tales of Boston. Old Boston marathoners often continued vicariously to pursue recruits to pursue victory. DeMar wrote a book. These inspirational trails left by ancient marathoners were easy to trace. The veterans talked a lot about their old marathoning days, and anyone within earshot could not help but be infected. Along with Ryan, another ancient Boston marathoner made a contribution to the 1949 field.

Runar Ohman, a Swedish immigrant who ran 8th in 1919 and 10th in 1920, went visiting in his homeland. He read about Karl Leandersson, a young groundskeeper in Valadalen, a resort town in the northern Swedish mountains, who could run well. The runner had three times been the Swedish cross-country champion. Friends and resort guests raised the funds to pay for the young runner's airfare to Boston as a next-best-thing to the Olympic Games. Ohman wrote to Ostersund Kamraterne Club and asked for Karl Gosta Leandersson to come to Boston to run the marathon. Leandersson was rapidly improving but was not well established as a marathon runner, so he had been left off the 1948 Swedish Olympic marathon team sent to London. In September of 1948 Leandersson won the Swedish marathon championships with a 2:31:12, and a month later he won the Kosice, Czechoslovakia, Marathon against the best of 12 nations with a dominating 2:34:46.4. He came to Boston ready to race.

Leandersson ran with some trepidation. He had not wanted to run as a favorite, but word of his time trial over the course 1 week earlier had leaked. He had run through 10 miles in 55:05 and 20 in 1:52:08 to post a final marathon time of 2:27:45. For a runner to test his fitness in such a long time trial so close to the designated race was akin to pulling up the carrots in the garden to see if they are ready. Leandersson was a man prone to bad luck. He had been bitten by a wolverine in 1946 while trying to feed the animal. The wound had become infected, and for 6 months Leandersson was not right. It might be suggested that he was a young man who had not yet developed a fine sense of judgment.

Lou White, who had won the time prize at the Cathedral run, looked ready to run the best race of his life. White, 34 years old, was black and small, 5'1/4" and 120 pounds. For work he swept out the Boston Arena. He was due at work the night of Patriots' Day. He had another job, too, as a shipper in a beer warehouse on Columbus Avenue. White was also the Class C handball champ at the Huntington Avenue YMCA, where a black man could not get a room. White was a skating champion as well. A graduate of New York University, he worked just enough to support himself and his eclectic athletic avocations.

Tom Jones, 32, of Pennsylvania, a history teacher at Lincoln University, led the 53rd Boston Marathon through Framingham and Natick, with Leandersson in second place. By Wellesley Leandersson passed Jones. Dyrgall moved into third with John Lafferty behind him. He had Leandersson and Dyrgall in sight.

Leandersson wore special shoes, with soles built up with sponge rubber. For traction he glued strips of rubber to their leather outsole. He wore no socks; he liked to train barefoot over golf courses and said barefoot running strengthened his feet. Today Leandersson was not as right or as strong as on the day of the time trial. As he ran with his long lean stride, the sunlight picked out copper highlights in his hair.

At Wellesley Square Leandersson ran 2:14 ahead of Yun Bok Suh's course-record pace. The weather was perfect for fast running. He had passed Jones after Natick and only Victor Dyrgall pursued him, although previous Boston winners Johnny Kelley, Gerard Cote, and Joe Smith chased him. Youngster

Jesse Van Zant ran in seventh place in Natick, but he began to learn his marathon lessons as the more experienced runners steadily marched past him for the duration of the race. This race was not as easy as had been his third place of the year before. But these lessons only made Van Zant hungrier.

Leandersson pulled away steadily. An aggravated Achilles tendon slowed him so that he did not run as fast as he had in his time trial, but he won easily. Had he had any tougher competition, running the time trial marathon so close to his race might have cost him the win at Boston. But it seems no one had a good race that day. The trailing runners spread out as they traveled the last part of the course. There were no dramatic stretch runs.

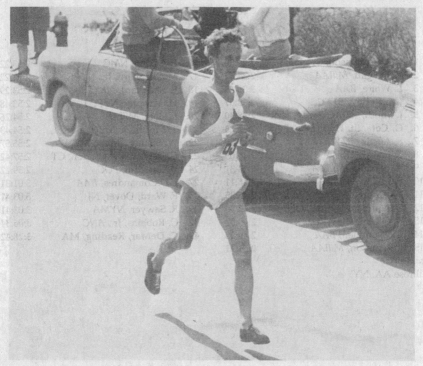

Karl Leandersson from Sweden ran a brilliant time trial on the course a week before the race, but would he have enough left to win? Photo courtesy of the *Boston Herald*.

The life fortunes of various runners changed from the days of the depression to the end of the war years: Clarence DeMar worked a Linotype machine at the *Boston Herald*, Fran Austin did pick-and-shovel work for the Quincy sewer department, Lloyd Bairstow worked in a restaurant in Cape Porpoise, Maine, where he had been stationed in the Coast Guard. As had been the case since the establishment of the marathon, the men who ran it by and large worked with their hands for a living. That was changing.

In the race Professor Jones struggled with blisters. Leandersson wanted to come back to Boston to win again with a time under 2:30. He set the goal of exceeding his time trial.

Milkman Joe Smith finished looking fresh. He told the *Globe* reporter after the race, "What's the sense of killing yourself? I could have done better, probably, but I'm still alive. That's what counts." Smith lived until January 25, 1993, when he died at age 77 in Pembroke Pines, Florida. Van Zant finished exhausted. He felt like he had nearly killed himself. His average pace was a minute per mile slower than the year before. The running had been so easy for the first 10 miles; maybe he needed to train more, he thought. Maybe that's what counts. He set to it.

1949 Results

1. K. Leandersson, Sweden	2:31:50	
2. V. Dyrgall, *MillAA*	2:34:42	
3. L. White, *BAA*	2:36:48	
4. J.A. Kelley, *BEEC*	2:38:07	
5. J. Smith, *RDAC*	2:38:30	
6. G. Cote, St. Hyacinthe, PQ	2:42:55	
7. F. Austin, *BAA*	2:43:28	
8. T. Jones, *LU*, PA	2:44:05	
9. A. Neidnig, *MillAA*	2:44:31	
10. P. Collins, *MillAA*	2:45:11	
11. W. Dupree, Foxboro, MA	2:45:35	
12. G. Norman, *GladAC*, ON	2:47:30	
13. K. O'Connell, *WRU*	2:48:52	
14. O. Manninen, *BAA*	2:49:38	
15. J. Kernason, *MillAA*	2:51:21	

16. L. Young, *NMC*	2:53:22
17. M. Shepherd, Jr., *NYPC*, NY	2:53:22
18. E. Shephard, *NMC*	2:53:29
19. H. Murphy, *NYPC*	2:53:48
20. L. Bolg, *MillAA*	2:54:26
21. T. Mederios, *NMC*	2:54:43
22. W. Steiner, Bronx, NY	2:55:57
23. G. Terry, New London, CT	2:57:42
24. J. Van Zant, *FOC*	2:59:22
27. J. DiComandrea, *BAA*	3:01:31
28. F. Ward, Dover, NJ	3:03:41
29. R. Sawyer, *NYMA*	3:03:41
32. C. Robbins, Jr., *ANC*	3:06:34
49. C. DeMar, Reading, MA	3:28:42

Team prize
Millrose AA, NY

Chapter 6

1950-1959
No More Plodders

Presidents: *Harry S. Truman, Dwight D. Eisenhower*

Massachusetts Governors: *Paul A. Dever, Christian Herter, Foster Furcolo*

Boston Mayor: *John B. Hynes*

1950 Populations: *United States, 151,325,798; Massachusetts, 4,690,514; Boston, 790,863*

Journalist I.F. Stone called the decade the "Haunted Fifties." The fear of communism, the fear of not conforming—for some the fear of conforming—cast a spell on nearly everyone during the period. Communists could be anywhere, and anyone acting strangely might be one. Yet in spite of, or perhaps causing, political and personal malaise, the people of America enjoyed unparalleled prosperity and mobility.

War opened the decade as 60,000 North Korean troops invaded South Korea in June of 1950. The decade closed with the election of a youthful president, John F. Kennedy. Eisenhower's landslide election victories in 1952 and 1956 showed that America preferred a genial president who played a lot of golf to "give 'em hell Harry" Truman. Nikita Khrushchev, the leader of the Soviet Union, on the other hand, said he would "bury" the capitalist states.

African nations decolonized. Africans born in this decade and the next would one day come to win the Boston Marathon. With the old colonial powers gone, the U.S. played the new Cold War game of favoring and disfavoring countries according to how anti-Soviet geopolitics fared.

A quick review of the '50s points up some characterizing events: People in January of 1950 talked about the Boston Brink's robbery of $2.8 million. J.D. Salinger published *Catcher in the Rye* in 1951. In 1952 a new reason for fear arose with the explosion of the first nuclear hydrogen fusion bomb in the Eniwetok Atoll in the Pacific. Soon the Soviets had their own H-bomb. A U.S.-aided coup installed Mohammad Reza Pahlavi as shah of Iran in 1953, replacing Premier Mohammed Mossadegh. Senator Joseph McCarthy imagined communists plotting everywhere and held hearings beginning April 22, 1954, to find them out. The communist conspiracy may not have been real, but Julius and Ethel Rosenberg were found guilty of such a conspiracy and executed. The censure of red-baiting McCarthy by Congress in December 1954 eased the paranoia somewhat.

In 1955 Rosa Parks, a black woman, refused to give up her seat on a bus to a white man, igniting the case that led to bus segregation being declared unconstitutional. The Federal Highway Act signed into law on June 29, 1956, inaugurated the interstate highway system and guaranteed that the United States would become a nation of the automobile. Those of the road-running subculture took to the roads in beat-up automobiles to travel anywhere every weekend for an ever-increasing number of races. Jack Kerouac published *On the Road* in 1957, and the Soviet Sputnik became the first man-made earth satellite in October of 1957.

Alaska and Hawaii were territories for their last year in 1958. In 1959 the music died when a plane crash killed rock-and-roll original Buddy Holly. Fidel Castro overthrew the Batista regime in January 1959.

In this world of the 1950s the Boston Athletic Association operated the marathon on just a few thousand dollars' profit from their indoor track meet. Marathon runners trained more than those of the '40s and followed bold, nonconformist notions of intense training from European schools of thought like the one fathered by Emil Zatopek. Fast, talented, college runners replaced the old "plodders." The new marathoners experimented with speed training. The world had shrunk and a worldliness invaded American runners. Yet ever-haunting was the fear that the Reds might take away all of America's prosperity. U.S. military advisors went to Vietnam. In the public mind athletic training and military training remained linked. There was no such thing as fitness running. One trained to race.

Prosperity brought the freedom to train for marathons. The malaise of the Cold War brought the need to escape to the roads and woods for long runs. For this small group of men trying to run faster than they had ever run before, running was their art, their poetry, their rock and roll. Communications made the sport global. Runners everywhere quickly knew what times runners elsewhere ran and wanted to know how they trained. They got to know each other through international communications and discovered that they liked each other. Runners from different cultures found that they had more in common than they had with some of their own neighbors. British runners Roger Bannister broke 4 minutes for the mile and Jim Peters broke 2:20 for a marathon. Runners wrote books about running.

Jet airline service began. Before that it would take 10 days by boat or 18 hours in a propeller-driven DC3 to come from Europe to run in the Boston Marathon. Nevertheless, except for one day during the '50s, foreign runners dominated Boston. But the pursuit of victory there dominated the thoughts of a new generation of American runners, track-trained and fast, who replaced the plodders of the decades before.

Van Zant, Choi, Ham, and Song

Korean Team in Town for Big Race

Uncoachable Jesse Van Zant, impulsive, talented, and restless, ran to defend Boston, and therefore American, distance running from a trio of Koreans. Van Zant worked as a laborer, or a groundskeeper, or in a paper processing plant. It didn't matter. He loved to run. He lived to run. All he wanted to do was to run as fast as a human being could. He fit his means of making a living around his life as a runner. He moved around a lot. He grew up in California. He moved to Boston to run. He moved back to California. He moved back to Boston. Two high school kids from Connecticut, one with the marathoner's name of John Kelley—John J. Kelley—and his pal, George Terry, idolized Jesse Van Zant. To them he was a saint. For months the two kids imagined they saw Van Zant everywhere. They had never met him, only read about him in the newspapers. They didn't know what he looked like, yet they thought of him daily, hourly. One day they saw a man they reasoned must be him on the streets of New London, Connecticut. They overcame their timidity and approached him to ask if he were Jesse Van Zant. He was not. So great were the talent and legend of Van Zant that high school boys bitten with the running bug saw him everywhere. The press and runners and officials expected wandering Jesse Van Zant to win the Boston Marathon one of these years.

Van Zant had won the 1950 Dilboy 20-miler in Medford with ease. He was big and strong like a woodsman. He could run fast. He did not come out of the plodder mold of DeMar or Kelley. He was not a skinny little endurance vessel. He proved that he of all Americans could run a marathon under 2:30. Uncoachable he was, but so had been his mentor, Jock Semple. Both were stubborn, independent men. American talent and courage seemed to ride along with streaks of independence. In the BAA race of 1948 Van Zant had worn new shoes that rubbed painful blisters on his feet, but still he hobbled to 3rd with a 2:36. In 1949 he staggered to 24th in just under 3 hours.

Jesse Van Zant was born in Costa Rica of a Costa Rican mother and a Dutch farmer father. When Jesse was 6 months old the family moved to San Francisco. Van Zant inherited his dark, dancing eyes from his mother. His

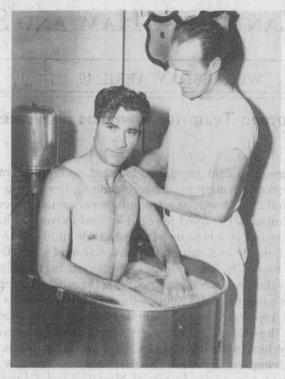

Jock Semple seems to be baptizing BAA Running Club hope Jesse Van Zant in the whirlpool bath. Semple pinned all his hopes on Van Zant to be the first BAA runner to win the Boston Marathon. Photo courtesy of the *Boston Herald*.

shy, taciturn nature may have come from his father. His hair curled, perhaps in response to a hybrid vigor. Like a saint he purely devoted himself to his passion. But his racing tactics, at least from the point of view of Semple, came straight from hell. He had difficulty settling down. During the war Van Zant served in the Pacific theater. In pursuit of running, in 5 years he moved across the country many times; he moved to New York and joined the Millrose Athletic Association, then back to San Francisco and came to New England to run the 25-kilometer championships in Gloucester, Massachusetts. There he met Jock Semple, the moving force behind the BAA running team, and moved to Boston.

Common streaks of stubbornness, independence, and unabashed love for running and road runners attracted Van Zant and Semple to each other. Van Zant happened to mention that he'd like to move to New England to train for the Boston Marathon. Semple thought that was a wonderful idea, that it would be good for Jesse to settle down and stop commuting across the country. Semple encouraged Van Zant to settle in Boston, not knowing what a vexation Van Zant would become. He seemed to be a pliable young man, ready to move anywhere to improve his running. He was shy. He was quiet. In Gloucester Van Zant appeared to be the pupil who would go anywhere and do anything. Semple saw in him the dedicated young man who would be the one to win the Boston Marathon. Jock saw Jesse winning, wearing the unicorn of the sponsoring Boston Athletic Association. The last BAA contender, Ted Vogel, had gotten so involved in his job that he could not make a comeback to contend for the Boston title. Jesse was Jock's man. But although Van Zant did not express himself often, and never as loudly as Semple, he had his own interpretations of what to do and when to do it.

Now Van Zant had trained to run faster than he had ever run before. He had learned the tricks of the trade. He wore old shoes so he would not have the same trouble as in 1948. He demonstrated his talent in countless victories in shorter races. And if he would only listen to Semple, Boston would be his, too.

Before the 1950 Yonkers Marathon Semple had told Van Zant to go out slowly and not burn himself out as he had the year before. As Charley Robbins told it, Semple carefully explained the folly of that. As Robbins and Semple slogged along near the end of the pack at about 8 minutes a mile, they assumed that Van Zant was way up in front, near but not ahead of the leaders. At 5 miles Jesse came up behind them. His arrival astounded Charley, but it made Jock livid: "What the hell arrrrre yuh doin?" "Starting slow," replied Jesse, proudly expecting the coach's praise for following orders. (That pace would yield a time of 3:30, an hour slower than Van Zant's ability.) Jock's reply came in a blast: "Well, get going!" Van Zant blasted off and finished second. Jock said to Charley, "Therrrr goes a million dollar rrrrrunnerrr with a five cent brrrrrrrrrain!"

By contrast, the trio of Koreans stayed put and trained full-time. They spent $9,020 to come to Boston to run Van Zant into the ground. They planned their strategy to target Van Zant from the outset.

The 1949 winner, Karl Gosta Leandersson, who had run a 2:27 time trial over the course a week before the 1949 race, came back to run in 1950. Most of the predictors discounted him, but Johnny A. Kelley picked him. Leandersson, however, had a high fever linked to a disease that had recurred since he was 19. His episode of erythema multiforme was a skin reaction to an infection. Leandersson was a sick man. Purple rashes spotted the pale skin of his legs. He had no business racing a marathon. Regardless, he ran.

Joe McKenney of the *Boston Post* wrote in his prerace story, "There is the slight, but fond hope that Johnny Kelley—the plodders' own Ponce de Leon—may find one final drop of his personal Fountain of Youth still left in his canteen."

Semple wanted to learn something about the abilities of the Koreans. In the days before the race they visited him often in his trainer room, what one reporter called "Semple's sunless solarium." Semple treated the Koreans as honored guests. They came to him complaining of injuries, and he would kindly offer a hot whirlpool bath. They accepted and kept coming back with more and more little injuries that they didn't really seem to have. Semple thought they simply liked the whirlpool and concluded that they had nothing like it in Korea. He watched the Koreans carefully and tried to gather intelligence that might be useful to Van Zant. But he could learn only a little: There were three of them and Coach Ki Chung Sohn, the runners were young, and they were all inspired by Yun Bok Suh's 1947 victory and world record at Boston. The youngest, Kee Yong Ham, had a bristle-brush haircut. The fastest was Yun Chi Choi. He was the reigning national champion. The third, Ki Yoon Song, could keep up with both in training. The coach was older. But Semple wanted to know how the Koreans ran. What was their strength? Their weakness? They trained out of sight. Semple complained, "They aren't running where any of us can get a line on them."

Ham would graduate from high school the next March. After this marathon he planned to visit American schools, for he wanted to attend college in the United States.

Semple picked Van Zant, "the most graceful runner I've ever seen," over the Koreans. Americans wanted an American to win. Yet the newspapers disagreed. "Favorite today—three tiny stained-skin men." America had won the war against "tiny stained-skin men" and was the most powerful nation on Earth, so American sports fans began to expect that one American was as good as 10 foreigners. An American champion had to emerge to take the Boston Marathon. The public was dismayed by the press predictions. Someone must save U.S. prestige. Semple reversed his earlier advice and told Van Zant to take an immediate lead.

Van Zant did. Under an overcast sky in ideal conditions Van Zant took the lead from the very first step. The Koreans lined up behind him. Leandersson dogged them. The 1936 Olympic gold medalist, Ki Chung Sohn, again coached the Korean team, but it was a younger team than the one in 1947. Choi caught Van Zant at 6 miles. Sohn's team answered every one of Van Zant's surges. Van Zant authored a surge into Wellesley. The Koreans hung on to him for 17 miles, eventually draining his surging. His talent, his strength, his aggressiveness all bled away under the tenacity of the Koreans. His willpower leaked away, too. Suddenly all the hope drained out of Van Zant. The big expectations and his physical feeling did not match. Victory grew into an impossible dream, then a nightmare. He dropped out of the race. Leandersson dropped out too.

No one pursued the Koreans. Kee Yong Ham led the bunch. At 17 miles he had felt for the first time that he might win. But by the 21-mile mark the fight with Van Zant had depleted Ham. He began to fall apart.

Ham stopped to walk 5 times in the last 5 miles. His sweat stung his eyes. He struggled to relax; fearing his leg muscles would cramp, he walked up the entire length of the last hill. He walked in terror of the gripping onset of a cramp that would paralyze his reaction to a runner coming up on him. But he held such a big lead that no one could catch him. Behind him his fellow runners suffered as much as he did. He ran past Boston College and down Beacon Street. No one came near. On to Exeter Street he ran alone. Twenty yards from the finish a college student on a prank, wearing a phony number, dodged the police and jumped in beside Ham to get into the finish line photo and fulfill the requirements for his sophomoric fraternity. The man suddenly appearing alongside him baffled Ham. But the buffoon did not baffle spectator Joe Smith. Within yards of the finish, Smith, the BAA winner from the spring of 1942, saw what had happened and seethed. He knew the student was a phony and was about to steal another young man's moment of glory. He knew Ham had given everything he had to get to that place, and no prankster should steal an accomplishment so painfully earned. Smith leaped out of the crowd and shoved the fraud into a bunch of spectators, who pummeled the imposter and left him seeking medical attention. Kee Yong Ham ran on to his deserved glorious finish. Ki Yoon Song soon followed.

Choi, a 2nd-year student at Chosen Christian College in Seoul, followed Song. Choi had led the London Olympic marathon to within 2 miles of the finish. He ran with a choppy stride and without a back-kick. Suddenly on Exeter Street, Choi stopped. He could see the finish line. He nonchalantly massaged his leg. He never looked back. John Patrick Lafferty, a first-class aviation mechanics mate in the U.S. Navy from Dorchester, could see Choi

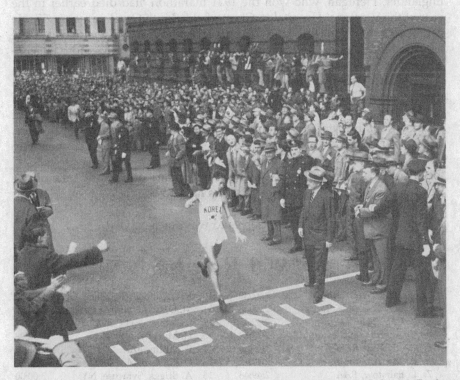

In 1950 Korean Kee Yong Ham continues the tradition of Yun Bok Suh's 1947 win. AP/Wide World Photos.

and the finish line. Lafferty wanted third place; he sprinted. He passed Choi on the far side of the road. Both men could see the finish line, but Choi could not see, or did not turn to see, the sprinting Lafferty. Lafferty saw the Korean trainer running in the opposite direction. Lafferty thought Choi was down and out and that third place was his. He relaxed. A Korean spectator screamed at Choi. Choi looked up and saw Lafferty across the road and ahead of him. That sight ignited a rocketing sprint in Choi. Lafferty had no rocket. With the din of the crowd he never heard Choi coming back. Choi swept by, leaving Lafferty no time to respond before the finish line.

Ham, Song, and Choi completed the first-ever 1-2-3 team sweep of the Boston Marathon. Ham told reporters after the race, "I am happy, but too bad I had to beat Choi. He is the champion." All Korea, a country that had been down too long, rejoiced for this sweeping victory on the heels of Suh's win of 1947.

In Seoul that year, electricity was usually shut off at night because of the military tensions with the North. But this night a special order decreed that the electricity be left flowing so the people could listen to the Voice of America broadcast progress reports on the three runners in Boston.

Lafferty received the Jimmy Henigan trophy for finishing as the first New Englander. Henigan, who won the 1931 marathon, had died earlier in the year at the Veterans' Hospital in Chesterfield, South Carolina, at age 57. He had been in ill health (probably a result of alcoholism) for several years. He left a wife, four sons, and three daughters in poverty in Medford, Massachusetts.

The Korean sweep extracted both respect and criticism from American marathoners. Clarence DeMar characteristically said, "That tells what you can do by hard work. We have too many machines in this country." But Charley Robbins sympathetically came to the defense of American runners. He said, "Get the A.A.U. or some other organization to give us money to do nothing but train for six months and it would be a pushover for us too." Jock Semple agreed: "They're good but how many of us could take off for Korea to train and run a race? Most of us have to beg for a *day* off from our jobs to rest on the day before a race."

Jesse and Jock resigned themselves to wait for next year.

1950 Results

1. K. Ham, Seoul, Korea **2:32:39**	10. K. O'Connell, Cleveland, OH 2:56:42
2. K. Song, Seoul, Korea 2:35:58	11. M. O'Hara, *MillAA* 2:57:37
3. Y. Choi, Seoul, Korea 2:39:47	12. J. Sterner, *NYPC*, NY 2:58:02
4. J. Lafferty, Dorchester, MA 2:39:52	13. H. Murphy, *NYPC* 2:58:08
5. J.A. Kelley, *BEEC* **2:43:45**	14. F. Austin, *BAA* 2:58:10
6. A. Mederios, *NMC* 2:47:15	15. C. Budd, *BAA* 2:58:29
7. L. Bairstow, *BAA* 2:49:46	16. A. Briggs, Syracuse, NY 3:00:00
8. P. Collins, *MillAA* 2:50:12	17. W. Steiner, *MillAA* 3:00:52
9. E. Romognoli, *NYCP* 2:52:50	18. F. Mulvihill, *GladAC*, ON 3:01:35

19. J. Ficcaro, *SH*, NY	3:01:42	
20. G. Gallant, Moncton, NB	3:01:58	
21. L. Davis, *NYMA*	3:03:07	
22. J. Semple, *BAA*	3:03:22	
23. J. Gray, Jr., *BAA*	3:05:12	
24. L. White, *NYPC*	3:05:56	

27. A. Scandurra, *MillAA*, NY	3:09:37
28. O. Manninen, *BAA*	3:11:50
29. R. Sawyer, *NYMA*	3:12:05
38. C. Robbins, Jr., *ANC*, CT	3:25:04
41. C. DeMar, Reading, MA	**3:28:13**

167 starters.
Team prize
Korea

HIROSHIMA

THURSDAY, APRIL 19, 1951

Japanese Marathoners Invade Boston

In 1950 three young Koreans had come and snatched BAA victory from Jesse Van Zant. This year four Japanese came to do the snatching. They planned to better the Korean sweep and take the top four. The Japanese marathoners felt that anything the Koreans could do they could do better. All that stood in their way were Van Zant and three Americans. The American press did nothing to hide their bias. Tom Fitzgerald of the *Boston Daily Globe* wrote about the previous year that "the little brown men whipsawed Van Zant back and forth." This year Van Zant resolved not to pay attention to his rivals. Jesse's coach, Jock Semple, said, "The one important idea I've tried to drum into him this spring is not to get maneuvered into running somebody else's race." But the Japanese came to run their own races and had something to prove. A peaceful, but competitive, national pride existed in occupied Japan. Soon the world would learn about it from their export of superior marathon runners drawn from the seemingly endless ranks of tough, disciplined young men. These young Japanese grew up in a world of war where the bombs fell on their own soil.

On the morning of August 6, 1945, 13-year-old Shigeki Tanaka had heard the American bombers high over Hiroshima. He had no indication that the raid would be any different from the hundreds of others. At times Johnny Kelley's younger brother, the late Eddie, had flown these missions. The Tanaka family owned a farm 20 miles outside the city. Shigeki saw the bright flash and the smoke and knew that this raid was more powerful, but none of his family were hurt by the fireball and fallout. A month later Japan unconditionally surrendered to General Douglas MacArthur. Thereafter, as commander of the occupation army, MacArthur had essentially become the ruler of Japan. Now young Tanaka, with a 2:28:15 victory in the Japanese team trials, came to Boston to win the marathon.

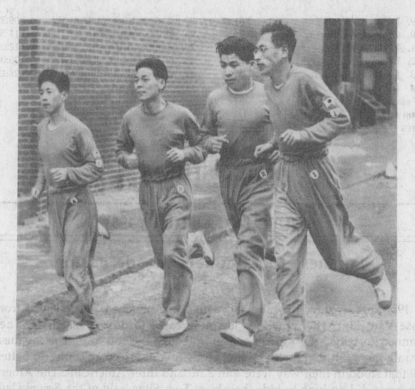

The 1951 Japanese marathon team invades Boston, planning to sweep the top four places: (from left) Yoshitaka Uchikawa, Fukuoka; Shigeki Tanaka, Hiroshima; Hiromi Haigo, Tokushima; and Shunji Koyanagi, Yamaguchi. Photo courtesy of the *Boston Herald*.

Kelley was the current American national champion. To get that title he outran a rapidly closing Jesse Van Zant at Yonkers. But Kelley, in his 20th BAA marathon, saw no chance of winning. He was having more fun than ever running and socializing now that he did not feel the pressure to win. Before the race Kelley made known his opinions on the chances of the Japanese:

> They could do it sight unseen because that's their whole life—the whole life, at least, for this particular four. They never ride, because there's little to ride in Japan. So they're always walking and running. As for this particular race and objective, they're privileged to make a career of it. They train a whole year. They come here and rest and train for three weeks. We working men, running only on weekends and in our spare time, must compete against that. It is unfortunate that the Korean sweep of last year should have been presented

before the whole world the way it was. People in other countries don't understand the full story. They conclude American athletics are soft. That is not true.

While Tanaka and the field passed about the 5-mile mark MacArthur began his speech to a joint session of Congress and to 30 million television viewers. President Truman had fired him in a test of civilian control of the military. Might MacArthur defy the president? Half the people who would ordinarily spend Patriots' Day lining Boston streets to cheer for the marathoners and wait for old Clarence DeMar planted themselves by their televisions and radios to listen to MacArthur. His story pushed marathon stories below the fold on the front pages of Boston papers. The general had come back to America after warring in the Pacific for 14 years. On April 19, 1951, the great general told the nation that old soldiers never die, they just fade away. Then he did just that. But Japan, militarily defeated, would not fade away. Four neat young Japanese men came to Boston wearing blue blazers with insignia on the breast pockets. Their plan of attack was to extract unconditional surrender from American marathoners by sweeping their marathon 1-2-3-4.

John Patrick Lafferty, who had finished fourth last year, had come to running rather late in life. In 1948 he had missed a bus that would take him to duty at the naval base. The navy penalizes tardiness, so to arrive on time for duty Lafferty ran the 5 miles. He liked the feeling. He found he was good at it. Lafferty was 33 and a 12-year navy man stationed in Quonset, Rhode Island, the father of three small daughters. He had graduated from Snyder High in New Jersey, class of 1933. In 1948 the navy stationed Lafferty in Newfoundland to watch the weather. Although there was plenty of weather to watch, Lafferty quickly bored. To him Newfoundland was little more than a big, foggy rock. Out of boredom he entered a 10-miler. He "half-killed" himself, but after another year on the rock he trained for the race and won it easily. As runners of the era go, Lafferty was big, 155 pounds and 6' tall. He was easy to spot amid the Japanese.

Shunji Koyanagi, of Yamaguchi, the 26-year-old Japanese national champion (2:30:10), took the early lead. He wore eyeglasses. He followed the plan of the team coach, Seiichiro Tsuda. Tsuda had placed just out of the marathon medals in the Amsterdam and Los Angeles Olympic Games of 1928 and 1932. He knew his sport. Koyanagi ran about a half minute slower than the course record to Framingham on the chilly day (31:04; the record of 30:23 was held by Ellison Brown, 1936). Van Zant ran his own race in sixth place. Tanaka ran just behind him.

But by Natick (51:06; record of 50:45 by Brown, 1936) the Japanese held the top three places. Their fourth man, Hiromi Haigo of Tokushima, ran in the top 10 despite a stress fracture in his ankle. X rays before the race had shown the break, but for the sake of Japan, Haigo ignored the pain.

Koyanagi, Yoshitaka Uchikawa of Fukuoka, and Tanaka led through Wellesley (1:07:38; record of 1:07:31 by Brown, 1936). Lafferty and Van Zant, both running for the BAA club, ran fourth and seventh. Their tactics seemed reasonable. Athanasios Ragazos, 38, of Athens, ran sixth. Ragazos had run at Boston before, placing sixth in 1947.

By Lake Street Tanaka had moved up to second. Once a 10,000-meter man, he had moved up to the marathon.

Kelley and Gerard Cote hovered just out of the top 10. They waited for the inevitable attrition, when they would pass the young fellows who had underestimated the enormity of the marathon. One of the harder men of American athletics was Bob Black, who ran in 10th place. Perhaps he was the speediest and most talented man of all. He was a wisp at 5'11" and 121 pounds. But he did not understand and respect the marathon the way the Japanese did. He said,

I think I can run the BAA in 2 hr, 20 min. I think the geography of the layout is ready made for lots of sustained speed—a speed greater than most BAA winners have shown. I think I have that speed. The first 18 miles is predominantly downhill. I figure the course requires high speed for the first 21 miles then a changeover starting the final five miles to speed combined with stamina. I think I have the stamina as well as the speed.

Black had spent 40 months in the army, 26 overseas, and then finished college. As a diploma-carrying runner at age 28, Black was just the sort of man who would lead the new generation of speedy, educated American marathoners. At Rhode Island State College, Black had won nearly everything in track and cross-country, up to two national collegiate and two Amateur Athletic Union cross-country championships. He had easily won a couple of recent 12-mile races. He was the heir apparent to the physical working men, the bricklayers, carpenters, miners, and ditch-diggers who had gone before. He and those like him would no longer have to exhaust themselves to make a living but could save their sweat for training. Black's talent was real, but he trained oblivious of the demands of the marathon. In January he ran a total of 50 miles (Cote did that in one day), in February, 100, and in March, 167—an average of less than 30 miles a week. But Black was Semple's pick to beat the Japanese four.

A hundred yards beyond Boston College Tanaka caught Koyanagi. Koyanagi did not resist. Tanaka got to Lake Street faster than anyone had, beating Brown's 1939 time by about half a minute. By Coolidge Corner Tanaka ran only 16 seconds slower than Suh's record. Black, Lafferty, and Van Zant never mounted a threat.

All the Japanese wore bifurcated footwear. The shoe uppers were canvas fashioned into a mitten of sorts, with a "thumb" for the big toe; the belief was that they could get a better grip with this shoe and a pure rubber sole.

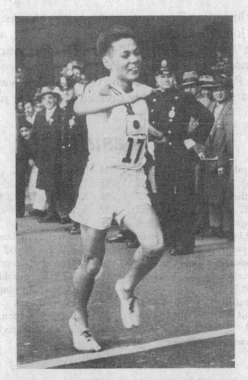

Shod in bifurcated footwear, Shigeki Tanaka wins the 1951 Boston Marathon. His shoes were made like mittens to allow a better grip. Photo courtesy of the *Boston Herald*.

The sole followed the "mitten" outline. Tanaka ran alone to the finish, where Mayor Hynes crowned him with the wreath of Greek laurel. On the victory stand baby-faced Tanaka talked and beamed. But his team did not get the sweep they wanted. Big Lafferty, Ragazos, and a tiny black American from New York named Lou White took the next three places.

Bob Black (who was white) walked the entire length of Exeter Street. "I have lots to learn. The heavy pounding that comes from hitting the roads for so many miles knotted the muscles highest in my legs. We can't let these foreigners keep showing us up every year." He decided to launch a full-scale training attack.

"I'm a couple of years away from my peak as a marathon runner," said Van Zant. Observers of the sport suspected that Van Zant suffered from a BAA mental complex. "Everybody seems to say I can do it yet. I'll sure keep trying."

"I'm not really in peak shape yet," said Lafferty.

Tanaka did not return to Boston; as of 1993 he was living in retirement in Tokyo.

A month later Jesse Van Zant won the American National Championship on a sprint over John Patrick Lafferty on the tough, hilly, accurate Yonkers course in 2:37:12. The next year would be an Olympic year and the foreign entrants would not be as formidable. Perhaps Lafferty would be Semple's great BAA hope. Perhaps it would be the year for Black, Van Zant, Lafferty, or Semple—or maybe an impeccably dressed accountant named Victor.

*1951 Results**

1.	S. Tanaka, Hiroshima, Japan	2:27:45	14.	J. Doherty, *NMC*	2:48:37
2.	J. Lafferty, *BAA*	2:31:15	15.	T. Corbitt, *NYPC*	2:48:42
3.	A. Ragazos, Athens, Greece	2:35:27	16.	A. Neidnig, *MillAA*, NY	2:49:20
4.	L. White, *NYPC*	2:35:53	17.	A. Confalone, *NMC*	2:50:31
5.	S. Koyanagi, Japan	2:38:36	18.	P. Collins, *MillAA*	2:50:58
6.	**J.A. Kelley, *BEEC***	**2:39:09**	19.	C. Farrar, New London, CT	2:51:05
7.	**G. Cote, St. Hyacinthe, PQ**	**2:41:15**	20.	C. Robbins, *NYPC*	2:51:44
8.	Y. Uchikawa, Fukuoka, Japan	2:41:31	32.	B. Black, Providence, RI	3:01:57
9.	H. Haigo, Tokushima, Japan	2:42:23	57.	M. Dukakis, Brookline, MA	3:31:00
10.	J. Van Zant, *BAA*	2:43:35	67.	**C. DeMar, Reading, MA**	**3:37:41**
11.	S. Koru, Istanbul, Turkey	2:43:41	75.	O. Spooner, MA	NT
12.	J. Marshall, *BAA*	2:43:49	81.	R. Packard, Boston, MA	NT
13.	F. Austin, *BAA*	2:46:07	85.	C. Bourdelais, Brockton, MA	NT

191 entrants, 153 starters.

Team prize
BAA

*This course was later found to be short. See page 248 for the story.

INFERNO II

SATURDAY, APRIL 19, 1952

Van Zant Leads Americans Against Foreigners

On April 19, 1952, Will Cloney of the *Boston Herald* nominated Jesse Van Zant, John Patrick Lafferty, and Bob Black the "American bulwark against foreign invasion." He didn't figure on Victor Dyrgall. Dyrgall was a Fort Lee, New Jersey, accountant. He looked like an accountant. He dressed like an accountant. He arrived at races dressed impeccably in a serious business suit. The other runners showed up in their sloppy clothes. After the race Dyrgall reclothed himself to look just as meticulous as when he arrived. A few young marathoners wondered how he got his suit from Hopkinton to Boston without a wrinkle. Where did he hang it? Dyrgall calculated a couple of things about his running. First he would win the Boston Marathon, then he would make the Olympic team. He was a small, thin, 32-year-old man with slight silver at his temples. He had finished second at Boston to Karl Gosta Leandersson in 1949. So why not first? Dyrgall's habit was to race only when he was ready. That meant that he did not race often. His fellow runners saw him as neat and mysterious.

Bob Black put action behind his new respect for the marathon distance. But he had trained so much that he injured his leg and could not start this year's race.

No foreigners entered except for three Guatemalans, Luis Velasquez, Guillermo Rojas, and Doroteo Flores. Other non-U.S. runners presumably stayed home to prepare to qualify for their countries' Olympic selection processes. But weather foreign to New England in April also entered the region. The temperature reached 76 °F in Hopkinton at starting time. It would climb into the low 80s before the race ended.

Velasquez, 32 and muscular, was the fastest of the three Guatemalans. He worked for the railroad as a time clerk. The cotton mill worker, 5'8", 130-pound, 30-year-old Flores was not muscular. He seemed to have skin painted directly over his bones, looking like a sun-dried fig. It was not that he looked emaciated, the way some highly trained, hollow, half-starved runners do with their skin appearing to be shrunken over their bones. Flores looked as if he had always been thin and always would be. Yet, he was darkly handsome, with a pencil-thin moustache. He finished his schooling at the 8th grade, then worked on farms and banana plantations, but at age 21 his big chance came. He got a $1.25-a-day job in the cotton mill. The employees there formed a track club; Flores ran the 1,500 meters but quickly found he was better at the longer distances.

Flores had run in Boston before. In 1947 he dropped out in Wellesley. He lived 12 hilly miles from the hot, humid cotton mills and frequently ran to work and back in the same day. Like Henri Renaud, who won the "inferno" Boston Marathon in 1909, Flores worked in an environment that prepared him for racing on a hot day. Flores did not mind the hard work in the mills as long as he had time enough to run. He remained unmarried and lived with his family, including many younger sisters. At work and at play he sweated. Daily he took gallons of water into his body and sweated them all out. The BAA offered a solid gold, diamond-studded medal to the winner of their race. Winning the marathon is what Flores came back to Boston to do.

Jesse Van Zant, newly wed and living in Quincy, Massachusetts, now worked as a temporary postal employee. He could use some diamonds and gold himself. Jerry Nason of the *Globe* picked Van Zant to win. Clarence DeMar did not. In a prerace article in the *Globe* (curiously, though DeMar worked as a compositor for the *Herald*, he wrote running articles for the *Globe*), he wrote this:

> The human body is such a wonderful machine that the subconscious intelligence seems able to dig up unexpected bits of endurance if a man is really interested and is concentrating on using what he

has. I have always believed that both Vogel and Van Zant might
have won the big race had they depended more on their inner
strength and less on the friendship and direction of a trainer
[Jock Semple].

Van Zant had won Yonkers in 1951 but still feared his Boston jinx. Representing the BAA, he might be the one to make Jock's dream come true and
wear the colors of the sponsoring club to victory, but Semple put his money
on another BAA runner.

On April 12, Semple guided the Guatemalans, John Lafferty, Van Zant,
and 20 others in a 2-hour training run. Semple picked Lafferty to win the
big race. He ran second in 1951, so winning would come next. Lafferty had
achieved all of his past BAA goals. Semple knew his sport. Who could argue
with a man with such a cantankerous love for road runners? The *Boston Post*
said that Semple puts "the good neighbor policy into practice by treating
and advising the Guatemalans just as he does his own charges. The guy
should be in the State Department."

In the race itself, the Americans started conservatively, respecting the heat.
Flores ran in the lead with Velasquez until Natick. There Velasquez slowed.
He had run Boston with an eighth place in 1948. He knew what was coming.
Flores, who had a policy of never looking back in a race, ran on. He didn't
see his lead lengthen. The crowds may have shouted that fact to him, but
he spoke no English so never understood that he was winning easily. He
ran along dumping water on his head and letting it drip onto his dark-blue
shirt with "Guatemala" printed across the chest.

Jerry Nason watched the race and wrote of Flores:

He looked almost fierce, like some bird of prey about to plummet
on a mid-day meal, as he now took complete mastery over the 56th
Boston AA marathon race and ruthlessly ran his opponents goofy
from there to the finish. There was a savageness to his performance
that had been unequaled on the course since the Indian Ellison
Brown dedicated his every ounce of heart and muscle to the task
of smashing the record in 1939.

No one came up to challenge Flores. Flores did not tire or dehydrate. He
won easily. After Flores finished, the spectators at the finish line had nothing
to do for a long time. Flores had the largest winning margin since Young
had won in 1937. The *Herald* writer, Joe McKenney, described "a weird period
of waiting before the faltering, spasmodic parade of runners-up entered the
stretch run of Exeter St." Dyrgall, in testimony to his superb conditioning
on a day that gave no help to long-distance runners, finished nearly 5 minutes
after Flores. Only 10 men broke 3 hours. None was under the age of 30.
Lloyd Bairstow dropped out at 8 miles, Les Pawson dropped out at 18, and
the third Guatemalan, Rojas, had to be rushed to the hospital for an emergency appendectomy.

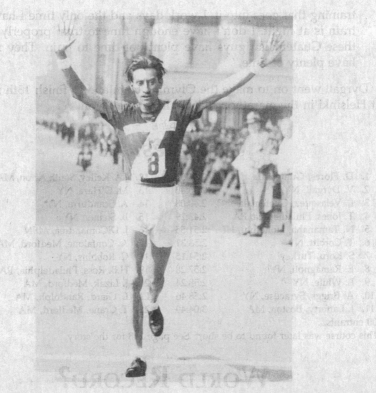

As lean and perfectly adapted to the heat as any desert dweller, Doroteo Flores, a worker in a steamy Guatemalan textile factory, beat the heat and all comers in the 1952 Boston Marathon. Photo courtesy of the *Boston Herald*.

When Harris Browning Ross, the Olympic steeplechaser who had won the Cathedral 10-mile race, thought there was a mile to go, there were seven. He said, "This is too far for anyone to run. Never again for me."

Lafferty said, "I can't understand it. Leg cramps at eight miles, stomach cramps at thirteen. I did not eat much breakfast, maybe that was it. I threw water on my head. Maybe that was it. Maybe it was the heat." Lafferty had been walking near the finish when he heard old Johnny Kelley coming and had to sprint the last 200 yards to beat him.

Van Zant walked in. He said, "This *is* my jinx race. The heat bothered me a lot and I got good and tired." He planned to run Yonkers to qualify for the Olympic Games; if he didn't qualify, he would quit running. Thereafter Van Zant's name never appeared in BAA entries.

Dyrgall knew he was in second place but could not see who led. He tried but could not catch him. He wondered (as reported in the *Globe*),

"Who is that guy?" Only at the finish did he find out. Then he said, "I think the whole secret of the thing is in the amount of training that goes into it. I work days and the only time I have to train is at night. I don't have enough time to train properly. But these Guatemalan guys have plenty of time to train. They must have plenty of time."

Dyrgall went on to make the Olympic team and to finish 13th in 2:32:52 at Helsinki in the marathon that Emil Zatopek won.

1952 Results*

1. D. Flores, Guatemala	2:31:53
2. V. Dyrgall, NY	2:36:40
3. L. Velasquez, Guatemala	2:40:08
4. T. Jones, Philadelphia, PA	2:43:29
5. N. Tamanaha, Honolulu, HI	2:51:55
6. T. Corbitt, NY	2:53:31
7. S. Koru, Turkey	2:54:15
8. E. Ramagnoli, NY	2:57:28
9. L. White, NY	2:58:24
10. A. Briggs, Syracuse, NY	2:58:46
11. J. Lafferty, Boston, MA	3:04:49
12. J.A. Kelley, South Acton, MA	3:04:59
13. M. O'Hara, NY	3:05:57
14. A. Scandurra, NY	3:08:39
15. B. Steiner, NY	3:09:41
16. J. DiComandrea, *MSN*	3:12:01
17. A. Confalone, Medford, MA	3:12:59
18. C. Robbins, NY	3:13:45
19. H.B. Ross, Philadelphia, PA	3:18:35
20. J. Lizak, Medford, MA	3:21:18
21. L. Giard, Randolph, MA	3:22:09
22. T. Crane, Medford, MA	3:22:54

200 entrants.
*This course was later found to be short. See page 248 for the story.

WORLD RECORD?

MONDAY, APRIL 20, 1953

Swede Vows to Break Marathon Record

In this post-Olympic year the foreigners came back to Boston. The 1949 winner, Karl Gosta Leandersson of Sweden, had recovered from his purple rashes and boldly told Jerry Nason of the *Globe*, "I will break the record and if anyone beats me he will have to break the record too." This was not an idle boast. Leandersson had done his training and in his 1949 solo training run of 2:27 over the course had proven that he could run alone at record pace. He had run a 2:28:11 marathon in October of 1952. He had spent the winter snowshoeing so was unaccustomed to training on pavement. To avoid a case of shinsplints while training in Boston before the race, he ran exclusively on the turf at the Belmont Country Club. He did run on the streets one day to travel 8 miles into Boston to buy a pair of slacks and moccasins. He ran back with them in his hands.

Gerard Cote, now age 39, came down from St. Hyacinthe, Quebec. He was the last North American to have won the race, in 1948, and had won three times before that. He placed in the top 13 eight times and was the only man at Boston to have run under 2:30 twice.

A fast Finn, Veikko Karvonen, the owner of four sub-2:30 marathons and the fifth-place Helsinki Olympian, came to prove himself at Boston. In what there was of his nonrunning life, this 26-year-old sorted mail.

The BAA itself had changed over the years. From an association that once possessed a grand clubhouse, the BAA had shrunken to an office in the Boston Arena on St. Botolph's Street. After the clubhouse was sold to Boston University in the 1930s, the club offices had been moved across the street to an entire floor in the Lenox Hotel. When rent in the hotel proved too expensive, BAA president Walter Brown moved a single office to the Boston Arena, where he was general manager and president. Brown set Jock Semple up with a physiotherapy clinic in the arena, and that room became the functioning BAA office. Without Brown's help, Semple said he might have become an aging man scraping along from hand to mouth with odd jobs. After a fire destroyed the arena, Semple and Brown moved the operation to the Boston Garden. By the late 1940s club members had thinned to a handful, who included Will Cloney, the *Herald* writer who had become race director in 1947 at Brown's request, R.H. Kingsley Brown, Ellery Kock, and Brown's brothers Tom and George. Semple had become co-director with Cloney. Walter often took a rubdown from Jock after his hard days in the office. Once he told Semple that he hoped to live long enough to see a BAA runner win the Boston Marathon. Semple made no comment, but he never forgot Brown's wish. It sparked Semple's drive throughout the 1950s to recruit talented runners to wear the BAA unicorn.

Other events indicated a change in long-distance running. Runners began to think more about their training. They began to study it—scientifically. Marathoner Charley Robbins, who used to work in an airplane factory, got drafted, went back to work, got married, went to medical school, and was now Dr. Charles Robbins, Jr. He wrote about training in the Amateur Athletic Union magazine, and the *Boston Globe* reprinted the article on April 17. Although Americans had begun to think about training, they still found reasons to do less of it. Foreigners had no such hesitations. Robbins wrote,

> For the optimum use of training time the distance should be put in with periodic sprints included—the more sudden and violent the better. Resting can be done while running between sprints. Training every other day is psychologically sound in that it avoids staleness. Unless a body system is taxed to its limit, it will not improve. Here is the art of training: to bring oneself just to the point of exhaustion periodically and not waste time training past that point.

Robbins went on to share some other insights:

> While living in the slums of NY and going to medical school on the G.I. bill, I noticed that after a run, the situation seemed brighter! Maybe in this sedentary civilization of ours most of us don't have the opportunity to thrash about enough and place our problems in their proper perspective!

The 1953 race was run on Monday, April 20, as had been the custom whenever the Patriots' Day holiday of April 19 fell on Sunday (except for the war years when the governor had requested that the race be held on Sunday so defense workers could watch). The day granted the best running weather yet in the history of the Boston Marathon. It was cool, 43 °F, and a big tailwind blew at the runners' backs. The wind blew from the northwest during the entire race at a steady 20 mph, with gusts up to 30 mph.

As he promised, Leandersson took the early pace. No one went with him. But striding a discreet distance behind ran Keizo Yamada of Japan. He had been undefeated since his 26th place in the Helsinki Olympic marathon. Yamada was a very little person; he weighed 108 pounds and stood only 5'2". He worked for $30 a month as a clerk in the Dohwa Mining Company. Jerry Nason described his face as merry-featured. Karvonen and a 22-year-old Boston University student named, of all names, Johnny Kelley (John J. Kelley), the same youngster who had idolized Jesse Van Zant, ran along with the tiny Japanese man in a black jersey. Young Kelley, although a scholarship-supported member of the BU track team, secretly trained with the BAA team. Semple wished Kelley would wear the BAA unicorn. This in itself did not mean that Kelley would have to quit college track and cross-country, but symbolically it did. A break would be inevitable. The BU coach saw no future in running long slow distances instead of endless rapid quarter miles. But Kelley saw no future in endless quarter miles. The Zatopek system impressed Kelley, but the application of Zatopek's methods would not pay off for years. On the early hills the youngster dropped back. Karvonen and Yamada caught up to the Swede. For miles they all stuck together.

On Heartbreak Hill Yamada spurted. Leandersson looked distressed. Karvonen looked surprised. Yamada looked, according to Jerry Nason, like "a porcelain doll caught up in a death struggle." But it was the big men who died. Yamada ran away, alone, "a wind blown leaf." He finished in 2:18:51 with his hand outstretched to shake the hand of Mayor John Hynes, who waited on the finish line for the winner. Good politician that he was, Hynes managed to get into the newspaper finish-line photos every year of the 1950s. Yamada would come to Boston several more times, in 1957, 1975, 1976, and as late as 1995. He ran over 150 marathons in his career. In later years he worked for the Fujita Tourist Company in Kawasaki.

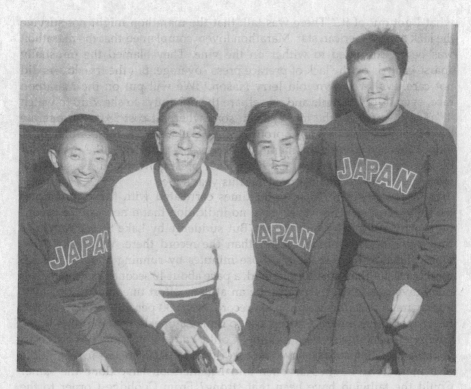

Tiny Keizo Yamada (left) sits next to his coach Yoshiaki Watanabe, Nobuyoshi Sadanaga, and Toyoshichi Nakata in this 1957 photo. Photo courtesy of the *Boston Herald*.

Karvonen, 2:19:09, caught Leandersson, and all three broke Jim Peters's world-best marathon time of 2:20:42 set on June 14, 1952, at Chiswick. That three runners in the same race could all break the course record by such a margin and the world mark besides seemed immortal. It seemed suspect.

Young Kelley survived to finish fifth. That impressed the old Quebec man, Cote. He told Kelley, "You are one good boy. You train hard, some day you are going to run away and hide from t'is people from Japan and places, you see."

The fast times astounded John A. (the elder) Kelley. He said, "He'd have beaten DeMar at his best by 1-1/2 miles. I don't believe it. Must be the course. Must be the watches. Must be something. Must be those guys are pros running against amateurs."

John Patrick Lafferty said, "I guess I'd better start living in Japan."

Clarence H. DeMar finished 81st. He complained about American mara-honers. "All they think about is money, money, money. They all ask me what I got out of it." There was talk that the marathon might not survive the lack of an American star. Marathon lovers complained that the marathon was being permitted to wither on the vine. They blamed the unusually sparse crowds on the lack of prerace press coverage. But the true lovers did not care. Walter Brown told Jerry Nason, "We will put on the marathon race, even if Jock Semple and myself are the only guys to show up to watch it." They would get the money from somewhere. It cost $3,000 to operate the marathon. Brown raided profits from ticket sales for the popular BAA indoor meet to pay for the marathon expenses. Worldwide, the prestige of the Boston Marathon remained high. That prestige would increase as the world heard about the fast times in this year's race.

Leandersson's early checkpoint times correlated with the record times (see chart on page 233). They gave no indication that a new course record by nearly 7 minutes would be set. But suddenly by Lake Street Yamada's time was about 5 minutes faster than the record there. Why? How? He would have to have made up those minutes by running about 7 miles 5 minutes faster than anyone ever had, a pace about 40 seconds per mile faster than anyone else ever. It would be an athletic effort unequaled in history. The average pace for the previous record was 5:30 per mile. Forty seconds faster would have been a pace close to Emil Zatopek's winning time in the Olympic 10,000 meters. Astounding. Could Yamada possibly have accelerated that much? Could he have run a world-class 10,000 meters in the middle of a marathon? Could Karvonen and Leandersson have done the same? Could the tailwind have been that strong? From Coolidge Corner to the finish the difference between the times recorded in previous races from checkpoint to checkpoint were again similar to Suh's times in 1947. Yamada slowed down. All of the time gained came only between certain checkpoints. Most of the other runners showed a similar acceleration between the same checkpoints. It was most curious. But then there was a gusty tailwind.

Jerry Nason of the *Globe* tried to explain why three men broke the course record. First, he said, Leandersson's fast early pace carried the field to such a performance (but his checkpoint times were not any faster than those in previous years). Second, a "booming baby hurricane pressing against the backs and buttocks of the men" pushed them to fast times in an erratic manner. Third, the quality of the field was incredible: Never before at Boston had six sub-2:30 men raced each other under such ideal circumstances. Clutching at straws, Nason also explained that the course actually drops 220 feet to sea level. (Nason's geography was wrong; Hopkinton is 463 feet above sea level, and the finish is 15 feet above sea level.)

Funny, no one suggested that the course might be short. But that explanation could make no sense. It was the same start and the same finish that had been used since the course was remeasured for the 1927 race. And everyone wanted to believe in an astonishing new record.

Comparative Split Times

	Checkpoint records	Suh's times, 1947	1953 race	
Framingham	30:23	33:04	Karl Gosta Leandersson	31:16
Natick	50:45	53:33	Karl Gosta Leandersson	51:16
Wellesley	1:07:31	1:11:47	Karl Gosta Leandersson	1:07:22
Woodland	1:31:40	1:35:24	Karl Gosta Leandersson	1:29:48
Lake Street	1:57:10	1:58:30	Keizo Yamada	1:52:33
Coolidge Corner	2:12:17	2:12:17	Keizo Yamada	2:05:49
Finish	2:25:39	2:25:39	Keizo Yamada	2:18:51

Finishing in second drove Karvonen to dedicate more of himself to the marathon and to return to Boston to improve himself. It seems nothing makes a runner crazier than to finish in second place. DeMar started in second place, and he'd been crazy about the marathon since 1910. Kelley finished second in the year before he won and later finished second six more times. He proved to be marathon-crazy for life. The marathon possessed Karvonen, and in it he found something larger to pursue than his own glory.

Karvonen wondered if a Finn could ever win at Boston. Enough of them had tried. Many men of Finnish descent had run well there: bald-headed Karl Koski, Willie Kyronen, tiny Willie Wick, Whitey Michelson, Otto Laakso, Gunnar Nilson, Nestor Erickson, Louis Tikkanen, David Fagerlund, and 1920 Olympic marathon champion Hannes Kolehmainen—all placed in the top 10. Kolehmainen's best was a fourth in 1917. Men born in Finland who had become North Americans had won Boston—Carl Linder in 1919 and Dave Komonen, the naturalized Canadian, in 1934. But Boston seemed to be a graveyard for Finnish champions. Finnish Olympic gold medalist Willie Ritola had placed second in Boston to DeMar in 1922. In 1926 Johnny Miles upset Albin Stenroos, another Finnish Olympic gold medalist. In 1947 Mikko Hietanen placed second behind Yun Bok Suh's record run. The Finns were a tough and hardy people, the best long-distance runners in the world. They owned plenty of Olympic gold. But none had brought victory back to Finland from Boston. Karvonen lived with the legend of Paavo Nurmi and his four Olympic gold medals. Karvonen thought a Finnish citizen *should* win the Boston Marathon. In fact, he thought that Finns should win many Boston Marathons.

*1953 Results**

1.	K. Yamada, Japan	2:18:51	14.	J. Cunningham, *PennAC*	2:41:57
2.	V. Karvonen, Finland	2:19:09	15.	A. Scott, *NYPC*	2:42:35
3.	K. Leandersson, Sweden	2:19:36	16.	G. Cote, St. Hyacinthe, PQ	2:42:40
4.	K. Nishida, Japan	2:21:35	17.	C. Robbins, *NYPC*	2:43:56
5.	J.J. Kelley	2:28:19	18.	A. Briggs, Syracuse, NY	2:44:47
6.	H. Hamamura, Japan	2:32:30	19.	W. Hackulich, *PennAC*	2:47:07
7.	J.A. Kelley, West Acton, MA	2:32:46	20.	J. Sterner, *NYPC*	2:47:48
8.	K. Hiroshima, Japan	2:33:33	21.	J. St. Clair, Jr., *PennAC*	2:47:59
9.	J. Lafferty, *BAA*	2:38:04	22.	K. Shinozaki, Japan	2:48:31
10.	N. Tamanaha, HI	2:38:36	23.	T. Mederios, *NMC*	2:48:35
11.	A. Neidnig, *MillAA*	2:38:53	24.	A. Scandurra, *MillAA*	2:48:42
12.	G. Mona, *BAA*	2:39:45	81.	C. DeMar	3:36:23
13.	A. Diamond, NY	2:41:50			

199 entrants, 157 starters, 92 runners under 3:56.

Team prize
BAA

*This course was later found to be short. See page 248 for the story.

BLUEBERRY JUICE

MONDAY, APRIL 19, 1954

World's Fastest Marathoner to Race Today

On April 18, 1954, U.S. Vice-President Richard M. Nixon said the country would have to send troops into Indochina if the French stopped fighting Vietnamese communist guerrillas at Dienbienphu. Senator Joe McCarthy found a communist under every rug in America. But the Korean War was over, and in this time of relative peace international marathoning flourished. Veikko Karvonen led this year's foreign invasion of Boston.

When Karvonen was only 13 years old, on November 30, 1939, the Russian army invaded Finland. His hometown of Sakkloa, on the eastern border, lay directly in their path. Veikko and his family fled to Turku, on the shores of the Baltic—the hometown of Paavo Nurmi. Young Veikko fell under the spell of Nurmi's spirit, as did thousands of other young Finnish boys. During the second world war Karvonen joined the Finnish army and set up telephone and radio communications. But by now he had a 10-month-old son, Pakka, and an urge to win the Boston Marathon to make up for his second place of the year before. Karvonen trained on skis twice a day all through the Finnish winter, in temperatures of 20 °F to –40 °F. Between workouts he still worked as a postal clerk to support his family. A group of Finnish-

Americans paid his way to come to try to win at Boston. The 1919 BAA champion, Carl Linder, who had emigrated from Finland in 1902, waited to greet Karvonen at the Boston airport.

But an Englishman came to prevent Karvonen's victory. After three Boston runners in 1953 broke his world-best time of 2:20:42, after he ran 2:18:40 in Essex, England—on a course remeasured and found to be 370 yards too long—and after he had beaten Karvonen by 7 minutes in a marathon in Karvonen's town of Turku, Jim Peters came to Boston to take a shot at Yamada's 2:18:51. The newspaper writers picked Peters as the overwhelming favorite. Back in England Peters worked as a dispensing optician. In Boston, it seemed victory would be automatic. The times of the new records were astounding to regular Boston marathoners. They were used to thinking of times like 2:30 as extraordinary, but suddenly there was talk about times 10 minutes faster. Here was a new generation that could beat the old generation by nearly 2 miles.

America's new generation did not have far to travel; they lived in student poverty a few blocks from the Exeter Street finish. John J. Kelley from New London, Connecticut, and top long-distance runners George Terry and Nick Costes lived together in a house in Boston's Back Bay. They had a hot plate but no refrigerator in their rented rooms in Evelyn Harrison's big house. Evelyn, about 80 years old, was a widow with a big empty house. Her boarders turned out to be distance runners on the BU team. John and his wife lived there. Dean Thackwray was a frequent guest. In the evenings they sat in Evelyn's parlor drinking tea and discussing Zatopek's training methods. Costes and Terry had met each other and Zatopek while they were stationed in the army in Germany. They traveled on a goodwill track team to show the Europeans that Americans were sportsmen, not barbarian conquerors. Evelyn quite enjoyed the discussions of training techniques. Kelley favored free and undisciplined speed-play training as a release from schoolwork or a job, but Costes disciplined himself in his training as he did in his academics. He would do workouts like 40 × 440 yards in 72 seconds with a 220-yard jog for rest. Evelyn especially liked the visits of reporters to the house around marathon time. She often accompanied her boys to road races.

Costes had graduated from Slippery Rock State College in Pennsylvania and now did postgraduate studies at Boston University. Terry, Kelley's brother-in-law, was a freshman at BU. Kelley and Costes had taken first and second in the recent 30-kilometer race in New Bedford, the hometown of Kelley's young wife, BU music major Jessie Braga. Kelley worked nights in the Hayes-Bickford cafeteria in Harvard Square to pay his way through school. Kelley was an IC4A collegiate champion but gave up college track and cross-country to run in road races. His early running hero was Clayton "Bud" Farrar, the New London Coast Guarder who led the 1945 Boston Marathon until the third Newton hill stopped him. A congenital heart valve deficiency led to Farrar's death from heart failure at age 42.

Jock Semple recruited an eclectic group of young men who shared an affinity for antiestablishment types of the late 1940s and early 1950s. Kelley led the pack of young college kids who were enamored of Emil Zatopek's iconoclastic training techniques and mildly rebelled against the training programs imposed by their college coaches. The Czechoslovakian Zatopek, the era's most rugged individualist, had struck a chord with these young runners after World War II. Zatopek employed no coach. He invented his own workouts. Reportedly, he even ran with a telephone pole on his back. Another story said that to train his mind Zatopek would hold his breath, then pick out a tree in the distance and walk slowly to it, not breathing or changing his pace until he touched the tree. No one else had ever talked about training the mind. To set his mind at ease that his training was complete, on March 13 Kelley ran a time trial over the entire BAA course in 2:29:39.

Kelley's dispute with his BU coach, Doug Raymond, centered on training. Raymond advocated fast quarters with lots of rest (like 60 to 65 seconds) with college teammates versus long easy runs with the old men of the BAA. College coaches generally held marathoners in contempt. The coaches believed they had no talent or speed and ran marathons because they had no skill for anything else. They saw the pursuit of a sub-four-minute mile as noble but the marathon as a circus, or even a freak show. Kelley felt

College coaches saw the pursuit of a sub-four-minute mile as noble but the marathon as a freak show.

squeezed into a difficult cranny. If he quit BU he would lose the track scholarship he needed, but if he joined the BAA and wore the unicorn, he might win the Boston Marathon someday. Kelley was no freak. The marathon was an Olympic event, taken seriously in the rest of the world. Only when talented Americans took the marathon seriously would they be seen to join Kelley, whom the press called "The only American hope."

Another man with an uneasy mind was the London (1948) Olympic champion, Delfo Cabrera from Argentina. At 5'7" and 135 pounds, he was what Will Cloney called a bundle of nerves, perhaps because he was 35 years old and knew he was not fit enough to be a contender. The Japanese team came without Tanaka or Yamada. Officials traveling with the new Japanese team said the old champions could not make the new team, implying that this new batch was so much better that they had to leave the old marathoners at home.

But the best marathon runner in the world was Jim Peters. He had the fastest times. He wanted to win Boston because the Americans considered it the unofficial world championship. No Englishman had won it, and he wanted to dispel the rampant rumor that his fast times had been solo efforts on short courses. He also, wrongly, believed that the course followed the route of Paul Revere and the beginnings of the troubles with the colonies. He thought, in good humor, that his victory might put the colonial rebels in their place—behind an Englishman. The British Amateur Athletic Association had received the BAA invitation for Peters but had no money to pay his airfare to Boston. There was no English community like the Finnish community in America to pay expenses of their countrymen to come to Boston. To Peters's rescue came the *Boston Globe* writer, Jerry Nason, and the man Peters called a grand Scotsman, Jock Semple. They raised $1,500 for Peters's expenses. Expenses would have been less, but the British athletics governing body insisted that a manager travel with Peters, and the manager insisted on traveling first class. He also insisted that they not arrive earlier than 48 hours before the race. Bad weather delayed their plane overnight at Prestwick in Scotland, and another delay took them to Goose Bay, Labrador. The donations in fact did not meet all the expenses, so Semple paid $300 out of his own pocket. For his efforts he got a tired marathoner.

Semple met the plane and gave Peters a thorough massage to loosen his legs, tight from the flight. A big rainstorm made it impossible to run over parts of the course. Semple took Peters to the Boston Garden, where he ran around between the seats for an hour. Then he took Peters sightseeing and to a fine restaurant for dinner. When Peters finally got to his room at 9:30, he had visions of the race dancing in his brain. After a fitful sleep he rose at 6:30 on race morning. Ted Vogel came by to drive him to the start. There he saw the well-rested Finns, who had been in town for 6 weeks.

The starter's pistol misfired twice. A nearby police officer saved the day: He took out his service revolver, pointed it skyward, and fired. They were off!

Nick Costes took the early lead, with Cabrera and Peters coming up to do some surge-filled racing. The rains stopped and the sun came out. The Japanese found it too warm at 70 °F. Japan had not had a warm day in the year yet. The cherry blossoms had not bloomed around Osaka Castle. Karvonen, Kelley (the younger), Finn Erkki Pulolakka, and Argentinean Ezequiel Bustamante joined the pack. The sun sifted hotly through the thin clouds. The pack thinned. By the start of the hills it was only Karvonen and Peters. Karvonen looked loose. Peters looked tight. Spectators shouted "Good luck, limey" as Peters enjoyed the clapping and cheering. The two men ran side by side and spoke not a word. Peters broke away on the hill. Karvonen held back. Blueberry juice and coffee upset his stomach. European cross-country skiers frequently drink blueberry juice for energy. It usually works well in the smooth, gliding world of cross-country skiing, but in the jostling downhill miles of the Boston Marathon the coffee and blueberry juice churned to a blue-brown froth in Karvonen's stomach. He ran along rubbing and poking his belly. The distress might have been a good thing.

Peters aggressively charged the hills. He expected to leave the Finn in his dust. Why not? Peters was 7 minutes ahead of Karvonen at Turku. Karvonen,

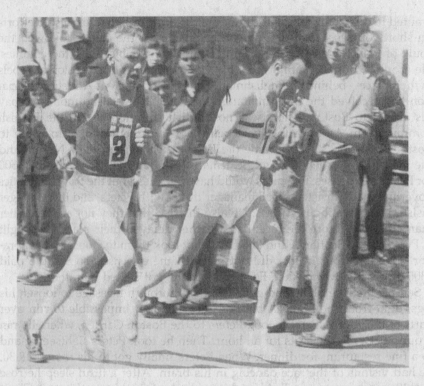

Jim Peters of England, #1—the fastest marathoner in the world—tries to break Veikko Karvonen, #3, of Finland on Heartbreak Hill in the 1954 race. Photo courtesy of the *Boston Herald*.

listening to his stomach, did not charge after Peters. But by the third hill Peters tired, and the pain in Karvonen's belly disappeared. The Finn caught the Englishman at the top of Heartbreak Hill just as a cold stiff sea breeze caught them both. Peters began to realize that he was up against a far different man from the one he had beaten the year before. Peters felt extraordinarily hot and tired. He realized to his horror that he could no longer hold on to Karvonen. As he watched him run away, he felt ashamed realizing that he would let down Semple and all the people who had been so kind to him; furthermore, he would sacrifice national prestige. Peters began to doubt if he could finish at all.

Karvonen steadily lengthened his lead over the remaining miles. He won by 2 minutes. Peters hung on for second place and fell across the finish line into Semple's arms. Running himself blind would become Jim Peters's legacy.

That summer at the Commonwealth Games in Vancouver, British Columbia, Peters entered the stadium with an 11-minute lead. He had 400 meters to go to win the championship of the British Empire. But the summer heat and his fast early pace destroyed him. He wobbled and spasmed down the track. The packed stadium watched in horror. With 200 meters to go he collapsed. Officials rushed to his aid. He never finished. For the Vancouver race, however, and not the Boston Marathon, Jim Peters will always be remembered in marathoning history.

The 1948 Olympic champion, Cabrera, said he underestimated the difficulty of the Boston course. People began to talk about an Olympic jinx. Olympic gold medal holders try to win Boston but can't: Hicks, Hayes, Kolehmainen, Stenroos, Kitei Son (Sohn), and now Cabrera. No Olympic gold medalist had yet won the Boston Marathon.

Nick Costes was not happy with his performance either. He had been with the leaders, and he felt he should have been able to stay with the leaders. At least he felt he should have been able to stay with his housemate, Kelley. Some American has got to teach those foreigners a lesson.

1954 Results*

1.	V. Karvonen, Finland	2:20:39	17.	N. Cirulnick, NY	2:50:58
2.	J.H. Peters, England	2:22:40	18.	M. O'Hara, NY	2:54:44
3.	E. Pulolakka, Finland	2:24:25	19.	D. Gott, Billerica, MA	2:55:10
4.	K. Hiroshima, Japan	2:25:30	20.	C. Quelimiz, Kearney, NJ	2:55:56
5.	K. Nishida, Japan	2:27:35	21.	T. Mederios, Lowell, MA	2:56:05
6.	D. Cabrera, Argentina	2:27:50	22.	J. Lafferty, Quonsett, RI	2:57:44
7.	J.J. Kelley, *BAA*	2:28:51	23.	J. DiComandrea, MA	3:01:15
8.	E. Bustamante, Argentina	2:33:40	27.	D. Fay, *BAA*, Quincy, MA	3:09:10
9.	N. Costes, Farrell, PA	2:35:17	28.	C. Robbins, *NYPC*	3:10:33
10.	N. Sadanaga, Japan	2:37:19	31.	J. Daley, Jr., *BAA*, Westford, MA	3:14:17
11.	T. Corbitt, NY	2:40:57	36.	D. Thackwray, *BAA*	3:22:12
12.	A. Diamond, Niagara Falls, NY	2:44:34	45.	O. Manninen, *BAA*	3:31:41
13.	N. Tamanaha, HI	2:45:45	59.	J. Daley, Sr., *BAA*, Westford, MA	3:46:16
14.	G. Norman, Toronto, ON	2:49:11	78.	**C. DeMar, Reading, MA**	**3:58:34**
15.	A. Scandurra, NY	2:49:57	83.	G. Mirkin, *HAA*	NT
16.	**J.A. Kelley, Arlington, MA**	**2:50:25**			

*This course was later found to be short. See page 248 for the story.

VICISSITUDES

TUESDAY, APRIL 19, 1955

Argentinean Olympian Set to Take Marathon

The medical profession annoyed Clarence H. DeMar. In his feature article in the April 20 *Boston Globe* he wrote about Dr. Charles Robbins taking the lead: "Perhaps I wasn't too anxious to have an orthodox medical man win until the profession learns a little humility. Forty-five years ago they used to warn us of the danger to our hearts. Now they tell us that we marathoners may outlive the average because of our exercise." DeMar, now officially retired and with an incipient cancer of the sigmoid (the intestine just above the rectum), rode in the press bus and wondered if Robbins's medical degree had conferred on him a special technological secret that would help him keep the lead.

In the rain of the 1955 Boston Marathon Nick Costes and Robbins ran side by side in the lead. Costes had predicted that he would run 2:25. The good doctor was not that good, but the excitement of the race caught him up; he enjoyed running ahead of the foreigners and making them wonder who he was. But Robbins had no secret. There are no secrets in long-distance running. He just prayed for the rain to keep him alive and grant him a miracle as the real race unfolded behind him, soon to gobble up the frolickers.

Perhaps Robbins frolicked in the lead because he wanted to be on television. For the first time the Boston Marathon was televised. WNAC-TV, channel 7, broadcast a 45-minute telecast from checkpoints, with 1942 winner Joe Smith doing commentary along with the station's regular play-by-play announcer. At the start a short, stubby, optimistic American master sergeant named Kurt Steiner elbowed his way to the front line. He sprinted into the lead for the first few hundred yards, but no one was fooled into thinking he would last. Steiner's enthusiasm and hope would continue for decades as his early burst became a ritual; Steiner's 60 seconds worth of distance run became his only minute of glory in an otherwise normal life. Costes knew that Robbins and Steiner were not contenders. But Costes knew who he was: this year's great American hope.

Before the race Costes said he was in excellent condition. He won the early spring Brighton 23-mile race by 6 minutes. But now, Costes said, the outcome depended on the *vicissitudes* of the race. He used that very word, vicissitudes. The word reflected the changed character of the BAA fields. Previously marathoners were laborers, bricklayers, miners, blacksmiths, mailmen, milkmen, soldiers. Now the marathon appealed to educated professionals, doctors and, like Costes, teachers. Costes taught sixth grade in Natick. He had a master's degree from Boston University, and of course Robbins had his medical degree.

His students cheered him as he ran through town. "Go, Mister Costes, go! Run, Mister Costes, run!!" He wore a "Natick High School Track" singlet with a dark diagonal stripe and the letter N over his heart. His hair he wore in a crewcut. He trained carefully; he recorded, charted, and graphed. He hadn't picked himself to win. But Costes was the only American with top-10 potential.

The press picked the 1952 Olympic silver medalist, Reinaldo Berto Gorno. He was a craggy-faced, wavy-haired, 38-year-old Argentinean from Buenos Aires. Gorno had recently won Japan's Kamakura Marathon. One paper called him a "loose-jointed" sanitation engineer. The real threats—another

Argentinean, Ezequiel Bustamante, who had run in Boston before, a Swedish woodsman named Gustaf Jansson, a Finn named Paavo Kotila, and a team of Japanese—ran along smoothly behind the morning glories. The third Japanese man, Hideo Hamamura, had finished far behind Gorno in Japan so did not consider himself any more than a possibility for the top 10.

Hamamura grew up on a rice farm in Yamaguchi, a village about 80 miles from Tokyo. His family worked the rice paddies in the same way as did the rest of the village. The village worked the rice paddies as did neighboring villages. All of Japan did the same thing at the same time. Plant the rice. Flood the fields. Transplant the rice. Harvest. As the season moved from the south of the islands to the north all farmers did what their neighbors did. The labor and the land necessary to produce rice meant that families had to live in small houses clustered together, with all the flat land surrounding them dedicated to food production. The labor-intensive nature of rice farming meant that families coordinate their work and do the various tasks consecutively and sequentially, following a precise and inflexible timetable. That agrarian life was a perfect model for training for long-distance running. Like rice cultivation, training must be done daily and in the proper sequence, under the authority of the old man of the village. It can be neither rushed nor postponed. An athlete must do what he must do when he must do it, not at any other time or in any other way. He must follow without question what the coach says. In this sense Japanese training for long-distance racing was the antithesis of the freedom and the liberty Americans considered natural. Young Hamamura had learned his lessons well.

Hamamura had a hero. In fact, he had many heroes. Shunji Koyanagi, the national marathon champion, came from the same village. And Hideo had run on the same team as Keizo Yamada, the Boston winner in 1953. Hideo's older brother had died during the war when an American submarine sank his troop ship. Now Hamamura worked in Fukuoka as a clerk in the office of the Prefector of Education. His co-workers raised the money to send him to Boston. Hamamura was 26 years old, 5'6", and weighed 132 pounds. In the race he wore a dark shirt with the flag of Japan on his chest. As he ran his grimace revealed a gold front tooth. His high back-kick muddied the backside of his white shorts. His rain-soaked socks rolled down around his ankles. He felt very good but did not want to take the lead too soon. In 1953 he had gone out too fast at Boston and paid for it. Today he did not want to pay. He wanted to collect.

The old American hope, now called Private John J. Kelley, had just returned from a tour of South America with the U.S. Army track team. He would not run the marathon because he was not in condition. Setbacks easily discouraged Kelley, and friends frequently had to talk him back into his sport.

Through Natick and Wellesley Costes got the distinct impression that the pace was too slow. He felt these guys were all walking. He decided to heat things up. The rain and the slight tailwind made for a day that would forgive a fast pace. Costes figured that the least he could do was to make the foreigner work hard for his victory. He led up the hills with Finnish Eino A. Pulkkinen following closely. DeMar thought the Finn would win. DeMar did not notice Hamamura slipping in behind Gorno as the hills began. Hamamura had been resting way back in 13th place in Framingham and moved gradually up to 6th place by Woodland Park. He felt strong.

Hamamura shadowed Costes and Pulkkinen at the crest of the hill at Boston College. He could see that they were tired. He was not.

Hamamura passed Pulkkinen. He passed Costes. He ran alone to collect his diamond-studded gold medal with the unicorn. Mayor John Hynes chased Hamamura over the finish line to place the laurel wreath on his head. Hamamura would not return to Boston. By 1992 he had retired from his job and lived in Yamaguchi and as a volunteer coach helped young marathoners.

After Coolidge Corner not one in the top 10 slowed. The rain made this a race remarkably free of attrition. Places in the top 10 remained unchanged. The final time of not only the winner but of the top 5 astounded everyone. Were they really 7 minutes faster than Yun Bok Suh in 1947? Would they have beaten Clarence H. DeMar, at his best, by 2 miles? How did they get to be that fast? Jerry Nason tried to figure it out.

Nason saw the structure of an athletic revolution in the philosophical approach to long-distance running. The old paradigm described marathon running in terms of pain, punishment, and toughness. Marathon running engendered adjectives like *grueling, arduous*, and *grinding*. The event itself was often called a grind and the participants were termed plodders—not racers, not runners, but plodders. These were men whose dominant trait was a stubborn courage rather than athletic ability. The image in the minds of the public and the participants themselves was of men hard as nails, heads down, shuffling along, refusing to quit.

But the new marathon runners were men of S-P-E-E-D. Nason spelled it out that way. Men like DeMar had little of it; DeMar's fastest mile was 4:48. DeMar had toughness, principle, and courage but virtually no inborn S-P-E-E-D. John J. Kelley and Costes ran many, many interval quarter miles faster than DeMar could have run a single quarter mile. Costes told DeMar that he had read his book and got a kick out of it, but he did not mean that literally. DeMar's form for training was only base work for the new marathoners. DeMar's individualistic discipline inspired Costes, but no one now could win the marathon training the way DeMar did. When speed men like Kelley and Costes got the basics of endurance running underneath their inborn speed talent—Kelley ran the fastest high school mile, 4:21, in the nation in 1949—Americans too would be able to do what the foreigners did at Boston. They would be able to sustain speed over the entire length of the marathon course. That's why these marathon times were so fast, Nason said, because these men had stopped thinking in terms of plodding and grinding. These new marathoners were prideful men of skill and talent. In his colorful descriptions of the race Nason called Hamamura the "nimble nip" and the "Honshu hotshot." Another foreign victory irked the Americans.

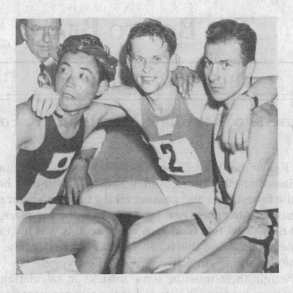

(From left) Hideo Hamamura, Japan; Eino Pulkkinen, Finland; and Nick Costes, USA, joyfully embrace at the conclusion of the fast 1955 race. Photo courtesy of the *Boston Herald*.

Costes said, "I'll end the foreign supremacy next year." He thought a bit, then Costes said, "If Johnny Kelley had been here he'd have beaten them all. Once he gets the proper training he'll be the boy to beat."

*1955 Results**

1.	**H. Hamamura, Japan**	**2:18:22**	15.	N. Tamanaha, HI	2:38:30
2.	E. Pulkkinen, Finland	2:19:23	16.	N. Cirulnick, Brooklyn, NY	2:39:01
3.	N. Costes, Natick, MA	2:19:57	17.	R. Dorion, Gardner, MA	2:40:23
4.	**P. Kotila, Finland**	**2:20:16**	18.	R. Eliberg, Upper Darby, PA	2:41:39
5.	R. Gorno, Argentina	2:20:28	19.	G. Wilcox, Newfoundland, NS	2:41:50
6.	G. Jansson, Sweden	2:21:40	20.	W. Welsh, *MillAA*	2:42:06
7.	Y. Uchikawa, Japan	2:22:40	21.	A. Confalone, Wakefield, MA	2:42:23
8.	T. Tanabe, Japan	2:26:08	22.	G. Waterhouse, Reading, MA	2:43:03
9.	E. Bustamante, Argentina	2:27:51	23.	**G. Cote, St. Hyacinthe, PQ**	**2:44:59**
10.	R. Mendez, *NYPC*, NY	2:28:30	24.	**J.A. Kelley, *BEEC***	**2:45:22**
11.	T. Corbitt, *NYPC*, NY	2:32:27	28.	J. Daley, Jr., *BAA*, MA	2:47:46
12.	J. DiComandrea, *BAA*, MA	2:37:08	37.	C. Robbins, *NYPC*, NY	2:56:20
13.	A. Scandurra, *MillAA*	2:37:49	42.	J. Daley, Sr., *BAA*	2:58:51
14.	L. Torres, *NYPC*, NY	2:38:00	53.	P. Donato, Lynnfield, MA	3:05:21

200 entrants.
Team prize
NY Pioneer Club
*This course was later found to be short. See page 248 for the story.

THE BOY TO BEAT

Foreigners to Dominate Marathon . . . Forever?

John Joseph Kelley met John Duncan Semple on a July evening in 1948 in Haverhill, Massachusetts. Young Kelley had won a 10-mile handicap race by running the fastest time and passing all the runners ahead of him, so he won two first-place trophies, one for time and one for place. Kelley had dropped out of his first two road race starts, so this was his first road race finish. No one had heard of this other, 17-year-old Kelley. The elder Kelley was off to the London Olympic Games with Ted Vogel.

Officials thought there must be some mistake in calculating the elapsed times of the slower runners who started at the gun compared with the times of the faster runners who ran with the largest handicaps from their later start at the scratch line. Officials tried to give the time prize to veteran racer Hawk Zamparelli. Semple intervened. He did more than intervene—he screamed. "For cripes sake!. . . Use yourr noggin, mon. Your head isn't just a hatrack. If he didn't win the time prize how the hell did he start five minutes ahead of your scratch man and finish seven minutes ahead of him? Answer me that!" In a moment Kelley had the coveted Hamilton wristwatch, the most frequent prize for the time prize winner in a road race. Kelley had done something unheard of: On his first time out he beat the experienced runners. He didn't really know what the game was all about, but he knew he was good at it. Semple had stepped in to protect a young, thin, frail, spindly, golden-haired, blue-eyed boy at just the moment in his life that he needed an old man to step in. The previous December Kelley's 57-year-old father had died of viral pneumonia. Young Johnny missed his father, but he knew that day he had made a friend.

By the spring of 1956 Kelley was done with the army and back at Boston University on the GI bill. He was not part of the track team. He found himself drawn to the side currents of the day. He read the beat poets like Gary Snyder and Jack Kerouac and followed the organic gardening philosophy of J.I. Rodale. Kelley adopted a vegetarian diet. He read Hemingway's *The Old Man and the Sea* and saw himself in the fisherman who engaged in a primitive sport. Kelley saw his life reduced to the moment, to long runs along the river or in the woods, to the weekly competitions. During an era when, in his own words, "the auto was the symbol of youthful aspirations and attainment," Kelley had not gotten his driver's license until he was 23. As part of his schooling he was practice teaching in Quincy, Massachusetts. He was fit and ready to run at Boston.

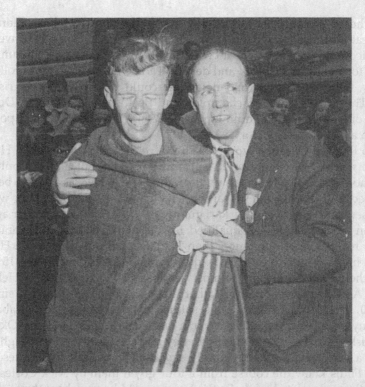

More than anything, Jock Semple wanted to see one of his BAA runners win Boston. Here he wraps his great hope, John J. Kelley, in the traditional finish line blanket. Photo courtesy of the *Boston Herald*.

Kelley's young friend George Terry took the 1956 BAA race out. Terry ran only 4 seconds slower through Framingham than Ellison Brown's checkpoint record set in 1936. By Natick Terry ran 14 seconds faster than Brown. Terry was a talent and a speed merchant; so must have been Brown, although he was two decades ahead of his time. In college Terry won the IC4A collegiate championship at 2 miles. Had Brown gone to college surely he would have won such championships too. At Kelley's first-ever road race, in 1947, he and Terry had run brazenly side by side for the first miles ahead of Olympian Vic Dyrgall. Then both dropped out.

But in Boston this brazen style got Terry into trouble halfway through. Until then he had felt like he was jogging. He had done so much speed work, so many interval quarter miles on the track that the checkpoint record pace felt slow. After 13 miles he began to pay. But thanks to Terry, at Wellesley Kelley and Costes had the lead at record pace.

The boy to beat, John J. Kelley of New London, Connecticut, and Boston University, took the lead in Wellesley. He broke Jim Peters's boisterous 1954 checkpoint record by a minute. Semple watched him run, and thrills rose in his heart. At long last a BAA boy might just win the Boston Marathon and beat all those foreigners, and with a record time, too. A man wearing the unicorn might win the medal with the unicorn pressed on it. But unfortunately for Kelley and Costes, and despite Terry's efforts, two Finns followed closely. Other contenders and defenders could not or would not risk the pace. The current Pan Am champion and Boston winner in 1952, Doroteo Flores of Guatemala, could no longer be seen. Only the Finns had position to stop a Kelley BAA victory.

Eino Illamari Oksanen worked as a police detective in Helsinki. He had set the world's best mark at 20 miles in Barcelona but had run only one marathon in 2:25:47. He was an undertrained talent. He was about to become obsessed with the Boston Marathon. His teammate, Antti Viskari, was an army sergeant. For 7 years Viskari guarded the bleak Finnish border against Russian incursion. He had qualified for the trip to Boston by winning an indoor marathon, running more than 242 laps on a 165-meter track. He was a man immune to tedium. He lived in the town of Lappeenranta, 15 miles from the Soviet border and almost as close to Leningrad as to Helsinki. When Antti was a year old his father died. At 27 and in the army since he was 20, Viskari was a stern, plain soldier, ever watchful and not about to take anything for granted—not even a fast early pace. Two Finns, Oksanen and Viskari, and two Americans, Kelley and Costes, ran in a straight line, not in a pack, under a partly cloudy sky at 50 °F with lively breezes.

The Finns knew the course from a tour given them by Nick Costes, who drove them along its length. So the Finns would know where they were on the course Costes arranged for someone they knew to be present at 5-kilometer intervals. Costes was only following the Semple/BAA tradition of local marathoners' offering help and hospitality to visitors. Even during the race itself BAA marathoners frequently shared water, sponges, and advice.

Terry's demise and dropout at 20 miles and Costes's slowing left Kelley and the Finns at the front. Oksanen fell back before the hills and Kelley and Viskari pulled ahead. On the second hill Viskari grabbed ground from Kelley. Thirty or 40 yards stretched to 75 by Lake Street but did not increase.

Coming into Coolidge Corner, Semple leaned out of the press bus window and shouted his desperate hope to Kelley: "Go get him now! Take a gamble, you can't possibly finish worse than second, now!" Kelley flailed away. He still thought he could win. He sucked in great gulps of air. Through the slits of his squint, he riveted his clear blue eyes on Viskari's neck. Kelley's world shrank as his peripheral vision vanished; now it seemed as if his life existed only to travel to the end of a long black tunnel, there to seize Viskari's neck. Viskari slowed to take some water. To Kelley this was a sign that the Finn was dying. Kelley pushed harder and Semple yelled louder. Kelley's clothes looked too large for him. Sweat darkened the unicorn. Viskari ran only seconds ahead, but with a mile to go through Kenmore Square, he heard the pleading screams of the crowd. He turned to see Kelley's pursuit. Dispassionately Viskari picked up the pace just enough to snuff out Kelley's hope. Kelley remained close enough to see the Finn finish first.

Again the winning times astounded everyone. Four men under 2:20. Had that happened before?

Costes said he'd never been suspicious about the distance. And before the 1927 race, Professor Edward Sheiry of the Massachusetts Institute of Technology had made a proper measurement of the course and found it to be 176 yards short. The distance was then adjusted. Jim Peters, second place in 1954, said that the downhill nature of the course, not shortness, accounted for the fast times. John A. Kelley said that of course Viskari ran the full marathon distance. (Kelley the elder himself dropped out and considered retiring—he was in his late 40s.) Nason concluded that the course was legal, but the runners were simply getting better.

The Boston Marathon attracted better athletic talent then in earlier decades. Gordon Dickson in seventh was a graduate of Drake University. Joseph Tyler in eighth place was a 4:14 miler. Fred Wilt had track speed, as did Thackwray and young Jimmy Daley, who was still at Newman Prep. Long-time AAU official Bob Campbell looked at this young crop and saw the future: "Only a matter of time—the schools have the runners with speed."

Not only were these young men talented, but they were students of the sport. DeMar was the first to make a careful study of the art involved in preparing for long-distance racing, but now came study with speed.

Comparative Split Times

	Old checkpoint records		1956 times	
Framingham	Ellison Brown, 1936	30:23	George Terry	30:27
Natick	Ellison Brown, 1936	50:45	George Terry	50:31
Wellesley	James Peters, 1954	1:07:07	John J. Kelley	1:06:06
Woodland	James Peters, 1954	1:29:35	John J. Kelley	1:27:29
Lake Street	Keizo Yamada, 1953	1:52:33	Antti Viskari	1:48:45
Coolidge Corner	Kee Yong Ham, 1950	2:05:49	Antti Viskari	2:01:45

These times were just too fast—3 minutes under the world's best. Perhaps someone should remeasure the course.

1956 Results*

1.	A. Viskari, Finland	2:14:14[CR**]	5.	D. Thackwray, *BAA*	2:20:24
2.	J.J. Kelley, *BAA*	2:14:33	6.	T. Corbitt, Brooklyn, NY	2:28:06
3.	E. Oksanen, Finland	2:17:56	7.	G. Dickson, Bronx, NY	2:28:45
4.	N. Costes, Natick, MA	2:18:01	8.	J. Tyler, San Diego, CA	2:29:17

9.	R. Cons, Los Angeles, CA	2:29:24	25. N. Tamanaha, HI	2:38:46
10.	F. Wilt, Lafayette, IN	2:29:27	26. L. Velasquez, Argentina	2:39:55
11.	T. Ryan, Atlantic City, NJ	2:29:35	28. R. Eliberg, Upper Darby, PA	2:40:11
12.	J. Daley, Jr., Westford, MA	2:31:25	29. A. Briggs, Syracuse, NY	2:41:20
13.	H. Ross, Philadelphia, PA	2:31:38	30. N. Cirulnick, Brooklyn, NY	2:42:22
14.	A. Scandurra, Great Neck, NY	2:33:34	33. T. Mederios, Boston, MA	2:44:59
15.	J. Lafferty, *BAA*	2:33:57	36. S. Kahainy, Israel	2:46:06
16.	L. Sebio, Jr., Los Angeles, CA	2:35:16	37. R. Sawyer, Concord, MA	2:46:06
17.	R. Dorion, Gardner, MA	2:36:35	43. J. Gray, Walpole, MA	2:51:49
18.	M. Allen, Fort Lewis, WA	2:36:40	48. C. Robbins, Brooklyn, NY	2:55:35
19.	L. Torres, Brooklyn, NY	2:36:47	61. J. Daley, Sr., Westford, MA	3:08:32
20.	A. Confalone, Wakefield, MA	2:37:17	67. G. Mirkin, Brookline, MA	3:16:24
23.	J. Green, Quincy, MA	2:37:56	87. E. Segal, *HU*	3:46:32
24.	G. Hillier, *BU*	2:38:30	97. K. Steiner, Fort Knox, KY	NT

201 entrants, 164 starters.

Team prize
BAA
*This course was later found to be short. See next story.
**Antti Viskari's winning time of 2:14:14 is considered a permanent record for 25 miles, 1,232 yards.

VICTORY FROM BEHIND
THE FINISH LINE

SATURDAY, APRIL 20, 1957

Boston Marathon Course 'Fixed'

Remeasurement of the Boston Marathon course failed to find 1,183 yards of roadway. They had disappeared. Where did they go? About 4-1/2 minutes had disappeared. Add it to the times. In the 1956 race, Viskari and Kelley ran legitimate sub-2:20 marathons, but no one else did. Runners indeed ran faster than they had ever run, but not as much faster as they would have liked. Some people wanted the course to remain short so that comparisons against earlier times could be made. But BAA Director Walter Brown said, "If a marathon race is supposed to be at a distance of 26 miles 385 yards, then let's race it at that distance." So they moved the start up the hill to the Hopkinton town green.

How could the course have shrunk, if the start and finish remained the same? During construction to cater to the automobile, the engine of suburban sprawl, 1,183 yards had disappeared as road reconstruction crews eliminated curves. Most of this construction occurred after 1951. All the Boston

Marathons between 1951 and 1957 were short, but not all by the same amount. No one can know just how short each was, but the preponderance of fast times by so many runners in the field forced officials to remeasure the course. The public works departments in the individual towns did not recognize the runners' holy path to Boston every time they had a street to fix; they could not be ex-

During construction to cater to the automobile, 1,183 yards of the Boston Marathon course had disappeared as road reconstruction crews eliminated curves.

pected to inform the BAA marathon officials of every road change. None of the runners in their yearly visits had noticed the piece-by-piece removal of pavement.

Everyone in New England noticed Johnny J. Kelley's presence at the Melbourne Olympic Games in November of 1956. Other New Englanders, Hal Connolly (the hammer throw) and Charlie Jenkins (the 400 meters), had their gold medals. Why not Kelley too? On November 27, 1956, Jerry Nason wrote, "If Kelley can win—Stop the Presses." Those kinds of expectations, that pressure of the press, put the squeeze on Kelley. There in Australia's late spring, as the sun approached the Tropic of Capricorn, Kelley felt obligated to take the lead in the Olympic marathon in 85 °F weather. He suffered with that lead for 12 miles. He cramped, walked, ran, and survived as a parade of the world's marathoners passed him: Alain Mimoun of France, who would win in 2:25; Franjo Mihalic of Yugoslavia (silver) who would one day come to Boston; Karvonen (bronze), who had won Boston in 1954 and came back in 1957. The great Emil Zatopek finished 6th, and Oksanen, the Finn Kelley beat at Boston in 1956, finished 10th; and finishing one place ahead of Kelley in his own private death march came Nick Costes. In all, eight past or future Boston Marathon winners ran in the 1956 Olympic marathon. John J. Kelley ran in 21st place in 2:43:40.

Kelley felt like quitting running. But simultaneously he wanted to atone for his miserable showing. His urge to atone overwhelmed his urge to quit. He trained harder and more thoroughly than ever to eliminate doubt from his atonement project. Kelley and his wife, Jessie, had spent the night before the race in the home of Laura Harlow, the fiancée of Johnny A. (the elder) Kelley. (The elder Kelley, now divorced, was about to be married for the third time and had decided in spite of his failure to finish last year's marathon not to retire from marathon racing.) John J. Kelley said, "By a fillip of teasing fate, I bore the monarch's name." He arrived in Hopkinton more fit than ever. At 11:30 on Easter Saturday, April 20, officials herded the entire field of 140 into a snow fence enclosure on the town green. There Kelley saw the favorite—Karvonen—Yamada, and Koreans and Mexicans along with two other Americans who just might be able to win the thing.

Kelley the younger's good friends George Terry and Rudolfo Mendez jiggled and stretched, warmed up and waited within the snow fence. Terry said he thought that one of them could win it. "Thing is, we have to decide who has the best chance. Then two of us are going to have to set it up for him." But Kelley paid no attention. He fidgeted, and his nervousness distracted him. But he had the speed, had worked hard, and had studied his sport. If only they would start the race so he could do the thing he trained to do. He had not trained for waiting around.

The lead pack took 3:43 to get from the new start to the old start. Kelley, Mendez, and Terry ran together into Framingham, 9th, 10th, and 11th. They planned to run their own race, not one where foreigners dictated the tactics. American runners did not resent the visits of foreigners. They did not even mind the foreigners winning the Boston Marathon year after year as much as the press implied. The American runners felt honored that the foreign visitation made the Boston Marathon the most important marathon in the world (except during Olympic years). The foreigners stimulated the competitive juices, brought out the best in the Americans, and forced them to prepare carefully. Gradually Kelley worked his way into the lead.

Kelley, Terry, Mendez, Costes, Joe Tyler, Fred Wilt, Gordon Dickson, Dean Thackwray, and Gordon McKenzie had adopted new ways of training. It was Wilt, a 29-year-old FBI agent, who came back from Europe with a new concept in training called *fartlek*, a Swedish word for speed-play. Fartlek training embraced long, untimed runs over the countryside where the pace varied whimsically. Later Wilt would write a book that became the training standard of the 1960s, called *How They Train*. But it was Zatopek who really made the difference. He combined the ideas of year-round training with the very fast quarter-mile repeats, which the American collegians were already doing, with high mileage. Not only would Zatopek run quarter miles in 62 to 68 seconds, but he would also go for 3-hour runs, or runs where he would sprint madly up hills or between telephone poles. (He never really ran, as the stories proclaimed, with a telephone pole strapped to his back.) Zatopek's training, which expressed individuality and encouraged experimentation, appealed to this new generation of runners, who felt a romantic power in creating their own training schemes. But, an element of rebelliousness poked through. Kelley read too much and thought too much. He studied literature. He wrote, and wrote well. He accepted inspiration but did not wait to be told what to do. Nor did he like being told what to do. This was a generation of running rebels, running with cause—to grow stronger and faster than they had ever been before.

Now, as Kelley ran along in the lead of the 1957 Boston Marathon, he knew he was stronger than ever. He could feel power seething within. He wanted to burst out and announce that he would win that day. On the other

hand he saw Finns as marathon gods, who descended to Boston every April
to run away from mere mortals.

Kelley knew Karvonen was the man to beat, so he never let him out of
his sight. Kelley was now 26 years old, 128 pounds, and a remedial reading
teacher in Connecticut. He dodged many spitballs in unruly classes. As he
ran gently, Kelley wanted to go hard. He wanted to just take off and wail
down the roads, but he contained his enthusiasm.

In Framingham a girl ran out and gave a bouquet of posies to Karvonen.
He took them, smiled, raised them to his face, and smelled them. The race
was young; there was time to smell flowers and smile at pretty girls. This
quiet man seemed to step out of the austere Finnish national character. But
his reverie did not last long. A discreet distance down the road, he discarded
the flowers and all came back to business. By 14 miles the lead pack had
dropped all other Americans but Kelley.

At Newton Lower Falls Semple jumped from the moving press bus.
"Johnny! How are you feeling?" he asked Kelley.

"Terrific, Jock! I can't believe it!" Semple gave him a water-soaked sponge,
then an orange slice.

Up the first of the Newton hills Karvonen forced the pace. It was here
that he had destroyed the great Jim Peters in 1954, and he intended to do
the same to Kelley. But the surge did not destroy Kelley. It did destroy the
other Finn, Olavi Manninen, and the two Koreans.

On the second hill Kelley took the offensive gamble. Karvonen looked a
little wobbly; he ran with hunched shoulders and sweated profusely. If

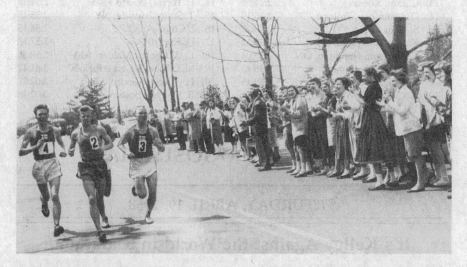

Wellesley College women of 1957 cheer #4 Olavi Manninen, of Finland; #2 Johnny
J. Kelley of the U.S.; and #3 Veikko Karvonen of Finland. Photo courtesy of the
Boston Herald.

Kelley was right, a burst here would do the trick. Kelley accelerated by about 10 seconds per mile. He could no longer see Karvonen in the corner of his eye. Kelley could hear Karvonen's footfalls receding. Karvonen clutched his sides as if lanced. He realized that this was Kelley's day and that no one was going to catch him.

Well, no competitor in the race was going to catch him, but Semple was going to catch him all right. Jock waited and sweated at the finish line. He wore a glen plaid jacket as he stood next to Walter Brown, a man to whom Semple owed much. Semple held an outstretched blanket in which to catch Kelley. He had promised Brown that someday a BAA runner would win the marathon. That was all both men really wanted. Semple waited with his blanket for his dream to come true. He was about to win the Boston Marathon from behind the finish line.

Kelley sprinted down Exeter Street alone. The ubiquitous mayor placed the laurel wreath on his head. Kelley broke the tape. Jock wrapped him in the blanket and Jessie kissed him. Reporters could ask questions without an interpreter.

The Boston hope came through. The city celebrated. Kelley's photo appeared everywhere that spring. His fame grew so great that one 8-year-old Boston boy confused the smiling Irish face and shock of blowing cornsilk hair of marathoner John J. Kelley with that of hatless Senator John F. Kennedy.

1957 Results

1.	J.J. Kelley, *BAA*, Groton, CT	2:20:05^{CR}	12. A. Scandurra, *MillAA*	2:51:35
2.	V. Karvonen, Finland	2:23:54	13. J.A. Kelley, Acton, MA	2:52:08
3.	C. Lim, Korea	2:24:59	14. L. Torres, Puerto Rico	2:54:58
4.	O. Manninen, Finland	2:25:19	15. T. Suito, Bayside, NY	2:55:45
5.	S. Han, Korea	2:28:14	16. J. Conway, *NYPC*	2:56:15
6.	K. Yamada, Japan	2:33:22	17. D. Fay, *BAA*	2:57:13
7.	G. Dickson, Hamilton, ON	2:37:04	18. L. Chisholm, Malden, MA	2:58:38
8.	N. Sadanaga, Japan	2:38:13	19. M. O'Hara, S. Ozone Park, NY	3:01:42
9.	R. Mendez, *NYPC*	2:39:45	20. H. Turcio, Mexico	3:02:21
10.	A. Confalone, Wakefield, MA	2:47:51	21. R. Sawyer, Boston, MA	3:02:38
11.	T. Corbitt, *NYPC*	2:49:14		

140 starters.

THE HOT YUGOSLAVIAN

SATURDAY, APRIL 19, 1958

It's Kelley Against the World in Marathon

The Russians launched Sputnik on October 4, 1957. As the artificial satellite beeped around the world it signaled communist bloc superiority to America.

A runner from a communist country came to Boston to demonstrate his superiority. The papers picked him as the favorite and again labeled John J. Kelley as the only American hope.

The newspapers picked the Yugoslavian, Franjo Mihalic. Because Kelley knew the course, Mihalic said he planned to run elbow to elbow with Kelley, then run away from him at the end. Mihalic had the credentials to support his plan. He had won the International Cross-Country Championships in 1953. He had won every marathon he entered except for one, placing second in the Melbourne Olympic marathon with a 2:26:32. That day under the hot Australian sun, he finished 17 minutes ahead of Kelley. Mihalic made his living as a printer in Belgrade. He was 36. He was tough, fast, and experienced. In his teenage years he raced on bicycles. He had blue eyes, black hair with a bald spot in back, and an enormous nose.

On the morning of the marathon Mihalic looked out his Lenox Hotel window and knew it would be a hot day—a day like the day of the Melbourne marathon. He wanted to protect his head from the hot sun, but he had no hat. He did have a white visor. He found a green napkin in his hotel room and stitched it to the visor so it covered the top of his head and the bald spot in back and then draped to his neck.

Jock Semple told Kelley to wear a head covering, but nervousness distracted Kelley. He worried that this might be another Melbourne. He decided that, regardless of what had happened and what might happen, he would jump into the race and make his presence felt. He remembered two lines from Shakespeare's "Hamlet":

> Beware of entrance to a quarrel, but being in,
> Bear't that the opposed may beware of thee.

If he withered in the heat while running in the lead and had to again suffer the indignity of staggering along while runners he had beaten marched past—so be it.

On hot days many runners commonly fashioned simple head coverings by tying knots in the corners of white handkerchiefs. As they ran along they tried to keep their handkerchief wet. From a distance they looked bald. But Kelley himself, like Jack Kennedy, never did wear a hat.

Eino Pulkkinen, a 32-year-old woodsman from Finland, was the other favorite. He had been second to Hamamura in 1955.

George Terry ran with Kelley and the other favorites in the lead pack. Their training averaged around 85 miles a week. Some runners did much more, notably, Ted Corbitt, who had run as much as 200 miles in a week. He commonly engaged in all-day runs around the island of Manhattan.

Pulkkinen and Mihalic passed cups of water to each other. Mihalic wore his makeshift hat. Mexican Pedro Peralta ran nearby. It felt like a Mexican day, one straight out of the Sonoran desert. At Natick the temperature hit 74 °F, in Wellesley, 78 °F. It climbed to 84 °F at the start of the hills. The

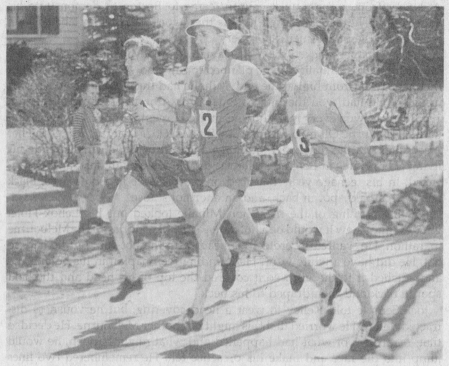

Johnny J. Kelley (left) raced #2, Franjo Mihalic, former world cross-country champion from Belgrade, Yugoslavia, in the heat of the 1958 race. Eino Pulkkinen of Finland wore #3. Upon hearing the day's weather report, Mihalic hand-crafted his white hat. Photo courtesy of the *Boston Herald*.

heat proved to be too much for Terry and Peralta. Only the three favorites remained in the lead. Soon Pulkkinen dropped off the pace. Kelley wanted to make the same move that had brought him to victory in 1957. He wanted to run away on the hills. But it was too hot for that. Kelley said the sun hit him on the head like an ax. It was Mihalic who made the move on Kelley on the hills.

When Kelley realized that he could not match the Yugoslavian's pace he adopted a defensive strategy. He told himself to be careful, to save second place, but to be ready in case Mihalic ran himself into trouble. It was a good plan. It half worked. Kelley did save second place. He saved it by more than 6 minutes, but Mihalic's blister problems and difficulties came only in the last mile, and by then he had built up an unbeatable cushion.

On this hot day all runners ran relatively slowly. Runners had been studying running, but now science began to as well. The public also began to show an interest. A story in the April 17 *Boston Daily Globe* told how the U.S. Army in their Natick laboratories took BAA marathoner and army private Kenneth Mueller, 21 years old, and ran him on a treadmill in condi-

Jock's Shoe Glue

Jock Semple knew that blisters destroyed more racers than anything else on hot days. He suggested to his BAA runner Jimmy Green that he spray his bare feet with a product Jock-the-trainer used on his Celtics basketball players to prevent blisters from forming under the athletic tape used to wrap their ankles. The product, called Tough-Skin, left an adhesive coating on the skin, the idea being that there would be no friction to raise blisters if everything was stuck together and could not move. Green and Semple had never used Tough-Skin in this way before, but they tried it now. Heat makes marathoners desperate.

But soon, Green, running in the top 10, began to have a terrible time with his Tough-Skin sticky feet. The spray glued his bare flesh to his shoes. Alone the gluing would not have been a problem, but with every stride his feet became unstuck, then when he landed became stuck again. He had to prevent the sticking. When he could no longer stand it, he stopped and removed his shoes. He removed his race number and placed pieces of it inside each shoe. But after a few miles the paper rotted with his sweat and wadded beneath his feet. The stickiness came back. If only he had something like petroleum jelly to grease his skin. He saw an automobile service station ahead. He pulled into it like a pit stop and asked the attendants for some axle grease. He coated his feet and had no further trouble.

tions varying from the desert to the arctic. Mueller, who would still be actively racing in 1993, volunteered for this duty. Similar studies went on in Utah at Brigham Young University. But the best "science" available was still the compiled experience of marathon runners themselves. One such compiler was an English military man named Robert Pape, who would come to run in Boston in 1959.

While in Her Majesty's service in 1955, Pape found himself in the summer heat of Hong Kong. He wanted to train, but common wisdom advised him not to run in the 90 °F heat with 90% humidity. Only mad dogs and Englishmen—and marathoners—go out in the tropical noonday sun. Pape went out, came back, and made notes. Here are his findings (condensed from "Long Distance Running In Heat and Humidity," an article that appeared as a clipping in Charley Robbins's scrapbook):

1. Have normal breakfast with lots of salt.
2. Salt tablets make you sick.
3. Drink four pints of fresh water before 10:30.
4. Run eight miles under the noon day sun.
5. Eat salad or fruit for lunch with plenty of salt.
6. Drink two or three pints of water early in the afternoon.
7. Evening run at 5-5:30.
8. Drink plenty of water.
9. Reduction in water and salt intake makes you dizzy.
10. Swimming and sunbathing make you sluggish.
11. Hot meals are bad.
12. Loss of sleep is bad.
13. Don't eat three hours before running.
14. Beer and brandy are OK but other spirits are bad.
15. Socks make your ankles ache.
16. Vaseline protects against chafe.
17. Better run without a shirt.
18. Head gear is no use.
19. Drinks during the run delay exhaustion.

Emil Zatopek, the 1950s god of running, also commented on hot-weather running:

> In my numerous races in India, I convinced myself that middle and long distance runners should take short rest pauses, and also because of the heat, train early in the morning and late in the evening. Hot sunshine is very disagreeable and, it may be said, dangerous. Tropical heat is breeding soil for the spreading of various infections. It is therefore necessary to pay special attention to personal hygiene and the cleanliness of the surroundings, and to avoid cold drinks, which have a harmful effect on the organism.

On the hot days the oldsters seemed to run relatively better.

Old Kelley, at age 50, placed a remarkable 9th. When asked how long he would keep running he said, "Until I am one hundred." But of course he was joking. And he was really 12th. The doctors rejected three serious, experienced marathoners before the start. The idea of physicians' approving of the health of entrants came from a need to save the uninitiated, the extroverts, the exhibitionists, the cranks, and the crackpots from themselves. But these rejected men were none of those. Doctors declared Ted Corbitt, Al Confalone, and John Patrick Lafferty ineligible because of heart murmurs. Back in 1903 John C. Lorden had anticipated the rejection of physicians and concealed the results of an unfavorable examination. A doctor told him he was unfit for the race, yet he won. Doctors told Clarence H. DeMar that he had such mutterings of the heart in 1910 and that all he should exercise was caution. Twenty years later he won the Boston Marathon for the seventh time at age 41, and for more than 20 years after that he still ran it. The three disqualified men, two members of the BAA, were true to the stubborn stock that has come to typify marathoners—they ran unofficially. They started 25 yards behind the official start and placed well within the top 10.

Clarence DeMar: 1888–1958

In May of 1957 Clarence H. DeMar, with advanced cancer and a colostomy following abdominal surgery, ran in the New England 30-kilometer championship, placing 21st with 2:39:30. DeMar died on his farm in Reading, Massachusetts, at 249 Forest Street on June 15, 1958. He worked until the end. An editorial titled "DeMar the Great" ran in the *Boston Daily Globe* under one about the French leader Charles de Gaulle. The editorial eulogized DeMar, comparing him to other sporting greats like Babe Ruth, Bill Tilden, Red Grange, and Jim Thorpe. "[DeMar] lived simply, always had a farm, and earned his living as a printer. He was a strict amateur: his expense accounts were small and exact. Occasionally, a career like his comes as a reminder of what human nature can achieve when great ability is united with strong character and single minded devotion to essential values." DeMar was 70 years old and his heart was in perfect shape.

1958 Results

1. F. Mihalic, Yugoslavia	2:25:54	
2. J.J. Kelley, *BAA*	**2:30:51**	
3. E. Pulkkinen, Finland	2:37:05	
4. T. Sapienza, *BAA*	2:39:46	
5. P. Peralta, Mexico	2:42:35	
Ineligible: T. Corbitt, *NYPC*	2:43:47	
Ineligible: A. Confalone, *BAA*	2:45:29	
6. S. Kahainy, NY and Israel	2:48:00	
Ineligible: J. Lafferty, *BAA*	2:48:48	
7. T. Ryan, Redondo Beach, CA	2:50:13	
8. G. Scotto, *BAA*	2:52:07	
9. J.A. Kelley, Watertown, MA	**2:52:12**	
10. L. Fauber, Boston, MA	2:53:17	
11. J. Green, *BAA*	2:55:32
12. T. Suito, Homer City, PA	2:57:52
13. N. Cirulnick, *NYPC*	2:58:26
14. J. Hughes, Boulder, CO	2:59:12
15. J. Bordan, *NYPC*	3:00:11
16. M. O'Hara, *SABC*, NY	3:02:07
17. J. Onus, *NYPC*	3:02:44
18. R. Packard, *BAA*	3:03:08
19. D. Fay, *BAA*	3:03:45
20. R. Cummings, Granby, MA	3:07:07
29. C. Robbins, *NYPC*	3:17:05
48. R. Ahti, *RpAC*, Fitchberg, MA	3:39:58

203 entrants.

Team prize
BAA

DETECTIVE SHARK FINN

MONDAY, APRIL 20, 1959

Kelley Top for U.S. in Today's BAA Grind

Like gunslingers in America's mythic Old West, marathoners from far away came to Boston looking to shoot down Johnny J. Kelley. And Johnny was the kind of guy who made a perfect target, an easy mark. He just stood still. His blue eyes full of trust and his hair all golden made him hard to miss. He ran for the sponsoring club in Boston—he had to run their marathon—and that unicorn on his chest offered a bull's-eye for any road-running sharpshooter on the planet.

On a cold and rainy day in April a stranger came to town looking for Johnny. The stranger had eyes set so deep into his skull that you couldn't tell if he blinked. It would not matter even if you could see his eyes. He rarely did blink. He was fast and he knew he was fast. Back in '56 Johnny had gotten the drop on him. The stranger wanted revenge. He wanted Johnny. He wanted to break Johnny's heart on the third Newton hill.

Once he caught sight of Johnny the stranger tailed him at arm's length. He followed in Johnny's wake like a hungry shark, just waiting for a mistake. The stranger tailing Johnny was a detective from Helsinki, Finland, by the name of Oksanen, Eino Oksanen. He had blazed a 2:18:51 at Pieksamaki, but he placed third to Kelley's second place in the BAA of 1956. Oksanen wanted to make good.

The detective wore brown cotton gloves to ward off the chilling 40 °F rain. They didn't help much. The chill settled to his bones. He wore a sweatshirt with "Suomi" (the Finnish name for Finland) printed on it. He tossed it off in Natick. Half a stride behind Kelley, he waited as they ran through mile after mile. Kelley could not see him, but he could hear his footfalls on the wet road for 24 miles. Kelley ran hatless and gloveless, his face twisted up in his wrinkled squint. The killer cold of this nerve-racking race settled into his bones, too. Oksanen followed Kelley like the black cloud of a term paper follows a college student. Kelley could not forget he was there no matter how much nip-and-tuck fun he had.

When Kelley slowed, Oksanen slowed. When Kelley pushed the pace, Oksanen followed. He always followed. Like the crocodile with the ticking clock that followed Captain Hook, Oksanen followed Kelley. It was a matter of time. Tick-tock, tick-tock. Oksanen followed.

Jock Semple watched the clock, and he watched his athlete. He shook his head. A foul and foreboding mood settled over him. Semple worried about Oksanen's tactic. The Finn looked too fresh. Then Semple saw something that made him explode in fury.

Down a side street came an intruder. He wore a white sweatsuit with his face covered by a clown's mask, and on his feet he wore gigantic flapping clown shoes. Semple snapped. Here Kelley and Oksanen were grappling in a struggle that would take every ounce of their energy and a fool jumps in to make a joke out of it! Semple leaped off the moving bus. This was a serious athletic contest, not an April Fool's parade. He sprinted to the clown and tackled him. Semple ripped off the clown's mask. In his rage he would have ripped more had the police not intervened. Semple returned to the press bus. So violent was his attack that reporters expected assault charges to be filed. None were.

Kelley knew nothing of Semple's fight. All Kelley knew was that there was a thing on his shoulder and he could not make it go away. Oksanen bided his time.

The time came on a temporary rude wooden bridge that arched over the railroad just before Kenmore Square. Only one man could cross at a time. There Oksanen struck. Like a striking praying mantis, like a closing Venus flytrap glistening in a marsh, Oksanen flew past Kelley and over the bridge. Kelley could not move on him. Oksanen had the power. He stretched his lead to 1 second past a minute as he swept into victory in front of the dilapidated Soden Building that had once been the BAA clubhouse on Exeter Street. He might be the last man to finish while the building was standing.

The Soden Building was the BAA clubhouse that the city had taken over for unpaid taxes in 1935. Boston University bought it for $35,000 and used it for classes until 1949, when the Boston Public Library bought it. The building would be razed later that year to make way for the new annex to the Boston Public Library.

Except for April 19, the BAA was only an idea held together by a few dedicated and unpaid men.

The wealth and power of the club that founded the Boston Marathon had long since dissipated. Except for April 19 of every year, the Boston Athletic Association was only an idea held together by a few dedicated and unpaid men who did not know where or if the Boston Marathon would start or finish the next year. The BAA could not properly be called an organization if it had virtually no membership and did only one thing on one day a year. It was Jock Semple who held the running club together and Will Cloney who organized the race; otherwise almost nothing remained.

1959 Results

1.	E. Oksanen, Finland	2:22:42	16.	T. Nakoa, Japan	2:41:50
2.	J.J. Kelley, *BAA*	2:23:43	17.	B. Smith, Hamilton, ON	2:42:30
3.	G. Dickson, Hamilton, ON	2:24:04	18.	R. McNicholl, Ridgefield, CT	2:44:33
4.	V. Karvonen, Finland	2:24:37	19.	A. Hatsuko, Japan	2:45:13
5.	O. Suarez, Argentina	2:28:24	20.	A. Hull, Jr., Brownsville, VT	2:46:34
6.	R. Pape, England	2:28:28	21.	R. Drake, Glendale, CA	2:47:20
7.	N. Sadanaga, Japan	2:29:30	22.	R. Packard, *BAA*, MA	2:47:31
8.	J. Green, *BAA*, Saugus, MA	2:29:58	23.	J.A. Kelley, Watertown, MA	2:47:52
9.	A. Confalone, *BAA*, MA	2:33:50	24.	W. Murphy, Warren, RI	2:48:09
10.	G. Watt, Australia	2:34:37	25.	J. Church, Toronto, ON	2:48:41
11.	T. Ryan, Redondo Beach, CA	2:37:03	26.	K. Mueller, *BAA*, MA	2:49:21
12.	T. Corbitt, *NYPC*	2:38:05	39.	A. Richards, Chicago, IL	2:56:22
13.	D. Pistenna, Bethesda, MD	2:38:47	49.	G. Scotto, *BAA*	3:05:24
14.	A. Sapienza, *BAA*, MA	2:40:41	55.	J. Daley, Jr., *NMC*	3:11:14
15.	J. Lafferty, *BAA*, MA	2:41:20	66.	C. Robbins, Middletown, CT	3:16:41

203 entrants, 151 starters.

Chapter 7

1960-1969
Times They Are
A-Changin'

Presidents: *John F. Kennedy, Lyndon B. Johnson, Richard M. Nixon*

Massachusetts Governors: *Foster Furcolo, John A. Volpe, Endicott Peabody, John A. Volpe*

Boston Mayors: *John F. Collins, Kevin H. White*

1960 Populations: *United States, 179,323,175; Massachusetts, 5,148,578; Boston, 789,439*

Numerically the '60s started when the '50s ended. But in spirit the 1950s ended for the United States on November 22, 1963, with the assassination of President Kennedy. I.F. Stone calls the '60s a Time of Torment. The era's zeitgeist extended through the deposition of Nixon in 1974. Politics began to mix with athletics. One Boston Marathoner wore a T-shirt proclaiming "Dump Nixon" at the 1972 Olympic trials.

It was a complex world in 1959 when Buddy Holly and the music died, but it was even more complex after the '60s, the decade when protest and counterculture became institutionalized. It was the decade of disaffected hippies, hair, and Vietnam. It was a decade of televised spaceflights and televised assassinations. Counterculture high priest Timothy Leary preached, Tune in, turn on, drop out. The Beatles and Bob Dylan wrote songs, and all the heroes were antiheroes. Ken Kesey wrote *One Flew Over the Cuckoo's Nest* and Rachel Carson wrote *Silent Spring* in 1962. James Brown sang it loud, I'm black and I'm proud.

The 1960s also became a decade of women. The second wave of feminism washed over America. When it touched the Boston Marathon, running changed forever. The women who touched it had to be extraordinary. This chapter contains the stories of two of them. Both were pioneers, and each made a difference, but their means and personalities could not have been more different. Roberta Gibb and Kathrine Switzer illustrate the great split down the center of America.

Early in the '60s fear gripped the world as President Kennedy, embarrassed by the failure of the Bay of Pigs invasion, confronted Soviet leader Nikita Khrushchev over the deployment of Soviet missiles in Cuba. The world froze as the superpowers glared eyeball to eyeball over Cuba. Fingers twitched over "the buttons" that controlled intercontinental ballistic missiles on both sides. Fortunately for the U.S., the Soviets blinked first, and life went on. But the fear remained. What if Khrushchev hadn't backed down? Children begged their fathers to build fallout shelters.

In 1965 black Americans living in the Watts area of Los Angeles rioted, killing 35 people and destroying $200 million in property. Riots followed in Newark and Detroit. Three years later James Earl Ray assassinated Dr. Martin Luther King on April 4, 1968. The long-standing annual Cathedral 10-Mile handicap road race, scheduled for 2 days later, included a stretch through a black section of Boston. It was cancelled and never held again. A month later Sirhan Bishara Sirhan assassinated Senator Robert Kennedy. Hundreds of civilians were massacred in 1968 by American soldiers in My Lai, South Vietnam, and a year later Neil Armstrong took a giant first step on the moon.

The sixties were a decade of a country divided on the basis of hair length. The movie *Easy Rider* (about a long-haired motorcycle rider blasted off his bike by a redneck's shotgun) rang true for both halves of the country, those for the Vietnam War and those against it. Young draft resisters became fugitives from their own government. The Peace Corps sent young Americans to do development work overseas, rock-and-roll was even better than in the '50s, and by and large Americans prospered further.

The numbers of runners in the Boston Marathon swelled—from 156 in 1960 to over 1,000 in 1969. The course record plunged from 2:20:05 to 2:13:49. The time for 50th place dropped from 3:18:10 in 1960 to 2:41:20 by 1969—a run that would have been 17th in 1960. The belief that running was bad for you and that men ran marathons at peril to their lives finally died. Physicians embraced running. President Kennedy and the astronauts endorsed a campaign for universal fitness in which running was basic. In the 1960s running became good, and that established the basis for the running boom of the next decades.

KELLEY'S LIMIT

TUESDAY, APRIL 19, 1960

Kelley, Finns Favored in Today's Marathon

April 19 headlines told of the hopeful candidate for the Democratic presidential nomination, John F. Kennedy of Massachusetts, accepting a debate with Hubert H. Humphrey of Minnesota. In Boston the marathon survived. It survived on Will Cloney's and Jock Semple's willpower. It had no sponsor but the BAA, and the BAA had no money. The pressure on Johnny J. Kelley to win again mounted as the day approached. He could not sleep. Beginning in 1956, Kelley had finished second, first, second, and second. Again of all American marathoners it was Kelley, only Kelley, who had a chance to win, and this time against two Finns. But John J. Kelley had problems that had nothing to do with Finns.

Every athlete has limits. There are physical and mental limits. The body can contain only so many stresses. If enough stresses accumulate, the effect on performance is catastrophic; the runner cannot go the distance. No one problem bothered Johnny J. Kelley, but lots of little ones harried him.

Kelley's stresses accumulated slowly. On a winter run he stopped to help push a stuck automobile. A little tendon in his ankle rubbed the wrong way against a bone, and the irritation continued for months. It worried him. The flu did a few orbits of his family. The local media pressured Kelley. For the newspaper writers it was fair-haired, blue-eyed Johnny against the world. This year's Boston Marathon was one of two compulsory U.S. Olympic trials; the other was the Yonkers Marathon a month later. To qualify for the team a man had to do well in both. The pressure prevented Kelley from simply running coyly to just make the team. He had to try to win the entire race. But his fitness was not what it could be. He had been doing the training, but he did not feel his usual zip and enthusiasm. His fast intervals came with too much strain, the long runs seemed chores, and in premarathon tune-up races he ran slower than in previous years and behind runners he had beaten before. Something was wrong, but not grossly wrong. Kelley was not bedridden. Nothing was bad enough to keep him from entering, but it was bad enough for him to want to hide from reporters.

In other years Kelley usually came into town from Connecticut to lodge with the elder John A. Kelley for the night. Everyone knew where to find him. Both Kelleys had always given generously to the press. But this time Kelley the younger would tell no one—not even his coach and father-confessor, Jock Semple—where he would stay. Semple did not want to know so he would not have to lie to the reporters. Kelley waited, on the verge of cracking, in an unnamed Boston hotel and not with old Kelley. One more press interview might break him. Better not talk . . . better hunker down and hide . . . better rest.

Kelley wanted every possible advantage. His nervousness drove him to take risks. He wanted the best shoes. Old Kelley had the best shoes. They were all light and magic, so young Kelley wanted a pair. Handmade by a retired Italian shoemaker in Cambridge, Louis Dell'Ambrosio, the shoes had uppers of stretch material and leather. Crepe rubber covered the soles. But the old man did not make many pairs of running shoes. Kelley coveted the light fantastic shoes so much that he finally begged Mr. Dell'Ambrosio for a pair. Kelley didn't run in the new shoes but walked around in them for a week. He wanted to allow time for his enormous bunions to press their unique form into the leather. But he should have run in them.

Kelley's competitors for the Olympic team, Alex Breckenridge and Gordon McKenzie, added more accumulating stress to Kelley by setting a quick early pace on a day perfect for running. A 15-mile-an-hour tailwind on a clear, brisk 50 °F day helped Breckenridge, a crew-cut Marine based in Quantico, Virginia, set course records past the Framingham and Natick checkpoints. Breckenridge was born a Scotsman like Semple, but unlike Semple and the Marine stereotype, he did not boisterously fill the halls of Montezuma with noise. He was a quiet person but a fast and furious competitor. He had a 10K personal best of 30:54, faster than Kelley. McKenzie was another 10K man, also faster than Kelley but not as fast as Breckenridge. He had run that distance for the U.S. in the Melbourne Olympics but had since moved up to the marathon. He worked as a civil engineer for the city of New York.

McKenzie was surprised by his pretty English wife, Christine, who popped out of the crowd to yell encouragement at every point on the course she could get to. In her excitement she kicked off her shoes and ran alongside her husband in her nylon-stockinged feet for distances as long as a quarter mile. Her uninhibited zeal and ability delighted and impressed reporters in the press bus. The next day's papers carried detailed accounts of her running and grabbing motorcycle, police car, and subway rides to keep up with her husband. She said they trained together. She had run races in Great Britain and had set records at distances from a quarter mile to 3 miles. The reporters called her good-looking, shapely, and feminine and wished that fetching blondes would run the marathon more often. Her intent, she admitted, was to make the U.S. Olympic team in the reinstated women's 800 meters. For that purpose she had taken out citizenship papers. The disproportionate attention by the press signaled that women runners in the early 1960s were still an odd sight, but they were on the verge of jumping into previously all-male events.

Some years later Christine McKenzie wanted to run in a 4-mile road race. The AAU required women to get special permission to compete at such long distances, the fear being that long-distance running would make women manly, unfeminine, and muscular. To disprove the theory, shapely Mrs. McKenzie attended an AAU meeting. Wearing only a fur coat over a bikini, at a crucial moment she stood up, threw off her coat, and asked the gentlemen officials if they thought she was unfeminine and too muscular. She made her point and got her permission.

Following Breckenridge and McKenzie and behind a small gap ran the two Finns, Paavo Kotila and Veikko Koivumaki, and Kelley. At 11 miles Kotila took the lead. Kelley forced himself into second place. Maybe the Finn would crack. Paavo Edvard Kotila, 32, at 5'7" and 142 pounds, had run fourth in 1955. He came from a family of 11 children raised in the farming town of Veteli in north central Finland, 300 miles south of the Arctic circle. This year he was not for cracking. He came to win the race. He did not have to worry about making an Olympic team.

Another American, Jimmy Green, in this complexity of an Olympic trial as part of a world championship marathon, did have to worry about making the U.S. team. Green, a small man with an impossible, and apparently imperfect, mode of running, wanted a place on that team. His unusual running style amazed his fellow runners. His arms and legs flayed to the sides as if he were continually swatting off a swarm of bees. He looked utterly feckless windmilling down the road. But where his feet met the road, they planted perfectly. Where it counted, deep in the heart, legs, and lungs, Green ran with perfection. He taught English in Saugus, a town near a saltmarsh a bit north of Boston, and ran for Jock Semple's BAA team. He ran slightly off the lead pace with a struggling young runner from Chicago, Hal Higdon. Green had hoped for a slow pace for 15 to 18 miles and then to make a break for it. But Breckenridge and McKenzie foiled that plan, so he fell back on his second plan. He would run with the pack and go for position.

Kelley could run for only one position. First place was his only thought. Victory or nothing. Kelley felt a hopeless blackness surround him. He did not feel well. The once reliable antigravity spring in his legs that had let him bound up the hills in previous years was gone. Kelley knew that his strength would not be there when he asked it to perform. At 3 miles one of his light fantastic shoes had begun to nibble a hole in his foot. He could not help but favor it. The blackness came from his knowledge of impending impossibility. Kelley ran in second place down the hill to where the 20-foot-wide Charles River passes under the marathon course in Newton Lower Falls. The downhill should have been easy running, but for Kelley, a man filled with self-doubts, the long downhill brought no relief. He knew the hills ahead. He knew too much. That knowledge depressed him.

Kelley's energy leaked away. He slowed to a walk. He quit fighting. After 17 miles he stopped pushing. He felt he had let himself, his family, his friends, and his fellow runners down. He felt unworthy. He wanted to find a hole, crawl into it, and draw the dirt in after him. He wanted to disappear. Blisters. He had half-dollar-sized blisters. He had run with blisters before, but never on top of the other burdens. They were too much. The blisters broke his will. Kelley dropped out of the race. The man possessed by divine enthusiasm walked ashamed; no race remained in him. At 21 miles he left the race course.

Kotila, remaining in the lead, felt a relief. Suddenly no footfalls pursued him. He had been positioning Kelley by the cheering of the crowds behind him, but now there was silence. Kelley was the only American he feared. Kotila relaxed and ran away to win. Gordon McKenzie, with Christine seeming to pop up everywhere, flashed into second place with a fast time. Jimmy Green flailed in next. He had done both of the things he wanted to do: He placed well overall, and he put himself squarely before the eyes of the Olympic selectors. It looked like McKenzie and Green had positions on the Olympic team. Kelley found his way to the finish. He talked to reporters.

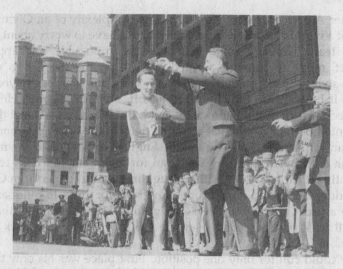

Ever so delicately, Paavo Kotila severs the finish line tape to win the 1960 Boston Marathon. Perhaps he was savoring the moment, trying to make it last. Photo courtesy of the *Boston Herald*.

Kelley said the perfectionist in him would not let him continue racing. The yearly pressure of Kelley against the world was too much. The Melbourne Olympic race had been a failure, and now it was impossible to make the U.S. team for the Rome games. What was the point of continuing? He had won the Boston Marathon, had won the U.S. National Championships many times, and had run the fastest times of any American—2:20:05, 2:20:55, and 2:21:00 at Boston, Yonkers, and Jersey City. He wanted to run a sub-2:20 on an accurate course, but he hadn't done it. Kelley talked without bitterness and blamed no one but himself. Maybe it was time to hang up the shoes and quit.

Old Kelley, aged 52, finished 19th in 2:44. He thought the requirement that marathoners run both Boston and Yonkers to be considered for the Olympic team was stupid. In 1948 they had to run *three* qualifying marathons. For the Olympic Games he said it was pointless to leave your firepower, John J. Kelley, the fastest American, in the states.

The absolute U.S. selection process dismayed Kotila, as he told John Ahern of the *Boston Globe*: "This is folly! In Finland we would not permit our very best man to be discarded because of one bad race. He is by far your best man. I knew that Kelley had foot hardships—problems during the winter and that he would not be at his best."

Johnny the younger Kelley said, "I ran my last race today."

Kotila said, "I'll be back again." But he did not come until 1983 when he ran 2:36 at age 55. But for Kelley, what he said was not what he did.

Checkpoint Splits

Framingham	33:56
Natick	53:39
Wellesley	1:08:54
Auburndale	1:30:48
Lake Street	1:53:24
Coolidge Corner	2:07:31

1960 Results

1.	P. Kotila, Finland	2:20:54	11.	B. Smith, Hamilton, ON	2:34:43
2.	G. McKenzie, *NYPC*	2:22:18	12.	S. Villa, *CCAC*	2:36:39
3.	J. Green, *BAA*, Saugus, MA	2:23:37	13.	J. Lafferty, *U.S. Navy, BAA*	2:36:55
4.	A. Confalone, *BAA*, MA	2:26:30	14.	A. Sapienza, *BAA*	2:39:26
5.	V. Koivumaki, Finland	2:28:30	15.	T. Corbitt, *NYPC*	2:40:13
6.	A. Breckenridge, Quantico, VA	2:28:44	16.	G. Scotto, *BAA*	2:40:26
7.	R. Carman, Pittsburgh, PA	2:29:06	17.	A. Vali, *VOC*	2:42:45
8.	R. Cons, *CCAC*, CA	2:30:39	18.	S. Tiernan, *NMC*	2:43:15
9.	T. Ryan, *LBSC*	2:32:49	19.	J.A. Kelley, Watertown, MA	**2:44:39**
10.	R. Drake, *CCAC*	2:34:12	20.	E. Brackett, Lynn, MA	2:45:31

156 starters, 83 finishers.

Team prize
BAA

Top Dog

WEDNESDAY, APRIL 19, 1961

Kelley Ready to Win Again

Ten days after the 1960 marathon the retired John J. Kelley, at age 30 with a wife, a child, a good job, and a house, mowed his lawn. It was a proper thing for a retired athlete to do. It was a spring day, the first mowing of the year. He thought it was time to grow up and give up the bohemian existence of a running-centered life. He had taken so many demeaning jobs in his younger days just so he could stick with his running; now it was time to become a solid citizen and a normal person. He had won the thing. He had the Boston Marathon course record. He remembered the poem "To An Athlete Dying Young," by A.E. Housman:

> *Smart lad, to slip betimes away*
> *From fields where glory does not stay*
>
> . . . .
>
> *Now you will not swell the rout*
> *Of lads that wore their honors out,*
> *Runners whom renown outran*
> *And the name died before the man.*

He had his job teaching English, a family, and a loyal dog. Should be enough for any man. Then his neighbor came and spoiled his plan. The old man leaned over the fence and locked Kelley in a conversation. Well, he told John, good thing you retired from running. You could damage yourself, at your age. You've got to face reality. Marathon running is a young man's sport, and you were wise to recognize that you just could no longer keep up. Better to quit, take it easy. You're not getting any younger. The words infuriated gentle Kelley. He thought, I'm not that old! Not as old as you, you old bastard! Maybe you've given up, but not me! Kelley left his lawnmower in midrow and his neighbor in midsentence and took off for Westerly, Rhode Island. OK, the old man didn't mean any harm, but still the words hurt. It was not good for Kelley that he retire from running; he missed it desperately. A 5-mile road race had been scheduled for Westerly later that day and he just might make it in time for the start. I'll show him who's washed up.

Kelley won at Westerly. He proved that running is not a part of reality. He did not retire gracefully like an old soldier, he did not fade away. He trained again and was happy. Perhaps the fury of vengeance against his 1960 dropout focused him. Once he gave up running, then came back, he no longer carried the fear that he might not fulfill expectations. As you focus on the things you fear, you tend to swerve into them. With his "retirement" the pressures of the press and those expectations he allowed to squeeze upon himself disappeared. Emotions other than fear powered his running. Revenge against his failure at Boston motivated him. The training clicked so that after dropping out of the Boston Marathon, giving up the sport, coming back to it, and now training hard and effectively, Kelley would feel gratification. Three weeks later he won big in the Olympic trials in Yonkers.

In the Olympic marathon at Rome Kelley defeated the Finns and placed a respectable 19th. Other runners included Franjo Mihalic, Boston winner in 1958, 12th; Eino Oksanen, Boston winner in 1959, 24th; Alex Breckenridge, 30th; Gordon McKenzie, 48th; and Antti Viskari, Boston winner in 1956, 53rd. Ethiopian Abebe Bikila won, running barefoot through the night streets of Rome.

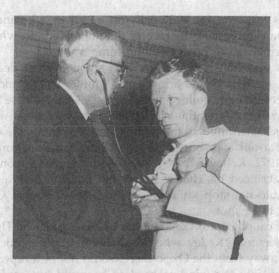

Through the 1960s medical examinations were required of all entrants. Here Eino Oksanen gets his. Photo courtesy of the *Boston Herald*.

Back in Boston in the spring of 1961, Kelley arrived ready to win again. The newspapers said so. On April 12 they reported that the first man to orbit the earth, Russian Yuri Gagarin, tumbled around the world in an hour and 29 minutes. That was about the time it took Kelley, Oksanen (now known as The Ox at 144 pounds), and 39-year-old Englishman Fred Norris to reach the hills. Snow spit through the 38 °F air as a mild northeast storm pushed a 10- to 12-mph headwind in their faces. The snow stopped by Framingham, but the wind had not. Kelley ran in perfect position to win, but so did Oksanen. Oksanen had had a better kick than Kelley in 1959 and probably still did. Fred Norris had a better kick than Kelley. Nearly everyone had a better kick than Kelley. Norris had the kick and he was fit, having run a 2:19:08 marathon in Liverpool, England, the previous autumn. But randomness in the form of a small black dog intervened. It had been following the action for miles. Kelley understood the dog and secretly liked that the dog liked staying with the leaders. The black dog only did what the leaders did—dog each other for the lead. A motorcycle cop chased the black dog away, but it came back. It was a front runner, a top dog—a dog after Kelley's own heart.

But suddenly the quick little dog darted in front of Oksanen; who jumped over it. Kelley couldn't see the dog and ran into it. He fell to the road and skinned his elbow. Norris stopped to help Kelley to his feet. That was the break for Oksanen and the breaking of Norris. The falling and skinning were not serious, and had they been earlier they would have been forgotten; but the timing proved critical. In the wind and cold and under such fatigue, stopping stiffened Norris. As Kelley scooted after Oksanen to reestablish contact, Norris lost contact. McKenzie ran a half mile behind and out of sight. Norris ran the rest of the race in the nowhere land where he could not see the men ahead of him or behind him.

Fred Norris was himself a person who spent a great deal of time in nowhere land. He was 39 and a former coal miner in England. He did the unusual thing of going to college at this late age. At McNeese State College in Lake Charles, Louisiana, this old British man on campus was indeed in a nowhere land as strange as the depths of a coal mine. He often trained with his 15-year-old son, Edmund, who became U.S. national marathon champion in 1972. Kelley felt that there was something wonderful about Norris, who sacrificed his chance for second place to help a friend. After the race he could not stop saying nice things about Norris. Oksanen said the dog ought to be shot.

After Kelley caught up to Oksanen the two ran together. The Ox had no need to run away from Kelley, whom he knew he could outkick. But Kelley wanted to get away from the Ox so there would not be a repeat of the 1959 race. Kelley ran into the wind as hard as he could but could not escape Oksanen anymore than he could escape his own shadow. Kelley's 122 pounds

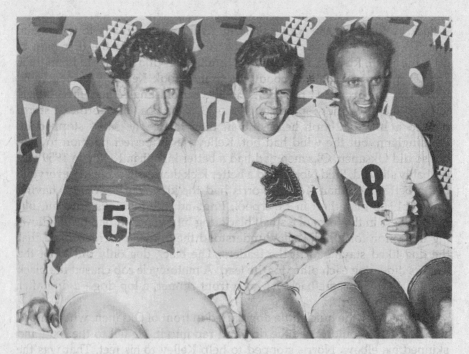

John J. Kelley (middle) fell over a black dog, Fred Norris (right) stopped to help, and Eino "The Ox" Oksanen (left) thought it should have been shot. Art Howard Photo/Courtesy of the *Boston Herald*.

provided little draft for Oksanen, but the Ox did not need to draft. All he needed was to stay in touch with Kelley. And wait. The physiology of the two men yielded the same result as in 1959. Oksanen of Finland won his second Boston Marathon by outkicking Kelley. The Finnish connection continued. It was not by chance that Finns had done so well in the Boston Marathon. They had a little help from their friends.

The Finnish-American Club of Foster, Rhode Island, had raised $14,000 since 1953 by holding raffles and dances to pay the expenses of Finns to come to Boston. The marathon was good ethnic public relations for Finnish-Americans. The newspaper writers began to run out of word plays—Finnish line and Finnagle and Flying Finns. In the years to come more flying Finns flocked fearlessly to Boston. And the Ox would come back too.

Checkpoint Splits

Framingham	Johnny Kelley/Eino Oksanen	35:22
Natick	Johnny Kelley/Eino Oksanen	56:02
Wellesley	Johnny Kelley/Eino Oksanen	1:12:05
Woodland	Johnny Kelley/Eino Oksanen	1:34:35
Lake Street	Johnny Kelley/Eino Oksanen	1:56:50
Coolidge Corner	Johnny Kelley/Eino Oksanen	2:10:18

1961 Results

1.	E. Oksanen, Finland	**2:23:29**	19. N. Higgins, *U.S. Army*	2:47:23
2.	J.J. Kelley, *BAA*	**2:23:54**	20. W. Squires, *BAA*	2:47:46
3.	F. Norris, Lake Charles, LA	2:25:46	21. A. Fletcher Hull, Jr., VT	2:48:05
4.	G. McKenzie, *NYPC*	2:28:40	22. A. Wooten, England	2:48:09
5.	O. Manninen, Finland	2:29:46	23. R. Packard, *BAA*	2:48:14
6.	G. Terry, Groton, CT	2:30:20	24. R. Cummings, Medford, MA	2:48:16
7.	G. Williams, Chicago, IL	2:32:22	25. J. Councill, Westerly, RI	2:51:34
8.	F. Gruber, Austria	2:32:49	26. G. Harvey, *BAA*	2:52:23
9.	J. Green, *BAA*	2:32:58	29. N. Cirulnick, *MillAA*, NY	2:54:45
10.	E. Duncan, *BAA*	2:33:46	30. D. Fay, *BAA*	2:55:17
11.	G. Parnell, Brockton, MA	2:37:32	31. R. Weeks, Lynnfield, MA	2:56:15
12.	T. Corbitt, *NYPC*	2:38:33	34. J. Garlepp, *MillAA*, NY	2:58:04
13.	J. Eblen, Baltimore, MD	2:39:09	35. R. Sawyer, Medford, MA	2:58:10
14.	A. Confalone, *BAA*	2:41:27	36. M. Bigelow, *BAA*	2:59:46
15.	R. McNicholl, *NYPC*	2:41:45	38. A. Scandurra, *MillAA*, NY	3:00:55
16.	D. Merchant, *BAA*	2:42:52	41. J. Kopil, *NYAC*	3:06:31
17.	**J.A. Kelley, Watertown, MA**	**2:44:53**	83. C. Robbins, *NYPC*	3:46:04
18.	R. Zollinhofer, *BAA*	2:47:18		

231 entrants, 166 starters.

WHERE'S KELLEY?

THURSDAY, APRIL 19, 1962

Finn and Friend Back to Defend

Eino Oksanen came back to Boston with a new personal marathon record, a 2:22:18 from Fukuoka, Japan. He brought another Finn with him, Paavo Pystynen, from Lappeenranta, the home of Antti Viskari, the 1956 Boston winner. Boston Marathon winners were great heroes in Japan and Finland. Because Finland bordered the Soviet Union, the U.S. government, in the midst of its Cold War with the communists, wanted good relations with Finland. The entire world bristled from the friction between Communism and capitalism. Two days before the marathon headlines in the *Boston Herald* told that "U.S. Combat Marines Enter Fray in Vietnam."

Pystynen had recently run a 2:23:11 marathon. Neither Finn had times to match Kelley's course record of 2:20:05 from 1957, but Oksanen had beaten Kelley twice before at Boston; however, Kelley had beaten him in the Rome Olympics. No American had come close to Kelley. Kelley ran to defend American prestige. Jock Semple told the *Herald* that "Johnny's going to put the pressure on early." The pressure was already on Johnny. Americans held a particular sensitivity toward being beaten at anything by other nations. Since Khrushchev had said in 1956 that Communism would bury the capitalist states, the Russians had beaten Americans into space, so Americans were sensitive about losing anything. President Kennedy had a physical fitness plan for the nation as well as a space program, but neither had had time to show results. So for another year, Kelley was America's best hope for victory in the Boston Marathon.

Kelley wanted to do more than win; he wanted to break 2:20. That number rang through his head. He said that internationally a marathon runner was nothing if he hadn't broken 2:20. In 1956, on the short course, Kelley's 2:14:33 Boston time might be corrected for the missing 1,183 yards by adding 4-1/2 minutes to get a 2:19; officially, however, he had not broken 2:20, and that deficiency bothered him.

Maybe Semple gave Kelley's race plan away to Oksanen. But maybe the plan stated was not the true plan and Kelley really planned to sit back and go on the hills. Regardless, Oksanen decided to go out hard to shake Kelley, but if Kelley survived until the hills, Oksanen would back off and wait to sprint away from him at the finish.

When Kelley failed to join the lead pack Oksanen worried. Where was he? Overcast skies covered the course. Once the leaders arrived in Natick, a headwind popped up. By the finish a steady drizzle fell. Alex Breckenridge, the Scotland-born Marine, in bright red shorts took the early lead ahead of the Finns in their flag's white and blue. Injury problems had kept Breckenridge to low training mileage, but the cool conditions let him use his speed. On a hot race day a runner would have to be much better conditioned to be able to deal with heat in addition to a fast pace. Cool days allowed a little leeway. Breckenridge appreciated his luck.

Breckenridge held on to the Finns while Oksanen kept looking behind. Where *is* Kelley? At last he asked a man on the press bus. Kelley was only 150 yards back, not feeling good but not feeling bad either. A surge from Oksanen and Pystynen through Newton Lower Falls disposed of Breckenridge, leaving Finns alone in the lead.

Oksanen and Pystynen ran together as they had for 3 weeks in the Arcadia State Forest in Rhode Island, where they had stayed before the race. In Finland they trained mostly on soft surfaces through the forest; as guests of American Finns they did the same kind of training in two daily sessions separated by a light meal. As they shared the lead of the Boston Marathon both could have gone faster, but they waited for Kelley's challenge. The hills passed and no Kelley challenge came. At the top of the hills Oksanen left Pystynen. Still, where was Kelley?

At the finish Eino accepted the laurel wreath and with it on his head went back to run in with Paavo. Both looked for Kelley. They saw that Breckenridge held on to third place. A minute later came Kelley. What had happened to him? Nothing. For a reason unknown to him or anyone else, he had run a mediocre race. Maybe this was his slide into oblivion. Maybe not. He didn't know. Sometimes races are disasters and sometimes they are glorious, but many are merely mediocre. On average one runs one's average. But Kelley maintained his enthusiasm and planned to come back next year. Maturity gave him a grip on his emotions. A mediocre race was not the end of the world—there was world and time enough.

The Finns, Eino and Paavo, took a hot bath together in a tub in their Lenox Hotel room. They invited press photographers in. Then they broke out the beer and had a good time, continuing their Finnish tradition of sublime postrace celebrations. Photos of two beaming Finns in a tub appeared in the next day's papers.

1962 Results

1.	E. Oksanen, Finland	2:23:48	10.	L. Damon, *BAA*	2:34:05
2.	P. Pystynen, Finland	2:24:58	11.	W. Schwab, *NYAC*	2:35:01
3.	A. Breckenridge, *U.S. Marines*	2:27:17	12.	E. Duncan, *BAA*	2:36:40
4.	J.J. Kelley, *BAA*	2:28:37	13.	D. Merchant, *BAA*	2:37:25
5.	O. Atkins, ON	2:31:49	14.	T. Corbitt, *NYPC*	2:37:42
6.	E. Kaunitso, Fitchberg, MA	2:32:26	15.	L. Ehler, *BAA*, Arlington, MA	2:38:30
7.	G. Terry, *EBAC*	2:32:48	16.	R. Bamberger, *NMC*	2:39:00
8.	A. Hull, Jr., *SpAC*	2:33:01	17.	R. Scharf, *BOC*	2:39:29
9.	R. Haines, *NCAS*	2:33:09	18.	R. Avery, Dedham, MA	2:39:40

19.	R. Cummings, *NMC*	2:40:46	25. J.A. Kelley, Watertown, MA	2:44:36
20.	W. Welsh, *MillAA*, NY	2:41:19	26. H. Higdon, *UCTC*	2:45:21
21.	R. Packard, *BAA*	2:41:46	33. G. Grasso, *BAA*	2:48:51
22.	W. Lamothe, *NMC*	2:42:05	34. G. Harvey, *BAA*	2:49:01
23.	A. Confalone, *BAA*	2:43:09	35. J. Adams, *BAA*	2:49:03
24.	M. Bigelow, *BAA*	2:44:08	47. A. Richards, *UCTC*	2:58:16

181 starters.

BIKILA

FRIDAY, APRIL 19, 1963

Gold Medalist Favorite in Race

The U.S. nuclear submarine Thresher, carrying 129 men, sank into 8,400 feet of water 200 miles off Boston on April 10, 1963. There were no survivors. Stories of the hull's breaking under the pressure of tons of water filled the Boston papers until race day. The papers reported that the Rome Olympic champion had been in Boston for several weeks. In Rome, Abebe Bikila, then an unknown, barefoot Ethiopian, ran away from the best trained long-distance runners of the world. Instantly the name Abebe Bikila and the image of his barefoot form racing down the nighttime Rome streets past the lamp-lighted symbols of Western civilization renewed the mystique of marathon racing to the Western world. (A marathon revival and mania also swept Japan, as would soon be apparent in Boston.)

Bikila was the hero and symbol of the Rome Olympics. No one had beaten him in a marathon since. That Ethiopia produced the first black African Olympic champion marathon racer should not have come as a surprise. Ethiopia, unlike the rest of Africa, had never been colonized by Europeans, and it had defeated a European power, Italy, in a war in 1880. In 1936 the Italians again invaded and stayed only 5 years until the British removed them. So was it not fitting that an Ethiopian should conquer Rome in a race celebrated by Englishmen? Yet Ethiopia was a strict and harsh country, politically as well as climatically. The Emperor Haile Selassie I had established a parliament and a judicial system but barred all political parties, including the Communist party. The U.S., wanting to encourage Ethiopia to keep the Communists out, was a major arms and aid source. Bikila's visit to Boston was not unconnected to the Cold War. The Ethiopian's visit to Boston came under the auspices of the State Department. Bikila, a member of the emperor's palace guard, spoke the country's soft, melodious official language, Amharic. The Ethiopians stayed with the family of Dr. Warren

Guild, the medical director of the marathon, in Lexington; the Guilds reported that their guests loved beef and simple foods but disliked ice cream and pastries.

Dr. Guild reported that Bikila's teammate, Mamo Wolde, complained of digestive problems but that they disappeared after he passed a gigantic tapeworm.

Bikila, Wolde, and Johnny J. Kelley waited on the scratch line of the 12-mile Hyde Shoe Race in Cambridge a couple of weeks before the marathon. They stood awaiting the handicapper's go-ahead as all the slower runners raced out ahead of them. Kelley had no chance. He stayed within calling distance as he ran in very last place. He had to let them go. People along the way who did not understand the inverted nature of handicapped road races made fun of Kelley. The Ethiopians ran with such speed that Wolde overtook every one of the competitors ahead of him and won the race outright. He ran through the streets of Cambridge with 4:40 miles. Bikila saved himself for Boston. Kelley did run faster over the course than he ever had before, but he was hundreds of yards behind Wolde and Bikila with his third-place time prize. For Kelley the challenge at Boston was third place. The Ethiopians were a talent apart. Nearly everyone conceded Boston to them.

Everyone conceded but Oksanen, the detective. He knew something. He predicted that Aurele Vandendriessche, a bookkeeper from Belgium, would win in a new course record. Vandendriessche had run stride for stride with Bikila for many miles in Rome before blisters forced him out of the race. He wanted another crack at Bikila. He had trained as much as 40 miles a day in three runs, at 4:00 a.m., noon, and night. He expected that his complete training would give him the strength and endurance to overcome the Ethiopians' speed and natural talent. In a marathon in Athens he finished a mere 100 yards behind Bikila. In the European championships Vandendriessche lost to an Englishman, Brian Kilby, because he made a tactical error on the last hill. Vandendriessche wanted to avenge those losses. He knew that Bikila was not as superhuman as most people thought.

At home in Waregem, Belgium, a farming town of 13,000 not far from Flanders, Vandendriessche worked as a bookkeeper. With his street clothes on, he looked like one. Each hair on his head seemed precisely accounted for. His looks reinforced the fact that he spent his days penciling precise numbers in ledger books. But when he changed into his racing clothes a transformation occurred. Vandendriessche's competitors could see clearly delineated muscles on his back. No subcutaneous fat mellowed their sharp contours. Obviously this man pushed more than a pencil. His enormous calf muscles bulged. The pace was what he planned to push. Of the rest of him there was little. A bookkeeper's precision stuck to everything Vandendriessche did.

A Footrace, Not a Parade

Sometimes the separation between spectators and participants blurs. This year one of the spectators became a participant. Her story needs to be told to illustrate how the symbolism of the marathon loomed larger in the public mind than a mere sporting event.

Near Centre Street in Newton, a 17-year-old girl detached herself from the spectators and slid into the race. She wore cut-off blue jeans, Keds sneakers, and a white T-shirt with the letters "MEEP" on the front and a large question mark drawn on the back. Jane Weinbaum was a senior at Newton South High School, where she and her eccentric friends called themselves *MEEP*. MEEP stood for nothing. The question mark explained it. Spectators thought she was part of a college sorority initiation. But really she was trying to prove to her father that she could finish the marathon. As she approached the finish line at the Prudential Center, police prevented her from crossing it.

Many people, whom Jock Semple called clowns, tried to use the marathon as their own personal publicity stunt. From Jimmy "Cigars" Connors, who wore pink panties and smoked cigars, to college fraternity boys trying to run into the victor's finish line photo to a girl trying to prove something to her father, they all demonstrated that the marathon attracted thrill seekers. Someone had to defend the race. The usurpation of the Boston Marathon for purposes other than running threatened to turn a simple footrace into a freak show. Semple and the BAA officials felt that if they did not enforce the rules the race would lose its prestige and become a parade of buffoons. Why would future Olympic gold medalists come to Boston if public attention went to the clowns? The girl got her picture in the next day's newspapers and even in *Life*, the national picture magazine, yet she had not run the entire race. The winner would not get his picture in *Life*. Semple saw such events as grossly unfair. Nearly 30 years later that same Jane Weinbaum, who claimed to have psychic powers that could be used for financial analysis, would call radio talk shows to boast that she was the first woman to run in the Boston Marathon. People who would join an event to undermine its intent infuriated Semple and BAA Marathon Director Will Cloney. Weinbaum did not go the whole distance, was not a trained long-distance runner,

was slow, and called undue attention to herself for her tres-
pass. Yet she felt she had made a cultural statement for
individualism. Semple, Cloney, and other BAA officials insisted that the marathon be an athletic event, a 26-mile, 385-
yard footrace, not a palette for free expression.

The race started with extra fanfare. The day was overcast with a threat
of rain, but the cloud ceiling was high enough to allow the WHDH radio
helicopter to beat overhead, carrying reporters in the air for the first time.
Alex Breckenridge ran 400 yards behind the Ethiopians as they broke his
checkpoint record through
Framingham. Everyone else
stayed well back of the unde-
feated Bikila and teammate *The WHDH radio helicopter*
Wolde. They ran 1:18 faster *beat overhead, carrying report-*
than the record. In an awe-
struck cluster 30 yards be- *ers in the air for the first time.*
hind Breckenridge ran Oksa-
nen, Kelley, Kilby, Fred
Norris, Tenho Salakka (another Finn from a little town up against the Russian
border), and Vandendriessche. By 10.5 miles in Natick, the Ethiopians ran
51:36 against Breckenridge's 53:59 checkpoint record. Kelley had been a
minute slower than the checkpoint record on the way to his course record
of 2:20:05 in 1957, but this time Kelley and the pack ran only 78 seconds
behind the leaders, or 52:54. Oksanen's prediction of a new course record
seemed to be coming true, but Bikila and Wolde looked unbeatable. They
ran expressionless, like tireless machines of ebony and sinew. By Wellesley
the pack ran 600 yards behind, but under Kotila's 1960 checkpoint record.
    As the race proceeded down into Newton Lower Falls and up over the
new Route 128 overpass, cold headwinds rose. The winds spun off a storm
that churned in the North Atlantic. These were not the thin winds of the
Ethiopian highlands; they came thick with dampness. The pack of pasty
men from Northern European stock picked up 29 seconds on the leaders.
On the hills, Wolde could no longer stay with Bikila. By the crest of the
hills, with the chill wind full in his face, leg cramps gripped Bikila. He
and Wolde still led the pack, but neither looked as smooth, as tireless, as
unstoppable as he had just a few miles earlier. Of course the pack following
did not know how the Ethiopians looked because they were so far ahead.
    Vandendriessche ran away from the pack toward the Ethiopians. Alone
against the hills and the wind, suddenly he did not feel well. On the Boston
hills Vandendriessche ran without the comfort of a pack. He did not expect
to catch the Ethiopians. He could not even see them.

Kilby raced with Kelley. Kelley described it as a "strained relationship." By running together each gained by the presence of the other, but eventually such cooperation would cease. Kelley gave chase to Vandendriessche and in doing so shook off Kilby. Kelley stole glimpses behind, hoping to no longer see Kilby or anyone. Vandendriessche looked ahead but listened behind. He wanted to hold on to third place. Neither Kelley nor Vandendriessche expected to catch the Ethiopians. For Vandendriessche, revenge against Bikila would have to wait. He had hoped to beat Bikila and Wolde, but now hope of victory shrank to a tiny thought. That thought hid beneath the need to get the thing over with and defend against Kelley. Kelley ran close to Vandendriessche and posed a threat. Vandendriessche had the consolation that Kilby ran well behind him.

Kelley himself had suffered from strep throat all the week before and had to teach school through a case of laryngitis. It was difficult to maintain classroom discipline with a whisper. That morning Kelley had told his wife, Jessie, that he did not want to run, but because they had come up to Boston she insisted that he give it a try. Perhaps his virus and the overwhelming presence of Bikila distracted him by decreasing his personal pressure to win. As the race progressed Kelley noticed himself feeling better and better. It still hurt to swallow, and as he ran Kelley said to himself that he really shouldn't be there in the pack, but the racing did seem to help.

Vandendriessche ran through the fog and mist when suddenly he saw Wolde walking with his hands on his hips. Then, like a miracle through the mist, he saw Bikila. On the descent into Cleveland Circle Vandendriessche saw that Bikila could be had. The little hope from way beneath his fatigue crawled out. The fates had delivered Bikila to him. Kelley had been getting closer. Vandendriessche surged away from Kelley. Kelley said he saw him take off "like a rocket to the moon." Now Vandendriessche looked to Kelley like the Ethiopians had looked to everyone else. All fatigue had suddenly vanished from Vandendriessche. His form perked up. He passed Wolde. He passed Bikila, who could only limp slowly. Bikila did not respond. Vandendriessche left Bikila far behind. Kelley passed Bikila. Kilby passed Bikila. Oksanen passed Bikila. As Kelley passed the Ethiopians he felt as if he passed fallen gods. Bikila was the seventh Olympic Gold medalist to try and fail to win the Boston Marathon. The race belonged to Vandendriessche. Now he knew he was going to win. He ran through Kenmore Square, smiling and waving to the crowd.

As joyous and legitimate Vandendriessche, now called Vandy by the press, finished he pushed off the official blanket, took his laurel wreath in his hands, and waved it to the thousands of cheering spectators. He plunged smiling and shaking hands into the crowd like a victorious politician already campaigning for his next win. Kelley sprinted in for another second place— for the fifth time. As he sprinted, a prankster jumped in and sprinted with him.

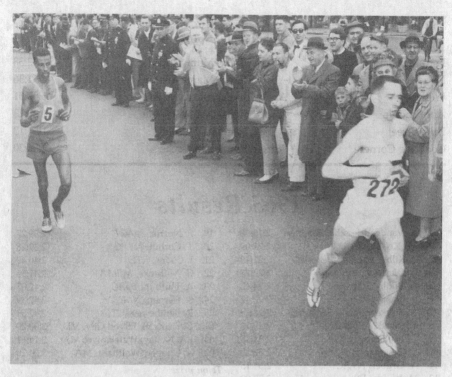

The moment of truth: Aurele Vandendriessche, #272, has passed the gold medalist, Abebe Bikila, #5. Photo courtesy of the *Boston Herald*.

The Most Perfect Marathoner

Bikila went on to win the 1964 Olympic marathon in another world-best time (2:12:11.2) and become an eternal hero of his country. In 1968 he dropped out of the Olympic marathon in Mexico City. His teammate Wolde won. One day in 1969 as Abebe Bikila was driving his Volkswagen, a gift of the Ethiopian government, it crashed, breaking his neck and destroying the nerves that directed his legs. He lived confined to a wheelchair until he died on October 25, 1973, at age 41. He was the most perfect marathon runner the world had ever seen. When the next generation of marathoners ran and their movement felt good and smooth and beautiful, they imagined they were Bikila.

Checkpoint Splits

Framingham	Abebe Bikila/Mamo Wolde	32:38
Natick	Abebe Bikila/Mamo Wolde	51:36
Wellesley	Abebe Bikila/Mamo Wolde	1:07:01
Auburndale	Abebe Bikila/Mamo Wolde	1:28:23
Lake Street	Aurele Vandendriessche	1:51:13
Coolidge Corner	Aurele Vandendriessche	2:06:30

1963 Results

1. A. Vandendriessche, Belgium	2:18:58^{CR*}	
2. J.J. Kelley, *BAA*	2:21:09	
3. B. Kilby, England	2:21:43	
4. E. Oksanen, Finland	2:22:23	
5. A. Bikila, Ethiopia	2:24:43	
6. J. Eblen, *SOC*	2:27:42	
7. A. Breckenridge, *U.S. Marines*	2:28:28	
8. T. Salakka, Finland	2:29:13	
9. G. Williams, *UCTC*	2:31:19	
10. L. Castagnola, *NCAS*	2:32:23	
11. A. Gruber, *NYAC*	2:34:15	
12. M. Wolde, Ethiopia	2:35:09	
13. H. Higdon, *UCTC*	2:36:13	
14. J. Green, *BAA*	2:36:38	
15. R. Buschmann, *SpAC*	2:37:06	
16. A. Sapienza, *BAA*	2:37:06	
17. G. Harvey, *BAA*	2:38:50	
18. J. Garlepp, *MillAA*	2:39:05	
19. F. Norris, *SpAC*	2:39:27	
20. T. Corbitt, *NYPC*	2:39:28	
21. J. Coons, *RTC*	2:40:49	
22. G. Muhrcke, *MillAA*	2:41:34	
23. A. Hull, Jr., *SpAC*	2:42:07	
24. S. Tiernan, *NMC*	2:42:39	
25. R. Bamberger, *CT*	2:42:53	
61. D. Heinicke, Ellicott City, MD	3:00:20	
84. J.A. Kelley, Watertown, MA	3:14:11	
102. K. Cooper, Waltham, MA	3:24:20	

Team prize

1. BAA: J.J. Kelley, J. Green, A. Sapienza
2. Spartan AC: R. Buschmann, F. Norris, A. Hull
3. Millrose AA: J. Garlepp, G. Muhrcke, V. Kern

285 entrants, 183 finishers.
*Permanent record for 26 miles, 385 yards.

THE RIGHT STUFF

MONDAY, APRIL 20, 1964

Belgian, Finns Favored in Today's Grind

An assassin's bullets had killed President Kennedy the previous November. The nation still mourned. Kennedy actively promoted physical fitness, so the Road Runners Club of America dedicated the 1964 Boston Marathon to his memory. Kennedy had pledged to put a man on the moon by the end of the decade, and those considered possessing the "right stuff" trained to go there. The right-stuff mood filled the nation. People read and reread Kennedy's book, *Profiles in Courage*. A big part of the space program and the right stuff was physical fitness. Astronauts trained for space. The National Aeronautics and Space Administration made sure the public had many opportunities to see their astronauts training. Training became an acceptable and patriotic thing to do. Even if you couldn't go to the moon, you could do push-ups or sit-ups or run a marathon. For most of the public a marathon was nearly as long as a trip to the moon, but in its extreme difficulty rested its magic. It might seem as unobtainable as the moon, but daily training put it within the reach of ordinary people, and ordinary people began to fall under its spell.

Men like the Reverend Ernest MacDonald and Dr. George Sheehan could not go to the moon, though had someone asked they would have happily become astronauts and gone into space. At first, mature men like them had trouble jogging around the block, but President Kennedy sanctioned physical training with his council on physical fitness and his fitness test for school-children as well as his publicized walks on the beach. So exercise and training seemed worth doing again and again, and to the surprise of millions daily physical exercise became easier as the days rolled on. And some, despite obligations of career and family, could not resist the challenge of the marathon. Many of the top U.S. marathoners of the future would cite the 600-yard run/walk in the president's physical fitness test as their initiation to long-distance running as well as their realization that they were good at it.

MacDonald had 6 children and Sheehan had 12, but they trained for the marathon and ran it for recreation—for fun. This notion of fun in training and racing spun directly off the space program and made it reasonable for grown-up men with serious careers to train for and race in marathons. A man alone, running, became a patriot instead of an eccentric. The paradigm shifted. No longer did the public and the participants see the marathon as a grueling brush with death. Now fitness for everyday life became a reasonable thing for reasonable people to maintain and enjoy; they had a national duty to do it. The citizen athlete became the new myth.

After President Eisenhower had a heart attack his physician, Dr. Paul Dudley White, became a celebrity himself by advocating a diet of low fat and the maintenance of low body fat through exercise. The public opinion that extreme exercise harmed a body prevailed until White championed exercise. After Clarence DeMar died in 1958, Dr. White wrote an article in 1962 debunking the fear of exercise by explaining the results of an autopsy done on DeMar's heart. "Nothing was found in the examination of the heart to indicate that the long-continued exercise had adversely affected it." Those two ideas—that running could prevent disease and that training for long-term goals was patriotic, not weird—combined with a steady increase in population led to an increase in numbers in the Boston Marathon. This year 369 runners entered the race. No women would run. Jerry Nason of the *Boston Globe* wrote,

> Naturally, the Boston AA does not permit the babes to complete in their bunion derby—possibly because they'd get 369 boy entries from Harvard, MIT and Boston U. alone, if they did. They might let down the bars though, for that Russian femme with the masculine muscles who flips the shot 54 feet.

The paradigms had changed, but only for men. Again the press played up a battle between John J. Kelley and the world, especially the Belgian and the Finns.

Two new Americans came to race. Together they represented the new American runner, college-educated, track- and endurance-trained along the lines of the very best Europeans, and well trained after college. One was a short, muscular, crewcut-topped chemist, Ralph Buschmann. He had been a varsity track and cross-country runner at the University of Massachusetts. He looked like an astronaut. Buschmann had not been a remarkable college runner, but he had since learned how to train. To him training was an applied science. Now it made all the difference because he had acquired the strength and power to challenge the best in the world. Hal Higdon was a professional free-lance writer who had just finished a book called *The Union vs. Dr. Mudd*, a serious investigation into the case against Dr. Samuel Mudd, the physician who treated Lincoln's assassin, John Wilkes Booth, for gunshot wounds. The American feeder system that poured high school athletes into colleges produced excellent track-and-field athletes in the events where athletes reached maturity at age 22, such as jumping and sprinting. But for those in technical throwing events and distance running there was no club structure after college as there was in Europe to develop skills and endurance into the peak years of the late 20s. Higdon saw the European system firsthand while in the army in Germany in 1955 and 1956. By 1964 he had joined a club and developed his endurance.

In Europe Higdon saw that European colleges only educated, they did not train athletes. Amateur clubs attached to professional soccer teams trained the marathon runners of Europe regardless of age. Youths in running clubs stayed in the clubs throughout their 20s and later remained on in coaching or advisory roles. American colleges cast off their athletes like milkweed seeds. Where they landed, in their hometowns or at their first jobs, was away from the rich soil of disciplined training with coach and training partners that had developed them in college. Their development stopped. Normal life absorbed them. Normal life did not absorb Hal Higdon.

In Germany two new ideas influenced Higdon and turned him toward the marathon. The first came from a German 3,000-meter indoor champion, Stefan Lupfert from Stuttgart. He trained by the interval method that breaks a race into segments and practiced the segments at paces at or faster than race pace with specific rest intervals. As training progressed the rest intervals became shorter or the fast parts got faster. Applied to track racing this interval training was not news, but for marathoners it was a revolution. Americans rarely did this kind of training for long-distance running and never did it methodically. Higdon already had speed. He had run a quarter mile in a relay in 52.2, a mile in 4:13, 5,000 meters in 14:43 That was a quickness superior to Kelley's. The other man Higdon met in Germany was Dean Thackwray, Kelley's friend who had finished fifth in Boston in 1956. Thackwray filled Higdon with stories of Kelley and the running scene around Boston. With Higdon's speed and talent and with Thackwray's endless promotion, New England became Higdon's promised land. He saw himself sweeping to victory after victory while touring the six New England states. Nowhere else in the country had all those races and all those runners. Nowhere else had Kelley. In 1964 Higdon came to Boston to win the biggest New England race of them all.

After graduating from Minnesota's Carleton College in 1953 Higdon attended graduate school at the University of Chicago, mostly so he could run for its track club. Higdon ran the 1959 Boston Marathon with the philosophy of a track race—maintain contact with the leaders at all costs. That tactic unsupported by long-distance training cost Higdon the supreme marathon sacrifice. He stayed with Kelley for half the race but dropped out at 18 miles. The next year he ran 22 miles, then dropped out. By 1962 Higdon at age 31 had learned his lesson. He went out slowly for the early miles and finished in 26th place with a 2:45. In 1963 he had consolidated his technique by again going out slowly. He finished in 13th, with a 2:36. Now in 1964 it was time to go with the leaders again. Higdon had done his consolidation. He had done his speed work in the form of dedicated interval training, and he had gotten his mileage up. He was now strong and fast. He had studied his sport, even creating the artwork to illustrate the bible of running training, Fred Wilt's *How They Train*. Nearly every aspiring runner in the 1960s took that book to bed at night. Wilt now coached Higdon by mail and induced him to double his mileage. He would get stronger and faster yet. A time very low in the 2:20s seemed reasonable.

Preparations were complete. Hal Higdon was ready to beat Johnny J. Kelley and become the best marathoner on the North American continent.

The effects of enforced amateur standards made unavailable the money necessary for top runners to maintain themselves and to travel to and from distant competitions. The best American marathoner of the early 1960s was a mysterious expatriate named Leonard "Buddy" Edelen, originally of Sioux Falls, South Dakota. Edelen never came to Boston. He wanted to race there, but to put himself consistently near the best long-distance competitors in the world he had to move to Europe. Jock Semple wanted him to come to Boston and wrote to him at his home base in England, but the world was too big. Travel to America was too expensive. Edelen could get $500 under the table to go to race in Europe; Semple and the BAA, in their quaint enforcement of amateurism, would offer him nothing. In 1962 he ran 2:18:56 in Japan to be the first American under 2:20—9 years after Jim Peters did it. Edelen ran 2:14 and 2:15 to win two major marathons in Europe. In 1963 Buddy Edelen, an American, had the fastest time of any marathoner in the world—the world record (2:14:28 on June 15, 1963, at Chiswick, England)—but he never ran in the Boston Marathon nor ever ran near his best times in his home country.

Finns Tenho Salakka and Paavo Pystynen, who ran in this year's lead pack, were fond of Johnny Kelley but still saw him as the man to beat. "Where's Kelley?" would be their watchwords again. Kelley had spent the spring in a nervous state, demonstrated by his susceptibility to a string of colds, probably incubated by his students. Vandendriessche, the Belgian, ran comfortably in that pack. No one, however, was actually comfortable, as a sleety wind blew in their faces. Snow melted as it blew through the 39 °F air and landed on their faces as little lumps of slush. Vandy came prepared. He had trained up to 200 miles in a week, but he thought the winds would slow the times by 5 minutes.

In Framingham Buschmann had a 50-yard lead on the pack. He still led through Natick, but later he ran side by side with Hal Higdon.

Higdon led slightly over Buschmann through Wellesley. He thought he could win. Higdon wore a special pair of lightweight Japanese running shoes from the Onitsuka Company. Other Americans had not yet discovered the bliss of running in Japanese shoes. The Japanese received a foot tracing from Higdon, then in their factory had custom-made his super shoes. They embossed his name on the back. The first pair he received did not fit, so he gave them to Fred Wilt. Wilt in turn gave them to Ron Wallingford, an assistant professor of physical education at McMaster University in Hamilton, Ontario. Higdon was shocked to see Wallingford at the start wearing those shoes, with "Higdon" on the heels. Higdon did not want to see those, or anyone else's heels.

Buschmann dropped back. Everyone else hung together. Nine men reached the hills together. Vandendriessche waited. He wanted to run away, but he waited. It is lonely to run out of the protection of the pack. Each man took inspiration from the others—if they can stick with this pace, so can I. Members of gregarious species can endure more pain in groups than they can alone. So Vandy stuck with the pack. He wore a bright red shirt with "WAC," the initials of his club, on it. Higdon wondered if he realized the meaning of that word in English. Vandendriessche thought that if he burst into the lead the way his body told him he could, then all those men could imagine the cross-hairs of a gun sight on the back of his head. Then they could gun for him with the strength of the pack. If he took off into a solo lead he could be as vulnerable as Bikila had been the year before. So Vandy stayed.

Of all the runners, Kelley alone did not seem to mind leading. The others jockeyed for protected positions in the slipstream of whoever led. Higdon thought the pack hung together like migrating geese. He took his turn leading the chevron into the wet wind. At 17 miles Higdon pushed himself up the hill and felt himself breaking free of the pack. He felt an exhilaration at leading the Boston Marathon at such a late stage. He ran over the emotional edge at escape velocity and on into free-fall. The moment etched into his memory and would stay with him for decades, playing like a movie on the blank walls of his office.

Vandendriessche remained with the pack until he was sure he was stronger than everyone else and he could no longer resist the urge within that said go. On the next downhill Vandy swept past the American experiencing his "moment of truth." Higdon looked at the red shirt and watched the smooth stride. The Belgian in the red shirt smiled. Higdon would remember forever the smile. The exhilaration left him. Higdon descended to earth. Photographers leaned over the tailgate of the photo truck snapping pictures of his breaking point. For Higdon life blurred; life moved on.

Vandendriessche went alone on the hills into the pressure of the wind. Instantly he opened up 55 yards. Only Salakka the Finn followed, but not closely enough to benefit from Vandy's slipstream. Two men dropped off the pack. The press bus loomed behind the pack of five remaining runners. Wallingford ran next to Higdon. Wallingford knew how Higdon felt—he ran in Higdon's shoes; Higdon's name was on them. Slowly the professor pulled away from the writer.

The other Finn came by Higdon. Higdon was still in the race. Second place was not far ahead. Higdon did not dare look around for Kelley. Higdon could sense that he was close. But Kelley's legs felt paralyzed from the cold. Vandy hid from the wind behind the photographer's truck and covered the hills faster this year than he had when he ran in pursuit of Bikila. But months before it had been Vandy who was paralyzed with sciatic nerve pain. In a month he had received 125 injections, but after 3 months of limping through training with no treatment, the pain departed, giving him time to train for Boston.

Vandy ran painlessly to an easy victory. He approached the finish line gingerly; Police Commissioner McNamara held the laurel wreath in the air a foot past the finish line. But Vandy wanted to cool down slowly; he pivoted on the line, ducked the descending wreath, and jogged back the way he had come, waving to the crowd. The commissioner stood dumbly with the laurels in the air and no victor to place them on.

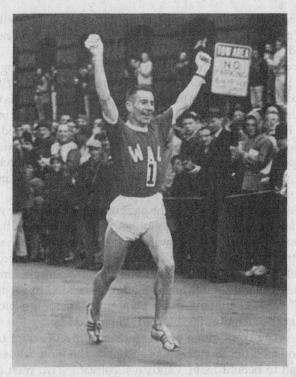

Aurele Vandendriessche victorious again in 1964. Photo courtesy of the *Boston Herald*.

Higdon finished his marathon in 2:21:55, 15 minutes faster than he had ever run. He was now the best United States marathoner. Inches past the finish line he dared to turn around: "Where's Kelley?"

Checkpoint Splits

Framingham	Ralph Buschmann	34:02
Natick	Ralph Buschmann	53:50
Wellesley	Hal Higdon	1:09:34
Auburndale	Hal Higdon	1:31:53
Lake Street	Aurele Vandendriessche	1:54:02
Coolidge Corner	Aurele Vandendriessche	2:07:19

1964 Results

1.	A. Vandendriessche, Belgium	2:19:59	3. R. Wallingford, Hamilton, ON	2:20:51
2.	T. Salakka, Finland	2:20:48	4. P. Pystynen, Finland	2:21:33

5.	H. Higdon, *UCTC*	2:21:55	23.	G. Muhrcke, *MillAA*	2:37:16
6.	D. Ellis, *TOC*	2:22:49	24.	W. Schwab, *NYAC*	2:37:30
7.	**J.J. Kelley, *BAA***	**2:27:23**	25.	J. Harlow, *PC*	2:37:49
8.	O. Suarez, Argentina	2:27:51	26.	T. Corbitt, *NYPC*	2:38:01
9.	P. Hoffman, *TOC*	2:28:07	27.	T. Durie, *PC*	2:38:18
10.	W. Allen, *EYTC*, ON	2:28:19	28.	S. Adams, *BAA*	2:39:11
11.	J. Green, *BAA*	2:29:21	29.	J. Coons, *RTC*	2:39:47
12.	C. Pell, *TOC*	2:29:53	30.	N. Marincic, *NYAC*	2:41:06
13.	A. Gruber, *NYAC*	2:31:10	31.	S. Gonzales, *BAA*	2:41:08
14.	H. McEleney, *GaelAAC*, NY	2:32:14	37.	R. Ahti, Lunenberg, MA	2:45:40
15.	R. Buschmann, *SpAC*, MA	2:32:36	39.	A. Williams, *NYPC*	2:46:46
16.	W. Hewlett, *HU*	2:32:44	43.	T. Osler, *DVAA*	2:47:26
17.	B. Drewett, *MtAC*, England	2:33:53	**48.**	**J.A. Kelley, Watertown, MA**	**2:49:14**
18.	H. Monck, *HOC*, ON	2:34:45	52.	R. Gaff, *BAA*	2:51:19
19.	J. Blake, *NHTC*	2:34:48	63.	E. Segal, *HAA*	2:56:30
20.	A. Hull, Jr., *SpAC*	2:35:17	76.	D. Heinicke, Ellicott City, MD	NT
21.	J. Kelley, *MillAA*	2:35:29	95.	G. Sheehan, *CJTC*	NT
22.	L. Smith, OH	2:36:49	96.	E. MacDonald	NT

369 entrants.

PRUDENTIAL

MONDAY, APRIL 19, 1965

New Start, New Finish, Same Old Marathon

As if from the sudden release of tectonic forces the Boston Marathon moved. The entire course moved west 1,159 feet and 6 inches. No longer would it finish on Exeter Street between the Lenox Hotel and the Soden Building (the former BAA clubhouse that had been sold to Boston University, then torn down to make way for an addition to the Boston Public Library). The lobby of the Lenox was now too small for the disrupting sprawl of exhausted runners. So the start moved uphill and around the Hopkinton town commons to start on Hayden Row. The BAA secured the cooperation of the Prudential Life Insurance Company, which occupied a new 52-story office tower—the tallest building in Boston—that was part of a $150-million complex. Thirty-two acres of aged, neglected railroad yards had occupied that spot. Now this new complex was Boston's showcase. It included hotels and a large civic auditorium named after former Mayor John B. Hynes, a great marathon fan. Across Boylston Street from the new finish line in front of the Prudential Tower opened the counterculture coffeehouse Unicorn, where protest folk-singers performed. This neighborhood was the cultural and countercultural hub of Boston. The move put the Boston Marathon on the far side of the ever-widening rift that separated it from its Victorian, amateur origins and pushed it toward commercialism, professional management, and professional racing. Yet, with the slow building of tectonic forces, it would take two more decades of subduction and collision before the upheaval would subside.

Race Director Will Cloney made the unilateral decision to move the race and to ally with Prudential based on a gentleman's handshake. He used no contract and no lawyers. Prudential agreed not to make any commercial tie-ins with the race and to install toilets and showers in their underground garage as a courtesy.

Vandendriessche came back to Boston to win for a third time. Since his Boston victory the year before he had placed seventh in the Tokyo Olympic marathon (Bikila won). Eino Oksanen, who had won Boston three times, had placed 13th in Tokyo. He brought another Finn, Eino Valle, with him, and Finnish-Americans again paid their expenses. Valle, the first Finn to have run under 2:20 since 1956, was a policeman in Lauritsala, a town in southeast Finland near the Soviet border. He was 33 and the national champion; the former national champion, the detective Oksanen, was the new national 10,000-meter champion. The best American and the country's only sub-2:20 runner, Buddy Edelen, who had beaten Vandendriessche in the Olympic Games, languished in England, an ocean away. A plane ticket and pocket money would have cured that, but the Boston Athletic Association had a policy not to pay expenses for amateur athletes and certainly not to slip them any cash. Kelley held his enthusiasm for running, but after failing to make his third Olympic team he had allowed himself to channel some of his passion to coaching and was not as fit as he had been in previous years. Jock Semple called it the poorest American field ever.

The Japanese had no such poverty. The U.S. had only one sub-2:20 marathoner, but the Japanese had a seemingly infinite number. To the Japanese, marathon runners were national treasures worthy of nourishment. The Japanese astounded and mystified the world with their postwar production of so many wonderfully fast marathoners. Just some of the names and times of the previous year's sub-2:20 performances by Japanese marathoners were impressive:

Toru Terasawa	2:17:48	Kokichi Tsuburaya	2:16:22
Kazumi Watanabe	2:18:44	Kenji Kimihara	2:19:49
Hidekuni Hiroshima	2:19:29	Toru Terasawa	2:14:48
Takayuki Nakoa	2:18:31	Takayuki Nakoa	2:15:42
Haruo Otani	2:18:41	Hidekuni Hiroshima	2:17:18
Kenji Kimihara	2:17:11	Masatsugu Futsuhara	2:17:23
Kokichi Tsuburaya	2:18:20	Morio Shigematsu	2:17:56
Toru Terasawa	2:19:43	Kimio Karasawa	2:18:10
Kenji Kimihara	2:17:12	Satoru Nakamura	2:18:31
Kokichi Tsuburaya	2:19:50	Ryoichi Masuda	2:19:01

Yoshikazu Funasako	2:19:15	Kazuo Matsubara	2:16:57
Mitsuo Minami	2:19:31	Hirokazu Okabe	2:17:05
Kazuo Matsubara	2:19:55	Satoru Nakamura	2:17:55
Hideaki Shishido	2:16:49	Isamu Sugihara	2:18:05
Hirokazu Okabe	2:16:59	Mitsuo Minami	2:18:38
Toru Terasawa	2:14:38	Seiichi Inagaki	2:19:27
Takayuki Nakoa	2:15:37	Rishu Kawabata	2:19:42
Hideaki Shishido	2:16:07	Takao Okamachi	2:18:04
Morio Shigematsu	2:16:15	Toshihiko Uehara	2:18:15
Yoshikazu Funasako	2:16:26	Masanao Haraishi	2:19:21

Twelve of these performances had occurred in the Beppu Marathon in February. At its expense the Japanese association sent the top five from Beppu—minus the winner, Toru Terasawa—to come to Boston. Marathoners from other nations stared at the Japanese statistics with a mixture of awe, frustration, and respect. The Japanese public and this young generation of Japanese marathoners in a postwar country took marathon racing seriously. These were young men born in wartime and raised under U.S. occupation. For them personal honor and national honor were one, making running more than a private recreation. The life of Kokichi Tsuburaya offered an example.

In the 1964 Olympic Games Tsuburaya ran into the stadium in second place, far behind Abebe Bikila. In the stadium Englishman Basil Heatley sprinted up to Tsuburaya. Regardless of a frantic home crowd he was too tired to respond, and Heatley passed him. Tsuburaya worked for the Japanese ground defense force and, apparently to improve his running, he was ordered to stop seeing his fiancée. He ran under 2:20 at least once after the Olympics but a series of injuries hospitalized him for 3 months. By January 9, 1968, Tsuburaya could no longer train. In a pit of depression he took a razor to his right carotid artery. His suicide note read simply, "Cannot run anymore."

The day for the 1965 Boston Marathon was overcast, 48 °F with a puff of a tailwind. Early in the going Kelley and Ralph Buschmann had kept the pack ethnically diverse. A mixture of Americans and Canadians—Ron Wallingford, Lou Castagnola, Dave Ellis, and Vince Chiapetta—tried to keep up North America's fight. But gradually each dropped off, leaving one Belgian and five identically dressed young Japanese men. For 22 miles Vandendriessche ran in a pack of Japanese: Hideaki Shishido, Takayuki Nakoa, Yoshikazu Funasako, Kazuo Matsubara, and Morio Shigematsu. Did the Japanese now have an advantage of team tactics, five against one, over the Belgian? Clearly the Japanese dictated the pace. First one and then the other would float gently to the front. To the westerners these Japanese seemed "inscrutable" and without minds of their own. They dressed identically in white gloves and neat uniforms with a tiny Japanese flag, and they moved as one tireless unit.

The youngest was Morio Shigematsu. At 22 miles he simply felt stronger than everyone else. Identical though these Japanese may have seemed to westerners and because of language and custom unable and unready to talk about themselves, they were nevertheless distinct individuals with unique histories. Shigematsu was one.

Morio Shigematsu was born in Hiraoka, Japan, 25 years earlier. As was a common custom in Japan, his mother gave him up for adoption to her childless sister. He grew up with both his adoptive mother and his biological mother in proximity. They lived in Fukuoka. Also in proximity was Hideo Hamamura from Yamaguchi, who had won Boston in 1955. Shigematsu had known and admired Hamamura since the age of 15. Now Shigematsu, full grown at 5'7" and 130 pounds, had been training 100 miles a week under his coach, the famous and highly competent Nobuyoshi Sadanaga. The entire team and the coach stayed with a Japanese-American family in Roxbury,

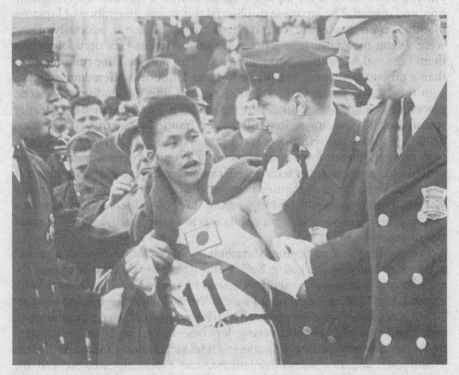

Jock Semple and police surround Morio Shigematsu moments after he crosses the finish line in 1965. Kevin Cole Photo/Courtesy of the *Boston Herald*.

Massachusetts. Shigematsu had gone for a training run in nearby Franklin Park and gotten lost. But there on the hills Shigematsu felt good, and thereafter he felt better. From 1 mile to go in Kenmore Square to the finish, he gained 30 more seconds on second place.

Five men broke Aurele Vandendriessche's 1963 course record of 2:18:58, and Ralph Buschmann proved he had the right chemical mix to become the new best marathoner in North America.

As Shigematsu sprinted to the finish line the puzzled crowds watched a man in a zippered jacket and tie, carrying a brown paper bag, run up behind him. Race Director Will Cloney saw him too. Cloney did not know what the man intended to do to the runner who was about to win. He did not wait to find out. Some crazed people still harbored wartime hatreds. With the instincts of his high school football days, Cloney sprinted at the intruder and threw a body block that would have made his old coach proud, bouncing the intruder into a police motorcycle and off the course.

Shigematsu would not come back to Boston. After retiring from international racing he became a director of a department store in Fukuoka. He kept up with his running and when contacted in 1992 said he hoped to come to Boston to run in the 100th running.

1965 Results

1.	M. Shigematsu, Japan	2:16:33^{CR}	21.	S. Quellett, Gorham, ME	2:32:34
2.	H. Shishido, Japan	2:17:13	22.	T. McCarthy, GaelAAC	2:32:59
3.	T. Nakoa, Japan	2:17:31	23.	G. Hodgam, Hamilton, ON	2:33:29
4.	A. Vandendriessche, Belgium	2:17:44	24.	D. Ashley, Rochester, NY	2:33:35
5.	Y. Funasako, Japan	2:18:18	25.	A. Burfoot, WU, CT	2:34:09
6.	K. Matsubara, Japan	2:19:17	26.	E. Ayres, CNJ	2:34:36
7.	R. Buschmann, Andover, MA	2:20:20	27.	T. Durie, PC	2:34:44
8.	E. Oksanen, Finland	2:21:13	28.	R. Scharf, Baltimore, MD	2:35:16
9.	E. Valle, Finland	2:21:52	29.	A. Gruber, NYAC	2:35:31
10.	E. Ostbye, Sweden	2:23:05	30.	V. Chiapetth, NYAC	2:35:55
11.	R. Wallingford, Hamilton, ON	2:23:36	34.	J. Wrynn, SpAC	2:37:31
12.	G. Williams, EH	2:25:06	38.	R. Darwin, Culver City, CA	2:38:49
13.	L. Castagnola, MD	2:25:12	39.	T. Corbitt, NYPC	2:38:51
14.	J.J. Kelley, Groton, CT	2:25:23	42.	D. Prokop, ON	2:40:15
15.	R. Daws, Twin Cities, MN	2:29:31	52.	T. Osler, SJTC	2:46:06
16.	L. Smith, OU, Athens, OH	2:30:33	59.	J.A. Kelley, Watertown, MA	2:48:32
17.	M. Kimball, Santa Barbara, CA	2:30:45	77.	L. Berman, MetAC	2:54:10
18.	J. Freeman, WA	2:30:53	113.	T. Mederios, NMC	3:09:30
19.	R. Hanck, Jr., Buffalo, NY	2:31:17	140.	S. Podlozny, NMC	3:26:12
20.	W. Schwab, NYAC	2:32:07			

443 entrants, 358 starters.

Team prize
NYAC

BOBBI

TUESDAY, APRIL 19, 1966

Japanese Team Set to Sweep BAA

An intruder hid in the bushes in Hopkinton, watching the men run by in the 1966 Boston Marathon. For a year she had been planning to inject herself into the race. When half of the runners had passed she emerged from behind her forsythia and slipped into the stream. She wore a black stretch nylon bathing suit. Her hair flowed long and blond. She had come by bus from California and looked every bit the surfing goddess. But what she looked like was not what she was. She covered the bottom half of her bathing suit with her brother's ill-fitting khaki bermuda shorts. Her only other clothing was a new pair of canvas running shoes. She had been doing her training in nurses' shoes. Roberta Louise Gibb called herself Bobbi. Because she had just married a sailor named Bingay, some called her Mrs. Bingay, but that was not an appellation that sat well with her. Once the world noticed what she was doing, neither her life nor the Boston Marathon would ever be the same. But for several miles no one noticed.

When she first got the idea to run in the Boston Marathon she had not intended to be stealthy. She had written to the BAA for an application to enter. She received a reply telling her that women were not able to run marathons and were not allowed to enter the race. But she wanted to do it. She liked to run. She was 23 years old, and she felt good and free when she ran. Fearing that someone would see her and prevent her from running, she hid in the bushes along the Boston course. Like a child listening to adult conversation and fearful of being sent to bed, she tried to call no attention to herself. But she would have to overcome her shyness to make her point.

Her point was not political. She did not concern herself with legal arguments, yet she would one day become a lawyer. After 69 highly publicized Boston Marathons, decades after women had swum the English Channel and flown solo over the oceans, this one particular woman decided to run the Boston Marathon. No others had tried. Why did she do it?

Bobbi Gibb both was and was not an athlete. She moved for slightly different purposes. Although Kelley and many men lost themselves in contemplation during long runs in the woods they were above all competitive athletes in training. Bobbi Gibb was not a competitor. Bobbi Gibb was an artist. When she ran she felt connected with everything. She felt an awe and sheer joy in being. Her context was different from that of the men around her. When she looked out from behind her bushes she saw in the stream of runners a stream of consciousness, not a race, not a competition. She slipped into the stream to join that consciousness, to be a part of the whole, not to prove anything political or to beat men at their own game, but to play. She was like a little sister wanting nothing more than to play with her brothers and their friends.

The running world had no hospitality for women in 1966. Myths abounded that kept them out. It is not surprising that the first woman to run in the Boston Marathon came obliquely to the event and slipped in unnoticed. The history of women's long-distance running is particularly disturbing.

The running world had no hospitality for women in 1966.

In 1752 a 4-mile women's race was promoted in London. Great numbers turned out to watch it. Part of the crowd came because the promoters intended to have the the women run nude, supposedly in the style of the ancient Greeks. But the women refused to run naked, interest waned, and the race was not repeated. Such exhibitions remained in the public mind in the place reserved for unimportant oddities like circuses and freak shows. Athletics as technically measured and timed events did not begin for men until the mid-1800s. At county picnics women ran races in full Victorian regalia but often in joke events like spoon races (carrying an egg in a spoon).

The first 70 years of worldwide women's marathoning can be detailed in a paragraph. In 1896, a Greek woman named Melpomene was said to have run in the first Olympic marathon. It took her 4-1/2 hours. In 1918 Marie Ledru ran in a French marathon and finished in 38th place. In 1926 Violet Piercy of the United Kingdom ran a marathon in 3:40:22; in 1964, Dale Greig, also of the United Kingdom, ran 3:27 and Mildred Sampson of New Zealand ran a 3:19. Two years later Bobbi Gibb hid in the bushes. That's all the history, or herstory, there is. Why had so few women tried the marathon, and why had no woman attempted the Boston Marathon before 1966?

There was ample inspiration for women in the form of splendid role models. Amelia Earhart, the first lady of the air, held press headlines for a decade as a "first woman." In 1928 she was the first woman to cross the Atlantic Ocean in an airplane. Alone that year she flew her airplane across the North American continent. Her 1932 solo Atlantic flight was second to Lindbergh's by man or woman. Earhart was a big media star. She had her own clothing line. Songs and books praised her. She wrote, "Women must try to do things as men have tried. When they fail, their failure must be but a challenge to others."

Women were highly regarded as long-distance swimmers. Surely there could be no doubt about a woman's capacity to endure when in 1927 Gertrude Ederle swam the English Channel 2 hours faster than anyone else, woman or man. In track and field there were heroines in Mildred "Babe" Didrikson and Francina "Fanny" Blankers-Koen from the 1932 and 1948 Olympics. But there were virtually no women long-distance runners.

In the face of inspiration and example a strong prejudice grew up against long-distance running by women. It was hysteria in the minds of male track-and-field administrators that can be traced to a single event in 1928. In the Amsterdam Olympics Lina Radke of Germany won the 800 meters in the world record of 2:16.8. That record stood for 32 years. It lasted so long because no woman could contest it: After the 1928 Olympics women were forbidden to compete in races longer than 200 meters.

That 1928 race was tight and exciting. Second place was less than a second behind and third was only two-tenths of a second behind that. Several women seemed to collapse after the race. They probably looked like the men did after their 800-meter race. But the sight of women sweating, gasping for breath, and bent over with hands on their knees was too much for squeamish male observers. The *London Daily Mail* quoted doctors who said that such "feats of endurance" by women made them "become old too soon." The president of the International Olympic Committee, Count de Baillet-Latour, wanted to eliminate all women's sports from the Olympics. The longest Olympic race for women was 200 meters until the 800 meters in Rome in 1960. Bobbi Gibb, though, knew none of this.

In her training she had run alone on beaches, over grass, or through the woods. Gibb had trained through the woods in the middle of Cape Ann in Gloucester, Massachusetts, where her relatives had a summer place and she spent her childhood summers. She ran through a strange and wild place there called Dogtown. Dogtown is on top of the granite rocks of the cape where the glaciers scraped off the soil; people have not lived there since 1600. The colonists had feared weather and Indian attacks along the coast, so they moved upland onto the thin, dry ground. By the 1700s people left for lands of rich topsoil and dependable wells. In 1968 you could, with care, find the foundations of their houses. With ease you could find blueberries, birds, and rabbits. It is a place where they said only dogs dwelled. Gibb liked to run there. She would run quickly up and down the hills and duck under the hemlocks. She imagined herself an animal and at one with the woods, the rocks, the cat briars.

As she ran, even the smallest grains of dust and the patterns in the road took on a beauty and a meaning to Gibb as she felt herself a part of the incomprehensibly wondrous whole. She liked to think of William Blake's poem "Auguries of Innocence":

To see a World in a grain of sand,
And a Heaven in a wild flower,
Hold Infinity in the palm of your hand,
And Eternity in an hour.

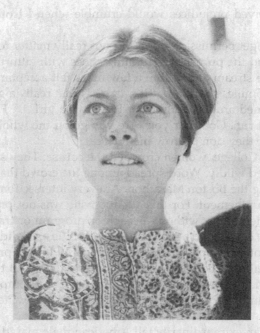

Roberta Louise Gibb was the first woman to run the Boston Marathon. Why after 69 marathons did this particular woman decide to run? Why had none run before? Photo courtesy of the *Boston Herald*.

Gibb had all the talent to beat most of the men, and in that regard she was indeed an athlete, but she had certainly not trained in a scientific way. She had no coach and was not part of a team. She had always been quick in school games like field hockey. She could sprint, she could jump, she could duck and dodge. She was a student at the Boston Museum of Fine Arts school when she had first watched the marathon a year earlier and decided to run. She had gone with her father and thought it was such a splendid celebration that she wanted to join. She ran with some men at Tufts University, where her father was a professor. That was where she met Bingay, who was a runner, who became a sailor, who became her husband. Before she went off to California to be married on February 5, she told her parents she would be back to run the marathon. Her only other long-distance running race was a 2-day 100-mile equestrian cross-country race. She did not know any better and tried to run against horses. Her knees gave out after 65 miles. At that point she was ahead of some of the horses.

Gibb was not in the mainstream of running, so she did not know that women were limited to racing a half mile or less. She had thought the marathon was open to every person in the world who signed up. But after her official rejection she would run as an outlaw. She had trained as much as 40 miles in a day. "My outrage turned to humor as I thought how many preconceived prejudices would crumble when I trotted right along for 26 miles."

Gibb did not get permission but it did not really matter to her. After a 4-day bus ride and the purchase of running shoes with gumrubber soles, she slipped into the stream and within a few miles felt acceptance by the male runners. After 5 miles she heard, "It's a girl. Is that really a girl? Pardon me . . ." Bobbi turned around laughing. "Hey, it is a girl . . . Fantastic. I wish my wife would run. Good for you. Are you going the whole way?"

"I hope so, if they don't throw me out."

At Wellesley College, women crowded the course. They saw one of their own and cheered wildly. Word spread among the crowd that a woman was actually running the Boston Marathon. At every intersection Gibb got more and more encouragement. For this attention she was not prepared.

She had trained alone, without a coach or program or training partners, and got to know herself and her own physical abilities; she did not know what to expect from other people. She was not prepared for the press attention at the finish line either. There is no "race" story to tell about the first woman in the Boston Marathon because she did not have any competition. She ran an even pace and had a pleasant time. For Gibb the excitement occurred after the race.

In Wellesley an extraordinarily tall American male marathoner ran in the lead pack surrounded by little Japanese men. It looked like 1965 again, but with a replacement for Vandendriessche. Vandy had entered and planned to come back to Boston to win for the third time or at least to prevent a clean sweep by the Japanese. He habitually arrived in Boston at the last possible moment. That scheme had worked every other time, and he was reluctant to change it. He waited in the Brussels airport for his flight to be called. When it seemed late he inquired, only to be told that it had departed. The precise accountant had missed the last plane that could get him to Boston in time. Vandendriessche could not take his place in the lead pack.

Norm Higgins, 29, at 6'3" ran surrounded by Toru Terasawa, Hirokazu Okabe, Kenji Kimihara, and Seiichiro Sasaki. Kimihara was born on March 20, 1941, the third child in a family of five whose father sold wholesale household products in Kitakyushu in the Fukuoka Prefecture. He lived not far from Morio Shigematsu, the 1965 winner, and had often dreamed of winning a trip to run in the Boston Marathon. He qualified to go there by winning the February Beppu Marathon in 2:15:28, defeating Shigematsu, who placed ninth. (The other three took the second through fourth places in Beppu to earn their trips to Boston.) The four Japanese runners had all broken 2:20 in various races, from Terasawa's 2:14:35 to Sasaki's 2:15:32. Higgins, in contrast, had run only 2:19:13 in Culver City, California, the previous November, making him the second fastest American marathoner ever, after Buddy Edelen. He was now the American male hope for the Boston Marathon. John J. Kelley, the former hope, decided that he was not in good enough shape to race this year. Yet in Norm Higgins resided a profound Kelley influence.

Norm Higgins grew up 7 years younger than Kelley in New London, Connecticut. In the same way that as a teenager Kelley had been awestruck at New London's Clayton Farrar, who had raced Kelley the elder for 18 miles of Boston in 1945, Higgins was awed by Kelley the younger. Both had Malcolm Greenaway as their high school coach. In 1954 when Higgins was 18, he met Kelley, who was then at BU, as Kelley won the Manchester, Connecticut, road race and Higgins won the high school division. Higgins had run a 2:07 half mile and a 4:44 mile in high school, whereas Kelley had run a national best of 4:20 in the mile. Kelley was the superior natural talent, but Higgins, though basically big and slow, possessed a relentless intensity.

As a young teenager Higgins would bet his friends that he could deliver 117 newspapers in under 15 minutes. He ran himself ragged to win the bets. He was bent on imposing difficult and tedious tasks on himself.

After high school graduation, Higgins joined Kelley for track sessions of 440-, 880-, 220-yard repetitions but not long runs. Kelley took Higgins to road races. Usually Kelley won and Higgins placed a distant second or third. After Kelley won Boston, Higgins joined him for long runs. While Kelley the English teacher ran, he talked in professorial ramblings that matched their peripatetic proclivities and in the process improved Higgins's vocabulary. Often the pace on these runs got severe in the last miles. Higgins wanted to learn more about how to train for long-distance running. He sought books about Vladimir Kuts, the great Russian 10,000-meter Olympic gold medalist of 1956, and of course about the Czechoslovakian Emil Zatopek. Higgins worked in the electric boat division of General Electric and eagerly accepted military draft because the chances were great that he would be sent to Germany and might meet his heroes.

Higgins did go to Germany, where he became a squad leader because of his height. As leader he had the liberty to tell the rest of his squad that he was going down to the post exchange (the sundries store) to round up the men who had "bugged out." But instead he would go to a nearby field, strip down to his shorts, and run barefoot laps on the grass. No one dared question him with no uniform. Wanting to make the army track team, he wrote miles of letters to Washington pleading for a chance. Higgins's unit, the 7th Cavalry, stood on alert in West Germany and faced the Communists on field maneuvers. Higgins volunteered to be the CQ runner, the man who runs from platoon to platoon or company to company delivering messages during times of critical radio silence. It was in essence the same mission that Tom Longboat (Boston winner in 1907) had performed in World War I. Higgins would do anything to run, even with the burden of combat boots and at the risk of being shot. One day a helicopter arrived in the field. The pilot had orders to take Private Higgins to a track meet in Mainz, Germany. Someone in Washington had read his letters.

The deal was simple: If Higgins could be the first American in a 1,500-meter track race he could stay in Mainz and train all summer. If not, the helicopter that snatched him from the frontier would take him back. A chance was just what Higgins wanted. He had kept himself fit in the field; he wanted to run with the Germans so he hung onto them from the first step. The commanding officer was impressed. No American military runner had ever stayed with the Germans. They all beat him, but he beat all the Americans. He received orders to report to the U.S. Army track team and spend the summer training with the German national team. From the German Olympic coach, Professor Vichmann, Higgins learned about running tempo and how to control it and, moreover, how to be patient in training and maintain a training consistency regardless of performance in individual races. A bad performance did not mean that one's training system should be scrapped.

Higgins met Max Truex, the U.S. 10,000-meter record holder with a 28:50 from his sixth place in Rome in 1960. Truex had a Hungarian coach, Mihaly Igloi, who had escaped the Communists and coached a group of dedicated distance runners in Los Angeles. Higgins resolved to find Igloi after he got out of the army.

In 1961 Private Higgins ran in Boston and placed 19th in 2:47:23. But as soon as he left the army he took off for California, arriving in Los Angeles with $14 in his pocket. He took a survival job with the Tidewater Oil Company, delivering mail to their executives. His only ambition was to learn more about training for long-distance running and to use that knowledge to become the best marathoner in America. As Jesse Van Zant had done a decade and a half earlier, Norm Higgins became bicoastal in his pursuit of the marathon.

In Wellesley in 1966, at the halfway mark of the Boston Marathon, Norm Higgins was the best marathoner in America as he led the four Japanese by a nudge. He had replaced Kelley, Higdon, Buschmann, and Edelen. He was ready to win. Four weeks earlier he had run a workout that demonstrated his readiness. He ran 4 × a half mile in 1:55 to 1:56. But Higgins ran beyond his experience in this marathon. In his past races he had either trotted along at 6:30 per mile or blasted away alone with a tremendous lead, running 5:10 miles. But now his competition clustered around him and raced him like Igloi had trained his athletes to do on the track. They would surge and fall back, surge and fall back, with a different runner leading each aggression. Higgins responded to each of them. The little men harried Higgins into fatigue greater than that inflicted by his strict Hungarian coach.

Igloi trained a cadre of runners. With his select vocabulary Kelley labeled Igloi's band as cabalistic, cultish, and even messianic to outsiders. Igloi, the survivor of a Russian concentration camp, felt no need to explain his methods or to cultivate public relations. He felt that the results should speak for themselves. His group included the top runners of the day: Bob Schul, Joe Douglas (who later became the coach and manager of sprint and long jump Olympic gold medalist Carl Lewis), Greg Magee, Jim Grelle, Bob Seaman,

Lazlo Tabori (who later became Jacqueline Hansen's and Mikki Gorman's coach), and Jim Beatty. The group trained by running hours of fast and slow intervals on the grassy fields of the University of Southern California. Their training was so regimented and strict that every day they ran on the same path in the fields, back and forth, around and around. They wore a rut in the field; to save it, groundskeepers asked them to find another one.

During a moment's inattention by Higgins on the Newton hills, the Japanese ceased to be a team. When Higgins's attention returned from his inner workings, the Japanese runners had strung out ahead of him, each man now surging to win the race from the others. Higgins snapped into focus and chased them, but could not catch them. Kenji Kimihara led the four-man sweep. The last of the Japanese finished only 15 seconds ahead of Higgins.

Kenji Kimihara went on to win the silver medal in the 1968 Olympic Games in Mexico City, finishing second to Mamo Wolde. Later he became athletic director of Kyushu Women's College in Japan. In 1993 he attended the Boston Marathon as race analyst for a Japanese television production and promised to come back to run in the 100th running in 1996.

Bobbi Gibb made big headlines and big photos in the Boston papers: "Hub Bride First Gal to Run Marathon" and "Blond Wife, 23, Runs Marathon." Yet she could not join the other runners for their traditional bowl of beef stew in the Prudential cafeteria: Women were not allowed. Photographers followed her home, and one of their shots showed her at home later on race day in the kitchen, making fudge with a friend.

What did Jock Semple and Will Cloney think about Bobbi Gibb's running the marathon? Not much. She was not officially in the race. She had not entered. She did not wear a number. Her progress was not monitored at the checkpoints. In their minds she had not participated, although she may have run on the public roads from Hopkinton to Boston. Because she did not interfere with the progress of the race they had no intention of throwing her out. In fact, they never saw her.

Seventh-place finisher Tom Laris, born in New York City of Greek parents and a graduate of Dartmouth College, finished with a resolve to take his track speed and apply it to next year's marathon. He was light and fast.

1966 Results

1.	K. Kimihara, Japan	2:17:11		11.	T. Salakka, Finland	2:25:19
2.	S. Sasaki, Japan	2:17:24		12.	G. Williams, Washington, DC	2:26:54
3.	T. Terasawa, Japan	2:17:46		13.	A. Boychuk, Toronto, ON	2:27:20
4.	H. Okabe, Japan	2:18:11		14.	Myung-Jong Yoo, Korea	2:27:52
5.	N. Higgins, Santa Monica, CA	2:18:26		15.	N. Kitt, SCS	2:28:33
6.	D. Ellis, Toronto, ON	2:19:47		16.	R. Wallingford, Hamilton, ON	2:30:06
7.	T. Laris, NYAC	2:21:44		17.	J. Duffield, Evanston, IL	2:31:26
8.	B. Scharf, Washington, DC	2:22:15		18.	E. Comroe, SCS	2:32:02
9.	R. Daws, Minneapolis, MN	2:24:27		19.	P. Hoffman, Toronto, ON	2:32:37
10.	K. Nae-Kim, Korea	2:24:44		20.	L. Castagnola, Washington, DC	2:33:48

21.	M. Kimball, Santa Barbara, CA	2:33:58	30.	P. MacDonald, *HRR*	2:38:11
22.	L. Carroll, *BAA*	2:35:20	42.	J. Daley, Jr., *NMC*, MA	2:46:28
23.	J. Brennand, Jr., CA	2:35:24	44.	T. Corbitt, *NYPC*	2:46:59
24.	R. Pratt, Toronto, ON	2:35:53	46.	L. Berman, *MetAC*	2:48:55
25.	L. Coppens, *PennAC*	2:36:10	57.	J.A. Kelley, Watertown, MA	2:56:10
26.	E. Ayres, *CNJTC*	2:37:06	74.	C. Ellis, *NMC*	3:03:08
27.	E. Winrow, *NYAC*	2:38:00	122.	P. Hoss, *UMass*	3:20:25
28.	J. Wrynn, *SpAC*	2:38:01	126.	Roberta Gibb Bingay, MA	3:21:40^CR
29.	J. Dockstader, *NYAC*	2:38:08	176.	S. Tiernan, *NMC*, MA	3:43:00

About 500 entrants.
*Unofficial.

KATHRINE

WEDNESDAY, APRIL 19, 1967

Japanese—Can They Sweep Again?

Tom Laris jumped into the Boston Marathon of 1966 because he had lived in Lynn, Massachusetts, and needed a long run. He usually ran 110 to 120 miles a week. But for 2 months he had trained specifically for the marathon with 130-mile weeks. During each of those 8 weeks he ran a 30-mile run. He ran 6-minute miles for the first 25 miles, then ran hard for the last 5 miles. That was a 2:38 marathon plus the hard five. In 1967 he worked for the finance department of General Electric in Palo Alto, California. Laris had talent and speed. He was genetically gifted. In high school he had run a 4:16 mile. In the BAA indoor games of 1967 in the Boston Garden he had run an 8:38 two-mile. Ralph Buschmann, the top American in 1965, was his army buddy. They trained together. It was Buschmann who had needled Laris into running in 1966. In that race Laris had ached to use his pent-up speed, but he did not dare let himself go without having done deep endurance training. He understood the science of long-distance running well enough to know his limits. Then he had speed; now he had endurance and speed. American track men took inspiration from Jim Ryun's new world record (3:51.3) in the mile, set during the summer of 1966. Laris was a fine track man. He was quicker than Kelley, faster than Buschmann, Higdon, or Higgins. The runner to match him had to come from the other side and the bottom of the world.

Dave McKenzie, a little (5'4", 119 pounds) freckle-faced redheaded runner from Greymouth, New Zealand, came to Boston with an impressive record over the previous 6 months: a 2:20:44 in his hometown in November, a dominating 2:16:02 in the Canterbury Marathon in January, and a 2:21:50 in Auckland, New Zealand, in March. He too had trained specifically. The

Auckland race was more of an effort than his time indicated because the last half of it was run headfirst into gale-force winds. But McKenzie thrived on such weather in Greymouth. The Grey River descended through the town to dump its load of snowmelt from the New Zealand Alps into the Tasman Sea, from which it evaporated and blew back into the Alps, and so on. It was nearly always cloudy and nearly always raining in Greymouth. The weather at Boston mimicked its turbulence. A scum of wet snow covered the lawns of the western suburbs in the morning, but by noon the wind-driven drizzle had washed it away. The drizzle itself fell nearly as cold as snow, colder in effect because it wet the exposed skin of runners' legs, hands, and faces, allowing the wind to suck the heat from their muscles in a way dry flakes could not. McKenzie liked to run in a small rain, but this east wind blew bitter.

The Japanese too loved rainy-day runs on their moist island homeland. Yutaka Aoki (2:18:11), Takashi Inoue (2:15:17 at Beppu), and Toru Terasawa (2:17:48 at Beppu) were not the fastest Japanese. Kimihara, Usami, and Sasaki had run faster but for various reasons had not come to Boston this year. But those three who did come were carefully prepared. They brought with them their own supply of instant noodles. When they trained in Boston's Franklin Park they carried cards with their host's address and phone number so they would not get lost as had Morio Shigematsu in 1965. Most observers expected a Japanese to win and just hoped that someone would break up their sweep.

McKenzie did not worry about the Japanese running as a team. He figured that eventually they would be trying to beat one another and there would be his chance. Terasawa, 8 years older than Inoue and Aoki, feared McKenzie. Or perhaps he said so just to be polite.

In the wet pack in Wellesley, McKenzie, Laris, Andy Boychuk of Canada, and five Japanese led. Laris fought to stay out of the lead. He felt so good that he had to keep his brakes on.

This year the Playboy Club of Boston offered its bunnies, waitresses at the men's club, to greet the marathoners at the finish line. (Bunnies were selected on the basis of breast size, cleavage potential, pouting lips, and legginess. They worked wearing strapless bathing suits, stockings, high heels, rabbit ears, and cottontails.) But Race Director Will Cloney refused the club's offer, saying the race was for racing, not for the promotion of nightclubs or girlie magazines. Or for political protests.

But the 1960s was an era of political protest, and hardly anything in American culture escaped criticism. The Boston Marathon was no exception. Two women came to run the marathon. Bobbi Gibb, now divorced, came back to run on the public roads, with no intention of applying for an AAU card or becoming an official entrant. For Gibb, to run was to be free, and all she wanted was to be free to run. As long as no one tried to throw her off the course, she was pleased to be part of it. Whatever she did would be done whether or not it was sanctioned by a bureaucracy. She told the *Boston Globe* reporter, ''Running is like getting back down to the core. It is like being wild again. It is basic. I'm running because a lot of my friends encouraged me to share the feelings of joy I get while I'm running. It is hard to explain. The other runners understand."

Kathrine Switzer of Syracuse, New York, felt the same things, but she wanted to be officially in the race and recognized officially for her effort. Whereas Bobbi Gibb might sit with a monk on a rock by a reflecting pool and meditate on the wonders of life, Kathrine Switzer might stand on a rooftop with Mario Savio, the Berkeley agitator in the free speech movement who said, "If you can seize the time, you can change the world." It was Switzer's intention to seize the time and shove the world a little further in the direction she thought it should move.

Kathrine Switzer went to George Marshall High School in Falls Church, Virginia, and then attended Lynchburg College, a 1,200-student liberal arts school that her parents picked for her. But in 1967, when she was 20 years old, she transferred to Syracuse University, where she became an English literature and journalism major.

To move the world Switzer bent the rules. She had gone to starting lines in men's races before. She had run a season of cross-country races, two track seasons, and indoor track in between. She had an AAU card and had sent the travel permits, required for competition outside an athlete's district, to the BAA with her entire—clearly female—name. Jock Semple had never bothered to look at them. At Lynchburg she ran a mile on the men's track team. It created an incredible fuss. The local newspaper got wind of the story, the AP bureau in Richmond picked it up, and then the papers in Washington got in on it. She received hate mail: "God will strike you dead." The campus of her southern religious school was divided between ardent supporters and those who considered her less than honorable. Their thinking could not extend beyond assuming that a woman who wanted to be on the track team wanted not to train and run races but to sleep around with the young men on the team. Women on campus looked askance at her because she did not wear a girdle. Her boyfriend at the Naval Academy thought women should participate in sports a little bit but that their function in life was to organize tea parties and look pretty when they came to visit Annapolis. Switzer did not see herself as an accessory to a midshipman. She did not visit him when she had track meets on the weekends. She trained and trained hard for athletics. On teams where the girls played she competed. She said, "When I played sports, I went out for the kill. Sports were never fun to me, although I did have fun. They were primarily an outlet for aggression or a catharsis for all my emotions." Aggressive women did not fit at the Naval Academy. When her boyfriend, the midshipman, told her, "I think of you as a freak," she turned wordlessly and walked away from him. She never looked back.

In 1966 at Lynchburg, Switzer wrote an article for the school paper about their team's 2-miler, Robert Moss, who had traveled to Boston to run in the marathon. He had run 3:45. Switzer, amazed to learn that Roberta Gibb had beaten him by over a mile, declared that someday she would run the Boston Marathon. The idea of running such a long distance fascinated her. She didn't know then that it would happen the next year.

At Syracuse she worked out with the men's team and met Arnie Briggs, a mailman and the unofficial distance coach at Syracuse. He had run 16th at Boston in 3 hours in 1950, had improved to a 2:41 in 1956, and had had a best place of 10th in the heat of 1952.

Briggs didn't believe the story about Bobbi Gibb's having run the Boston Marathon; he thought women incapable of doing such distances. His skepticism provided all the more motivation for Switzer, who wanted to follow in Gibb's footsteps and prove to Briggs that women could indeed run marathons. Ultimately Gibb was her inspiration.

When Switzer told Briggs of her intention, he said, "If you can show me in practice that you can run that kind of distance, I'll be the first one to take you to Boston." Despite his doubts, Briggs agreed to train her. Later he concluded that if any woman could finish the Boston Marathon, Switzer could. During runs of ever-increasing length, Briggs filled Switzer's head with "tales of the ancient marathoner." Switzer went 31 miles with Briggs in practice although she had never run a road race.

Switzer filled out an application under the name K. Switzer. For this BAA officials later accused her of bending the rules to the breaking point. (She didn't tell them she was female, but then they didn't ask.) She took the required medical examination in Syracuse and mailed it in with her entry, and her coach picked up her number, 261, in the gym with the numbers for the rest of the team. Switzer pinned it on herself. It was cold, so she went to the starting line in a hooded sweatshirt and sweatpants, like most of the men.

They knew what they were doing was unusual and they were proud of it, but they did not believe it was against the AAU's and the BAA's rules. Thus the BAA officials had no idea that a woman had defied the rules and gotten a number by apparent subterfuge.

Briggs and Switzer's new boyfriend, a hammer thrower named Tom Miller, ran with her between 2 and 4 miles when the press bus and the photographers' truck caught up with them. The photographers had noticed that a woman was running wearing an official race number, and they snapped to attention. Will Cloney ran

Semple tried to rip the number off Switzer. He shouted, "Get the hell out of my race and give me that number."

up and began to argue that she should not have a number. Briggs argued back. "Arnie, you know better than that," said Cloney.

Jock Semple ran past Cloney and tried to rip the number off Switzer. He shouted, "Get the hell out of my race and give me that number."

Semple ripped off a tiny corner of the number. He came back for the rest but only grabbed some sweatshirt. Switzer felt confused and frightened. Her aggressiveness did not help her now.

Briggs argued with Semple. "Leave her alone, Jock. She's trained for this." "Arnie, you stay out of this," Jock said.

Switzer did not understand. She saw only an angry man with a snarling face, but Arnie apparently knew him. Big Tom the hammer thrower, looking even bigger in an orange sweatshirt, felt no confusion. A footballer's instinct took over. To protect the quarterback, he knocked Semple out of the way. The big man hit the old man hard. Old Jock went sprawling.

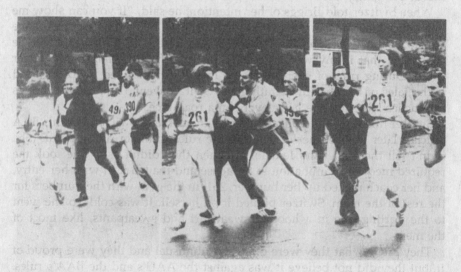

Jock Semple, seeing that a woman had broken the rules to receive a number, tried angrily to retrieve it. Blocked by the runner's hammer-throwing boyfriend, he failed. Kathrine Switzer went on to finish in about 4:20, an hour after Bobbi Gibb. Photo courtesy of Harry Trask.

Arnie yelled, "Kathy! Run like hell!" The photographers and reporters captured everything. Semple picked himself up and got back on the bus. As it zoomed off he shook his fist: "You're in deep trouble." Without incident a few miles later, the bus passed Bobbi Gibb, who wore no number.

Dave McKenzie did not feel in deep trouble as he ran in the lead pack through Wellesley. He earned just $55 a week in his job running a printing press back in rainy Greymouth, but he felt rich and at home on the descent into Newton Lower Falls. There Laris caught a stomach cramp. He nursed it down the hill as his competition filed past. It must have been those scrambled eggs he had for breakfast. He did not usually have scrambled eggs before racing. By Auburndale and the start of the hills he ran in 11th place. When McKenzie and his pack reached the first hill McKenzie felt a click. He felt as if every part of his body ran in place and in perfect function. If a chiropractor could have examined him at that moment he would have felt every bone, joint, and tendon in perfect alignment. McKenzie had never felt better in his life. He lifted up and away, and no one could catch him. Not even Laris. But he tried.

The Laris belly stitch disappeared as suddenly as it had come. His change in body angle on the hill might have done it. But where there had been pain was now a rush to catch up and use his splendid fitness to make up for lost time. No finer stretch run had ever been made at the Boston Marathon.

Laris ran in eighth place by Lake Street. He swooped down through Cleveland Circle and over the trolley tracks, past runner after runner, to Beacon Street. By Coolidge Corner only Yutaka Aoki ran between him and McKenzie. Laris streamlined himself and looked for McKenzie's head. The 130-mile weeks paid off. He felt no fatigue. If only the race would last long enough. He passed Aoki in Kenmore Square. Laris ran faster than McKenzie at this point. The race was not over until it was over. McKenzie ran a palpable distance away. Laris had gained 40 seconds on McKenzie since Boston College. But suddenly Hereford Street, Ring Road, and the Prudential Center rose into view, and McKenzie had stopped running at the finish line. Laris had 300 yards to go. He had flown over the last mile, but the race had ended. McKenzie had won in a new course record. Laris finished out the race nearly breaking Shigematsu's record from 1965. In the summer after this marathon Laris ran the fourth fastest 10,000 meters in the world for the year. Two weeks after the BAA he ran an 8:36 two-mile. In 1972 Laris ran his personal record of 28:12 for 10,000 meters. McKenzie went on to run a 2:12:25 personal best at Fukuoka in December and as of 1992 still worked at the same job for the *Greymouth Evening Star*.

But K. Switzer made the big headlines.

Will Cloney said, "I'm terribly disappointed that American girls force their way into something where they are neither eligible or wanted." K. Switzer forced her way to the finish through the cold rain, fatigue, and fear that police might pull their team from the race at any time. She wore no watch, and reporters did not note a time. Officials had left. Few spectators remained from when the race began at noon. She may have finished between four and five o'clock, perhaps earlier. Bobbi Gibb had finished an hour earlier and her time was accurately recorded. Gibb had stopped with a cramp at a house in Newton to call her father for a ride home. She had decided that running through pain was not what she ran for, so she had decided to drop out. But her cramp vanished so she jumped back in. One has to wonder just how fast Gibb may have run had she begun her running only a few years later when women's running had become much more organized.

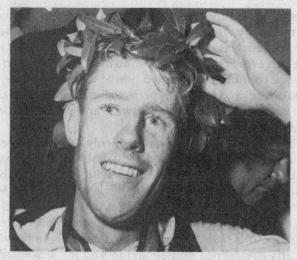

Redhaired, freckle-faced, tough little New Zealander David McKenzie smiles warmly after winning in a cold rain in 1967. Gene Dixon Photo/Courtesy of the *Boston Herald*.

The next day everyone else in the race became an also-ran to the Switzer flap. The UPI photo of the shoving match appeared everywhere. Press coverage grew out of proportion to Switzer's athletic performance as the media brouhaha eclipsed Gibb's genuinely impressive running. Switzer helped it grow. When she saw that the *New York Times* story reported that she had not finished, she was furious. She *had* finished. The conditions of cold and apparent assault were difficult. She was proud of her athletic accomplishment, and she wanted to make it clear that she was a real marathoner, not the kind of publicity-seeking feminist who bashes her way into all-male barrooms. She thought it was wrong of Gibb to run without a number. She called the *Times* reporter to clarify matters. What followed was a larger story, including photos of Switzer when she ran on the men's track team at Lynchburg. For the rest of the week her dormitory mates at Syracuse answered the phone for a celebrity. But as much as the process celebrated Switzer, it radicalized her. She'd entered the race positive and proud to be an athletic woman. She emerged still proud but also obligated to use her experience to insure that other women should not be treated the same way. She wanted to get as many women as possible into running. She became an organizer, an agitator. She also became determined to become a better marathoner.

As had happened before, both John Kelleys ran in this race. But John J. (the younger) took part in what both would come to describe in later years as a figurative torch-passing as he ran part of the way with a youngster he had coached in high school. The youngster was now a college junior. But the youngster had some difficulties in the race. It seems that the night before he had eaten some apple butter that during the race desperately wanted to escape from his body. He had to stop at a service station. The restroom was locked. Time ticked away. He had to ask an attendant for the keys. He took the keys in his drizzle-numbed hands and fumbled at the locks. Time ticked, and his bowels rumbled. At last he slipped in, and then quickly he was out and running down the road. He passed runners he had passed earlier. Five miles down the road it happened again. Again the same frozen-fingered fumbling. Again he passed the same runners he had passed twice before. All in all he lost 5 minutes to the apple butter. The runner was Ambrose Joel Burfoot. And he would be back.

Checkpoint Splits*

	Old records	New records
Framingham	34:28	34:20
Natick	53:53	53:26
Wellesley	1:09:09	1:08:51
Lake Street	1:52:12	1:51:31
Coolidge Corner	2:05:53	2:04:39

*Times unavailable for Woodland

1967 Results

1. D. McKenzie, New Zealand	2:15:45	

1. D. McKenzie, New Zealand 2:15:45^CR
2. T. Laris, *NYAC* 2:16:48
3. Y. Aoki, Japan 2:17:17
4. L. Castagnola, Washington, DC 2:17:48
5. A. Ambu, Italy 2:18:04
6. A. Boychuk, ON 2:18:17
7. T. Inoue, Japan 2:20:41
8. T. Terasawa, Japan 2:21:17
9. D. McFadzean, England 2:22:06
10. K. Ihaksi, Finland 2:22:07
11. E. Comroe, CA 2:25:16
12. J.J. Kelley, *BAA* 2:25:25
13. E. Carmona, Mexico 2:25:59
14. M. Kimball, Santa Barbara, CA 2:26:26
15. L. Buendia, Mexico 2:27:23

16. S. Matthews, Denver, CO 2:27:52
17. A. Burfoot, *WU* 2:28:05
18. R. Daws, *TCTC* 2:28:42
19. T. Osler, NJ 2:29:04
20. W. Harvey, NY 2:29:22
21. T. Clarke, Quantico, VA 2:29:44
22. J. McDonaugh, *MillAA* 2:30:26
23. O. Atkins, CA 2:30:26
24. J. Colpitts, *KAFB* 2:31:01
25. K. Weiser, *KTC* 2:31:05
44. K. Mueller, *BAA* 2:36:09
72. G. Muhrcke, *MillAA* 2:43:51
98. J. Henderson, IA 2:49:48
135. J.A. Kelley, Watertown, MA 2:58:13
266. Roberta Gibb 3:27:17*

Kathrine Switzer (her own estimate) 4:20.
*Unofficial.

KELLEY'S PUPIL

FRIDAY, APRIL 19, 1968

Top Mexicans in Town for Marathon

One fall day at Fitch High School in Groton, Connecticut, coach and English teacher John J. Kelley could not free himself of his teaching duties long enough to paint arrows on the cross-country course. But come meet time, according to Kelley, the course magically had signage fit for an expressway. Amby J. Burfoot's father, Amby W. Burfoot, Jr., had painted the big beautiful arrows around all the turns of the course. Kelley described the elder Burfoot as a "galvanic" local figure who doted on sports and especially supported his sons, who were cross-country runners on Kelley's team.

Kelley remembered young Amby J. as an inner-directed boy and a loner. He was amenable to suggestions, and Kelley did not have to repeat coaching instructions. While riding back from the state championships of Amby's junior year, Kelley moved to the back of the bus to talk with Burfoot. The coach wanted to congratulate the boy for having come out of nowhere to run a great season. Burfoot put down his book and said quietly, but uncharacteristically, "Yeah, coach, I'll eat 'em up next year." Kelley was surprised by such aggressive talk from a bookish boy. He concluded that Burfoot listened to his own internal timetable and that his time would come. Moreover, Burfoot loved to run. But there was a time before he knew that.

Before he discovered running, Amby loved to play baseball. He played third base, hit good line-drive doubles, and batted .461 in Babe Ruth League. As a junior varsity basketball player he was the worst kid to make the team. One day after the team had played poorly the coach punished the players by making them run the cross-country course. The punishment proved an epiphany for Burfoot. It was the singular moment when he discovered he could effortlessly run long distances and that it felt good to do it. He easily outdistanced the entire J-V basketball squad. It was good to be good. The next spring he went out for track. There he discovered Mr. Kelley—as he was called because he was primarily an English teacher rather than a coach—and had another epiphany.

Kelley was a greater sports hero than any man Burfoot had ever met. Kelley was world-famous. But he was not the big-shouldered, sullen, aggressive, swaggering male that Burfoot had encountered in other sports. Kelley was little and excitable; he used big words and talked of books. Kelley admired Jack Kerouac and Bob Dylan. He championed the underdog and railed against authority, talked of politics and big ideas. On weekends and off-season, runners gathered at Kelley's house for runs. George Terry would be there. Sometimes Norm Higgins. They would run single file through the

Johnny J. Kelley was Henry David Thoreau at 6 minutes a mile.

woods and apple orchards of the Haley Farm, or out to Wolf Neck Road for a looping 14-mile run that ended with a brutal half-mile charge up Cliff Street from the flatlands along the Mystic River, or maybe to Bluff Point to run barefoot on the beach. Always they ran loosely and easily, without regimentation. They might quickstep on fallen trees across streams, sprint up wooded hills. Kelley was Henry David Thoreau at 6 minutes a mile. After the runs Burfoot would hang around; Kelley's wife, Jessie, would cook, they would eat, and Kelley would talk. Burfoot sat transfixed at these lectures. He saw himself sitting at the foot of a wise and learned man.

Burfoot's high school days produced a 9:39 two-mile and acceptance to Wesleyan University. There his coach, Elmer Swanson, quickly perceived that Burfoot would train hard; Swanson made no attempt to direct his training but merely facilitated Burfoot's own initiatives. In the winter of 1968 Burfoot put together a perfect 2-mile race in the Knights of Columbus indoor track meet in Boston Garden. He ran an effortless 8:44. He was training 15 miles a day at 7:30 per mile.

In mid-March his Wesleyan team went south for a 2-week spring break. There they could escape the New England weather at the Quantico, Virginia, marine base. To prepare for Boston, Burfoot ran a marathon a day for the 2 weeks (175 miles per week). One day he took his younger roommate, Billy Rodgers, for what they thought would be 10 miles in the forest. Three hours and 22 miles later they were still running. Rodgers dragged himself along, but Burfoot felt only mildly tired. His mileage for the day was 39 miles. A 10-mile run at 6 minutes a mile was effortless. He was keenly aware that he was more fit he had ever been in his life. He floated on a physical and emotional high. Back at school he went on Sunday morning 25-mile runs, where sometimes late-rising roommate Rodgers would join him for the last hilly 10 miles in 65 minutes.

One Sunday Burfoot cajoled his sleepy roommate into joining him for a full 25 miles. The first 15 passed at 7 minutes a mile, and the roommate still hung on. College boys tend toward establishing pecking orders and hierarchies. Burfoot, 21, was not immune to a desire to put the youngster in his place. He cranked the pace down to 6 minutes a mile. The kid hung on. Burfoot ran intensely. Rodgers looked around. On his runs he would often find money. Burfoot never found money. Not until 2 miles to go, when Burfoot tossed in a couple of 5:20 miles, did he manage to dump Rodgers.

The kid was pretty good, but no match for Burfoot with such a high level of endurance training. In earlier years Burfoot ran with Wesleyan teammate Jeff Galloway, who became a U.S. Olympian in the 10,000 meters in 1972.

Slowly Burfoot began to feel that he could win the Boston Marathon. He felt empowered by that feeling but thought it prudent not to speak it aloud. He told no one except his younger brother, Gary.

Burfoot went to bed on the night before the Boston Marathon obsessed with the importance of awakening at exactly 6:00 in order to drink tea and honey. He feared that if he did not consume them at the proper time he would have the same expulsive bowel problem that the apple butter had caused the year before. He was staying at the house of a girlfriend's parents, and the clock in his room had no alarm. Burfoot feared that if he overslept all his training would be wasted. He awoke sure that he had ruined everything by oversleeping. He looked at the clock. The sweep hand had just moved from 5:59 to 6:00. He had done it. He had awakened perfectly. He had done the hard part. He drank his tea and honey. Every preparation was now complete.

The lead group through Wellesley included John J. Kelley, Bill Clark, Bob Deines from Occidental College in California, and others to total half a dozen runners. It was a warm, clear day. Three Mexicans ran a safe distance behind the pack but never threatened the lead as expected. Burfoot felt like he was jogging. He wore a Pittsburgh Paints painter's cap to keep off the hot sun. Deciding that the pack was too big, he threw in a surge to drop one or two runners. To his horror he dropped all of them except Clark—who Burfoot knew could outkick him. Burfoot's own impudence horrified him. This wasn't supposed to happen. It was not supposed to be a two-man race. It was supposed to be a pack. The plan was to break away from the pack on the hills. Burfoot ruined his own plan with one slight surge. The need to drop Clark on the hills began to consume Burfoot. Clark followed him. Clark planned to hang on and kick. Burfoot felt caught in a spider's web. Just as Oksanen's predatory clinging had snared Burfoot's coach, Kelley, in 1959 and 1961, Burfoot feared he too was set up to be the victim. The sun at their backs threw Clark's shadow ahead of Burfoot. He looked down at Clark's shadow skimming the ground. It did not look tired. Burfoot could not stop looking at the shadow. He pushed as hard as he could up the hills, but the damn shadow stuck. Peter Pan didn't have a shadow, why should Clark?

When they crested the hills by Boston College, Burfoot knew it was all over. There were no more hills. Clark could coast downhill, then pop a sprint whenever he pleased. There was nothing Burfoot could do. There he was, Amby Burfoot—victim. The marine's killer instinct could devour him at will.

Jock Semple came by on the press bus. "Give it hell on the downhill, Amby!" he shouted. Suddenly on the downhill Burfoot saw only sunshine. The shadow and Clark were gone. Cramps in Clark's thighs prevented him from striding fully with the grace of gravity. The kick, the kicker, the spider, the killer marine, the tireless shadow—all the demons vanished like magic.

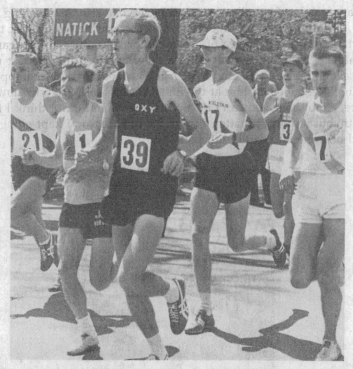

Californian and later draft resister Bob Deines, #39, leads in Wellesley, with marine Bill Clark (#21), John J. Kelley (#1), college senior Amby Burfoot (#17), and Ralph Buschmann (#7). Photo courtesy of the *Boston Herald*.

With 3 miles to go the crowds crushed into the road ahead so tightly that Burfoot could see nothing. The spectators bent away like tall marsh grass allowing a boat to pass, then folded back behind him. Burfoot could not see behind. Other races had not been like this. Last year's sparse crowds in the cold rain were not like this. Burfoot could not see if anyone was gaining on him. The noise of the crowd gave no hint as it sometimes would—listening for the cheers directed at the runner behind you, you could judge his proximity. Burfoot ran blind down Beacon Street. A side stitch stabbed him. He bent over. He tried to massage it out. He worked at it as if trying to pull an arrow from his ribs. He was sure he had slowed and that half of the 900 runners in the race would go by. He had done everything right, and now he thought he was going to pieces. They were going to get him.

Burfoot panicked. The paranoia of the leader grabbed him. It was the fear of someone sneaking up from behind, the fear that makes dictators execute their underlings. That fear gripped Burfoot. He thought he could not breathe. "I am a sitting duck. If only I had a kick. They are coming to get me."

But there was no one there. No one came up on Burfoot. No one kicked. No one executed him or assassinated him. He did not die. He did not trip, fall down, or stumble. None of these gremlins came alive. He did slow in the heat of the last few miles, but so did everyone else. Astonishing himself, Amby Burfoot won. Of course he always thought he would, but that had been the essential arrogance of a competitor speaking—an arrogance that most athletes rationalize away after a defeat. But during the last miles of the race it all seemed too good to be true. Burfoot called it the happiest day of his life. Kelley joined him at the finish. Kelley said, "I know how happy you are, Amby. But you can't be any happier than I am. I think I finished fifteenth, but it doesn't matter. I think the only reason I kept going was so I could be in here to exult with you."

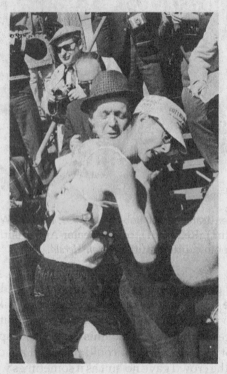

After outrunning Bill Clark's shadow, Amby Burfoot, Mister Kelley's pupil, finishes in the arms of Jock Semple—Kelley's father-confessor—after winning the 1968 race. Photo courtesy of the *Boston Herald*.

1968 Results

1.	**A. Burfoot, *WU*, CT**	**2:22:17**	8.	M. Ala-Leppilampi, Finland	2:31:35
2.	W. Clark, Quantico, VA	2:22:49	9.	D. McFadzean, *RNAC*	2:32:27
3.	A. Penaloza, Mexico	2:25:06	10.	A. Muhrcke, *MillAA*	2:34:15
4.	P. Garrido, Mexico	2:25:07	11.	E. Winrow, *NYAC*	2:35:12
5.	R. Daws, *TCTC*	2:29:17	12.	B. LaBudde, *GSU*	2:35:47
6.	R. Deines, *OccC*, CA	2:30:13	13.	R. Wallingford, *HamAC*	2:37:03
7.	J. Gaspar, Mexico	2:30:29	14.	A. Coolidge, *BAA*	2:37:03

15.	J.J. Kelley, *BAA*	2:37:03	31.	P. Stipe, *BAA*, Wellesley, MA	2:47:34
16.	J. Daley, Jr., *NMC*	2:38:05	32.	T. Gallagher, *UK*	2:47:56
17.	R. Hall, *ConnCAA*	2:38:09	33.	A. Wooten, Willimantic, CT	2:49:08
18.	M. Aarbo, *EOC*	2:39:02	34.	P. Thompson, *TU*	2:49:37
19.	J. McDonaugh, *MillAA*	2:39:34	35.	P. Wood, *Marin AC*, CA	2:49:40
20.	J. O'Connell, *SABC*	2:40:45	37.	N. Weygandt, *SJTC*	2:49:45
21.	W. Harvey, *NYPC*	2:41:41	41.	G. Comroe, *SCS*	2:51:09
22.	J. Colvin, *PennAC*	2:42:02	43.	T. Corbitt, *NYPC*	2:52:00
23.	T. Osler, *PennAC*	2:42:15	45.	L. Castagnola, Washington, DC	2:52:15
24.	R. Ashley, *RTC*	2:43:14		R. Gibb	3:30*
25.	R. Gaff, *NMC*	2:44:43			

*Unofficial.

THE SELF-MADE MARATHONER

MONDAY, APRIL 21, 1969

Very Fast Japanese to Race Today

Two days before the Boston Marathon of 1969, the courts found Sirhan B. Sirhan guilty of assassinating Robert Kennedy. The movie everyone had to see was "2001: A Space Odyssey." The real space odyssey, the Apollo mission to put men on the moon, waited in its final phase. The political folly of yet another president peaked the number of U.S. forces in Vietnam at 534,000. The Boston Marathon was about to see the biggest marathon field in the history of the sport. Some young men took the marathon as their personal odyssey.

Ron Daws of the Twin Cities Track Club was a bit faster than most, but unlike the marathon gods like Abebe Bikila, he exemplified the young men in wild pursuit of the unicorn. Daws was meticulous nearly to fanaticism in his pursuit. He trained for every contingency. The improvement was in the details. For example, because every ounce counted, Daws made his own ultralight racing shoes out of parts of beach thongs. Daws could tell by looking at their tans which runners were not trained for the heat. To prepare for another hot day at Boston, like the year before when he finished fifth, Daws wore his winter running clothes late into the spring. Often he wore two sweatsuits and a wool hat when shorts and a long-sleeved T-shirt would have been enough. Coming off his Minnesota winter, Daws was tempted to peel down, but he disciplined himself to stay dressed. Sweat! Prepare! Suffer now so you won't have to suffer later. It would have felt good to let the sun fall on his pasta-pale skin. Only with two sweatsuits could he simulate in March in Minneapolis the effects of an 80 °F day. He had to pass great volumes of water down his throat and out through his sweat glands to prime them for the race. Daws felt that runners with tans could not have been as thorough as he in their preparation.

Daws described himself as a self-made runner. It was an accurate assessment; he had to have been made, because he wasn't a born runner. Daws needed to be thorough in his preparation because he had little natural talent. He made the 1968 Olympic team with a 3rd-place 2:33 marathon under the difficulties of the high altitude in Alamosa, Colorado, and ran the same time for 22nd place in the thin air of the Mexico City Olympics. He frequently raced wearing a white painter's cap to which he attached a white handkerchief to shade his neck. With the handkerchief flapping behind him, he looked like a gallant member of the French foreign legion. He had never run any elite track times. His fastest mile was only 4:25. Nearly every high school had a kid who could do that.

Yet Daws decided that he would dedicate himself without compromise to the pursuit of marathon racing. He said and later wrote in one of his books about running, *Running Your Best*, that

> unless you go all out for something, you may conclude your life
> without actually having lived it. It doesn't have to be running, but
> it should be a quest for excellence, and it need be for only that
> period of your life that it takes to fully explore it. That's how you
> find out what you are made of. That's how you find out who you
> are. To live your life your way, to reach for the goals you have set
> for yourself, to be the you that you want to be, that is success.

Daws could not run one mile as fast as Burfoot or Laris could run two in a row, yet it was Daws who made the Olympic team, not Burfoot, not half of the 129 runners who started the Olympic trials and dropped out. Now it was Daws who was fit and ready to race and not Burfoot.

Burfoot was not the same superman that he had been in the spring of 1968. He had run 2:14:28.8 in December in Fukuoka to make up for his quitting the Olympic trials at 18 miles. His time was sort of an American record. Buddy Edelen had run 2:14:28-something at Chiswick, England, in 1963, but the Japanese timed their races to the nearest tenth of a second. So Burfoot was the second-fastest American ever. That, however, was in December of 1968, not in the spring of 1969. Having taken a job teaching school, he had no time to train as he had during his 2 weeks of leisure at the Quantico marine base last spring. He did not expect to do well and said so. The marathon is not a race that can be won with skill, experience, or desire without recent training.

Bob Deines had finished sixth in Boston in 1968, fourth in the Olympic trials. He had not cut his hair since. A student at Occidental College, Deines ran with a black and orange shirt with the word "OXY" on it. He was tall and thin. In 1969 he was drafted into the army to fight in Vietnam. Deines had profound moral objections to a war that he felt was to help save Vietnam from the Vietnamese. He appeared for his preinduction physical within days of having run in a marathon and had not eaten or hydrated himself. At 6'2" and 130 pounds and walking with postmarathon stiffness, he looked wretched, hardly a fighting machine. The army rejected him for military service for being underweight—precisely the desired effect.

Daws, Deines, Burfoot, both Kelleys, a Japanese team, a Mexican team, several women, a Finn, and a Greek joined more people than had ever run in a marathon anywhere before. There were 1,152 official starters. The numbers overtaxed Jock Semple, Will Cloney, and the systems and volunteers who put on the race. They talked of instituting qualifying times. They were in no mood to throw the thing open to women, yet more women than ever came to run. If women jumped out of the bushes, that was fine, because the roads are free; but, to discourage additional women, Semple said, "We won't show them any privileges." But statements that Semple and Cloney were against women belied the fact that they were so much *for* marathoners that for the last 2 years they had arranged a special showering and changing area in the Prudential Center garage for Bobbi Gibb.

Stylianos Kyriakides, the Greek winner from 1946, could not stay away from Boston. He brought Demitrious Vouros from Athens to win it. Kyriakides had just retired from his work with the electric company of Athens. Vouros had run a 2:23 marathon. But the speed king of the field was the Japanese runner Yoshiaki Unetani, a physical education teacher who had run 2:12:40.6 at Fukuoka. He blasted out of Hopkinton with 4:43 miles to Framingham. His coach, Kazusuke Nishitani, watched carefully. Mexicans Alfredo Penaloza and Pablo Garrido, who had been third and fourth the year before, followed closely, but they never made contact with the runaway leader. The Finn, Pentti Rummakko, followed them. He had run brilliantly the year before with a 2:17:53.8 in the Karl Marx Stadt Marathon and a 2:17:47.2 in Reykjavik, Iceland, but he seemed to have no energy and gradually dropped back. A brilliant 2:17 was still a mile behind a 2:12; Rummakko really had no chance against Unetani at his best. Rummakko needed no extra harassment, but it came regardless. A crazed spectator attacked him. He used his arm to ward off the blows, then continued his uninspired race. He would return the next year in the best shape of his life.

At the start of the hills Unetani felt that the Mexicans ran too close. They knew the course and worked together hungrily. Unetani unleashed a furious frontal assault on the hills that left no one within a half mile of him. At the crest of the hill he could see no one behind him. He asked the riders on the press bus if anyone followed. They laughed. They held no doubt about his winning. No one followed; Unetani went on to win by nearly 4 minutes—the largest margin since 1952 and a course record. Daws ran in 18th place in Framingham. He said Boston was a sucker's course. The early downhill had seduced many a runner into committing himself to an impossible pace. Daws would have none of that. After Framingham Daws worked himself up through the destruction left in Unetani's wake to fourth place. In the closing miles Daws knew the Mexican, Penaloza, was a short distance ahead,

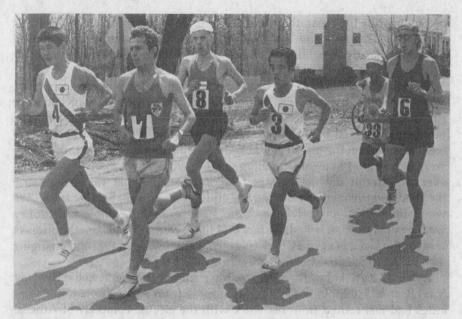

Yoshiaki Unetani, #4, of Japan left this pack far behind as he smashed the course record in the 1969 race. Other top finishers included Patrick McMahon of Ireland (#7), Pentti Rummakko of Finland (#8), and Bob Deines of California (#6). Photo by Jeff Johnson.

but he could not see him through the crowds. Daws finished fourth, the first American. Daws would come back to Boston again and again and he would later coach and marry Lorraine Moller, who would win the Boston Marathon. At age 55 on July 28, 1992, three days before his by-then former wife would win the bronze in the Barcelona Olympic marathon, Daws would die in his sleep of heart failure.

Pat McMahon, an Irishman, BAA member, and a schoolteacher in Lowell, Massachusetts, who finished eighth, would also come back. McMahon had actually been the favorite in 1968 but never showed up. Yoshiaki Unetani never came back to Boston. He became a high school teacher in Hiroshima, Japan.

And back would come Sara Mae Berman—this year's first woman, who finished hand-in-hand with her husband, Larry. And also to return was a man who ran, and finished, but whose name does not appear in the results. He ran hard for the first 20 miles just to get a feel for the course, then jogged to the finish in a respectable time, but he didn't bother to cross the finish line. There was no point. He planned to come back the next year and run tremendously fast. He was as meticulous and careful as Daws, but he had run a 4:01 mile. He had a rare combination of intelligence and talent. His name was Eamon O'Reilly. He had already run a 2:16:39.8 marathon in Santa Rosa, California, but he missed the Olympic team. He thought *he* was the best marathoner in America.

1969 Men's Results

1.	Y. Unetani, Japan	2:13:49^{CR}

1. Y. Unetani, Japan	2:13:49ᶜᴿ	18. J. Colvin, Harrisburg, PA	2:29:58
2. P. Garrido, Mexico	2:17:30	19. W. Yetman, *UWO*	2:30:23
3. A. Penaloza, Mexico	2:19:56	20. F. Pflagina, *BOC*, MD	2:30:43
4. R. Daws, *TCTC*	2:20:23	21. D. McFadzean, *RNAC*	2:30:54
5. R. Moore, *TOC*	2:21:28	**22. J.J. Kelley, *BAA***	**2:31:36**
6. R. Deines, *OccC*, CA	2:22:49	23. P. Stipe, *BAA*	2:31:50
7. J. García, Mexico	2:23:16	24. R. Gaff, *NMC*	2:32:42
8. P. McMahon, *BAA*, Ireland	2:23:24	25. P. Thompson, *TU*	2:33:22
9. P. Hamilton, *RNAC*	2:23:46	26. J. Kneen, Australia	2:33:27
10. P. Rummakko, Finland	2:24:14	28. J. Dirksen, *TCTC*	2:33:40
11. J. Reneau, *TCTC*	2:24:42	31. R. Wallingford, *HamAC*, ON	2:34:05
12. M. Ande, *OccC*, CA	2:26:58	49. H. Higdon, *DTC*	2:41:18
13. G. Muhrcke, *MillAA*	2:27:53	65. S. Gachupin, NM	2:44:42
14. D. Vouros, Greece	2:28:40	85. T. Derderian, *NMC*	2:49:33
15. J. McDonaugh, *MillAA*	2:29:07	100. A. Williams, *NYPC*	2:52:36
16. J. Clare, *RNAC*	2:29:16	**186. J.A. Kelley**	**3:05**
17. A. Burfoot, *CConnAA*	**2:29:07**		

1969 Women's Results*

1. S. Berman, Cambridge, MA	**3:22:46**	3. N. Kuscsik, NY	3:46
2. E. Pederson, CA	3:43		

1,342 entrants, 1,152 starters, 678 under 4 hours.
*Results unofficial.

Chapter 8

1970-1979
The Boom Years

Presidents: *Richard M. Nixon, Gerald Ford, James E. Carter*

Massachusetts Governors: *Francis Sargent, Michael S. Dukakis, Edward King*

Boston Mayor: *Kevin H. White*

1970 Populations: *United States, 203,302,031; Massachusetts, 5,698,170; Boston, 641,000*

Men had landed on the moon. Now it seemed that people would forever be saying, "We can land a man on the moon, but we can't [fill in any complaint]." The Apollo program's trips to the moon did not distract the country from the distasteful and divisive war in Vietnam. The country split in half over the war, and so did marathon runners. Some actively protested the war and resisted the draft; others felt that if the protesters did not support America, right or wrong, they should take their long hair, beards, and blue jeans and leave it. Two conscientious objectors—those who would not serve in arms but would perform alternative services—Jon Anderson and Bill Rodgers, won the Boston Marathon during the 1970s.

Brutal murderer Charles Manson and heiress Patty Hearst, whose kidnapping and subsequent metamorphosis fascinated the American public, symbolized the bizarreness of this decade in American life. Manson was found guilty in 1971 of murdering actress Sharon Tate and six others with the help of his cult followers. Hearst, the victim of kidnapping in February 1974, was by March of 1976 a convicted bank robber and self-proclaimed revolutionary. Throughout the '70s an urge to align oneself with a subculture, in most cases a beneficial one, seemed strong among young people. Runners were not immune to it.

Young people in the 1970s came together to generate the "Age of Aquarius," full of the feeling that love and happiness could come to the world while war and hunger could be overcome if only people would give peace a chance. Every city had its enclave of hippies, with long hair, beads, and bellbottoms, greeting each other with the two-fingered V of peace. They believed that if only the world's consciousness were to lift—just a little bit—all would be harmony. Of course no one knew what consciousness-raising was. Every city also had its growing enclave of runners pursuing their own version of harmony. Often the two groups borrowed terminology from each other. A listener might have overheard either a runner or a hippie talk about "doing speed," "LSD," and "feeling high." The hippie would be referring to amphetamines, a hallucinogenic drug, and the effects of marijuana, whereas the runner would mean speed work, long slow distance, and the good feeling that comes from running well. Memberships among the groups of runners, hippies, and prowar militants often overlapped. Nationwide, runners banded together through the spread of national publications like *The Long Distance Log* and *Distance Running News* (which became *Runner's World*).

The world, too, began to band together in the beginnings of what would become known as the global economy. In 1972 President Nixon traveled to Peking, China, and later to Moscow. The U.S. began selling wheat to Russia. These acts gave the first signal to Americans that the Cold War might eventually end.

In June of 1972 police arrested five men for breaking into the Watergate offices of the Democratic National Committee. That break-in and the subsequent cover-up led to President Nixon's resignation in August of 1974. Gerald Ford, his successor, pardoned Nixon the following month. The next April the U.S. officially lost the Vietnam War with the evacuation of Saigon. To help ease the bitterness of the divisive war, in 1977 President Jimmy Carter pardoned 10,000 draft evaders.

Fields in the Boston Marathon increased from what had once seemed an astounding 1,000 to an unimagined 7,000. Rodgers, who lived in poverty and wore a hand-lettered shirt for his first victory, by the end of the decade owned several running gear stores and his own clothing line.

Faith in technology slipped with the 1979 accident at the Three Mile Island nuclear power plant. An unprecedented bailout of a private company by the government occurred with a $1.5-billion loan guarantee to Chrysler Corporation. Faith in capitalism slipped. The decade closed with the capture of 63 Americans on November 3, 1979, in Tehran by supporters of Ayatollah Khomeini. Their intention was to humiliate America. They demanded return of the ruling Shah of Iran, who was in New York City for medical treatment, so they could imprison him.

In spite of the decade's turmoil, the 1970s saw a running boom. A little athletic shoe import company called Blue Ribbon Sports became Nike. Runners themselves began to make money directly, albeit under the table, from their sport, and the era of the megarace arrived. Runners as a group ran faster than ever. The New York City Marathon, begun only in 1970, blossomed into numbers of runners so great that it seemed more like a mass migration than a footrace. The numbers of races blossomed, too; it seemed that every major city had to have its marathon. The Boston Marathon rode the crest of the wave.

Women arrived officially at Boston's starting line in 1972, and by the end of the decade they had achieved times that would have challenged Clarence

DeMar, John A. Kelley, and Gerard Cote. The 1970s also began an era of a long-sought American domination of the Boston Marathon.

HARD RAIN

MONDAY, APRIL 20, 1970

Canadian, Englishman to Face Off in Marathon

A hard rain fell in Boston on Patriots' Day 1970. The counterculture, antiwar, hippie-freak movement muddled in a confusion of rock music, drugs, and ideology. The U.S. government muddled in its own confusion about how to handle the protesters. Shoot them or defer them? Four student protesters at Ohio's Kent State University would be shot by national guardsmen 2 weeks after the Boston Marathon. Two months earlier the "Chicago Seven" had been found innocent of conspiring to incite a riot, but five of them had been found guilty of crossing state lines to incite a riot. The Nixon administration developed a lottery scheme to diffuse the antidraft protest by letting chance defer great numbers of potential protesters. Three days after the Boston Marathon came Earth Day, the sweet, innocent celebration of the planet. An explosion on the lunar excursion module forced Apollo 13 to limp back to Earth without succeeding in its third mission to land astronauts on the moon. On the Wednesday before the marathon 6,000 young people rioted across the Charles River in Harvard Square. About 170 rioters and 35 police officers were injured. On race day a literal hard rain pelted the marathon runners. One bearded antiwar runner tried repeatedly to give the peace sign to spectators, but he could not uncurl his cold fingers. Instead he gave them the peace claw.

A few days before the marathon, U.S. Olympian Kenny Moore of Eugene, Oregon, now an army information specialist, sat in the living room of a house behind a funeral home in Wellesley, Massachusetts, talking with other runners. They joked that it would be fun to hear the radio announcers talk about Ken Moore leading into Kenmore Square. Moore thought that it was not Burfoot or Daws or Higgins or Laris but Moore who was the best American marathoner. Of course he didn't say so aloud. When he spoke he selected his words carefully. In December he had run to seventh place in Fukuoka with an American record of 2:13:27.8. He had led the Olympic marathon in Mexico City from 3 to 6 miles until a combination of petroleum jelly and perforated tape that he had used to prevent foot blisters loosened to betray him, bunching up and creating blisters. Moore wanted to improve on these performances and knew that he could. He nurtured a plan to win Boston. He had attended law school at Stanford briefly until he decided that he would rather be a writer, so he planned after the army to pursue a master's degree in fine arts. Moore said that he had been misled when he was told that Boston was an easy course. He saw nothing easy about it. But he was young and fresh off some tough European cross-country races. He sat on the sofa with a quiet confidence.

Another young man, with a black beard and long tied-back hair, sure that it was he who was the best marathoner in America, stopped by for a visit with Moore and the assembled runners. The house was rented by a runner-photographer named Jeff Johnson, who operated the east coast division of a running shoe company called Blue Ribbon Sports. That company would later become Nike, and Johnson would become a multimillionaire. But for now he dressed in jeans and Tiger running shoes and hoped that he would always be able to dress that way rather than in suits and ties; Johnson, Moore, and other runners in the room—including other Blue Ribbon Sports employees—cared more about the next day's run than about the things money could buy.

Egos did not clash in that living room as Eamon O'Reilly, 4:01 miler and 2:16:39.8 marathoner, dropped in for his brief visit. His first marathon, the year before, had come to him under harsh and hot conditions, so he knew he could run much faster. But no one else knew. O'Reilly did not tell them. He was studying for a PhD in mathematics at Georgetown. He possessed a quiet brilliance, demonstrated by long pauses in his sentences during which he searched his mind for just the right word. There was no strutting, posing, innuendo, or braggadocio, only a silent steeling of resolution against the coming contest. There is much more silence in a room of marathoners before a race than after.

Running is such a blatantly performance-dominated sport that coordination, finesse, and psychological warfare play only a small part. In a marathon you don't fake left and go right. You just go. Each man held a confidence in his own abilities. Each had prepared to the limit. Each made his own resolutions. He said to himself about the other, You may be a fine and intelligent person and I may like you very much and enjoy your company and respect your intellect and athletic abilities, but tomorrow . . . I'm going to kick your butt. The impending race makes a runner flicker from the cerebral to the reptilian. Runners don't show up at internationally competitive marathons having trained to win without expecting to win, and therefore they expect everyone else to lose. An arrogance is essential. Logic and intellect say that it is entirely possible that someone else may run faster or that you could have a bad day, but to play out your own race to the fullest extent of your emotions you must believe that you are better than everyone else and deserve to win. You must buy that illusion in its entirety. Because of the enormity of the task ahead and its potential to generate pain, embarrassment, and psychological devastation, because of its simple hardness, because in every race it is much more logical to see why you will lose, a quiet arrogance must take root.

Out of the rain in the Hopkinton gymnasium, an hour before the start, Kenny Moore waited in a long line to use the toilet. His own nerves agitated him. They made him say and think things he never would otherwise. He wanted to warm up properly, but instead he had to wait. In his prerace temporary insanity, he complained that since he was a contender to win he should not have to wait in line behind all those slow losing runners. His slower friend in the line reminded him that the country was a democracy. Moore's gentility and sense of fair play returned, and he replied that it was indeed a democracy—until the race starts.

Staying the nights before the race several miles away in Winchester had been the second best marathoner in the world, Ron Hill of England. He, like Moore and O'Reilly, was extraordinarily well educated. He held a PhD in textile chemistry from Manchester University in England and since leaving the university in 1964 had worked as a research and development chemist in the dyeing research department of Courtaulds Ltd. He had run a mile in 4:10 in 1965; he clearly had the necessary speed, but not the killer speed of O'Reilly. Hill was the 1969 European champion with a 2:16:47.8 and runner-up on the dead-flat Fukuoka course with a 2:11:54.4. The winner of Fukuoka had slipped out quickly and run away. Hill had mustered a painful final effort to catch the leader, but he had waited too long and had to race instead for second place.

Now he had a personal score to settle with that winner. Hill felt that Jerome Drayton, a Canadian, had beaten him with tactics, not fitness. When Hill heard that Drayton was coming to Boston, he wanted to race his best for first place. Hill had prepared for a victory with weeks of training mileages well over 120 miles and races on Saturdays until 3 weeks before Boston, when he eased down to a mere 107 miles for the week. He trained through a dreadful, dreary-cold winter in the north of England by running to work and home again via a long route. He raised two boys at the time and had household chores like tiling the bathroom as well as reading to the lads. The British Road Runners Club took up a collection to send Hill to Boston. Ordinary blokes chipped in. He had training trouble, ranging from a thick-ened Achilles tendon to blood in the urine, but he survived to arrive in Boston ready to race.

Hill began a special and somewhat secret two-part prerace diet, with a high-protein, low-carbohydrate phase starting about 5 days before the race and a high-carbohydrate regimen in the final days before the marathon. Hill thought that he was the first marathoner to use "the diet" until in preparation for Boston he read DeMar's 1937 book, *Marathon*. DeMar described a similar diet, what he called an "elimination" diet, composed of a week of eating only fresh, nonstarchy fruits and vegetables. Later when DeMar reintroduced bread, potatoes, and bananas he was amazed at how fast he could run without tiring. Hill experienced that same amazement.

From Jim Peters's accounts of the race in *The Long Run* and from Brian Kilby (third place in 1963), Hill learned of the potential that Boston had to be fast under cool conditions. Upon seeing the course Hill was dismayed by the many early course "undulations," but he thought a 2:12 marathon was entirely possible, if everything went right.

Spoilers for Hill might be the Japanese, a team of Kunio Fujita (2:17:37.6), Kokichi Uchino (2:16:55.8), and Teruo Yoshida (2:13:21). Or it might be the man who beat all the Japanese. Somewhere in Boston stayed the 1969 Fukuoka winner, Jerome Drayton. With his 2:11:12.8 Fukuoka defeat of Hill, Drayton had to be considered to be the best marathoner in the world, although Derek Clayton and Akio Usami had run 2:08:33.6 and 2:11:27.8 at Antwerp in 1969. The press portrayed Drayton as a dark and brooding personality. If that picture was true, then the brooding came as much from his circumstances as from himself. His boyhood passed in a defeated world. His misfortune was to be born Peter Buniak in Kolbemoor, Germany, in the closing days of World War II on January 10, 1945. He grew up in poverty. Authorities and his parents shifted him from foster home to foster home. The poverty and deprivation of postwar Germany prevented the young boy from seeing his parents often. The Buniaks were not German but Ukrainian. To be a Ukrainian boy in a defeated country where the Nazi government had despised all persons non-German and tried largely to exterminate Ukrainians to make living space for Germans, to be poor and slight of stature and unprotected by parents was to grow up a friendless, scrappy kid who got beaten up frequently. Young Peter Buniak's defense was to retreat to his fortified inner self.

Buniak's parents separated. His mother left Germany, and Peter remained in foster care. But by 1956 Sonia Buniak had moved to Toronto, remarried, and sent for her son. By 1965 Peter had discovered his fantastic talent for long-distance running. He made the Canadian squad for the Mexico City Olympics after a long and bitter struggle with the selectors—he had to break the Canadian record in the 10,000 meters and the marathon in special time trials to convince them of his worthiness—but he contracted dysentery and dropped out of the Olympic marathon. Everything came hard for Peter Buniak.

In March of 1969

> he startled friends and family with a bold symbolic act declaring his new identity to the world. He changed his name. By the stroke of a lawyer's pen he expunged his old name and became Jerome Drayton. . . . Buniak was not a name to which he had ever felt attached. For as long as he could remember, back to the hostile days of the German foster homes, it had been a liability. Even in Canada it marked him as an immigrant, something less than a full member of society. "Peter Who?" people would ask. He resented having to spell and pronounce it.

In October of 1969, with his new name, Drayton won the Motor City Marathon in Detroit by 15 minutes over the university professor, Ron Wallingford, in 2:12:00. That time got him his invitation to Fukuoka, where he beat Hill and became (perhaps) the best marathoner in the world. On a rainy day in Fukuoka Drayton took the lead going out of the stadium and never looked back.

Ron Hill would not let Jerome Drayton get away with that trick again. Hill planned to stick to Drayton. O'Reilly, the mathematician, calculated that Drayton would use the same fast starting tactic as he had in Fukuoka and that Hill would go with him, insuring a screaming pace. O'Reilly planned as Drayton's pace destroyed Hill, to keep Hill in sight, then go like hell on the hills. Moore planned the inverse—to go like hell on the downhills.

At the starting line Peter Lever, a Bolton Harrier like Ron Hill but now living in Toronto, delivered a bit of news to him. "Drayton tried for the 10-mile track world record 2 weeks ago and he dropped out after 4 miles."

"Oh," replied Hill, but he thought, Good news.

Looking about the starting line, Hill was surprised to see about 10 women set to run. Men and women did not race against each other in England. He saw Kenny Moore in a white vest lettered "Army" and noticed how youthful Moore looked. He saw Drayton in a yellow T-shirt, wearing race #2. Hill wore #1. After what seemed like ages to Hill, they were off. After they passed the usual fast starters, it was Drayton straight to the lead. Hill went after him as did a pack of Bob Moore (transplanted from Yorkshire, England, now of Canada), Kenny Moore, Pat McMahon (a transplanted Irishman now of the BAA and thus Jock Semple's hope), a couple of Japanese, Finnish Pentti Rummakko, and a few others. O'Reilly was one of them, but Hill had no idea who he was.

At a mile Drayton accelerated and Hill tucked in behind him. The others dropped behind. At 4 miles Hill felt Drayton ease off the pace. Instinctively, Hill took the lead to put the pressure on. Then suddenly he was alone. He could no longer hear Drayton behind him. The ease of it bewildered Hill. Four miles into a big marathon and he was alone and with an easy pace. It was curious. But at 6 miles Hill heard footsteps on the wet pavement. When the yellow T-shirt pulled into his peripheral vision, Hill knew Drayton was back. Hill thought this was odd; why let me go if he was just going to come back? But, feeling chipper, Hill turned to Drayton and joked, "Where have you been all my life?" Drayton said nothing.

By 7 miles the hard rain drove numbness into Hill's hands. When he raised them to his mouth to blow the exhaust of his breath on them his elbows ached from the cold. Yet the pace did not slow. In fact, it increased. Hill thought it was "bloody suicide." He wanted to tell Drayton so, but he had learned to keep his mouth shut.

At the Natick checkpoint, about 10.3 miles, a designation kept by tradition but useless to most runners because of its inaccuracy, Drayton's coach, Paul Poce, shouted, "The pace is fast; you're running fast and looking good!" Hill wondered if Drayton really looked good. He took a look and was not impressed. Just after that Drayton faltered a little on a rise. Hill moved ahead slightly, but he thought of the lonely 16 miles ahead, slowed, and waited for Drayton. "Are you OK?" Hill asked.

Drayton snapped back, "Yeah, I'm OK." But on the next hill he faltered again.

Meanwhile, O'Reilly kept Hill in sight. McMahon suffered a massive stitch and the heat drained from Kenny Moore's body. He ran too efficiently to keep warm. Far from his expectations of victory, he now felt hopeless.

Drayton walked as O'Reilly passed him. Drayton never appeared at the finish line. A green helicopter hovered overhead. Hill heard reports on the radios of spectators that he was a half mile ahead. How did they know? Of course, reports from the helicopter! Well, Hill thought, take no risks. He eased up the Newton hills, passing a legless racer in a wheelchair who wore a shirt reading "Jesus Saves." The wheelchair racer was Eugene Roberts, who had lost his legs to a land mine in Vietnam. He had been a 10:04 two-miler at Forest Park High School in Baltimore. He had started the marathon earlier and would finish just after six o'clock. He had not officially entered in a wheelchair division because none would exist for 5 more years. He said, "Praise the Lord!" or "Run for Jesus!" to Hill and later every other runner who passed. He had to finish, he explained later, because his brother was waiting with his artificial legs at the finish line.

The Japanese team felt as if their legs had stiffened to prosthetics in the cold. They ran poorly. Whereas Moore felt like hell on the hills, O'Reilly gave it hell on the hills. O'Reilly liked the rain. He felt refreshed. Or that is what he told himself to extract something positive from the misery of the hard running. By the crest of Heartbreak Hill he imagined he could reach out and touch the right shoulder of Ron Hill. The plan had worked! Now to hang on and kick.

Hill had heard Jock Semple shouting, "You're 2 minutes up on the record. Don't let up! You are 26 seconds up on O'Reilly and he's coming up on you."

Here history repeats: Like when old Kelley in 1936 had come up on Ellison Brown in the same way at the same spot, the arrival of the second man ignited a panic in the leader.

Hill thought, Christ, who the hell is O'Reilly? I never heard of him—O'Reilly? In his fatigued brain he began repeating, Old Mother Riley. Hill forced himself to run away. Propelled by fear, he jammed himself against that razor's edge when a cramp threatened to grab the back of his thighs.

O'Reilly had trained to go the distance and had trained his speed because he believed that it was a kicker's world. O'Reilly had arrived in position at the top of the hill. The spectators shouted, "It's all downhill from here." Hang on and kick, he told himself. It should be easy. O'Reilly followed along, a perfect predator, talons at the ready. Down the hill by Boston College and on past Lake Street, O'Reilly ran as a contender. Then just past Lake Street, the unevenness of a patch of bulldozer-scarred pavement triggered a cramp in his leg. The cramp would have come regardless of the footing. In a flicker O'Reilly was in, then out, talons or no talons. He could not stay close enough to use them. O'Reilly had to run defensively for second place. Should he charge forward and catch Hill again, risking getting the cramp and having to walk? Under the weight of his fatigue, second place did not look so bad.

Hill listened for the applause behind him, the sounds of clapping for Old Mother Riley. He could not hear it. He ran to keep his cramp at bay. Both men now ran as much against their own inner twitchings as against each other. Hill made the turn onto Hereford Street and on alone to Ring Road in front of the Prudential Center. At the line he snapped his fist above his head in a victory salute—take that, Old Mother Riley! Hill's time of 2:10:30 filled him with joy. He turned and waited to clap in O'Reilly, who congratulated Hill. They waited for the third-place runner. Suddenly they were no longer fighters but two cold, weary men. The cheering stopped. There was no public address system. For 3 minutes all was quiet, dark, cold, and wet.

At last, bearing down on the finish line ran Irishman McMahon and the tall Finn, Rummakko, the 8th and 10th men of 1969. They ran shoulder to shoulder with a few hundred yards to go. The cheers came back up. McMahon had outkicked Rummakko in the Wellesley 10-miler a few weeks earlier so expected to do it again, but now as McMahon accelerated, Rummakko would not fall back. He would not give up. It had been so easy to dust Rummakko in sprint at Wellesley, but now he would not unglue himself from McMahon's shoulder. It became clear to McMahon that this would come down to a chest-to-the-line finish; perhaps judges would even have to consult a photo timer line as in a 100-meter dash. A single image drummed

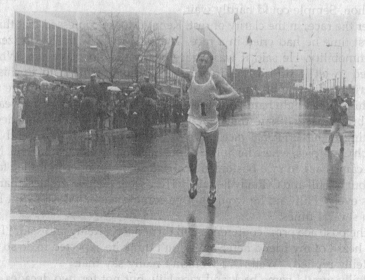

Ron Hill brings Boston Marathon performances straight into the contemporary with his 2:10:30 on a cold, raw day in 1970. Photo by Jeff Johnson.

in Rummakko's mind—the shining finish line. McMahon explained later that the Finn's tunnel vision was his undoing. With only a few yards to go they reached a crosswalk. It shined from the rain, and Rummakko saw its broad line across the blacktop as the official finish line. He wanted to beat McMahon and feel the end of this hardness and rain. Rummakko threw himself at the crosswalk. McMahon kept going the few yards to the real finish line and looked back at Rummakko, sprawled and bewildered on the pavement.

Pat McMahon, born in County Clare, had left Ireland because there were no jobs. He moved to London to work and took up running at age 21. His talent was not instantly apparent. His first race was an 880-yard handicap that he did not win. It took him 2:40. McMahon did run cross-country well enough to go to an international meet in Belgium, where he got the idea of going to college in America. He wrote to Fred Wilt, the FBI agent and author of *How They Train*, the book with illustrations by Hal Higdon. Wilt had run Boston himself back in 1956, placing 10th. Wilt put McMahon in touch with people at Oklahoma Baptist College. He got a teaching degree from there and moved to Boston, the mecca of road running and home to some of his relatives. Jock Semple promptly found him and signed him up for the BAA. Semple had a new BAA hope to win the marathon. McMahon promptly won a well-publicized 20-mile race and through the ensuing publicity was able to advertise that he needed a job. Within weeks he had a job teaching physical education in Lowell, Massachusetts. With the quota for Irish immigrants decreased, McMahon needed Congressman Tip O'Neill's help to get permanent residence, then citizenship. McMahon set about to win every New England road race he entered. The next year would be his big Boston Marathon. Semple could hardly wait.

After the race, in the clarity of rest, Kenny Moore confessed that this was the first time he had cried in a race. The sleet-filled wind had frozen him into immobility. He said it was a race he should not have run. When he planned to let it rip on the downhills, he did not mean to rip his own hamstrings. Coming off the Newton hills into the hard rain, he tore something high in his right hamstring that, when it healed, developed a weakness and abrasive scar tissue that plagued him for the next several decades, including in his 2:11:35.8 race the next December in Fukuoka and in the Munich Olympics, where he finished fourth, two places ahead of Hill. Moore never came back to race Boston and carried that reminder in his leg forever after, but of Hill and O'Reilly he said, "They were the two greatest marathon efforts ever." Hill said he would not be coming back to Boston, but he did return several times.

At the postrace press conference Hill turned to O'Reilly and said, "I really never heard of my friend here, and I don't think he expected to do so well." O'Reilly replied, "Well . . . I wouldn't really say that."

O'Reilly would come back and race Hill, but not for two decades.

1970 Men's Results

1. R. Hill, Cheshire, England	2:10:30^{CR}	
2. E. O'Reilly, *AthAC*	2:11:12	
3. P. McMahon, *BAA*	2:14:53	
4. P. Rummakko, Finland	2:14:59	
5. K. Hakkarainen, Finland	2:19:42	
6. K. Moore, *OTC*	2:19:47	
7. R. Moore, *TOC*	2:20:07	
8. A. Boychuk, Toronto, ON	2:21:06	
9. W. Clark, *PP*	2:22:17	

1. **R. Hill, Cheshire, England**   2:10:30^{CR}
2. E. O'Reilly, *AthAC*   2:11:12
3. P. McMahon, *BAA*   2:14:53
4. P. Rummakko, Finland   2:14:59
5. K. Hakkarainen, Finland   2:19:42
6. K. Moore, *OTC*   2:19:47
7. R. Moore, *TOC*   2:20:07
8. A. Boychuk, Toronto, ON   2:21:06
9. W. Clark, *PP*   2:22:17
10. W. Yetman, *TOC*   2:22:32
11. G. Harrison, *VOS*   2:23:18
12. E. Walkowitz, *MPAA*   2:23:26
13. K. Ragg, *HTC*   2:23:45
14. W. Speck, *PC*, RI   2:24:43
15. R. Deines, Oakland, CA   2:24:50
16. **A. Burfoot, *CConnAA***   **2:25:27**
17. K. Fujita, Yamaguchi, Japan   2:25:50
18. H. Balthis, Jr., *DTF*   2:27:29
19. S. Dean, *SSC*   2:27:37
20. J. Garcia, Gaspar, Mexico   2:27:42
21. R. Perez, Costa Rica   2:28:06
22. J. Colvin, *SC*   2:28:09
23. M. Mayfield, Jr., *PP*   2:28:14
24. F. Best, *CJTC*   2:28:20
25. V. Yehnert, *ARR*   2:28:27
26. P. Stipe, *BAA*   2:28:31
27. D. Cole, *PA*   2:28:35
28. G. Muhrcke, *MillAA*   2:28:37
29. J. McDonaugh, *MillAA*   2:28:49
30. S. Adams, *NCTC*   2:29:09

31. T. Derderian, *NMC*   2:29:57
32. R. Will, ON   2:30:08
33. G. Williams, Washington, DC   2:30:23
34. J. Leydig, *WVTC*, CA   2:30:52
35. P. Ryan, *BAA*   2:31:07
36. J. Mowatt, *TOC*   2:31:14
37. K. Mueller, *BAA*   2:31:16
38. W. Harvey, *NYPC*   2:31:27
39. P. Bernstein, *BAA*   2:31:47
40. L. Paul, *CSU*   2:31:57
41. G. Teal, ON   2:32:00
42. N. Coville, *MFA*   2:32:21
43. L. Fuselier, LA   2:32:27
44. K. Kling, *SJTC*   2:32:34
45. E. Walther, *SABC*   2:32:38
46. V. Lopez, Guatemala   2:32:44
47. R. Daws, *TCTC*   2:33:04
48. C. Hereford, *NCTC*   2:33:09
49. C. Cuque, Guatemala   2:33:31
50. A. Haas, CA   2:33:35
55. K. Uchino, Hiroshima, Japan   2:34:53
63. **J.J. Kelley, *BAA***   **2:36:50**
65. A. Massaquoi, *BAA*   2:37:10
66. J. Pagliano, *STC*, CA   2:37:17
68. T. Fleming, *WPC*, NJ   2:37:36
71. L. Berman, *CSU*   2:38:03
74. R. Thurston, Washington, DC   2:38:29
163. **J.A. Kelley**   **3:03:00**
      T. Leonard   3:18:00

1,173 entrants, 1,011 starters.

A COLD AND LONELY WOMAN

MONDAY, APRIL 20, 1970

Gals to Show a Little Leg in Marathon

As Sara Mae Berman finished running the Boston Marathon in the same cold, hard rain as a thousand men and well ahead of the other four unofficial women runners, a big, fat, male reporter stuck a microphone in her face and asked, "Why did you do it?" Even if she had not been tired and cold his question would have annoyed her. As if she had just committed a crime, he asked her why she did it. He did not ask that of any of the men who had just finished the race. To Berman the questioner represented an attitude displayed by too many reporters and broadcasters, who either patronized women runners or treated them as freaks. She remembered headlines referring to "girls," puns about "figures" in the marathon, and requests for cheesecake photos ("Show a little more leg, gals"). One headline read "Housewife Wins Race." She thought, You'd never read "Husband Wins Race" in a headline! She thought of the photo of Bobbi Gibb after her race in 1966, at home making fudge. The photographer had to follow her home to be sure to get her back in the kitchen. "Why did you do it?" As Berman sought to get warm, she rolled the reporter's question over and over in her mind. Why *did* she do it?

In the race itself, cold gave her the biggest problem. Her hands suffered from the near-freezing rain. She needed gloves. About halfway through she begged a pair off fellow runner Julian Segal. Her hands had stiffened to uselessness, so she had to use her teeth to pull the gloves on. She never saw another female runner during the race as she ran with various male acquaintances or with members of her club, the Cambridge Sports Union.

Sara Mae Berman, born in 1936, attended high school in Manchester, New Hampshire, and graduated from the Rhode Island School of Design in 1958 with a degree in interior design. At the time of her Boston Marathon running she had three children and a husband named Larry. He ran long-distance races before they married in 1955 and interested Sara Mae in the sport. The idea of running would never have occurred to her otherwise. At first she tried to be a sprinter, or rather she had to be a sprinter because the only competitive running events open to women were no longer than 220 yards. She was a bad sprinter. Then in *Life* magazine Berman read about Julia Chase, whom officials barred from running in the Thanksgiving Day road race in Manchester, Connecticut. Chase ran regardless.

Sara Mae Berman ran her first long-distance race in Marlboro, Massachusetts, in 1964. It was a 5-mile handicap race. She was the first woman in Massachusetts to show up to run such a long event. She felt strange, a young matron (age 28) with three children in the care of a baby-sitter, wearing shorts in the middle of the city. But the men in the race smoothed the way for her with encouragement and helpfulness. She started on the scratch line, the one reserved for the slowest of runners, along with old Fred Brown, one-armed Siggy Podlozny, and some little boys. She ran 38:37.

Two years later with mixed feelings Berman watched Bobbi Gibb run in the Boston Marathon. She was pleased that Gibb showed "those old fuddy duddies" in the BAA officialdom that a woman could run long distances, but she was disappointed that she had not done it first.

By 1969 Berman trained 60 miles a week and regularly ran New England road races. She usually beat half the men in a given field. Jock Semple frequently saw her at these races and considered her a fixture, so it did not disturb him to see her on the starting line in Hopkinton. Of course she wore

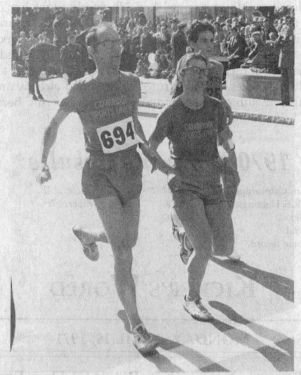

Three-time first-place female winner Sara Mae Berman, shown here finishing the 1969 race with her husband, Larry, was asked by a fat reporter after the 1970 race why she ran, but he didn't ask the same question of the 1,173 male racers. Photo by Jeff Johnson.

no number to ignite his temper. She did, as she later said, "stay out of his face" on race day, but she believed that what infuriated Semple about women in the marathon was that they appeared to be strangers to the sport, using it only to make a feminist statement—like marplots, those people who join organizations in order to change them. But Semple saw Berman as one who had paid her dues to running by showing up at the little races.

When Sara Mae Berman reached Kenmore Square, Larry, having finished his race, jogged back to meet her and run in with her. But just past the finish line they lost each other. Although women were not official entrants, the BAA had taken pains to reserve a place for them. Officials directed Berman to the special area.

The top men took hot showers in the Prudential locker room before moving next door for their traditional bowl of beef stew. They filed through the employee cafeteria, where they ate as much as they wished. The women, in contrast, could use the ice-skating changing room, a cold room of nothing but lockers and benches. Berman rested on a bench for an hour. No one came to collect her. No one joined her. No one brought her dry clothes, warm food, or anything to drink. Larry had no idea where Sara had gone.

As she waited cold, lonely, hungry, and thirsty on the hard wooden bench, she thought more about that fat reporter's question: Why did she do it? Why did she suffer miles of hills and cold, not to mention all the daily training and the weekend 15-mile runs? But she had already answered the question with something better than words—with her run: Because I am a woman and because I can.

1970 Women's Results*

1. S. Berman, Cambridge, MA	3:05:07^{CR**}	4. D. Fournier, ME	3:32:00
2. N. Kuscsik, S. Huntington, NY	3:12:16	5. K. Switzer, NY	3:34:00
3. S. Zerrangi	3:30:00		

*Results unofficial.
**Unofficial course record.

KICKER'S WORLD

MONDAY, APRIL 19, 1971

Irish Runner Favored in Patriots' Day Footrace

Pat McMahon held the vision of the finish line of the Boston Marathon in his mind as he lined up to race from Hopkinton on a hot April day in 1971. He knew the course well. When he closed his eyes he could see the entire playing field, a yard wide and 26.2 miles long. He especially knew the turn from Commonwealth Avenue to Hereford Street and the little rise and swing to the last downhill shot over Ring Road for the finish line in front of the Prudential Center. He had beaten Pentti Rummakko in 1970 by knowing that finish so well. If it came down to it, he could do it again. It looked to McMahon as if it would. Hill did not come back. Burfoot was not in top form because of his tour with the Peace Corps in El Salvador. O'Reilly was injured. Moore nursed bad memories of Boston. The Boston press had ignored the winner of March's Burlingame, California, marathon, Alvaro Mejia (2:17:22.2). The reporters didn't know who he was and did not pick him as the favorite. They chose McMahon.

But McMahon knew of this Colombian, Mejia, from the pre-Olympic 10,000 meters in Mexico City in 1966. McMahon was there; he saw Mejia, a 4:04 miler, win that race against some highly regarded runners, including the world record holder, Ron Clarke. Mejia was a deadly fast 10,000-meter man moving up to a marathon. McMahon knew that meant trouble. McMahon himself had run 2:18:47.4 in February, so he knew he was ready. At last he had money, a job, and time. Mejia, on the other hand, had only time. He had lost his job as a metal spinner in California and simply ran a lot. He had married American Olympic swimmer Terri Stickles after he had met her in Colombia, where she worked as a Peace Corps volunteer. They had had a son in mid-February. He had a job offer back in his native Bogotá, Colombia, as an administrator. But it was the Boston Marathon that needed an administrator.

The BAA field had grown too big to handle. More than a thousand runners taxed the BAA's system to its limit. It certainly taxed Jock Semple to his limit. The prerace phone calls frazzled him. He tried to do therapeutic massage on athletes in his "salon de rubdown" at the Boston Garden, where he attended to Bruins hockey players and Celtics basketball players. But the tiny room with its wall covered by framed photos of athletes also served as the BAA office. The phone would ring and Semple would answer, "So you want to run the marathon? Where are you calling from? Your home? Good-bye." He had no tolerance for those he considered to be fools.

On race day he lost his civility. In 1970 BAA rule #3 attempted to free the field of interlopers, of unprepared runners:

> A runner must submit the certification of either the Long Distance Running chairman of the AAU of his district or his college coach that he has trained sufficiently to finish the course in less than four hours: This is not a jogging race.

But they interloped anyway. Coaches and pseudocoaches freely signed certifications. In 1970 1,173 runners entered, the year before, 1,342, but this year new qualifying standards limited the field to 1,011 entries. Semple received dubious entries, argued with the hopefuls, and ultimately accepted them. In spite of his exasperation he did have a soft spot for marathoners. Will Cloney had a soft spot for the marathon too. He did not collect a salary for his administration of the race; he made his living at first as a newspaper reporter and a journalism teacher at Northeastern University and later as a public relations officer for a financial firm. He called the marathon a labor of love, but he said love affairs pay off in more ways than money.

The new qualifying times required a runner to have run a marathon in under 3-1/2 hours or in the last year to have run 10 miles in 65:00 or better, 15 miles in 1:45, or 20 miles in 2:30. Of all the entries, Semple had no doubt about who would win: It would be Pat McMahon of the BAA.

Hal Higdon came to Boston for a party celebrating the publishing of his new book, *On the Run from Dogs and People*. Much of the book was about the Boston Marathon, so this Patriots' Day was a good time to introduce it. Higdon explained his addiction to the Boston Marathon: "Every runner wants to come here at least once before he dies. . . . It is sort of an ego trip. It is one place where people line the streets to see you; you feel loved, wanted." Another runner and author, Erich Segal (who wrote the novel *Love*

Story) expressed his love of the marathon: "for me running is a spiritual affirmation." Higdon had almost won the race in 1964, but now he was in shape only enough to complete the course respectably. Segal at his best barely broke 3 hours, yet now as a wealthy, famous, and undertrained man, he felt as compelled as Higdon to run again and subject himself to the indignity of racing beneath his abilities. Higdon said about his dropping out one year that he had to live with the fact that he quit as if it were a prison record. Segal not only ran slowly and in distress, but during the race he had to put up with comments from spectators critical of his writing. As he slogged along the lowest blow was "Hey, Segal, you run better than you write."

Early in the 1971 race, in Ashland, Finnish Markku Salminen (2:16:36 in Mantsala, Finland, in March) ran ahead of everyone as he burst out to a 70-yard lead. No one went with him. McMahon and Mejia waited. It looked as if it would be a hot day. By Framingham Mejia's West Valley Track Club teammate, Bill Clark, who had finished second in 1968 to Burfoot, took the lead with a slow pace. Another Finn, Seppo Nikkari (2:16:35.4 in Mantsala), waited in the pack with recent graduates John Vitale from the University of Connecticut, Art Coolidge from Ohio's Kent State, and Byron Lowry from San Jose State in California. The Japanese had not sent a team. Except for 30-year-olds McMahon and Mejia, it was a young pack. There was such a growing interest in marathon racing among college runners that there was serious talk about instituting an intercollegiate (NCAA) national marathon championship. Vitale had run a 2-mile in 8:48, so he had the speed to stay with this group. He thought that if Burfoot could win, why couldn't he?

In fact it was Burfoot who had planted the idea of winning the Boston Marathon in Vitale's head. Early in 1968 the two, friends who had frequently competed against each other in college, went on a training run on the University of Connecticut campus. Burfoot told Vitale that he would not be running in the UConn vs. Wesleyan meet because he would be running in the Boston Marathon. Vitale listened but made no comment. As Burfoot explained his training, Vitale began to sense from his tone of voice and excitement that not only did Burfoot intend to run, but he intended to win. That a Connecticut college student could be the first American to win the Boston Marathon since Kelley 11 years earlier seemed a little unlikely to Vitale, but he listened politely as they ran along. Of course Burfoot did win in 1968, and again Vitale said nothing; he began to train for a marathon.

He had never run a marathon, but his coach, Bob Giegengack of Yale, who had coached Frank Shorter, promised Will Cloney that Vitale would finish in the top five. Cloney, although dubious, let Vitale into the race without a qualifying time.

Vitale pushed his hopes into play at 17 miles as he led the pack. The hills and the heat killed off Nikkari and he dropped out. But as the miles rolled past, Vitale did not have the strength of the older men. His eagerness left him. The hills and the heat squashed Vitale's hopes, too. He had to give up the lead and let it wait for another year. But he would not drop out, and he would not let the fifth-place man pass him. The hills disintegrated the pack. By their peak only McMahon and Mejia remained.

They suffered. Mejia looked for puddles to run through to cool his feet. He wore a wrinkled black outfit and looked out with sad eyes over a sweaty moustache. McMahon's feet suffered, too, as his socks and shoes raised bloody blisters. He quietly cursed himself for wearing stupid shoes and stupid socks. Both men ran with feet a bloody mess. McMahon saw ahead his nightmare of another sprint to the finish. He'd rather not have to do that, so he pushed as hard as he dared up the hill. Mejia stuck to him. The sudden-death duel was set. It would come down to a sprint—two men sprinting and grinding their feet into hamburger. The two men ran shoulder to shoulder in the bright sun, each looking at the shadow of the other on the road ahead. They raced each other, yet they shared sponges to wash the salt off their necks. McMahon knew that Mejia under most circumstances would have a better kick, but the end of a marathon has a way of dissolving kicks, and McMahon knew the snakey configuration of the last two turns. He saw a dotted line in the map of his mind of how he would cut from the inside turn onto Hereford Street and kick hard before Mejia could see the finish line. McMahon planned to open a sudden gap up the little incline, then with the advantage of space and surprise, angle to the last corner and be gone down the little swoop to the tape before Mejia could respond. McMahon set himself to do exactly that, with every detail vivid in his mind.

At the turn onto Hereford Street McMahon put his plan into action. He sprinted. But, in the road, dead in front of him, was a screaming crowd of spectators. They stood exactly where he planned to run. The line of cheering people along Hereford Street had bellied out into the middle of the road, changing the straight road into a reverse curve and covering the straight dotted line McMahon held in his mind's eye. He could not run where he had planned to. In his fatigue he was inflexible. Like Rummakko in 1970, who dove for a crosswalk thinking it was the finish line, McMahon was a prisoner of his preconceptions. He hesitated. He lost the element of surprise. Mejia seized the moment and the momentum and reached the crest of the little hill first. From there he could see his clear shot to victory. He took it and hit it dead on.

Observers at the finish line, looking into the glare of the western sun, saw McMahon in his light colors first. Mejia seemed to materialize out of thin air and shadows from the camouflage of his dark clothes against the dark crowd until at the last moments observers could distinguish motion. All the crowd could tell was that two men ran very close to each other. Then they could see that the dark one was running slightly ahead, sprinting madly.

Mejia and McMahon sprinted in the closest-ever finish of the Boston Marathon—only 5 seconds apart. The loss disappointed McMahon but did not devastate him. He understood the nature of sport and loved to compete, and he believed there would be another day. Always before defeat had

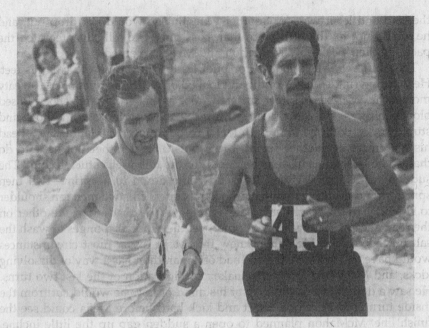

Pat McMahon and Alvaro Mejia suffer together in the heat of 1971. Photo by Jeff Johnson.

made him train harder, made him improve and race more effectively. He thought it would be no different this time. He would be back, he thought, and be back faster.

But Pat McMahon never raced Boston again. In fact, he never raced anything again. A series of injuries culminating in a chronic sciatica prevented him from training. He remained a member of the BAA, continued teaching physical education in Lowell, and coached and helped the club manage things on marathon day, but the Boston Marathon of 1971 was his last race.

Vitale, however, placing fourth in his debut marathon, saw that all he needed was just a little more strength. He quietly set out to get it. He wanted to be the American who beat these foreigners.

Checkpoint Splits		
Framingham	Bill Clark	33:12
Natick	Pat McMahon	52:33
Wellesley	Pat McMahon	1:08:18
Woodland	John Vitale	time unrecorded
Lake Street	Pat McMahon	1:53:46
Coolidge Corner	Pat McMahon	2:06:51

1971 Men's Results

1.	A. Mejia, *WVTC*	2:18:45	30.	J. Brennand, CA	2:32:21
2.	P. McMahon, *BAA*	2:18:50	31.	C. Keating, Natick, MA	2:32:27
3.	J. Halverstadt, *OS*/South Africa	2:22:23	32.	A. Massaquoi, *BAA*	2:32:55
4.	J. Vitale, *NHTC*	2:22:45	33.	R. Ashley, *RTC*	2:33:09
5.	B. Lowry, *SFOC*	2:23:20	34.	J. McDonaugh, *MillAA*	2:33:14
6.	A. Coolidge, *BAA*	2:23:23	35.	A. Taylor, ON	2:33:34
7.	W. Speck, *PC*	2:23:54	36.	G. Peal, ON	2:33:48
8.	M. Salminen, Finland	2:24:02	37.	G. Harrison, Vancouver, BC	2:34:00
9.	R. Wallingford, ON	2:25:21	38.	W. Harvey, *NYPC*	2:34:49
10.	B. Clark, *WVTC*	2:26:19	**39.**	**A. Burfoot, *CConnAA***	**2:35:11**
11.	J. Galloway, *FTC*	2:26:35	40.	E. Horst, *CVAC*	2:35:29
12.	**J. Fultz, *USCG***	**2:27:12**	41.	M. Staw, CA	2:35:45
13.	R. Bayko, *NMC*	2:27:37	42.	W. Renaud, ME	2:36:14
14.	J. Gubbins, *GU*	2:28:03	43.	E. Ayres, VA	2:36:14
15.	F. Best, *CJTC*	2:28:24	44.	W. Van Dyke, *CSU*	2:36:26
16.	M. Ande, *OccC*	2:28:27	45.	T. Osler, *PennAC*	2:36:40
17.	A. Calle, Colombia	2:28:31	46.	J. Howell, *WVTC*	2:36:47
18.	J. Lesch, *UC*	2:28:50	47.	C. Lopez, Guatemala	2:36:56
19.	R. Kochan, *US*	2:28:53	48.	R. Will, *TOC*	2:37:22
20.	R. Fitts, *MillAA*	2:29:15	49.	R. Crow, *WVTC*	2:37:25
21.	P. Stipe, *BAA*	2:30:08	50.	E. Walther, *SABC*	2:37:39
22.	P. Thompson, *NMC*	2:30:23	64.	J. Green, *BAA*	2:39:17
23.	K. Mueller, *BAA*	2:30:38	70.	N. Weygandt, *PennAC*	2:40:02
24.	M. Alonso, NY	2:31:02	94.	H. Higdon, *DTC*	2:43:56
25.	O. Atkins, *STC*	2:31:07	**96.**	**J.J. Kelley, *BAA***	**2:44:10**
26.	S. Adams, *NCTC*	2:31:21	100.	C. Fortier, *NMC*	2:44:54
27.	T. Ratliffe, *MillAA*, NY	2:31:30	210.	B. Squires, *BS*	2:57:51
28.	R. Thurston, *WSC*	2:32:07		**J.A. Kelley**	**3:45:47**
29.	J. Mowatt, *TOC*	2:32:19			

1,011 entrants, 877 starters, 588 under 3:30.

Team prize
BAA: P. McMahon, A. Coolidge, P. Stipe

SHE ROLLS SEVENS

MONDAY, APRIL 19, 1971

A Few Girls to Run in Today's Marathon

When a high school boy saw a woman dressed to run but without a number slinking around the starting line of a New England road race, he poked his older buddy. "Hey, who's that?" "That's Sara Mae Berman. She's pretty good." Fear seized the high school boy's heart. "How good?" "She rolls sevens." [Long pause.] "What do we roll?" "We roll sixes." "Oh, uh, OK."

Heads turned when Sara Mae Berman showed up at races. Her husband, Larry, who had gotten her started running races, said she would be a pioneer. So she was—and a troublemaker too.

At the Claremont, New Hampshire, 10-miler officials presented Berman with roses at the finish line. That was fine recognition for a pioneer. Yet in another race she passed a barroom in the company of a pack of men running halfway deep in the field of runners. A bunch of "beer bellies," as she called them, rumbled out of the dark to squint and shout at the passing runners. As Berman passed they yelled bad things at her—the kind of things drunken men yell at passing women—and in reaction the men in Berman's pack peeled off to go fight the drunks. She persuaded them not to go fight because it would hurt their overall times. She felt well protected running in a convoy of men who understood and accepted what she was doing. The trouble she made was not with her fellow runners. It was nonrunners, drunken or otherwise, who became enraged at the sight of a woman in a man's race.

The sport of running lends a clear understanding to the winners and the losers that a runner who is beaten by another, man or woman, had a simple recourse. You would have won except you got tired and slowed down. No argument. No referee's call to dispute. Men who were beaten by a woman understood what had happened and had no argument. Running competitors understand one another and accept the differences in performance. A race is as much cooperation as competition.

> *To give women official numbers and allow them to run with the men would threaten the entrenched bureaucracy.*

Sara Mae Berman and her "co-conspirators," adult women long-distance runners, caused serious dissension with the AAU administrative and coaching establishment. Used to coaching pliable girls, the men didn't know what to make of these troublesome ladies. They wouldn't do what they were told as would the teenage females who had heretofore comprised the national teams for cross-country and track. They did not fit into the hierarchy of the AAU club system, where the coach with the winningest girls got to go on international trips as an official of the AAU. Teenagers needed chaperones on team trips to other countries; adult women did not. Berman, with children of her own, did look conspicuous competing in a sport that had been restricted to girls. Yet no one suggested that the sport be limited to participation by teenage males. As Berman saw it, AAU officials feared losing their power and their perks to full-fledged women athletes. To give women official numbers and allow them to run with the men would threaten the entrenched bureaucracy. Berman saw the drive to get women marathoners official recognition as a basic struggle for power.

A primal power struggle played itself out at the crest of Heartbreak Hill when, for the first time in the short history of women running the Boston Marathon, two women raced each other in the latter stages of the race. Berman had been leading when suddenly Nina Kuscsik swept past her and on to a 60-yard lead by Cleveland Circle. Berman said to herself, My God, 21 miles and suddenly this has become a race. She had been content to run her pace and push one foot in front of the other at the rate her physiology allowed. She did not want to be rushed; however, official or not, this was a race. Berman surged in response.

She caught Kuscsik on Beacon Street and squeaked past her. Berman won by about 30 seconds to a minute. Because the women's race was not official, no exact time has been preserved.

Only three women started and finished the 1971 Boston Marathon. Berman, Kuscsik, and Kathrine Switzer began immediately afterward to agitate for official inclusion of women in long-distance races. A strong bond grew among these and the few other women involved in long-distance racing. In fact, an unwritten pact among them required that as a matter of honor they enter a marathon only if they were fit enough to finish well. They felt that the AAU was looking for an excuse—like a woman dropping out of a race, or worse yet collapsing, and worst of all being photographed doing so—to continue to ban women from long-distance racing for their own good and the good of future generations. A patronizing attitude presumed that a woman's womb was societal property and had to be preserved as such.

A ban against women's running longer distances had occurred in 1928 when spectators saw women runners in the Olympic 800 meters collapse in exhaustion. This event for women did not return to the Olympic Games until 1960. These women marathon pioneers acutely understood that images of exhausted males, giving their all to try to win, were heroic, yet such symbols for women did not yet exist and could in fact be detrimental to their efforts to being accepted as competitors in the sport of long-distance running.

On May 30 Berman went on to set a world best in the marathon with a 3:00:35 clocking in a marathon in Brockton, Massachusetts.

*1971 Women's Results**

1. S. Berman, *CSU*	3:08:30	3. K. Switzer	3:28
2. N. Kuscsik, NY	3:09		

*Results unofficial.

FINNISH PRECISION

MONDAY, APRIL 17, 1972

Mexicans, Finn to Race Today; No Top Americans

At the last minute Alvaro Mejia decided to jump on an airplane and come to Boston to defend his title. He came with some other Colombians, mostly because he was the only one of the group who could speak English. Victor Mora was one of his companions. He had never finished a marathon but had dropped out of a race in Colombia at 9,000 feet of altitude at 15 miles. He had a respect for marathons, so he started slowly. He would hang back with Mejia, who was not as fit as he had been but could not stay away. Mora was the fastest and most talented runner in the field, but his fear of the distance seemed to force a tactical mistake.

Old Don Heinicke from Maryland came back to run his 30th Boston Marathon. Ted Corbitt, Orville Atkins, Gar Williams, Kurt Steiner, and Arnie Briggs all had run over 20 times at Boston. John A. Kelley was back for his 41st marathon. All this attention to the Boston Marathon brought some controversy about the accuracy of the course.

How Short Is It?

Discussion arose about the accuracy of the course that these men ran on. To stop the speculation some local runners had set out to measure it with the latest degree of accuracy. Precision had not been important in the early years of marathon running, but more and more frequently course lengths were being questioned. If someone ran a good time, listeners commented, "How short was it?" The Boston course distances had changed by design or accident over the years:

1897 to 1923	24 miles, 1,232 yards
1924 to 1926	26 miles, 209 yards
1927 to 1950	26 miles, 385 yards
1951 to 1956	as short as 25 miles, 962 yards
1957 to present	26 miles, 385 yards

In 1972 literature about the Boston Marathon said that the course started at 220 feet elevation, dropped to 50, went back to 220 again at the crest of Heartbreak Hill, then descended to near sea level at the finish. A group of area runners, John Booras of Winthrop and Larry and Sara Mae Berman and Rick Levy of Cambridge refuted that statement by a careful study of topographic maps and altimeter readings, which revealed that the net drop in elevation was not 210 feet, but over twice that—about 480 feet. Levy wrote,

> What I did was consult US Geological Survey maps of the entire course. My altimeter readings cover the last 10 miles. The starting line is at 491 feet above sea-level, the finish only 10-15 feet. The course then has a downward tendency that would help account for fast times to the first checkpoint (6.72 miles) [they used odd, traditional checkpoints in those days whose reported exact distance kept changing instead of the now standard kilometer and mile marks], if not all the way. Sorry if this contributes to the de-mystification of the Boston Marathon!

Booras and the Bermans had measured the course in 1967 for AAU certification. They found the total course distance to be 26.27 miles, not the standard 26.22. Levy calculated that the course was long by about 15 seconds at a 5:00 per mile pace. The course was downhill and by much more than runners and officials had thought. No one seriously suggested running it in the other direction.

But technicalities did not matter to the men while they raced. The year before John Vitale had taken a taste of the lead. This year he swallowed it whole. He led in Wellesley under perfect running conditions—clear sky, no wind, 50 °F. His time of 1:06:56 felt good, easy, and relaxed. At times he had a 300-yard lead. With ease he had won his last marathon in Connecticut over a hilly course with no competition. Now he wanted to push the pace and run away from any potential kickers.

In November Norm Higgins had run a 2:15:21 personal best at Culver City, California. He was now 36 years old. This would be his last chance to

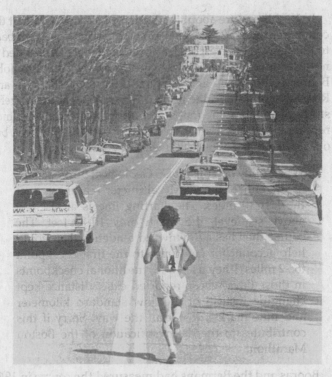

There's fear, panic, and glory when you leave the comfort of the pack, as John Vitale does in 1972. You can't see your competitors, but each contender can draw a bead on the back of your head like a sharpshooter. Photo by Jeff Johnson.

win at Boston. Higgins was back living in New London, Connecticut, working as a door-to-door Fuller Brush salesman. He lived alone in an apartment with little but a mattress on the floor. Higgins had dedicated himself to the task of sculpting his body to squeeze out every drop of ability to help him run 26 miles. With his gray hair and the slack-jawed strain on his face, he looked ghostly as he ran through Framingham. He sweated profusely, running in a trance behind Vitale. For Higgins it was now or never. Vitale could hear Higgins making various effort-filled noises.

Olavi Suomalainen of Finland waited back a distance too. He was small and fair, with straight blond hair spilling over his ears. This was his first marathon. He was an engineer by schooling, and with an engineer's love of precision and control he had measured every aspect of his training. Food, sleep, training distances, and pace were all planned and recorded. He wore two pairs of socks and jammed his feet into tight racing shoes. He knew that movement allowed friction to generate heat that raised the blisters. He would not allow any unplanned movement to occur. Suomalainen ran comfortably and did not sweat.

Jacinto Sabinal, Alfredo Penaloza, and Pablo Garrido, all swarthy Mexicans in red, raced in the lead pack. Penaloza and Garrido had been to Boston before, in 1968 and 1969. Sabinal was new. He pursued Vitale. Just before the downhill into Newton Lower Falls, Sabinal passed Vitale and seized a 50-yard lead. Suomalainen carefully moved closer, passed Vitale and two Mexicans, and moved up the hill. Vitale had been seduced by the ease of the downhill first miles. Again the course rejected him. He lapsed into survival pace.

Suomalainen ratcheted his climb, clicking off the yards as he cranked his way closer to Sabinal. At the top of the hill, at Boston College, Suomalainen pulled even. At that moment the press bus passed. It was too close. Suomalainen feared that he would fall under the giant wheels. As each tried to avoid the bus, the runners collided. Both staggered off-balance and held the other up so neither fell. Danger avoided in a moment of instinctive camaraderie, they got on with the race.

On the hills Victor Mora realized that he'd better get moving. It had been a mistake to stay with Mejia, who was having a bad day. He passed Higgins. He passed Vitale. Ahead Mora could see the light Finn and the dark Mexican. He put his great speed to task and chased them. He had beaten Ron Hill and Mamo Wolde in the San Blas half-marathon in Puerto Rico (1:04:22). He had the speed, but fear had kept him from contention. Mora sped through sub-5-minute miles. If the race lasted long enough he would catch the Finn. He flickered past Sabinal. Mora ran the last 2.2 miles in 10:40. But the race ended too soon for him to catch Suomalainen, who charged the finish line yarn, grabbed it with his hands and—not carefully, not precisely, not meticulously—ripped it apart.

Ten minutes later a big guy finished. He was the son of a 6'2", 235-pound former Chicago Bears tackle. The son stood 6'1/2" and weighed only 145 pounds. His name was Tom Fleming. On the wall of his room hung this sign: *Somewhere in the world there is someone training when you are not. When you race him, he will win.*

1972 Men's Results

1.	O. Suomalainen, Finland	2:15:39	12.	C. Hatfield, WVTC	2:22:07
2.	V. Mora, Colombia	2:15:57	13.	T. Hoffman, UCTC	2:22:19
3.	J. Sabinal, Mexico	2:16:10	14.	J. Vitale, NHTC	2:22:57
4.	A. Penaloza, Mexico	2:18:46	15.	H. Barreneche, Colombia	2:22:58
5.	P. Garrido, Mexico	2:19:50	16.	R. Thurston, WSC	2:23:03
6.	B. Mortenson, RTC	2:19:59	17.	J. Gubbins, GU	2:23:28
7.	J. Galloway, FTC	2:20:03	18.	R. Bayko, NMC	2:23:32
8.	A. Mejia, WVTC	2:20:06	19.	G. Hayes, NCTC	2:23:51
9.	S. Dean, Sacramento, CA	2:20:29	20.	L. Fidler, FurTC	2:24:49
10.	M. Salminen, Finland	2:20:42	21.	J. Mowatt, TOC	2:24:53
11.	D. Tibaduiza, Colombia	2:21:58	22.	J. Leydig, WVTC	2:25:15

23.	T. Fleming, *WPC*	2:25:26	39. J. Green, *BAA*	2:29:58
24.	J. McDevitt, Jr., *WVTC*	2:25:28	40. M. Sabino, *BOC*	2:30:07
25.	M. White, *BAA*	2:25:31	41. J. Witkowski, *CJTC*	2:30:13
26.	T. Derderian, *NMC*	2:26:06	42. K. Mueller, *BAA*	2:30:41
27.	B. Hannula, *MT*	2:26:09	43. L. Seethaler, *PennAC*	2:31:03
28.	N. Higgins, New London, CT	2:26:14	44. M. Graham, *US*	2:31:08
29.	P. Stipe, *BAA*	2:26:53	45. D. Fish, *OH*	2:31:37
30.	R. Wayne, *BAA*	2:27:02	46. W. Renaud, *MA*	2:32:12
31.	R. Tadeo, Mexico	2:27:18	47. D. Anderson, *HdC*	2:32:31
32.	D. Kennedy, Fort Benning, GA	2:27:33	48. G. Teal, *ON*	2:32:51
33.	R. Wallingford, *LUTC*	2:27:53	49. P. Ryan, *BAA*	2:33:38
34.	P. Pearson, *TOC*	2:28:08	50. G. Williams, *WSC*	2:33:44
35.	P. Thompson, *NMC*	2:28:25	**79. J.J. Kelley, *BAA***	**2:40:05**
36.	D. Brown, *RTC*	2:28:29	168. T. Corbitt, *NYPC*	2:49:51
37.	C. Coeppen, IN	2:28:34	J.A. Kelley	3:35:12
38.	A. Williams, CT	2:28:39		

1,220 entrants, 1,081 starters.

Team prize

1. North Medford Club:
   R. Bayko, T. Derderian, P.
   Thompson

2. BAA: M. White, P. Stipe, R.
   Wayne

WOMEN, OFFICIAL AT LAST

MONDAY, APRIL 17, 1972

BAA Bows to Ladies

The AAU at last decreed that women could *sort of* run in marathons. On February 2, 1972, Pat Rico, the women's track-and-field chairman, wrote to Will Cloney, "The women cannot start with or run against the men." She suggested that the women start an hour or a half hour before so as to create in effect a separate event. But such an addition would not be really the same thing as running in *the* Boston Marathon. A month later Aldo Scandurra, a frequent competitor at Boston and an AAU official, wrote to Cloney with his ideas about women running in the Boston Marathon. Bob Campbell of New England, Ken Foreman of Seattle, and Dr. Nell Jackson from the midwest had all attended a meeting at Lake Placid, New York, the previous October at which at last the principle of women starting at the same time as men and on the same starting line was accepted as a women's race if the women were scored separately for place and for prize. Regardless of the contradictions and controversies, the BAA opened the marathon to women.

Actually, the BAA said that "special women" could run its marathon—those who met the new men's qualifying time of 3:30. Half a dozen special women qualified to run the first official women's section of the Boston

Is It OK for Grown Women to Run?

In her early adult life Nina Kuscsik felt guilty about competing in ice-skating races and bicycling races because the prevailing expectation was that adults must spend their time
engaged in serious things, not sports. Only when President
Kennedy supported 50-mile hikes did she feel that it was
OK for an adult to engage in difficult endurance events.
When she trained in the rain, people—often police—stopped
to give her a ride. One day the police stopped her because
they had a report that a woman had been seen running
down the road with an arm cut off and covered with blood.
In fact she ran with her arm in a cast and wore a white
sweatshirt with red letters—the blood. When Kuscsik explained to the police that she was training they wouldn't
listen, but told her to call her loverboy to come pick her up.
In those days special running clothing was not available to
signal that a person was out training. Nice girls didn't do
that. The neighbors who saw her regularly thought she was
an eccentric, a weirdo. But that weirdness was training, and
it paid off.

Marathon. From 1969 on, the women's division of the Boston Marathon had
been the most official, unofficial group there could have been. The unofficial
women did go upstairs to the Prudential cafeteria to have the traditional
beef stew with the official men. BAA officials Cloney and Jock Semple had
become, if not supportive, at least hospitable. It would take them another
year to fully become fans of women's marathon running. But for now the
BAA stipulated that special—that is, well-trained—women could run in the
Boston Marathon, but only if they were scored separately and awarded
separate prizes and started at a separate starting line. This separate but
equal treatment meant that they would have to draw their own starting line
somewhere, but that proved impractical so the women started in the road
with the men. They felt they deserved a fair and equal start.

In the spring of 1972 for the first time in New England, women received
official numbers to run with the men in a 15-kilometer road race. The race,
run from Lexington, Massachusetts, to Cambridge in March, included half
a dozen women. Jock Semple watched the women run quite well. The first
woman, Charlotte Lettis, beat most of the men and received acclaim in the
press. As Semple watched, he knew he had seen the future and that these
women would be impossible to resist. He never again complained about
women runners.

As she waited on the starting line, Nina Kuscsik realized that, in her own words, she "deserved" to win the race. She had already been involved with the AAU concerning women in marathons in New York and Boston so from a political point of view she felt she had a right to be there on the line, free and equal with the men. But from an athletic point of view she realized that her only competitive threat was Beth Bonner—the only other sub-3:00 woman marathoner who might come to Boston. Kuscsik and Bonner had both broken 3 hours in the New York City (Central Park) Marathon the September before with 2:55:22 and a 2:56:04. These were the first two American women to break 3 hours, the second and third in the world. But Bonner did not come to Boston, so Kuscsik thought that no one in the field had trained as much as she had. But maybe someone she didn't know about had trained more. Could she be sure? Regardless, as she stood there she suddenly felt she deserved to win. It was important for Kuscsik to tell herself that she deserved to win.

Kuscsik found the lead easily. Kathrine Switzer had trained harder than ever and expected to run 3:20. For this special, official day she selected a white tennis outfit with a skirt. Under it she wore a black leotard and tights. She wore her hair up and took care to keep it neat. Photographers caught her in a moment of fixing her hair, and subsequent pictures showed her appearing to be more concerned with preening than with racing. She had in fact been doing the training, but she felt obligated to appear feminine and attractive as well as to run quickly. She wanted to counter the public image of women athletes as necessarily unfeminine and unattractive. The point she wanted to make was that a woman did not have to look like a man to compete well. Unfortunately, it was a hot day, and Switzer suffered from the heat. She had thought the frictionless tights would help her; her other years at Boston were bitterly cold. But the tights, held on by the leotard, were a big mistake. She was trapped in her clothes. When she could stand it no longer she stopped at a service station to chop the legs off her tights. She lost so much time hacking at the fabric that it cancelled the benefits of her increased training. She would have to come back to Boston another year to run a fast time.

Kuscsik ran in Danskin shorts and a dacron-and-cotton blouse with buttons down the front. Later, in the light of so much special running apparel designed for women, Kuscsik would laugh at her selection of a buttoned blouse for marathon running. As she ran she felt good and under control and right on sub-3:00 pace, until she felt intestinal rumblings at 13 to 15 miles. She knew from the feelings of these spasms that they would result in diarrhea within a few miles. But if she stopped she would lose any chance at 3 hours and might lose the race. If she only had to stop once she could do it, but she knew that her condition would call for multiple stops. Besides, there were no convenient pitstops. She knew she deserved to win. She had

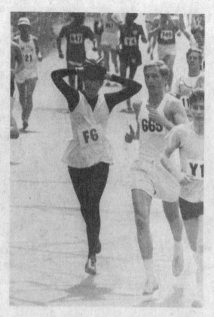

To illustrate that women need not look like men to run fast, Kathrine Switzer wears tights and a skirt in the 1972 race, but as the day turned sunny and hot she found herself a prisoner in her own clothing. Photo by Jeff Johnson.

the lead. She had argued that women have the right—she couldn't stop. She decided not to. While still running she just let it go.

Suddenly great embarrassment replaced her competitive feelings. Could the crowds see the diarrhea dribbling down her legs? They cheered wildly for her as she approached but stopped as she passed. Were they disgusted by the brown streak on her legs? She was sure she was revolting thousands of people as she passed. But then crowds usually do stop cheering after the runners pass. Would the newspapers write about her diarrhea? Surely the runners behind her could see. What did they think? Yes, I deserve to win, but will this accident set women's running back 10 years? she wondered. The closer she got to the finish line the more she worried, not about winning but about how to conceal what had happened. No longer was breaking 3 hours important. She did not want to embarrass all of women's running. It was a great responsibility being at the vanguard of a movement as well as a race. If only she could wash it off.

Kuscsik's friend Ben Malkasian held her sweatpants and planned to meet her at the finish, but what if the officials whisked her off to the awards platform before she could get her pants on? She would not let anyone photograph her in that condition and did not want to answer questions.

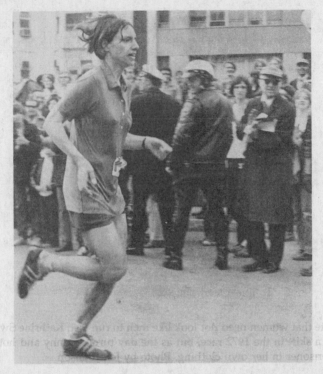

Running in a dacron-and-cotton blouse, Nina Kuscsik is the first official woman to reach the finish line in 1972. Photo courtesy of the *Boston Herald*.

The only greater embarrassment would have been not finishing. She decided on a plan. She would cross the finish line and take three steps. If Ben wasn't there she would sit down. She would just sit down until he found her, even if it took the rest of the afternoon.

In the last half mile to the finish she could not thoroughly savor the cheers of the crowds; she worried. But she need not have. As was the custom at the finish for all the official male runners, a man wrapped her in a large brown blanket, and Ben was there too. She was saved. At last she could relax and enjoy the glory of being the first woman to officially win the Boston Marathon.

1972 Women's Results

1. N. Kuscsik, Huntington, NY	3:10:26*	4. P. Barrett, NJ	3:40:29
2. E. Pederson, CA	3:20:35	5. S. Berman, *CSU*	**3:48:30**
3. K. Switzer, Syracuse, NY	3:29:51		

*First official course record.

A CONSCIENTIOUS OBJECTION

MONDAY, APRIL 16, 1973

Finn Favored for Today's Race

There was little in Tom Fleming's room but the sign telling him to train, inspirational posters of runners, and inspirational running books. He had been running steady 100-mile weeks since 1969. Some days he went for 15 miles in the morning and did it again at night. In the Boston Marathon of 1970 he had run in 20th place for a while but had died on the hills and finished with a 2:37, in 68th place. That summer of 1970 he was accepted to the U.S. Olympic marathon training camp in Pullman, Washington. He was the youngest (age 19) and slowest marathoner there. He followed the older, faster guys around. He would do whatever they said was necessary to run faster. If they had told him to strap a refrigerator to his back and run up a mountain, he would have. He was everyone's eager little brother. In 1972 at Boston he finished in 23rd place. In contrast to his willingness to run vast mileage alone, he was not a quiet person.

Tom Fleming from New Jersey was "everything New Jersey"—big, boisterous, the Cassius Clay of distance running. In a sport of tight-lipped introverts, Tom Fleming was pure lip—brash, big-shouldered, grinning, a verbal brawler. He would argue any point of view with anyone. He could not keep his opinions to himself. He considered himself the favorite to win Boston this year. And why not? He had trained more than anyone else in the world.

Everyone else's considered favorite was Tom Fleming's houseguest, Olavi Suomalainen. Olavi drove Fleming's mother crazy with his meticulousness. Tom was the opposite. While Olavi ate only crisp vegetables, fresh fish, and wholesome breads at set mealtimes, trained in measured amounts, and met a precise schedule of sleep, Tom ate whatever was handy or tasted good, trained as much as possible, then crashed for the night whenever he had to. It made no common sense, but they became good friends. The Finnish community of Massachusetts was outraged that Olavi chose to spend his time in New Jersey with a non-Finn, but such is the nature of running friendships, that they transcend national and ethnic boundaries. In an odd sense, the runners of the world consider themselves a distinct tribe apart from nationalities, politics, and governments. Fleming and Suomalainen were a strong example of that international community of "runnerhood."

In January of 1973 Fleming won the Jersey Shore Marathon in 2:19:16, then only 3 weeks later beat Olympians Jon Anderson, Jeff Galloway, and

Lasse Viren in the San Blas, Puerto Rico, half-marathon. He went on a pleasant run in Puerto Rico with Anderson, Galloway, and Suomalainen. They talked about how they would meet again in Boston. Fleming was a 4:16 miler, so he had speed enough and had done the training. Who else was running 160 miles in a week? As a student teacher of brain-injured kids, he had to get up at 5:30 a.m. to train. Although Fleming hated early morning running, he did it. If he didn't, somebody else might.

Fleming feared only the 10,000-meter Olympian, Jeff Galloway, because of his well-known ability to run what Burfoot called his "rock steady" pace. Fleming had reason to fear West German Lutz Philipp, a 32-year-old math teacher from Darmstadt, near Frankfurt. He had beaten Ron Hill by 1 second with a 2:12:50 in the Maxol Marathon in England in 1972.

Philipp led through Natick in 52:55, a reasonable pace for a hot day. Fleming ran in second place with Welshman Bernie Plain, Anderson, Galloway, John Vitale, and Suomalainen close behind. He glanced constantly around the group, studying faces. It was 77 °F. Philipp led through Wellesley in 1:08:26 with Fleming 10 yards behind. Fleming's number came unpinned. He casually pinned it back on as he ran. Winning seemed quite a reasonable thing to him at this point. Fleming believed that if you wanted to be someone in this sport, you had to win the Boston Marathon.

> *Fleming believed that if you wanted to be someone in this sport, you had to win the Boston Marathon.*

Here in the early miles Philipp made his big burst. It looked like he was trying to "pull a Frank Shorter," to run away from the field early and hold a big lead the way Shorter had done to win the previous year's Olympic marathon. Fleming coolly did not respond. Philipp, 32nd in 2:24 in Munich, was no Frank Shorter. Fleming ran with his friend, Suomalainen. By the beginning of the hills it became clear that Philipp could not win. Suomalainen took over the lead through 17 miles. No sweat showed on him. He looked like a winner again. Fleming and Anderson followed. Anderson had been hanging with his friend, Galloway, from the beginning. Anderson did not look good. On the downhills he placed his hands on his hips. It looked like he was having some trouble.

Anderson had had a down period in his running during the previous winter. In 1972 he was an Olympian, but 3 weeks before Boston he had been depressed and nearly quit running. The training was not going well, and he had just married and thought perhaps he should join the real world and give up running. He called his father, the mayor of Eugene, Oregon, who had agreed to finance his trip to Boston, to say he didn't want to go. But the elder Anderson said he would like to see Jon run at Boston. He left the decision to Jon. On looking back Anderson later could see that this period was not a life crisis, just a few poor workouts, but at the time a major race seemed like an insurmountable task. No pressure, no expectations, just do it. By the end of March he had put in a 130-mile week, including a 30-mile run. He felt better. Anderson had planned to run Boston ever since he had taken up running as a teenager. He decided not to wait and to do Boston this year.

Jon Anderson lived in San Mateo, California, where Alvaro Mejia had lived in 1971. As a conscientious objector to the war in Vietnam, Anderson felt he was spinning his wheels in his alternative service, washing dishes in a hospital. He felt that as an accomplished person, a graduate of Cornell University, he had more to offer society than cleaning its dishes. The Olympics 7 months earlier had been exciting. Travel to road races was exciting. The training and the racing were a chore and a challenge. His job was not. Until this moment on a Monday afternoon leading the Boston Marathon, his weekdays had been dull. Anderson rose at 5:30 a.m., ran 5 miles as if in a dream, washed dishes all day, slept for 15 minutes on returning home, went for a run, ate, settled down, went to sleep at 9:00 p.m., and did it again the next day. With his Olympian status he could have joined the army track team like fellow Eugene Olympian Kenny Moore, but because he did not believe in war he had decided back in 1971 to seek conscientious objector status rather than enlist or wait to be drafted. His father supported his decision to apply for CO status by writing a letter to the local draft board. Two days before the race Jon Anderson took the red-eye flight out of San Francisco to Boston.

When Anderson took the lead even so late in the race, Fleming was not impressed. Fleming had beaten Anderson in the San Blas half-marathon, and because Anderson was a 10,000-meter man it did not seem likely that he could hold a strong pace for a whole marathon. When he drifted into the lead, Fleming let him go—let him burn himself out like Philipp had. There is time enough. Give him the rope . . .

Anderson uncoiled nearly a half mile of rope and showed no sign of choking. When Fleming and Suomalainen looked up, Anderson had 2-1/2 minutes on them. Fleming thought, Stupid! I should not have been content to stay with Olavi. Olavi thought that he should not have stayed with Fleming. Both went after Anderson.

Anderson, whom reporter Dave Prokop described as having a drooping moustache that did not quite conceal his dimples, asked Prokop, who rode in the press bus, how Fleming looked. Prokop said he looked OK. Anderson, alert and calculating, increased his pace. His appearance of fatigue had been deceiving. He especially wanted to beat Fleming because Fleming was a road runner and thereby a member of a slower subset of runners who merely stacked up the miles. Personally Anderson liked Fleming, but it was the principle of the thing—to a track runner, speed is king. Suomalainen got a stitch coming off the hills. He clutched grotesquely at his side. Fleming passed him. Fleming was closing on Anderson, but would there be race enough to catch Anderson?

Anderson had started the day expecting to break 2:20 and be the first American, but on feeling the heat he revised his prediction to 2:25. Contrary to most big marathoners, Anderson, 6'2" and 165 pounds, had run well in heat. At the Olympic trials in Eugene, Oregon, he had made the team for 10,000 meters on an extraordinarily hot day—so hot that before the race, officials had to wet the track to cool it. Galloway had made that team, too, and before the race he jumped into the steeplechase pit, emerged wet, and went to the starting line. It had helped. In Hopkinton both Galloway and Anderson had gone to the marathon starting line wet. Anderson's hair was matted down and his Oregon Track Club racing vest clung to his body. Just because he had run well in the heat didn't mean it would be easy this time. As Galloway ran rock-steady through the pack, picking off the faster starting runners, Anderson in the lead had to contend with emotional shakiness. He fought back tears. Here was his boyhood dream coming true. Tingles ran up and down his spine. But this feeling was weird. The race was not over yet. Anderson put his head down and ran. Fleming stalked him. Fleming ran with all the power he could squeeze from his body. But it wasn't enough. On average Anderson gained 8 seconds every mile.

As Anderson approached the finish line he realized that he would likely win. With every step toward the finish the chance that Fleming or Suomalainen or rock-steady Galloway would catch him decreased, but the level of discomfort in his body rose. Anderson thought that to run a marathon you have to love it, but for a little while at the end you hate it.

As he ran toward the finish line Anderson saw a wall of people. He saw faces and hands moving, with no space to run through. He ran into a dead-end canyon, with no room for himself beyond the finish line. He knew the crowd would smother him, leaving him no room to cool off and stretch his cramping legs. He crossed the line, escaped the crowd, and found the cool water of the reflecting pool beneath the statue in front of the Prudential Center. He jumped in. The press closed around clicking pictures, but he didn't mind being surrounded then. He was cool, he was relaxed. He had realized his boyhood dream and won the Boston Marathon. He couldn't wait to call his father.

After interviews in the press room, Anderson wanted to make his call. Jock Semple found a telephone for him. As he picked it up the ever-frugal Semple said, "Hey, Jon, call collect."

After a party with the Finns in the Lenox Hotel, Anderson walked alone to his room at the Sheraton. Early the next morning he walked alone down the endless flights of stairs to the subway. His thighs screamed at him. The descent took forever. Later in his career he would learn that walking backward down stairs eased postmarathon thigh pain. He took the blue-line subway to the airport and went home . . . to go back to washing dishes in the hospital kitchen. Anderson fulfilled his service obligation and went back

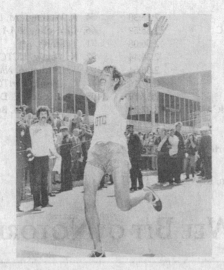

Jubilant in victory, Jon Anderson throws up his hands at the finish of the hot, steamy 1973 race. AP/Wide World Photo.

to Eugene, where he took up the family business of publishing a newsletter for the forest products industry. He would, however, come back to Boston in 10 years and run approximately the same time to finish well back in the field.

Fleming went home to read the writing on his wall and train much harder than anyone on Earth.

1973 Men's Results

1. **J. Anderson**, OTC	**2:16:03**	20. R. Pate, *OTC*	2:29:26
2. T. Fleming, *WPC*	2:17:03	21. D. Spitz, *MCS*	2:29:30
3. **O. Suomalainen, Finland**	**2:18:21**	22. B. Fitts, *SLTC*	2:30:47
4. B. Plain, Wales	2:21:10	23. **J. Fultz**, *WSC*	**2:30:55**
5. J. Galloway, *FTC*	2:21:27	24. M. Graham, *US*	2:31:12
6. D. Spencer, *UG*	2:22:31	25. W. Bragg, *NJS*	2:31:18
7. B. Moore, *TOC*	2:23:57	26. J. Butterfield, *BAA*	2:31:24
8. P. Leiviska, Finland	2:23:57	27. D. Slusser III, PA	2:31:25
9. J. Vitale, *NHTC*	2:24:06	28. M. White, *BAA*	2:31:40
10. R. Daws, *TCTC*	2:24:09	29. P. Bastick, *MillAA*, NY	2:32:22
11. L. Philipp, Germany	2:25:04	30. W. Van Dyke, *CSU*	2:32:56
12. J. Mahurin, *NCTC*	2:25:31	31. F. Best, *CNJTC*	2:33:23
13. S. Hoag, *TCTC*	2:25:36	32. P. Lever, *TOC*	2:33:57
14. N. Sander, Jr., *MillAA*	2:25:50	33. R. O'Connell, TX	2:33:57
15. R. Wayne, *OTC*	2:26:25	34. J. Cederholm, Boston, MA	2:34:12
16. U. Hakansson, Sweden	2:27:26	35. C. Kim, Korea	2:34:15
17. L. Olsen, *NMC*	2:27:31	36. R. Jones, *BAA*	2:34:38
18. J. Gubbins, *GU*	2:28:33	37. C. Hatfield, *WVirTC*	2:34:58
19. R. Bayko, *NMC*	2:28:40	38. G. Teal, ON	2:35:13

39. A. Taylor, ON	2:35:30
40. G. Guins, *SummAC*	2:35:59
41. J. Boyle, *RTC*	2:36:08
42. G. Holliday, PQ	2:36:44
43. J. Carmody, NJ	2:36:54
44. W. Renaud, MA	2:37:16
45. M. Sudzina	2:37:19
46. P. Thompson, *NMC*	2:37:32
47. D. Larson, *Yale*	2:37:38
53. J. Skaja, *TCTC*	2:38:48

54. R. Wallingford, *LUTC*	2:38:53
66. J.J. Kelley, *BAA*	**2:41:13**
71. T. Smith, *MS*	2:41:53
97. K. Young, *UCTC*	2:45:47
103. T. Derderian, *NMC*	2:46:43
141. C. Dyson, *HartTC*	2:51:09
1105. J.A. Kelley, E. Dennis, MA	**3:35:02**
W. Rodgers, A. Burfoot, DNF	
at 21 miles	

1,574 entrants, 1,398 starters.

Team prize

Oregon TC: J. Anderson, R. Wayne, R. Pate

A WEE BIT O' NOTORIETY

MONDAY, APRIL 16, 1973

Kuscsik Back to Defend Title

At the starting line of the second year of women-officially-in-the-marathon, the notorious Kathrine Switzer moved to her position on the starting line. Celebrated sportscaster Howard Cosell worked from atop a large platform 100 feet in front of the runners. Spectators gazed up at him. Jock Semple focused his critical eye on Switzer. It had been agreed that one woman would start with her toe to the line and the others would file in behind her. The honor of being the woman to toe the line would go to last year's winner, Nina Kuscsik. Semple approached Switzer. She wore a number. The cameramen were ready. She thought he was going to yell at her, to tell her to get back. He was yelling at everyone else, chasing the high-numbered runners away from the starting line. But instead of yelling at Switzer, he smiled and said, "Come on, lass, let's get a wee bit o' notoriety." In front of the clicking cameras he gave her a giant kiss. With that symbolic act, women racers in the Boston Marathon were at last celebrated in spirit as well as in the letter of the law.

In 1972 BAA officials had begrudgingly allowed women into the race; now at last they welcomed them. Semple and Will Cloney were beginning to come around. They began to appreciate that women marathon runners were not out to pull stunts and get publicity, nor were they merely trying to use the marathon to make a feminist statement. These women were real long-distance runners, and not only did they qualify for and run the Boston Marathon, they ran the other races in the circuit (except for Bobbi Gibb, who was off doing other things like sculpting and attending law school and would not return to run a marathon for 10 years, when she would run her best time in New York City). They trained hard and turned in respectable times. They liked running and liked runners. Semple began to like them because they liked and supported the sport he loved. He said these women were a lot better than the men. Semple complained about the "very strange people out there; they'll be coming in at six or seven o'clock. For cripes sake, I once *walked* the entire course in 4-1/2 hours. To be honest, I'd be much happier if, when the race started, many of these guys would run in the other direction, to Worcester." Switzer thought Semple was now acting as if *he* had invented women's running. Women's running, however, was still quite primitive, perhaps on a par with men's running before 1900. Women lacked participants, organization, teams, clubs, and competitive opportunities. But for this moment, after years of organization and agitation, little of the politics and administration of the new sport of long-distance running for women mattered to Switzer. She had a race to run.

So did defending champion Kuscsik, who held her lead out of the narrow chute of women. By the middle of the race a young track runner from California stalked her.

The people of Granada Hills, California, raised the money to send Jacqueline Hansen to Boston. She had won California's Culver City Marathon in December with a 3:15. She had extraordinary talent, the speed that Berman, Kuscsik, Switzer, and Gibb could only dream of. She had run a mile in 4:54 to win the previous year's national collegiate title. At last a very fast woman came to race at Boston, but unfortunately talent is not everything. Just as willpower alone cannot create the ability to run fast, neither can athletic talent without preparation, proper coaching, and experience.

Jacqueline Hansen had a coach and had done preparation, but both were lacking; however, at the time she did not know it. Her clothing alone could tell how little she knew of what to expect. Because it was Boston, the cradle of liberty, and Patriots' Day, Hansen decided that she should look appropriately patriotic. She selected a pair of red-and-white checkered terrycloth shorts. She thought the soft terrycloth would be a good fabric to wear for a marathon. Her top was red, white, and blue. On her feet she wore two pairs of socks because she knew from backpacking that a thin pair of socks covered by a heavier pair of wool socks would prevent blisters in hiking boots. She thought that strategy should work well for a marathon, too. But it was a hot day. She suffered. Her feet were hot. To cool herself she let a spectator dump a bucket of water on her head. The water flowed over her shoulders and down to her shorts. The terrycloth soaked up the water like a towel, weighing her shorts down. To keep them on she had to reach down and squeeze the weight of the water out of them. The wool socks held water, too. Hansen squished down the road in pursuit of Kuscsik, leaving little puddles in her wake.

Hansen had coaching of a most extreme kind. Her coach was Lazlo Tabori, a Hungarian who had trained under Mihaly Igloi, the coach of Norm Higgins,

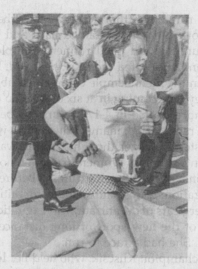

Jacqueline Hansen's red-and-white terrycloth shorts look patriotic, but they absorbed so much water in the 1973 race that they nearly fell off. AP/Wide World Photo.

the first American to finish Boston in 1966. Like Igloi, Tabori kept his athletes under strict control. He had rules. Train on the track and grass, not on the road. On off-days, that is, non–track interval days, run for no more than an hour on grass. Hansen strained against that control, but she followed his one foolish rule for marathon running (more to come on that).

Jacqueline Hansen started running at Granada Hills High School in Los Angeles, but in the mid-1960s, girls were limited to distances of 440 yards. She tried the sprints and jumps but was not inspired. Not until the presidential physical fitness tests did she discover her ability at fast long-distance running. She learned in the 600-yard run/walk that she could really run and she enjoyed it. This single event made the difference. The revelation was what eventually made Hansen into a marathoner, because otherwise the schools were indifferent to girls' athletics. When it rained the boys got the gym and the girls hung around in the locker room, listening to the radio. Girls were not expected to take athletics, and especially not running, seriously. But young Jacqueline wanted to run. After high school she went to Pierce Junior College and tried to do just that.

But the Pierce track coach was really a golf instructor, with the notion that track-and-field training amounted to week after week of the whole team dedicated to one event at a time until the season ended. The team was composed of mostly Hansen's friends from high school and was not very effective in training anyone for anything, but at least the longest event was now the 880 yards.

Hansen was allowed to race as long as a mile after she transferred to San Fernando Valley State, where she ran with the boys. But running with the boys' team did little except satisfy the school physical education requirement. While out running one day Hansen encountered a rare sight—another woman running. Instantly she saw a comrade. She ran up to her to get acquainted. From this chance encounter she learned about the Los Angeles Track Club and Tabori.

Under Tabori's rigorous, disciplined training Hansen pared down to the 4:54 mile that won the women's collegiate national championships. In Tabori's club she met Cheryl Bridges, who had run a 2:49:40 marathon in Culver City in 1971. Bridges provided the inspiration for Hansen to step up to the marathon. But Hansen had only inspiration and a miler's speed and training. She had done no marathon training. Twice she had sneaked off to do 10-mile road runs with a bunch of runners in Balboa Park, including the talkative 66-year-old Monty Montgomery. She enjoyed road running. Unlike during Tabori's rigid workouts, these road runners joked and told stories. They told stories of the Boston Marathon. They hooked her.

On a December day Hansen told her family that she was going out for a run and would be back in time for the big family dinner. They did not think much of her taking this running stuff so seriously. Her family did not understand; they expected young ladies to participate in athletics for the sake of health and recreation, but the ambition they detected in Jacqueline unnerved them. They feared she might hurt herself, set herself up for failure, or at best engage in folly. She did not tell them or her coach that she had been planning for months to run the Culver City Marathon. She had asked Tabori's permission to run, but only a week before the race. Tabori's athletes had to ask his permission before doing almost anything. Hansen was surprised that he did not forbid her to run; instead he said mysteriously, "There are things I never did when I was younger that I will always wonder about. You are very stubborn; you will go very far." Hansen found her coach's statement not an endorsement but a conundrum. Did "very far" mean that he expected her to go 18 miles and drop out and thereby learn her lesson and give up road running foolishness? Was he being sarcastic, or did he mean something prophetic? But instead of going for a mere run that day, she entered and ran the Culver City Marathon.

When she returned home late for the family dinner, no one had eaten yet; everyone waited for her. They watched her walk in the door. She thought she was in big trouble for making them wait. She didn't know that an aunt on the Culver City Marathon course had watched her pass by and alerted the family, who then tuned in to the race on television to watch their Jackie win. Suddenly they understood. She had not hurt herself, and she had won, and moreover she appeared on television. She was a heroine. A winner. They broke into applause. At last her family accepted her running.

Winning the Culver City Marathon had not been easy. Hansen's 3:15 marathon came at a great cost. Lots of track intervals and only two 10-mile road runs were hardly a basis for marathon training. Her last 6 miles were a death run. That is when she decided to train for the Boston Marathon with 100-mile weeks. With the encouragement of her boyfriend, a Yale student, she set her sights on the Boston Marathon because it was the biggest and most famous marathon in the world.

Now in striking distance of the Boston lead on a hot day, Hansen still followed Tabori's rule: no drinking while running. She would dump water on herself but would not drink any. From backpacking she knew a person should take water before thirst called for it, but the coach's rule was law. Not a drop passed her lips. As Hansen passed Kuscsik to take the lead, Kuscsik said, "Go, Jackie; good luck." Hansen was surprised that the famous Nina Kuscsik knew her name. But of course Kuscsik, who was as much political promoter of women's marathon running as racer herself, knew Hansen's name. Kuscsik also realized it was a hot day and expected the California runners would do better, but she was secretly relieved that some-one else would have to put up with the pressure of the press. In 1972 they had followed her home. This year her homelife itself was stressful enough; she had separated from her husband before a divorce and did not need television cameras and reporters at her door. Good luck, Jackie, she said, referring as much to the media pressure as to the miles ahead.

Back at Yale, Hansen sat with her boyfriend. The Boston Marathon first-place trophy and laurel wreath rested on the table. The boyfriend said that only two of those had been given out today. She took him to mean the laurel wreath, which she pressed and preserved. The trophy she gave away, or "recycled," for use as a prize in another race. After Boston Jackie Hansen trained for one 100-mile week after another, learned to dress properly and drink water, and ran a world record marathon not once but twice—in Culver City with a 2:43:54.6 the next year and in 1975 with a 2:38:19 in Eugene, Oregon. She became central in the movement to establish women's Olympic marathon, 5,000-meter, and 10,000-meter races, including bringing a lawsuit against the Olympic Committee, but such things would not happen for another 10 years. She would come back to race at Boston in 1978 and 1984. She married another Igloi-trained runner, Tom Sturak, and they lived in a house perched above a canyon in Topanga, California. By age 43 in 1991 she could still run a quarter mile in 65 seconds.

1973 *Women's Results*

1.	J. Hansen, Granada Hills, CA	3:05:59^{CR}	5.	S. Berman, Cambridge, MA	3:30:05
2.	N. Kuscsik, Long Island, NY	3:06:29	6.	G. Reinke, West Germany	3:30:20
3.	J. Taylor, Newton, MA	3:16:30	7.	S. Nadon, OH	3:30:40
4.	K. Switzer, NY	3:20:30	8.	M. Cushing, Amherst, MA	3:36:06

THE LIMERICK

MONDAY, APRIL 15, 1974

Fleming Favorite for BAA

In Boston, old marathoner Mike Dukakis, who had finished 57th in 1951 with a 3:31, announced his intention to run for and win the governorship of Massachusetts. Tom Fleming announced his intention to run for and win the Boston Marathon. Running and winning are the same for runners and politicians; to win takes all you've got.

Fleming had built his progression to Boston Marathon victory with seeming perfection. This would be his fourth run at Boston. He had come a long way from being the youngest and slowest kid at the U.S. Olympic training camp in 1970 to, in 1974, ranking better than or equal to every U.S. marathoner except Olympic gold medalist Frank Shorter. Because Shorter wasn't coming to Boston, the road looked free for Fleming. He had logged another year's worth of 100+ mileage weeks, including many 30-mile days and 160-mile weeks. Until the Thursday before the race everything in his life waited pending his supreme effort in Monday's event. Then, while running easy mileage in New Jersey with his frequent training partner, Hugh B. Sweeny III, Fleming twisted his ankle. There it went. All that preparation—gone to a New Jersey pothole.

How bad was the sprain? Would it heal in time? Fleming simply did not know. To give the joint maximum time to heal he would not run a step until those first steps in the race itself. The injury pushed him away from a complete confidence to nothingness. He withdrew his announcement that he would win. He felt no lack of confidence, just an agnosticism about whether or not he would run at all. Any pressure to win evaporated because he did not know if he would even get to compete.

While Fleming wondered how his ankle would hold out, Pat McMahon bumped into another Irishman in the Hopkinton gym. McMahon still could not run because of injuries, and he had not run a race since his second place in the BAA of 1971, but as a BAA member he volunteered to help out on race day. Neil Cusack from Limerick, Ireland, just 2 miles from McMahon's Clare, waited amid the smell of liniment and the prerace chatter. Cusack was another great Irish runner recruited for an American college from the apparently endless supply of Irish talent. From Ron Delaney, who went to Villanova, to McMahon to at least a hundred others, Ireland stocked American colleges with fast men. Cusack had run the 10,000 meters in the Munich

Olympics. When McMahon asked him how he expected to run, Cusack answered, "Oh, Patrick, to be honest, I think I can win the thing."

Cusack's collegiate cross-country season had been good, and indoors he had run a 4:04 mile and half a dozen 2-miles in 8:30. In March he had run well in the World Cross-Country Championships in Italy with a 66th place. Cusack looked over the lads in the gym and saw them as endurance road runners, plodders, not "crispy and fast" track men. He had been running 95 to 100 miles a week, but his longest run had been only 16 miles—just a morning workout for Fleming.

At the hotel in Boston, Fleming had the room adjacent to Cusack's. Cusack noticed all the journalistic buzz and flurry around Fleming, whom reporters regarded as the favorite, although Fleming no longer did. Cusack said to himself, If this man is the favorite, I'm going to win.

Other previous contenders had little to compare with Cusack. Daws was back, but running more out of habit and for a good place. Drayton was back, but he was considered erratic and had been plagued by injuries and employment problems, though he may have put those problems behind him with his 2:13:26.8 at St. John, New Brunswick, in September.

Bernie Allen of England and Maryland shot off to an early lead. This act and subsequent similar early shots into the lead would earn him the title *Morning Glory*, one that would follow him for several decades. With his 2:16:34.6 runaway win in Rotterdam, Allen was a serious contender. Cusack followed with Fleming, Lucian Rosa (another fast collegian, imported from Ceylon to Wisconsin), and a Boston runner named Bill Rodgers who had been Amby Burfoot's college roommate. Rodgers had dropped out in 1973, but in the autumn he had learned how to pace himself in a marathon, though he ran only a little bit faster than 2:30. He appeared to be over his head in this competition. He was not running an even pace scheduled to allow him to finish well; he boldly ran with the lead pack, so apparently was running to win, not just place well. Cusack snorted with each step. The snorting drove Rodgers crazy. It was like running in a herd of buffalos. Fleming ran like a buffalo with lumbering thighs. His ankle felt stiff on the downhill start, although he started as slowly as he dared, but once it warmed up it worked perfectly. But he labored against the handicap of his slow start. He chased the dust of the herd.

Cusack had the lead by Natick with Rosa, Fleming, John Vitale, and Drayton pursuing. Cusack wore a mesh singlet with a single shamrock on it. On his face he wore a wispy moustache and a goatee. He felt sharp, relaxed, and clever. He was not bothered by his own noises.

Fleming felt frustrated. He ran in second place and played catch-up, but he could not catch up to Cusack. Fleming put his head down and charged, but when he looked up Cusack was just as far ahead. Steve Liquori, a Boston College freshman and younger brother of miler Marty, followed on a bicycle and pleaded with Fleming to speed up. He pedaled up to Cusack, examined him, then fell back and reported his findings to Fleming. Cusack overheard the reports and kept himself ahead of Fleming. Cusack judged Fleming's pace with an ear cocked to the rear and adjusted his own pace to maintain the gap. He ran hard enough to keep the shouts of "Go, Tom Fleming" well behind him. The harder Fleming tried, the faster Cusack went. The tactic was very clever—to judge one's pace from the pursuing runner, or in essence to follow from the front.

Fleming ran through a gauntlet of spectators who had narrowed the road to a path through a prairie of screaming people. At one point Fleming wished those people would go home, but at the next he tried to extract energy out of their enthusiasm—"Go get him. You're in second place." Fleming thought, Yes, I know I am in second place—shuddup! Then he tried with every ounce of strength to obey. All the emotions from hate to love flowed through him. His father told him to be the best he could be at what he did. He was being the best he could be, but Cusack was being better.

A cramp grabbed Fleming. He stopped and bent over to rub it out. A spectator ran over and dumped cold Coca-Cola on his head. The spectator meant well, and in a rational moment Fleming could have appreciated the gesture and even seen the humor in it, but now it annoyed him. He did not need to be sticky and have flies follow him to Boston.

Cusack hit the finish first. Fleming hit the finish and burst into tears. Second again. "Two years in a row! It's hard to take. I thought I was really moving in on Neil when the cramp hit me. I had my heart set on winning, especially after what happened to me last year."

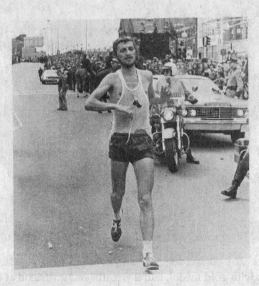

On the wall of Tom Fleming's room hung this reminder: "Somewhere in the world there is someone training when you are not. When you race him, he will win." Here Fleming finishes second in 1974 for the second year in a row. Photo by Jeff Johnson.

Bill Rodgers had his heart set on winning, too. He hung on to 4th place at Lake Street but lost his grip and slipped to 14th by the finish. But he did finish the Boston Marathon. On his second attempt he did, at least, finish.

Sportswriter Jerry Nason could not resist typing out a limerick about the man from Limerick:

> *A young man from the Emerald Isle,*
> *With a beard mostly framing his smile,*
> *Took the bit in his teeth,*
> *Looking limber and lithe,*
> *From the first to the twenty-sixth mile.*

Cusack lives again now in Limerick and is the director of a computerized printing firm. He trains 100 miles a week at age 40 and plans to win the Boston Marathon masters division sometime in the 1990s.

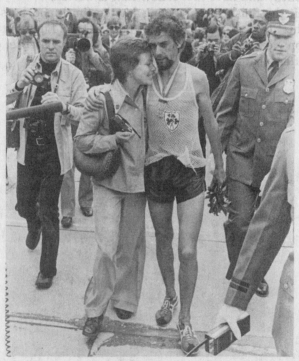

Irish Neil Cusack with gold medal, laurel wreath, and girlfriend at the finish in 1974. Photo by Jeff Johnson.

Checkpoint Splits

Framingham	Bernie Allen	31:26
Natick	Neil Cusack	42:46
Wellesley	Neil Cusack	1:04:29
Woodlawn	Neil Cusack	1:25:06
Lake Street	Neil Cusack	1:46:46
Coolidge Corner	Neil Cusack	1:59:27

1974 Men's Results

1. N. Cusack, *ETS*	2:13:39	
2. T. Fleming, *NYAC*	2:14:25	
3. J. Drayton, *ON*	2:15:40	
4. L. Rosa, WI	2:15:53	
5. V. Paajanen, Finland	2:16:15	
6. S. Hoag, *TCTC*	2:16:44	
7. B. Moore, Toronto, ON	2:16:45	
8. R. Wayne, *OTC*	2:16:58	
9. B. Allen, MD	2:17:02	
10. C. Hatfield, *WVirTC*	2:17:36	
11. J. Vitale, *NHTC*	2:18:54	
12. D. Moynihan, *TU*	2:19:13	
13. R. Harter, *SMTC*	2:19:15	
14. B. Rodgers, *GBTC*	2:19:34	
15. H. Kubelt, West Germany	2:19:50	
16. D. Kennedy, TX	2:20:22	
17. R. Bayko, *NMC*	2:20:56	
18. L. Fidler, NC	2:21:27	
19. R. Hughes, Beverly Hills, CA	2:21:45	
20. M. Sudzina, PA	2:22:11	
21. R. Daws, *TCTC*	2:22:16	
22. B. Eiermann, West Germany	2:24:10	
23. G. Logan, *TS*	2:24:38	
24. W. Schamberger, *DBC*	2:24:50	
25. P. Span, AZ	2:24:52	
26. K. Nutter, *WVirTC*	2:24:53	
27. W. Roggenbach, W. Germany	2:24:54	

28. J. Pasternack, NJ	2:25:03
29. W. Speck, *BAA*	2:25:08
30. T. Derderian, *SMtAC*	2:25:23
31. T. Antczak, IL	2:25:37
32. K. Young, *UCTC*	2:25:46
33. B. Thurston, *WSC*	2:25:46
34. R. Bourrier, AR	2:26:02
35. P. Farwell, *UCTC*	2:26:04
36. K. Scalmini, San Francisco, CA	2:26:10
37. J. Bowles, *WVTC*	2:26:17
38. K. Hartman, Finger Lakes, NY	2:26:29
39. B. Bragg, NJ	2:26:35
40. J. Cederholm, *BAA*	2:26:38
41. T. Smith, *MS*	2:26:42
42. U. Schuder, West Germany	2:26:57
43. P. Peeters, West Germany	2:26:58
44. A. McAndrew, *BAA*	2:27:03
45. M. Steffny, West Germany	2:27:11
46. M. Cryans	2:27:18
47. R. Rouiller, *WVirTC*	2:27:29
48. R. Pate, *OTC*	2:27:50
49. G. Schmitt, West Germany	2:27:52
50. S. Molnor, *JAC*	2:27:54
69. H. Sweeny III, NJ	2:31:37
78. J.J. Kelley, *BAA*	2:32:18
150. P. Caruccio, Winthrop, MA	2:38:13
1266. J.A. Kelley, E. Dennis, MA	3:24:10

"A LITTLE BIT OF A THING"

MONDAY, APRIL 15, 1974

Top West German Women in Today's Marathon

The 1974 women's Boston Marathon story began in China in 1935, the year John A. Kelley won Boston for the first time, with the birth of a Japanese doctor's daughter in the port city of Chinwangtao, near Manchuria. Japan occupied China, and the doctor was stationed at a hospital there. In the last year of World War II, the family and their 9-year-old daughter moved back to Tokyo, but the threat of American bombing was too great and the family fled to safety in the countryside. American firebombing destroyed their Tokyo home. The girl, Michiko Suwa, reached college age during the American occupation of Japan and received a student visa to study secretarial skills at a college in Pennsylvania. In the late 1960s she married an American businessman named Gorman and settled in Los Angeles, California. She worked as a secretary. In 1974 she was 38 years old. She did not seem to be an athlete or an iconoclast.

Michiko Gorman's businessman husband thought his quiet Japanese wife should become more outgoing and get acquainted with a wider circle of people. He was a sportsman and member of the Los Angeles Athletic Club so he persuaded Michiko to join. She felt that she was not an example of feminine beauty; beautiful Japanese women are not dark and thin, but plump and white. Perhaps, she thought, exercise would help her put some weight on—even muscles would be better than this skinniness. She weighed 89 pounds. Gorman was 33 years old in 1969 when she started to run for health and beauty. One run led to another, and by December of 1973 she had run what was proclaimed to be a women's world marathon record of 2:46:36 in Culver City, California. An Australian woman was said to have run 6 seconds faster in 1971 but had never come close to that time again, so with no official course certification process the distance was suspected of being short. Only two other women, both of them Americans, had run under 2:55, and neither entered Boston this year, so Michiko Gorman at age 38 overwhelmed the field. She believed she would win. She had no doubt that she would win. So did the LA Athletic Club that paid her way to Boston.

In her quiet way Gorman had prepared herself like no other woman who had come to Boston in this year's field of 42 women or in any other. Perhaps her lack of athletic experience, her smallness, her shyness made her prepare so thoroughly. After running some promising times a few years earlier she had met Cheryl Bridges, who held the top U.S. time for the marathon. Gorman saw Bridges as the ideal of feminine athleticism. Bridges looked down at Gorman from her athletic height and through shocks of blond hair and said, "Oh, you're such a little bit of a thing." Gorman said nothing, but the comment infuriated her, especially coming from one whom she had admired. Gorman vowed to get Bridges's record for that crack. Her 2:46:36 in Culver City came to her as sweet revenge.

Gorman passed Kathrine Switzer and a woman from Texas early in the race and held a commanding lead by 10 miles. Gorman won the race easily by pure physical domination. No one came close, yet several of the runners far behind her would become the best in the world in a few years. She won by about a mile over Christa Kofferschlager of West Germany, who would, after her last name became Vahlensieck, run the 2:34:47.5 world record in Berlin in September of 1977, breaking the record of another future international star, Chantal Longlace of France, who would later improve to a personal best of 2:35:15.4 in Spain in May of 1977 but finished 18th in Boston on *this* day. In 1974 Michiko Gorman had no challenger, no equal, and no trouble on the Boston course.

Michiko Gorman would be back to Boston two more times and watch the world of women's marathoning change, requiring her to train to extraordinary lengths to remain in the same place. Kathrine Switzer came very close to breaking 3 hours and establishing herself as a marathon racer of accomplishment rather than an agitator. She left Boston hellbent to return the next year as a sub-3:00 marathoner.

In a single year the women's record at Boston had dropped 18:48. It is safe to assume that will never happen again. From this date there would remain no doubt about a woman's ability to run a marathon well.

1974 Women's Results

1.	M. Gorman, LAAC	2:47:11[CR]	10.	I. Rudolph, San Francisco, CA	3:12:13
2.	C. Kofferschlager, W. Germany	2:53:00[1]	11.	K. Loper, SATC	3:14:30
3.	N. Kuscsik, SuffAC	2:55:12	12.	M. Cushing, SMtAC	3:16:37
4.	M. Pruess, West Germany	2:58:46[2]	13.	J. Ullyot, San Francisco, CA	3:17:10
5.	K. Switzer, NY	3:01:39	14.	M. Bevans, BaltAA	3:17:42
6.	L. Ritter, West Germany	3:05:18	15.	L. Kralick, CA	3:18:25
7.	R. Kieninger, West Germany	3:08:45	18.	C. Longlace, France	3:24:45
8.	V. Rogosheske, MN	3:09:28	28.	P. Butterfield, BAA	3:54:14
9.	L. Bunz, San Francisco, CA	3:10:57	30.	N. Viamides, TX	3:58:35

[1]Married name became Christa Vahlensieck.
[2]Married name became Manuela Angenvoorth.

If I Only Had a Brain

MONDAY, APRIL 21, 1975

Hill, Drayton Head Field for 79th BAA Classic

Since childhood Bill Rodgers's favorite song had been "If I Only Had a Brain," sung by the scarecrow in "The Wizard of Oz." Rodgers knew all the correct words. Like the scarecrow, he would while away the hours, looking at flowers or conferring with the rain. But inside his head thoughts would be busy hatching. Bill Rodgers looked skinny, loose, and flaky, with a head topped by long straw-colored hair—like a scarecrow. But his head was not stuffed with straw, although he often acted as if he had no brain, as he lost track of time or misplaced small objects. He ran with his right arm flapping and free of muscular strain. That was because he had virtually no muscles. When he ran he floated rather than powered along. No one would call him a buffalo as they might Fleming. Often Rodgers was late for things or lost things—but never things that mattered. He seemed constantly surprised and easily distracted. John J. Kelley, the schoolmaster with the giant vocabulary, might have stuck the word *insouciant* on him to describe his lighthearted unconcern. Billy Rodgers did not look like a young man with ambition. He did not look like a fierce competitor. He did not look like an athlete. But like the scarecrow in Oz, who proved after all to have the most brains, Bill Rodgers was not really what he looked like or acted like. At the starting line of the 1975 marathon, Tom Fleming, ever the wiseguy, handed Rodgers a headband with the name of the New Balance athletic shoe company on it. "Here, Billy; this will keep the hair out of your eyes so you can see where you are going." Rodgers now knew exactly where he was going. But things had not always been so clear for him.

In March he had been in Rabat, Morocco, the site of the World Cross-Country Championships. There he had been beating the best runners in the world until the last mile, when only two of them passed. Olympic gold medal marathoner Frank Shorter finished second on the U.S. team, far behind Rodgers. Such a feat shocked Rodgers's teammates on the Greater Boston Track Club. They considered Billy a very good runner—sub-2:20 at Boston the year before—and maybe a national class runner, but almost the best in the world? His teammates said, in a comic-book dialogue, "Our Billy? He is just a regular guy. No? Yes. Wow!"

The status of the World Cross-Country Championships had never been high in the U.S., but worldwide its status was on a par with the Olympics.

Cross-country in its simplicity is difficult to appreciate. Often the overall pace is slow because race organizers go to the trouble of collecting mud and building barriers on the course. Because there were no records, because courses and conditions were so different and the race is held without pageantry and in strange places, the American public had heard little about the international cross-country championships. So the Boston public did not realize how great Rodgers had become. Rodgers was pretty nearly the best runner in the world, but at home he was barely known. To the newspaper readers, if they knew him at all, he was a guy who had won some local races.

Among the subculture of runners, it was a different matter. Rodgers had become an instant hero and the favorite to win the Boston Marathon. Rodgers's coach, Bill Squires of the Greater Boston Track Club, did not want the pressure of being the favorite to weigh on Rodgers. So he thought the lack of press attention was just as well. Squires and Rodgers told the reporters that they thought maybe a 2:15, 2:16 would be reasonable. The press wasn't interested. But with his teammates, Billy was the clear favorite. The only leak came from Jock Semple, who told reporters to watch out for a runner named Bill Rodgers. But his comment was taken as local boosterism. Rodgers had been a member of the BAA before the Greater Boston Track Club formed. Of course Semple would like to have another Kelley or Burfoot instead of foreigners or Americans from the west coast. Wouldn't it be wonderful for a Boston runner to win the Boston Marathon! That hadn't happened since Arthur Roth's victory in 1916. Because Rodgers had an apartment in Melrose, Clarence DeMar's former town, technically he did not reside in Boston proper, but he would wear a Boston shirt that would endear him to fans.

There was also good reason not to expect much from Bill Rodgers and to expect a great deal from the course record holder, Ron Hill, who at age 36 came to Boston intent on winning again. He hoped he might get a tailwind and break 2:10. In contrast, Rodgers had barely broken 2:20 the year before. In the fall he had tried to win the New York City Marathon in Central Park and break Tom Fleming's course record of only 2:21:54. He had led for a while but finished with a 2:35:59 in fifth place. But in November he won the Philadelphia Marathon with a time in the low 2:20s.

Ron Hill was an Olympian and an international star with every right and reason to be the race favorite. Rodgers by comparison traveled to races in old cars filled with his fellow runners. When they went to Philadelphia two runners rented a hotel room with two double beds. Six other runners came up the back stairs. They took the mattresses off the box springs and put them on the floor so that the room accommodated all eight runners—two on each mattress and two on each box spring. When Rodgers and his friends returned to Boston, no one had a single dime left; they had to return via back roads because they could not afford the turnpike tolls.

In April Ron Hill flew to Boston; he was met at the airport and escorted to his lodgings with Jeff Johnson in New Hampshire. Hill intended to visit the Nike research and development factory in Exeter because Ron Hill Sports Ltd. imported Nike shoes to the United Kingdom. No longer did Ron Hill cook up dye formulas for the textile industry. He was now a running gear entrepreneur. To Rodgers, Hill was awe-inspiring, a giant among marathoners. He was comfortable, established in a business, and 36 years old—rather unlike Rodgers.

Through the early 1970s Bill Rodgers had lived a life full of what Alan Watts called "the wisdom of insecurity." After graduating from Wesleyan, Rodgers thought that he might have to leave the country to avoid the draft, maybe take a freighter to New Zealand, but like Jon Anderson, he applied for and received conscientious objector status. That meant he had to find himself a job in a nonprofit business. Raised as a Roman Catholic, Rodgers held strong religious beliefs against killing. He admired the nonviolent philosophies of Martin Luther King, Jr. and Mahatma Gandhi. Rodgers gave up running after his graduation with a personal best of a sub-9:00 two-miles at Wesleyan, where he roomed with Amby Burfoot during the semester that Burfoot won Boston.

Burfoot liked having a younger guy as a roommate and a pliable training partner. Rodgers even joined Burfoot for part of an indoor marathon. But on weekends when the elder roommate returned from visits home, beer bottles and lingering cigarette smoke told him that young Billy had not spent the weekend training. Rodgers barely completed his degree requirements.

Rodgers smoked Winstons. He borrowed money to buy a used 650-cc Triumph motorcycle. He would buy half a pint of gin, a mixer, and some cashew nuts and ride around. Bill spent a long time unemployed; he was in turn aimless, happy, confused, angry, and frustrated. He wandered between rebellion and destitution, like many from the graduating classes of 1970.

When he got a job it was in the Peter Bent Brigham Hospital, wheeling patients around for $75 a week. When they died Rodgers took their bodies to the morgue. Quickly he became disgusted with the way people ignored their health and deteriorated. Before this he had always been around young people who retained their vigor despite excesses of drinking, smoking, and sloth. In the hospital he saw a man who had lost his larynx and part of his trachea to cancer and still smoked by inhaling through a hole in his neck. Rodgers decided he didn't really like smoking that much and quit. He watched the 1971 Boston Marathon and saw old friends Burfoot, John Vitale, and Jeff Galloway racing. Realizing that he missed running, he joined the YMCA and began jogging on their indoor track. He would think about the time he accompanied Burfoot for part of the indoor marathon as he trotted around and around inside the YMCA.

After someone stole his Triumph motorcycle Rodgers jogged to work. At work he tried to organize a union. He would stand on the grounds after hours and hand out flyers to other employees. The management did not like his rabble-rousing ideas so they fired him. They posted his photo in the lobby so security officers would know to keep him off the grounds. Rodgers spent 1972 unemployed, which gave him more time to train. In 1973 he got a job at the Fernald School, became involved with a girlfriend, and got some constancy in his life. He also started running 100 miles a week and discovered that running was something in his life that he could control. Rodgers knew he had some talent and that if he trained hard he would succeed; in the world of minimum wage jobs, talent and hard work did not directly produce success. In the early 1970s running had no potential to earn any real money, but neither did minimum wage jobs.

Bill Rodgers's training miles in weeks before the 1975 Boston Marathon

January   201, 136, 85, 140, 96

February   80 (trials for International Cross-Country team), 117, 143, 125

March   135, 107 (World Cross-Country Championships in Morocco), 113, 139

April   140, 128, 14 Friday, 5 miles easy Saturday, 3 miles easy Sunday, Boston Marathon

---

Hill wasn't the only talented, hard-working runner who came to race Boston. Jerome Drayton was another of many. While one could say that Fleming trained madly and Rodgers trained hard, Drayton trained madly, methodically, and hard. He had been third in 1974 and wanted now to beat Hill, Fleming, and Tom Howard from Ontario, who had run a 2:14:33.8 in Vancouver the year before. Drayton lived a solitary life so that nothing would interfere with his training. In this sense selfishness is essential to get the most out of a human body. Drayton, at 5% body fat, weighed 130 pounds at 5'9". He applied his reclusive logic to a rigorous interval training cycle.

[Drayton] trained in disciplined phases, six in all that can last up to eight weeks each. The first consisted solely of long, slow runs to build up his aerobic base. Occasionally he travelled more than thirty miles in an outing. Hill work followed. Three times a week he picked out a hill on his training route and assaulted it repeatedly to toughen the workload. In the third phase he varied the routine not with hills, but timed quarter-mile intervals in the track. Twelve, fourteen, sixteen times he circled the track at a pace that took him to the edge of his anaerobic threshold, the point at which the body begins to slip into oxygen debt from the stress. This usually occurred with laps of about sixty-five seconds, a 4:20 mile pace.

In the fourth phase he deliberately pushed his body into oxygen debt, running quarters at maximum effort with almost no pause in between. So stressful is this form of training that it can exhaust an athlete of Drayton's stature in fewer than half a dozen laps. At least two, often three, track workouts a week are included in his schedule. Then follows the fifth and most taxing phase in which Drayton combined both aerobic and anaerobic intervals in the same session. Quarters that previously took sixty-five seconds to cover without going into oxygen debt he flew through in just fifty-seven seconds, the pace of a world class miler. Through all these phases his total training rarely dropped below one hundred and thirty miles a week.

The sixth and final phase came when Drayton "rested" by tapering to about seventy-five miles a week and substituted short weekly races for the speedwork of the track.

Drayton said,

I like the solitude. I like this one or two hours to myself once a day when I don't have to do speedwork and I can go for a long run. This mental activity has helped shape my attitude toward life. I've come to the conclusion that people who are involved with a high degree of consistency, in an activity such as sports, just seem to enjoy life more. They seem to have a zest for life.

By the 6-mile mark in Framingham, morning glory Bernie Allen was finished leading, and Drayton took over. He wore dark glasses and a maple leaf singlet. Hill ran a few steps behind wearing a mesh singlet of Ron Hill design and a pair of Ron Hill "freedom" shorts bearing the Union Jack. As he ran he noticed that bits of paper and plastic cups blew ahead of the runners, propelled by a following wind. Later he would write in his training log that this was a 2:08 day if he ever saw one. Next to Hill, Fleming wore a singlet with the armholes so exaggerated that his nipples showed. He wore #2. Always cavalier and talkative, he said to Hill, "How're you feeling, Ronnie boy?" to which Hill gasped, "Bloody knackered; I'm hanging on to you." Richard Mabuza from Swaziland wore all white, which contrasted with his glistening black skin. A. Gylling of Finland wore a blue cross on his shirt. Rodgers wore a white mesh T-shirt with "Boston GBTC" printed on it in black marking pen, the headband from Fleming, and white gardening gloves. It was Drayton who decided to break up this oddly attired bunch.

Rodgers went with Drayton. Rodgers felt feisty. He was sure he would not let Hill win. At age 36 Hill was too old; it would not be right. Rodgers made up names for the runners he raced against. He chanted "Ronald the Hill" until the footsteps of the pack were far behind. Then a spectator began to cheer for Canada: "Go, Jerome! Go, Jerome!" The cheering infuriated Rodgers. It irritated him that a Boston spectator would cheer for a Canadian and not him, especially after he had gone to the trouble of branding himself

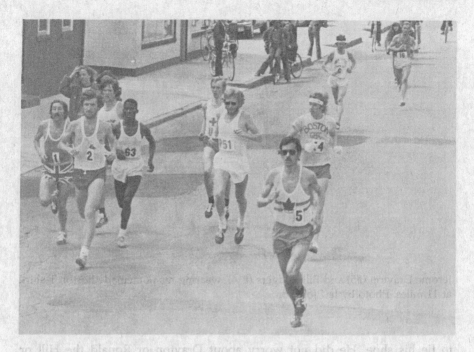

Those among the 1975 pack in Framingham include Ron Hill (#1), Tom Fleming (#2), Richard Mabuza (#63), Jerome Drayton (#5), Bill Rodgers (#14), and Steve Hoag (#6). Photo by Jeff Johnson.

"Boston" with letters as big as his shirt would allow. Rodgers poured it on. He saw it as a midrace duel to the death, man on man. He intended to increase the pace until the other runners died and then hang on for the rest of the race. Kill or be killed. He felt that fierce.

Fleming did not feel that fierce. There was plenty of race to go and Rodgers wasn't that good of a marathoner—only 2:19:34 and 14th last year. He'll kill himself, thought Fleming. They'll both kill each other. Good for me.

But Fleming did not figure on the inspiration factor. Rodgers liked running in the lead. He liked seeing the press truck and the police motorcycles. He liked the attention. He was thrilled. Drayton disappeared. In a twinkle. Gone. When Hill passed him Drayton stood on the side of the road. "Come on Jerome, bloody finish it, if you have to walk." Drayton just answered, "Good luck." Hill noticed that the vest Drayton wore had come from Ron Hill Sports.

With Drayton gone Rodgers figured if he pushed the pace until the top of Heartbreak Hill he'd have it in the bag. He realized that he could trash himself with too furious a pace, so he tried to calm down. A boyhood friend, Jason Kehoe, popped out on a bicycle. After they greeted each other Rodgers tried to relax by pretending that he was just out on a training run. He stopped twice to calmly drink water. He did not spill any and stopped once

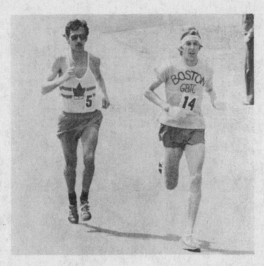

Jerome Drayton (#5) and Bill Rodgers (#14), wearing his homemade Boston T-shirt, at 11 miles. Photo by Jeff Johnson.

to tie his shoe. He did not worry about Drayton or Ronald the Hill or Fleming. If they came up on him he would just start running again. But no one came up on him.

For Rodgers the last several hundred yards came to him and lingered like a dream. He funneled down Ring Road through the vortex of the crowd, who with nearly one voice were shouting "Boston, Boston." He thought about Amby Burfoot, about his wife Ellen who had given him stability, about his brother Charlie who jumped up and down, about coach Squires, and about his Greater Boston Track Club teammates. All of it seemed swirling and timeless.

Fleming tried with all the hardness that was in him to catch Rodgers. Fleming had been second twice. He could not stand to be second again. But Rodgers would not die. Now on Hereford Street the race was over for Rodgers, but Fleming had a minute to run. You can't catch a runner who has already finished, so Fleming went soft. Steve Hoag caught him. Fleming did not care. He waved Hoag on. Fleming went on to the finish line because there was nowhere else to go. The crowds lined the street. There was no escape. He had to finish. Numbly he did so. When he found out his time (2:12:05) he was elated and wished he had kicked it in to get under 2:12. He had gone far faster than he imagined he could run. Fleming felt no shame to lose to a 2:09:55 course and American record.

The day produced the fastest mass finish in marathon history to date. Amby Burfoot, in 32nd place, ran nearly a minute faster than when he had won in 1968. Twenty-two runners broke 2:20—faster than John J. Kelley's best—and more than 100 ran faster than 2:30, John A. Kelley's best. And not only did the men run astoundingly fast, so did the women.

1975 Men's Results

1.	W. Rodgers, *GBTC*	**2:09:55**CR,AR*	33.	R. Bayko, *NMC*	2:21:28
2.	S. Hoag, *TCTC*	2:11:54	34.	C. Karthauser, NE	2:21:30
3.	T. Fleming, *NYAC*	2:12:05	35.	E. Vera, Puerto Rico	2:21:43
4.	T. Howard, Canada	2:13:23	36.	L. Olsen, *NMC*	2:21:45
5.	**R. Hill, *BH*, England**	**2:13:28**	37.	R. Blackmore, NY	2:21:56
6.	J. Stanley, *SummAC*	2:14:54	38.	K. Mueller, *BAA*	2:22:26
7.	R. Pate, *ColTC*, SC	2:15:22	39.	R. Mabuza, Swaziland	2:22:34
8.	P. Fredriksson, Sweden	2:15:38	40.	M. Sudzina, PA	2:22:45
9.	M. Quezas, Mexico	2:16:03	41.	D. Spitz, MI	2:23:18
10.	A. Boychuk, Canada	2:16:13	42.	A. Sidler, Switzerland	2:23:22
11.	L. Fidler, *ATC*	2:16:51	43.	E. Fuchs, CO	2:23:27
12.	T. Brien, *MC*, KS	2:17:20	44.	R. Thomas, ME	2:23:30
13.	A. Gylling, Finland	2:17:32	45.	R. Fitts, MO	2:23:39
14.	H. Lorenz, *PennAC*	2:17:43	46.	B. Heinrich, CA	2:23:49
15.	D. Kennedy, Fort Worth, TX	2:18:31	47.	C. Copp, KS	2:24:03
16.	R. Wayne, *WVTC*, CA	2:18:55	48.	B. Hance, IL	2:24:12
17.	J. DeJesus, Puerto Rico	2:19:02	49.	R. Conn, CT	2:24:18
18.	T. Derderian, *SMtAC*	2:19:04	50.	P. Stipe, *BAA*	2:24:19
19.	J. Bowles, *WVTC*	2:19:25	55.	J. Vitale, *HartTC*	2:24:49
20.	T. Antczak, IL	2:19:36	101.	P. Thompson, *NMC*	2:29:08
21.	T. Hoffman, *UCTC*	2:19:38	114.	R. Frankum, Huntington, NY	2:30:00
22.	P. Stewart, *WSC*	2:19:58	**169.**	**J.J. Kelley, *BAA***	**2:34:11**
23.	P. Farwell, *UCTC*	2:20:09	**177.**	**K. Yamada, Japan**	**2:34:51**
24.	E. Strabel, *NCTC*	2:20:12	179.	T. Clarke, *CapTC*	2:34:53
25.	W. Bragg, *NYAC*	2:20:18	396.	M. Parker, Stamford, CT	2:44:39
26.	K. McDonald, NJ	2:20:24	422.	J. Babington, *NMC*	2:45:54
27.	C. Hatfield, *WVirTC*	2:20:26	840.	R. Paffenbarger, CA	2:59:13
28.	W. Schamberger, Canada	2:20:31	842.	H. Cordellos, CA	2:59:15
29.	M. White, VA	2:20:40			(blind)
30.	L. Austin, England	2:20:51	1075.	G. Sheehan, *ShoreAC*	3:08:38
31.	P. Reiner, West Germany	2:21:18	1306.	J. Fixx, *FS*, CT	3:15:54
32.	**A. Burfoot, *MS*, CT**	**2:21:20**	1633.	**J.A. Kelley, E. Dennis, MA**	**3:22:48**

2,340 starters; 22 under 2:20, 113 under 2:30, 887 under 3:00, 1,817 under 3:30.

AR*denotes American record.

Team prize

1. San Blas, Puerto Rico:
   J. DeJesus, E. Vera,
   P. Santiago

2. West Valley TC
   R. Wayne, J. Bowles,
   J. Loeschhorn

3. Greater Boston Track Club:
   B. Rodgers, S. Graham,
   V. Fleming

4. Bolton Harriers, England:
   R. Hill, K. Mayor,
   G. Bennison

"BILLY, I'D REALLY LIKE A BEER"

MONDAY, APRIL 21, 1975

Biggest Women's Field Ever for BAA

This year Kathrine Switzer presented herself on the starting line with no regrets. She could say to herself that she had trained as well as she could. She did not wish for another 2 weeks to train. She was ready. She wanted to show that she was an athlete, not merely an agitator. She wanted her name in the paper for a victory in her best time ever, not fighting with Jock Semple or kissing him or fixing her hair. All that agitation was done. Now was the time for athletics, for racing, for winning the Boston Marathon.

But she also knew that Liane Winter had come to Boston from West Germany. Winter, coached by Dr. Ernst Van Aaken, had run a 2:50:31 at Waldniel in September the year before. A 2:50 did not seem likely for Switzer, but marathons were unpredictable.

Winter took the lead from the start. Though big for a marathon runner (5'9" and 145 pounds), she had trained well with Van Aaken's method of long-distance training with kilometers of solo runs through the forest trails around her native Wolfsburg. Winter was 33 and worked as an accountant for the Volkswagen company. Switzer took second place from the start, but she could not see Winter. Both had a few difficult stretches but felt good most of the way. Because they never saw each other they had little sense of racing against one another, so each ran according to her own physiological needs and abilities. Winter won the race in a new women's world record time, beating Jacqueline Hansen's 2:43:54.6 that had been set in Culver City, California, in December.

Switzer finished jubilantly in second place, 10 minutes faster than her best previous Boston Marathon. Although 9 minutes behind the winner, she ran fast enough to prove to herself and everyone else that she deserved to be counted not only as a pioneer, but as a performer.

Switzer ran the eighth-fastest time in the history of the women's marathon. From this peak she semiretired from running and applied herself to a career in journalism, race promotion, and later broadcasting. Fueled by her own improvement, she developed a circuit of races for women only that traveled to 30 countries, involved over a million women, and, along with the work of Jacqueline Hansen, Nina Kuscsik and others, sparked the inclusion of a women's marathon in the 1984 Olympics. Switzer now broadcasts the sport on television.

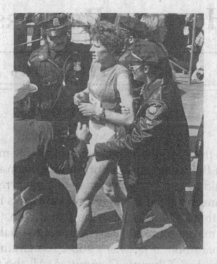

Liane Winter towers over Boston police officers who felt duty-bound to escort her to the victory platform after her world record run in 1975. Photo by Jeff Johnson.

At the awards ceremony Bill Rodgers looked up at Winter standing above him and told her that she had run a great time and that she must be very happy. He smiled his best smile. She said, "Thank you, I am. But could you get me a beer? I'd really like a beer."

Gayle Barron, a great beauty, a former University of Georgia cheerleader and a journalism major, stood nearby. She had just finished 3rd in the 13th-fastest marathon time in history. She would not dream of retiring. She had fun! She wanted to keep doing this forever. Coach Van Aaken took an interest in her and began a pen-pal coaching relationship that would pay off 3 years later.

1975 Women's Results

1.	**L. Winter, West Germany**	**2:42:24**CR,WR	14.	K. Smith, Baltimore, MD	3:13:20
2.	K. Switzer, NY	2:51:37	15.	M. Glenney, Ft. Lauderdale, FL	3:13:34
3.	**G. Barron, *ATC***	**2:54:11**	16.	P. McSwegin, OH	3:16:48
4.	M. Bevans, Baltimore, MD	2:55:52	17.	J. Heinonen, *OTC*	3:19:00
5.	M. Cushing, Amherst, MA	2:56:57	18.	W. Geller, Canada	3:19:05
6.	K. Loper, Wurtsmith, MI	2:59:10	19.	K. Magnuson, St. Paul, MN	3:20:49
7.	M. Paul, Portland, OR	2:59:37	20.	P. Price, TX	3:21:35
8.	J. Ullyot, *WVTC*	3:02:20	21.	S. Weiner, Canada	3:21:38
9.	J. Gumbs, *WVTC*	3:02:54	22.	S. Williams, MD	3:21:47
10.	J. Arenz, *TCTC*	3:03:03	23.	S. Davis, Canada	3:22:51
11.	H. Yamamoto, Japan	3:08:35	24.	V. Moore, Kailua, HI	3:26:45
12.	E. Turkell, Plattsburgh, NY	3:10:00	25.	P. Stafford, WI	3:27:40
13.	J. Haas, *CharTC*	3:11:23			

52 starters.

HOSE THE RUNNERS!

MONDAY, APRIL 19, 1976

Heat Wave Hits Hub

Nobody had to run this marathon. In fact most top U.S. marathoners, including 1975 champion Bill Rodgers, did not run in Boston in 1976 because the Olympic trials would be run a month later in Eugene, Oregon. In an Olympic year American runners trained for their Olympic trials race, not for Boston or any other marathon. The problem was that a man (there would be no women's Olympic marathon until 1984) first had to qualify for the Olympic trials with a 2:23 marathon; if he was a sub-2:20 marathoner, he would get his way paid by the U.S. Olympic Committee. All the top Americans had already qualified by this late date. Jack Fultz had not met the trials standard of 2:23, but it was not for lack of trying. He had not lost hope of running in the Eugene trials. He wanted to get his way paid from his home in Washington, DC, and a sub-2:20 at Boston would do it. He knew he could do it only if conditions were right for a fast time. He had been told by top runners that if you are going to run a good marathon, do it in Boston—the epitome. He had tried to get the qualifying out of the way sooner, but weather conditions were against him. It had stormed during one marathon, with winds and rain so strong that a fast time was impossible, so he dropped out and hoped for better conditions at Boston. Boston was his last chance.

Fultz had been trying to run well in the epitome of marathons since 1971, when he placed 12th, and 1973, when he placed 23rd. He had been in the Coast Guard then. He had quit the University of Arizona at Tucson, where he had been a miler in 1968 and 1969, and had been drafted into the military while transferring to Georgetown. He thought the Vietnam War was unjust and did not want to die there for nothing. He did believe in defending his country from real threats. With tongue in cheek he said that in order to defend America from North Vietnamese invasion, he joined the Coast Guard, which stationed him near Washington, DC. When the Coast Guard released Fultz he enrolled at Georgetown University with a track scholarship to study finance. He won his first marathon in the Washington's Birthday Marathon of 1971. He was the sixth of seven children. His father worked as a shipping clerk for the Joy Manufacturing Company of Franklin, Pennsylvania. Winning the Boston Marathon seemed unlikely for Fultz, but not impossible. At the start of Boston another Georgetown runner, Eamon O'Reilly, second in 1970, told him to begin slowly, run comfortably for the first half, then pick it up. A runner asked Bill Rodgers for advice. He said, "Don't run, but if you must run, go slowly." The reason for all this caution was the extremely high temperature.

A thermometer at a Hopkinton corner gas station read 100 °F. On the opposite corner another station's thermometer read 101 °F. The official reading for Hopkinton, the one in the shade, was 90 °F. In Ashland it was 96 °F, in Wellesley 93 °F. The temperature had never been this high on marathon day. Not in 1909, the first inferno when Henri Renaud came from 53rd place in Framingham to win; not in 1927, when Johnny Miles's shoes picked up smears of melted tar; not in 1952, when Doroteo Flores of Guatemala won; not in 1973 when Jon Anderson sweated his way to victory. The heat had been beating on New England for days, during a month when snow was not unusual. Everyone talked about the heat. Runners fashioned shading headgear and spent their prerace moments cutting holes in their shirts.

Those who knew marathon running thought a man from North America could not win in such heat. A man from a hot country was sure to win. Those who came from hot climates were Mexicans, Puerto Ricans, a Costa Rican, and the man who had run with the lead pack in the cold of 1975, Richard Mabuza of Swaziland. He saw this day as his kind of day. The year before the cold had ruined his race. Mabuza liked to sweat when he ran; hills and heat did not bother him. Mabuza, little and bouncy, worked as a policeman in Swaziland. He had run 2:12:54.4 in Christchurch, New Zealand, for third in the Commonwealth Games in 1974. He saw this day as right out of Africa and just for him.

Mabuza took the lead. Through Framingham he ran 2 minutes slower than last year. He felt good. The sun and the sweat felt good. This would be a cool day near the Tropic of Capricorn. Radames Vega of Puerto Rico followed him. Two foolish North Americans, Jim Bradley and Ron Kurrle, led Mexican Mario Cuevas, Vega's teammates José DeJesus and Eduardo Pacheco, 42-year-old Jack Foster of Rotorua, New Zealand, and Rafael Perez of Costa Rica. Bill Rodgers said Foster was the class of the field with his astounding 2:11:18.6 in the 1974 Commonwealth Games. But that was before Rodgers realized how hot it would be.

Jack Fultz followed Amby Burfoot, who was back and training well after his service in the Peace Corps in El Salvador. They ran in the top 20. Perhaps Burfoot now considered himself a hot weather runner, or perhaps deep inside he harbored hopes of stealing the race again in an Olympic year like in 1968. Fultz tried to stay wet. At one point he tried to pick up a 5-gallon bucket of water from the ground to dump it on himself. He thought he'd just scoop it up without slowing—and the 40 pounds of water nearly pulled his arm out of its socket. He dropped the bucket. Fultz planned on a race of attrition, but not his own. He planned to gradually pass the dropouts. Fultz abandoned all hope of a fast time and instead hoped for a top-10 finish.

But maybe he could squeak in under 2:20 to get his airfare to Oregon. He thought he'd let the runners come back to him—let them tiptoe back to me. He kept his pace steady as a machine. The sun beat down on the street, but the unprecedented numbers of spectators prepared to help the runners.

Someone had taken a marking pen to cardboard to make a sign that read "Hose the Runners" and taped it to the front grill of the leading press bus. The people rallied with garden hoses, lawn sprinklers, trays of ice cubes, buckets of water, sopping sponges, and millions of cups of water. On one lawn a table with brightly colored cups of drink waited for runners with a sign: 1% saline Kool-Aid. People rushed up to runners and dumped water on their heads. Kids gleefully aimed hoses full bore on runners and blasted them with cold water. Homeowners set their hose nozzles on fine spray, giving runners rainbows to run through. Grandmothers pressed ice cubes into runner's hands. Water was everywhere. For years and maybe generations these residents of Boston's western suburbs had watched the marathon. On this hottest day, dressed in Bermuda shorts and bikinis instead of minks and mackinaws, they knew exactly what to do.

Halfway passed in 1:09:32 for Mabuza. Fultz ran 1:10:02, in 10th place. From Wellesley to Woodland, Fultz passed runner after runner: Kurrle, DeJesus, Perez, Cuevas, Pacheco. Then only one remained: Mabuza.

Bill Rodgers, like Clarence DeMar before him, followed the race in the press vehicle and prepared to write his observations for the *Boston Globe*. He thought a 2:25 would win it. He noticed the glide had gone from Mabuza's stride. Fultz noticed it too. They were in Newton on the hottest section of the course, the treeless uphill overpass above Route 128. The hill is long and not advertised as a heartbreaker, but it comes after the long and refreshing downhill out of Wellesley into Newton Lower Falls. That hill breaks down other parts of a runner's body, like the quadriceps muscles, in preparation for later uphill cardiac cracking. Mabuza's racer instincts told him to keep that downhill speed on the uphill. In doing so he overheated and presented himself at the foot of the real hills a mile later in no condition to mount them aggressively. Fultz ran amazed that he did so well. True to his intentions, Mabuza had come tiptoeing back to him. But Fultz had run well in hot weather marathons before, Boston of 1971 and a fourth in the national AAU championships in 1972, on a steamy summer day in Liverpool, New York. Fultz thought that if he could get to the top of the hills in first place he might actually win the whole thing.

Fultz wanted to surprise Mabuza by passing on the opposite side of the road. No need to encourage him. As he sneaked across the tangent, Will Cloney leaned out of the press bus with a bullhorn announcing "make way for another runner." Cloney spoiled Fultz's surprise. He passed Mabuza anyway. Mabuza did not respond. Fultz moved on. The crowds shouted "Georgetown, Georgetown" as they read his racing shirt. They looked up his #14 in the newspaper and shouted "Fultz, Fultz." But just before Fultz took the lead, he found the constant dousing of water had dissolved his number and it fell away. As he pulled even with the photo truck the reporters and photographers asked him who he was. He smiled and would not tell them. All except Jeff Johnson, the Nike executive/runner/photographer, had used up their film on Mabuza and were passing around six-packs of beer. Fultz worked hard doing his job, and he thought the press should do theirs, finding out who he was instead of having a party right under his nose. He was not about to tell them. He made them guess. Reading his shirt they guessed, Justin Gubbins from Georgetown. Fultz had to laugh. That was his roommate who had passed up the race. He shook his head. Guess again.

But Fultz knew that it was not over yet. If Mabuza could die on the hot hills so could he. Fultz looked back once. No one was coming. He crested the hill in the lead. At the peak at Boston College a sea breeze caught him. Cool as air conditioning off the wintry North Atlantic, the wind dropped the temperature 10 degrees every 15 minutes. At the finish line flags pointed straight west, and the temperature was 60 °F. Now the gamble for Fultz was much smaller. It would be difficult for runners following to accelerate at such a late stage in the race, and in the coolness Fultz's collapse or a drastic slowing was much less likely. In the new coolness Fultz held his

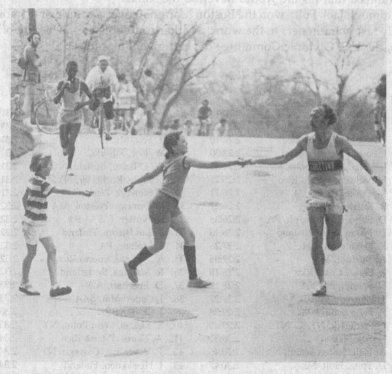

Jack Fultz accepts a drink after passing Richard Mabuza of Swaziland to take the lead on the hottest day in the history of the Boston Marathon. Photo by Jeff Johnson.

place. He felt a bit of a calf cramp between Lake Street and Cleveland Circle and backed off the pace. He knew no one he had passed could come up on him, but what about someone stalking him using the same strategy? Cuevas, DeJesus, and Foster moved up through the pack. Burfoot moved into ninth at Coolidge Corner. Fultz began to think. He began to think too much.

Jack Fultz began wondering as he ran through the biggest crowds ever gathered to watch the Boston Marathon how he would respond to victory. What do you do when you have won the epitome of marathons? In the past he had let defeats overwhelm him, but he did not have a great deal of experience with victories. What would he do for an encore? Surely the Olympic trials only a month away were too soon. What if he won the Boston Marathon in a time slower than 2:23—would the Olympic Committee let him into the trials? If he ran under 2:23 but slower than 2:20, would they give him a plane ticket? He felt as if he were watching himself win the Boston Marathon, his dream come true that he hadn't expected to come true. He wondered if he was having an out-of-body experience. Wow, he realized. People would be asking him questions. What would he say? He tried to think of a victory speech but could not. Useless thinking aside, Fultz ran on to a deafening crowd at the finish line. On crossing the line he guaranteed that his life would never be the same.

Although Jack Fultz won the Boston Marathon over a couple of extraordinarily fast marathoners in the worst weather conditions in the history of the race, the U.S. Olympic Committee did not give him a ticket.

1976 Men's Results

1.	J. Fultz, *GU*	2:20:19	24.	B. Robinson, *WashRC*	2:31:10
2.	M. Cuevas, Mexico	2:21:13	25.	G. Pfeiffer, Stamford, CT	2:31:14
3.	J. DeJesus, Puerto Rico	2:22:10	26.	T. Fox, MI	2:31:33
4.	J. Foster, New Zealand	2:22:30	27.	W. Roe, *WashRC*	2:31:47
5.	J. Berka, Minneapolis, MN	2:24:32	28.	W. O'Brian, Buffalo, NY	2:31:51
6.	E. Pacheco, Puerto Rico	2:25:11	29.	J. Boyle, Rochester, NY	2:31:56
7.	M. Burke, *BAA*	2:26:11	30.	P. Stewart, *WashRC*	2:31:57
8.	R. Kurrle, CA	2:26:21	31.	R. Duncan, Weston, MA	2:32:05
9.	D. Slusser, Pittsburgh, PA	2:26:38	32.	K. Nutter, *U.S. Army*	2:32:21
10.	D. Fiskin, New Zealand	2:26:43	33.	R. Lindstrom, Finland	2:32:25
11.	P. Talkington, OH	2:27:26	34.	S. Molnar, PA	2:32:37
12.	**A. Burfoot, *MS***	**2:27:56**	35.	A. Aponte, Puerto Rico	2:32:42
13.	R. Perez, Costa Rica	2:28:15	36.	R. Mabuza, Swaziland	2:32:46
14.	N. Sander, *MillAA*	2:28:19	37.	D. Eberhart, AZ	2:33:22
15.	T. Wilcox, *SMtAC*	2:29:27	38.	J. Cederholm, *BAA*	2:33:27
16.	P. Thompson, *NMC*	2:29:38	39.	J. Bradley, PA	2:33:30
17.	L. Frederick, *NYAC*, NY	2:29:40	40.	S. Maizel, West Point, NY	2:33:48
18.	H. Seki, Japan	2:30:31	41.	A. Flores, Puerto Rico	2:34:05
19.	A. Hall, Staten Island, NY	2:30:46	42.	F. Verdoliva, Oswego, NY	2:34:16
20.	D. Spitz, Holt, MI	2:30:47	43.	J. Heiskanen, Finland	2:34:23
21.	K. Mayer, WI	2:30:56	44.	C. Mericle, Corpus Christi, TX	2:34:35
22.	B. Fraser, WI	2:30:57	45.	F. Mueller, NY	2:34:38
23.	**Y. Unetani, Japan**	**2:31:08**	46.	J. Friel, Toronto, ON	2:34:49

47.	H. Wiegand, NC	2:34:56	154.	J.J. Kelley, *BAA*	**2:46:43**
48.	R. Gerard, CO	2:35:09	163.	T. Derderian, *SMtAC*	2:47:17
49.	R. Conn, MS	2:35:36	215.	**K. Yamada, Japan**	**2:50:42**
50.	J. Grabowski, MI	2:35:38	416.	M. Kazama, Ondekoza, Japan	3:00:01
53.	K. Randall, Hanover, NH	2:36:14	538.	J. Wallace, *BAA*	3:04:53
55.	L. Olsen, *NMC*	2:36:39	808.	J. Babington, *NMC*	3:15:43
56.	K. Uchida, Japan	2:36:40	884.	R. Paffenbarger, Berkeley, CA	3:18:40
60.	E. McGilvery, *NMC*	2:37:13	973.	W. Shrader, Albany, NY	3:22:43
64.	K. Young, *UCTC*	2:37:33	1013.	N. Bright, Seattle WA	3:24:34
77.	K. Nakada, Ondekoza, Japan	2:38:55	1524.	**J.A. Kelley**	**3:28:00**
137.	G. Muhrcke, *MillAA*	2:45:10			
146.	R. Swan, Bermuda	2:45:47			

1,898 starters.
Team prize

1. San Blas, Puerto Rico: J. DeJesus, E. Pacheco, A. Aponte
2. Washington RC: B. Robinson, W. Roe, P. Stewart
3. North Medford Club: P. Thompson, L. Olsen, E. McGilvery

THIG SMASH

MONDAY, APRIL 19, 1976

Winter, Gorman, Merritt Head Women's Field

Soon after the start of the 1976 Boston Marathon, Kim Merritt of Kenosha, Wisconsin, passed former winner Michiko Gorman. The women's field attracted higher ranking competitors than did the men's field because there were no women's Olympic marathon trials to distract them—there was no women's Olympic marathon.

Merritt never saw another woman runner for the rest of the race. She ran in a pack of men who chatted with each other. Some were faster runners who had either already qualified for the Olympic trials or conceded the race to the heat but still wanted to participate. She said nothing to them. Frequently someone in that pack, a spectator or her husband, Keith, who popped out of the crowd at intervals and ran for miles alongside her, would dump water on her head. At 5'4" and 114 pounds, with two blond pigtails and a red shirt and shorts, she ran continuously wet.

Back at the University of Wisconsin, Merritt trained with Lucian Rosa, who had placed fourth in 1974 at Boston. From him she had heard tales of the Boston Marathon. She had run 2:46:13.8 in New York in September of 1975 to beat Michiko Gorman's 2:53:02. On distance training only this spring she had run a personal best in the mile of 4:50. That pleased her. Back in Kenosha Merritt added new words to the runners' jargon. That aching feeling of having been drained of energy, what Bill Rodgers called *zapped*, she called *runner's sickness*. As this race developed she realized that she had contracted a severe case of it.

Merritt wanted to get the thing over with. Actually she wanted to drop out, but she dared not while still leading. She wanted to win, but almost as much she wanted to quit. She was just plain hot and tired and she wanted to stop. Her competition was herself, time, and the heat. She told herself that she would run one more mile, then quit. The deception was essential to her. She had never hurt this much in a marathon. She knew that if she kept at it she might win. But if some woman passed her, then she would quit. She told herself these sweet lies to keep herself going for the moment.

Merritt had beaten Gorman by 7 minutes in New York City, so she felt that she could only lose the race if something went wrong with her. She could only be defeated by herself, a fact that created enormous pressure. Merritt denied the pressure by telling herself that she would soon drop out. She could not employ tactics against a runner she could not see or hear and who could not see or hear her. Any information she got about her competition came secondhand and from spectators who had not yet seen the pursuing competition. She felt as if she raced against ghosts. "She's 2 minutes behind—5 minutes—400 yards—800 yards—way back," came the reports, all sketchy and unreliable. Husband Keith during his poppings from the crowd ran alongside her and urged her to run faster. She urged him to shut up and go away. She ran on the frazzled edge of mobile domestic altercation. They argued. He didn't want any woman to come up out of the pack and catch her. But she said she was running as fast as she could—Husband, you don't know how it feels. Realizing she was flat-out, he withdrew his advice and offered only encouragement. She ignored all advice, accepted encouragement and cheers, and just ran to get the thing over with.

Her thighs hurt. On the downhills pressure built in her legs. She coined a new term—*thigh smash*. After the race she would repeat it to herself for the next 2 weeks as she approached any situation requiring her to sit down. Her quadriceps muscles could not control her descent into a chair. She had to simply position her buttocks and fall into the seat. Thigh smash. Boston Marathon thigh smash. She did not like the Boston Marathon.

In the last 3 or 4 miles she stopped to walk every half mile. Still no woman caught her.

When Merritt finished all wet in the 60 °F sea breeze, she rapidly chilled. Now cold was her enemy. Officials carted her off to Massachusetts General Hospital for treatment for hypothermia. Ultimately she suffered no ill effects. She knew she could run faster on a cool day and planned to come back the next year to do just that if she could get someone to pay her way from Wisconsin.

The next year both Fultz and Merritt would come back to do it again. After the Olympics everyone else would be back too. Fultz had to prove his victory wasn't just a fluke of hot weather against a weak field.

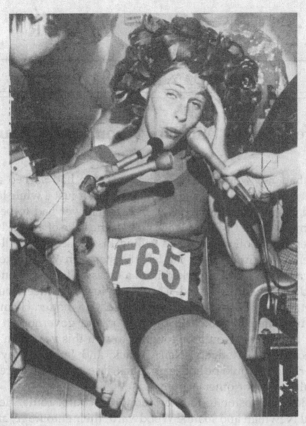

The hottest Boston race ever sent Kim Merritt from heat exhaustion into hypothermia. She tried to answer reporters' questions but eventually wound up in Massachusetts General Hospital. AP/Wide World Photo.

1976 Women's Results

1.	**K. Merritt, Kenosha, WI**	**2:47:10**	14. J. Ullyot, *WVTC*	3:15:57
2.	**M. Gorman,** *LAAC*	**2:52:27**	15. T. d'Elia, Ridgewood, NJ	3:16:56
3.	D. Doolittle, Austin, TX	2:56:26	16. P. DeMoss, *WVTC*	3:17:24
4.	**G. Barron,** *ATC*	**2:58:23**	17. K. Gervasi, Wallingford, CT	3:17:59
5.	N. Kent, Conshohocken, PA	3:00:53	18. M. Gallagher, Brookline, MA	3:18:53
6.	M. Bevans, Baltimore, MD	3:01:22	19. C. Allison, *HETC*	3:19:28
7.	C. Spawei, Holland	3:04:46	20. K. Switzer, *CPTC*	3:19:35
8.	H. Yamamoto, Japan	3:05:36	21. R. Anderson, *NCS*	3:20:24
9.	L. Lorrain, *ATC*	3:11:01	22. E. Turkel, Plattsburgh, NY	3:20:44
10.	**L. Winter, West Germany**	**3:12:44**	23. N. Lindsay, NY	3:21:12
11.	J. Gumbs, *WVTC*	3:13:24	24. E. DeMendonca, *CSU*	3:21:57
12.	K. Obata, Ondekoza, Japan	3:14:46	25. M. Cutsforth, MA	3:22:01
13.	G. Gustafson, CA	3:15:26	26. **N. Kuscsik,** *SuffAC*	**3:23:08**

78 entrants, 73 starters.

THE ANGRY VICTOR

MONDAY, APRIL 18, 1977

Rodgers Set to Win His Second BAA Marathon

Jack Fultz had not worked in the past year. He had earned a degree in finance, but he wanted to pursue the marathon for just a while longer. How good could he get? He didn't know, but the answer had to be—better. In the meantime he didn't want to work just for the sake of a weekly paycheck. He had been living off savings and selling his possessions. All he had left was his stereo and his Toyota. He left the stereo in Washington, DC, and drove the car to Boston. He parked it on a crosswalk on Beacon Hill. When he returned it was gone—towed. The Olympic Committee would not give him a ticket, but the Boston police would. Well, no matter. He might be able to clear it up when he talked to the mayor and governor on the victory stand after the race. It would be tougher to win this year than it had been in 1976 because Bill Rodgers, Neil Cusack, and Jerome Drayton had all entered. Perhaps it would be hot again. Luck, it seemed, had a greater affinity for Jack Fultz than for other people.

Fultz rode from Boston to the start along the course route. He saw chaos. Actors Paul Newman and Joanne Woodward, their entourage, and hangers-on clogged up the road. Newman was making a movie starring Woodward about a woman marathon runner, and they intended to film some live scenes. Everybody wanted to get in on that. Fultz needed to get through to the gym a mile beyond the start at the common and back again before the start. There was no way he could get through. Fultz thought his luck had evaporated. He could not officially run without a number. He ran the remaining mile to the gym to pick up his number. He had less than 15 minutes until the start. When he got to the gym Jock Semple's assistants said that the top 100 numbers had already been taken to the start. He ran a mile back to the start and found Semple. No, he did not have the numbers. Someone else did, but Semple said that he'd give Jack his number at the first checkpoint and not to worry. Fultz thought, Am I supposed to stop and pin it on? No one showed up at the first checkpoint or any other with a number for Jack. He wore a plain shirt and had shaved off his characteristic moustache. He ran the entire race without a number, lost in the crowd. He looked like an unofficial runner, a drop-in, a bandit, or perhaps even to some people a cheat. Few people recognized him to cheer for his defense. The race did not go as well as last year.

The Olympic trials had not gone well for Fultz either. He had trained very hard after his Boston win of 1976 for the trials that came only 6 weeks later. By the last half of the race he had no energy and had to shuffle to the finish at survival pace. Bill Rodgers, on the other hand, had easily made the U.S. Olympic team but the Olympics had not gone well for him. He placed 40th in 2:25. But in the fall Rodgers had rebounded in New York with a win over 1976 silver medalist Frank Shorter in 2:10:09.6. In December he won the hilly Maryland Marathon in 2:14:22 over Tom Fleming. In February he won the Kyoto Marathon in a costly 2:14. He paid for his victory with fatigue that forced him to slow over the last six miles. In March he fell, hurting his knee, and missed 3 weeks of quality training. On the Tuesday before the Boston race he managed to complete an interval session of four 1-mile runs in 4:50 to 4:55 each with a quarter-mile jog in between. Rodgers did not feel very well. He lied to himself that he was just tired from high (slow) mileage. These uncertainties combined with something that had become Rodgers's great phobia. Like the scarecrow made of straw from the Wizard of Oz, who feared nothing but a lighted match, Rodgers feared having to race a marathon on a hot day. Rodgers's fear was not irrational. He had dropped out of Boston in 1973 on a hot day. He had dropped out of the hot Enschede Marathon in the Netherlands in 1975 after his Boston victory. For weeks before this year's race he scanned newspaper weather reports trying to figure out some weather pattern that would predict race day temperatures. He knew that in New England such a thing was impossible, but he tried anyway. Rodgers desperately wanted "good" weather.

In the Hopkinton gym before the race Rodgers encountered Jerome Drayton. Drayton had beaten Rodgers soundly at Fukuoka in 1975, winning with a 2:10:08.4 to Rodgers's third in 2:11:26.4. In the Olympics Drayton ran sixth with a 2:13:30. In Fukuoka, the unofficial world marathon championships in those days, Drayton beat the Olympic gold medalist Waldemar Cierpinski of East Germany by 2 minutes. Rodgers had been hoping that Drayton would not show up, but there he stood. He had solved his employment and injury problems. He had trained logically and consistently. He looked like the Drayton of 1970—the fittest marathoner in the world. Rodgers could not help but notice that Drayton looked as good as he had on that day at Fukuoka when he used the Rodgers tactic of a long sustained surge to break the field in the middle of the race. Although he wished it were not so, Rodgers had the gut feeling that he, himself, could not run such a race that day. Drayton told Rodgers that he hadn't been planning to race Boston until he heard that the weather would be "good"—from his point of view, that meant warm. All of this was bad from Rodgers's point of view. As the sun notched higher in the clear sky and the temperature rose past 70 °F, Rodgers felt impending doom. But maybe, Rodgers reasoned, ignoring his intuition, Drayton would drop out again as he had in 1970 against Ronald the Hill and against himself in 1975. Maybe. Maybe. Maybe.

But Drayton came to Boston out of curiosity rather than hometown necessity and pressure to atone for a bad Olympic-year effort, as Rodgers and Fultz did. Drayton had won Fukuoka again in December of 1976, and as an experiment for the winter he converted himself to an indoor 3-miler. He thought about racing at Boston but had trained during the winter for indoor track to see if the speed thus acquired would convert to a good marathon. The indoor season ended 4 weeks before Boston, and he had trained with hard long-distance running for only 4 weeks. Would that strategy produce a good marathon race? So Drayton came to Boston to find out if he could run a marathon off track training and how well. Drayton saw Neil Cusack in the entries but knew he was not the runner he had been a couple of years earlier. Drayton saw Fultz but knew he was not capable of a 2:11, at least not yet, so that left only Rodgers. That Rodgers was beatable Drayton had proved, however much respect he held for Rodgers.

Drayton said that Rodgers could set a fast pace from the start, maintain it, and then at the 25-, 30-, 35-kilometer marks put in an all-out effort and just *gut* the bloody thing the rest of the way if necessary. To Drayton, Rodgers's unpredictable tactics produced a danger.

Drayton stood in the first row at the Hopkinton starting line. He heard no warning that the gun was about to fire. Just suddenly it *had* fired. Someone grabbed his shirt and pulled him. Someone kicked him. He thought he would fall and had the vision of 2,000 feet trampling all over him. Before he could recover and rock himself forward into a stride, the first two rows of runners passed him. Runners pushed Rodgers several times before he could get up enough speed to run free of any fear of falling. The two top contenders came close to mob-induced injury. They expected controlled starts like those in the elite Olympic and Fukuoka fields, not the hydraulic pressure of 7,000 nervous runners at their backs. Marathon running had never been a contact sport before.

After a quarter mile of frantic downhill running the lead pack began to coalesce. By 3 miles it had formed. As temperatures reached 77 °F, the runners looked around for water. Rodgers felt a stitch in his side. He tried to settle into the pack to rest and relax. Rodgers's wife, Ellen, handed him a water bottle at the Ashland checkpoint. He shared it with the other runners, but no one really got as much water as was needed. There weren't many spectators in the early stages, and the ones who did watch were not inclined to participate by passing out water. Because the weather in the days before the race had been seasonal, spectators did not bring water with them; to them the day seemed perfect—for watching. Approaching Framingham Drayton expected an official water stop with a table and full cups for everyone. When he got to the main town he saw none.

Drayton turned to Rodgers and asked half jokingly, "Bill, don't they have any official water stations in this race?"

"No, you're sort of on your own here. You have to depend on the spectators."

Rodgers looked at Drayton carefully. Drayton's dark glasses stymied Rodgers because he could not see Drayton's eyes to determine his level of fatigue. Inscrutable, thought Rodgers, using one of his favorite words.

Bill's brother Charlie popped out of the crowd with a water bottle for him. Drayton watched. Bill shared the water with Drayton. Suddenly it hit Drayton that this was Rodgers's hometown; there would be plenty of water offered to him, but if Drayton were to break away, where would he get water? You never know what is in the cups offered by spectators. Many runners have inadvertently dumped soft drinks on their heads or slowed to accept cups of fluids that were not what they wanted—like beer or whiskey. The prospect of an all-out duel with Rodgers in 80 °F heat when they were already past the first checkpoint and Drayton was desperately looking for water presented a grim and frightening picture. As Drayton ran along he became enraged. He saw before him a hard two-man race that was unfair because of the race organizers' laziness. Was he to come to Boston to run a world-class race and at the same time find his own water? Did he have to be dependent on his competitors for it? The next time Rodgers offered some water Drayton said no.

Drayton later said had he seen Will Cloney or one of the Boston officials along the side of the road he would have run over and squeezed his throat for a couple of minutes. Later Cloney said, "We had eight Gatorade stations and about a million kids with water." When told that Drayton does not like -ade drinks, Cloney said, "Well, he wears those sunglasses, and he probably can't tell the difference between water and Gatorade." Drayton angered the normally unflappable Cloney. Anger fueled Drayton as he ran at the raw edge of jangled emotions. Marathon races are, at the end of it all, emotional things. Drayton's usual temperament was shy, and friendly with his close friends; he was not normally the Boston Strangler.

Rodgers tried to observe other runners during the pack phase of the race—seeing how much they were sweating, listening to their breathing. He talked to them—a runner who could respond with a full sentence at a 5-minute-per-mile pace at 15 miles on a hot day was in control of the situation. But Rodgers liked to go early. When Drayton refused the offer of water, Rodgers wasn't quite sure who controlled this situation.

By Natick, Rodgers and Drayton had clearly broken away from Tom Fleming and the rest of the field. The crowds grew bigger and more boisterous than ever before. For many the race offered an excuse to party. Hal Higdon, who came as a reporter for *Runner's World*, observed "pot smokers, drunks clutching beer cans, girl-huggers and boy-huggers." Rodgers heard the crowd call his name again and again. He was glad to hear it but knew that the crowd support would do him no good. They partied, but Rodgers ran blistered and dizzy, feeling empty and exhausted—that feeling he called zapped, really zapped. Ellen handed him another bottle at the halfway point. He gave her a thumbs-down. Drayton pulled away, breathing easily. If either of them had looked back he would have seen no one.

The photo truck pulled alongside Rodgers. It had a flatbed with benches arranged along the sides and back like bleachers around an athletic field. Banks of photographers examined Rodgers in his moment of failure. He had no spring in his legs and no will left to race. The cameras did not care. Like so many disinterested snakes, the battery of them blinked at his weakness. He could do nothing. He had hit the wall, the thing he trained to avoid. He had gambled on two points: that Drayton would not show up and that it would be cool. He had not prepared well enough and lost both gambles. He thought of himself like Dorando Pietri in the 1908 Olympics or Jim Peters in the 1954 Commonwealth Games stumbling along to the finish line. Of course those two had been leading their races when they hit the wall. Rodgers had a tireless Canadian in front of him and a hungry field behind him. Rodgers resolved that he should not enter marathons on hopes and prayers instead of uncompromised training. At that moment he could do nothing other than make resolutions. After a mechanical slog up Heartbreak Hill he dropped out of the race at the very spot where he had dropped out in 1973. He had come full circle. Would this be the way his career ended? He scrounged a ride to the Eliot Lounge, sat down, and drank a beer as he listened to radio reports of Drayton's victory and waited for Ellen and Charlie to find him.

When the photo truck caught up to Drayton, the riders met a different runner. He had spring and bounce in his stride and anger in his voice. He directed his wrath at this official-looking truck and the men in it. Though these photographers and reporters were not the race officials who had been negligent in Drayton's eyes, he blasted them with criticism simply because they were in the way. He ran along livid and tirelessly venting his anger. He ran and he complained. He did not receive sympathy. On the contrary, here he was winning the greatest marathon in the world and complaining about it! As he realized the secret dream of these reporters and photographers of winning the Boston Marathon he ran coldly, complaining about the very thing he was winning. He did not try to run fast. He just wanted to get the unpleasantness of this race behind him. He no longer cared about his time. He ran as if it were an ordinary Sunday run at the park with the guys back in Toronto. Rather than concentrate on the race, he ran through the congestion of crowds looking at everyone's hands to find a cup. There weren't many cups around. No one had put a sign on the lead vehicle telling people to water the runners. Drayton expected the treatment he received at marathons like Fukuoka and the Olympics, and when he did not get it he stopped caring.

The press and the public held victory in the Boston Marathon as a great fantasy—a dream come true—but in the view of the Boston press Drayton committed a heinous crime—a crime of omission. He won their marathon without elation, without joy. On top of that he dared criticize a Boston institution. He said the race administration was amateurish and that the race could turn into a disaster if it was not handled more professionally.

In the next day's papers the reporters blasted him without mercy for his joylessness and candor. No one bothered to examine the logic of what he said.

Jack Fultz likewise felt no elation; he failed again to break 2:20 and to get the ranking that he so much wanted as a serious or world-class marathoner. Other marathoners regarded Fultz not as a talent but as a guy who got lucky on a hot day and won Boston when no really good runners showed up. He was not happy about that evaluation. He did not want to be an Henri Renaud, who had won by default in 1909 by wading through a field of dehydrated runners to a laurel wreath, then never ran well again. He did not want to be dismissed as a no-talent. Fultz believed that he could run a truly fast marathon against a truly fast field. He promised himself that some day he would do just that. And his impounded automobile? He got Boston Parks Director Peter Meade to pay the parking fines and the towing charges. Boston people seemed to like Jack Fultz and take care of him. His luck might be returning. They did not like Jerome Drayton, and they felt bad for Bill Rodgers. Yet in the future the BAA administration would have to answer Drayton's questions. Drayton saw the future.

1977 Men's Results

1.	J. Drayton, TOC	2:14:46	30.	A. Usami, Japan	2:25:28
2.	V. Bally, Turkey	2:15:44	31.	C. Griffin, OH	2:25:40
3.	B. Maxwell, CA	2:17:21	32.	T. Donovan, Peoria, IL	2:25:56
4.	R. Wayne, NOTC	2:18:18	33.	B. Robinson, WashRC	2:25:59
5.	V. Fleming, GBTC	2:18:37	34.	G. Mason, Lawrence, KS	2:26:07
6.	T. Fleming, NYAC	2:18:46	35.	K. Mayer, Milwaukee, WI	2:26:14
7.	G. Tuttle, TSdr, CA	2:19:42	36.	M. Murphy, Cromwell, CT	2:26:22
8.	C. Berka, WVTC, CA	2:19:48	37.	D. Landriault, PQ	2:26:39
9.	J. Fultz, PA	2:20:44	38.	J. Bowles, WVTC	2:26:41
10.	R. Pate, SC	2:21:16	39.	A. Hall, Staten Island, NY	2:27:12
11.	C. Hatfield, WVirTC	2:21:16	40.	W. Yetman, TOC	2:27:39
12.	J. Wells, TX	2:21:42	41.	S. Maizel, West Point, NY	2:27:42
13.	B. Varsha, ATC	2:21:44	42.	K. Kule, Ohio	2:27:46
14.	V. Anderson, Australia	2:21:51	43.	L. Olsen, NMC, MA	2:27:52
15.	P. Stewart, WashRC	2:22:00	44.	J. Vitale, HartTC	2:28:02
16.	C. Burrows, TCTC	2:22:24	45.	C. Conejo, GA	2:28:09
17.	P. Dolan, Scotland	2:23:00	46.	R. Hodge, GBTC	2:28:45
18.	S. Curran, England	2:23:19	47.	D. Reed, Corning, NY	2:28:50
19.	D. McDaid, Ireland	2:23:25	48.	G. Pfeiffer, Stratford, CT	2:28:55
20.	L. Fidler, ATC	2:23:42	49.	R. Currier, Manchester, NH	2:28:58
21.	R. Kurrle, CA	2:23:49	50.	T. Allison, Pittsburgh, PA	2:29:16
22.	M. White, WashRC	2:23:56	54.	G. Muhrcke, MillAA	2:29:32
23.	E. Vera, Puerto Rico	2:24:05	57.	B. Thurston, WashRC	2:29:52
24.	R. Hughson, Toronto, ON	2:24:15	58.	P. Farwell, WRR	2:29:56
25.	N. Cusack, Ireland	2:24:25	79.	F. Mueller, CPTC	2:32:12
26.	T. Antczak, WI	2:24:34	113.	J. Green, BAA	2:34:56
27.	B. Durden, ATC	2:24:39	230.	G. Goettleman, WVTC	2:41:44
28.	G. Fanelli, PP	2:24:55	239.	J. DeJesus, Puerto Rico	2:42:20
29.	K. McCarey, NYAC	2:25:03	353.	J.J. Kelley, BAA	2:46:26

362.	A. Burfoot, *MS*	2:46:37	1704.	O. Pilkey, *NCTC*	3:25:18
932.	R. Paffenbarger, *NCS*	3:02:24	1892.	J.A. Kelley	**3:32:12**
1383.	T. Grilk, *GBTC*	3:13:45	2154.	R. McGregor, Concord, MA	3:47:35
1420.	G. Sheehan, *ShoreAC*	3:16:30		B. Rodgers, DNF	

MICHIKO AGAIN

MONDAY, APRIL 18, 1977

141 Women Set to Race 26-Miler Today

The favorite, Kim Merritt, dropped out in 1977. General overwork, overracing, and overdoing it did her in. She did not like the Boston course and it did not like her. That left the road free for Michiko Gorman. She had increased her training tremendously since her last win in Boston in 1974. She trained on the track under Lazlo Tabori and piled on the distance to as much as 140 miles a week.

She ran with a thin gold chain around her neck, a San Fernando Track Club green singlet, and blue shorts. At the start a couple of men near her fell. In the madness someone kicked her. Gorman was terrified. In any encounter her 89 pounds was likely to lose.

Gorman survived the start, but the hot weather did not let her run a time that could show off her training. Her increased training in the last 3 years

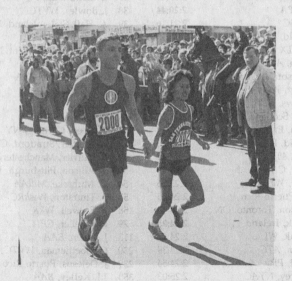

"Such a little bit of a thing," 89-pound Michiko Gorman, won in 1974 and here in 1977. Photo by Jeff Johnson.

produced the same first place and a time a minute slower than in 1974, but in the heat and the chaos of this disorganized race, it was enough to win.

1977 Women's Results

1.	M. Gorman, Los Angeles, CA	2:48:33	17.	E. DeMendonca, CSU	3:06:45
2.	M. Bevans, Baltimore, MD	2:51:12	18.	J. Greaney, LAC	3:07:33
3.	L. Lorrain, ATC	2:56:04	**19.**	**N. Kuscsik, SuffAC**	**3:08:12**
4.	G. Olinek, Canada	2:56:55	20.	M. Cushing, SMtAC, MA	3:08:28
5.	A. Forshee, MI	2:58:54	21.	C. Bravakis, HartTC	3:08:35
6.	L. Matovcik, HETC	2:58:54	22.	M. Cutsforth, MA	3:09:21
7.	J. Ullyot, WVTC	3:01:04	23.	M. Burns, DesMoines, IA	3:09:45
8.	P. DeMoss, WVTC	3:01:16	24.	R. Anderson, Oakland, CA	3:11:20
9.	J. White, VA	3:03:33	25.	T. Hom, Los Angeles, CA	3:11:28
10.	S. Sullivan, HartTC	3:03:46	27.	K. Obata, Japan	3:12:38
11.	S. Petersen, CA	3:04:22	31.	E. Wessel, Arlington, VA	3:13:31
12.	T. d'Elia, NJM	3:04:56	39.	G. Gustafson, CA	3:20:36
13.	K. Fady, DCRRC	3:05:11	44.	D. Butterfield, Bermuda	3:22:11
14.	L. Pedrinan, WSY	3:05:49	**61.**	**S. Berman, CSU**	**3:28:45**
15.	J. Killion, WSY	3:05:52	72.	H. Yamamoto, Japan	3:34:18
16.	D. Doolittle, ARC	3:06:05			

141 entrants, 102 finished under 4 hours.

THE JINX!

MONDAY, APRIL 17, 1978

Frank Shorter to Race in Boston Marathon

The big news at Boston this year was that the 1972 Olympic champion, Frank Shorter, would race in Boston for the first time. He had previously complained about the BAA policy of refusing to pay expenses to top runners. Whereas other major marathons around the world invited the top runners and paid their airfare and lodging (and maybe some under-the-table appearance money), Boston did not. In fact Boston officials were quite proud that they did not have to "bribe" runners to come to their race. Tradition brought them. Shorter said that the BAA officials expected top runners to hitchhike to Boston.

What brought Shorter to Boston if the race directors would not pay his way? A mixture of reasons: exposure for his shoe sponsor, Tiger; exposure for his own line of running apparel, Frank Shorter Sports; and probably most importantly, the fact that Boston was the next big prestigious marathon that Shorter had not won. At the heart of it all, Shorter was a man who liked winning races.

The Boston press made a big deal of what they called "The Jinx"—the fact that no Olympic gold medalist had ever won the Boston Marathon, though many had tried. To Frank Shorter that was a fine fact for journalists to play with, but neither that nor the inverse fact, that no Boston Marathon winner had ever won an Olympic gold medal, much interested him. Each race was a new contest, as

No Olympic gold medalist had ever won the Boston Marathon, though many had tried.

divorced from the previous one as a coin toss. For Shorter this would be not an attempt to break a jinx but a test of his fitness, to see where he stood since recovering from a metatarsal injury.

For Bill Rodgers this Boston would be a makeup for 1977 and would pave his way to Olympic gold in Moscow in 1980. He had resolved after the previous year's race never to run a marathon unprepared, and for this one he had prepared unmercifully. But to friends, the press, and even himself he played the underdog. Questioned about his readiness, he told his old roommate, Amby Burfoot,

> No, not as ready as I could be. I'm about 90%. I'm a little leery of the distance because I haven't been doing many long runs. I've averaged only 133 miles a week over the last 10 weeks. Last week I did seven times a mile in 4:47 to 5:00 with [Greater Boston Track Club] teammates including Randy Thomas [as well as the author of this book, on an extremely windy day], and it felt tough. I suspect Shorter is in better shape than he is letting on, and Jeff Wells is ready for a good marathon too. He's very dedicated. On the way back from the International Cross-Country race in Edinburgh, Scotland, he went out with me for a training run from one of the airports. You've got to be fairly fanatical to run at an airport.

The fact was that Wells ran with Rodgers in the airport in order to be with a runner he greatly admired. Wells would have followed Rodgers anywhere. But it was ironic that Wells could maintain his reverence for Rodgers when it was Wells who finished in 29th place in the international championships and teammate Rodgers only 44th and Randy Thomas 99th. (John Treacy of Ireland won that race, but he does not figure into the Boston story for another decade.) In the repeat-miles workout Randy Thomas had run with more apparent ease than did Bill Rodgers. Fortunately for everyone, the weather in Boston registered ideal—overcast, windless, and 47 °F.

Not a fanatical trainer but a methodical one, Jerome Drayton came back to Boston. He did have a leg injury that worried him, but he thought he was fully recovered. He was quite pleased that the BAA had adopted suggestions he had made the year before. For one thing, to keep runners from bunching up and pushing over the starting line early, the start would be separated into sections according to time, with space between sections. Five minutes before the gun the ropes holding the runners in each section were withdrawn, and they could ease into the new space and alleviate the pressure on the front. This system worked well, and there was no pushing panic like the one in 1977 that had caught Drayton and Rodgers.

The race officials moved the start from narrow Hayden Row to Route 135 to eliminate the 90-degree right-hand turn after only a few hundred yards. Drayton's comments were heeded, although the BAA did not admit to it at the time. But there was still more work to be done to answer his complaints about crowd control, as became evident to runners like Jack Fultz in the later stages of the 1978 race.

Drayton dropped out at 3-1/2 miles. His leg was not functioning well, so there was no point in continuing. His point was to race to win—that was the fun of it—not to finish at all costs. The old idea that for men the marathon is a test of manhood measured by the ability to endure pain and discomfort was finally gone. Drayton anticipated the Canadian National Championships in 4 weeks and figured that his leg would be healed by then if he dropped out early now. Better to run away and live to fight another day.

Shorter tested his fitness to fight at 5 miles with a surge of about 200 yards. Rodgers went with him. No one else did. Then Shorter eased up and the pack closed. There were actually two packs. In the first one ran New Zealander Kevin Ryan, Esa Tikkanen of Finland, Tom Fleming, and many others. The second pack included Don Kardong, wisecracking Randy Thomas, Ric Rojas, and many more. Jack Fultz, like a vulture, ran a steady pace, waiting for the inevitable abrasion of the miles to bring the field back to him. A steady-pace tactic seldom leads to a marathoner's victory in a major race, except in hot weather as Fultz had faced in 1976, but it does frequently result in a good finishing time and position. Shorter, for one, said that if he were going to "die" in a race he would rather die from the front.

The inevitable strains of racing drained Shorter, and he did die from the front. He wore samples from his new apparel line. Sales promotions and marketing had reached the lead packs at Boston. Rodgers wore a Bill Rodgers Running Center shirt; he had his stores and planned to also start a clothing line. Actually Rodgers sold Shorter's clothing in his stores. But soon he would compete with Shorter not only on the roads but in stores for shelf space. Commercialism came to the runners in the Boston Marathon before it came to the administrators.

Boston University graduate student Randy Thomas had no clothing line, but he did have a deal. Two days before the marathon he had agreed with the Nike promotional manager, Todd Miller, that he would wear a pair of Nike shoes in the race for $1,000. If Thomas ran those shoes to the first American finish, Nike would pay him $2,500; he would get $1,500 for second and $500 for third. Nike had made special shoes for Thomas in their Exeter, New Hampshire, research and development factory. They were made from the nylon uppers of one model combined with the outsoles of another. Wearing these shoes, a Labatt's Beer singlet, and hopes of an improving bank balance, Thomas ran with a roguish bravado. Through Wellesley he felt a surge of strength and left the second pack just as the first one broke up. People called his name and toasted him with Labatt's as he picked his way through the human fatigue of the first pack.

But Kevin Ryan had not been picking his way, he had been pushing and pushing the pace from 10 miles to the beginning of the hills with Rodgers and Tikkanen hanging on. But Thomas moved on and up.

As Thomas passed Shorter they slapped hands for luck, but Shorter's luck was gone. Ellen Rodgers offered water to Thomas. He declined. "She doesn't like me," he thought, and imagined that she might have put some vile potion in the bottle. Thomas's passion produced a paranoia; he saw Ellen as a Lady Macbeth, willing to stop at nothing to see her husband become king. He was wrong—the bottle contained pure water. By the top of the hills near Boston College, Thomas had passed everyone but his training partner, the would-be king of the roads, Bill Rodgers, who ran only 30 to 40 yards ahead. Thomas had visions of a throne and a crown of laurels and the $2,500 from Nike. Now to depose the king. Thomas had waded through slaughter to sneak up behind him. Like Kelley and Tarzan Brown in 1939, like O'Reilly and Hill in 1970, Thomas ran a step away from the kingdom. From there the course ran all downhill on roads he had trained on a hundred times.

When Thomas reached Cleveland Circle, right where he shared an apartment with several Greater Boston Track Club teammates, he began to lose his sense of balance. As if a spell had been cast, the fine muscles in his legs did not work the way they were supposed to. He began to lose ground, as well as balance and a sense of proportion. Jeff Wells, the man studying to be a reverend, came up on him.

"Randy, how far to go?"

To where? The promised land? The magic kingdom? Thomas knew he himself was out of the race for first. He withheld wisecracks.

"Two and a half miles. You'd better get going."

Wells got going. Thomas thought, OK, I've still got $500 left.

Near Kenmore Square, Finnish Esa Tikkanen passed Thomas. That was fine with Thomas. Tikkanen was not an American, and he had run a courageous race with the leaders. On Hereford Street, Jack Fultz passed Thomas. That was not fine. "Chickenshit," Thomas thought. He despised Fultz's sneaky tactic of not racing bravely with the leaders, as had Tikkanen and Ryan, but pacing himself as if in a detached time trial. To Thomas, Fultz was a great pretender, not a real racer. But Fultz had run a fair race, and with his finishing time of 2:11:17 he finally dispelled the curse that he was just a lucky runner, not a fast one. There went Thomas's $500.

But Fultz had had problems getting up through the pack. His major opponents seemed to be the press bus and the police cars. Just past Lake Street the crowds were so thick that they stopped a police car dead in the road and closed in around it like quicksand. The driver, the crowds, no one knew what to do. Fultz quickly decided that if he could not run around the car he would run over it. He visualized how he would put his foot first on the bumper, then the trunk, the roof, and the hood and leap like a steeple-chaser for the open road. But at the last moment the crowd opened a little gap on one side of the cruiser and Fultz side-stepped through.

A half mile later the press bus got in Fultz's way. It squeezed him against the crowd as he pounded on the side with his fist and choked on the exhaust fumes. He feared for his life as well as his race. Both the bus and Fultz tried to go through a single-file slot in the crowd. Three times Jack and the bus leapfrogged through the crowd. One time the door opened in his face and a national guardsman jumped out into Fultz's path. Fultz had to quick-step and leap to avoid a fall. This was like football, not marathon racing. Drayton was right. Something had to be done to control the crowds. With each pass Fultz had to turn his shoulders to squeeze through a little slot to freedom and running room.

Rodgers looked back and thought he saw teammate Thomas. "Oh, God, he's going to beat me," he thought. "I'll never hear the end of it." Rodgers wanted to savor victory and cruise in under control and smile to the crowd. He wanted to ham it up, lifting his arms in the air to signal victory and thanking the crowd for their support. He wanted the last quarter mile to be the marathon equivalent of a victory lap. Rodgers had run the last half-marathon in 1:04:39, faster than any winner in history and yet here was someone coming up on him. He had run the hills faster than anyone, breaking Morio Shigematsu's record from 1965 by 21 seconds and running away from Ryan and Tikkanen—so he thought. He had put all his best moves on those guys at what was a truly crazy pace; they should be all done, so it must be someone else coming up on him now.

He did not want to sprint like some gasping, desperate maniac. When he saw the pursuer was Wells, not Thomas, he worried even more. Rodgers thought, Wells is quicker. Wells is a fanatic, he trains in airports. Wells beat me at Edinburgh.

Wells had run the last half of the Boston Marathon in 1:04:22. Like Victor Mora in 1972, he had moved too late. He had too much energy left. As he ran through Kenmore Square and saw the big Citgo sign and knew there was a mile to go, Wells thought two simultaneous and contradictory things: Thank God the race is almost over, and God, I wish I had more time to chase Rodgers.

God was Wells's life. He grew up in Madisonville, Texas, and after running at Houston's Rice University he went to graduate school at the nondenominational Dallas Theological Seminary. He wanted to become a pastor. During the summer between high school and college he had made a decision to yield control of his life to Jesus Christ. He said, "My life began to change in many ways. One of those ways was running. I began depending on God rather than on myself. I prayed about workouts and races and God met my needs." Soon God would decide if the king should be deposed by Wells. Obviously He had already decided against Shorter, Fultz, and Thomas. Was

Jeff Wells the anointed one? Someday he wanted to have his own church. So did his Rice roommate, John Lodwick. But before that both of them wanted to win the Boston Marathon. In college Wells had run a mile in 4:06 and a 10K in 28:27 and had qualified for the Olympic trials with a 2:17 marathon in his first serious attempt. In 1977 he had finished 12th at Boston but ran in second place up Heartbreak Hill behind Drayton until the procession of runners led by Turkish Veli Bally marched by. In the heat Wells had gone out too fast and had to walk and jog the last 5 miles, but this year, under ideal conditions and in better personal shape, he had been too cautious. He trained under coach Harry Johnson of Athletics West in Eugene, Oregon, and could do workouts like 4 × 800 meters at 2:10 to 2:08, then leave the track to run 5K of fartlek and return to the track for 8 × 200 meters at 28 to 31. He had gone out too slowly and for a while there was time enough.

After 26 miles and 285 yards it came down to a 100-yard dash. Wells ate up the ground. Only with 15 yards left a policeman's motorcycle came between Wells and Rodgers. It became clear that Wells could not catch Rodgers. The motorcycle made no difference. People later said it did, but it did not. A protester with a big sign proclaiming Israel to be an outlaw state jumped out of the crowd. First Rodgers, then Wells passed him. People later

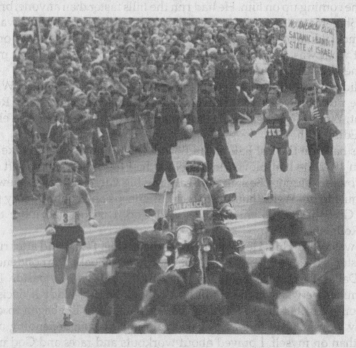

Jeff Wells (#14) had to dodge a motorcycle and a protester with a sign reading "satanic bandit" in his pursuit of Bill Rodgers (#3) at the finish of the 1978 marathon. Photo by Jeff Johnson.

said the protester foiled Wells's kick, but he did not. Wells sidestepped both the motorcycle and the protester and finished 2 seconds behind Rodgers. It was the closest Boston Marathon finish to date. Rodgers's gap gambit had paid off, just barely.

The fastest mass finish in the history of marathoning followed, with an unprecedented 32 men breaking 2:20, 160 under 2:30, and 4,000 under 4 hours. Never had six men run under 2:12 in the same race, and 170 men ran faster than the best times of Johnny Kelley, Gerard Cote, and Clarence DeMar. This was a new era, there was no doubt about it. Yet the jinx continued: No Olympic gold medalist had yet won the Boston Marathon.

1978 Men's Results

1. W. Rodgers, *GBTC*, MA	2:10:13	31. R. Peres, Costa Rica	2:19:46
2. J. Wells, Dallas, TX	2:10:15	32. J. Bowles, *WVTC*, CA	2:19:57
3. E. Tikkanen, Finland	2:11:15	33. C. Burrows, *MAFB*, NJ	2:20:03
4. J. Fultz, *GBTC*	2:11:17	34. J. Yurkovich, Salem, OH	2:20:14
5. R. Thomas, *GBTC*, MA	2:11:25	35. T. Nickevich, Berkeley, CA	2:20:23
6. K. Ryan, New Zealand	2:11:43	36. B. Klecker, Long Prairie, MN	2:20:28
7. D. Kardong, Spokane, WA	2:14:07	37. S. Flanagan, East Lansing, MI	2:20:36
8. J. Lodwick, Dallas, TX	2:14:12	38. F. Mueller, New York City, NY	2:20:47
9. Y. Taketomi, Japan	2:14:34	39. L. Curran, Salina, KS	2:20:56
10. T. Fleming, *NYAC*	2:14:44	40. J. Callaci, Ireland	2:21:25
11. B. Durden, *ATC*	2:15:04	41. B. Hensley, Milford, CT	2:21:33
12. B. Doyle, Central Fall, RI	2:15:37	42. T. Brien, OK	2:21:50
13. J. Dimick, Brattleboro, VT	2:15:58	43. R. DiSebastian, PA	2:21:52
14. L. Fidler, *ATC*	2:16:14	44. W. Gavaghan, Indianapolis, IN	2:21:54
15. J. Vitale, *HartAC*	2:16:17	45. A. Hall, Staten Island, NY	2:22:07
16. R. Pate, Columbia, SC	2:16:39	46. M. Cohen, Brighton, MA	2:22:12
17. R. McOmber, OH	2:17:01	47. A. Kean, England	2:22:27
18. M. Suzuki, Japan	2:17:10	48. M. Duggan, Reading, MA	2:22:35
19. E. Strabel, Ft. Leavenworth, KS	2:17:12	49. S. Yeagle, Baltimore, MD	2:22:42
20. T. Donovan, *GBTC*	2:17:49	50. W. Haviland, Athens, OH	2:22:51
21. A. McAndrew, *BAA*	2:18:01	**161. A. Burfoot, New London, CT**	**2:30:04**
22. B. Robinson, Silver Spring, MD	2:18:02	164. T. Derderian, *GBTC*	2:30:10
23. F. Shorter, Boulder, CO	2:18:15	744. P. Kane, Needham, MA	2:45:00
24. R. Currier, *BAA*	2:18:18	1011. B. Squires, *BAA*	2:48:29
25. B. Heath, Norfolk, VA	2:18:24	1121. P. Wallan, Troy, NY	2:50:01
26. W. Sieben, Rahway, NJ	2:18:29	2430. Cowman X	3:07:25
27. M. Murphy, Cromwell, CT	2:18:44	3241. J. Fixx	3:24:02
28. R. Zimmermann, Kenmore, NY	2:18:55	3561. D. Costill	3:32:22
29. L. Olsen, *NMC*	2:19:23	**3729. J.A. Kelley**	**3:42:36**
30. B. Wilson, Troy, VA	2:19:34		

4,764 entrants: (57 from Japan); 4,189 starters; 4,067 finishers under 4 hours (plus 1,491 bandits).

Masters

1. F. Mueller, NY 2:20:47
2. K. Mueller, *BAA* 2:25:23

Team prize

Greater Boston TC: W. Rodgers, J. Fultz, R. Thomas

JUST WANTIN' TO BE UP THERE FOREVER

MONDAY, APRIL 17, 1978

Merritt Vows Repeat Victory

Kim Merritt came back to Boston prepared to win again and this time under good racing conditions. She pushed her memories of runner's sickness and thigh smash from Boston 1976 to the back of her mind. She had pushed the pace at the women's Avon World Championships in Atlanta, Georgia, in March and suffered for it with a dropout. She did not like the Boston Marathon course, but she had demonstrated superior fitness with a 2:44:44 in Honolulu in December of 1976 and a 2:37:57 marathon in Eugene, Oregon, the fall of 1977. Gayle Barron of Atlanta had run second in Eugene with a 2:48:34, placed fifth in the Avon marathon with a 2:53:05, and placed third in Honolulu with a 2:52:16. In Waldniel, West Germany, Barron had run 2:47:43.2 for third to Merritt's 2:47:11.2. Barron had never beaten Merritt, yet they had traveled around the world together racing marathons. It seemed as if Barron was improving faster than Merritt, but regardless they and their husbands had become friends.

Both Merritt and Barron were tired. Merritt was the race favorite, but her heart was not in this race. On Saturday she said, "I'm 3 minutes off my normal 10-mile time. Instead of hitting 57:00 I'm doing 60:00, and it feels terrible. I've just been incredibly sluggish. I make this huge effort in every race and it seems to get me nowhere." She and Barron had raced too much and came to Boston mostly because their husbands wanted to race. They thought that since they would be in town they might as well run, but neither had actually pointed for it. At least that is what they said outwardly and might have actually believed until the gun went off.

Barron had been to Boston before, placing third in 1975 and fourth in 1976. It was in 1975 that she had met Dr. Ernst Van Aaken of Waldniel. He coached winner Liane Winter but had never heard of Barron. He said through a translator that he wanted to coach her. So began a long and useful relationship between the two, conducted by mail. Barron would receive her workouts written in German; she then had to have them translated so she could execute them. The training emphasized long, slow distance running.

Merritt and Barron ran at personal record pace through the first checkpoint. Merritt led Barron by about a minute. Kim ran with her husband Keith, but Gayle led Ben, who had a bad day. Gayle had a good day and

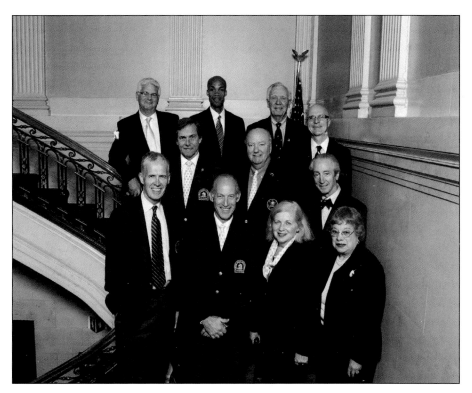

BAA board of Governors: Tom Grilk front row on the left. Front on the right, Gloria Ratti, next to president Joanne Flaminio.

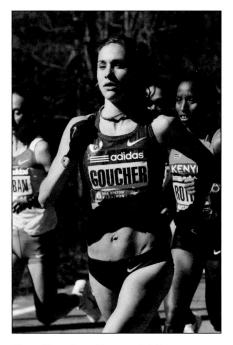

Kara Goucher, Boston 2011.

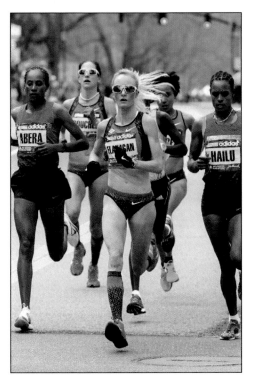

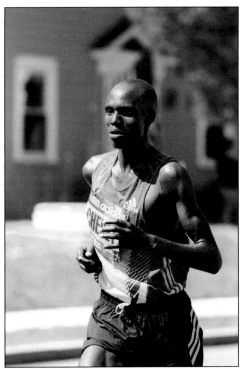

Flanagan leading Boston 2014, pushing the pace to record speeds. Kara Goucher in matching sunglasses.

Wilson Chebet in 2012 tried to chase down Meb Keflezighi in 2014.

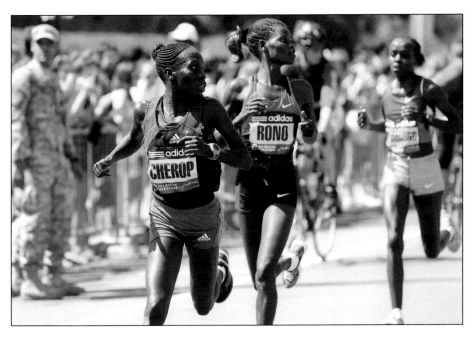

Boston 2012, Sharon Cherop and Georgina Rono look back to check on Jemina Jelagat Sumgong. Sumgong would go on to win the Olympic Marathon in Rio 2016.

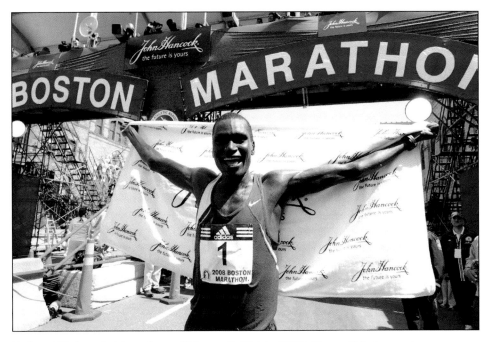

Robert Kipkoech Cheruiyot of Kenya 2:07:4 in 2008: One of his four wins.

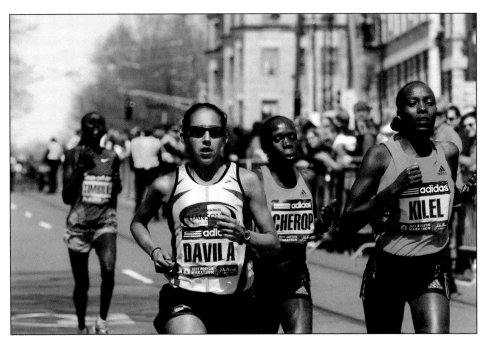

Desiree Davila (Linden) leading Boston in 2011 with Sharon Cherop and Caroline Kilel. "Desi put America back on the boards big-time."

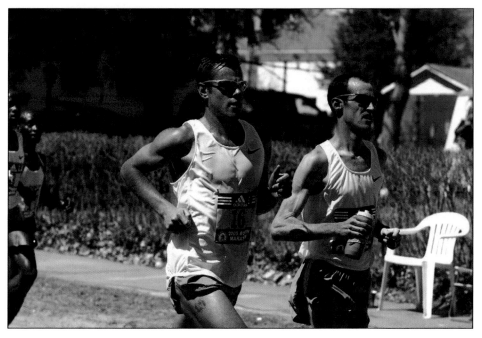

Ryan Shay, #16, and Alan Culpepper in 2005.

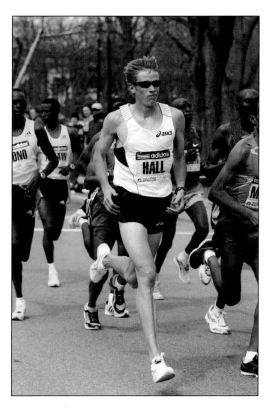

Ryan Hall racing and pushing the pace in 2009.

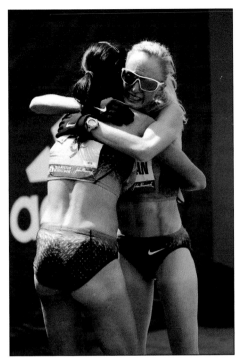

Comfort after an emotional race in 2013:
Training partners Shalane Flanagan and
Kara Goucher hug.

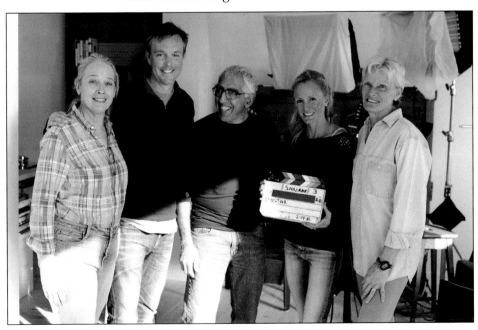

Boston: The Story of the World's Greatest Marathon in California studio for an
interview with Shalane Flanagan. L-R, Megan Williams, Producer, Jon Dunham,
Director, Tom Derderian Executive Producer, Shalane Flanagan, and her mother
Cheryl.

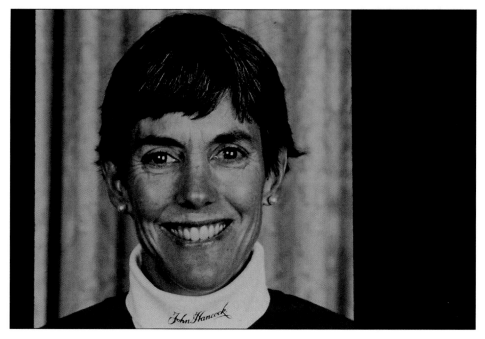

Joan Benoit Samuelson.

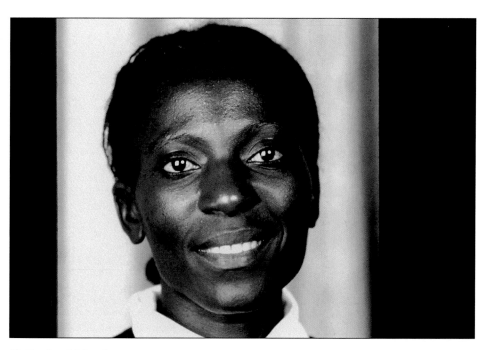

Catherine Ndereba.

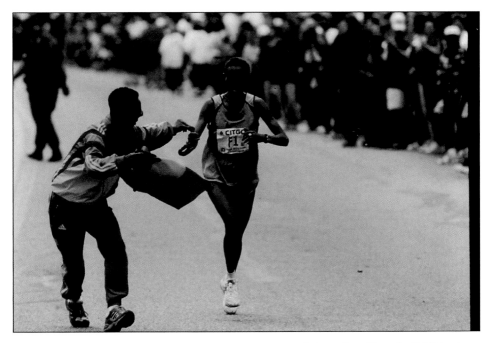

Long-time Boston Ethiopian runner gives Fatuma Roba a headband of Ethiopian colors and an Ethiopian flag.

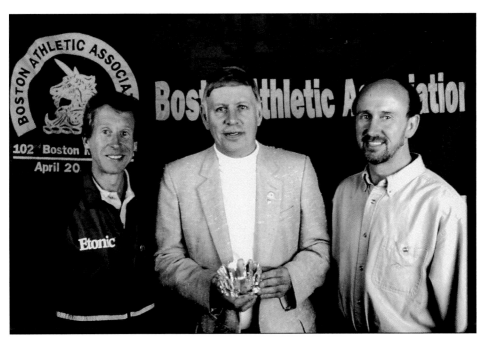

Bill Rodgers, Greater Boston Track Club original Coach Bill Squires, and 1983 Boston Winner Greg Meyers in 1999.

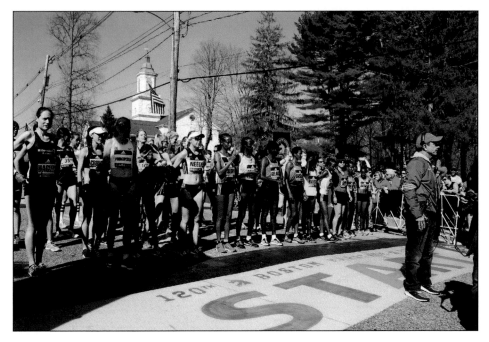

Elite women ready to start in 2015.

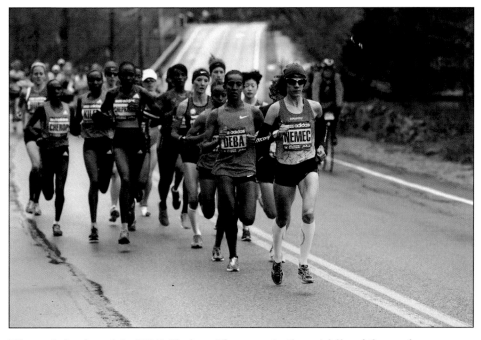

Women's lead pack in 2015. Shalane Flanagan in the middle of the pack.

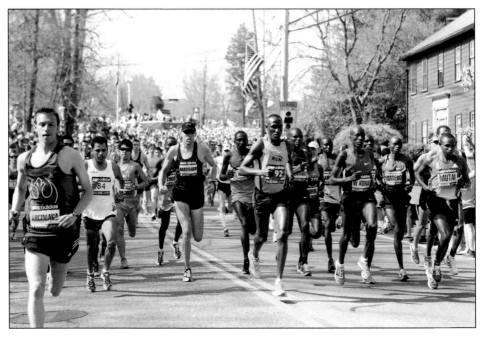

Start 2012. Jason Hartmann in red, Geoffrey Mutai on the far right, with Wesley Korir on his right.

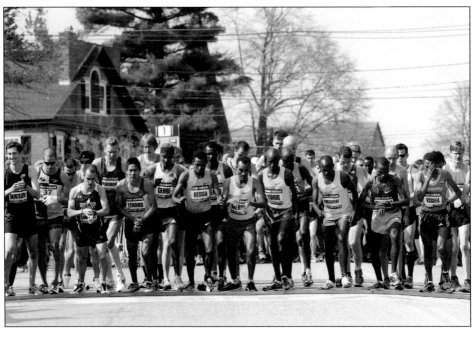

Men's start 2013.

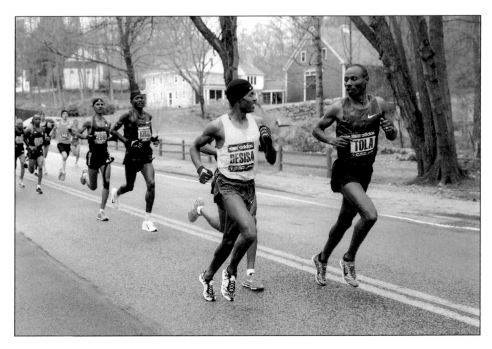

Desisa and Tola Chatting in the early miles in 2015.

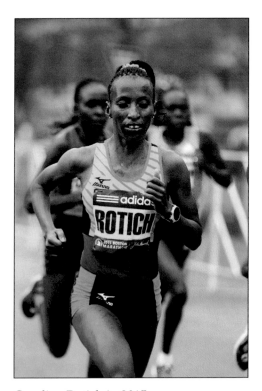

Caroline Rotich in 2015.

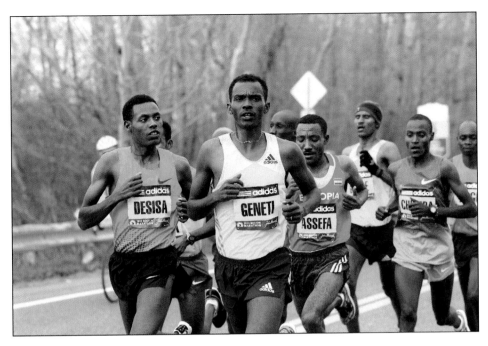

Lelisa Desisa and Markos Geneti leading the pack in 2013.

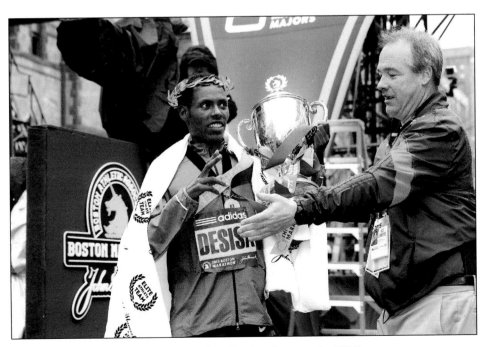

The BAA's Jack Fleming shows Lelisa Desisa the way in 2015.

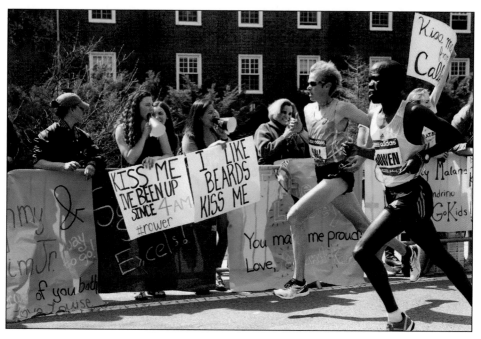

Ryan Hall and fans at Wellesley College.

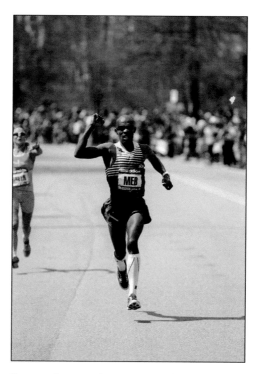

Boston Strong: American Meb Keflezighi,
the first American winner since 1983,
celebrates Boston Strong a year after the
bombing.

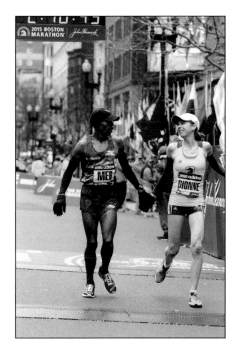

Meb and the BAA's Hilary Dionne
cross the line hand in hand in 2015,
showing Boston is united.

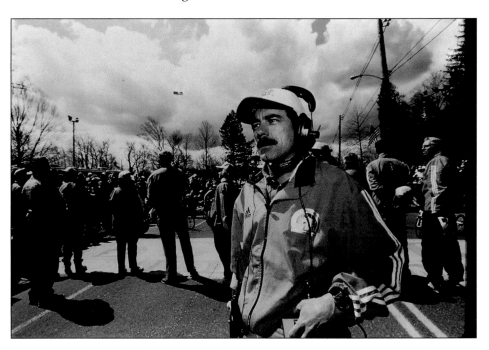

Race Director Dave McGillivray on the line sometime in the last century. For
many years he would finish directing the race, then go back and run the entire
course in the dark, thus unofficially finishing last in his own race.

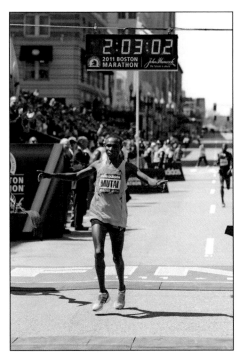

Geoffrey Mutai runs the fastest marathon
in the world at Boston, but it is not a
world record.

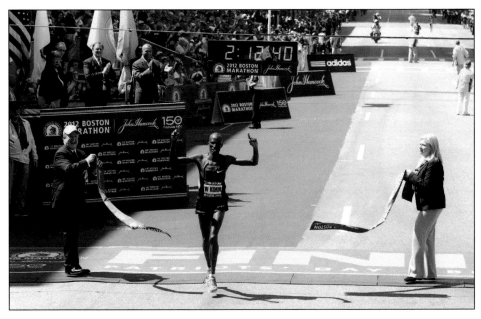

Wesley Korir won the Boston Marathon in 2012 and later won a seat in the
Kenyan Parliament. Applauding in the stand is BAA's Gloria Ratti, Guy Morse,
and Massachusetts governor Deval Patrick. Holding the right side of the finish
line tape is BAA president Joanne Flaminio.

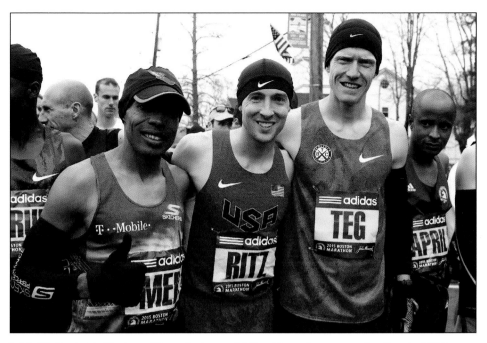

Meb Keflezighi, Dathan Ritzenhein, and Matt Tegenkamp on the line in 2015.

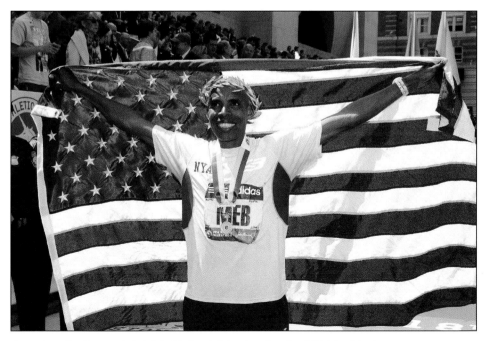

America the Beautiful: Meb Keflezighi wins for the USA in 2014.

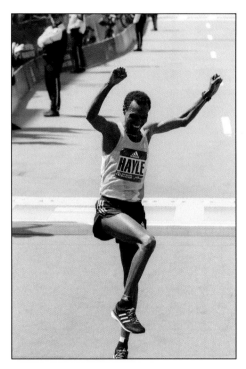

Hayle dancing over the finish line in 2016.

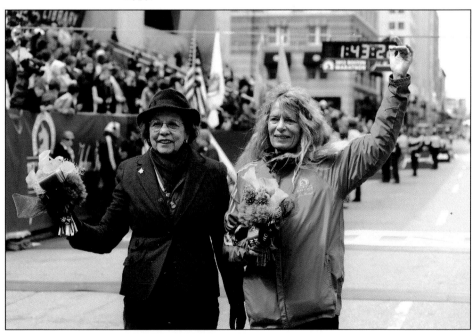

Sara Mae Berman and Bobbi Gibb, women running pioneers, celebrated about a half-century later.

caught the Merritts by Natick. They told her that there was another woman up ahead. She was Gayle Olinek, a Canadian with astoundingly muscular legs, suitable for anatomy book illustration.

Through Wellesley Keith slowed, leaving Gayle and Kim alone. They looked ahead for Olinek's remarkable legs. They talked and encouraged each other and speculated on rumors about who, if anyone, ran ahead of them. Rumors were what Barron called them. These were not accurate reports, and she wanted accurate reports. She had studied journalism at the University of Georgia and had begun work at the CBS affiliate in Atlanta 6 months earlier. Now 33, she had been a cheerleader in college, not a track runner like Merritt. Barron was darker, taller, and more muscular than Merritt. She did not consider herself Merritt's equal; she thought she was undertrained and out at a pace too fast for her ability. She felt so strong and so good that she expected something to go wrong.

Merritt and Barron caught Olinek, whose muscular legs began to fail her at the beginning of the Newton hills. They passed and received no resistance. Olinek was all done racing, relegated to survival shuffle. Barron thought she herself would soon be in that state. Merritt gained a quick 25 yards on the first hill. Barron caught up on the flat. They ran together until the last hill, where Merritt fell back. Barron assumed Merritt would use her superior speed to catch up on the downhills, but it was those downhills that had produced the thigh smash of 1976. The smash set in again. Kim Merritt did not catch up to Gayle Barron again.

Meanwhile Ben Barron had caught up with Keith Merritt. They discussed their wives' race. They too passed Olinek. Gayle Barron received reports that she held first place and a woman in pigtails ran in second. Kim Merritt wore pigtails, but so did Olinek and so did Penny DeMoss. Gayle Barron did not know who pursued her. The husbands also wondered who was in second. Later they learned that DeMoss was the one who closed on Barron. Barron still felt well except for a numbness in her big toe. For the women and all runners far behind the leaders, crowd control did not exist. Not only was there a crowd of spectators, but Barron ran in a crowd of runners. The spectators narrowed the road to a winding trail through their screaming midst. To pass a tiring runner Barron had to develop a special technique. She would tap him on the shoulder, say "Excuse me," and hope he would brush out of the way. Usually he did, but she knew that her time, and everyone's times for that part of the field, would have been several minutes faster had the running road been wider.

Barron was never sure she was winning until she sprinted over the finish line and Boston police officers took her arms and escorted her through the finish chute and up to the victory platform. The mayor had left, but the mayor's wife remained to place the laurel wreath of victory on Barron's head. She waved and smiled to the crowd. In a few minutes a man said to her, "It's time to get down, ma'am." But she did not want to get down. It had taken her 2-3/4 hours to get to the victory platform—couldn't she stay just a tiny bit longer? Later, in her sweetest southern accent she said, "But I was just wantin' to be up there forever."

Winning the Boston Marathon changed Gayle Barron's life. As she said, it opened doors. She got more air time at the TV station because she was no longer merely a reporter but the Boston Marathon Winner. She got contracts to endorse Brooks running shoes and Head sportswear. Race directors paid her $1,000 in under-the-table appearance money. She went on speaking tours. With ghostwriter Kim Chapin she did a book published in 1980, *The Beauty of Running*. She became a corporate spokesperson and started a business called Fitness Management Group to coordinate personal and employee fitness programs. She worked as color commentator for WNEV-TV in Boston during the marathon. One year she ran in the marathon carrying a microphone to broadcast the sounds of the race as the film crew followed her; other years she sat at the anchor desk giving expert commentary. But she did not finish the race the year she ran with the microphone, nor did she race Boston again.

Perhaps she recognized that faster women, younger than 33, were entering the sport of marathon running and that it was time to get on with a career and go where the money was. One could say she saw the handwriting on the road. Young women who had the opportunity to spend their college days running fast track intervals instead of cheerleading would soon dominate the sport for women as track-trained runners had for men. The women's marathon racing population followed in 7 years the same progression the men had followed in 50—from exclusively endurance-trained road racers to much

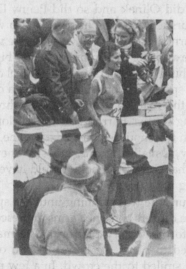

TV broadcaster Gayle Barron accepts the laurel wreath from Race Director Will Cloney and the mayor's wife for winning the 1978 marathon. Photo by Jeff Johnson.

faster athletes who were track-trained as well. From Bobbi Gibb to Kathrine Switzer to Nina Kuscsik—no longer would any woman win the Boston Marathon who could not break 5 minutes for the mile. The women's records were about to crash.

1978 Women's Results

1.	G. Barron, *ATC*	2:44:52
2.	P. DeMoss, *WVTC*, CA	2:45:36
3.	J. Killion, *NYAA*	2:47:23*
4.	**K. Merritt, Racine, WI**	**2:47:52**
5.	L. Pedrinan, *NYAA*	2:48:42
6.	K. Obata, Japan	2:52:34
7.	E. DeMendonca, *CSU*, MA	2:52:49
8.	L. Donkelaar, AZ	2:52:58
9.	N. Lindsay, NY	2:53:07
10.	G. Olinek, Canada	2:53:20
11.	D. Butterfield, Bermuda	2:53:51
12.	C. Bravakis, *HartTC*, CT	2:54:13
13.	G. Andersen, Sun Valley, ID	2:54:21
14.	S. Petersen, *SFernTC*, CA	2:55:12
15.	G. File, *OH*, New Zealand	2:56:29
16.	J. Lutter, St. Paul, MN	2:56:34
17.	E. McEvily, Larchmont, NY	2:56:43
18.	L. Petronella, Boulder, CO	2:57:10
19.	**N. Kuscsik, *NYAA***	**2:57:22**
20.	K. Smith, Baltimore, MD	2:57:45
21.	D. Riley, Tulsa, OK	2:57:50
22.	N. Dragoo, Waterford, NY	2:57:58
23.	S. Kahler, Auburn, NY	2:58:43
24.	J. Ullyot, *WVTC*, CA	2:58:43
25.	N. Johnson, Wynnewood, PA	2:59:17
26.	G. Jones, Unionville, CT	2:59:36
27.	B. Kleve, NY	2:59:36
28.	L. Cunningham, Penfield, NY	2:59:55
29.	M. Pugh, Dallas, TX	2:59:58
30.	M. Wright, Arlington, MA	3:00:28
36.	T. d'Elia, *NYAA*	3:04:26
37.	E. Wessel, Arlington, VA	3:05:03
53.	F. Madeira, Sherborn, MA	3:10:21
115.	M. Schwam, Ossining, NY	3:26:14
133.	S. Lupica, Brighton, MA	3:32:30
154.	M. Moline, Cambridge, MA	3:38:00
	J. Hansen, Topanga, CA, DNF	

202 starters; 186 official finishes under 4 hours.

*Lynn Jennings, later to become many-times world cross-country champion in the late 1980s and early '90s, finished in an unofficial 2:45 for third place. She was not allowed to enter officially because she was only 17 years old.

INSCRUTABLE, INSCRUTABLE

MONDAY, APRIL 16, 1979

Can Boston Billy Win #3?

If Bill Rodgers could win the Boston Marathon for a third time he would rank in the record book alongside four-time winner Gerard Cote and three-time winners Leslie Pawson and Eino Oksanen. He had no illusions of matching Clarence DeMar's seven wins. He thought he would not run in 1980 because it was an Olympic year, so three victories would be just enough. But one thing stood in his way—the inscrutable Toshihiko Seko of Japan. Seko had beaten Rodgers soundly in Fukuoka and unleashed a humiliating kick on him in a 10,000-meter race in Stockholm. In each race Seko figuratively sat on Rodgers's shoulder and literally ran away from him. Rodgers was powerless against Seko's kick, and both of them knew it.

After the Olympics and Fukuoka, people said Rodgers was vulnerable. After the 1978 squeaker past Wells, they knew he was beatable. That just made him train harder and more carefully. He had gone out to California for the winter to get in a lot of mileage and decided not to travel as much and not to race as often as he had in the previous year. He planned to train as if Boston were the big one—the Olympics. He wanted the sub-2:12 that had eluded him in New York and Fukuoka. He wanted to appear invulnerable, and more than that, invincible.

Seko was not the only other quality runner in the field. This year it contained 10 sub-2:12 marathoners; it was the fastest marathon field ever assembled. With such quality there was a danger that the race might become a slow-paced tactical event, where everyone waited for someone else to take out the pace. But Tom Fleming waited for no one. He wanted running room.

What did he care about cat-and-mouse games? Fleming ran like a large mammal, not a small one, and he had already taken second twice and third once at Boston. There was only one other place he wanted, and his tactics in other years had failed because he was cautious and cagey. In 1973 against Anderson, in 1974 against Cusack, and in 1975 against Rodgers, Fleming had not aggressively seized the lead. He had expected those runners to come back to him but they never did. Perhaps this time in the windless, cool mist he would not come back to them. He blasted away to a 50-yard lead by 2 miles. He thundered his way through 5 miles in 23:40 (exactly a 4:44 pace; that is, a 2:04:06 marathon). Kevin Ryan of New Zealand, who had pushed the pace early in 1978, had promised himself that he would not do it again. But like a wolf on seeing running deer, he lost control of himself and had to put Fleming to the test. So through Framingham an observer could see Fleming out 100 yards on the cunning pack while a lone wolf in New Zealand black chased him.

Fleming ran 40 seconds ahead of the pack that hit 10 miles in 47:55. In the huge pack a remarkable group ran shoulder to shoulder. Four members of the Greater Boston Track Club—Rodgers, Randy Thomas, Bob Hodge, and Dick Mahoney—ran surrounded by the best runners in the world. They ran together toward their familiar training grounds around Boston College. Hodge had been the yearly winner of the Mt. Washington 8-Mile Road Race for the past 3 years. When he heard the 10-mile split he turned to Mahoney and said, "This is crazy." He looked around at everyone's waist to check their stride efficiency and saw that they all looked great. Hodge and Mahoney, a mailman in a nearby town, felt privileged to be in such company. Fleming had often talked about a 2:06 marathon, and Rodgers began to worry that today might be his day to do it.

In the pack behind Fleming and Ryan ran 1976 Olympian Don Kardong, Garry Bjorklund, Esa Tikkanen of Finland, Chris Stewart, and Herm Atkins, and following as closely as possible at Rodgers's heel ran Seko in deep-stealth mode. He tried to make himself invisible in Rodgers's slipstream. Rodgers wore a big woolly hat that made him look like a gnome and white gardening-style gloves. It was 42 °F.

Kardong led a charge through Natick that absorbed Ryan and closed on Fleming. At first startled by the ferocity of Kardong's attack, the pack strung out, making each runner distinct except for Seko, who clung to Rodgers like a lamprey. Kardong's aggression cramped his calves and he did not make it past 17 miles.

It was Bjorklund who actually led the downhill surge into Newton Lower Falls that caught Fleming. When Rodgers and Seko caught Fleming at the 17.5-mile mark, Fleming turned to Rodgers and said, "Hi, Bill, nice to see you, we'll catch B.J. [Bjorklund] on the hills, but why did you have to bring him along?" Rodgers asked, "Who?" Fleming said, "Behind you." Rodgers was quite surprised to see silent Seko on his heels. He had forgotten that Seko was in the race. This was not what he wanted—another two-man race down to the wire. He had to get rid of Seko.

But Seko passed Rodgers after they both passed Fleming. Still Bjorklund led them both. Rodgers worried. He tucked in behind Seko and watched him. Up the hills Rodgers adopted a shorter stride. It made him feel better, but still Seko had to be shaken off. Rodgers feared a Fukuoka replay.

Seko had run a 27:51 10K. Rodgers had to move hard and constantly to take the kick out of Seko, preferably building up a couple minutes' lead so he could coast in and savor the victory. Rodgers did not hear any times during the race, but his time to Woodland at 17.5 miles was a minute slower than his record. Everyone had slowed. Rodgers began the push to catch Bjorklund. Again like a shadow Seko settled in behind him.

Four miles later as Rodgers and Seko came off the hill past Lake Street they ran only 17 seconds behind the record. They had made up 43 seconds on the toughest part of the course. The record hovered within reach. A sub-2:10 began to seem possible.

As they passed Bjorklund, he said, "Go for 2:08."

Past his store at Cleveland Circle Rodgers had everything going for him. He ran in familiar territory, and the crowds wildly supported him. He poured on the effort and got a little lead over Seko. "Good," he thought, "give me an inch and I'll take a mile." But all down Beacon Street several official vehicles obscured Rodgers's view to the rear so he could not see where Seko ran. So out of fear of another sprint like that with Wells last year, he poured it on even harder. As Rodgers passed the Eliot Lounge he caught a glimpse of Seko, safely 200 yards behind. Now Rodgers had his cushion. All down Hereford Street he could savor his victory. In the last quarter mile Rodgers removed his hat and waved it to the crowd. He felt flamboyant, like the Kenyan miler Kip Keino. But as he turned the corner on to the last downhill he saw that the clock read 2:09:22. He knew Ron Hill's age-31 record was 2:09:28. He wanted it and sprinted like a maniac.

With his hat in his hand, teeth bared and lips pulled back in a nasty snarl, he broke the finish line tape to win the race, break the course record, and break Hill's world age-31 record.

Seko followed. And so did the rest of Rodgers's Greater Boston team. Not only did the Greater Boston Track Club beat all the other clubs entered in the race, they beat all the other countries. President Jimmy Carter, a cross-country runner in college, personally invited Rodgers to a state dinner at the White House. Even the president of the United States was about to take up road racing. Things were beginning to look very good for the sport. Top runners made money in appearance fees and contracts with shoe companies, opened running-shoe stores (as did Rodgers, Kardong, Vitale, Shorter, and Bjorklund), or got jobs with running shoe companies (as did Thomas and Ryan).

But within a year, politics a world away would steal the dreams of these men.

Checkpoint Splits

Framingham	31:54
Natick	50:08
Wellesley	1:05:01
Woodland	1:25:28
Lake Street	1:46:20 (record 1:46:03, 1975)
Coolidge Corner	1:58:39 (record 1:58:41, 1975)

1979 Men's Results

1.	B. Rodgers, *GBTC*, MA	2:09:27^{CR}	19.	N. Takao, Japan	2:16:10
2.	T. Seko, Japan	2:10:12	20.	F. Richardson, Ames, IA	2:16:20
3.	R. Hodge, *GBTC*	2:12:30	21.	G. Mielke, West Germany	2:16:30
4.	T. Fleming, Bloomfield, NJ	2:12:56	22.	C. Kirkham, England	2:16:34
5.	G. Bjorklund, Minneapolis, MN	2:13:14	23.	S. Palladino, CA	2:16:41
6.	K. Ryan, New Zealand	2:13:57	24.	W. Sieben, NJ	2:16:44
7.	B. Doyle, Central Falls, RI	2:14:04	25.	J. Lodwick, Eugene, OR	2:16:46
8.	R. Thomas, *GBTC*	2:14:12	26.	D. Babiracki, CA	2:16:49
9.	H. Atkins, Everett, WA	2:14:17	27.	D. Hooper, Ireland	2:16:50
10.	R. Mahoney, *GBTC*	2:14:36	28.	R. Wayne, Alameda, CA	2:17:02
11.	**J. Drayton, Canada**	**2:14:47**	29.	R. Sayre, Akron, OH	2:17:17
12.	D. Matthews, Clemson, SC	2:14:48	30.	C. Alitz, West Point, NY	2:17:25
13.	D. Greig, New Zealand	2:14:49	31.	D. Harper, San Diego, CA	2:17:31
14.	C. Stewart, NY	2:14:56	32.	T. Wright, England	2:17:35
15.	T. Sandoval, Eugene, OR	2:15:23	33.	T. Nickevich, Berkeley, CA	2:17:38
16.	D. McDonald, CA	2:15:28	34.	L. Fidler, Stone Mountain, GA	2:17:44
17.	J. Norman, England	2:15:44	35.	K. McCarey, Eugene, OR	2:17:50
18.	E. Tikkanen, Finland	2:16:00	36.	W. Gavaghan, Indianapolis, IN	2:18:00

37. K. Brown, Newtonville, MA	2:18:04	
38. T. Howard, Canada	2:18:09	
39. K. Takami, Japan	2:18:10	
40. R. McOmber, OH	2:18:15	
41. D. Clark, England	2:18:28	
42. C. Karthauser, New Brunswick	2:18:31	
43. W. Saeger, Dayton, OH	2:18:40	
44. J. Rafferty, Flushing, NY	2:18:54	
45. K. Lazaridis, Greece	2:18:57	
46. B. Robinson, MD	2:19:03	
47. K. McDonald, Greenville, SC	2:19:10	
48. F. Will, Germany	2:19:23	

49. R. Pate, Charlottesville, VA	2:19:28
50. C. Burrows, *MAFB*, NJ	2:19:33
51. R. Tabb, Houston, TX	2:19:41
52. T. Stanley, PA	2:20:06
75. F. Shorter, Boulder, CO	2:21:56
94. G. Goettleman, CA	2:23:19
113. K. Randall, Hanover, NH	2:24:29
127. R. Rojas, CO	2:25:01
J. Foster, New Zealand	2:39:10
3032. A. Burfoot	**3:00:24**
3577. J.A. Kelley	3:45:12

7,357 entrants.

Masters

1. H. Lorenz, NJ	2:24:41
2. F. Mueller, NYC	2:26:00

Team prize

Greater Boston TC: B. Rodgers, R. Hodge, R. Thomas

MICMAC PATTI AND THE STOREKEEPER'S DAUGHTER

MONDAY, APRIL 16, 1979

Boston Woman Leads Field for Today's Marathon

The favorite for the women's race, Patti Lyons from Boston, arrived strong, well trained, and experienced. She had been running and winning marathons since 1976. She had run 2:47:20 to win in Newport, Rhode Island, in 1977, and had run 3 marathons between 2:40 and 2:45 in the three months before the 1979 Boston Marathon. She had been running 100 to 140 miles a week in preparation for Boston. No one could be more ready. She was the hope of Boston and Jock Semple. She ran for the BAA. She took rubdowns from Jock on Tuesdays between 11 o'clock and noon.

Patti Lyons was born on April 6, 1953, in Chelsea, Massachusetts, on a Navy ship in Boston Harbor. Her father was an All-Navy boxer in the lightweight division for which his 5'1-1/2" and 112 pounds qualified him. Her mother, from Antigonish, Nova Scotia, home of 1898 Boston Marathon winner Ronald MacDonald, was a Micmac Indian, half an inch taller than her husband. Patti looked Micmac like her mother but was taller at 5'4". Patti wore her straight hair parted in the middle. She was linked to the long line of native Americans trying to win the Boston Marathon. From Mohawk Bill Davis, second to Caffery in 1901, to Onondaga Tom Longboat in 1907, to Penobscot Andrew Sockalexis in 1912, to Narragansett Ellison (Tarzan)

Brown in the 1930s and dozens of others from many other tribes, Micmac Patti Lyons might be the last of them.

Lyons went to high school at Sacred Heart in Weymouth Landing on Boston's south shore, but there were no athletics there for the girls. It would be years before the idea of running came to her. Like everyone else at Sacred Heart, she wore a plaid uniform and saddle shoes. She tried to blend in and disappear. She rarely spoke and would rather not be spoken to; her nickname was Still-Mouth. To avoid being called on in class, she picked the last desk in the middle row, the one with the high top and low seat; then she would slouch to be sure she was out of the nun's line of sight. She would never raise her hand. She stole her name out of the nuns' calling cards so they would forget to call on her. She was quiet, withdrawn, and afraid. The nuns did forget about Patti. Her picture never appeared in the yearbook. She started working after school hours in Quincy Hospital as a candy striper volunteer and later full-time as a nurse's aide. After high school she continued working at the hospital; planning to go to nursing school, she took courses at Quincy Junior College. But her father had a heart attack and subsequently open heart surgery. He died 13 months later. By age 23 Patti Lyons had reached the top of the nurse's aide pay scale at $5.25 per hour.

Stuck living at home and caring for her eight younger siblings, Lyons floated. She hated school. She hated work. She smoked Parliament cigarettes. Then came conflict with her mother. With 152 pounds on her 5'4" Patti was the biggest in the fatherless house. The children followed her lead instead of her mother's. That infuriated her mother, so she threw Patti out. Patti moved to Cape Cod, got a job as a

Lyons ate donuts by the dozen, smoked Parliaments by the box, and drank beer by the six-pack.

nurse's aide, then quit, then moved back to Quincy. She ate donuts by the dozen, smoked Parliaments by the box, and drank beer by the six-pack. She was in and out of school and work, fat, poor, and unhappy, so she decided she had to do something about her life. She decided to take some time out for herself—to, as she called it, be nice to Patti.

At first she went window shopping or took bubble baths during her be-nice-to-Patti time. Then she decided to lose weight. She bought Ken Cooper's Air Force aerobics book. She learned that there were 3,500 calories in a pound and that running would burn them off the fastest. The first day she ran she lost 3 pounds. It was all sweat, but she did not know that, so she kept running. The unease that made her eat donuts and drink beer drove her to run. She rapidly lost weight. The more she ran, the better she felt, so she ran more. The thin woman inside Lyons leaped out. She met some men who ran out of the Quincy YMCA in March of 1976 and began to run with them. They told her that they planned to run the Boston Marathon. The idea amazed her just as her running ability and her monstrous appetite for training amazed them. By May Lyons had decided to run the Boston Marathon too, but she learned that she would have to run another marathon to qualify. In October Lyons not only ran in the Newport, Rhode Island, marathon, she won it. She ran under the name LaTora, the result of a 4-month marriage that was subsequently annulled. The Newport race came a mere 5-1/2 months after she started running, yet she ran 2:53:40, the 10th-fastest time so far that year in the country. (The fastest was Kim Merritt's 2:47:10 at Boston.) At the time of her Newport victory she still smoked the Parliaments. That dark side of her troubled upbringing stayed with her.

As Lyons demonstrated her physical talents to her newfound running community, she appeared to have overcome her personal difficulties. She had in fact substituted one obsession for another. Her binge donut-eating turned to binge running. She developed anorexic and bulimic habits wrapped in emotional mileage that ranged within minutes from rapture to tears. She became insistent that everything and everyone cater to her training for running; she clung to anyone who might help her run better. As her fame grew everyone had to "be nice to Patti."

By October of 1978 Lyons was a member of the BAA and coached by BAA runner Joe Catalano, whom she would later marry and divorce. All the mileage made her very fit, but a painful bursitis in her foot threatened. She took a cortisone injection hoping to calm the inflammation. She *had* to run the Boston Marathon and she *had* to win.

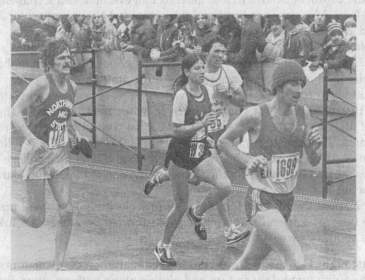

Patti Lyons, running for the BAA, entered the race as the hometown favorite but ran with a painful bursitis in her foot. Photo by Jeff Johnson.

Lyons's competition on this day would come from a Bowdoin College student named Joan Benoit. Benoit had run her first marathon in Bermuda. The day before that race she had raced the 10K in Bermuda and told friends that she would do part of the marathon as a long training run. She said she wasn't racing and wouldn't run hard. At the turnaround friends saw her wearing a pale blue turtleneck. It was raining and through the wet turtleneck her friends could see an official marathon number pinned to the singlet underneath. After the turnaround Benoit threw off the turtleneck. From the start she'd intended to run the whole thing and that she wore a number meant that she knew it would count. She did it in about 2:50—some training run. She may have run all the way, but she did not run hard. She had secret marathon plans.

Benoit came down from Cape Elizabeth, Maine, a wealthy suburb of Portland where the Benoits owned a prestigious men's clothing store. Although her family had means, they did not live in opulence. The family valued hard work and modesty. They lived well but plainly. Her father had graduated from Bowdoin and her mother from William and Mary. They summered on an island that the family owned. The cottage there had no heat, no telephone, and no electricity. In the winter they shared an old house near Sugarloaf Mountain in Kingfield, Maine, with four other families. The object was to ski as much as possible.

When Joan worked in the store selling men's suits, she always tried to sell the customer an extra pair of pants with each suit. The family was based in firm traditions and full of athletes. Her dad was an excellent skier. Her two older brothers, Andre Jr. and Peter, set an example and a challenge for young Joan. Her younger brother, John, provided the incentive for her to try and try again to keep up. The family skied, hiked, and swam. At 15, Joan played field hockey, performed on the track team, and could slalom down a ski run well enough to harbor serious national ski team ambitions. Her childhood and adolescence were wealthy, athletic, and happy.

Benoit loved to ski. Years later she wrote, "Great speed is an opiate, and speed that is under your control, open to your manipulation, is the best high of all." That love of speed and occasional control transferred readily to running. She came to running by the channel that male runners followed. She ran on an organized high school track team and later on a college team. She was the first contender for the women's division of the Boston Marathon to come up in this "normal" fashion.

Benoit spent the night before the 1979 race sleeping on a small mattress on the floor of a friend's apartment in Boston. At breakfast she told her friends about her weird dream.

> Last night I dreamed I was running the marathon on escalators. I was going up and up and up and gliding along with no effort. But I couldn't see the other women so I didn't know what I was doing. Right behind me on the escalator was my mother.

At the start Patti Lyons began slowly. Joan Benoit took the lead quickly and held it through a 5:42 mile. But soon Lyons took over and ran in a pack including her coach, Joe Catalano. They passed 5 miles well under 28 minutes. By Natick at 10 miles Lyons and Catalano had a 40-second lead on Benoit and Sue Krenn of California. But then the bursitis began to hurt Lyons. She could do nothing about it. Catalano could do nothing about it. By Wellesley Benoit ran only 15 seconds behind them.

At the bottom of Heartbreak Hill Benoit caught Lyons. They ran together for a mile. Lyons tried to make the pain in her foot go away. She tried not to think about it, but her body noticed it and limped slightly with each step. The training didn't count; the amount of it probably had caused the problem. Wanting the victory and needing the victory didn't count. In the cold and rain no one awarded an *A* for effort. The cold reality set in, and Patti Lyons realized that she could not win. But still she kept on, because a chance remained that Benoit could still lose.

At 23 miles a fellow Bowdoin student came out of the crowd and gave Benoit a Red Sox baseball cap. Now she had two things to please the crowd, her black Bowdoin shirt and her baseball cap. They could shout, "Go Bowdoin," "Go Red Sox," or "Go Boston." The cap reminded her that the Red Sox, her favorite team, had often held huge game leads and blown them. But she felt good and at ease with her pace. Over the last several miles the applause deafened her. She remembered little else about those miles but the noise of the crowd and the ear-splitting finish.

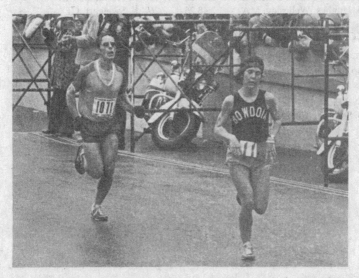

Wearing a Red Sox hat and the shirt of her alma mater, Joan Benoit of Maine races through the rain of the 1979 Boston Marathon, getting cheers for Boston and Bowdoin. Photo by Jeff Johnson.

Her 2:35:15 established a new American record, destroying Liane Winter's course record of 2:42:24 from 1975. It put her third on the world all-time list behind Grete Waitz and Christa Vahlensieck. This Boston Marathon women's field ran the fastest yet, with 520 women entered, four ran under 2:40, 15 under 2:50, and all of the top 25 under 2:56.

Patti Lyons finished second. She had broken the record too. The inflamed bursar sack throbbed in her foot. She had run as hard as she could. It hurt too much to go faster. Her eyes found her coach. She looked for a nod, a smile, anything to say that the pain was worth it, but she saw only that Catalano was not satisfied. Lyons resolved to try harder and train more. She would show him. She would show everyone. She would be back again and again.

1979 Women's Results

1. J. Benoit, ME (477th overall)	2:35:15^{CR,AR}*	15. M. Bevans, Baltimore, MD	2:49:56
2. P. Lyons, *BAA*	2:38:22*	16. D. Butterfield, Bermuda	2:50:13
3. S. Krenn, San Diego, CA	2:38:50*	17. B. Guerin, Wyomissing, PA	2:50:25
4. E. Hassell, Australia	2:39:48*	18. P. Robinson, Brighton, MA	2:51:03
5. S. Petersen, Laguna Beach, CA	2:43:02	19. S. Silsby, FL	2:52:11
6. K. Merritt, Racine, WI	2:44:28	20. C. Bravakis, Windsor Locks, CT	2:52:33
7. C. Dalrymple, Seattle, WA	2:45:30	21. S. Barbano, Yonkers, NY	2:53:27
8. K. Doppes, Cincinnati, OH	2:45:45	22. K. Jackson, AZ	2:53:41
9. G. Olinek, Fort Lauderdale, FL	2:47:30	23. S. Swannack, CA	2:53:58
10. L. McBride, New York City, NY	2:47:37	24. E. Tranter, IL	2:54:35
11. D. Lewis, Solana Beach, CA	2:48:00	25. K. Heckman, MD	2:54:55
12. S. Hughes, Wellesley, MA	2:48:26	26. K. Sweigart, CT	2:55:23
13. L. Binder, San Diego, CA	2:48:35	30. M. Wright, MA	2:57:15
14. J. Gumbs-Lydig, San Mateo, CA	2:48:44	234. S. Berman, *CSU*, MA	3:28:04

520 entrants, 296 under 3:35:04.

*The top four broke the old course record.

Masters

1. T. d'Elia, NJ	2:58:11
2. S. Stricklin, CA	3:00:23

Chapter 9

1980-1989
The Last Amateurs, The New Professionals

Presidents: *James E. Carter, Ronald Reagan, George Bush*

Massachusetts Governors: *Edward King, Michael S. Dukakis*

Boston Mayors: *Kevin H. White, Raymond Flynn*

1980 Populations: *United States, 226,542,580; Massachusetts, 5,737,093; Boston, 562,994*

The most famous nonmarathoner of all time emerged in the 1980s. Rosie Ruiz proved symbolic of her time; any study of the decade cannot avoid the illusions, imagery, and fraud. We cannot sidestep Ruiz. The public remembers her name. Its chintzy, ersatz ring sticks in the mind. In 1980, by dint of the sound bite and the photo opportunity, the country elected a former actor to be their president. The film star of the 1980s was not a person, but special effects. Even prosperity proved an illusion as the national deficit increased and the U.S. became a net debtor nation. It was easy for people to wonder whether they felt genuine, original feelings or merely selected their hopes and fears from the ones packaged and articulated by spin doctors and media specialists. The difference between wishes and reality blurred. Michael Milken went to jail for making millions of dollars on illusions by selling "junk" bonds to finance leveraged buy-outs made by people who only imagined they knew how to make a company profitable enough to pay for the money they borrowed. In 1981 a Boston attorney named Marshall Medoff sold his own illusions to Will Cloney and, for a time, looked to be the sole owner of the Boston Marathon. Runners in pursuit of Boston sacrificed more and changed their bodies on a scale that would have been unimaginable to their predecessors. The best-known name associated with the marathon belonged to a fraud and a cheat, yet despite such ignominy, the marathon changed more in this decade than in the seven before it.

Of all the vicissitudes the Boston Marathon had survived since 1897, including two world wars, two lesser wars, and a major economic depression, it was the 1980s, peace, and money that nearly killed it. By the middle of the decade other marathons offered prize money that attracted the top racers while the Boston officials insisted on retaining a race that was pristine, pure, and poor—an amateur event. The top marathoners, like their forerunners

411

who preferred merchandise prizes to trophies in amateur races, followed the money. Until a pivotal point in the mid-'80s, all the money led to marathons other than Boston. One wag said of the time that "money is the marijuana of the '80s." Money certainly changed the Boston Marathon, making the race of 1989 utterly different from the race of 1980. The changes pivoted on 1986.

Before 1984 world-class fields came to contest the Boston Marathon, but in 1984 only Geoff Smith came; he beat an excellent but not world-class Connecticut runner by 4 minutes. The next year Smith ran out alone, blew up, staggered, threw his arms up into the sky, then walked across the finish line. Still no one challenged him. All the potential challengers prepared for payday races elsewhere. People wondered, What if they gave a marathon and no one came?

In an attempt to remedy the lack-of-money and thereby the lack-of-competition problem, Boston Athletic Association President and marathon Race Director Will Cloney in 1981 quietly signed a deal with attorney Marshall Medoff, a vilified and perhaps nefarious character, the heralded and mysterious villain of this story. The deal made Medoff the sole agent of the marathon, entitled to "sell" sponsorship in perpetuity. Cloney may have had good intentions, but he made a bad deal for the BAA. Like the Grinch who stole Christmas, Medoff seemed to have stolen the Boston Marathon. Or perhaps Cloney had given it away. Perhaps they even conspired on it. The city rose up to claim its marathon. Newspapers and their columnists attacked Medoff and Cloney. The mayor of Boston and the governor of Massachusetts involved themselves in the issue. Off to court went the BAA and Medoff. Passionate, painful, and bitter years passed before the race took its present form.

After Will Cloney was forced to resign, Tim Kilduff became director for the 1983 race. A vicious dispute shook the BAA board of governors. Guy Morse started the same year with the BAA as an administrator and became director in 1988, a role he retained as of 1993.

The John Hancock Financial Services company became race sponsor in 1986 and offered cash prizes; the best runners in the world flocked to Boston, and one from Australia broke the course record.

The 1980s began with Bill Rodgers's last of four victories in the Boston Marathon. But Rodgers influenced most of the Boston Marathons of the decade. He often finished in the top ten and he became a prominent masters competitor.

ANGRY YOUNG MAN

MONDAY, APRIL 21, 1980

Can Boston Billy Make It 3 in a Row?

After Bill Rodgers's third Boston Marathon victory, in 1979, President Jimmy Carter invited Rodgers and his wife, Ellen, to a state dinner on the west terrace of the White House on May 2, 1979. Joan Benoit sat at the same table with the Rodgerses, the Carters, and Prime Minister Ohira of Japan. When Rosalynn Carter said she worried about a demonstration by antinuclear activists, Joan remarked that she herself worried about problems concerning the long-term storage of nuclear wastes. The Carters advocated nuclear power; they had no answers for Benoit and adroitly changed the subject.

They ate avocado with a seafood salad and chose among entrees of chicken, buffalo, or suckling pig with the option of Georgia or Texas barbecue sauce. Rodgers and President Carter discussed running as they ate. Carter had had troubles with an adductor muscle during his 5-mile runs and asked Rodgers's advice. Rodgers liked the president; he admired Carter's sincerity, straight-forwardness, and honesty. But later, in 1980, Jimmy Carter's presidential actions thoroughly angered Bill Rodgers. Rodgers had had no intention to run the Boston Marathon in 1980; he planned to save himself for the Summer Olympic Games. But the USSR had invaded Afghanistan in 1979, and on April 12, 1980, after little debate, the U.S. Olympic Committee had voted by secret ballot to endorse President Carter's boycott of the Moscow Olympic Games. The boycott, which Carter intended as a protest of the Soviet invasion, infuriated Rodgers. His world had collapsed. The Olympic dreams that had driven him evaporated. He could stand to lose the Olympic race or to not make the team if another runner outraced him or if he were injured—that was part of the running game. Every experienced runner knows how to lose. But to not be allowed to play? The rebel and the revolutionary arose in Rodgers. Feelings of the early 1970s returned.

Rodgers wanted to wear a black armband in this 1980 Boston Marathon to protest the boycott. He railed long and loud about the decision. He left no ambivalence about his position. He may have acted disorganized, but he did not hesitate to tell people his feelings. However, just as people back in the early 1970s had thought Rodgers's antiwar position was unpatriotic, some people now saw Rodgers as un-American. Threats were made against him and his brother Charlie because of his public statements.

On a busy premarathon sales day in the Bill Rodgers Running Center, a phone call rang in the hectic air. A worker took the call amid the jostling of customers buying souvenir T-shirts and shoes. The worker froze, turned pale, and looked across the room at Bill and Charlie. The caller said that Billy would never make it alive past Coolidge Corner. Charlie knew how the crowds pressed against the runners, leaving them perhaps inches from someone carrying a con-

> *The caller said that Billy Rodgers would never make it alive past Coolidge Corner.*

cealed gun. Charlie had visions of Jack Ruby's having shot Lee Harvey Oswald at point-blank range. The employees at the running center called the state police to report the threat. (It would be later in 1980 that Mark David Chapman shot and killed Beatle John Lennon; the next year John W. Hinckley, Jr. shot President Reagan.)

Race Director Will Cloney also worried about assassination attempts during the race. Events on the other side of the world created a nasty twist in the Boston Marathon. Could speaking up and running a marathon be unpatriotic, especially on Patriots' Day in Massachusetts? Could it incite murder? The police decided they would make any attempt on Rodgers's life difficult to accomplish by forming a phalanx of motorcycles around Rodgers during the race. All this struck Rodgers as bizarre, so he backed off on his criticisms of the boycott in the last days before the race.

President Carter said that the boycott was necessary because national security was threatened (by the invasion), but he said that a team would be selected for honorary purposes. Honor alone did not interest Rodgers; he wanted to race in the Olympic Games. He wanted that chance and he felt he deserved it. Greater Boston Track Club teammate Bobby Hodge proclaimed that the Olympic trials offered a road to nowhere. Tom Fleming said that Boston meant more than the Olympics anyway. Vice President Mondale drew parallels between the Soviet Union's Olympic Games in Moscow and the 1936 games in Berlin, used by Hitler as a showcase to garner international acceptance of Nazism. He said, "The American people do not want their athletes cast as pawns in that tawdry propaganda campaign." But most of the athletes who trained for the Olympic Games saw the games as an alternative to war. They believed in the Olympic ideal and wanted to run in Moscow.

Les Pawson, another three-time Boston winner (1933, 1938, 1941), disagreed with Rodgers and supported the boycott. Pawson had been selected for the 1940 Olympic Games, which were scheduled first for Tokyo, then switched to Finland because of the war in the Pacific, and finally cancelled because of the Russian invasion of Finland. Rodgers thus was the second Boston Marathon winner to be denied a chance to run in the Olympic Games because of a Russian invasion. Pawson agreed with Rodgers that the Olympic Games were not to be seen as a political event, but he disagreed with the Soviet government in both 1940 and 1980, and so felt the U.S. team should *not* go to Moscow this year. Pawson thought he could have it both ways—an apolitical Olympics but still a boycott to make a political statement. It did not follow logically, but such were the emotions of patriotism.

Rodgers decided at the last moment not to wear the armband, which would in itself have made a political statement. But how could he make a political statement through sport to say that sport should not be used to make political statements? He tried to reconcile within himself this paradox, his disappointment, and his anger with his president. Tom Fleming said of Rodgers, "The one thing you don't want to do is get Bill angry. You see how well he runs when he's meek and mild and spaced out. When he's running angry, he'll crush you so fast that you'll think he's in a 15K race instead of a marathon. And Bill is angry no matter what he says."

With his fury and a vision of someone leaping out of the crowd to slug or shoot him, Bill Rodgers went to the line. Will Cloney had received the same death threats against both Bill and Charlie Rodgers. The anonymous caller warned again that Bill would not make it alive through Coolidge Corner. There was no way the entire course could be made secure. It was a warm day in an unusually early spring that had brought the forsythia to bloom before the marathon. Rodgers saw the prerace temperature of 67 °F, turned to Ellen, and said, "Uh, oh." His biggest enemy, heat, was back. Would this be a replay of 1977, when Drayton and the heat had forced him to drop out? Would he be able to match DeMar in winning three straight Boston Marathons? Would someone slug him? Would someone shoot him?

Without the boycott, the Boston Marathon of 1980 would have been less of a contest. With the Soviet invasion and subsequent boycott, the attention of American marathoners was diverted from the May Olympic trials to Boston; the typical weak field of an Olympic year became highly competitive. Good heat runners came to race, runners like Ron Tabb (2:11) from Houston, Benji Durden (2:13:48) from Atlanta, and Kevin Ryan (2:11:43) from New Zealand. Fleming and Hodge came to race. They had trained with Rodgers for several weeks in Florida to adapt to the heat. A couple of runners from under the Mediterranean sun, Italian Marco Marchei and Greek Michael Koussis, were capable of 2:11 or 2:12.

Puerto Rico's Eduardo Vera and Koussis took the early lead. They passed the easy downhill 5 miles in 24:15. By Framingham Marchei joined his neighbor from across the Ionian Sea and Vera dropped back. Tabb lead a pack of 11 runners that included Rodgers, Ryan, Hodge, Durden, Dick Mahoney, Steve Floto, and Kirk Pfeffer, a young runner from Colorado. Pfeffer had led the New York City Marathon the previous fall for 24 miles before succumbing to Rodgers. Pfeffer had since had a bout with hepatitis and minor knee surgery, so experts questioned his basic fitness. But Rodgers saw him as a wild card.

Hodge, Mahoney, and Fleming soon dropped out of contention and later the race. They had inexplicably bad days.

At 12 miles Ryan, Rodgers, and Pfeffer caught Tabb and Marchei. Those two and Ryan formed a pack while Rodgers and Pfeffer stormed ahead. They passed the Wellesley checkpoint (13.75 miles) in 1:05:49. Rodgers still did not know what to expect from Pfeffer. Rodgers planned to wait until the hills to make his move.

On a slight downhill in Wellesley Rodgers let his friendliness with gravity carry him down the little hill. He seemed to go for the fall line with the unerring grace of a downhill ski racer. With hardly a flicker or clue revealing strain, he fell away from Pfeffer. Sometimes he didn't realize he was doing it and surprised himself to see that he suddenly ran ahead of his competition. Just such a thing happened on that little downhill in Wellesley. Suddenly Pfeffer disappeared—no footsteps. Brother Charlie on the photo truck told Billy he had 60, then 150 yards. A mile later the pack passed Pfeffer and he walked. He never finished. Now Rodgers had only time and distance to worry him.

The other runners suffered. Marchei suffered from the hot sun. After 20 miles no one could race against anyone else. They all tried merely to survive, to get the thing ended. Fortunately for Rodgers he had 48 seconds on Tabb and Marchei at the Woodland checkpoint (17.25 miles), which he passed in 1:26:07.

In other races Rodgers had won against competition, but to win this one he would have to overcome his own disintegrating body. He wanted to drink. The wedge of state police motorcycles may have kept away would-be killers or angry "patriots" who wanted to attack Rodgers, but they also kept away spectators with water cups. Rodgers pointed at his mouth, but no one could get near enough to him to give him water. He might as well have been running in a desert. Charlie in the press truck saw him pointing, but he could do nothing. Rodgers ran on, parched. Twenty miles passed in 1:38:37, 4:56 per mile—a new American record, if he could hold it.

Larger-than-ever crowds lined the course. People leaned out of windows and off of balconies; they danced on rooftops. Some had signs: "Boston Loves Billy." The enthusiasm helped, because Boston Billy hurt going up the hills. On the downhills he got leg cramps. He fell apart, yet he held the lead. He got no boos from the crowd for his outspokenness against the president's Olympic boycott, so although he had slowed drastically, he knew he could not drop out; all those people would not let him. They would push him back onto the road if he tried to leave the course. He had to run or collapse. He expected to collapse.

At Kenmore Square, Rodgers thought about the death threat. On the brink of collapse he felt oddly invincible. As is true for many runners in this state of extremity, a little craziness possessed him. After hours of pushing at the ragged edge of oxygen debt, he detached from the real world to live in one of pulse, push, and rhythm. In his imagination he taunted the assassin: Come

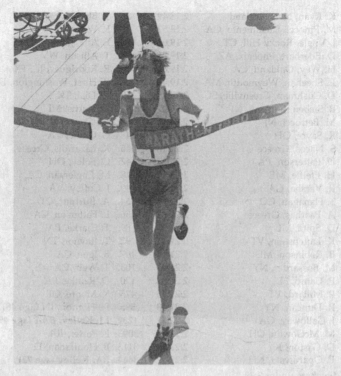

"Bill Rodgers will never make Coolidge Corner alive," threatened an anonymous caller in 1980, outraged that Rodgers spoke out against President Carter's Olympic boycott. Photo by Jeff Johnson.

on, you son of a bitch. Like Clarence DeMar, Rodgers would have socked anyone who interfered with his running, even someone with a gun.

When at last the race ended, Rodgers's 48-second advantage increased by 21 to just over a minute (1:09), only 2 or 3 seconds per mile. By the finish line Rodgers's anger had dissipated. He felt only relief that the thing had ended. He had won the Boston Marathon for a fourth time. He had matched the Great Cote. But he would not go to the Olympic Games. The thought left him with no joy. He would take the time instead to consolidate the business side of marathon running. Amateur, shmamateur—Bill Rodgers wanted to make money.

1980 Men's Results

1. B. Rodgers, MA	2:12:11	5. P. Friedman, NJ	2:16:46
2. M. Marchei, Italy	2:13:20	6. B. Durden, Atlanta, GA	2:17:46
3. R. Tabb, Houston, TX	2:14:48	7. J. White, Sacramento, CA	2:17:58
4. M. Koussis, Greece	2:16:03	8. S. Floto, Boulder, CO	2:18:19

9.	K. Ryan, New Zealand	2:18:49	36. T. Blumer, OH	2:22:29
10.	M. Pinocci, Sacramento, CA	2:18:52	37. R. Wayne, CA	2:22:33
11.	J. Vitale, Rocky Hill, CT	2:19:01	38. F. Abe, Japan	2:22:39
12.	D. Eberhart, Phoenix, AZ	2:19:21	39. T. Allison, WV	2:23:13
13.	H. Wey, Oakland, CA	2:19:34	40. R. Rodriguez, Jr., TX	2:23:17
14.	E. Sheehan, Weymouth, MA	2:19:42	41. R. Hirst, Washington, DC	2:24:06
15.	D. Cushman, Greenville, SC	2:19:46	42. D. Dial, TX	2:24:18
16.	B. Sieben, Rahway, NJ	2:20:07	43. D. Kurtis, MI	2:24:25
17.	M. Petrocci, NJ	2:20:11	44. W. Devoe, NY	2:24:47
18.	R. Sayre, OH	2:20:15	45. G. Crane, VA	2:24:52
19.	S. Nacos, Greece	2:20:16	46. K. Lazaridis, Greece	2:24:57
20.	D. Patterson, PA	2:20:27	47. G. Foley, OH	2:25:14
21.	H. Pfeifle, ME	2:20:34	48. M. Engleman, CA	2:25:14
22.	R. Varsha, GA	2:20:37	49. J. Coffey, VA	2:25:19
23.	S. Flanagan, CO	2:20:42	**54. A. Burfoot, CT**	**2:25:47**
24.	A. Paathas, Greece	2:21:01	56. L. Patterson, CA	2:26:04
25.	D. Spitz, MI	2:21:03	89. T. Clarke, PA	2:28:38
26.	K. Lauenstein, VT	2:21:11	92. T. Raynor, TN	2:28:49
27.	B. Robinson, MD	2:21:15	107. B. Igoe, CA	2:29:52
28.	M. Bossardet, NY	2:21:41	108. T. Weir, CA	2:29:58
29.	P. Camp, FL	2:21:52	120. D. Reinke, PA	2:30:43
30.	P. Millard, VT	2:21:55	475. K. Moore, OR	2:42:24
31.	R. Duncan, NY	2:21:58	595. H. Higdon, IN (age 48)	2:45:02
32.	J. Galloway, GA	2:22:02	**1232. J.J. Kelley, BAA (age 49)**	**2:55:45**
33.	M. McGowan, OH	2:22:08	3093. F. Porter, BAA	3:25:25
34.	D. Gaston, KY	2:22:10	3113. B. Honikman, FL	3:25:46
35.	P. Oparowski, NH	2:22:17	**3444. J.A. Kelley (age 72)**	**3:35:21**

3,428 finishers under 3:30.

Masters

1.	B. Heinrich, CA	2:25:25
2.	R. Swan, Bermuda	2:27:29

THE ROSY RUSE

MONDAY, APRIL 21, 1980

Lyons Favorite in Today's Marathon

The women's division of the 1980 Boston Marathon will live in infamy. That day a soft, untrained, unprepared imposter jumped into the marathon with a mile remaining to steal the cheers, the laurel wreath, and the medal that belonged to the real runner who raced from Hopkinton to Boston faster than any woman that day.

The story of Rosie Ruiz is larger than she is, and it represents what the marathon had become and how people saw the marathon and many other things in this decade. Did Ruiz plan a careful hoax that she intended to reveal later to prove her cleverness, or did she intend to profit from her notoriety, or was she crazy? Why did she do it? What did she hope to gain? What did it cost the real winner and the public?

Patti Lyons wanted to win the Boston Marathon—she had started racing in order to run it. She had no interest in the Olympics. They held no women's marathon, so her dream remained to win Boston. Lyons's first marathon victory, in Newport, Rhode Island, in October 1976 qualified her to run in Boston. She knew the Boston Marathon would be run every year, and after her second place in 1979 she would rather be nowhere else in 1980. Her second place at Boston had brought her more fame than her three wins in Newport or her win in the Honolulu Marathon. For her coach (and now fiancé), Joe Catalano, she planned to win Boston. She would do it to be nice to Patti and as a wedding gift for Joe.

The press anointed Patti Lyons their favorite as they matched her against Ellison Goodall, the daughter of a wealthy doctor, a former medical school student from North Carolina who had taken up residence in a big house in Wellesley with four other top women runners. Goodall had run well in shorter races, winning the Falmouth road race in course record time. Joan Benoit could not race in Boston in 1980 because she had recently had her appendix removed. She had planned to do radio commentary, but acute disappointment about not being able to race kept her in Maine. The second- and third-place runners from the New York City Marathon, Gillian Adams of England and Jacqueline Gareau of Quebec, had run under 2:40. The Boston press had ignored Gareau. A shy, petite, dark-haired 27-year-old French Canadian, Gareau wore W22, which was supposed to indicate the twenty-second fastest qualifying time. Few people knew that her previous marathon best was the third fastest of the field.

Only 3 years earlier Gareau had graduated from recreational jogging to casual long-distance running. Any idea of racing lingered only vaguely in the back of her mind. Raised on a dairy farm in the northern Laurentian Mountains near the town of L'Annonciation, Gareau had skied and skated as a child but had otherwise busied herself with schoolwork and her daily farm chores. Only boys competed seriously in athletics. Gareau grew up in a culture similar to the one that raised Gerard Cote, four-time Boston Marathon winner in the 1940s. But she was no roistering female version of the flamboyant Cote. The fourth of seven children, Gareau moved into Montreal and began working toward a college degree in allied health services. She studied respiratory technology, kept irregular hours, attended late-night parties, and smoked half a pack of cigarettes a day. In short, she lived a rather typical life for a young adult. In that respect she was not much different from Bill Rodgers, and like him she gave up smoking after seeing its results in hospital patients. Only after Gareau's tours of the pulmonary wards at the Hôtel-Dieu did she convince herself to "run for good health."

But it was not Gareau or Patti Lyons who controlled the race through the early miles. Goodall led the women through 8 miles. Kenny Moore, 1968 and 1972 Olympian, ran by her side to cover the women's race for *Sports Illustrated* from the ground rather than from the press truck. He wanted to see every nuance. But in fact he would miss the biggest news of all. Moore had last run in Boston on a cold day in 1970. He had had a miserable time then and would have a miserable time again, but for entirely different reasons. Lyons ran conservatively with the first 5 miles in only 29:55 and a 10-mile split of 59:58. The year before she had been much faster, but in this day's heat she seemed to be doing the right thing. But at 8 miles Gareau grabbed the lead from Goodall. By 15 miles Lyons ran only 16 seconds in arrears. Gareau passed 20 miles in 1:56:50, but Lyons ran 30 seconds back.

At 18 miles Jacqueline Gareau held up her index finger to the spectators to ask if she was first. They told her yes. Kathrine Switzer rode a press bus just ahead of Gareau. Switzer flashed a grin at Gareau, held up her index finger, and said, "You're #1." A wave of applause followed Gareau to Boston. At times the noise racked her eardrums to the threshold of pain. Cries of "first woman!" preceded her to the city. Lyons could hear the din as she tried to accelerate; she wanted those cheers for herself. Gareau looked, as Lyons would say, "catchable, definitely catchable." But mile after mile, Lyons could not draw any closer. The two ran in lock step, 150 yards apart. They ran a hard and honest race.

Gareau led with a mile to go. Both she and Lyons knew Gareau would win and Lyons would finish second unless something bizarre happened to Gareau. A quarter of a mile later something bizarre did happen. Just where the crowds are thickest, they quieted. The frenzy stopped. The calls of "first woman!" stopped. Suddenly it seemed as if Jacqueline Gareau ran through a wake.

"You're second," a man called—she was running in another runner's wake. But Gareau knew she was first.

But neither Gareau nor any other runner knew that a woman born Maria Rosales in Havana, Cuba, plowed through ahead of Gareau, taking the glory with her. Rosales had come to the U.S. in 1961. In 1973 and again in 1978 she underwent brain surgery for the removal of benign tumors. She wore white shorts with blue trim and a bulky yellow T-shirt with the letters M.T.I. screened across the front, the initials of her New York City employer, Metal Traders, Inc., who had paid her way to Boston after she showed her New York City Marathon certificate with a 2:56:29 printed on it. On the basis of that certificate she received number W50 for the Boston Marathon. She had changed her name to Rosie Ruiz and entered races under it.

Ruiz stood 5'8" and weighed 130 pounds. She had grown up in Florida and claimed she graduated from Wayne State College in Nebraska in 1973 before settling in New York City. She lived with two roommates in an apartment at Manhattan Plaza in the west 40s. She had friends who liked her and appreciated her intelligence. In Boston from near Kenmore Square she had watched the top runners go by.

In the square Ruiz selected her moment to stumble out of the crowd and onto the race course, her arms flying about. She ran awkwardly, almost out of control. No one nearby took her seriously as they watched her come onto the course. Some joker clowning for her friends, maybe, or an enthusiastic spectator jumping in for a few yards. A couple of Harvard students, who later told their story to the *Boston Globe*, watched her; one noticed that she wore a number. Just a few yards down the road the leaning crowds, eager to shout for the first woman, caught sight of Ruiz and hailed her as the women's leader. The first cheers legitimized others. All the way to the finish the big cheers followed her.

When Gareau finished no one received her. She crossed the finish line alone, then stood there. She had run what she hoped. Her plan had worked so well that she broke Joan Benoit's course record with a 2:34; that should have been enough to win, but did she win? She thought so. In the Boston Marathon tradition officials quickly ushered the winners up to the victory platform to award the prizes while the politicians and race officials could bask with the winners in front of the full finish-line crowd. The custom produced immediate gratification for the crowds, photographers, and television cameras.

But no police escort, no race official met Gareau. No one ushered her to the winners' platform. It puzzled her. She looked up to see a woman she did not recognize up on the victory platform with Bill Rodgers. The woman Gareau did not know and had never heard of had finished 3 minutes earlier. Rodgers and the woman wore laurel wreaths on their heads and first-place medals around their necks. Gareau thought, Who is she? How fast could she have run to beat me? She knew that she herself had run well. She had beaten Patti Lyons, and if anyone had run faster than 2:34:28, she deserved to win. But who was this woman? Everybody else wanted to know too. Bill Rodgers studied this Rosie Ruiz. She perplexed him. He had been around the road race circuit and knew his sport, but he had never heard of her. She didn't look like a runner to him. Gareau felt herself drawn into a growing controversy.

What did Gareau do? What could she do? She was too tired to argue. She wanted to meet Rodgers, shake his hand, share a victory kiss, and sit together to talk to the reporters about the race. Hadn't she earned that? But she had to stay away. At first the reporters didn't want to talk to her about her race, only about Rosie Ruiz. Gareau didn't know anything about Ruiz. She didn't know how or with whom to file a protest. All she knew was what *she* had done. Frustration, self-doubt, and fatigue filled her. She felt stupid standing there alone in a cold, underground garage. She wanted to board a plane and go home. She had never experienced anything like this before. Not having run races for very long, she didn't know who was who. Maybe that

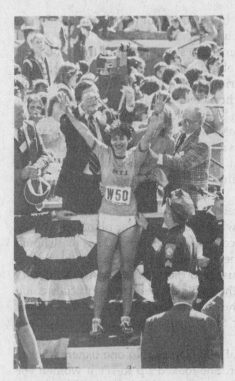
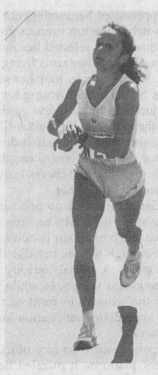

Rosie Ruiz basks in glory accepting the victor's medal from Will Cloney and Governor Ed King, while the real winner, Jacqueline Gareau (right), is ignored. Photos by Jeff Johnson.

woman did not cheat. Gareau's thoughts raced in French, but articulate, argumentative English would not come to her. Self-doubt did.

Reporters rushed around the new winner of the women's race. It was *possible*, if unexpected, that someone with a number like W50 could win. To win the 1926 race Johnny Miles had come out of nowhere, but he had been the last unknown to do so, 50-some years ago. In the fairly new sport of women's marathon racing, though, a new star could fall from out of nowhere. Someone with an accomplished track or cross-country background could be new to the marathon but have run an easy qualifying race and then go all-out in Boston. A runner could have trained well under Zatopek's methods of timed intervals on the track. The possibility did exist. Following that idea, Kathrine Switzer, now a television reporter, asked Ruiz how many miles she had trained. She said about 65 miles a week. Hearing such a low figure, Switzer asked if she had been doing a lot of intervals. Ruiz answered that it was a funny thing, but that was the second time today that someone asked her about "intervals." Ruiz asked Switzer, "What's an interval?"

Charlie Rodgers didn't need to ask any questions: "The first thing I did was look at her legs, and I said to myself, 'Uh, oh, we have a problem here.' I mean it was cellulite city." Other observations added to the suspicions. The patterns of sweat on Ruiz's T-shirt denied that she had just run 26 miles. After 2-1/2 hours, any runner's T-shirt would be soaking wet. Ruiz's shirt was too dry, especially under the armpits, and it was too heavy to begin with. It was impossible that the shirt, not to mention the runner, had gone the full distance. A marathon race changes a person.

Ed Ayers of *Running Times* elaborated:

> Runners are intimately familiar with these changes and recognize them in others. They may not be able to say what those changes are (any more than one can accurately describe the face of a friend), but the signs are unmistakable nevertheless: a characteristic pattern of sweat on the clothing; a residue of salt left by the continual evaporation of sweat on the face; traces of foam or incrustation around the mouth resulting from dehydration of saliva; sunburn patterns which include whitish "squint" marks from running into the sun, and from the characteristic facial tension (which reporters so often confuse with pain) of a marathoner; tautness of the leg muscles resulting from hours of repeated contraction with full extension; and the peculiar finishing chute walk of a person whose legs are usually strong but temporarily depleted of glycogen—the walk of an exhausted athlete, which is quite different from the walk of someone whose fatigue is due to a lack of conditioning. These and many subtler signs make up the "gestalt" of the runner who has just finished two hours of physiological struggle. There is no way this gestalt can be faked.

Ruiz said to the press and the television cameras, "I really didn't expect to win. I came across in 2:31, that's all I have to say. I know I ran the course. I did the best I can. What else can I say? How would you feel? I just wanted to finish. I didn't know I was the first woman until I crossed the line. To be sincere, this is a dream." She seemed genuinely pleased, surprised, and proud. Tall, dark-haired, trim, but not particularly fit-looking, she seemed believable to the uninitiated. From the victory platform she smiled and waved to the cheering throng.

Jock Semple went on a rampage. He sputtered around the press room, declaring Ruiz a fraud. Semple glared at Ruiz: "She's a bloody thief." Rodgers had made up his mind that she was an imposter, so he glared at Ruiz too.

As the doubts grew, however, Rosie would not confess. She had the laurel wreath. She had the medal. They had given it to her. She would not give it back.

Race Director Will Cloney had awarded her the victory. In fact he had actually clipped the medal around her neck himself. Now it was up to him to take it back. He had to investigate the entire incident, line up the provable facts, and, if they were as they seemed, disqualify her. People muttered possibilities of a lawsuit on Ruiz's behalf. Cloney had not bargained for this. He had been working gratis as race director since the BAA track meets had ended in 1972 (before that George Brown of the Boston Garden had paid Cloney $1,500 to direct the two track meets and the marathon). Cloney was nearing retirement age. Since 1931 he had been involved with the Boston Marathon, first as a reporter, then the director. Mostly by default he had acquired a proprietary attitude toward the race.

Cloney had become as much a victim as Gareau in this deceit. Had he directed the race sloppily so that an imposter could easily fool him, or would he be trying to take a victory away from a winner whose only crime was being unknown? The press and the public waited for Cloney's decision. William B. Tyler, an attorney on the BAA board of governors, advised Cloney to be careful because Ruiz was a woman and a minority; dealing with her with even the appearance of unfairness could attract a lawsuit of the worst kind. Extricating himself and the marathon from this sudden mess would be difficult. A mess engulfed Gareau, too.

Reporters surrounded Gareau. If Rosie Ruiz would not confess, perhaps Jacqueline Gareau would condemn her as a cheat. Howling for a story somewhere, reporters surrounded Gareau like hyenas after scraps. Every reporter wanted a quotation to scream across a banner headline. The group tried to rile Gareau. But she had run as hard as she could, and she wanted to go home. What emotions she had for the day had already been used up. She gave to reporters only a flat, factual sentence devoid of accusations or bitterness: "I supposed I was first, then I arrived at the finish line."

Cloney issued his own statement, a masterpiece of spontaneous diplomacy in a day of passionate charges, countercharges, and fear of compounding error:

> There is an obvious problem with the determination of the women's winner. At this moment we have no proof one way or the other that would cause us to reverse the decision immediately. But we will try to do everything possible within the next week to check whether there was a discrepancy. If this proves to be the case we will invalidate the final results and adjust the places accordingly. If the medal had not already been awarded it would have been held up. I have not talked to the young lady in question. I have no reason to accuse her of anything. We do have grave doubts.

The Boston papers went to press with Rosie Ruiz's name atop the list of women runners and questions about her authenticity in the main body of the story. That day and for 3 days following a photograph of Ruiz appeared on the front page of the *Globe*. The story went on the wires and around the world. Rosie Ruiz became the most famous marathoner in the world as debate raged for a week. Did she or did she not run the whole Boston Marathon? Her name entered the household vocabulary. The whole affair became a big mockery. The irreverent enjoyed it. The jokes flew. Did you hear that Rosie Ruiz is writing a book? It starts on page 425. Have you seen the new Rosie Ruiz panty hose? Guaranteed not to run. Or the Rosie Ruiz doll? Wind it up and it just stands there.

The *Boston Herald* published a photo of the start of the race with the headline "Win $1,000: Find Rosie in this photo of the start." To some she became a folk hero, a Jesse James of the fad of running, a symbol of someone who put one over on the establishment.

Carefully Cloney accumulated the evidence. He wanted to be sure not only that justice would be done but that it would appear that no decision to disqualify Ruiz was made in haste. This was the evidence he gathered:

Nowhere in the entire marathon distance did any official checkpoint register the passage of W50. No journalist showed her on film until the finish. She did not appear in any one of the 10,000 frames taken by the official race photographers. Could she have passed a million people and been noticed by no one?

A single witness came forward on Ruiz's behalf. The one person who said he saw her at the start had himself been banned from the New York City Marathon for cheating. Out of the mold of Jimmy "Cigars" Connors, he sought publicity by wearing a costume. A friend of Ruiz's had called to ask him to help, and he came rushing to the rescue, dressed in the Superman suit he wore to run road races. He would strut around before and after races, his red cape aswish. As the fantastic scene unfolded, there stood Rosie Ruiz, Superman at her side, with wide-eyed innocence and wonder at all the controversy. But her Superman had no X-ray vision, no superpowers, and no facts. One by one Cloney gathered facts.

With sensitivity and generosity Cloney met with Ruiz in her hotel room later in the day, accompanied by the BAA attorney, William B. Tyler. They behaved gently toward her, and she listened agreeably and attentively. Cloney and Tyler expected Ruiz to confess, but when Cloney asked her to return the medal, she broke down in tears. She would not give the medal back. She said the lack of evidence baffled her too, so she could understand how Cloney might have to disqualify her, but she had won the Boston Marathon. Cloney left the meeting thinking that Ruiz had not intended to win, only to show up in the official results. Reporters asked if he thought she was a liar, a fraud, a cheat. Cloney replied that he would never use those words to describe another human being.

In the week following the race the New York Marathon officials gathered some facts to help Cloney. Rosie Ruiz had entered the New York City Marathon after the application deadline by claiming that she had a terminal brain tumor and might not live to run the next year. On that basis she was granted special entry. But she never finished the New York City Marathon in October 1979—in fact, she never ran it at all. Yet she obtained an official finishing certificate and appeared in the official results, which she used to qualify for Boston. How did Ruiz do it?

After the Boston controversy, the New York City Marathon officials tried to find Ruiz on the videotape of the New York finish, but she did not appear. The New York race director, Fred Lebow, and marathon officials investigated, and they unearthed how Rosie Ruiz had really finished their race. During the race Ruiz was supposedly running, freelance designer and photographer Susan Morrow happened to meet her on the subway at Fourth Street Station at Eighth Avenue at 11:30—an hour and a half after the start—and rode with Ruiz to the finish area. Ruiz, claiming injury, made her way to the chutes and told an official that she had hurt her ankle. The official assumed she had finished, took her bar code, and rushed her to the medical area, then gave the bar code to an official messenger, who stood in Ruiz's place in line in the chutes so the number could be recorded in sequence and later matched with the finishing times.

Because Ruiz had never passed under the video camera at the finish, Lebow disqualified her from the New York race. The jokes continued. T-shirts appeared with "Rosie Ruiz Track Club" on the back and a picture of a subway token on the front (because of the way the New York City Marathon officials found she had arrived at their finish line). In May, comedian Johnny Carson quipped on national television: "Last Saturday, Genuine Risk became the first filly since 1915 to win the Kentucky Derby. However, there has been an inquiry. Another horse is claiming that she and Genuine Risk took a subway together to the finish line."

Because of Ruiz's disqualification at New York, technically her qualifying time for Boston was invalid, so her very entry was fraudulent. But Cloney did not want to use that method of disqualification because the New York decision came after the Boston race. Doubt might linger if he used that line of reasoning.

What reasoning had Ruiz used? Or did she simply get caught up in the booming popularity of running? Marathon running seemed to confer a status of immortality, even deity, on those who completed one. In the New York City culture a person could be neither too rich nor too thin; marathon runners, thought to be immune to heart disease, looked tanned, rich, and thin. Central Park became the place to jog and be seen jogging. Rosie Ruiz jogged there. Running clothes became a fashion statement. Participation in the New York City Marathon best made that statement about thin, rich, fit, and fashionable. Tens of thousands applied to run it. Perhaps for Ruiz, error slipped in and turned to opportunity. Perhaps she was oblivious to the error that led to her "official" finish. But the next day, when co-workers who had seen her name in the newspaper began to congratulate her, she did not deny finishing. She believed what she wanted to believe. The newspapers and everyone else believed she finished, so she said nothing. She came to enjoy accepting congratulations. But then she had to live up to a lie.

When her company offered to pay her way to the Boston Marathon, Ruiz felt trapped. She couldn't say no. She wanted to go. She liked the attention. So she went. But her employer expected too much of her. Her boss wanted to see her name in the papers again. Perhaps that pressure inspired her to slip into the stream of runners. Maybe Ruiz hadn't wanted to win, just to make a showing, but in her ignorance of the sport became impatient after watching 300 men run by. She had never seen the finish of a marathon before. She did not want to miss placing high enough to get her name published to validate her trip to Boston at company expense, so she slipped in among the men and blundered to the victory platform.

On her way there the lie locked itself into her brain. Just as alcoholics often deny having a problem by believing they can quit drinking at will, just as entire families with severe problems of violence or incest may maintain that everything is fine, Rosie Ruiz denied she had a problem. The deeper she sank into her lie, the more difficult and ultimately impossible it became for her to summon the courage to tell the simple truth.

Ruiz possibly slipped into what Dr. Daniel Goleman has called a lacuna, a black hole of the mind, diverting attention from select bits of subjective reality—specifically, certain bits of anxiety-evoking information. She wanted to run the marathon to be noticed, important, respected, but the momentum of events got away from her and she did not have the strength of character to stop them. Then she retreated and ultimately acted puzzled, truly baffled at why she didn't appear in any of the checkpoint videos. She apparently repressed the memory of not running. She "forgot" she didn't run and she forgot that she forgot. In the sense that she believed she had run the race, Ruiz was not a cheat, but she *was* an imposter. And because she did not know right from wrong pertaining to the marathon, she was, at least in that aspect of her life, insane. She may also have been criminal. Certainly her act, done in a race with prize money, could be seen as having criminal intent.

Ruiz continued to have difficulties after her Boston brouhaha. She was fired from her job at Metal Traders, and she was charged with writing bad checks totaling $1,000 to New York department stores. (The stores settled the matters out of court.) Half an hour before the start of the Boston Marathon in 1982, a police detective named John Kelly and his partner arrested Ruiz on charges of grand larceny and forgery for stealing $15,000 in cash and $45,000 in checks from her employer. The courts sentenced her to 5 years probation. In 1983 undercover agents arrested Ruiz and two others for agreeing to sell them 2 kilograms of high-grade cocaine for $52,000. She was convicted and sentenced to 3 years probation.

Writers Sam Merrill and Marc Bloom offered another explanation of the Rosie Ruiz story in their investigative article in the July 1980 issue of *The Runner* magazine. After the Boston race they visited Ruiz in her apartment; the woman they saw was not in the usual sense crazy or criminal. They found her intelligent and charming. They checked her medical records and found that the operations to remove brain tumors in 1973 and 1978 had succeeded in every way, leaving no brain damage. She appeared completely normal, except she said she had won the Boston Marathon.

Merrill and Bloom came to favor the term *sociopath* to describe Ruiz. They concluded that she intended to do exactly what she did in both the New York City and Boston marathons. She had even told her mother before the Boston race that she had to win it. She had acted rationally, with no commonly accepted symptoms of psychosis—no neurotic anxiety or unease in situations that would unsettle the average person, no sense of responsibility, guilt, regret, or shame. The social pathology of her behavior exhibited itself in a cavalier attitude about telling the truth and an unflappability about lies being detected. Merrill and Bloom saw a woman with poor judgment, who failed to learn from experience or punishment. Not only did Rosie Ruiz not follow the rules, but she could not even see them. At the end of the entire affair, when no doubt existed in anyone else's mind that she had cheated, Ruiz still would not give the medal back.

And what of Jacqueline Gareau? What cost did she bear for Ruiz's actions? Gareau had to make three trips from Montreal in the week following the race back into Boston's preposterous controversy. Will Cloney assembled his information and at last disqualified the imposter. Observers congratulated him on the fairness and tact with which he conducted himself, single-handedly protecting the prestige of the Boston Marathon. About Ruiz, Gareau said without animosity, "I feel sorry for her because I think she didn't run. I think she doesn't want to lose face. I think she is afraid to say, 'I did not run.'" Gareau had to wait 7 days, 23 hours, and 25 minutes to be awarded her victory ceremony, to be awarded her new, bigger medal and a new laurel wreath, to stand on a victory podium with Bill Rodgers and share a victory kiss. At last she was crowned. When she walked into the runners' bar, the Eliot Lounge, the patrons and runners who were waiting sang "Oh, Canada." They opened vintage bottles of Dom Perignon. Gareau smiled and thrust her fist into the air. She would be back, Patti Lyons would be back, again and again. Lyons finished second, for the second time. For the next year she thought weekly, daily, hourly about victory in the Boston Marathon.

1980 *Women's Results*

1.	J. Gareau, PQ (201st overall)	2:34:28^{CR}	11.	J. Robinson, Seattle, WA	2:47:04
2.	P. Lyons, Boston, MA	2:35:08	12.	L. Donkelaar, AZ	2:48:33
3.	G. Adams, Bromley, England	2:39:17	13.	C. Dalrymple, WA	2:48:36
4.	L. Binder, San Diego, CA	2:39:22	14.	L. Jorgensen, CO	2:50:05
5.	K. Samet, Albuquerque, NM	2:41:50	15.	D. Slater, New York City, NY	2:50:24
6.	E. Goodall, Wellesley, MA	2:42:23	16.	S. Hughes, MA	2:51:02
7.	T. Bernhard, Houston, TX	2:44:40	17.	S. Henderson, CO	2:51:15
8.	D. Eide, Salem, OR	2:45:36	18.	S. Durtschi, OR	2:51:33
9.	E. Campo, Santa Barbara, CA	2:46:44	19.	D. Butterfield, Bermuda	2:51:46
10.	K. Sweigart, Darien, CT	2:46:47	20.	F. Madeira, MA	2:52:10

21.	D. Burge, TX	2:53:41	25.	M. Bevans, MD	2:55:26
22.	J. Buch, OH	2:54:21	40.	E. Mendonca, MA	3:00:48
23.	C. Young, CA	2:54:46	124.	M. Atamanuik, MA	3:17:53
24.	D. Riley, CA	2:54:48	211.	S. O'Hagan, MA	3:30:23

Masters

1.	A. Lee, CA	3:01:48
2.	K. Scannell, CA	3:03:47
3.	J. Lutter, MN	3:05:38

ZEN AND THE ART
OF MARATHON RUNNING

MONDAY, APRIL 20, 1981

Japan's Champion Here for Record

Bill Rodgers prospered in the running business. Gone were his days of enduring unemployment and existing on food stamps while hoping for a $10,000-a-year job. Now he could get $20,000 for just showing up at a marathon—almost $10,000 an hour! He said he did not want to end his days like Ellison Brown, penniless in a tar-paper shack. After a fight in 1975 outside of a bar in Rhode Island, the man Brown had been arguing with ran Brown over with his car. Quickly, unimportantly, and poor, Brown died. He had always lived on the edge of desperation. Rodgers wanted to stay clear of the edge; he did not want to wind up a footnote to history like Brown. Rodgers had a $25,000 deal with *The Runner* magazine and a 3-year deal with Puma at $80,000 for the first year, $100,000 for the second year, and $120,000 for the third. His Bill Rodgers Running Centers, as many as four at one point, with a gross of $1.5 million, and his clothing line with an $8-million maximum, kept him far from the ragged edge. He bought a big house surrounded by big trees in a prestigious suburb of Boston, out among people who owned horses and rode them along stretches of green grass between white rail fences, out where the land was inherited, not subdivided. No longer did he have to scrounge rides to races and share beds and box springs with his teammates in low-budget motels. No longer did he live in a cheap apartment where the floors sloped.

Before one of his New York City Marathon victories, Rodgers stayed in an opulent suite in the Sherry Netherlands Hotel. United Artists' movie stars stayed there. Maids scurried up the back stairs at midday; paintings and paneling covered the walls. The bathroom fixtures sported heavy polished brass. Way up on the 20th floor above the big city of New York Rodgers had it his way, with room and money to spare. Bill and his brother Charlie laughed like cowboys at the irony of it all.

Emil Zatopek, Czechoslovakia's Olympic gold medal marathon runner in 1952, came to visit Rodgers in his suite. He marveled at the dishwasher in the kitchen, amazed that the hard life of running could bring a man so many soft comforts. Zatopek lived a different life in Czechoslovakia. Bill asked for Zatopek's autograph on one of his trademark running gloves. He knew that the foundation of his own intense training methods could be traced back through Amby Burfoot and Johnny J. Kelley to Zatopek himself—the father-coach-inspiration of them all.

Despite his material success, other aspects of Rodgers's life spun in disarray. He and Ellen split after 6 years. Divorce awaited. He traveled and lived out of a suitcase before settling into an apartment in Stoneham, Massachusetts, with a professional singer named Gail Swain; the two later married and had two children.

Before the 1981 Boston race Rodgers tried to break the Japanese national champion Toshihiko Seko with psychological pressure, but the burden would not bend Seko's mind. Seko had been the shadow on Rodgers's shoulder in 1979. After that race, where Seko drove Rodgers to a new course and personal record, Rodgers marveled at Seko's performance: "He's so young, at only 22. In a few years, I'll probably have to step out of his way or get run over." Since 1979 Seko had won the Fukuoka Marathon for the third time, with a 2:09:45. Seko announced that at Boston he would go for Derek Clayton's 1968 marathon world record of 2:08:34, a time that when it was run had been considered unbelievable.

Seko's psyche stood as sturdy as a sumo wrestler. He did not fall for Rodgers's trick of transferring pressure to the competition by depicting himself as the underdog. With his solid but light 5'6" body, Seko ran 10,000 meters in 27:43.5. But his mode of operation seemed bizarre to Rodgers. One day in Boston Seko's coach, 67-year-old Kiyoshi Nakamura, wanted him to run on a track. Seko and the Japanese federation official who traveled with him did not know where in Boston to find a good track that they could use, but the official knew that Bill Rodgers would know. They drove out from their downtown hotel along the marathon route. When they came to Cleveland Circle, they stopped at the Bill Rodgers Running Center. They parked and the official went inside to ask the whereabouts of a suitable track. Seko stayed in the car; he did not go into Rodgers's store. Rodgers directed the official to a nearby track and as he left Rodgers could see Seko waiting in the car. Rodgers was unnerved by the idea of his competitor waiting in a parked car outside his store. Was Seko shy or hostile? Why not come inside and say hello? Rodgers's experiences in Japan had taught him that politeness and formalities ruled there. Wouldn't it be the polite Japanese thing to do to come into the store for a greeting? It would be all formal and distant, with bowing on both sides. Seko would call him Will-san, they would smile and say the ritual nice things. But Seko stayed in the car.

Rodgers expected Seko to win the Boston Marathon. He predicted it from Seko's second place in 1979, when Rodgers ran 2:09:27 to beat Seko's 2:10:12. Seko's performance since 1979 indicated that he indeed could race faster than anyone in the world. But this year Rodgers, at age 33, did not feel quite as fit and sharp as he had in other years. He had prepared well, but not as thoroughly as in previous years. At least the weather—overcast, windless, cool, 49 °F—promised fast times. It looked like a good day to get run over, but Rodgers would not stand still while Seko did it. Seko had come to Boston with his parents and siblings; they all dressed immaculately. Seko wore a blue blazer and shined shoes. He felt he came to Boston not just as an individual but representing his country. Well groomed, neat, and prepared to the tiniest detail, Seko well represented all Japanese.

Five years earlier Seko had graduated from Kuwana High School near Nagoya. He ran Japan's top high school 800- and 1,500-meter times. His parents urged him to train harder. When he flunked his entrance examination to Waseda University his parents sent him to the University of Southern California. He went there with two other Japanese runners. They did not train very hard and, by Seko's admission, mostly sat around and ate. When Seko came back to Japan he had gained 20 pounds. His friends started calling him by the names of famous sumo wrestlers. He studied hard and on his next attempt passed the Waseda entrance examination. Discipline did not come to Seko naturally or at an early age. The matter and mode of his acquisition of discipline, dedication, and courage to become the best possible marathoner could not have been more different from Bill Rodgers's. It was half a world and 10 centuries different. His passion, *jonetsu*, to do his best at all times was inspired from a combination of Zen Buddhism and the Christian Bible.

Seko's world became his coach, Kiyoshi Nakamura, perhaps a Japanese version of Pete Gavuzzi, who coached Gerard Cote and Walter Young in the 1930s and '40s, or of Bill Rodgers's coach, the affable and approachable Bill Squires. All three men devoted themselves to long-distance running, almost beyond reason. Gavuzzi ran with his runners and talked, Squires talked a lot, but Kiyoshi Nakamura lived with them.

After the war Nakamura had earned millions in several businesses. He had retired in 1965 and could live off his fortune. Now he received a token salary of $150 a year from Waseda University as the track coach. He lived in a small historic house on the campus, where he led a simple life. Nakamura gave himself and his fortune entirely to running. Once a runner himself, he had held the Japanese 1,500-meter record of 3:56.8 for 16 years. Every night 4 or 5 of the 90 runners he coached came to his house for dinner. He spent $15,000 a year on steak, vegetables, and fruit for his athletes. He served as their father, brother, friend, coach, and master. Nakamura loved his runners as if they were his own family. Their attitudes differed toward him in return.

Until the mid-1970s Nakamura had beaten his runners. They nicknamed him Satan because of his brutal practices. He gave up the beatings when he learned that he could get the same results with words. Traditional Japanese samurai wielded lethal weapons such as swords, but an understanding of Zen controlled the weapons. Nakamura, the sensei, the master, taught his athletes to hold the teachings of Zen in their hearts and minds so they could control their every emotion and thought. For 40 years he had studied Zen Buddhism, other forms of Buddhism, Christianity, and other religions. He told Seko that he must study the Bible, Buddhist scriptures, and all famous works. He must study nature: mountains, rivers, stars, the sun and moon. All could teach him. Nakamura saw relaxation as the key to strength. At first Seko rebelled. He ran away, but his father returned him to Nakamura, saying, Do with him whatever you must.

Nakamura wanted to mold the best characteristics of the best runners in the world into Seko. That way Seko, with a part of his competitors in him, could beat them. Nakamura said, "God gave me Seko, and I want to thank God by making Seko the best marathon runner in the world." Seko and his parents thought that a middle-distance runner could not become a marathoner, but they decided to give it a try. In time Nakamura came to control every aspect of Seko's life. Some people claimed that Nakamura transformed Seko into a robot through daily brainwashing. Seko said, "Everything in me, down to the smallest detail, has changed since I met Nakamura-sensei. I am what I am and who I am because of him. I believe everything he says."

At night Seko sat cross-legged on a tatami mat before a knee-high table while Nakamura read aloud from religious works. Nakamura often read a quote from Buddhist monk Daruma-taishi: "Welcome the hardships when they come. Be patient and work through the burdens. Only then can you overcome them and grow stronger." In other words, whatever doesn't kill you makes you stronger. The outgrowth of this philosophy was ultimately not much different from that produced by the quote on Tom Fleming's wall. The art of the marathon was to outrun the other guy because you outtrained him, uncompromising in your preparations.

Will Cloney had compromises of a different sort to manage before the 1981 Boston Marathon. The mayor of the city of Newton, Ted Mann, threatened to close the roads unless the BAA or the state provided additional security to handle the huge crowds that lined the course. The mayor feared that if the crowds squeezed together and pinched off the race at some critical juncture, thousands of runners finding their way blocked would pile in a confused and growing mass into frightened spectators pushed into the course by the pressure of curious crowds behind them. A panicked mob could lead to violence and injury. Cloney asked Governor Edward King for support. King ordered the National Guard to ensure safety along the route. And if that were not enough, the Boston Police Patrolmen's Association, angry about the layoff of 200 officers, threatened to disrupt the marathon at Cleveland Circle. Skillful negotiation averted a demonstration. In this competition without the protection of a stadium, such fears continually haunted race directors.

At the gun a game runner named Gary Fanelli, wearing the Disney cartoon character Goofy on his shorts, immediately sprinted to the front. No morning glory, he had run a 2:14 marathon, but now ran at a pace far faster than that. He planned not to race well himself but to set a pace that would insure a world record by someone else. The weather, the course, and Rodgers's and Seko's presence made plausible Fanelli's presumption to be the sacrificial race-maker. Charlie Rodgers rode on the press truck. Fanelli's move annoyed him.

> I thought that what Gary did was ludicrous and irresponsible. He's out there blowing kisses and waving to everyone on the truck and making a joke of the whole thing. He was out in front by so far that he screwed up the media coverage of the race. If you think you can win, fine, go ahead and race, but don't make a joke out of it. This is Boston.

Fanelli still led at the checkpoint in Wellesley. He no longer blew kisses. He passed in 1:04:50 for 13.75 miles, but Kirk Pfeffer, Craig Virgin, and Dave Chettle, an Australian living in England, moved up on him. However, it was Greg Meyer who caught Fanelli first. Meyer took a 10-yard lead on Rodgers, Seko, Virgin, Chettle, and Pfeffer. The ferocious pace began to extract its toll.

When Rodgers ran down the long incline into Newton Lower Falls, a weird feeling filled his chest, and he had trouble breathing. The pace had been hard and he pushed it like crazy. He had not run under 2:12 since 1979 in New York City. He had been dropped from the top 10 of the world rankings. At 15 miles Rodgers faded to sixth place. Greg Meyer still led. Could this mark the beginning of the end of a career? Could he be just too old for this any more?

On the hills Rodgers began to loosen up. It is a funny thing that sometimes the changes brought by the hills make running easier. The slower cadence, the use of different muscles, a change in the angle of the body, softer footfalls—all could allow a highly trained runner to relax. Rodgers started to feel some strength. He had been thinking he would run a 2:14 and finish between 6th and 10th. But then he caught back up to Seko and Virgin.

In only his third marathon, Greg Meyer looked like he would win at 16 miles. Rodgers admired his courage. But before the race Meyer had said that there were 10 runners in the race who were better than he was. Rodgers, watching Meyer, thought he was going to "bust open the race going for the whole ball of wax." But as much as Rodgers admired the gutsy effort of his teammate and training partner, he knew not to go early. Virgin pulled alongside Rodgers to ask if Meyer was catchable. Rodgers remembered Jim Peters, who when asked by Zatopek in the 1952 Olympic marathon whether the pace was too fast, cavalierly replied "Not fast enough!" and took off. Rodgers, annoyed by Virgin's question, replied noncommittally that yes,

Meyer could be caught. As Rodgers loosened up he caught Meyer and told him to hold back, run steady, and not push. Rodgers knew Seko would stick to Virgin until about 23 miles then go himself. Rodgers wanted to be there when Seko made his move.

But Rodgers could not be there. He thought Seko and Virgin might be running world-record pace. He feared that Virgin would bring down his American record of 2:09:27. Rodgers slipped past Chettle, Meyer, and Pfeffer. Rodgers saw Chettle die and Seko and Virgin duel neck and neck. He didn't see Pfeffer disappear again. Virgin had just set an American record of 28:06 for 10K on the roads. He had run 27:29.16 on the track in Paris just 9 months before, faster than Seko.

From Rodgers's point of view, Craig Virgin, the only American to win the World Cross-Country Championship (twice, most recently 3 weeks before Boston in Madrid), emerged as the likely winner of the 1981 Boston Marathon. Virgin tried psychologically and physically to break Seko, but Seko was not to be bent or broken. Seko had run Boston before; Virgin ran it today for the first time, in only his second major marathon. Could his greater speed make up for his lack of marathon experience?

Virgin grew up in the midwest farming community of Lebanon, Illinois. Runners, writers, and fans described him as the most professional and media-conscious of all the top runners. But as he grew famous he did not grow worldly; he assumed instead the costume and manners of what he thought constituted a successful athlete and businessman. But he misinterpreted those mores and became a caricature of a politician. To postrace gatherings he wore a cream-colored three-piece suit, his hair coiffed into a bouffant. He worked the crowd of runners and friends who dressed in casual clothes, blue jeans, or running clothes. He overcompensated for his typical long-distance runner's introversion with an extreme and awkward extroversion. In his attempts to overcome shyness, Virgin treated fellow competitors like fans, friends like political contributors. He shook too many hands and smiled too much as he gazed over the head of the person before him to find another, apparently more important, hand to shake. His oppressive friendliness did not gain him many friends. Virgin incorporated himself into a business that he called Front Runner, which sold its only product, himself. He raced in a yellow adidas singlet, perhaps to help his fans locate him in lead packs and to celebrate himself after the fashion of the Tour de France, where the previous winner traditionally wore a yellow jersey. He represented adidas running shoes. Despite his distasteful self-promotion, Virgin trained with a maddeningly fastidious, aggressive, intelligent plan. Craig Virgin sprang as much from the values of the American midwest—God-fearing, hardworking, and honest in the face of adversity—as Seko rose from the disciplines of the samurai.

When Seko made his move—he got laughs when he described it in the postrace press conference as "at Bill Rodgers's store in Cleveland Circle" (the same spot where he sat in the car waiting for direction to a track)—Virgin could do nothing. Virgin could not defeat Nakamura's pupil. Seko beat Virgin by an even minute and beat Rodgers's course record by 1 second. At the press conference Seko put on a big grin as he told Bill Rodgers, "I'm sorry that I broke your record." Rodgers countered that Seko must now be regarded as the #1 marathon runner in the world.

Virgin never came back to Boston, but Rodgers, Seko, and Meyer would return. Now that Meyer had tasted the lead, had come through the corridor of cheers while leading the race, had felt the rhythm of the hills, and had blown up in a valiant attempt to hold the lead, he knew what it would take to win the Boston Marathon. A hunger drove him to come back to Boston after that little taste of glory to devour the whole city.

1981 Men's Results

1.	**T. Seko, Japan**	**2:09:26**^{CR}		
2.	C. Virgin, Lebanon, IL	2:10:26		
3.	**B. Rodgers, Boston, MA**	**2:10:34**		
4.	J. Lodwick, Dallas, TX	2:11:33		
5.	M. East, Pittsburgh, PA	2:11:35		
6.	J. Toivola, Finland	2:11:52		
7.	D. Rinde, Orangevale, CA	2:12:01		
8.	D. Chettle, England	2:12:23		
9.	K. Heffner, Boulder, CO	2:12:31		
10.	V. More-Garcia, Colombia	2:12:55		
11.	**G. Meyer, Holliston, MA**	**2:13:07**		
12.	J. Kortelainen, Finland	2:13:14		
13.	N. Wilson, England	2:13:16		
14.	W. Saeger, Dayton, OH	2:13:30		
15.	R. Thomas, Wellesley, MA	2:13:48		
16.	K. Louis, Johnson City, TN	2:13:51		
17.	M. Pinocci, Lake Tahoe, CA	2:14:09		
18.	R. Serna, Anaheim, CA	2:14:16		
19.	D. Patterson, Norristown, PA	2:14:18		
20.	B. Maxwell, Berkeley, CA	2:14:57		
21.	H. Alvarez, Mexico	2:15:05		
22.	R. Holland, McKees Rocks, PA	2:15:07		
23.	**N. Cusack, Ireland**	**2:15:20**		
24.	D. Smith, Rancho Cordova, CA	2:15:29		
25.	R. Parra, Colombia	2:15:50		
26.	D. Sanders, NY	2:15:53		
27.	D. Kurtis, MI	2:15:55		
28.	B. Klecker, MN	2:16:01		
29.	R. Davide, RI	2:16:03		
30.	D. Paul, CA	2:16:04		
31.	J. Johnson, WA	2:16:11		
32.	J. Vitale, CT	2:16:34		
33.	R. Bogaty, PA	2:16:35		
34.	S. Podgajny, PA	2:16:45		
35.	R. Callison, OH	2:16:47		
36.	T. Baker, MD	2:16:49		
37.	J. Zetina, TX	2:16:59		
38.	P. McNeill, NY	2:17:15		
39.	J. Ellis, CA	2:17:23		
40.	G. Mason, CA	2:17:24		
41.	C. Hepburn, MA	2:17:26		
42.	M. Petrocci, Canada	2:17:34		
43.	R. Clifford, MA	2:17:39		
44.	A. Maravilla, Argentina	2:17:43		
45.	H. Barksdale, Jr., DC	2:18:06		
46.	A. Rodiez, WI	2:18:07		
47.	M. Bossardet, NY	2:18:31		
48.	J. Roscoe, IN	2:18:34		
49.	R. Larsson, CA	2:18:38		
50.	M. Matsuo, Japan	2:18:45		
64.	G. Deegan, Ireland	2:19:51		
65.	G. Wallace, MA	2:20:01		
97.	G. Fanelli, Oreland, PA	2:22:25		
191.	T. Derderian, Exeter, NH	2:26:46		
250.	**J. Drayton, Canada**	**2:28:49**		
326.	P. Stewart, Alexandria, VA	2:30:50		
527.	P. Thompson, Providence, RI	2:35:32		
5074.	**J.A. Kelley (age 73)**	**4:01:25**		

Masters

1.	B. Hall, Durham, NC	2:21:19
2.	R. Swan, Bermuda	2:26:37

DOWN UNDER ON TOP

MONDAY, APRIL 20, 1981

Maine's Benoit Versus Patti Catalano

Racers develop a keen, almost animalistic sense of how other runners are doing. Sometimes they don't even have to look. It is a sense akin to a wolf's ability to scout herd animals; the wolf gives feint chase to get the herd running and watches for subtle weakness, for an unsure step or a slow response. Racers develop the same sort of predatory sense in feeling how nearby runners are faring and sensing the time to attack with a surge.

I am breaking format for this particular narrative to step out in front and describe this race in the first person, because I was there. In 1981 I ran near the lead woman all the way. In other Boston Marathons I ran, but never with the leaders; in this race I could observe the lead woman and watched as the lead changed three times. From my precious vantage point I could hear breathing, observe facial expressions, watch cramps being massaged, see who took water, tell who sweated and when and how much. I could watch a single drop of sweat track its way down the leader's neck. I could look for telltale worried glances to the back. I could see the next leader coming. I had the best spot on the playing field, inches away from world-class action.

On a day cool and perfect for running I ran as if I were in the wolf pack. I expected 1979 winner Joan Benoit to come up quickly to dispatch the women's field. I did not expect to be able to keep up with her when she did. I knew she was in better shape than me. So I waited and ran along near Julie Shea, the early leader, knowing it was only a matter of time before my friend Benoit would blow by.

Benoit looked unbeatable in training. I knew because I had I trained with her before this year's marathon when we both worked in the Nike research laboratory in Exeter, New Hampshire. Benoit had a tedious job of inputting biomechanical data, frame by frame, from films of runners in various designs of motion control shoes. She would sit alone in a dark room watching the film, plotting limb lengths and joint centers, then punching the data into the big computer. My job was designing the shoes. After work we went running with most of our co-workers in a situation that seemed like a runner's paradise. I dated Joan's roommate's best friend, Cynthia Hastings, whom I later married—Cynthia had run the Boston Marathon twice already. Everything came together in Exeter: work, friends who were also training partners, and all the Nike shoes we could wear-test. We could run in new experimental models every day.

On a long run with Benoit a few weeks before the marathon I could not keep up. I hitchhiked back. Usually running with her had been trivial for me. In those days I was running a 10K in about 31 minutes, but on this day Benoit was running too fast for me. I knew I could beat all the women in the Boston Marathon, and if Benoit could beat me she was unbeatable by the women's field. In early 1980 Benoit had run the Choysa Marathon in Auckland, New Zealand, in 2:31:23. It was a hot day and still she ran a fast time. On a cool day like this she should really be able to fly. There had been big changes in her life since her Boston victory in 1979. But she still had the demanding problem of making a living. Running was not her job—not yet.

Joan was a substitute teacher at Cape Elizabeth High School in Maine right after graduating from college. It was difficult to see herself as a teacher rather than a student. When she went into the teacher's lounge she felt out of place; she expected a real teacher to come along and order her out. But she didn't know if running alone could support her. Should she develop a nonrunning career or gamble on running? A lot of runners finished college and instead of pursuing a career just ran, winning what they could and eking out a living with odd jobs that allowed time to train. But that choice was a big risk. If the running didn't pay off, the runner was left with just the eking—a sparse resume.

In November of 1980 Benoit moved to Exeter to work in Nike's lab. On the coldest days she could do her workouts on their treadmill. Benoit would do hill sprints—she'd jump on, run uphill for a minute or two, then jump off. There never was a downhill to jar her shins. Sometimes she would take turns on the treadmill with a partner, almost like a track session, one resting while the other ran. She couldn't resist the challenge the treadmill offered. One day she adjusted it to an absurdly high 45° angle and jumped on to run. Like John Henry swinging a hammer, she tried to beat the machine. The angle was so steep that she had to touch only the tips of her toes to the moving belt. The pressure on her toes levered her heels right out of her shoes and she fell face down flat on the belt. The machine shot her off the back and onto the floor. Her friends stood horrified for a second, expecting to see a bloody face. Benoit simply picked herself up, lowered the angle— slightly—and continued her workout. Her training was indeed rigorous and complete that winter. She was superbly fit for Boston. The entire Nike R & D lab could vouch for it.

In my role as voyeur, a peeping Tom of the marathon, I ran and chatted with the Olympic track racer, Mary Decker, who rode on the electric cart leading the women's field as a news announcer. The news centered on the favorite, #2 from the year before, Patti Lyons (also second in 1979), who had since married Joe Catalano. She had set American records for every distance from 5 miles to the marathon. Grete Waitz was the only woman in the world to beat her in her last 33 races. Waitz wasn't in Boston. Patti was picked to win. Joe had his heart set on it.

Joe had been characterized as a bad guy by the press, a Svengali, an opportunist. He tried to shield Patti from the press to conserve her energy, and anyone who for any reason keeps someone from the press is labeled a bad guy. Perhaps he also shielded the press from Patti, who in her own dealings with the media and race directors often played the brat. But Joe Catalano had been running long before he met Lyons and was quite a good and dedicated New England–level club runner.

Patti Catalano took the lead from Shea shortly after the start. She held it for 10 miles. She had perfect running style. Her straight blue-black hair blew straight out behind her. She ran concentrated and relaxed. The roads seemed lined with people giving advice and encouragement. Catalano seemed to have a million fans. At times she acknowledged friends, but mostly she concentrated on her race. She paid strict attention to her pace. She held her emotions in check. In 1979 she had gotten too excited and gone out too fast. This year her pace and relaxation looked perfect. She wore her red-and-white Athletics West uniform and Nike shoes. That pace seemed easy for her, but I expected Benoit to soon come up and make a race of it, eventually leaving Catalano to finish second again.

But it was Julie Shea of North Carolina State University who came up. This was Shea's first serious marathon. She had run one in Bermuda in 1979 with a time in the 2:50s. She was the current women's collegiate champion at 3K, 5K, 10K, and cross-country. She had a gangly, spread-out running style. I once wrote that she ran splay-legged, like a colt saddled too soon. She had grown into a woman who wore tan leather cowboy hats and fresh leather boots with pointed toes and curlicued stitching. One time on a run she told me that she took umbrage at that image of a colt. She said I should never have written it. She thought of herself as smooth, fit, and fast, as indeed she was. She led Catalano until the hills. There in a burst of emotion and opportunity, Catalano took over again.

Catalano sprinted up the hills. Shea chose to maintain her pace and not respond to Catalano's sudden and erratic tactic.

Catalano crested the hills looking every bit as good as she had an hour earlier. I thought Benoit had better hurry up. There wasn't much race left, and it was all downhill from here. It looked as if it would be a speedster's race from the hills to the finish. I knew that Shea and Benoit had better track times than Catalano. I figured Joan was saving herself for a track-style kick. It was a risky strategy, but it proved effective. The crowds had gotten frighteningly thick; their screams were deafening. A high-energy roar followed us along. I could see what Bill Rodgers meant when he talked about getting energy from the crowd's enthusiasm. Suddenly as Catalano began the descent past Rodgers's store and into Cleveland Circle, I heard a second roar of the crowd behind us and coming closer. Just as I expected—here comes Joan, or maybe Julie. But I turned to see a tall, blond woman runner, wearing black, approaching us, a woman a head taller than Joan. It was not Julie. Where was Joan?

The blond was Allison Roe, a woman I hadn't met, but whom I had heard of. She was from near Auckland, New Zealand. She was born Allison Deed and had married Richard Roe, a chiropractor, a year earlier. As a teenager she had run in the 1975 World Cross-Country Championships in Morocco, where Bill Rodgers had first come to worldwide attention. She had finished second to Benoit in the 1980 Choysa Marathon in Auckland but with a slow 2:51. The following September she ran in the Nike/Oregon Track Club Marathon with a 2:34:29. The next time around at Choysa she ran 2:36:16. She had been running 10Ks regularly in under 33 minutes. She stood 5'8" at 129 pounds. Roe's interests and talents were eclectic. She had been a good high jumper, tennis player, swimmer, and water skier. She descended full of advantage from a wealthy family. She worked as a secretary for an architectural firm and was coached by Gordon Pirie, himself one of the pioneering world milers in the 1950s. It should have been no surprise that Roe was running so well. She had a plan. Everything she did she did well. She was intelligent, astute, and beautiful. A reporter on the scene called her the Renaissance woman of running.

Roe's plan had been to follow Catalano and Benoit because she felt confident that they would run a reasonable pace to produce a 2:28. She knew that Joe Catalano would run with Patti for 16 miles. She first followed Benoit, staying about 10 meters behind, then after Benoit slowed she settled in behind Catalano by the same sort of margin, using Patti and Joe as "rabbits." On Roe's way down the hills, she watched Catalano and realized that she could "have her" right there because Roe had been watching her for a mile from 10 seconds back.

On the downhill along the trolley tracks past Rodgers's store into Cleveland Circle, Roe approached Catalano, several male runners, and an electric car carrying Mary Decker. The crowds pressed so close that there was room enough for only two runners abreast. A police officer on a big horse tried to control the crowds, but their sudden shouting upon seeing the first woman sent the horse side-stepping into her path. Catalano ran smack into the horse's buttocks. Its hooves banged and slipped on the steel trolley tracks. Catalano bounced off the horse into me. The horse did not fall and Catalano did not fall. Instinctively I supported her for the split second it took her to regain her balance. In the strictest sense I influenced the outcome of the race. Had I not been there, Catalano would have fallen, perhaps been injured, perhaps not, and Allison Roe might have taken the lead.

That crisis and the downhill passed. Catalano knew someone was coming. For the first time she showed fatigue. I could sense the hesitation in her stride. Her arm carriage shifted. At the 23rd mile Roe pulled even. She did not look directly at Catalano. Catalano did not look directly at Allison Roe.

Neither spoke to the other. I watched both carefully. The skin on Catalano's face tightened over her high cheekbones. She looked gaunt, hollow. She seemed to be digging down as deep as she could go. Like the crew of a steamship out of coal she threw her own decking into the furnace. She wanted to win this race.

Roe's face, by contrast looked peaceful, in control. She looked like an actress coming onstage to take the leading role. Other than sharing commandingly beautiful running form, the two could not have looked more different—blue-black hair versus blond, brown eyes versus blue, a dark face with chiseled features versus a pale baby face. As Roe tossed in the gentlest of surges I looked at Catalano and saw her face frozen like a department store mannequin. Again she would be a loser after coming so close so often. She could not respond to Roe's challenge. Roe took a downward, backward glance at Catalano, then looked forward and smiled. The smile came involuntarily. No one but me could see that Mona Lisa smile sneak across her face as contact broke.

Roe ran on to win, breaking the women's course record by 7:42. It is safe to assume that will never happen again. She finished full of energy and talk. The Boston press triumphed at her victory.

Catalano never gave up. She strained to the very last step. I had expected Benoit to come along, but she never showed up. Benoit finished third. Head

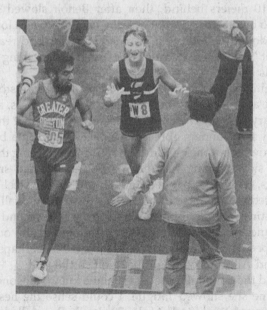

Allison Roe and author Tom Derderian at the finish in 1981. Photo courtesy of the *Boston Herald*.

case, I thought. She was physically fit enough on that day to have run 2:23-2:24, but she didn't do it. She had psyched herself out, or perhaps she had run too hard in completing a 20-mile run a week earlier. Perhaps her confidence had disappeared. Fear and worry weighed her down. She couldn't handle the pressure of her own expectations. That's it, I thought. The courage is gone. Fear has won. She won't improve anymore. She won't dare to run really fast. But that's not the sort of thing you can tell a friend. Happily subsequent events proved me wrong. Yet in 1981 I didn't believe she would win a major race again. Benoit said,

> I really can't explain my disappointing finish at Boston. I had high hopes of winning for a second time, but they were quickly dampened when I found myself as far back as eleventh in the first half of the race. . . . I didn't expect so many other runners to show me their backsides in the early stages. . . . My biggest asset, my fluid stride, abandoned me that day.

When that sort of weakness without cause strikes an athlete, that paralyzing fear of failure, that despair, there is nothing a friend, a coach, or a training partner can say or do to bring back the confidence. Most athletes never recover from such psychological burnout; they just disappear. Benoit felt depressed because she could not figure out what was wrong. A relative unknown had beaten her, and Patti Catalano, whom she had beaten before, defeated her as well on this ideal day for fast times.

The 1979 winner, Joan Benoit, finished third in 2:30:16, a personal record. Under ideal conditions she had not improved as much as everyone else had. Perhaps this was a time for her to regroup, maybe even give up. Jacqueline Gareau finished fifth. She was the only woman in the top 11 who did not register a personal record.

When Catalano finished she searched the finish area for Joe. He had planned to get a ride from the 16-mile mark. She didn't know what to feel. Had she done something wrong to finish second for the third time? She had tried hard. She had run a personal record, an American record, and she was tired. She had wanted to win, to win for Joe. She wanted to make him love her. She wanted a hug. She had given up everything—she had lost so much weight since she became a marathoner. She had eaten so little, had forced the food out of herself that she swallowed during the weak moments that led to eating binges. A dozen donuts could go in and out quickly. She would run for hours while Joe and his friends watched television sports. Now, though she was sweaty and cold, she wanted a hug. When she found Joe he had his arms crossed over his chest. He did not uncross them. Crowds of people watched. He said, "I don't know what to do with you, Patti. You ran an American record. I just don't know what to do. Please stop crying." Through the crowd Patti found her sisters. They all cried together.

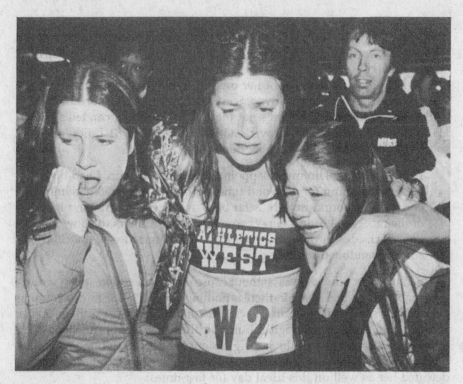

Crying Patti Catalano and her sobbing sisters after the 1981 marathon. Joe Catalano, Patti's husband, looks on. UPI/Bettmann.

1981 Women's Results

1.	A. Roe, New Zealand	2:26:46^{CR}	
	(192nd overall)		
2.	P. Catalano, MA	2:27:51^{AR}	
3.	J. Benoit, Exeter, NH	2:30:16	
4.	J. Shea, Raleigh, NC	2:30:54	
5.	J. Gareau, Canada	2:31:26	
6.	S. Grottenberg, Norway	2:33:02	
7.	N. Conz, Easthampton, MA	2:34:48	
8.	L. Dewald, Arlington, VA	2:35:57	
9.	K. Sweigart, Darien, CT	2:36:55	
10.	L. Dierdorff, San Diego, CA	2:38:03	
11.	J. Wipf, UT	2:38:27	
12.	L. Binder, San Diego, CA	2:39:35	
13.	N. Sasaki, Japan	2:41:47	
14.	J. Horns, MN	2:41:49	

15.	R. Longstaff, Australia	2:43:03
16.	C. Cook, St. Louis, MO	2:43:08
17.	S. Silsby, FL	2:44:59
18.	K. Consolo, OH	2:45:08
19.	M. Hulak, NY	2:45:57
20.	J. Isphording, OH	2:46:40
21.	J. Kerr, NY	2:47:07
22.	J. Welzel, NH	2:48:26
23.	F. Madeira, MA	2:48:56
24.	S. Given, NY	2:49:15
25.	S. Kainulainen, Canada	2:49:25
29.	J. Taylor-Tuthill, MT	2:50:51
30.	A. Chiappetta, NY	2:51:07
35.	D. Israel, NY	2:52:45
82.	K. Cossaboon-Holm, NY	3:04:45

Masters

1.	S. Stricklin, CA	2:56:46

THE ROOKIE AND THE FARM BOY

MONDAY, APRIL 19, 1982

NYC Winner, Salazar, to Run Boston

Seko did not come back to Boston in 1982. Rodgers looked like the most experienced runner of the favorites. But at age 34 Rodgers heard time's winged chariot hurrying near. In fact, the chariot had arrived, and on it rode two marathoners in their early 20s, Dickie Beardsley and Alberto Salazar. Two young men could not be more different in their origins and outlooks, yet they were powerfully influenced by the same man who influenced Rodgers. They developed athletic abilities that in the end only the tiniest difference would separate. On this day they would fight like gladiators.

Alberto Salazar, born in Cuba, grew up in Wayland, Massachusetts, not far from the start of the Boston Marathon. After college at the University of Oregon he stayed on to live in Eugene. Alberto and his family had fled from Castro's revolution. Batista was bad, but Castro turned out to be worse for the Salazars, so after initially supporting Castro, José Salazar brought his family to the United States. José was a man who would go back to his native Cuba at the drop of a beret to drag Fidel Castro kicking and screaming into the sea. But rather than launch a solo Bay of Pigs invasion, José Salazar worked as a civil engineer on high-rise buildings and fathered a large family: Christine, Ricardo, Alberto, and Fernando.

Ricardo had the running talent of the family. In high school he ran a mile in 4:24 before going on to the naval academy and then on to fly in navy fighter planes. In his early teens Alberto tried to play basketball, but he was not good at it. Like most adolescents he wanted to be good at something. Ricardo wanted Alberto to be good at running. In their neighborhood another kid had the record for running about a half mile around the block. Ricardo of course broke it. A classic powerful, smooth stride carried his lean muscular body. Ricardo boasted to the kid that even his little brother could break the record. He talked Alberto into trying. Ricardo started his watch and cut across the block to cheer for Alberto. Alberto passed, looking gawky, awkward, and tired. He would never have Ricardo's silky smooth, ground-eating stride. Ricardo dashed back to the finish. He waited. After far too long Alberto showed up walking, looking at the ground. Time and again Ricardo tried to coach Alberto into breaking the other kid's record, but Alberto always wound up walking and looking at the ground. Ricardo concluded that his little brother had a low pain threshold and would never be any good at long-distance running. Fortunately Ricardo never told that to Alberto.

Bill Rodgers knew Salazar well. Back in 1973–74 Alberto had at last followed his brother's footsteps to run for Wayland High School. He joined the North Medford Club, old Fred Brown's club and the nemesis of Jock Semple's BAA. Salazar eagerly signed up to go to any race he could. When Jack McDonald formed the Greater Boston Track Club, including runners like Rodgers, Randy Thomas, Bob Hodge, Vinnie Fleming, and Dick Mahoney, Salazar eagerly joined. Bill Squires coached the club and Salazar tagged along. McDonald founded the club for college-graduate runners, not bag-of-bones 15-year-olds. Squires and his teammates called Salazar The Rookie. He just kept hanging around.

The club met on Sundays for long runs through the quiet country around Sherborn. Tommy Leonard, the bartender at the Eliot Lounge who would become the official "greeter" of the Boston Marathon, would be there running, not in a pair of tights or sweatpants but baggy slacks. The rookie thought Leonard had rather strange habits. But Salazar's new habit of long runs on Sunday mornings seemed strange to his mother, who would rather he be in church. On one of these runs, Salazar remembers, Bill Rodgers saved his life, but Rodgers has no memory of the incident.

Alberto, the skinny, gangly rookie, hung on to the back of the pack as they proceeded along a country road bordered by a ditch. Daydreaming, he did not see the Great Dane bound up. Suddenly the big silent dog attacked Salazar and knocked him to his knees and into the ditch. The dog had followed a million years of hunting instincts to cut the youngest, weakest member out of the herd. The rest of the runners continued down the road, oblivious to the rookie's fate. The dog commanded the situation. His bared fangs gleamed level with Salazar's face. If he tried to move the dog snarled. Salazar froze in place. At the instant he resigned that he would be eaten, the dog suddenly let out a yelp and ran away. Above him and grinning stood Bill Rodgers, the savior. It seems he often carried his car keys with him when he ran; otherwise in his absentmindedness he would lose them. When he saw what had happened to Alberto, he doubled back. He whipped his keys like a Ninja warrior spinning into the dog's rump. In that way, Salazar says, Bill Rodgers saved his life, or at least his good looks, or the nose on his face.

When Rodgers had finished third in the World Cross-Country Championships in March of 1975, he impressed the Salazars. Alberto went with Ricardo and his father to watch the marathon as Rodgers won. That day sealed it; Alberto would become a marathoner, and he would run the Boston Marathon.

When Alberto left Boston to go to college in 1976, Squires stopped coaching him. Squires had a marathon plan for Salazar, but that plan paradoxically required that he limit his training mileage. Squires said Salazar must not run more than 60 or 70 miles a week. After a trip to the National Junior

Cross-Country Championships Alberto got ideas from the two runners who beat him. He did not tell Squires, but he started running 100 miles a week. Soon he felt flat and stale. Finally he confessed to Squires, whose anger flared. Squires knew that Salazar's running style, or lack of it, predisposed him to overuse injuries.

Squires had a talk with Alberto's new coach at the University of Oregon, Bill Dellinger. In 1955 Dellinger had won the NCAA mile championship by beating Squires. Squires told Dellinger not to try to change Alberto's admittedly ugly running style. He is just built that way; he doesn't do it on purpose. Keep Salazar's mileage low for the first 2 years; after that, do whatever you want. Squires predicted that Alberto would be a good 5K man and a great 10K man in college but that his best event would someday be the marathon.

In a flicker Salazar moved from high school rookie to college runner and, while still in college, an international contender.

On March 21, 1982, Salazar finished second to Mohamed Kedir of Ethiopia in the World Cross-Country Championships in Rome—one place better than Rodgers had done in 1975. On April 10, on a rainy day in Eugene, Oregon, he ran the fifth fastest 10,000 meters in the world, 27:30.0. Virgin had run less than a second faster, and the world record was only 8 seconds faster. Salazar already had the world marathon record of 2:08:13 set in New York City the previous fall. He had run the fastest-ever first marathon with his win in New York City in 1980 with a 2:09:41. He wanted to be the best runner in the world. He had nearly realized it. He promised himself he would do whatever it took to win.

Since the best long-distance runners in the world lived in Kenya, Salazar went there to live and train. He stayed only weeks in what proved for him an alien environment, but his commitment was clear. Another time he adopted a mode of training with a breathing device that reduced the amount of oxygen he could breathe, thus simulating altitude training. The device looked like a lightweight Aqua-lung, complete with corrugated tubes and a mouthpiece. He could not speak. When he trained in that thing through suburban American streets he looked and sounded like a visitor from another planet.

In contrast, Dickie Beardsley grew up in the midwest American farming town of Wayzata, Minnesota, blending into its population of 4,000. As a boy Beardsley often walked his dog through a nearby swamp. As the going got deeper and muckier he liked it more and more. He spent his free time trapping and hunting. He liked the excuse it gave him to wander alone over the countryside. Yet his ambition for running came slowly. He ran in high school and college but did nothing notable. After college he stopped serious racing to take a job on a dairy farm. A chance invitation for a run set him dreaming of the 1980 Olympic marathon trials, but his subsequent success at running surprised him. The Olympic boycott postponed his ambitions, so he looked forward to the 1984 Olympic Games and the 1982 Boston

Marathon. He entered the top ranks of the sport of marathon racing in its last days of amateurism.

Nothing remarkable had happened in Beardsley's life until he ran a 2:09:37 in Grandma's Marathon in Duluth, Minnesota, in June of 1981. People did not take his Grandma's time seriously. Most runners continue to regard reported fast marathon times with skepticism, to ask upon hearing of a good time on an obscure course, "How short was it?" So Beardsley still had something to prove before he pursued his real-life ambition to be a dairy farmer. In the spring of 1982 he went to Georgia to train in the heat with Dean Matthews.

Bill Squires said that Beardsley ran with fluid motion in his free-floating, relaxed stride and that to watch him was like watching a natural dancer take the floor with God-given talent. Squires thought God had made Dick Beardsley for long-distance running. Salazar and Beardsley represented the vanguard of post–Rodgers era runners, but a lot else had changed with the race.

In the 1950s it had cost Will Cloney, Jock Semple, and Tony Nota about $3,000 to put on the marathon. But times had changed. By 1982 it cost a reported $150,000. But the biggest change had not yet arrived. A scandal broke in February 1982 that Will Cloney had sold the marathon to an agent named Marshall Medoff. The resolution of that scandal would take 2 years. (We will revisit it in detail in 1985.)

Ron Tabb led through the first 3 miles of the 1982 Boston Marathon; then Beardsley's training buddy, Dean Matthews of Atlanta led the pack through the Framingham checkpoint in 32:35. (The two trained together under the tutelage of Bill Squires.) The sun warmed the day and energized the spectators into a vernal frenzy, but that same pleasant sunshine burdened the runners with the threat of dehydration. On a cool day in 1970 Jerome Drayton had run through that same checkpoint in 31:26. It did not look like a record day. Salazar, Beardsley, and Rodgers ran patiently in a big pack. Salazar thought that Tabb and Matthews were constantly pushing the pace with lots of stupid surges, acting like a couple of jerks to accomplish nothing but destroying their own rhythm. Salazar sat back laughing at the two fools. Burn baby, burn yourself up.

At 10 miles Beardsley, feeling a little restless, threw in a 200-yard surge. As Matthews responded Beardsley said, "Hey, Deano, I'm just doing a fake. Don't get too excited." Matthews had foot problems that would eventually force him out of the race, but he and Rodgers led the pack through Natick, though well off Ron Hill's 1970 checkpoint record. Doug Kurtis and Matthews flanked him, with Salazar and Beardsley tucked into the air pocket behind them. Bobby Hodge followed alone, smeared with his sweat in a procession of sticky, tired men. The few spectators between Natick and Wellesley seemed quiet, perhaps out of respect for how difficult this race would be. It did not look like a day for fast running.

But something happened between Natick and Wellesley. Suddenly the pace had picked up enough to burst through the half marathon in 1:04:04. The crowds in Wellesley showed their respect by erecting a wall of noise. Rodgers, aging or not, still led with Ed Mendoza, who had arrived in the lead pack, joining Matthews, Salazar, and Beardsley. Salazar wore a white Nike Athletics West singlet; Beardsley wore a dark New Balance singlet and a painter's cap with the visor flipped up. Their average pace had been 4:53 per mile. No one could be quite sure who it was who pushed the pace. They all looked intense and grim, but each harbored eagerness to cut loose and make a run for it. Salazar planned to make his move at 20. But something Bill Rodgers had said ate at him. Rodgers had told him that someday the marathon would humble him. As Salazar could feel a knot growing in his hamstring he wondered if this would be the day. Could he hang on that long? Matthews's day neared an end as he dropped back because of the foot problem that would force him to drop out.

The hills waited ahead—four of them. The first, a sunny climb over Route 128, the second, Brae Burn, named for the country club that sits halfway up it. A nameless quarter-mile hill hides the one *Globe* writer Jerry Nason had long ago labeled Heartbreak. But the hill does not do the breaking, it merely offers the stage where winners break losers. This pack of four approached those hills. Not all would survive.

When Beardsley hit the turn by the fire station to begin the Brae Burn Hill he took the initiative. Salazar squinted and held on. Salazar's macho

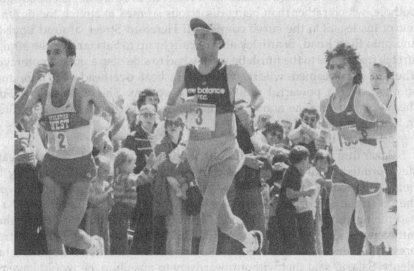

Alberto Salazar (#2) takes a rare drink while Dickie Beardsley (#3) cruises alongside with Ed Mendoza running just ahead of Bill Rodgers in the middle of the 1982 Boston Marathon. Photo by Bill Boyle.

prerace assertions that he considered no one in the field to be a threat annoyed Beardsley. Beardsley thought that as long as somebody is human, he's beatable. Beardsley resolved that nobody was going to win this race having a bad day. Rodgers broke first. Then Mendoza's grip slipped, first a little, then a lot as he fell permanently behind. Spectators with amplifiers trumpeted the theme from the movie "Chariots of Fire," which seemed to follow the race from start to finish. The glorious music mixed with the cheers made Mendoza's slipping and Rodgers's breaking seem surreal.

Salazar and Beardsley fought each other like boxers. Salazar had decided with his current coach, Bill Dellinger of the University of Oregon, that he would never lose a marathon during his entire career. The fight took the style of, Hit me, then I'll hit you. By the top of the fourth hill neither man had fallen. On the contrary, the pace had picked up. By Lake Street they ran only 27 seconds behind Rodgers's course record.

Beardsley ran in the lead. The sun cast Salazar's shadow ahead of him. Every time the shadow moved up, Beardsley pulled away. He wanted to run his own race, not Salazar's. But Salazar decided to change his tactic, to not run from the front but just hang on to Beardsley and outsprint him at the end. He didn't like to use that strategy, but he had no choice. Beardsley was much tougher than he had imagined. Salazar told himself that there was no way he would allow himself to lose this race. Together they ran very fast, yet even in this deadly serious duel they passed a water bottle back and forth. Beardsley drank more than Salazar. Salazar only sipped because he worried about cramps.

Near the Eliot Lounge Salazar took the lead as Beardsley stepped into a pothole, which rather than being disastrous seemed to stretch the tightness out of his legs. On the curve coming off Hereford Street, around Boylston and onto Ring Road, Beardsley almost caught up to Salazar. On the straight stretch from there to the finish Beardsley had to side-step a police motorcycle. The crowd screamed wildly. Helicopters beat overhead. An announcer shouted over a powerful public address system. The "Chariots of Fire" theme played on: The announcer proclaimed this the most exciting finish in marathon history.

And it was the most painful.

Salazar dug into his pain threshold, found a toehold, and sprinted. Beardsley sprinted. Both broke Seko's course record by a giant margin. By the finish Alberto Salazar had six steps on Dick Beardsley. Twenty yards beyond the finish they embraced. Beardsley said, "You ran a hell of a race." "You had me hurting," Salazar answered. Hurting so much that he needed three intravenous feedings to replace body fluids; he appeared at the postrace press conference with bandages on his arms. The marathon had hurt; it hurt plenty. Salazar said that without Beardsley to push him, he would have run only 2:10. This was the same little brother that elder Ricardo concluded had a low tolerance for pain.

Neither Salazar nor Beardsley ever came back to race Boston. Salazar made the 1984 Olympic team but placed 16th in Los Angeles. Beardsley did not run the Olympics. Injuries plagued them both. They tried to come back to world-class marathoning, but injuries ended their careers early. Both men pointed to this 1982 Boston race as the beginning of their physical demise. Neither ran well again. Salazar opened a restaurant and a tanning salon in Eugene, Oregon, and later went to work for Nike. Beardsley started a dairy farm in Minnesota that he named "Marathon Dairy Farm." In 1989 Beardsley suffered a mangling accident when caught in a piece of farm machinery. He recovered from that, but a few years later a car hit him during a training run. He was still recovering in 1993.

Checkpoint Splits

5K	Ron Tabb	14:44
5 miles	Doug Kurtis	23:55
15K	Dean Matthews	45:08
10 miles	Alberto Salazar	48:50
20K	Dean Matthews	1:00:28
20 miles	Dick Beardsley	1:38:14

1982 Men's Results

1.	A. Salazar, Eugene, OR	2:08:52^{CR*}	24.	R. DiSebastian, PA	2:20:02
2.	D. Beardsley, MN	2:08:54	25.	R. Hintz, WI	2:20:04
3.	J. Lodwick, TX	2:12:01	26.	J. Westlund, Sweden	2:20:16
4.	B. Rodgers, MA	2:12:38	27.	M. Green, MD	2:20:19
5.	K. Stahl, Sweden	2:12:46	28.	E. Hulst, CA	2:20:22
6.	D. Rinde, CA	2:15:04	29.	B. Gavaghan, IN	2:20:32
7.	T. Baker, MD	2:16:32	30.	C. Holm, NY	2:20:35
8.	R. Callison, OH	2:16:35	31.	K. Lauenstein, VT	2:20:51
9.	R. Wallace, NE	2:17:18	32.	M. Bossardet, NY	2:20:58
10.	B. Morturi, TX	2:17:30	33.	S. Podgajny, ME	2:21:10
11.	E. Sheehan, AL	2:17:43	34.	T. Nickevich, OR	2:21:15
12.	T. Antczak, WI	2:17:48	35.	S. Molnar, PA	2:21:24
13.	L. Kenny, TN	2:17:50	36.	C. Hewes, VT	2:21:25
14.	H. Spiik, Finland	2:17:53	37.	S. Jenkins, NE	2:21:37
15.	G. Mason, CA	2:17:55	38.	M. Petrocci, Canada	2:21:46
16.	B. Maxwell, CA	2:17:58	39.	H. Barksdale, Jr., DC	2:21:50
17.	J. Stuckey, NJ	2:18:08	40.	K. Jezierski, MI	2:21:54
18.	I. Ray, England	2:18:11	41.	J. Miller, VT	2:21:54
19.	B. Fisher, FL	2:18:19	42.	L. Frederick, NY	2:21:56
20.	R. Davide, RI	2:19:18	43.	J. Wellerding, IA	2:22:06
21.	B. Coates, PA	2:19:48	44.	M. Whelan, NY	2:22:17
22.	T. Howard, Canada	2:19:57	45.	J. Roscoe, IN	2:22:20
23.	J. Zetina, TX	2:20:00	46.	Y. Karni, Israel	2:22:26

47.	L. Parker, LA	2:22:26	109.	D. Kurtis, MI	2:27:13
48.	P. McNeill, NY	2:22:36	111.	J. Vitale, CT	2:27:29
49.	D. Byrnes, Australia	2:22:39	156.	L. Supino, CO	2:29:59
50.	B. Boyd, CA	2:22:42	1621.	J.J. Kelley, CT	2:55:50
61.	R. Treacy, RI	2:24:03	2027.	T. Congdon, NH	3:00:00
63.	P. Dones, Puerto Rico	2:24:17	4560.	T. Hersey	3:34:59
71.	Y. Wantanabe, Japan	2:24:53		J.A. Kelley	4:01:30

6,689 starters, average time 3:04:06.

*Permanent record for the course (1965-1985) with race finish in front of the Prudential Building.

Masters

1.	B. Hall, NC	2:24:20
2.	R. Jenkins, VA	2:25:14
3.	R. Zimmerman, NY	2:25:41

THE INCIDENTAL VICTORY

MONDAY, APRIL 19, 1982

Norwegian Woman Eyes Marathon Record

Everyone hailed the three-time winner of the New York City Marathon, Grete Waitz, as the outstanding favorite to take the 1982 Boston Marathon. She wanted to win; not only that, she wanted to set a new world record. She already had the second fastest marathon time in the world. She had run a half marathon in a world-record time of 1:09:19 in Stramilano, Italy. She figured a world-record marathon came next. By the 17-mile mark of the Boston race she had a 2:23 marathon going. Second place, Charlotte Teske, a 32-year-old pediatric nurse from West Germany, ran far behind, as if she were in her own race. No one doubted that Waitz would win; the question was by how much. It looked like she would run 3 minutes under Allison Roe's new world record of 2:25:28 from New York City. Waitz ran surrounded by male runners. Teske had no hope of catching her. She didn't even think about it. Teske was not a heat runner, but otherwise she felt particularly good in the hills. But she had won the Miami Marathon in 2:29:01 in January. She felt easy. She ran alone, hugging the side of the road, minutes behind. But she did not know how painful it would get for Waitz.

Heartbreak Hill felt good to Waitz. She liked hills and ran them well. She had won the World Cross-Country titles in Limerick, Glasgow, Paris, and Madrid. It looked like nothing could go wrong. She expected the running would be easier on the downhill into Boston. But pain in her quadriceps muscles, which had begun in Wellesley on the long downhill into Newton Lower Falls, became unbearable. She wanted to stretch those constricting muscles, but to do that she would have to stop. They hurt so much that she did stop, while still leading at 23 miles. She stepped off the course. Spectators rushed to her side. No, she would not continue. No woman had passed her. She could run no more. Waitz had plenty of cushion, but she could not even jog to the finish line. It was not another runner who beat her, but the course itself. Someone called an ambulance, and it wisked Waitz off to the hospital. From there she took a taxi to her hotel.

Teske never got the word that she was the first woman. It is hard to believe that no one in the crowd shouted "First woman," but with a limited command of English, perhaps Teske did not understand the announcement. She ran the last half mile to wild cheering, and the last 100 meters with the roar of the crowd—a crowd roaring for first place, but she thought she was finishing second. She could not savor the moment as it occurred. Charlotte Teske won, but she hadn't seen Waitz drop out and didn't know she was first. Just past the finish a policeman told her that, incidentally, she had won. She really had had no idea. Suddenly elation filled her, but she said she felt "very sorry" for Waitz and that "I didn't really beat her."

1982 Women's Results

1. **C. Teske, West Germany**	**2:29:33**	
	(148th overall)	
2. **J. Gareau, Canada**	**2:36:09**	
3. E. Claugus, CA	2:38:48	
4. K. Sweigart, CT	2:39:49	
5. S. Durtschi, OR	2:40:47	
6. K. Molitor, TX	2:41:12	
7. J. Isphording, OH	2:43:31	
8. Z. Shmoeli, Israel	2:44:00	
9. S. Finken, NJ	2:44:09	
10. N. Mieszczak, NY	2:44:17	
11. H. Fena, Austria	2:44:45	
12. S. Quinn, NY	2:45:06	
13. C. Lorenzoni, VA	2:46:02	
14. A. Ray, KS	2:46:40	
15. L. Edgar, WA	2:47:23	
16. M. Hulak, NY	2:47:24	
17. K. Burns, AR	2:47:26	
18. K. Cossaboon-Holm, NY	2:47:58	
19. K. Consolo, OH	2:48:14	
20. K. Cosgrove, OH	2:48:49	
21. J. Turney, Australia	2:49:12	
22. S. Lupica, Boston, MA	2:49:37	
23. S. Barbano, Boston, MA	2:50:20	
24. M. Harmeling, NY	2:50:34	
25. B. Dillinger, VA	2:50:40	
28. M. Schwam, MA	2:53:08	
31. E. Rochefort, Canada	2:54:04	
36. F. Madeira, MA	2:55:58	
63. A. Igoe-Maguire, CA	3:01:54	
112. J. Emmons, GA	3:08:17	
115. J. Ullyot, CA	3:08:43	
136. K. McIntyre, NY	3:11:56	
201. **N. Kuscsik, NY**	**3:26:38**	
484. R. Waters, CA	3:34:58	

750 starters, average time 3:17:27.

Masters

1. P. Thomas, WA	2:58:55
2. H. Bedrock, NJ	3:02:41
3. A. Bing, NJ	3:07:01

Don't Let the Wise Guy Lead

MONDAY, APRIL 18, 1983

Michigan Marathon Man Favored

Greg Meyer had done some fancy work before his marathon at Boston in 1983. He'd run a 46:13 ten-miler at Cherry Blossom in Washington and a 27:54 solo 10K at the Colonial Relays practicing Coach Bill Squires's surge technique. At Boston he ran with a pack including Bill Rodgers, Jeff Wells, John Lodwick, Duncan McDonald, Tom Fleming, Jon Anderson (10 years after his victory), Ron Tabb, and Benji Durden. Meyer knew he would win, his coach knew he would win, and the rest of the pack knew he would win. He had run a sub-4:00 mile and had done all the necessary work. He had moved to Boston from his native Michigan to train with Bill Rodgers and the astoundingly strong Greater Boston Track Club. They passed 10 miles in 49:11. A jovial pack surrounded a foregone conclusion. Everyone just knew that Meyer would win. Abraha Gebrehiwet Aregha, an Ethiopian living in Decatur, Georgia, led. Durden, the leading jokester of the pack, pointed ahead to Aregha, "See, he's wearing headphones—a Sony Walkman."

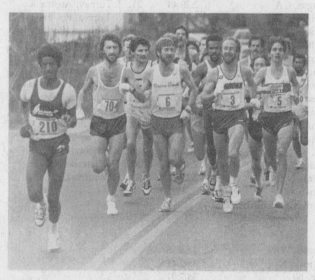

Benji Durden (#6) jokes with Greg Meyer (#3) about what Abraha Aregha (#210) might be listening to. Tom Fleming is #704. Dan Schlesinger is #5. Photo by Jeff Johnson.

"I bet he's getting $5,000 to be seen in the lead wearing it on TV," Rodgers retorted.

Another guy asked, "What do you think he is listening to?"

"Mozart, to run that fast."

"Naw, disco."

"Betcha he can't hear us coming."

Aregha would ultimately finish 110th, provoking the quip that the guy with the Walkman had only a 45-minute cassette in his machine. Even before the race, something had angered Durden: The Boston papers did not pick him for the top 10. He'd show them. But now in the early miles he did not want to be too serious. He wanted to keep it light. The pace was fast, but everybody stuck to it. An aid station offered a large piece of cardboard smeared with Vaseline. The runners speculated about what they were expected to do with the goop.

At each water stop Durden felt the pack slow. He just kept going and built up a lead through Wellesley. He floated ahead. He waved to the camera truck. Meyer usually beat him in the shorter distances, but Durden had been telling him to wait until the marathon, that things would be different. For that reason Meyer especially wanted to nail Benji. Durden projected a self-assured presence, a cockiness to some; he was outspoken—a wise guy. Some runners compared him to Zonker Harris in the "Doonesbury" comic strip. He often said things other people did not understand. He read a lot of science fiction.

Checkpoint times showed they still ran fast. Downhill into Newton Lower Falls Durden ran a 4:18 mile to build a frightening lead. Meyer had to go after Durden; he could not let the wise guy get too big a lead. Meyer knew not to be so cool so late in the race. Meyer concentrated on Durden's back. He willed Durden toward him. When Meyer caught Durden midway up Heartbreak Hill, Durden turned, put his palm up, and said, "Greg, did you feel the rain? I think it's raining. Did you feel it?"

No answer.

"At least we are going to have a fast time."

"Yeah," Meyer replied.

He dumped Durden with a well-practiced Squires pseudosurge and passed 20 miles in a world-record pace of 1:37:11. On a day that couldn't be more perfect for running, he still had a 4:40-mile *real* surge left in him. He ran 4:49 from mile 21 to 22 and 5:09 from 22 to 23. No one pursued. He tried to look back to see for sure, but the press bus blocked his view. People yelled that he had a chance for the course record, but he had relaxed. He enjoyed winning. Meyer said later, "I tried to maintain and savor the lead."

Ron Tabb often started fast and then faded. Some people thought that since DNF followed his name so frequently in race results, perhaps it was the name of his track club. But this time he did not start fast; he had a new coach. He came up on Durden. For months Tabb had carried a newspaper clipping in his wallet with a quotation about himself from Durden. Reporters after the Houston Marathon had asked Durden, the winner, if he had been worried about Tabb's large early lead. Durden said no, he had not worried, that Tabb always went out fast and always lost with that tactic. Tabb felt Durden tossed him off as a flyweight. Furious, he confronted Durden. Durden asked Tabb if he had ever won a marathon that way. Tabb said no. Durden asked if what he had said was true about Tabb's never winning with that tactic. Tabb said yes, but that Durden didn't have to say it to reporters.

Tabb got a coach, Salazar's coach Bill Dellinger, who told him that he must not start as fast in a marathon as he liked. Dellinger gave Tabb direction, purpose, confidence, and camaraderie. Tabb had also ended his 2-year marriage to American middle-distance Olympian Mary Decker. He had spent most of his time training with her and putting his own career on hold. The split was congenial, and he had no regrets about the past 2 years, but Decker's running to the pinnacle of her ability forced her to balance on a peak where there was no room for anyone else.

When Tabb came up on Durden in the last couple of miles of the race, he patted Durden on the butt, said, "Ta, ta, Benji," and ran away with the last laugh. He ran his last mile in 4:35. He wanted to catch Meyer next. But nobody caught Meyer, who cruised his last mile waving to the crowds and, according to Squires, missing his chance to break Salazar's course record.

1983 Men's Results

1.	G. Meyer, MA	2:09:00	26. J. Dimick, VT	2:15:23
2.	R. Tabb, OR	2:09:31	27. B. Allen, CO	2:15:36
3.	B. Durden, GA	2:09:57	28. E. Castellanou, Venezuela	2:15:40
4.	E. Mendoza, AZ	2:10:06	29. L. Barthlow, MA	2:15:43
5.	C. Bunyan, IL	2:10:54	30. M. Mesler, MI	2:15:44
6.	D. Edge, Canada	2:11:03	31. M. Pinocci, CA	2:15:50
7.	M. Layman, WA	2:11:24	32. P. Cummings, UT	2:16:05
8.	D. Schlesinger, MA	2:11:36	33. J. Hope, CA	2:16:10
9.	J. Wells, OR	2:11:42	34. J. Anderson, OR	2:16:19*
10.	B. Rodgers, MA	2:11:58	35. R. Serna, CA	2:16:26
11.	D. Hinz, MI	2:12:05	36. J. Thomas, MA	2:16:28
12.	J. Lodwick, OR	2:12:49	37. F. Stonecipher, MO	2:16:35
13.	D. MacDonald, CA	2:12:49	38. A. Azocar, Venezuela	2:16:38
14.	B. Coates, PA	2:13:02	39. S. Molnar, PA	2:16:41
15.	D. Gorden, OR	2:13:11	40. M. Patterson, PA	2:16:45
16.	H. Schulz, CA	2:13:37	41. B. Hensley, CT	2:16:50
17.	D. Rinde, CA	2:13:48	42. J. Metcalf, OK	2:17:02
18.	R. Sayre, OR	2:13:49	43. R. Hagemann, TX	2:17:05
19.	G. Vega, NY	2:14:01	44. F. Torneden, KS	2:17:08
20.	K. McCarey, CA	2:14:09	45. A. Cendejas, CA	2:17:15
21.	T. Fleming, NJ	2:14:14	46. P. Friedman, NY	2:17:17
22.	C. Law, NC	2:14:21	47. D. Ryberg, NC	2:17:18
23.	D. Matthews, GA	2:14:46	48. G. Fanelli, PA	2:17:29
24.	T. Shibutani, Japan	2:15:12	49. A. Treffinger, PA	2:17:30
25.	D. Patterson, PA	2:15:20	50. R. Fritzke, CA	2:17:31

55.	G. Tuttle, CA	2:17:40	943.	A. Ratelle, MN (age 58)	2:42:27
77.	B. Maxwell, CA	2:19:13	**1283.**	**A. Viskari, Finland (age 55)**	**2:46:30**
83.	T. Ratcliffe, MA	2:19:51	1641.	W. Schultz, PA	2:50:01
87.	B. Igoe, NH	2:20:20	1887.	S. Lyons, MA	2:52:38
110.	A. Aregha, GA	2:21:57	**2127.**	**J.J. Kelley, CT (age 52)**	**2:55:30**
303.	J. Berit, MA	2:29:41	2588.	J. Best, VA	3:00:00
370.	J. Parker, NJ	2:31:56	4486.	R. Lewis, CA	3:30:00
561.	**P. Kotila, Finland**	**2:36:42**	4753.	S. Sotir, MA	3:46:26
789.	G. Cochrane, ME	2:40:00		**J.A. Kelley (age 75)**	**4:23:22**

5,415 starters, average time 3:02:41, 84 finishers under 2:20.

*16 seconds slower than his 1973 winning time.

Masters

1.	B. Hall, NC	2:23:19	3.	J. Weston (age 50), Canada	2:24:05
2.	G. Muhrcke, NY	2:23:33	4.	T. Gerrity, PA	2:24:27

"I'D RATHER BURN OUT THAN RUST"

MONDAY, APRIL 18, 1983

Roe's Opposition Is an Ocean Away

World record holder Allison Roe came back to win Boston again. She had to be considered the favorite for the 1983 race. Since her victory at Boston in 1981 she had gone on to win the 1981 New York City Marathon in the world record time of 2:25:29. The *Boston Globe* ran a headline that, "Roe's Opposition Is an Ocean Away." Tall, blond, and beautiful, she looked unbeatable, but the attraction of her attractiveness became her undoing. For companies in need of product endorsements she looked too good to pass by. For race directors she was the photogenic archetype of the Greek goddess of the hunt. For publishers she was the perfect cover photo—she looked as good as any model but she was a real athlete, so the magazine could not be accused of descending to cheesecake to sell copies. For reporters she was the ideal interview. Various reporters went ga-ga over such a curvacious lady's describing the Boston course, with its curvacious hills, as undulating.

Roe became a spokesperson for the New Zealand tourist board, represented Onitsuka Tiger Athletic Shoes (latter Asics), and frequently flew to California on promotional tours. Her husband ran a successful chiropractic practice in Auckland and would have liked for her to stay put. All these distractions pulled Roe away from the quintessential element that made her a great runner. With the fame, travel, attention, and stress, she neglected to train as diligently as before. For a time her natural athletic talents allowed her to continue performing well on less training. While her base training held her fitness, the resting allowed her to race "sharp" and actually improve her performances—for a time. But away from her New Zealand hills, relaxed running partners, and the structured training that created her, she began to break down. Too often she tried to squeeze in a run when she was half a world away from the Waiatarua run in the Waitakere range. Sloppy preparation for racing led to injuries that decreased training, giving rise to pressure to come back quickly, causing more injuries. The cycle continued throughout 1982.

In any runner less than the best in the world, such deviation from perfect training would not be noticeable, but when you already are on the edge, there is no other path. In the spring of 1983 Roe stayed with runners in Wellesley. Her real opposition was an ocean away; Grete Waitz planned to break Roe's world record in the London Marathon, the day before Boston. Roe said it would be very exciting if Waitz broke the world record on Sunday and the Boston runners were out doing their thing on Monday. Surprisingly, Waitz exactly tied Roe's marathon record. Quickly, on the night before the Boston race, Allison Roe telephoned Joan Benoit. Roe had heard that Benoit was in great shape. She had run a 2:26:11 marathon in Eugene, Oregon, for the third fastest time ever and had a pending American record of 31:44 for 10K. Two weeks before Boston Benoit ran 122 miles. Four days before she ran 3 × 440 at 69, 68, and 66.5; 2 × 330 at 50 and 50.5; 2 × 220 at 31.13 and 30.49; and 1 × 440 at 65, all after an 11-mile run and a Nautilus workout! Still, before the race she said that she was worried. When told that Roe had said that Benoit was the favorite, Benoit herself replied, "How can she say that? She's the world record holder. She's the favorite."

In the telephone call Roe suggested that the next day they race together for the record. Benoit had spent the previous day in pouring rain on the University of Massachusetts track, coaching her Boston University women's team. Benoit declined to run with Roe for the record. She thought it would be fine if they wound up running some parts of the race together, but she did not intend to alter her prerace plans. She told Roe that usually there was somebody she wanted to run into the ground, but this year she just wanted to run the best race that she could. She did not admit to Roe that the world record was what she had in mind. She thought she could run under 2:25. She thought 2:24 would be possible, but she did not want Roe to be any part of it. She wanted that record for herself.

Many observers regarded Benoit too lightly. She had won Boston in 1979 but in 1981 could not manage better than third. The Oregon time looked good, but it had been done on a flat course. Boston had hills, and Benoit had had problems with her heels. The experts predicted she would not do well and looked toward Jacqueline Gareau or Mary Shea if Roe faltered.

Joan Benoit had come a long way since 1981, when she had the habit of overtraining with the much faster men runners at the Nike laboratory in Exeter. It had taken her awhile to learn her lessons.

The school of hard roads began for Benoit in the summer of 1981. In the Old Kent River Run in Michigan she had set a 1:26:10 American record for 25 kilometers, won the TAC National 10K in 33:37.5, won the prestigious Falmouth road race, and ran the Avon International Marathon in Ottawa in 2:37:24. So far so good, but she also teetered on that narrow cliff's-edge. In the Columbus Bank One Marathon in November of 1981 Benoit had raced dismally; she ran out of energy and barely survived the thing to finish in 2:39. (To runners painful marathons become "things.") Her legs had cramped. She had been anemic and her heels had hurt. The race taught her a couple of lessons: You cannot go into a marathon unprepared, and anything can happen in such a long race.

After the Columbus Marathon a fear of marathoning crept up on Benoit. She had to learn to channel that fear the way her parents had taught her to fear the ocean; it is a mighty and beautiful thing, but it is big and cold and it can kill you. Training mileage became her life raft; for her the basic feeling that the race can be run quickly rested on the arithmetic. She could not give up those miles. She had to have them. On training runs she would madden her training partners by always taking the longest possible route around a curve. With just a change of pronouns Tom Fleming's warning could fit neatly on her wall: "*Somewhere in the world there is someone training when you are not. When you race her, she will win.*"

In high mileage lurks great risk. Like medieval sailors on the edge of the world reading their charts ("Beyond this place there be dragons"), runners pursuing personal bests could expect to be devoured. By December of 1981 Benoit's heels bothered her so much that a surgeon had to remove bone spurs and bursa sacs from both heels. Her torn right Achilles tendon had to be repaired. She had clearly crossed the line from perfect training to overtraining. Instead of making her body better she was making it worse. The miles added up, but they subtracted from her performance. During the 1982 Boston Marathon she could not run so she did radio commentary on Boston's WCVB with Randy Thomas. It drove her crazy to watch Charlotte Teske win so easily by so much.

But by the summer of 1982 Benoit was back training hard, but not too hard, and set an American record of 53:18 in the Bobby Crim 10-Miler. By September of 1982 she had won the Oregon Track Club Marathon in Eugene in 2:26:11—the third fastest marathon ever by a woman. Benoit worked on her speed until November of 1982, when she turned in a 31:44 10K American record in the Rosemont Turkey Trot in Illinois. The peak sharpness of her speed came in February of 1983 with an indoor mile personal record of 4:36.48. In March she placed fourth in the World Cross-Country Championships in Gateshead, England. Yet she nonchalantly threw in a 125-mile week 2 weeks before the marathon. Her body's ability to change air and food into energy developed tremendously. She became a dynamo. In the Nike research lab, scientists measured Benoit's $\dot{V}O_2$max and found that her body consumed 79 milliliters of oxygen per kilogram of body weight per minute at full effort, the highest rate ever recorded for a woman. In contrast, Greg Meyer's muscles consumed 80. The balance between speed, fear, and preparation fit just right. Benoit came to Boston in unheralded but perfect shape.

At the starting line Benoit saw New Zealander and Boston resident Kevin Ryan, sixth in 1978 in 2:11:43, attaching himself to Allison Roe. He was assigned by a radio station to run alongside the first woman and report on her condition. He carried a small radio transmitter. He obviously thought Roe would win. When Benoit saw that Ryan did not even glance her way, she reformulated her plan. She would go out quickly and get as big a lead as possible because she thought Roe wanted to race on her shoulder and outkick her in the last miles. Benoit vowed that Roe not only would not outkick her but would never even come close enough to try.

With this detached grimness Benoit waited at the start. Suspecting that Roe planned to sit on her tail, she decided not to wait around and play cat and mouse—with herself as the mouse. She blasted away at the gun, and before she knew it she passed the mile in 4:47. It was downhill, but that was still 45 seconds faster than the average she planned to run. The move was deliberately meant to discourage Roe. It was a premeditated, aggressive strategy. All marathoning wisdom also said it was stupid. A few miles out an experienced male runner turned to Benoit and said, "You'd better watch it, lady." The year before Waitz had run at a reckless pace and paid the price by dropping out. Was Benoit planting herself as a feckless morning glory from Maine? The history of the pursuit of the Boston Marathon is full of runners who unhinged themselves with a rapid early run only to crash and burn in the Newton hills. The 10K passed a second slower than Benoit's best. Her philosophy led her to prefer burning to rusting. She even expressed that out loud: "I'd rather burn out than rust."

But as Benoit heard her splits that old devil fear rose. She heard a 2:17 pace reported, but she didn't believe it because she felt so good. So much had been invested that she dared not back off. She pushed the devil away. Kevin Ryan abandoned Allison Roe, who appeared unwilling to give chase. Ryan caught Benoit at 10K and posted himself, a mobile radio station, at her side. His big New Balance shirt loomed in all the photos of the race dominating the little Nike logo on Benoit's Athletics West shirt. Later all sorts of charges upwelled against Ryan. Did he pace Benoit? Did she have unfair advantage? Did he interfere with her? Was he a billboard? He did offer water to Benoit, and she did accept, but most runners do that for each other. Benoit had no watch; Ryan gave her split times and offered encouragement. There was no clock on the women's lead truck. The men's truck had a digital clock that gave the times and the projected finish time; the truck itself functioned like a pacer. The women did not have this digital advantage of constant split times. Magazines and newspapers ran articles criticizing Benoit and Ryan, but no rule was ever passed against this kind of pacing.

Ryan was officially entered in the race and had every right to run wherever he pleased. This question of pacing could never be resolved in any mixed race. In fact, Benoit considered his presence a nuisance. She tried to ignore him. She had a difficult race to run. She hammered 10 more miles.

A cramp had grabbed Roe's calf muscle at 10 miles, but it did not slow her. Roe had her fastest training times on her home loops, including the long, undulating run in the Waitakere range that every New Zealand runner from Peter Snell and Murray Halberg to Rod Dixon and John Walker had trained on. By 13 miles she caught 1976 winner Jack Fultz. He ran along with her. That she could not see Benoit discouraged her. Fultz tried to console her with the reminder that she had a 2:25 marathon going. It did not work. Roe could not concentrate on her own racing because she could not see Benoit. The pressure of not winning squeezed her. In 1981, as an unknown, she had had nothing to lose. Now she had everything to lose.

In Wellesley a side stitch grabbed Benoit. She slowed. She reached the hills relatively rested.

Partway up the hills Jacqueline Gareau passed Roe. Roe suddenly slowed to a jog. She walked. She gave up. By 17 miles she dropped out. She went with Fultz to a house of his friends. They were in the midst of a marathon party when Fultz and the favorite dropped out of the race and into their party. The friends offered her a shower, food, and drink. In her rebound from the tensions of the race Roe became the hit of the party. When she wanted to go back to Wellesley, Fultz borrowed a car to give her a ride back to Randy Thomas's house, where she had left her stuff. Roe said she still had a good marathon inside her.

Gareau held second place. This time she knew full well she was in second place and just how distant she was from the flying Benoit. Benoit survived the hills, but the raw bottoms of her feet hurt on the downhill. Her legs wobbled alarmingly on one downhill stretch, and she thought it might be the end. She ran the second half of her race 6 minutes slower than the first half. In Coolidge Corner she broke her concentration for the first time when she heard her name shouted from the rooftops. Most of her Boston University track team had gathered on top of the transit station roof to chant her name.

Only in the last few seconds did Benoit's concentration break again. She knew she had run much faster than she dreamed—not just barely under the record, not 2:24, but 2 minutes and 46 seconds under the old world record and about 4 minutes under Roe's course record! She ran 2:22:43. A great grin of relief and affection for the Boston crowds splashed across her face. Women's marathon racing had come a long way.

Since Liane Winter had set the women's world marathon record of 2:42:24 in Boston in 1975, various women, all of whom ran in Boston at one time or another, had lowered the record (in this progression, at various races):

2:40:16, Christa Vahlensieck, West Germany, 1975

2:38:19, Jacqueline Hansen, United States, 1975

2:35:16, Chantal Longlace, France, 1977

2:34:48, Christa Vahlensieck, 1977

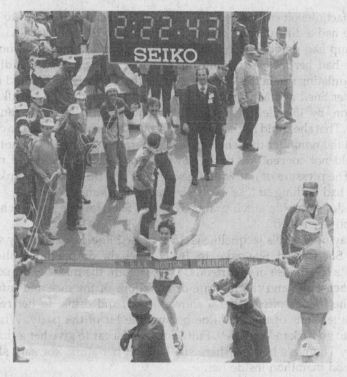

Joan Benoit sets a new course record, American record, and world record for women in 1983. Photo by Jeff Johnson.

2:32:30, Grete Waitz, Norway, 1978

2:27:33, Grete Waitz, 1979

2:25:42, Grete Waitz, 1980

2:25:29, Allison Roe, New Zealand, 1981

2:22:43, Joan Benoit, United States, 1983

In 1984 Joan Benoit went on to Los Angeles to win the gold medal in the first women's Olympic marathon. In October of 1985 she won the Chicago Marathon in a personal best of 2:21:21. The number 2:20 began to ring in her mind. She wanted to be the first woman to break it for the marathon. Of course so did Grete Waitz and Ingrid Kristiansen. Waitz had already tried and failed in Boston to break 2:20. Kristiansen had not come to Boston yet, but for the next 2 years the Boston Marathon would become inhospitable to potential world record–breaking fields. Benoit would come back to race Boston several more times as Joan Benoit Samuelson (after her marriage to Scott Samuelson), but not until the Boston Marathon had changed drastically.

A week later at the Rome Marathon Allison Roe begged out of the race at the last minute, claiming a stomach disorder. She never ran another fast marathon. Injuries nagged her. She tried competing in the triathlon with some success, but she never regained world-level stature. She returned to North Auckland and her chiropractor husband (ironically, the injuries that troubled her were back problems) and eventually became a mother, but she never stopped being a heroine and a public figure in her native New Zealand.

The 1983 Boston Marathon produced a women's world record, and three world-class times in the men's race, and the highest quality overall marathon race ever. Eighty-four runners broke 2:20. That had never happened before, not even in an Olympic marathon. And it would not happen again at Boston. But the Boston Marathon was about to enter its darkest years—years when its very existence descended into doubt.

Checkpoint Splits

10K	Joan Benoit	31:45
10 miles	Joan Benoit	51:38
Half marathon	Joan Benoit	1:08:22
15 miles	Joan Benoit	1:18:56
20 miles	Joan Benoit	1:46:44
25 miles	Joan Benoit	2:15:47

1983 Women's Results

1.	J. Benoit, Watertown, MA	2:22:43CR,AR,WR*	19.	T. Martland, RI	2:49:06
		(121st overall)	20.	K. Heckman, VA	2:49:08
2.	J. Gareau, Canada	2:29:27	21.	S. Zimmer, CT	2:49:52
3.	M. Shea, NC	2:33:23	22.	J. Millspaugh, FL	2:50:15
4.	K. Dunn, NH	2:33:35	23.	N. Suarez-Blackwood, FL	2:50:32
5.	S. King, AL	2:33:52	24.	F. Madeira, MA	2:50:37
6.	J. Wipf, UT	2:37:18	25.	P. Meade, MA	2:50:55
7.	K. Cossaboon-Holm, NY	2:37:40	26.	S. Lupica, MA	2:50:55
8.	M. Ireland, CA	2:39:07	27.	P. Barnett, MA	2:50:58
9.	M. Trujillo, AZ	2:39:45	28.	K. Beaulieu, ME	2:51:15
10.	K. Burns, AR	2:42:10	29.	S. Moen, TX	2:51:37
11.	S. Henderson, CO	2:44:13	30.	C. Matsuda, Japan	2:52:22
12.	A. Peisch, MA	2:44:41	60.	C. Myers, PA	2:59:58
13.	E. Oberli-Schuh, CA	2:45:33	208.	N. Kuscsik, NY	3:17:24
14.	B. Dillinger, VA	2:46:46	344.	E. Mendonca	3:25:53
15.	W. Ng, NY	2:48:17	421.	P. Duckworth, MA	3:32:05
16.	C. Gilroy, CA	2:48:33	498.	G. Chapin, NV	3:40:00
17.	P. Deuster, MD	2:48:35		B. Gibb	about 4:00
18.	B. Filutze, PA	2:48:45		A. Roe, DNF	

555 starters, average time 3:20:57.

'Permanent record for the course (1972-1985) with race finish in front of the Prudential Building.

Masters

1.	T. Hayward, MI	3:02:35

WHERE IS EVERYONE?

MONDAY, APRIL 16, 1984

Weak Field for Big Race

The Los Angeles Olympic marathon overshadowed the Boston Marathon in 1984 and drained its talent. The remaining weak field masked the problems facing the Boston Marathon. Strong fields had stayed away from Boston every Olympic year since the 1960s—except for 1980, the boycott year—so the BAA board of governors simply saw this year's field as the usual undermining of an Olympic year, not as the beginning of a trend. They could not see trouble coming. They refused to see trouble coming. Other races had shown that prize money and expense money would attract a world-class field regardless of Olympic proximity. The 1983 race had been terrific with Meyer's 2:09 and Benoit's world record. Those winning times and the fast times for the rest of the field clearly marked Boston as the apotheosis of marathons. So why worry?

The BAA governors did not care to see that other marathons and road races around the world used money to attract top athletes. Even if top competition, not money, was the motivation of specific athletes, they would still have to go to the "money" races because that was where all the top runners would go, except for the Olympics. But of course lucrative product endorsements would go to Olympic winners. The Olympic year gave the Boston Marathon a reprieve, a breathing space of one year. But the BAA steadfastly refused to become a commercial, professional road race. They felt that since the race had always been an amateur event, it should always remain so. Public debate was aired in the Boston newspapers on the subject.

Anthony Notagiacoma, whom everyone called simply Tony Nota, summed up the feeling of the BAA board of governors. Nota had worked as a volunteer at the marathon for 47 years. He had given selflessly to the sport, working at track meets, helping with timing, giving advice to young runners. He had never married and lived with his sister in Somerville. At over 80 years of age he worked at the Boston finish line, carrying time sheets from the timers to the officials. In the dark days Tony Nota stood by Will Cloney and Jock Semple as the three of them held the marathon together from year to year on a tiny budget. "The world is changing so much, but the Boston Marathon should be an amateur event forever. That is the makeup of the race. It is a tradition that we should keep," said Nota.

Jerry Nason, the *Boston Globe* sportswriter, supported Nota and the governors; he wrote that he worried that Boston would sell its "priceless" traditions, prestige, and heritage for a price. When told that famous runners would bypass the race, Nason said, "Let them." He saw the marathon not as a race for established runners but as an opportunity for runners who "seek names." He thought that previously unknown runners would surface at Boston. His long historical view of the Boston Marathon made him think that it could be the last amateur stop for runners who would become the new professionals who would thereafter race elsewhere for prize money. But others of equal stature disagreed.

Amby Burfoot, the 1968 Boston winner and editor for *Runner's World*, wrote a long rebuttal to Nason's argument printed in the *Globe*. Burfoot said that if the marathon didn't change it would lose its grandeur, and furthermore that traditions could be improved and still remain traditions. He observed that amendments had improved the U.S. Constitution 26 times. "The Boston Marathon should not be a petrified relic of a bygone era; it should be a vibrant, changing footrace." Later he characterized the BAA board of governors as "insular, timid and paranoid."

The Chicago Marathon offered prize and appearance money of $350,000. Boston offered nothing. The financial value of marathons had already been proven by the commercial success of the Chicago and New York City races. The cost of the Boston Marathon had grown tremendously since the days when Jock Semple, Will Cloney, and Tony Nota managed it on $3,000 of profits from the BAA indoor track meet. In those days George V. Brown had paid Cloney $1,500 to direct two track meets and the marathon, but those payments had stopped in 1971 with the end of the track meets. Cloney had received no salary since. Now the marathon appeared to have a budget of $150,000. The Prudential Insurance Company paid for the finish line costs of $80,000. Honeywell paid $70,000 to publish the results book, and the New Balance Athletic Shoe company in turn contributed some money against that $150,000 for getting its name on the numbers. The commercial potential was there, and everyone but the BAA governors saw it.

Volunteer race director Tim Kilduff, age 38, in his second year after replacing Will Cloney, would resign out of frustration after the 1984 race. His relationship with the marathon had become an obsession. Kilduff thought a love affair would have been natural and appropriate, but when the race became an obsession he started to lose perspective on all the other things in his life, such as family and career. Kilduff worked as vice president of public affairs for the Bank of New England.

The BAA board of governors was the source of Kilduff's distress. They wavered between myopia and paranoia. Shortsighted, they could only look backward, and they feared the rise of a sharp entrepreneur who might steal the race from them. The board desperately wanted the marathon to retain its worldwide importance, but as volunteers with no full-time staff or office, they could not manage details and policy simultaneously, nor did they realize the enormity of the task before them. It would take 4 more years to appoint a full-time race director.

Americans Greg Meyer, Bill Rodgers, and Alberto Salazar prepared for the Olympic trials; the proximity of the Boston Marathon and the trials meant that no runner could race at Boston and recover sufficiently for an all-out race for a position on the Olympic team. The American system used one trial—one race—to pick the top three marathon runners, with no appeals or exceptions. Other countries employed selection committees to choose representatives based on a judgment of multiple performances. Thus the British Olympic selectors saw Geoff Smith's second-place finish in his only marathon, the New York City Marathon, as a fluke. He had to prove to them that it was no accident that he had run 2:09:08. He had to do it again, and he knew it would impress them not just to run a fast time but to win to boot.

Smith had begun running relatively late in life. Before age 20 he played soccer. Born in 1953 in Liverpool, England, birthplace of the Beatles, he had worked for 10 years on fire brigade. As a fireman Smith rode on clanking trucks, then ran into burning buildings to save people's lives at the risk of his own. The job required courage and a wary aggressiveness. Timid firefighters rescue no one, but those who take too many risks eventually burn. Smith's running attracted the services of the venerable coach Eddie Sones, who had been the national cycling coach. Sones said that at first he didn't really want to coach a marathoner, but he was impressed that this one had so much courage.

Smith came to Rhode Island's Providence College at age 26 on scholarship hoping to run in college competition, but new NCAA rules prohibited older runners from running against college-age runners, so he could only run in a few non-NCAA meets. Smith was without an extreme physique; he stood 5'9" and weighed about 135 pounds. He ran with a miler's vigorous arm pumping. He trained hard.

Smith could have gone to England to race in the London Marathon, but he felt it would take him 4 weeks of training there to adapt. He had spent 4 years studying business at Providence College and did not want to skip 4 weeks of school and perhaps have to make up the semester to go to England to satisfy the British Olympic selectors. At age 30 he did not want to interrupt his education. He had run second in the world at 10,000 meters with a time of 27:43 in 1981 and had run a mile in 3:55.8, 2 miles in 8:23, 5K in 13:22, 10 miles in 46:23, half marathon in 1:01:38. Geoff Smith arrived in Boston clearly the fastest man that year to attempt to win the marathon, but, the British selectors thought his history unsound and his performance a fluke. He had to prove them wrong.

Smith's New York City run had made him famous by virtue of the television cameras. While winner Rod Dixon alternately lifted his arms in triumph and kissed the ground in gratitude, viewers could see Smith collapsing onto the finish line, having apparently given the supreme sacrifice. They had watched Smith leading for miles as Dixon stalked him. The symbolism seemed perfect and simple. It looked like life and death. The drama of it all made the "People in the News" sections in both *Time* and *Newsweek*. People from all over the world wrote to Smith to applaud his courage and to tell him that he was a winner in their eyes. Smith could run himself nearly to death. He had proved that to the world. But still the British selectors wanted proof that he could do it again before they would invite him to join their Olympic team.

Given his notoriety after the New York race, Smith attracted media attention at the press conference before the Boston Marathon. Reporters asked him countless questions, which he answered patiently and at length. When he finished, Coach Sones said, "You talk too much. Save some of your wind for the race."

Race day dawned dark, wet, and windy. A big storm stalled off the coast of Massachusetts and swirled drizzle in the runners' faces. On a day like this runners did not sweat, nor did they dehydrate. The wind would slow them a little, but all things considered the runners faced a decent day for racing. Because the low cloud ceiling prevented helicopters from going airborne to relay television broadcasts to their studios and transmitters, the cameras dependent on them waited uselessly on the lead truck and at the start. Smith stood nervously in the front row. Tom Fleming, now 32, stood stoically nearby. He had been hammering at the Boston Marathon for over a decade, except for the years when he was outlawed as a professional after accepting $25,000 in 1981 for winning the Jordache Marathon in Los Angeles. This could be his year. He had trained harder than ever for it. He looked leaner than ever.

The leaders reached Framingham at 6.75 miles in the reasonable time of 32:45. Smith led, with Domingo Tibaduiza of Colombia on his heels. Fleming led the second pack looking calm and reserved.

By Wellesley Smith had extended his lead to over a quarter mile. Fleming dropped back, out of contention, but would finish respectably. He would be back in 8 years to contend for the masters title. In the meantime he would tend his shoe store in New Jersey, Tom Fleming's Running Room. Smith reached the half-marathon point in 1:04:14 as the drizzle turned to rain.

Smith ran hard but under control. Like a seasoned firefighter he fought but took only a professional degree of risk. He did not get too excited, as he had in New York when he threw in a 4:28 mile in the middle of the race. He would not collapse at the end of this race, and no one would catch him and take his lead in the last miles as Dixon had done. Inexorably Smith extended his lead. Soon no one else in the race could see him.

Geoff Smith won easily, with the next runner nearly a mile behind in a cold rain. His time of 2:10:34 looked excellent for an essentially solo performance against a buffeting headwind. Smith's victory impressed the British selectors. He proved that he could run fast and win under unfavorable conditions. They selected him for their Olympic team.

A 23-year-old substitute teacher from New Milford, Connecticut, named Gerry Vanesse moved up through the ranks of tiring top runners. He wore #5933. The public and the press had never heard of him. Bill Squires, who had coached Rodgers, Salazar, and Meyer, coached Vanesse. Squires knew how fast he could run. Squires's plan called for Vanesse to run the second

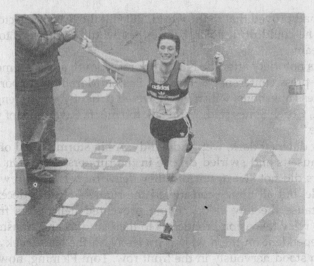

Geoff Smith wins the 1984 Boston and a place on the British Olympic team. Photo by Jeff Johnson.

half of the race faster than the first. The night before the race Squires called Vanesse and told him, "Get your pen out and write this down: Don't go out too fast." While Smith, still pumping his arms, won by a 4-minute margin, Vanesse had passed everyone he could see. But he never saw Smith. Vanesse finished second, nearly a minute ahead of Tibaduiza in third place. Coach Squires's advice had worked perfectly. But for the man who said the Boston Marathon should forever remain an amateur event, everything stopped.

In the hubbub of the finish area, timekeeper Tony Nota rushed from the finish line with his hands full of time sheets for the officials. Suddenly he stopped and fell to the ground. The time sheets scattered in the rain. A blood vessel had burst in his brain. Officials and bystanders rushed to him, but they could do nothing. Tony Nota died at 3:40 p.m. His contemporary, Fred Brown, said, "But you know, if Tony wanted to pick a day to go, he'd pick this one. He loved the Boston Marathon. As far as I'm concerned he always was and always will be part of it. We lost a very fine person, a gentleman and a kind man."

1984 Men's Results

1. **G. Smith, United Kingdom**	**2:10:34**	7. D. Olds, MI	2:17:05
2. G. Vanesse, CT	2:14:49	8. J. Correa, Colombia	2:17:12
3. D. Tibaduiza, Colombia	2:15:40*	9. P. Ballinger, New Zealand	2:17:39
4. J. Zetina, TX	2:15:41	10. D. Freedline, PA	2:17:46
5. K. Johansen, Denmark	2:16:36	11. R. Lanzoni, Costa Rica	2:17:50
6. M. Kiilholma, CA	2:16:56	12. D. McDonald, VA	2:17:51

13.	D. Northrup, NY	2:18:07	35.	T. Fleming, NJ	2:20:36
14.	J. Kruse, NJ	2:18:26	36.	T. Wunsca, FL	2:20:39
15.	R. Ferguson, VA	2:18:42	37.	L. Parker, LA	2:20:43
16.	D. Skarda, IL	2:18:56	38.	P. McNeill, NY	2:20:51
17.	K. Judson, PA	2:18:57	39.	R. Leland, WA	2:20:57
18.	G. Minty, MD	2:19:03	40.	S. Snover, MA	2:21:02
19.	M. Tibaduiza, Colombia	2:19:05*	41.	C. Pilone, New Zealand	2:21:07
20.	M. Skinkle, RI	2:19:09	42.	D. Hulme, NY	2:21:09
21.	B. Hinzmann, CA	2:19:15	43.	H. Chavez, Mexico	2:21:21
22.	J. Holzman, KY	2:19:21	44.	P. Dodd, WI	2:21:42
23.	J. Kallio, IL	2:19:29	45.	Y. Karni, Israel	2:21:43
24.	J. Reis, Mexico	2:19:39	46.	C. Carl, NM	2:21:44
25.	M. Bossardet, NY	2:19:52	47.	T. Dooling, NE	2:21:50
26.	M. Sandlin, MS	2:20:02	48.	E. Heurga, Argentina	2:21:53
27.	K. Hartman, CO	2:20:04	49.	J. Hopkins, NJ	2:22:06
28.	L. Arana, Mexico	2:20:09	50.	A. Azocar, FL	2:22:09
29.	R. Murdock, CT	2:20:10	59.	S. Murakoshi, Japan	2:22:44
30.	J. Gonzalez, Puerto Rico	2:20:14	194.	R. Taylor, AR	2:29:59
31.	R. Robinson, New Zealand	2:20:15	2121.	J.J. Kelley, CT	2:58:35
32.	N. Blair, NC	2:20:16	4236.	L. Tomasetti, RI	3:29:48
33.	L. Supino, CO	2:20:26	4708.	D. Ellis, MA	3:59:56
34.	T. Downs, KY	2:20:27		J.A. Kelley (age 76)	sub-5:00

6,086 entrants.

*Domingo and Miguel Tibaduiza are brothers. Their sister, Rosalba, ran 2:54:09 in the women's race for 37th place.

Masters

1.	R. Robinson, New Zealand	2:20:15	3.	J. Bowers, CA	2:26:29
2.	T. Gerrity, PA	2:25:12			

THE BODYMIND CONNECTION

MONDAY, APRIL 21, 1984

New Zealander Top of Field

Allison Roe came back. She needed a fast time to make the New Zealand Olympic team, and so did her teammate and friend, Lorraine Moller. The New Zealand Olympic selectors gave the two of them a last chance to qualify for the final spot on the team. A Roe victory did not seem as likely as her win in 1981. She had been injured and had not run well since then. She had dropped out of Boston in 1983, when as world-record holder she faced Joan Benoit. Moller knew Roe's tendencies. She had trained with her. Moller knew Roe could not hold back, because she had a precedent on the course. From the beginning of her running career Roe had needed help with pacing or she would forget and run away with her enthusiasm. In the 1980 Oregon Track Club Marathon in Eugene, Moller had had to caution teammate Roe with unequivocal language: "I know how to pace, you don't; if you pass me I'll hit you." The threat worked, and both ran excellent times that day. But things had changed in 4 years. You cannot use such language with a former world-record holder and race winner and a woman whom the public considered a favorite.

People expected Roe to win Boston again, so Moller expected Roe to forget that a cautionary early pace had allowed her that win in 1981 and that she would "jump out," then try to "hang on." Moller intended to counter by starting slowly and working her way up. Moller used her inside information to decide her strategy. But Moller at age 28 had established her own unique training and racing philosophy. She had given a great deal of thought to athletic competition and to the mental and spiritual aspects of training and racing long distances. Since she started running she had traveled a long way geographically and emotionally to come to stand at the Boston Marathon starting line. Symbolism mattered to Moller. She wore silver earrings in the shape of the fern leaves on the all-black official New Zealand national team uniform.

Moller had started her running at an early age, racing over 60 yards with the neighborhood children in Putaruru, New Zealand, for a chocolate fish at Easter. By age 17 she had finished fifth in the 800 meters in the Commonwealth Games with a 2:03.6 lifetime personal record. She ran on the same team with Roe in the World Cross-Country Championships in Morocco in 1975, when Bill Rodgers had made his first international appearance. She earned a degree in physical education from Otago University but gave up teaching to move to the U.S. in 1979, settling in Minneapolis. She came at the invitation of Ron Daws, whom she met at the 1978 Choysa Marathon in Auckland.

Daws had finished as the first American in 1969 with fourth place in Boston. He called himself the self-made Olympian, having begun with little talent but a boundless capacity for hard work. His marathon in Choysa closed his international racing career, but he had developed an interest in coaching. He coached Moller after she came to the U.S. She ran her first marathon in Duluth in 1979 at Grandma's Marathon; an astounding 2:37:36 win ranked her sixth in the world all-time list. She had begun it as a training run, but she felt so good at 20 miles that she told Daws she would go all the way. She won her next eight marathons. In 1981 she went all the way again and married Coach Daws.

Daws coached Moller like he coached himself. Her 20-mile training runs became 28-mile runs, and her weekly mileage rose from 90 to 120 miles. The extra work did her no good other than to prove that she could survive it. She threw up during runs and found herself crying for no reason. "Ron was coach and I was athlete so I acquiesced."

But after a year Moller could no longer tolerate the oppression, so she divorced Daws and moved back to New Zealand. Under the gentle guidance of Olympic 5,000-meter silver medalist Dick Quax, she won bronze medals in track races in the Commonwealth Games in Brisbane, Australia, in 1982. The hard work had not destroyed her ability to run short and fast.

Thereafter Moller coached herself with advice from Quax, arranged her training so she would enjoy it, and allowed the racing to take care of itself. Other runners and would-be coaches suggested she could run faster if she trained harder and followed a structured, disciplined, scientific program. But Moller disagreed. She maintained that it was a far greater discipline to understand and follow one's inner self than a plan from a book or instructions from a coach. Ultimately she said a plan generated from within would take her further and faster. She wanted to keep playfulness in her running.

Moller saw herself as a creative performing artist, expressing herself through running much as a dancer does through dance or a singer through song. The body is the expression of the mind and spirit. She wanted to explore the boundaries of herself and her potential and urged others to see sport in the same way. She wrote,

> In the greater game we strive not for winning, but to extend our personal boundaries of who we are and what we can be, not as much to become faster as to become more, not to punish but to enjoy, not to beat someone else, but to become the best we can be, not to destroy others, but to create ourselves in motion as a celebration of our creaturehood. True excellence is achieved only in playing the greater game.

Moller's revelations about her running brought to mind Bobbi Gibb, but it was Kathrine Switzer who lent important influence in Moller's development.

On the strength of Moller's Grandma's Marathon performance, Switzer invited Moller to the Avon all-women's marathon in London. Switzer managed the races and worked in public relations for the Avon cosmetics company. Moller won the Avon Marathon three times and in the process became the "Avon Queen." The queen represented the company and followed a code of conduct with such regulations as always wearing a dress in public. Moller often had to make promotional appearances in New York City on behalf of Avon cosmetics. Life became a cosmopolitan whirl for Lorraine Moller, who saw herself a pigtailed country girl. Lorraine did not know how to apply sophisticated makeup until Kathrine, the worldly older woman, taught her. Switzer became Moller's mentor; she helped her develop the composure to present herself publicly with femininity and confidence without compromising herself athletically.

Women's running had been modeled on men's running. Even the shorts were the same. Switzer told Moller that it was OK to be feminine—you didn't have to be "a jock." You didn't have to be masculine to run fast. Switzer took Moller shopping in the best stores in New York. Moller did not know how to spend her money; Switzer taught her. Moller made as much as $10,000 to $20,000 in prize money in a single race, yet she hesitated to buy a $100 dress. Switzer's counseling abolished those inhibitions. Moller arrived in Boston clear, professional, well dressed and ready for what Switzer called a "celebration of physicality."

In the 1984 Boston Marathon celebration, Roe did jump out to a 27:41 first 5 miles, just as Moller expected. But Moller herself did not run in the top 10 at that point. She had decided that to run a marathon she would rely on her own self-awareness, and by doing so she would have to let other runners go. By 10 miles Moller ran third, by 15 she ran second, only 60 seconds behind Roe. Faith and patience appeared to be working for her. By this time Roe, again as Moller predicted, merely hung on. Moller waited until the 20th mile to pass her. In passing Moller could say nothing. She liked Roe. She did not want to be patronizing, but each of them knew nothing could be done at that point. Moller knew she had the race. She knew she could run the downhills well. Moller had learned that running the marathon is an act of faith. Roe dropped out with only 2 miles to go. Moller ran easily to victory.

Moller ran fifth in the 1984 Olympic Games marathon in Los Angeles, placing behind Joan Benoit, Grete Waitz, Rosa Mota, and Ingrid Kristiansen—all (except Waitz) to be major players in future Boston Marathons. In 1989 Moller opened a shop in Boulder, Colorado, called The BodyMind Connection, to sell books and learning tapes, whole-grain technologies, and information on the psychological aspects of sport and performance. In 1992 she won the bronze medal in the Barcelona Olympic marathon.

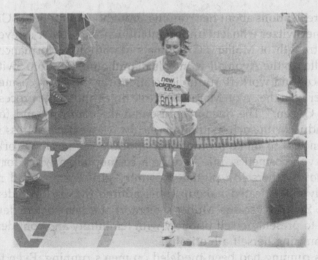

Lorraine Moller's BodyMind connects with the finish line tape in 1984. Photo by Jeff Johnson.

1984 Women's Results

1. L. Moller, New Zealand	2:29:28	2. M. Hamrin, TX 2:33:53
	(180th overall)	3. S. Grottenberg, OR 2:36:07

4.	A. Hird, RI	2:37:11	18.	A. Igoe-Maguire, MA	2:48:23
5.	T. Toivonen, Finland	2:37:43	19.	D. Magnani, NY	2:49:14
6.	G. Andersen, ID	2:39:28	20.	V. Smith, TX	2:49:27
7.	L. Dybdal, Denmark	2:43:12	21.	S. Crowe, PA	2:49:58
8.	B. Moore, New Zealand	2:43:47	22.	S. Chiong, FL	2:49:59
9.	S. Mewett, Bermuda	2:44:07	23.	S. Beugen, NY	2:51:01
10.	L. Hollmann, PA	2:45:33	24.	A. Ingalls, CA	2:51:38
11.	L. Geraci, GA	2:45:55	25.	S. Given, NY	2:51:51
12.	A. Ray, KS	2:47:44	37.	R. Tibaduiza, Colombia	2:54:09
13.	K. Culla, NY	2:47:47	60.	H. Hoyt, NJ	3:00:02
14.	**J. Hansen, CA**	**2:47:48**	381.	M. Jackson, UT	3:30:01
15.	W. Ng, NY	2:48:14	582.	C. Klingman, OH	3:58:50
16.	K. Wagner, MD	2:48:15		**A. Roe, DNF at 24 miles**	
17.	S. Wurl, MN	2:48:16			

838 entrants.

Masters

1.	J. Ullyot, CA	2:54:17

THE WALKING WOUNDED

MONDAY, APRIL 15, 1985

Smith to Go for World Record

For the first time ever the outcome of the Boston Marathon meant nothing in the worldwide scheme of the sport. Anyone who gave importance to the outcome of this year's Boston race did so out of respect for its passing. All but one of the world's best runners ran elsewhere. To them Boston had no value. If they were going to risk injury by running a marathon, they might as least have a chance of being paid for it. Runners never know which race might be their last. Better not waste one against a flimsy field without a payday.

Other marathons throughout the world had surged past Boston in size and quality and threatened to push the Boston Marathon from a global event to a mere local road race. The background for this decline was complex. It had taken nearly 100 years for the slow-to-change, traditional Boston Marathon to collide with the rapid changes in economies, technologies, and athletes' role in an instantaneous and commercial world. The collision course began with the 1887 founding of the BAA as a men's social and athletic club by a special act of the Massachusetts legislature. The legislation provided the purpose of the association: "maintaining a club-house for social purposes and for the encouragement of athletic exercises, and maintaining a reading room." Wealthy, powerful men joined—so wealthy that they would never have to sweat for money, wealthy enough to persuade the legislature to enact laws for the establishment of their athletic club. They owned things. Other people in 1887 sweated for money because they had to, but not these wealthy men; they were amateurs who could compete for the pure love of the sport or could sponsor the search for astounding natural talent. The BAA first lost its building during the Great Depression, then gradually lost power and prestige as the meeting place for the movers and shakers of Boston, then slowly abandoned its other tasks and holdings until only its marathon remained. Through the 1950s and 1960s Jock Semple and Will Cloney held the club together with sheer love of the event. But in the early 1980s the Boston Athletic Association revived and formed a new board of governors. They served with an arrogance like that which had characterized the original elite founders.

In 1982 an amendment to the BAA charter added to its purpose: "With particular emphasis on the sponsorship of long distance running events (especially the annual BAA Marathon) and of track and field teams and meets." The collision of tradition and commerce essentially arose when sponsorship of the marathon became the sole function of the BAA, for the board of governors did a poor job in securing sponsorship because an amateur event, both in its management and participation, had little to offer potential sponsors. It also offered little to runners, who could no longer rely solely on natural talent but had to train full-time to compete at an international level. But before dissecting the reasons for the board of governor's failures—a story that had begun in 1981—let's look at the magnitude of the fall of the Boston Marathon and the relative rise of other marathons through the first half of the 1980s.

In the spring of 1985 many performances that in other years would certainly have been executed in Boston went elsewhere: In Rotterdam, Holland, Carlos Lopes ran 2:07:11 to set a new world record, and 5 men ran under 2:14; in Hiroshima, Japan, Ahmed Saleh of Djibouti ran 2:08:09, and 17 men ran faster than U.S. Olympian Pete Pfitzinger's 2:12:28; Dean Matthews, who led the 1982 Boston Marathon, ran 2:11:48 for 13th place; in London Steve Jones ran 2:08:16, 10 men ran under 2:14, and Ingrid Kristiansen ran 2:21:06, with 7 women running under Lisa Weidenbach's 2:34 winning time at Boston. Why did none of them come to Boston?

Not only did fast runners stay away from Boston, the entire field shrank by 1,329 participants to 5,595. What was the attitude behind it all? Had the race outgrown its logistics under part-time management and limited sponsorship? Did the baggage riot of the year before signal the need to change? In 1984 wet, tired, cold marathoners had rebelled in the Prudential garage as confused high school volunteers forced them to wait shivering in line for their bags of dry clothes. The Prudential had secured the underground garage as the only place available out of the wet weather for 7,000 runners. But the cold, gray concrete walls, the oil spills, the puddles, the dank drafts, and the residual smells of auto exhaust gave the garage the air of a dungeon, replete with spills of sweat, Coca-Cola, and vomit. As runners cooled and overcooled to the point of hypothermia, as stiffness set into their joints and the so-called runner's highs vanished, they could no longer wait for the volunteers to check their numbers and fetch the correct labeled bags. The runners rushed the volunteers to rummage through the bags themselves, grabbed their fresh clothes, and escaped the hellish garage. Money could cure those and other problems, but the Boston Marathon didn't have it.

In large part it was the reputation of the Boston Marathon as the most famous footrace in the world that engendered the arrogance and inertia of the BAA officials. Harold Carroll, one of the four BAA members charged with organizing the 1985 race, was proud that for the first time they had provided hotel rooms for special runners. But other marathons also provided airfare and appearance and prize money. The Boston Marathon had moved an inch. Tradition, mystique, and the weight of its past success made change for Boston difficult and painful. The process began early in the decade; it played out in years of drama that, in the story's climax, forced huge changes, ushering in the appearance of the new professionals in 1986. The drama—"Who Owns the Boston Marathon?"—started over a dinner table in the winter of 1981.

On March 11, 1981, Will Cloney, R.H. Kingsley Brown, William B. Tyler, and Marshall Medoff met for dinner at Boston's uptown Harvard Club on Commonwealth Avenue. They hoped that the papers they were to examine would save the Boston Marathon. They arrived at 5:30 p.m. and would stay and talk past brandy and leave at about 10 o'clock. They wanted to change the marathon for the better, to insure that it would have the financial power to compete with the growing number of well-financed marathons world-wide, in cities like New York City, Chicago, Rotterdam, and London. But their actions had the opposite effect, initiating a chain reaction of emotional events that nearly killed the marathon.

Tyler and Brown sat on the newly revived BAA board of governors, of which Cloney had been elected president and Brown was secretary-treasurer. Tyler was a real estate attorney. Tyler and Brown had never met Marshall Medoff, but Medoff had a deal to propose involving more money than either had dreamed of.

The private Harvard Club was restricted to Harvard alumni, of which Cloney and Tyler were two, and their guests. Cloney introduced Medoff as influential in an organization called the Société de Monte Carlo, a personal friend of Prince Rainier of Monaco, and a man with a Boston sports promotion background. Tyler had done research on Marshall Medoff but learned only that he had graduated from Tufts University and the University of Chicago law school and had an office at 27 State Street, all of which Tyler regarded as perfectly respectable. Tyler's doubts about Medoff arose because he did not practice law per se but engaged in various business activities, including brokering deals. Echoing the sentiments of many others, Brown (no relation to the Hopkinton Brown family of George V., Walter, and Tom) supported Cloney in anything he might want to do regarding the marathon. He felt that since Cloney had taken all the decisions and work upon himself for all those years since the 1950s—years when no one but Cloney, Jock Semple, Tony Nota, and a handful of others cared much about the marathon—Cloney should still be in charge now that marathon running had become popular and attracted big business.

By default Cloney had had carte blanche over Boston Marathon business for years. Tyler acknowledged Cloney as czar of the marathon, but he came along to offer legal advice. But Tyler knew that Cloney disliked lawyers as a breed and was not loathe to say so. Tyler felt that Cloney had always made sure to denigrate any role Tyler might attempt to play as legal advisor. Cloney felt that lawyers got in the way, and he regarded contracts and legalese documents as just so much mumbo jumbo. (When asked to define legal mumbo jumbo Cloney said that it is what lawyers write.) As a good and professional writer himself, Cloney saw legal writing as largely deliberate obfuscation, as a conspiracy against the laity. Cloney preferred gentlemen's agreements sealed with an understanding human handshake, like his long-standing and successful agreement with Prudential.

Medoff got the instant attention of his dinner companions by claiming he could raise a million dollars for the Boston Marathon. Cloney, by now in his early 70s, wanted to remove himself from the day-to-day workings of the race. Most men had retired by age 70. The strain of the Rosie Ruiz affair in 1980 had proven to be too much for an old man working a volunteer job in addition to his paid one. Cloney had handled the crisis deftly, with the best possible result, but at an emotional expense he

> *The BAA needed $400,000 to put on the marathon, and Cloney saw Medoff as a supersalesman. . . . Others would come to see Medoff as malicious . . . , the bad guy of the marathon.*

did not want to repeat. He felt he could no longer direct the marathon from his kitchen. He wanted to see a full-time race director in an office run year-round by a professional staff. To hear Medoff talk about a million was a possibility too good to be true. Cloney knew that as president of the BAA and race director of the Boston Marathon he stewarded a valuable sales commodity. He had thought that perhaps someone could raise $300,000, $400,000—$500,000 tops—selling sponsorship of the marathon, but not a million dollars.

The BAA needed $400,000 to put on the marathon, and Cloney saw Medoff as a supersalesman, a perennial optimist. Cloney felt the job needed such a personality, one distinct from his own. Others would come to see Medoff as malicious and acquisitive, the bad guy of the marathon. Though Cloney wanted to leave the daily operations of the marathon, he wanted to always be a part of it, preferably as senior management, perhaps to supervise the supersalesman. He felt Medoff was the man to sell the sponsorship to raise the money to make the marathon financially sound, but with Cloney giving the last word. Medoff sat at the Harvard Club and sold hard, bubbling with the push and enthusiasm of a potent salesman.

Marshall Medoff, 44 years old the night of this dinner, lived in Weston, Massachusetts, a community wealthy, arborous, and sparsely populated by large estates with winding drives. He said he was so confident of his ability to raise sponsorships that he would guarantee the first $400,000 to the BAA out of his own pocket.

Cloney did not know that Medoff's seemingly generous "guarantee" was nothing more than hot air. Cloney did not know that the Société de Monte Carlo organized gambling junkets to Monaco and had been under scrutiny by FBI investigators looking for reputed New England Mafia boss Raymond Patriarca.

Everyone except Medoff ridiculed the idea of a million-dollar sponsorship deal, but they discussed advertising, marketing, public relations, and who would control the event, the BAA or the sponsors. As the group talked, Tyler's dislike and distrust for Medoff grew.

Tyler reviewed the draft of Medoff's legal contract and rejected it. Medoff agreed to strike the word *sell* from his contract language about the marathon. He began to talk about "just licensing some rights." They discussed what kind of sponsors they might want and not want. They did not want beer or cigarette sponsors. They did want solid Fortune 500 companies. Tyler took notes. Medoff—who had designed his plans around the idea—voiced strong support for moving the race to Sunday to take advantage of the advertising that national television would attract.

Tyler said he thought it unreasonable to expect a million dollars or even $700,000. In light of Medoff's guarantee of $400,000, Tyler said that if Medoff raised only that sum he might end up a hero, having possibly raised money for the BAA but being paid nothing for his efforts. "You really don't want to be that kind of hero," said Tyler.

The group suggested instead that Medoff get 15% if he raised less than $400,000 and, if he raised more, he could keep all the excess money.

Tyler also lived in Weston, so Medoff offered to drive him home. Tyler resisted, knowing that the purpose of the drive would be to secure his support, but then accepted. On the ride in Medoff's Mercedes Tyler said that he agreed it was high time the BAA got themselves organized and on the right footing, but he did not accept the contract Medoff proposed. Medoff said Tyler seemed stiff in his resistance, that as a real estate attorney he did not fully understand promotional activities, that he should leave such decisions to those like Medoff who had experience and knew better. In a later telephone conversation Medoff said to Tyler, "Do you know that by your negative attitude, you are threatening an arrangement which is important to the BAA? You people need this money for the future." Then suddenly Medoff changed tack in a personal direction. "I know what the problem is. You just don't like my kind of people." Medoff's accusation of anti-Semitism dismayed Tyler. He simply thought the contract was bad.

After the dinner at the Harvard Club Tyler and Brown thought they had seen the last of Medoff. Tyler heard nothing about him from Cloney or anyone else. He assumed the idea of a contract with Medoff was rightly dead. But it lived on—between Medoff and Cloney.

A month after the Harvard Club meeting, Cloney secured for himself broadly drawn and documented authority from the BAA board of governors. He got in writing the power he had exercised de facto for the past 25 years. His deal with the Prudential, sealed with only a handshake, worked well for 20 years. The board voted full authority to Cloney on April 27, 1981.

> That William T. Cloney as President of the Association be and hereby is authorized and directed to negotiate and to execute in the name of and in behalf of this association such agreement as he deems in the best interest of the association for the perpetuation, sponsorship or underwriting of the Boston A.A. Marathon.

Only one board member, Rod MacDonald, an employee of Prudential, voted no. Medoff incorporated IMI, International Marathons Inc., a few days later with the Commonwealth of Massachusetts. Cloney signed a contract with IMI on September 23. Did Cloney get board authority to sign the contract? Cloney said he was only doing what he felt was best for the marathon. He never told any board members that he intended to sign the contract with Medoff or that he did. But he had to tell someone.

Susan "Dusty" Rhodes, whose company, Conventures, operated the Boston Marathon exposition, where running-related companies—mostly shoe companies—displayed goods and services, felt she had a father–daughter relationship with Will Cloney. The new contract gave Medoff control of the expo along with the race and in early 1982 Cloney introduced him to Rhodes as a man nationally famous and respected as a sports promoter. Rhodes had never heard of Medoff, despite her work in sports promotions for the National Football League. She grew uneasy as she sat through several hours with him. She asked pointed questions that he evaded. He called her "little girl" and told her that she would do this or that. Cloney emphasized that Rhodes must keep the entire arrangement secret. Uneasy, Rhodes called her friend Will McDonough, sports columnist at the *Boston Globe*, to ask if he had ever heard of Marshall Medoff, sports promoter. He had not. His suspicions aroused, he launched a journalistic investigation.

No board member knew of the deal between Medoff and Cloney until McDonough revealed the story of their signed contract in his column on February 26, 1982. Upon reading the column, Rod MacDonald promptly resigned from the board of governors. The contract had rendered the board powerless. Cloney said he never intended such a thing.

Cloney said he had read every word of the contract with IMI. Cloney understood writing; he taught a course in journalism at Northeastern University and had written for the *Boston Herald* for years. Yet when he read every word of Medoff's contract, he did not see that he was selling sponsorship rights. What Cloney saw was legal mumbo jumbo. He saw that he was agreeing to a partnership whereby the BAA would conduct the race and get the first $400,000 raised and IMI would promote the race and keep the rest of the money. Cloney did not notice that the details the four men had discussed in their dinner meeting were nowhere reflected in the contract, now that the discussion was translated into legalese. Medoff had pulled a fast one.

Cloney had also missed a double negative in the contract language. The BAA kept rights "not inconsistent" with IMI. That meant that the BAA kept no rights. The BAA could not get sponsors on its own. The contract assigned IMI exclusive rights to the name and logo of the BAA and its marathon. According to the contract the BAA could assert its right only to *refuse all* sponsorship money. It could put on the marathon with no money, or it had to use Marshall Medoff's IMI as agent.

The Boston Marathon became the legal property of Marshall Medoff in perpetuity, unless the contract could be declared null.

The contract provided no way to terminate the relationship. The Boston Marathon became the legal property of Marshall Medoff in perpetuity, unless the contract could be declared null.

In 1981 and 1982 Medoff had raised $712,000. His expenses came to $312,000. The board of governors hired the law firm of Ropes and Gray to press the court to declare the contract between IMI and the BAA illegal.

The proceedings were not pleasant. Cloney received a subpoena at 10:00 at night. Medoff said the court tried to deliver its summons to him in temple on Yom Kippur. Both felt harassed by the board of governors.

The Supreme Judicial Court of the Commonwealth of Massachusetts ruled on February 13, 1984, that the duties vested in the Boston Athletic Association board of governors could not be abdicated. Such an abdication would constitute a breach of fiduciary duties, so that if the vote of April 27, 1981, was to give Cloney full discretionary power, the board would have acted illegally.

The court said that a board of directors cannot vote itself out of business by giving its authority away; the law obligates it to vote on major decisions. The BAA board of governors could not delegate control of its major asset, the name and logo of the Boston Marathon.

The court further ruled that even the board of directors of a nonprofit organization could not sell its name and logo to a for-profit organization. In the words of the court, such a sale would "create at least the possibility that the name and logo of a nonprofit corporation, the BAA, will be utilized to create a potentially enormous profit for International Marathons Incorporated. . . . It is unlawful for a public charity such as the BAA to be converted into a vehicle for private profit." The court concluded that the effect of Medoff and Cloney's agreement was to put the BAA into a partnership with IMI. The wheels of justice rolled slowly, but by 1983 and 1984 the BAA secured declarations from the Massachusetts courts that the contract with IMI was illegal and invalid. Cloney no longer involved himself with the marathon, and for many years he seemed estranged from the board as well as the race. The incident produced bitterness, mistrust, and massive legal fees over the question of who owned the Boston Marathon. The $712,000 raised by Medoff probably went to pay lawyers to pursue legal action for several years, although such figures are still confidential. The legal documents alone amounted to a stack of paper 4 feet high, yet for the runners who ran and the people who watched, no doubt existed about who "owned" the Boston Marathon: They did.

A marathon is not much of a thing to own. Without the people running in it and the people lining the road to watch, there is no marathon. The city of Boston and the communities of spectators along the route in Hopkinton, Ashland, Framingham, Natick, Wellesley, Newton, and Brookline felt they owned the Boston Marathon, as did the runners who had run it or wanted to. Obviously, people were the marathon and no one owned them. All felt ownership for the race, spectators and runners saw the BAA as caretakers of a public trust, burdened with the responsibility to manage the race, not vested with the right to cash in on it. But there was fear that a commercial Boston Marathon might destroy the tradition that had made the race so endearing. By 1985 the BAA had recaptured the marathon from Marshall Medoff, but it had done little to improve it relative to other world marathons. In fact the one world-class marathoner who came to race in Boston in 1985 faced no competition, only destruction of his own making.

In 1985 Geoff Smith ran in the lead again, but this year the race day temperature reached 70 °F. Smith reached for something. Perhaps as the Boston Marathon event itself seemed to be committing suicide, Smith tried suicide by running himself to death. Perhaps he wanted a world record. Why not? There was nothing to lose. In the 1983 New York City Marathon, where Smith had run his first half in 1:03:23, he felt that he had not made a mistake in going out too fast for the first half, but then had run too slowly for the second half. He thought that one day he would just keep going and that today was the day.

Smith had failed to renew his promotional contract with a shoe manufacturer, so he needed a fast time as a bargaining chip. The British selectors had placed him on the 1984 Olympic team because he had won the Boston Marathon that year, but in Los Angeles he had taken sick before the race, started hopefully, but had to quit at 14 miles. In Boston this year he faced a weak field. He'd won the year before; go for the record now, he figured. No runner anywhere near his caliber stood on the starting line. He could win nothing if he beat a poor field with a slow time, he could lose nothing if he tried to go fast because he had already handily beaten everyone in the field in other races. He could trot along next to whomever ran in the lead, then use his 3:55 mile speed to outkick him and win, but why bother? To win the race in a slow time would not earn him a cent or even a trifle of prestige. The Boston Marathon offered no money. Winning did not challenge Geoff Smith; running phenomenally fast did. It would partly atone for his missed Olympic opportunity. For him this was not a race in the usual sense but a public time trial; by the end, though, it seemed more like a public execution. In a sense he raced in a postal competition against the runners in London, Hiroshima, and Rotterdam. (Postal competitions were races held in the 1950s and '60s; runners ran track races on the same day in different cities and mailed their results to a central official, who compiled the results and mailed back the new list of all participants by time, saving travel expenses for everyone.)

A fast time would impress the rest of the world, especially those top Americans who had skipped Boston to run in the World Cup Marathon in Hiroshima the day before. In Hiroshima 18 runners broke 2:12:30, with Ethiopian Abebe Mekonnen running 2:09:05, Italian Orlando Pizzolato 2:10:23, and Tanzanian Juma Ikangaa 2:11:06; all of them would one day come to Boston (as would Welshman Steve Jones, who ran 2:08:16 in London a few days later).

Smith blasted out 5K in 14:15 as if he were racing against ghosts. That go-from-the-gun strategy had gotten Joan Benoit a world record. His coach, 73-year-old bald and paunchy Eddie Sones, said in his blunt, pithy way, "You don't set a world record by running slowly, now do you?" But the coach looked at the 3-mile split and saw three sub-4:40 miles. He said, "Geoff has the heart and courage of a great champion, but those first 3 miles are a little crazy." Smith calmed a bit to pass 10K in 29:05. No other runner had him in sight. He ran 1:02:51 for the first half. Was he planning a 2:05:42? That would show those guys in Hiroshima. If Geoff Smith could run faster, that would show them—so he attacked. He could afford to attack. No one clipped his heels or had the talent to catch him, as had Rod Dixon in New York in 1983 when Smith ran his 2:09:08 for second place. So he did not have to worry about tactics.

But it is not nice to fool Mother Nature. She does not like to give up world records without extracting a payment in pain. The day grew hot and muggy. At 20 miles Smith's split was still 18 seconds under the world record pace Steve Jones had set in Chicago on October 21, 1984. But Smith ran his 21st mile in 6:17. He stopped. He rubbed cramping hamstrings. Under the skin the muscles boiled, then relaxed. He began to run again. He staggered as the muscles cramped again. "I had to put one foot in front of the other and grit my teeth," Smith said. It hurt.

Downhill and far behind him word reached the two runners in second place, Dan Dillon and Gary Tuttle, that the leader walked. A spectator had heard about Smith's cramping on the radio and yelled to Dillon and Tuttle that one of them could win the whole race. The possibility had not occurred to either of them that day. They could not see Smith. For Dillon the idea came as a bolt. He was not an experienced marathoner, but he was a terrific cross-country runner who had run on the U.S. national team for many years. He was from Massachusetts and had run for the Greater Boston Track Club. It would be a tremendous thing if he could win the Boston Marathon. To follow the tradition of his GBTC teammates Rodgers and Meyer would be the running accomplishment of his life. His hopes and dreams bubbled up, and he bounded away from Tuttle to charge up the hills. In full-blown pursuit, Dillon looked ahead for Smith's walking figure. He had chased that shape before. He knew Smith well because they had been teammates at Providence College. In fact before the race he had posed with Smith in a publicity photo with Boston mayor and marathoner Ray Flynn, also a graduate of Providence College, who ran about 10 miles behind them.

But Smith's form did not pull into view. Under a hazy sun in temperatures in the low 70s on the gentle hills of Newton, the same thing happened to Dillon as to Smith; both struggled toward the finish at a minute per mile slower than their earlier pace. The gap between them did not change. Tuttle and others slogged past Dillon. Dillon faded to eighth place. His Boston Marathon dream of victory, short-lived, faded as had similar dreams of so many others. By 1993 Dillon had married Patti Catalano; they live in Boston with their young son. No one ran anymore; everyone slogged. Still, no other runner pulled Smith into sight. He had run so far ahead that he could walk and jog and not be caught. He would have dropped out of the race had the crowds let him. Like a reluctant gladiator in the coliseum, Smith was not free to quit the fight although the fight had quit him. At 2:14:05 Geoff Smith crossed the line on Ring Road at the Prudential Center. Tired and dehydrated, Smith did not run but walked across the finish line—not so much out of fatigue as frustration. He held his palms out and shrugged apologetically to the crowd. He had tried so hard to run fast. He had won the race by the largest victory margin since 1937, when Walter Young beat Johnny A. Kelley on a warm day, but Geoff Smith lost the time trial. And Boston may have lost its international marathon and become a mere local road race. The first non-U.S. resident finished sixth.

The year before Smith had won by 4:15. Added to this year's 5:06, that yielded a greater victory margin (9:21) in Smith's two wins than Bill Rodgers had in four wins (3:55) or Cote in his four (5:46). The gap illustrates the weakness of the field during these years. Smith's winning time was the slowest since Jerome Drayton had jogged through the heat in 1977. Without Smith the winning time would have been Gary Tuttle's 2:19:11, a finish that

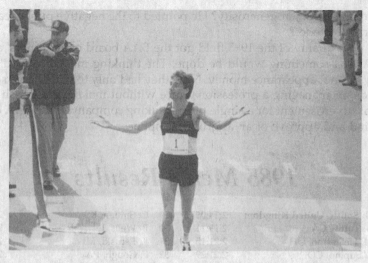

Though he won by 5 minutes, Geoff Smith apologizes to the crowd for a slow time in 1985. © Victah/Agence Shot.

would have placed 77th in 1983, 20th in 1982, and 19th in 1975. The best runners no longer came to Boston. The race was dying.

Many of the top runners could not consider traveling to a race that paid neither travel expenses nor appearance or prize money. Many with established reputations wanted appearance payments. The dark horses and ingenues wanted cash prizes. The BAA could not decide what to do. It looked like its marathon from here on would be a mediocre event with a rich tradition but only local importance. International professionals would ignore it. Unless the Boston Marathon began paying winners, it would be bypassed on the international circuit. It would have no future. It would become insignificant. Someone with lots of power, prestige, and money—someone besides Marshall Medoff—had to come along to pull Boston from the quaint past of amateurism and push it to catch up with the rest of the world.

Hints of change originated from various sources. Joe Catalano, who coached Lisa Weidenbach, the 1985 women's winner, and worked on the race committee charged with recruiting top runners to Boston, said, "Prize money wouldn't hurt. I think the BAA will make the changes that need to be made." BAA member Harold Carroll said that if someone could guarantee a good field just for prize money, they would consider it. He feared that elite runners' demands for appearance money and escalating prices would produce a beauty contest rather than a race. Race administrator Guy Morse wondered what would be lost if the race offered prize money. Would the community refuse to support the race with volunteers if they saw it as a commercial venture? Would they refuse to help if they thought someone made money off their generosity? He pointed to the negative public reaction to Marshall Medoff.

The poor quality of the 1985 field got the BAA board of governors' attention. At last something would be done. The thinking moved toward prize money but not appearance money. Now they had only to find a large source of funds for managing a professional race without making it a garish commercial advertisement for a single profit-making company. If the BAA could only find and approve of an appropriate sponsor.

1985 Men's Results

1.	G. Smith, United Kingdom	2:14:05	29.	C. Sniffen, KS	2:29:51
2.	G. Tuttle, CA	2:19:11	30.	B. Wells, IN	2:30:15
3.	M. Helgeston, OH	2:21:15	31.	L. Peruski, MI	2:30:29
4.	L. Supino, CO	2:21:29	32.	F. Gough, PA	2:30:47
5.	B. Doyle, MA	2:21:31	33.	E. Cohn, NY	2:30:54
6.	T. Mimura, Japan	2:23:35	34.	B. Beach, MD	2:30:55
7.	C. Hewes, NH	2:23:35	35.	Y. Yamamoto, Japan	2:31:15
8.	D. Dillon, MA	2:23:50	36.	B. Kuprewicz, ME	2:31:18
9.	C. Fletcher, FL	2:24:29	37.	D. Coyne, NY	2:31:21
10.	N. Blair, NC	2:25:23	38.	R. Wunderlich, FL	2:31:21
11.	R. Dyson, TX	2:25:36	39.	D. Smith, CA	2:31:25
12.	M. Amway, PA	2:26:22	40.	H. Suzuki, Japan	2:31:39
13.	W. Jacob, CT	2:26:59	41.	D. Gavoret, France	2:31:50
14.	M. Slavin, MA	2:26:59	42.	C. Trayer, PA	2:31:53
15.	S. Grygiel, MA	2:27:04	43.	R. Staback, IL	2:31:53
16.	M. Lohman, OH	2:27:11	44.	C. Fallon, Australia	2:31:56
17.	P. Kanfer, CA	2:27:12	45.	J. Hopkins, NJ	2:31:56
18.	J. Zupanc, WI	2:27:13	46.	S. Johnson, PA	2:32:11
19.	J. Worden, PA	2:27:20	47.	W. Nakai, NM	2:32:17
20.	E. Hurlow, MA	2:27:58	48.	K. Hicks, MA	2:32:23
21.	M. Novelli, TX	2:28:23	49.	G. Braun, WA	2:32:23
22.	B. Clifford, MA	2:28:27	50.	T. Loftus, TX	2:32:24
23.	P. Corrigan, OH	2:28:33	66.	G. Foley, MA	2:33:56
24.	K. Retelle, MA	2:28:36	197.	N. Weygandt, PA	2:42:10
25.	F. Schneck, PA	2:28:39	901.	P. Root, Canada	3:00:00
26.	J. Kallio, IL	2:29:26	2511.	R. Gorham, AZ	3:30:00
27.	J. McGuire, Canada	2:29:34	3428.	R. Flynn, MA	3:57:50
28.	R. Bayko, MA	2:29:35		J.A. Kelley (age 77)	4:31

4,894 starters.

Masters

1.	J. McGuire, Canada	2:29:34
2.	C. Fallon, Australia	2:31:56
3.	H. Goforth, CA	2:33:52

Team prize

Etonic A: N. Blair, W. Jacob, D. Hammond

TO PAY THE RENT

MONDAY, APRIL 22, 1985

Few Stand Out in Women's Field

Lisa Larsen Weidenbach, formerly of Michigan and who now lived in Marblehead, Massachusetts, took the 1985 lead at the start. Her mostly local competition proved ineffectual; she won by a gaping 8 minutes. Years earlier Weidenbach had swum competitively, specializing in the butterfly; in 1980 she had competed in the Olympic swim trials. But President Carter's Olympic boycott destroyed her enthusiasm for spending 5 hours a day staring at the bottom of a swimming pool. She took up running.

In the 1984 Olympic marathon trials Weidenbach had placed fourth. (She also would place fourth in the 1988 and the 1992 trials.) Her victory over the weakest women's field of the last 10 years did not impress her. At 23 years old she had run a 2:31:31 marathon. The second-place time nearly matched the world record winning time of Liane Winter in 1975, but in the rapidly evolving history of women's running, hundreds of women had run that fast.

At the finish she apologized for her slow time. She had hoped to run at least under 2:30. She ran nearly 12 minutes off Benoit's course record. Weidenbach entered the Boston Marathon because her sponsoring shoe company, Saucony, gave a bonus for a Boston win. She said, "My career is running and I follow all the amateur rules, but I have rent to pay and a car, and it's just very difficult to go to a race for a handshake. I'll probably be shot for saying that, but . . . sorry." She won the race, but she did not really outrace anyone. She won Boston because the best runners went elsewhere.

For runners like Bill Rodgers, Greg Meyer, Geoff Smith, and Lisa Larsen Weidenbach, the Boston Marathon could not remain on their competitive schedules. Runners of international caliber intended to race for prize money, for their ego as well as for money. The prize money assembled the talent. Runners who wanted to race against the best did it in prize money races. Top runners in nonpaying races would likely run furious solo time trials signifying nothing. The results of the 1985 Boston Marathon declared that it meant less to place well or even win Boston than it had in previous years. Without a decision from the board of governors to award prize money, the Boston Marathon would fall precipitously from its status of second in importance to the Olympic marathon. The board's intransigence might lead to a forfeit of Boston's most precious athletic possession. Will McDonough of the *Boston Globe* wrote, "The BAA board of governors is out of touch with reality. . . . They are on a self-destruct course and completely out of control."

A Consequence of Chasing Cash

New priorities overtook marathon running during the 1980s. Runners picked their races according to money, a practice that produced a strange hollow in the field in Boston. Before prize money became widely available, racers with the talent and training to run 2:15 to 2:25 all came to Boston to race against the best in the world. But once the Boston Marathon and most marathons offered prize money, the top runners in the world still came to Boston, but the 2:15 to 2:25 runners went to local prize money races to pick up paychecks. As a consequence, from 1986 on fewer (male) runners finished between 2:15 and 2:25 compared to the first 3 years of the 1980s, leaving a hollow, a sparseness in the field. Fortunately women came along to fill the gap. From 1986 on the women ran in a relatively traffic-free part of the race.

Note the progression of the first woman's finishing place across the decade—in 1980, Gareau ran in 201st place; 1981, Roe, 192nd; 1982, Teske, 148th; 1983, Benoit, 121st; but in 1986 the first woman ran 38th; in 1987, 40th; in 1988, 63rd; in 1989, 26th. Now, after the elite runners thunder past, a quiet time follows where the field loses the density of the early '80s; with few runners passing in the time interval for a 2:15 to 2:25 marathon, the course has an eerie feel for 10 minutes. While the excellent men and women come to Boston, where do all the pretty-good men go? Not to Boston— they're gone chasing cash.

1985 *Women's Results*

1.	L. Larsen Weidenbach, MA	2:34:06	5.	V. Smith, TX	2:46:33
		(67th overall)	6.	K. Northrop, NH	2:46:43
2.	L. Huntington, TX	2:42:15	7.	K. Moody, ME	2:46:51
3.	K. Dunn, NH	2:42:27	8.	M. Hynes, MA	2:48:57
4.	D. Butterfield, Bermuda	2:43:47	9.	E. Bulman, MO	2:50:16

10.	B. Dillinger, VA	2:50:36	19.	E. Portz, PA	2:58:33
11.	P. Wassik, CO	2:52:42	20.	M. Ireland, CA	2:59:11
12.	S. Lupica, MA	2:53:33	21.	L. Walmer, PA	2:59:44
13.	C. Andrew, NY	2:53:35	22.	K. Gilbert, MI	2:59:55
14.	S. Langlais, GA	2:55:34	23.	E. Brim-Snodgrass, OR	3:00:51
15.	B. Nelson, IN	2:55:38	24.	P. Burkes, CA	3:00:59
16.	P. Brown, CA	2:56:08	25.	D. Sottile, NY	3:01:14
17.	S. Zimmer, CT	2:56:53	221.	J. Kurk, UT	3:30:14
18.	N. Munroe, MA	2:58:19	458.	P. Bloom, MI	3:59:40

701 starters.

Masters

1.	M. Ishigami, Japan	3:03:47
2.	H. Walters, CA	3:10:56
3.	D. McDonald, MA	3:12:16

MONEY, MONEY, MONEY

MONDAY, APRIL 21, 1986

Aussie Marathoner Comes to Boston

To continue as a world-recognized race, the Boston Marathon had to find a rich friend. Top runners needed pay. But the acquisition of money and its dispersal had to be done fairly and properly. Runners nearly 50 years earlier had complained about money paid under the table to certain athletes. In a letter dated July 27, 1937, from a frequent back-of-the-pack Boston Marathon runner, A. Monteverde, to Clarence H. DeMar (because of DeMar's activism on behalf of amateur athletics), Monteverde said, "We athletes should govern ourselves, make our own laws, conduct games and have jurisdiction over sport, instead of a bunch of dishonest, arrogant racketeers who have long dwelt in the luxury of power, prestige and financial reward. Go after them. We are all with you."

Monteverde wrote to DeMar because DeMar spoke out against athletes' accepting money to appear at races. Monteverde had seen envelopes with cash passed from the meet committee to competitors in a track meet at Princeton, New Jersey. He listed the committee members and the athletes, who received sums like $1,300 and $300. He listed middle-distance runners Glenn Cunningham and Gene Venzke. Monteverde and DeMar maintained that it was fraudulent to tell the public that a track meet was among amateurs when money was being paid, making the race professional. "When the AAU, incorporated solely to govern the conduct of amateurs, openly violates the articles of their incorporation they are subject to investigation by authorities. And they have used the mail to continue their fraud," Monteverde's letter continued.

Few people in the world believed that top milers or marathoners, whether in 1937 or 1986, lived purely amateur athletic lives. Yet the debate continued about what was proper. In the 1940s and 1950s DeMar and old Kelley had actively sought gas money, meals, and lodging from race promoters. Overwhelmingly the public and runners themselves thought that runners did not need to be pure amateurs, but many members of the Boston Athletic Association held to the pro-amateur sentiments that Monteverde and DeMar held in the 1930s. Some said that only money for travel, meals, or lodging was OK. Others wanted to award prize money but not appearance money. In 1986 the BAA finally accepted that top athletes received money for top performances. How the money came, who provided it, what they expected in return and why is part of the story that follows. It is a story about a corporate sponsor within the story of an extraordinarily fast marathon. It must be told now because money, more than the essential athletic talent, won the 1986 Boston Marathon.

Without the good fortune of Geoff Smith's appearance in Boston in 1985, no world-ranked marathoners would have run. In 1986 other U.S. marathons—Houston, New Jersey, San Francisco—offered prize money. The best runners would go to one of them, not Boston. The BAA board of governors had to do something or the last and only reason for the existence of their association would disappear. Without top runners there would be no Boston Marathon as it had been known, and without the Boston Marathon there would be no Boston Athletic Association. Many companies wanted to plaster their names all over the marathon and would pay a great deal of money for the privilege, but the governors knew that the wrong sponsor might do more harm than no sponsor. The year before they had sold space on the runners' numbers, and they did so again, for $125,000. But to pay prize money they needed much more than that. What would they have to give up for more? Board member Harold Carroll wanted to keep finish line signage to a minimum. He wanted the finish banner to read "Boston Marathon," not to advertise a product, especially if the advertiser would change every year. He wanted to offer an attractive package of prize money to attract a top field. He did not want the marathon to become a garish billboard, looking like an automobile race, with the course and the runners papered with advertisements.

The potential sponsor had to want something more than ad space. The needs of the sponsor and the race had to mesh. The sponsor could not be transient and trashy. Not many candidates happened to have corresponding needs. But one old Boston company filled the bill.

The John Hancock Insurance Company had been in Boston since 1862, longer than the marathon. The company had built the tallest building in the city in 1976, slightly taller than the Prudential tower, and moved from its old, short, fat building to a new, slim, shining one. The new building symbolized the new company, or so they intended. The 62-story tower of steel and reflective glass, 790 feet high, dominated nearby Copley Square. Some say the building overpowered the square, but everyone could see the city reflected in its steep glass walls. Its sheer weight altered the geology of the land-filled Boston Back Bay where it stood; the foundation of the nearby Trinity Church had to be reinforced. The height of the building sucked air down to form a vortex around the base of the building on seemingly windless days. During construction in 1972 and 1973, the flex and sway of the building popped the glass out of the windows and carried it spinning and smashing to the pavement. The building that was supposed to symbolize modernity and progress had become a hazard. Plywood patches had to replace the popped windows, making the building appear to be a large bandaged mistake. It became the butt of jokes. The building had become an architectural and design nuisance and a public relations nightmare.

In the mid-1980s John Hancock wanted to change their business from predominantly insurance to the broader and lucrative field of financial services. They had assets of $38 billion. They spent $20 million a year on advertising. They wanted to change their image from a sleepy old stodgy company to an aggressive, modern, diversified, competent, dependable one. They wanted to increase their international business. But the bad building made the company look like a stodgy old fool.

With such a history in mind, the new head of corporate communications, David D'Alessandro, heard of the Boston Marathon's search for a sponsor. Instantly he saw the parallels. Both Hancock and the marathon had a rich and patriotic history linked solidly to the city of Boston and the American Revolution. John Hancock the patriot had lived in Boston, and the marathon had come to celebrate Patriots' Day and be associated in the minds of the public with Paul Revere and his famous ride. The link became as clear as red, white, and blue. Both institutions needed change. Both were old and needed something new.

D'Alessandro did what all fast-thinking executives do—he telephoned. He set up meetings. He presided over those meetings. He was a short man, aged 35, with a small moustache and a big cigar. He insisted all arrangements for this first Boston Marathon sponsored by John Hancock go smoothly. He saw to that personally. D'Alessandro said that a page of advertising in *Newsweek* cost $48,000 and, being advertising, created a credibility problem. But the one page *Newsweek* story on September 5, 1986, about BAA President Frank Swift's announcing the John Hancock sponsorship made the company look good and credible and cost nothing.

John Hancock's agreement with the BAA would cost $10 million over 10 years. In front of the Boston Public Library on Copley Square D'Alessandro wrote out the check for the finish line setup that cost $175,000 to $200,000, not including $25,000 for the two-story Diamond Screen video display. Other minor sponsors made donations of goods or services or bought advertising space in programs or on the racers' numbers.

In 1986 new numbers appeared beside the finishers' names and times—numbers preceded by dollar signs. At last winners and top finishers would get paychecks at the Boston Marathon. But first someone had to win the race. At least someone had to try.

Pete Pfitzinger, a U.S. Olympian from 1984 and 1988 pressed to the front guiding the leaders through the first mile in 4:37. He wore a faint, scruffy beard. Pfitzinger lived in Wellesley, had coached at the University of Massachusetts, and had been a member of the Greater Boston Track Club, where he trained with teammates Salazar, Meyer, Thomas, Hodge, and Rodgers. He worked for the New Balance Athletic Shoe Company. The pressure to race the Boston Marathon overwhelmed him. Continually, new Boston acquaintances, hearing that Pfitzinger raced long distances, would ask if he had run the Boston Marathon. When he replied no, but he had run in the Olympic marathon, people looked skeptical. Why not Boston? Pfitzinger saw the marathon course daily, yet year after year he had avoided entering for one good reason or another. But this year the inevitability of his running Boston caught up with him. You can't be a marathoner and live in Wellesley and not run the Boston Marathon. Perhaps in this year's run his emotions led him to race counter to the tactics that had worked for him in the past. His best strategy had been to run off the pace for the first miles, then work his way through a tiring pack to a striking position. He had won the Olympic trials that way, beating Salazar, and he had led all Americans in the Los Angeles Olympic marathon with his careful, cautious tactics to finish 11th in 2:13:53. But at Boston enthusiasm overpowered his common sense and carried him in front of the group through 10K in 30:08. It felt good to be there, grand perhaps.

But Pfitzinger faced a field almost as formidable as the Olympic one: the winner of the last two New York City marathons, Italian Orlando Pizzolato; Australian Rob de Castella; the 1983 Boston winner, Greg Meyer; Canadian Art Boileau; first-time Mexican marathoner, Arturo Barrios; Japan's Kunimitsu Ito; Kenya's Joe Kipsang. These men all ran with Pfitzinger through 10 miles. A terror began to creep into him as he realized that none of them was about to slow down.

De Castella took over in Wellesley. Pfitzinger could no longer imagine himself maintaining such a pace all the way to Boston. His faith evaporated. Depression replaced his enthusiasm. Sadder and wiser he stopped at his house, but he had tasted the lead of the Boston Marathon. He learned the lesson that would help him to make the 1988 Olympic team. Henceforth he would contain his enthusiasm, store it up for the last miles, and run his own race, not everyone else's.

Safe in his house in Wellesley, Pfitzinger had no idea that de Castella ran at world record pace. Sportswriters had picked de Castella to win Boston, but they had picked him to win the Olympic marathon too, and he had failed in Los Angeles. But in Boston no one could stay with him. Kipsang hung on the longest, but fatigue degraded his perfect stride into an anaerobic twist, with his upper body rotating to counter his fatigued legs; he too would drop out. De Castella ran on alone to a fast half-marathon time of 1:03:38; although not as fast as Smith had run the year before in his suicide race, it still presented the possibility of collapse in this less-than-ideal weather. De Castella, not a pretty runner but a bull who refused to get tired, ran through a humid day—rain would fall just after he finished—but he had every intention of racing the course to a new record.

De Castella came to Boston to race against the best. In previous years when asked if he would run Boston, he said that since the race did not attract elite athletes, he could not see a reason to go there. Now he saw the reason—and the dollar signs. He wanted to look back at his career and be able to say that he had run well not just on one race course year after year, but in every major marathon in the world. Had Boston offered no prize money and attracted no elite field, de Castella would have gone back to Rotterdam or on to London to win money and race against the best, but since he trained in Colorado, once Boston decided to offer prize money, his

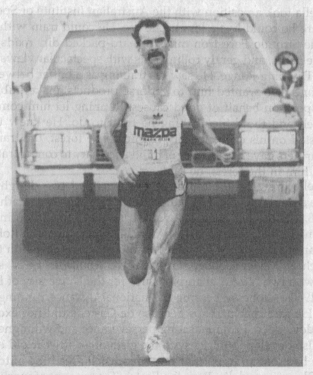

All alone on a course record pace, Rob de Castella still dares not look back. © Victah/ Agence Shot.

manager, IMG (International Management Group of Cleveland) advised him to go to Boston. D'Alessandro and John Hancock wanted de Castella to race in the Boston Marathon because he ranked as the best marathoner in the world. D'Alessandro had to have de Castella in his race, to reestablish Boston as the world's best marathon. D'Alessandro made it easy for de Castella to accept Boston's invitation with an appropriate amount of appearance money.

In Australia Rob de Castella commanded national fame. His handsome outdoorsman's face and trademark moustache appeared and reappeared in newspapers in every territory. No other athlete on the continent received more public attention. In Sydney and Melbourne de Castella could not finish a meal in a public place without being pestered by autograph seekers. Announcement of the birth of his daughter took front-page space in several of the nation's newspapers. He had finished a gratifying 10th in the Moscow Olympic marathon, but after his win in Fukuoka in 1981 with an astonishing 2:08:18, his life changed. He won the Commonwealth Games Marathon by 12 seconds over Tanzanian Juma Ikangaa in 2:09:18. Australians expected him to win the gold medal for them in Los Angeles, but in the cloying heat he placed 5th in 2:11:09. Some Australians called him a "dolebludger," someone who is lazy and self-indulgent. That characterization hurt de Castella; he trained hard, raced hard, and worked hard.

De Castella took a position with the Australian Institute of Sport in Canberra, where he could live a less hectic life. He could train with long runs through the Stromlo Forest on miles of hard-packed dirt roads, forgiving pine-needle paths, and gently rolling hills with spectacular views of Australia's Great Dividing Range. He saw his training as a buffer between himself and everyone who wanted him to endorse products, make public appearances, or speak on behalf of good causes. Running let him come to terms with himself and the difficult thing he tried to do. He knew that all his success rested on his diligent daily training. The forest, the trails, and his training partners gave him a peace of mind necessary to concentrate. Nobody could find him in the forest, he said.

De Castella grew up the oldest of five sons and two daughters in the Melbourne suburb of Kew. His father, Rolet, ran over 20 marathons with a best of 2:58. His brother Nicholas would run a 2:15 marathon in the fall of 1983, making him the second fastest Australian marathoner to Rob that year. As a 12-year-old Rob joined his father for morning runs. He didn't like them. Rob's coach at Xavier College, an exclusive Jesuit-run boys' school, Pat Clohessy, won two NCAA championships for the University of Houston in the early 1960s. Clohessy became the national distance running coach for Australia. He said that perhaps because de Castella did not excel at other sports, he developed a compensating perseverance and willingness to work hard. He also developed thighs with the girth of an 18-year-old eucalyptus.

After he had lost an important race, de Castella read the autobiography of British Olympic medalist Brendan Foster. The amount of work Foster put into his running impressed de Castella. Foster wrote, "All top international athletes wake up in the morning feeling tired and go to bed feeling very tired." De Castella had not yet realized the difficulty and the singlemindedness of the training. He did not have the talent to approach international marathon racing frivolously. To be the best runner he could be, he had to devote himself monastically to the task. Once he adopted a singularity of purpose, everything in his life, from his spouse to his education, related to running.

After Xavier, de Castella earned a double degree in biophysics and instrumental science from Swinburne College in Melbourne. A biophysicist at the Sport Institute, de Castella saw himself and his year's worth of 130-mile weeks as a one-subject experiment. With the foundation of a scientific, meticulous, almost instrumental approach to the study of his own body in his preparation, de Castella took the lead in the Boston Marathon.

Barrios ran in third. Many expected Barrios with his superior speed to challenge de Castella. De Castella expected any one of the pack to come up to his shoulder to challenge him at any time. He did not dare back off the pace or relax. His strength was his strength, not his speed, relative to other runners of his accomplishment. He could tell himself that he had been the most consistent marathoner in the world for the past 6 years. He had won the Commonwealth Games Marathon, Fukuoka, and the inaugural World Championships in Helsinki, Finland. But he also knew he was not infallible; he had run poorly in the Olympic marathon. So he did not dare look back. He had tried to leave nothing to chance. He had trimmed all the excess paper from his racing number, judiciously leaving only the sponsor's name, Ricoh (a Japanese company that made photocopying machines), and his number, 1.

Boileau moved up on Pizzolato, and settled in behind him. Boileau's drafting annoyed Pizzolato. He waved to Boileau, indicating that he should pass. Boileau would not pass. He reasoned that it was Pizzolato who had the bigger name so it was OK to draft off him. De Castella extended his lead. He had written the split times for a 2:08 marathon in waterproof ink on his palm. He was 29 years old.

De Castella lived in two places: Canberra and Boulder, Colorado. He trained full-time for running. Yet his apparent jet-set lifestyle contrasted with the stoicism necessary for marathon training. He drove an Alfa Romeo and a Toyota, in Colorado a Subaru. Friends called him "Deek." Neighbors said they could set their watches by his regular training on the same loops at the same times and at the same pace. He suppressed opportunities for flamboyance.

De Castella married a woman named Gayelene Clewes. They met and fell in love in Limerick, Ireland, in 1979 when both were members of the Australian national cross-country team. Together they lived wandering, freelance athletic lives in two hemispheres. They had a 2-1/2 year old daughter, but both remained active competitors; Clewes traveled the American triathlon circuit and won several major races. Later she ran the Boston Marathon herself, although she never emphasized marathon racing. But this year while Rob raced, Gayelene sat in their Boston hotel room, nervously knitting a sweater for their daughter. By end of the race she had finished it.

At 18 miles Barrios ran 45 seconds behind de Castella. Barrios had extraordinary talent but didn't show it in this, his first marathon. A precise and patient young man who graduated from Texas A&M in chemical engineering, he would have to wait for another day to run his marathon. Boileau ran away from Pizzolato. Boileau, a 28-year-old native of Edmonton, Alberta, lived and trained in Eugene, Oregon, after graduating from the University of Oregon. Alberto Salazar's coach, Bill Dellinger, coached Boileau, too. Boileau had never earned any significant money as a runner, although he had a small contract with the Tiger athletic shoe company.

De Castella charged up the hills. Running up slopes in the thin air of Colorado prepared him well; he powered up Heartbreak Hill. The *London Daily Express* once described de Castella as running as "if he was tearing jungle undergrowth out of his way." The hill miles fell away behind him in 4:56, 4:54, 4:57, and 5:13. He broke all checkpoint records from 20 miles on. Barrios faded, his thin thighs constricted by cramps. Bill Rodgers gained on him. Rodgers had been running with Greg Meyer when Meyer turned to him and said, "I'm beat as a dog; go along." Rodgers had been feeling bad for 15 miles but now felt fine, so he did move along, but he suffered in the last miles in his pursuit of Barrios. Boileau passed Pizzolato near Coolidge Corner. He could not see de Castella and knew he could not catch him, but he also knew that no one would catch him. Rodgers electrified the crowds as he caught Barrios in the final mile. But for Rodgers there was no savoring this little victory. Eleven years after his first win at Boston, Rodgers could still be a factor, but not without running himself to his limit. Three minutes behind de Castella, Art Boileau ran on to the biggest paycheck of his life for second place. De Castella powered through the finish line tape with his thighs flapping and his fists in the air.

For his running at Boston, Rob de Castella earned several paychecks, in addition to money from adidas for wearing their shoes and shirt and from the Mazda automobile manufacturer for displaying their name prominently on his chest as he broke the finish line tape to win $60,000 and a dark blue Mercedes-Benz. He ran a course record of 2:07:51 to break Salazar's course record of 2:08:52. Only the Olympic gold medalist, Portugal's Carlos Lopes, with his 2:07:12 in Rotterdam in April 1985 and Great Britain's Steve Jones in the previous fall's Chicago Marathon with 2:07:13 had run faster. For his 2:07:51, "Deek" won $30,000, another $25,000 for breaking the course record, and $5,000 for a sub-2:10. His "personal services" contract with John Hancock was $75,000, with the promise to double it if he won. (Personal services contracts paid for perfunctory talks and promotional activities at "clinics" where members of the public could meet contracted athletes.) All told, de Castella earned over $250,000, and he negotiated an appearance guarantee of $150,000 for the next year. The Boston Marathon would never again be an amateur event. It would not fade away, but it would never be the same.

Someone suggested to Bill Rodgers that he might train a little harder to win in 1987. But Rodgers realized that the race and the sport had reached new levels—levels beyond his talent. At age 38 he was not about to take 2 minutes off his personal record, but neither was he about to quit the marathon just because he could not win against the new generation. He answered, "That's ludicrous. I just want to keep in shape to set masters' records when I turn 40 in 2 years." As much as Rodgers enjoyed depositing ever-larger and more frequently offered checks for appearances at races, his love remained the pleasure of running well.

Checkpoint Splits

5K	Pete Pfitzinger/Rob de Castella	14:55
5 miles	Pete Pfitzinger/Rob de Castella	24:11
10K	Pete Pfitzinger/Rob de Castella	30:08
15K	Rob de Castella	45:22
10 miles	Rob de Castella	48:42
20K	Rob de Castella	1:00:23
half marathon	Rob de Castella	1:03:38
25K	Rob de Castella	1:15:16
30K	Rob de Castella	1:30:20
20 miles	Rob de Castella	1:37:08
35K	Rob de Castella	1:45:51
40K	Rob de Castella	2:01:05
25 miles	Rob de Castella	2:01:51
one-to-go	Rob de Castella	2:02:54
finish	Rob de Castella	2:07:51
last mile	Rob de Castella	4:57

1986 Men's Results

1.	R. de Castella, Australia	2:07:51ᶜᴿ	12.	G. Meyer, MI	2:17:29
2.	A. Boileau, Canada	2:11:15	13.	H. Nagashima, Japan	2:17:38
3.	O. Pizzolato, Italy	2:11:43	14.	G. Huggins, PA	2:18:11
4.	B. Rodgers, MA (age 38)	2:13:36	15.	B. Doyle, RI	2:19:03
5.	A. Barrios, Mexico	2:14:09	16.	M. Hurd, England	2:19:04
6.	B. Hodge, MA	2:14:50	17.	T. Fieldsend, OK	2:19:19
7.	D. Tibaduiza, Colombia	2:15:22	18.	M. Patterson, PA	2:21:14
8.	P. Cummings, UT	2:16:05	19.	K. Johnsen, Denmark	2:21:19
9.	D. Schlesinger, MA	2:16:29	20.	N. Cusack, Ireland	2:21:24
10.	K. Ito, Japan	2:17:02	21.	S. Liuttu, VA	2:22:12
11.	P. Tiainen, VA	2:17:04	22.	P. McGovern, MA	2:22:18

23.	M. Bossardet, NY	2:22:29	41.	M. Meyers, WI	2:26:16
24.	P. Kanfer, CA	2:22:42	42.	H. Chavez, Mexico	2:26:34
25.	L. Lopez, Costa Rica	2:22:42	43.	S. Grygiel, MA	2:26:42
26.	C. Hewes, NH	2:23:16	44.	J. DeJesus, Puerto Rico	2:26:57
27.	C. Carl, NM	2:23:17	45.	J. Loeschhorn, CA	2:27:03
28.	J. Molloy, TX	2:23:27	46.	R. Taylor, PA	2:27:06
29.	M. Skinkle, RI	2:23:59	47.	R. Blatt, CT	2:27:13
30.	D. Coyne, NY	2:24:06	48.	B. Igoe, MA	2:27:25
31.	B. MacGillivray, Canada	2:24:09	49.	R. Bayko, MA	2:27:36
32.	S. Molnar, PA	2:24:15	50.	M. Pringle, MA	2:27:41
33.	M. Whelan, NY	2:24:27	74.	C. Policarpio, Bolivia	2:30:23
34.	J. Flores, TX	2:24:32	**354.**	**J. Fultz, Weston, MA**	**2:43:41**
35.	J. Sheridan, Ireland	2:24:35	1227.	M. McCusker, MA	3:00:34
36.	T. Augat, IL	2:24:43	**1274.**	**J.J. Kelley (age 55)**	**3:01:40**
37.	R. Bieber, PA	2:24:44	1703.	M. Roach, MA	3:09:28
38.	L. Roberts, England	2:24:59	2651.	B. Crow, FL	3:30:00
39.	M. Slavin, MA	2:25:16	3211.	R. Flynn, MA	3:52:47
40.	J. Sipploa, VA	2:25:46		**J.A. Kelley (age 78)**	**4:27:00**

40-49

1.	M. Hurd, England	2:19:04[MCR]
2.	J. Sheridan, Ireland	2:24:35
3.	L. Roberts, England	2:24:59

60-99

| 1. | F. DiMarco, CT | 3:05:31 |

50-59

| 1. | J. Weston, Canada | 2:35:22 |

[MCR]denotes masters course record.

HEGNE NORGE

MONDAY, APRIL 21, 1986

Norwegian Woman Comes to Crack 2:20

Born on March 21, 1956, in Trondheim on Norway's northwest coast, Ingrid Christiansen (later to become Kristiansen) grew up a beaming snow-child who cross-country skied every weekend with her parents and older brother. Ski racing followed. Christiansen excelled. She joined the national ski team, placed second in the national championships three times from 1976 to 1980, and skied to many fourth and fifth places. She loved to ski and skied long and fast. But she never won a national title on skis.

Christiansen could not pursue skiing after college when she left Trondheim to work as a cancer researcher in Stavanger, on the coast 500 kilometers to the south. Working allowed her less time to find good skiing snow. She tried running and liked it because it met the same needs for movement and competition as skiing and ski racing. In 1981 she married Arve Kristiansen, a 2:34 marathoner who worked as an engineer for the Norwegian National Oil Company planning oil production in the deepest parts of the North Sea. By the mid-1980s the family, including son Gaute born in 1983, moved into a spacious pine house in a quiet residential district of Oslo.

Within 9 days of Gaute's birth Ingrid began hard training; 5 months later she won the 1984 Houston Marathon in 2:27:51 and 3 months later set a European marathon record of 2:24:26 in the 1984 London Marathon. "She is an enigma, a woman who keeps her intense dedication successfully segregated from the rest of her life, shrugs off setbacks and belies her strength with a genuine happy-go-lucky demeanor," said Cliff Temple, a British coach and writer. Ordinarily Kristiansen was jolly, but when she raced she was fierce.

Ingrid Kristiansen blasted out of Hopkinton with a 26:00 for the first 5 miles of the 1986 Boston Marathon. She wanted to run a sub-2:20. She had already run the fastest marathon in the world; now she wanted to run faster. Perhaps all her life she had been preparing for the coming 2 hours.

Johan Kaggestad, Norway's national distance running coach, met with Kristiansen at least once a week. She frequently trained on hills. Coach Kaggestad said, "Her hill training involves no more than one-minute intervals because she has quite a low anaerobic threshold and when she passes it she gets much slower and runs with poor form. High-level intervals on the track just don't work for her." Kristiansen had managed to avoid many of the injuries that plagued other top marathoners. Kaggestad said she listened well to her body, so if she felt awful one day she would simply take it off.

At the 5-mile split she ran 11 seconds faster than had Joan Benoit in her course record run in 1983. "A woman can break 2:20. I want to be the one to do it," both had said. The idea especially obsessed Benoit, now Samuelson, who had to watch Kristiansen run. Benoit Samuelson thought, with remorse, that surely Kristiansen would break 2:20 and snatch the honor of being the first to destroy that barrier. Benoit Samuelson was not fit to race; having had a second operation on her heels, she had not done enough training to run a fast marathon. Without Benoit Samuelson, who had run 2:21:21 in Chicago to beat Kristiansen, there was not a woman in the field who could run within a mile of her.

Kristiansen's pace would yield about a 2:17 marathon. After her world record of 2:21:06 at London, a sub-2:20 seemed like the product of reasonable arithmetic. She had run a world record of 14:58.89 for 5,000 meters and held the world record for 10,000 meters. She could have simply raced to win, collected the money and the Mercedes-Benz with no risk. A tactical race looked like a sure thing to grant Kristiansen victory. Another Norwegian, Grete Waitz, the role model of all Norwegian women distance runners, had tried for a world record sub-2:20 on the Boston course in 1982 and had been forced to drop out. To run for a tactical win made good business sense. A sensible, even pace would allow considerable profit-taking.

But Ingrid Kristiansen ran for more than business reasons. Although she had a contract with Nike to wear their clothing and shoes, she came to race, not advertise. But she did wear Nike's bright yellow Sock Racer, a shoe with an all-elastic fabric upper that certainly would have impressed S.T.A.R. Ritchins back in the 1930s. To advertise the shoes further, Nike promotional executives hung

For women, 2:20 had become a barrier, as the 4-minute mile had been for men.

two multistory-long inflated models from a building in sight of the finish area. Like de Castella, Kristiansen had a contract to wear the Mazda name on her chest. She wanted to break the 2:20 barrier for the marathon before any other woman in the world. Also, D'Alessandro and John Hancock had paid her well and arranged all her expenses for the trip, and she knew they would like a world record or a course record for their money. A world record run would declare that the Boston Marathon had reclaimed international importance. Sponsors' and athlete's interests meshed; art and business merged. The beauty of running fast would also make money for her sponsors. Kristiansen also knew that to deliver a record she would have to gamble. For women, 2:20 had become a barrier, as the 4-minute mile had been for men. It could not be broken by a mere decision to do so.

Kristiansen also raced against the ghost of Benoit Samuelson's course record of 2:22:43. Beating her course record might be good revenge for the loss at Chicago. For Kristiansen to train to race against Benoit Samuelson, to train to beat her record, showed respect. Above the treadmill where she trained to escape Norway's winters, Kristiansen kept a photo of Joan breaking the tape in the 1983 Boston Marathon, with the electronic timer reading 2:22:43. Temperatures in Oslo's January average −5 °C, so Kristiansen ran up to 150 kilometers a week on the treadmill, alternately looking into a mirror to check her form and at Benoit's photo, then setting to running with infused intensity. Like the sign on Tom Fleming's wall, the photo reminded Kristiansen that her friend Joan might be out there training when she was not.

Samuelson sat out the race in front of television cameras, contributing color commentary to the broadcast. She watched with a mixture of excitement and apprehension. She mildly preferred to see her course record remain, she wanted her friend Ingrid to win, and she wanted to see an exciting, newsworthy race, but more than anything she would liked to have been in the race, pushing the pace under 2:20 herself. But she could not have that. She tried to suppress her disappointment as she commented on the air.

By the halfway mark Kristiansen still ran a sub-2:20 pace with a 1:09:44, but she knew that the early downhills made the Boston course easier and faster for the first half than the second.

As Kristiansen approached the Newton hills she gradually realized that sub-2:20 would have to wait for another day but she might have a shot at the course record. She did not run herself into a wall, but she sensed that the even apportionment of her speed and endurance under these somewhat warm conditions would not allow her Norwegian body to sustain sub-5:20 miles over the remaining distance. By the top of the hills she realized that she could not break Benoit Samuelson's course record either. Only then did she slow and run conservatively to insure that she would finish ahead of the other women. She won the race in distress. In a curious detachment of her self and her body she said she felt fine; her mind was in the race but her body was not. "Am I disappointed? Yes, I am. . . . I won a race, and I am glad for that. But I will have to wait for another time to break the 2:20 barrier. . . . That was my goal for today."

Kristiansen said that her body had played an awful trick on her. The problems started the day before as a result of menstruation, which caused more physical symptoms than usual and painfully upset her stomach to the distraction of running sub-5:20 miles. But her disappointment did not last long. Her husband said that above all she was a happy runner. "If she aims for a record and doesn't get it, she may be annoyed for an hour but that's it. She doesn't take it too seriously. She will come back to Boston and try to break 2:20 again."

Kristiansen won in 2:24:55, ahead of Carla Beurskens from the Netherlands. She won a car and $35,000. Lorraine Moller never seemed to be able to get herself going that day, but she would be back too. The first woman masters

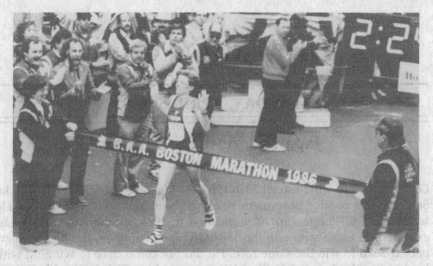

Ingrid Kristiansen blasted out of Hopkinton in pursuit of Benoit's record, but Kristiansen would have to come back again. © Victah/Agence Shot.

runner was a 44-year-old elementary school cook from Lidkoping, Sweden, named Evy Palm. She earned $12,000 for her record-breaking fourth place.

1986 Women's Results

1.	I. Kristiansen, Norway	2:24:55		16.	E. Guevera-Mora, FL	2:47:37
		(38th overall)		17.	O. Bruni, CA	2:49:22
2.	C. Beurskens, Netherlands	2:27:35		18.	G. Speery, VT	2:49:34
3.	L. Bussieres, Canada	2:32:16		19.	M. Ballentyne, MA	2:50:30
4.	E. Palm, Sweden	2:32:47		20.	D. Sottile-Mastalli, NY	2:51:24
5.	S. Keskitalo, Finland	2:33:18		21.	B. Dillinger, VA	2:51:26
6.	J. Isphording, OH	2:33:40		22.	N. Munroe, MA	2:51:51
7.	C. Vahlensieck, West Germany	2:34:50		23.	M. Anderson, MA	2:53:19
8.	L. Moller, New Zealand	2:35:06		24.	P. Sher, FL	2:54:11
9.	E. Claugus, CA	2:38:23		25.	S. Dianat, NH	2:54:22
10.	E. Rochefort, Canada	2:40:00		26.	M. Schwan, Wellesley, MA	2:54:59
11.	H. Stewart, New Zealand	2:41:12		42.	L. Downey, WY	3:00:14
12.	M. Hynes, MA	2:41:50		276.	B. Zolldan, CA	3:30:00
13.	S. Grottenberg, OR	2:43:00		456.	K. Dailey, MN	3:59:57
14.	B. Rothman, FL	2:43:36			P. Catalano, DNF	
15.	A. Kemp, CA	2:46:52				

642 entrants, 593 starters.

40-49

1.	E. Palm, Sweden	2:32:47[MCR]
2.	B. Rothman, FL	2:43:36
3.	B. Nelson, IN	2:58:06

50-59

1.	W. Yu, NY	3:18:23

60-99

1.	M. Miller, CA	3:23:38

THE WAITING GAME

MONDAY, APRIL 20, 1987

Japan's Finest Back for #2

On a humid and windy April 20 in 1987, the Japanese marathoner Toshihiko Seko ran in a pack of 19 runners. Seko had been to Boston twice before. He was second to Rodgers in 1979 and first in 1981. As the Australians had expected de Castella to win the 1984 Olympic marathon, the Japanese expected Seko to win the same race. He did not come close to winning with his fourteenth-place finish. That failure stung him. The death of his coach several months later hurt him too. Kiyoshi Nakamura died in a drowning accident that some speculated was a ritual suicide to atone for his charge's failure. On days before the race in Boston, Nakamura's widow prepared Seko's meals. He wanted to win the Boston Marathon for the memory of his coach. He had already won the London Marathon and the Chicago Marathon (Chicago in a personal best of 2:08:27 in October of 1986). For his country he wanted to amend his poor Olympic showing. Seko said to himself as he ran in that big Boston pack that he *must* win. The humid weather and the headwind turned the race into a big waiting game. They ran through 10 miles in 50:28, 2 minutes slower than in 1986. De Castella and the Olympic silver medalist, John Treacy of Ireland, waited too.

Born June 4, 1957, in Waterford, Ireland, Treacy, like Geoff Smith, came to Rhode Island's Providence College. He earned a degree in accounting and a master's degree in business administration in 1980. He had watched the Boston race in 1986 and saw it as the greatest in the world. Of all the world's races, Treacy most wanted to win the Boston Marathon. He had already won the World Cross-Country Championships twice, in 1978 in Glasgow, Scotland, and in 1979 in Limerick, Ireland. He had run under 2:10 in his first marathon, the Olympic marathon. As he waited for his second marathon to begin, he knew he was fit and fast because he had run a 28-minute 10K 2 weeks earlier. The starter, however, had waited for no one.

As the seconds closed on noon, two BAA officials and a police officer lingered in front of the starting area. The rope used to hold back the runners and define the starting line remained in place. The race starter, former BAA president Tom Brown, intended to begin exactly at 12:00. He held the starting pistol at his side. Tradition dictated that the race start at the stroke of noon, ready or not. Brown, of the same family as his predecessors George V. and Walter, held to that tradition—but he did not know that a restraining rope remained in place at waist height in front of the runners. He did not count down the start or give the runners any instruction to get ready. While looking at his watch he raised the pistol and fired it. The field of 5,315 charged, engulfing the BAA officials and the police officer. The runners did not know the restraining rope remained in place. It caught Rob de Castella. He tripped and fell to the ground. Thousands of runners moved to trample him. The press made a big show of it, but de Castella had fallen in other races and had always gotten up and back into the race. He did not ponder the idea of staying on the ground. Reflexively he rolled and quickly bounced up to follow the leaders. He suffered only scratches. The much-reported incident did bring to mind Jerome Drayton's criticism of the unprofessional start 10 years earlier. De Castella said that the fall did not influence the outcome of the race.

De Castella, however, had raced too much, and that did influence the outcome. The fall offered a good excuse to drop out and take his $150,000 appearance money, but he got back into the race. He had come to town to race and he would race, tired or not. As he rolled off the ground he found himself in 50th place. He gradually worked his way up to the back of the lead pack of 19. Unlike the year before, he had no urge to break open the race. Last year he felt omnipotent. Now he did not have the unbeatable strength or fitness to run away. A lack of attention to details by the race organization annoyed him. He expected water stops every 5 kilometers, as is the case in most international marathons. But Boston tradition placed them at 1.9 miles and at 2.3, then none for 6 miles. Without omnipotence de Castella had to rely on tactics, so he conserved his energy waiting for others to fall off the pace.

All the others did the same thing. No one seemed to want to race. Everyone wanted to wait. Why? The thick headwind did not refresh the runners as had the wind from an ocean storm some other years. Instead the air flowed in their faces like some animal's hot breath. Humidity approached 100%. The stickiness killed the usually irrepressible macho urge in someone to break the race open. Water splashed on runners' heads did not evaporate to cool them, nor did their own sweat evaporate effectively. Sweat pooled and each runner stewed in his own, waiting.

Juma Ikangaa of Tanzania pressed his little body against that wind. He insisted on staying at the head of the pack, but the ever-present wind whittled away at his strength. De Castella watched him and knew he would eventually pay the price for his bravery. All the others, stingy with their energy, tried to hide from the wind.

But another reason might have accounted for the reluctant pace. Many of these runners, not in peak condition, received appearance money from John Hancock in excess of the potential prize money that their level of fitness suggested that they might win. The director of the Chicago Marathon, Bob Bright, told the *Boston Globe* that the ratio of appearance money to prize money looked so out of line that it encouraged not-in-top-shape runners to play it safe. It seemed ironic that if Hancock's involvement the year before had produced a high-quality race by injecting cash for prizes and appearances that the same injection of cash could now have the opposite effect.

Of course this accusation made no sense to the men and women who stood to win races or had accomplished enough to receive appearance money. Bright and the Chicago Marathon had set the market and now resented that D'Alessandro, the Boston Marathon, and Hancock had taken leadership. Top runners knew that their creditability was on the line every time they were, and if they had agreed tacitly or overtly not to compete they would be seen through, found out, and dropped from the invitational running circuit.

Hancock had recruited top runners through clinic fees, personal services contracts, and appearance fees, deals that ranged from $1,000 to $50,000, with individually negotiated time and performance incentives and bonuses. Money to marathoners clearly helped the sport, but since the practice had so recently developed no one had found a balance among the possible sources of money to athletes. The balance remained somewhere between a risky all-prize money scheme and an all-salary scheme. In the common professional team sports, players earned salaries as team members. They did not win prize money for every game, but they did get bonuses for winning championships. In a way Hancock provided a team, but it had no team to compete against. Future races would have to sort the options in a way that recognized the unique nature of athletics where performance can be absolutely measured against a standard compared with games where physical performance is relative to the talents and tactics of the other team.

Everyone in the lead pack had talent and knew tactics. The half marathon passed in 1:06:22, a 2:12:44 pace. The 15th mile passed in a slow 5:17, a common training pace for everyone in the pack. John Treacy, the Olympic silver medalist, waited too. He had trained for 11 months, thinking of the Boston Marathon every day.

Treacy planned to stay with the pack until 20 miles, then go. Still Seko waited, the only runner seething with any urge to go. All the others surveyed the surrounding talent and, each man feeling he had no superior speed or strength, decided to exercise only caution.

Seko looked around the pack at his competition. He saw sweat on all their faces. He thought that Steve Jones sweated too much. He thought Treacy appeared to have problems with his back. He watched Smith labor. *Globe* columnist Leigh Montville watched from the press bus and described Seko: "He looked as if he could run across fire and through steam and deep into the center of the earth." But to everyone else Seko looked calm, rested, and analytical. He felt calm and in control. Seko looked at Geoff Smith. Smith looked at Seko and shot him a cavalier smile. Seko did not smile back; he just took off.

Smith and Jones felt honor-bound to go with him. This showed the courage that Smith's coach Eddie Sones admired. But courage or no, with miles of

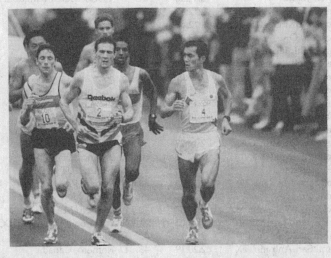

Toshihiko Seko took a long last look at the pack, including Geoff Smith (#10) and Steve Jones (#2), and said *sayonara*. © Victah/Agence Shot.

4:49, 4:52, and 4:40 from 20 through 22, Seko shrugged off the Britons. Smith thought maybe he shouldn't have smiled at Seko. Smith lost contact last. Jones caught back up to Smith. They forged an alliance to work together to catch Seko. Seko might yet fail. Treacy rallied to join Smith and Jones. They shared water. Treacy had beaten Seko by a lot in the Olympic marathon. He pressed after Seko. Seko had failed at the Olympic marathon in this kind of weather. But this time he would not fail. He had prepared fiercely for this kind of weather after his Olympic disappointment. It was Treacy who failed. On the downhills he felt as if his legs had been whacked. At 22 miles he walked. He had lived for this race for nearly a year; with bitter disappointment he jogged to the finish, managing to cross one place ahead of 39-year-old Bill Rodgers.

Seko completed the second half faster than the first, with a 1:05:28; he finished with a clenched fist in the air and gruesome concentration on his face. When he saw Mrs. Nakamura the gruesomeness drained from his face; he bowed. Seko won $40,000 and a $31,000 Mercedes-Benz. Smith and Jones made the turn onto Hereford Street together. After their working together for all those miles to catch Seko, it remained to see who would take second and who third. They talked about the wisdom of tying, but that would only fuel the argument that appearance money took the racing out of marathoners. After all, they had come to race. Friends or not, racing resided in their bones. Pride and honor mattered as much as dollars. They shook hands as they decided to sprint for it. Jones beat Smith.

1987 Men's Results

1. **T. Seko, Japan**	**2:11:50**	
2. S. Jones, United Kingdom	2:12:37	
3. **G. Smith, United Kingdom**	**2:12:42**	
4. D. Gorden, OR	2:13:30	
5. T. Taniguchi, Japan	2:13:40	
6. **R. de Castella, Australia**	**2:14:24**	
7. D. Vanderherten, Belgium	2:15:02	
8. E. Hellebuyck, Belgium	2:15:16	
9. H. Kita, Japan	2:15:23	
10. K. Martin, Phoenix, AZ	2:15:41	
11. J. Ikangaa, Tanzania	2:16:17	
12. A. Aregha, Decatur, GA	2:16:23	
13. R. Umberg, Sweden	2:17:01	
14. J. Treacy, Ireland	2:17:50	
15. **B. Rodgers, MA (age 39)**	**2:18:18**	
16. J. Padel, France	2:18:49	
17. B. Bickford, Wellesley, MA	2:18:57	
18. Y. Takahashi, Japan	2:19:03	
19. E. Eyestone, Orem, UT	2:19:19	
20. R. Yara, San Antonio, TX	2:20:19	
21. K. Souminen, Finland	2:21:10	
22. D. Tibaduiza, Colombia	2:21:35	
23. G. Fanelli, PA	2:21:36	
24. D. Clark, United Kingdom	2:21:37	
25. B. Clifford, MA	2:21:40	
26. G. Pezerat, France	2:22:10	
27. M. Patterson, PA	2:22:21	
28. L. Lopez, Costa Rica	2:22:25	
29. A. Oman, NY	2:22:38	
30. B. Bobes, France	2:23:52	
31. M. Cobb, CT	2:24:22	
32. J. Eastman, VA	2:24:23	
33. T. Latincsics, NJ	2:24:23	
34. E. Lee, United Kingdom	2:24:39	
35. F. Weber, NJ	2:24:45	
36. J. Zupanc, WI	2:24:46	
37. N. Segura, UT	2:24:51	
38. I. Meyers, PA	2:24:59	
39. M. Hunt, New Zealand	2:25:19	
40. J. Madden, MA	2:25:28	
41. R. Robinson, Washington, DC	2:25:31	
42. D. McDonald, VA	2:26:04	
43. D. Romero, Canada	2:26:21	
44. F. Schuler, IL	2:26:26	
45. B. Klecker, MN	2:26:36	
46. T. Abbott, PA	2:26:44	

47.	T. Mikata, Japan	2:26:46	2304.	J.J. Kelley, CT (age 56)	3:08:46
48.	G. Hageman, WI	2:26:49	3283.	H. Short, VT	3:22:38
49.	G. Guillemette, RI	2:26:56	4266.	R. Flynn, MA	3:54:54
50.	L. Bandt, MO	2:26:58	4490.	J.A. Kelley (age 79)	4:19:56
71.	B. McClement, WA	2:29:49			

4,576 starters.

40-49

1.	D. Clark, United Kingdom	2:21:37
2.	E. Lee, United Kingdom	2:24:39
3.	M. Hunt, New Zealand	2:25:19

50-59

1.	B. Spratt, FL	2:47:25
2.	S. Light, TN	2:48:18
3.	D. Seagrave	2:48:58

60-99

| 1. | J. Start, NJ | 3:13:24 |

ROSA AND JOSÉ FROM PORTUGAL

MONDAY, APRIL 20, 1987

No Threats to European Champ

Rosa Mota, from Portugal, had run 2:26:57 to win the bronze medal in the 1984 Los Angeles Olympic marathon. She had improved on that with a 2:23:29 for another third place in Chicago behind Benoit Samuelson (2:21:21) and Kristiansen in 1985. Without those two, Lorraine Moller, and Lisa Martin (later Ondieki) in the field, reporters, athletes, and race-watchers overwhelmingly favored twice (1985 and 1986) European marathon champion Mota to win the 1987 Boston Marathon. Her coach, agent, and lover Dr. José Pedrosa told her to go out and have fun—smile to show the people how much you enjoy their race. She ran; she smiled; she blew kisses. The people smiled back. Americans of Portuguese descent waved red-and-green Portuguese flags. Rosa Mota liked that. Even her ever-distant competitors liked her. None of them could say anything bad about her. She was little— 5'1-3/4", 99 pounds—and smiling.

The Japanese liked her, too. After Mota won the Tokyo Marathon in November of 1986 Pedrosa had said,

> They like her in Japan. They know her from the Olympic perfor-
> mance, of course. And when Rosa won the European Champion-
> ships for the second time, more than one Japanese television
> network covered her race. Then when she ran in Tokyo, the race
> was live for three hours. Marathon running is a big deal in Japan,
> and not just in Tokyo. It's a different sport there. You know how
> much the Japanese love the Boston Marathon.

But the sports federation back in Portugal did not like her. They especially did not like Pedrosa. In fact, they nearly prevented Mota from coming to Boston. Rosa Mota came from the wrong town in Portugal. The powerful clubs and the federation were in Lisbon, in the south. Mota lived in Portugal's second largest city, Porto, in the north. In Portuguese athletics two things mattered: soccer and men. The federation wanted Mota to move to Lisbon. She would not. They wanted her to join one of the three power clubs in Lisbon. She would not. They wanted her to get rid of her coach. She would not. Her coach was more to her than a source of workouts. She had met him when she was a 20-year-old, 7 years after she started running. José Pedrosa had changed her life.

When Mota was 13, her schoolteacher in Porto had made everyone run around the soccer field. Mota beat them all, including the boys. The teacher soon had her running on the boys' cross-country team. That same year she ran in the national championships in Lisbon. By age 20 Mota ran faster than any woman in Portugal (although that was no great distinction given the few women running).

The federation told Mota they did not send women to compete in international competitions. She experienced physical problems, but the federation told her they were psychological. Mota began to train with men from Pedrosa's club. They sent her directly to Pedrosa, a general practitioner, for her physical problems. He quickly ran some tests and found that she had severe anemia and asthma. He nursed her back to health. He decided that she would eventually rank highest worldwide in the marathon. Mota first ran a marathon in the European Championships in 1982. She started slowly and won in 2:36:04. Regardless of her victory, the federation hassled her.

Before the 1984 Olympic marathon Mota had trained with Pedrosa in the clear air of Boulder, Colorado. Because of the poisonous automobile exhaust in traffic-choked Porto and Lisbon, Mota had run endless loops around a small park. Colorado's big sky and clear, thin air helped her train to her best. She did not want to leave Colorado, but the federation called her daily, insisting that she return immediately to Portugal. Pedrosa explained the reason: "They said they wanted us to return to Lisbon from the USA so the entire Portuguese team could fly together to the USA, but really they wanted Rosa in Lisbon so the Portuguese federation officials could pose for photographs with her."

At the Olympic Games Pedrosa angered the federation because he would not allow Rosa to march in the opening ceremonies—the women's marathon was one of the first events and he did not want to tire her. He would not allow her to go to Disneyland with the officials. They retaliated by not allowing her out of the Olympic Village to go to Santa Monica to train. Pedrosa explained the obvious:

They didn't like me. . . . They said Rosa's only problem was José.
The federation wanted her to move to Lisbon. They didn't like her

to live in Porto or in Boulder. They didn't like me to coach her. I had friends who were important people, but the guys in the federation and Olympic Committee were too old, and they didn't understand world-class athletes. For them, the most important thing was to have their pictures taken at the airport. They never helped us, but once they saw that Rosa did so well they gave us money so we could train and live.

Not withstanding fights with her federation, Mota trained, lived, and led the women's 1987 Boston Marathon from the start to the finish in 2:25:21. No woman ever ran close to her. She had no worries. The headwind and humidity did not seem to bother her. She ran closer to her best than did most of the men. When she ran, she said, she did not like to suffer. She said she could not run that way. Maybe she did not try to fight the wind so did not feel the frustration of its pressure. But she did not have to push herself. She took away $40,000 and a car. Belgians Agnes Pardaens and Ria van Landeghem each ran under 2:30 for second and third. The thick air prevented former winners Gareau and Weidenbach from racing effectively.

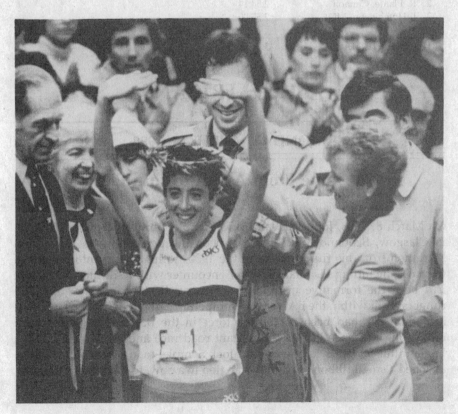

No woman could come close to Rosa Mota in 1987. © Victah/Agence Shot.

1987 Women's Results

1.	R. Mota, Portugal	**2:25:21**	15.	C. Iwahashi, CA	2:49:42
		(40th overall)	16.	K. Moody, WA	2:49:46
2.	A. Pardaens, Belgium	2:29:50	17.	A. Wehner, GA	2:50:21
3.	R. van Landeghem, Belgium	2:29:56	18.	L. Dobkowski, MO	2:52:31
4.	O. LaPierre, Canada	2:31:33	19.	C. Boessow, AL	2:52:43
5.	S. Keskitalo, Finland	2:33:58	20.	C. Ciavarella, WI	2:54:02
6.	E. Palm, Sweden	2:36:24	21.	K. Culla, NY	2:54:03
7.	E. Rochefort, Canada	2:36:42	22.	R. Plante, Canada	2:54:14
8.	L. Hayer, Greenfield, MA	2:37:58	23.	C. Gibbons, NJ	2:54:22
9.	**J. Gareau, Canada**	**2:40:40**	24.	J. Hutchinson, MO	2:55:00
10.	**L. Larsen Weidenbach, MI**	**2:43:06**	25.	P. Donovan, NH	2:55:38
11.	E. Guevera-Mora, Peru	2:44:38	36.	K. Beebee, MA	3:00:05
12.	T. Jousimaa, Finland	2:44:39	343.	M. Merton, West Germany	3:30:00
13.	N. Corsaro, MA	2:46:10	706.	J. Howell, TX	4:00:09
14.	C. Skarvelis, PA	2:46:52			

Over 790 finishers.

40-49

1.	E. Palm, Sweden	2:36:24
2.	R. Plante, Canada	2:54:14
3.	J. Hutchinson, MO	2:55:00

50-59

1.	C. Capetta, MA	3:17:24

60-99

1.	A. Reinhard, WI	3:53:19

THE AFRICANS

MONDAY, APRIL 18, 1988

36 Come From Africa to Join Field

On March 8, 1988, John Duncan (Jock) Semple, born on October 26, 1903, in Glasgow, Scotland, died. He had been the personality of the Boston Marathon from his first running in the 1930s to his crusty enforcement of the rules, including his infamous 1967 encounter with Kathrine Switzer. He had been the formative inspiration for many Boston and New England runners, both within the BAA and in competing clubs, to train for the Boston Marathon. He had been not only a force in the Boston Marathon, but a motivating presence in every important road race and track meet in New England for 50 years. In memory of Jock Semple, many marathon runners attached a small ribbon of plaid, tartan tied in a bow, to their racing singlets.

At Last a Professional Race Director

The BAA board of governors searched for the first time for the 1988 race for a full-time, professional race director, partly to maintain good relations with the seven municipalities along the route. Several had functioned as race directors, but like Will Cloney they received no pay and did not work full-time, or like Tim Kilduff they functioned like a director but had no title. For many years now the race had been of a size and influence that demanded complete attention. A great deal of that attention had to go to the cities and towns along the marathon route.

On June 17, 1987, the BAA appointed Guy Morse the marathon race director. There was nothing extreme about Guy Morse. He graduated from Marlboro, Massachusetts, High School. He did not run there or at Northeastern University in Boston, from which he graduated in 1974. After college he worked for Prudential, where volunteer work for the marathon attracted him. The marathon appealed to him because of an accident of residence. Until age 5 Morse had lived with his family in Hopkinton, and he was baptized in the church that overlooked the starting line. From his earliest childhood memories he was quite aware of the Boston Marathon. By 1988 he was 36 years old and had served as a race administrator since 1984. In contrast to the impassioned, personally involved, and amateur service of Will Cloney, the late Tony Nota, and Jock Semple, Morse managed a cool, detached, and professional staff.

Africans came in the 1988 Olympic year to race to the closest-yet finish of the Boston Marathon—closer than Tim Ford and Dave Kneeland's 6 seconds in 1906, closer than Mejia and McMahon's 5 seconds in 1971, closer than Rodgers and Wells's 2 seconds in 1978, closer than Salazar and Beardsley's 2 seconds in 1982. In Olympic years odd things happened at Boston. Often the field had been weak as in 1968 (Burfoot, 2:22:17) and 1976 (Fultz, 2:20:19). Americans usually stayed away from Boston in Olympic years in favor of their Olympic trials, but other countries' teams had often used the Boston Marathon as their own Olympic trials. Foreign federations often saw the strong field in Boston as most likely to imitate an Olympic marathon and thus be a good site for selecting their teams.

To the race of 1988 came Africans to make their contribution to Boston Marathon history. The idea of Africans coming to Boston would have astounded the original founders of the BAA, men who grew up acclimated to segregation. Although the wealthy did not actually run in the marathon, working-class white men ran their race, with maybe a few native North Americans. Some African-Americans had run well in Boston, Lou White in the 1950s and Ted Corbitt in the 1960s, but no black man had ever won. A few Africans had come before, like Ethiopians Abebe Bikila and Mamo Wolde in 1963 and Richard Mabuza from Swaziland in 1975 and 1976, but in 1988 Africans came en masse. They came from a poor continent of a billion people, 40-some countries, and a thousand tribes. Africa was a continent of contrasts, of deserts and jungles, of poor people who struggled for a future and rich leaders who callously amassed personal wealth, of Animists, Moslems, and Christians. Africa was a continent of colonial rape, revolution, economic collapse, and starvation as well as tremendous natural wealth and beauty. It had been ruthlessly exploited by European colonial rulers, who destroyed the old tribal governing structures, and when the mercantile colonial system no longer profited them, abandoned a ravaged continent to chaos. At the end of the 19th century wealthy members of the Boston Athletic Association, in imitation of the colonial British, went on safari to Africa, then returned to their clubhouse on Exeter Street to mount their rhino and wildebeest trophies—Teddy Roosevelt style—on the dark-paneled walls of rooms where members could sit and smoke in overstuffed leather armchairs and tell stories of the hunt. Nearly a century later events had turned full circle: Africans safaried to Boston to take a different kind of trophy— money and a Mercedes-Benz—back to Africa. In Kenya families and orphanages survived on the earnings of runners in America. This year 3 dozen Africans trekked to Hopkinton to run on April 18. Each one had something to prove.

Kenyan Ibrahim Hussein, at 120 pounds and 5'8", looked pleasant and moved with the demeanor of a relaxed and hospitable tour guide. Strangers felt instantly at ease with him. Teammates followed his example. Polished, bright, articulate in English and Nandi, passable in Arabic and Swahili, Hussein earned a degree in economics from the University of New Mexico in 1984. Everyone who met him liked him—a nice guy. At 29 years old he spoke modestly about everything except himself as a runner. When he raced he ran aggressively and fiercely—not a nice guy. Hussein told New York City Marathon director, Fred Lebow, a week before the Boston Marathon, "If I'm in sight of the finish line, I'm going to win it." Hussein had a secret weapon that few marathoner runners possessed: speed enough to have run a quarter mile in 47 seconds—a speed bordering on world class for just a quarter mile, once-around-the-track sprinter's talent. With that speed, that talent, and a worldliness that travel and education brought him, Hussein thought his dreams had come true and that he should be considered the best marathoner in the world. As a boy he had even pretended to be the best runner in the world.

In 1968 9-year-old Hussein had watched on television as Olympic gold medalist Kip Keino, a fellow Nandi, arrived to waiting crowds at the Nairobi airport. When Keino, wearing a Mexican sombrero, stood in the doorway of the plane about to descend the stairs, the Nandi danced and sang in joy and tribute to his accomplishment. They presented him a calabash filled with fermented milk, the traditional drink given to returning victorious warriors. Jomo Kenyatta, the Kenyan president, came to greet Keino.

Hussein decided as he watched that he too wanted to come home an Olympic champion. The next day on his 3-mile run to school he pretended to be Kip Keino as he ran. When he ran 2 miles to his grandmother's house for lunch he pretended to be Keino. When he ran back to school he pretended to be Keino. And on the 3-mile run back home he pretended to be Keino. He ran all but the final 3 miles quickly. At the end of the day Hussein was in no hurry to get home early because his family might find extra chores for him to do.

Hussein's family, including two younger brothers and two older sisters, lived in a tiny Moslem section in the center of the village of Tilawa. Moslems were a minority in Tilawa, but they operated the businesses of the village, on the outskirts of the town of Kapsabet in the Rift Valley at about 5,000 feet above sea level. Hussein's father, a sometime carpenter, owned and operated a variety store that sold paraffin, sugar, tea, and whatever else villagers might want. The family also managed a 13-acre farm where they raised corn, vegetables, tea, and cows. Cows indicated status for the Nandi people.

A few days before the 1988 Boston Marathon, Hussein held court in the lobby of the race headquarters at Copley Plaza, giving lessons in Kenyan child-naming to a circle of reporters and fans. According to Hussein, each Kenyan baby would get a name that indicated something about the circumstances of its birth. The given name *Kipcoghi*, for example, meant that the mother had a hard birth. (The *Kip* part just meant boy baby—if you shouted "Kip" to a group of Kenyan men, they all would answer.) Lots of Hussein's countrymen came with him to race at Boston. Hussein was the only Moslem on the team.

Ibrahim's father taught his children Islam, and they gained strength by meeting its requirements. He raised his family in strict adherence to the five laws of Islam: There is no God but God, and Mohammed is his prophet; pray five times a day facing Mecca; give to charity; fast during the holy month of Ramadan; make the pilgrimage, Hajji, to Jedda and Mecca at least once in your life if you can. Young Ibrahim fasted through Ramadan. He learned the discipline of Islam and how to surrender to God. This discipline helped him to train for running. Ibrahim's father wanted to make the Hajji, but he could never afford it. He supported many relatives as well as his immediate family. By 1988 Ibrahim had earned enough money from running in America that he could have paid for his father's pilgrimage. It would have given his father great joy to go to the holy places, but he had died 10 years earlier.

In 1978 Hussein was attending Catholic boarding school 60 miles from home at St. Patrick's, academically and athletically Kenya's best school. He ran the 400 meters at first, but for the district qualifiers he entered the steeplechase. He had never run a steeplechase before, but he knew that the Rift Valley was a very hard zone in which to qualify for the nationals. He ran 9:04 for the 3,000-meter steeplechase and qualified. He won a scholarship to the University of New Mexico.

In college Hussein ran 800 meters with a best of 1:47. By 1984 he watched the New York City Marathon on television. He saw the runners running so slowly and saw them stop. He had tried some long-distance races— Bloomsday in Spokane, Washington, and the Bay to Breakers in San Francisco—and had won them easily. He thought he would never have to stop in a marathon. He tried New York in 1985, expecting it to be easy. He got a leg cramp and moved from fourth to ninth. He indeed had to stop running during the race. The realization that the marathon takes more preparation than other races enabled Hussein to begin a string of three Honolulu Marathon victories only a month later. He started the string with a 2:11:42. In 1987 he won the New York City Marathon on a hot day. He thought he could run much faster, maybe 2:08, and said so. Why not?

American men and women stayed away from Boston in 1988 to save themselves for the Olympic trials, to be held for the men in Jersey City a week later and for the women in Pittsburgh 2 weeks after the Boston Marathon. Officials of the BAA and John Hancock encouraged the Americans to seek Olympic berths and come to Boston the following year. The top three in the trial marathon made the team—no exceptions. Other countries had selectors, or sometimes kings, who made exceptions.

The Olympic team selectors for Kenya, Tanzania, Italy, Finland, England, Ireland, and Mexico would all, to some degree, use the Boston Marathon results to select—or more accurately reject—runners for their Olympic teams. The British runners especially had something to prove. Geoff Smith and Welshman Steve Jones passed up the official British trials in London to run Boston. Both had run well at Boston before and hoped to run so fast that the British selectors would be forced to choose them.

Some watchers remembered the recent World Cross-Country Championships where Kenya and Ethiopia had taken all the top 10 places. Some expected that this year's Boston Marathon would resemble a dual meet between Kenya and Tanzania. The first-place finisher would win a Mercedes and $45,000. The total prize purse was $270,000, double the entire budget for the race just 8 years before.

Hussein had won the New York City Marathon the previous November and later won his third straight Honolulu Marathon on December 13, but few picked him to win at Boston. The popular prerace favorite was the rich field. Juma Ikangaa had won the Beijing Marathon in the fall of 1987 and had run second to Ethiopian Abebe Mekonnen in Tokyo on Valentine's Day with a 2:08:42. But his Boston of 1987 had not shown his abilities. Ireland's John Treacy, 1984 Olympic marathon silver medalist, entered the Boston Marathon at the last minute, leaving everyone to wonder about strategy. His race the year before had left him bitterly disappointed.

A pack of 22 cruised through the damp 5-mile checkpoint in 23:41. Smith's record of 23:18 stood. Perhaps this would be a tactical race, but unlike 1987 it would be fast. Everyone was there: British Smith, Jones, and Mark Roberts; Tanzanians Gidamas Shahanga, Zakariah Barie, John Makanya, and Ikangaa; Italians Gianni Poli and Gelindo Bordin; Kenyans Hussein, Gabriel Kamau, and Joseph Nzau; Mexican José Gómez; and Irishman Treacy. In the second pack lurked Kenya's Joseph Kipsang and the two-time winner of the New York City Marathon, Italian Orlando Pizzolato, who hoped to exercise his clever come-from-behind tactic. But it was Hussein, smiling and relaxed, who led the race so early.

At 10 miles Hussein still sat comfortably in the pack. It had thinned, but not much. Another African, Nechchadi El-Mustapha of Morocco, joined the pack. They all passed 10 miles in 47:57. Everyone—on the press truck, along the course, watching on television, even those in the pack—speculated. Who would emerge? What were the clues? They all looked good. The almost perfect running weather made a fast second half seem likely. There would be no sun-baked suffering in this race, only the high drama of barely re-strained speed.

The pack, an international juggernaut, rolled through the half marathon in 1:03:12. Upon hearing the split time some runners in the pack must have doubled it to imagine breaking Ethiopian Belayneh Dinsamo's day-old world record of 2:06:50, set in Rotterdam. But most of them knew better. The Boston course has a seductively easy first half—and a heartless second.

Bordin ran in that pack, but he did not plan to win. He came to Boston to run in the year's most competitive marathon as part of his plan to win the Olympic gold medal in Seoul at the end of the summer. Now he felt quite pleased that his partial preparations enabled him to stay up with the leaders with such ease.

After a 20-mile split of 1:37:36 the pace had whittled the field to an impul-sive Irishman and two Africans. Treacy had said he was not going to run the marathon, but reported, "I asked my wife on Thursday night what she thought about me running. She thought I was joking." Yet there over the Newton hills on the heartbreaking second half of the race, Treacy locked himself in a battle to the bones with Hussein and Ikangaa. The Africans repeatedly broke Treacy, but he kept coming back time and again, to be

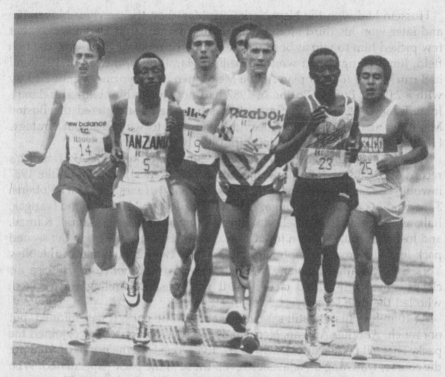

Ibrahim Hussein (#23) leads the ever-dwindling pack. Next to him is Steve Jones (#1), Gianni Poli (#9), Juma Ikangaa (#5), and John Treacy (#14). © Victah/Agence Shot.

broken in another East African surge. Treacy saw the two Africans talking and looking back. He felt they were working together against him. But mostly it was Ikangaa pushing and pushing. Always he pushed. Even his training runs went with a militant intensity. He was a little man who could not relax. In conversation Ikangaa was sweet, always carefully choosing his words to meet the expectations of the listener. He referred to his competitors as "the other friends." But when he ran he gave his opponents no quarter, no chance to relax and stride.

Regardless of Ikangaa's hammering, Hussein ran blithely, with a childlike joy to his stride. Treacy agonized while Bordin followed dispassionately. But between Hussein and Ikangaa the drama swelled.

Robert Ouko, the secretary of the Kenyan federation of marathoners, held the Kenyan flag as Hussein prepared to use his superior speed to sprint past Ikangaa. Both runners could see the finish line. But Ikangaa, though full of pushing and surging, did not possess the rocket speed to run a quarter mile in 47 seconds, and he knew it. Hussein lifted his knees and flickered his elbows. He flashed away from Ikangaa. He ripped the finish line banner with his chest. Before the banner had reached the asphalt, Ikangaa finished as well. The two runners from neighboring countries finished closer to each other than any winner and runner-up in Boston Marathon history, but Hussein expected it. Another race, another victory. Although polite, Hussein seemed workmanlike toward his win.

Other Kenyans, however, let their emotions carry them away. Ouko said, "I should be there at the finish line with my country's flag. It is a tradition for Kenyans, and we have done it since we have entered the Olympic Games and the Commonwealth Games, all games we have done it. It is an honor to win a race, and the country must repay the honor with its flag." He wrapped Hussein in the Kenyan flag. Ibrahim Hussein from the Kenyan village of Tilawa wrapped in the the black, green, red, and white flag of Kenya with its shield and crossed spears accepted the laurel wreath of Boston.

Hussein said, "I was the first African to win New York; it's great to be the first African to win this race." Hussein would next run the Olympic marathon in Seoul. He expected to win that too. On this day in Boston Hussein felt invincible and indeed proved it, but the race in Seoul and subsequent Boston Marathons would lift powerful emotions. He felt it a

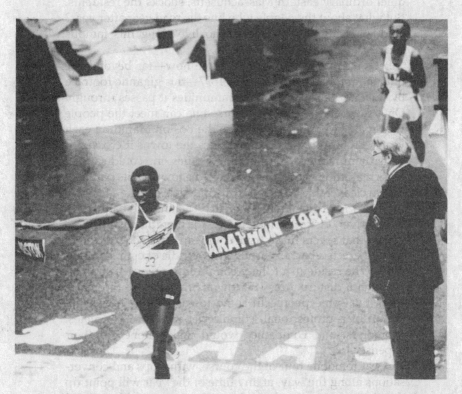

At the last possible moment, Hussein unleashed his kick to devastate Ikangaa.
© Victah/Agence Shot.

great honor to represent his country in the Olympic Games and a great personal honor for his teammates to select him captain—not of the marathon team, the track-and-field team, but of the entire Kenyan delegation. Ibrahim Hussein would carry Kenya's flag into the Olympic stadium.

By the Roadside

Twenty-five miles of the Boston Marathon actually passes through towns and cities other than Boston proper. Boston Marathon runners and the people who follow their fortunes focus their attention one day a year on a narrow strip of road from Hopkinton to Boston. Runners come from all over the world to run the Boston Marathon, but they think little about how their presence, along with 10,000 other runners in a wild charge through the quiet ordinary hometowns of quiet ordinary eastern Massachusetts, shocks the residents. But what about the people who line the road year after year? And what about the people who live along this famous route?

Let's examine the course and see how—far beyond the imagination of the founders in 1897—this gigantic footrace by the late 1980s rends the communities it passes through. On a slow drive along the course one can meet the people who make it possible to operate the Boston Marathon each year. The Boston Marathon fatigues the towns it crosses. It costs them money. In a flurry of similes one could say the mass marathon yearly dismembers the towns in its path like a meat cleaver, like Moses parting the Red Sea, like a tectonic fissure, a fault line, a snow melt breaching the banks of a leveed river. Pick your metaphor—the marathon is a human glacier that severs north from south; an avalanche; a freight train. It erects a barrier through the middle of eight communities. The residents of these communities never bargained for such a disturbance. The towns must endure the marathon, but some people in some towns did not relish the notion of a professional, commercial race where athletes, promoters, and companies would make money at their expense.

An automobile tour of the course, with stops and conversations along the way, at any time of the year will point up the Boston Marathon's lasting effect on the citizens and businesses of the towns it passes through. The marathon's duration is shortest in Ashland and longest in Newton—the length within the city of Boston is actually less than 2 miles. (The race might be more accurately called the Newton Marathon!) On race day police officers can't get from one side of any town to the other. Ambulances cannot move north to south from an accident scene to the hospital. A ladder truck cannot move from south to north to get from the station to a fire. Populations double, even triple. Cars park where they are never seen the other 364 days of the year. Whole towns virtually shut down for a day.

An Ashland police lieutenant said that helicopters, biplanes, and blimps nearly block out the sun on marathon day. For his police force it is the biggest day of the year; they mobilize every person they can recruit. Months of planning go into the few hours the runners invade the town.

Ashland's fire station is on the south side of town and the hospital is on the north. On race morning an ambulance is moved to the south side and a fire engine to the north of the marathon "wall" in anticipation of an accident during the race. Police officers must patrol streets far from the course to keep confused motorists from wandering onto the course. The runners, obsessed with their race, of course know nothing about these preparations and inconveniences.

Ashland residents and employees have to pick up odd items along the course after the race passes through, especially when temperatures were cool at the start but warmed up later. Runners litter the roadside with discarded hats, gloves, shirts, trash bags worn as cheap rain gear, and old socks used as mittens. This debris and thousands of paper cups remain for the highway department to gather. Patriots' Day is a legal holiday, so the town must pay overtime to the employees who work that day. Town crews spend a good part of the winter months repairing cracks and potholes along the marathon course to assure the safety of the athletes. Repairs to roads in other parts of town have to wait until after marathon day.

But Ashland's police officers are just a fraction of the 1,500 law enforcement and public safety officials who line the 26-mile, 385-yard section of road that stretches from Hopkinton to Boston. State, registry, and metropolitan police and officers from Massachusetts Bay Transportation Authority—even the National Guard—go to work.

And while the communities may feel the race is part of their civic duty, scores of private businesses also have a say in the matter.

Most businesses that are open do well on marathon day. There's always a party at T.J.'s bar on the Ashland/Hopkinton line and a bash at LaCantina in Framingham, town No. 3 in the marathon convoy, where patrons eat pizza while watching the marathon on the big screen TV. Ever since Prohibition ended, Framingham marathon revelers have gathered at the Happy Swallow Cafe on the curb of the course for their annual Patriots' Day party. The owner says that the same folks come back every year. Some of the regulars have even run the race; their fellow patrons cheer hard as they pass, and party in their place.

One year, a thirsty competitor stopped for a happy swallow from a tavern mug, ran another block, returned for another swallow, and stayed—his number still pinned to his chest. The parties and the tales are similar in Natick at the V.F.W. and the American Legion Post.

The marathon is also good business for the Massachusetts Turnpike. For every mile run in the marathon, probably hundreds are driven on the Pike. There's a rush on toll booths for the 2 hours before and the 2 hours after the race. It's bigger and quicker than the usual weekday commuter crush; the extra traffic would be a serious problem if it were a workday. The spectators drive madly to get to sites along the course, then rush on to Boston.

In 1987 the seven gates at the Interstate 495 exchange took in $9,282 on marathon day, $4,500 more than a regular Sunday or holiday. The turnpike averaged $15,000 to $20,000 in tolls from marathon runners and watchers—and that's not including income from speeding tickets. Total revenue attracted to Boston exceeded $60 million during the marathon weekend, proclaimed the Greater Boston Convention and Visitor's Bureau.

Halfway to Boston, on the rolling roads of Wellesley, students at Wellesley College watch the marathon. The bigger the race, the easier the crowd control. Police in Wellesley, the fifth town in the marathon parade, usually had to rope off a half mile of the course to control the crowd, but as the race grew larger, the mass of runners itself kept the spectators off the road. No one dared try to wade across the raging torrent.

Usually the Wellesley women cheer extra hard for the female athletes, but from time to time they give an extra cheer to young men. One warm marathon day, a fellow sweated along in a heavy crimson sweatshirt displaying a big white Harvard *H*. It was dumb to wear such a heavy shirt on such a hot day. The Wellesley students cheered wildly for "John Harvard," who perspired and beamed with joy. Just yards past the women, he peeled off his sweaty top, tossed it to the side, and confessed to a nearby competitor that he'd never been to Harvard, but he'd also never in his life been cheered so strongly.

The crowds are easy and good-natured—not wildly spontaneous, as if the Red Sox had won the World Series— yet the police still have to use miles of rope to insure the safety of spectators and runners.

The courseside Armenian rug merchants of Newton Lower Falls know that the marathon is not good for business, so they go up on the roof—not to jump off, but to watch. Instead of selling rugs, as they have since 1951, they relax and have lots of fun watching the race pass by the store. They invite their friends, set up a watering station, and call it a gala day.

At the Newton firehouse, at the corner of Route 16 and Commonwealth Avenue where the course eases toward Heartbreak Hill, the firefighters have to park their engines across the street. One faces up the hill and the other down— just in case. It's either that or stop the marathon if there's a fire.

While the trucks wait across the street, firefighters pass out water, attend to various runners' aches and pains, and watch over the long line at the station's only bathroom.

"Newton has the longest stretch [6 miles] and our participation costs us," a mayor of Newton has admitted. One year Newton threatened to bill the race for costs incurred during the marathon but decided against it. "We have a historical commitment to the marathon," said the mayor.

1988 Men's Results

1.	I. Hussein, Kenya	2:08:43	11.	Z. Barie, Tanzania	2:14:32
2.	J. Ikangaa, Tanzania	2:08:44	12.	H. Kita, Japan	2:14:40
3.	J. Treacy, Ireland	2:09:15	13.	J. Kipsang, Kenya	2:15:05
4.	G. Bordin, Italy	2:09:27	14.	M. O'Reilly, Ireland	2:15:27
5.	G. Poli, Italy	2:09:33	15.	A. Altun, Turkey	2:15:48
6.	J. Campbell, New Zealand	2:11:08	16.	J. Charbonnel, France	2:15:58
7.	O. Pizzolato, Italy	2:12:32	17.	V. Kahkola, Finland	2:16:17
8.	J. Makanya, Tanzania	2:14:04	18.	G. Smith, England	2:16:34
9.	S. Jones, England	2:14:07	19.	J. Madelon, France	2:16:42
10.	T. Taniguchi, Japan	2:14:18	20.	J. Burra, Tanzania	2:17:11

21.	G. Shahanga, Tanzania	2:17:33	42.	A. Kipkogei, Kenya	2:20:58
22.	T. Ekblom, Finland	2:17:34	43.	A. Lind, CO	2:20:58
23.	R. Soler, TX	2:17:46	44.	A. Tulu, MN	2:21:21
24.	S. Salazar, Colombia	2:17:49	45.	T. Moriguchi, Japan	2:21:34
25.	R. Marczak, Poland	2:17:53	46.	S. Kykkanen, Finland	2:21:41
26.	D. Kavuu, Kenya	2:18:03	47.	T. Tounsi, France	2:21:55
27.	J. Assamet, France	2:18:16	48.	J. Otieno, Kenya	2:21:58
28.	**B. Rodgers, MA**	**2:18:17**	49.	P. Holmnas, Finland	2:22:26
29.	M. Vainio, Finland	2:18:37	**92.**	**N. Cusack, Ireland**	**2:28:42**
30.	S. Kogo, Kenya	2:18:47	93.	J. Suarez, Colombia	2:28:45
31.	M. Kudo, Japan	2:18:50	94.	L. Ristaino, MA	2:28:50
32.	G. Kamau, Kenya	2:18:59	95.	R. Marion, VT	2:28:55
33.	G. Hogberg, Sweden	2:19:37	95.	R. Abbott, TX	2:28:55
34.	G. Miranda, Mexico	2:20:11	97.	R. Moore, MD	2:28:55
35.	S. Harjamki, Finland	2:20:12	98.	D. McGillivray, Canada	2:28:58
36.	N. El-Mustapha, Morocco	2:20:18	99.	F. Rivas, MA	2:28:58
37.	A. Masong, Tanzania	2:20:23	100.	M. Roberts, United Kingdom	2:29:02
38.	L. Torres, Peru	2:20:32	109.	R. Jarzynka, Netherlands	2:30:05
39.	R. Lanzoni, Costa Rica	2:20:37	**1532.**	**A. Burfoot, PA**	**2:59:45**
40.	I. Vaanenen, Finland	2:20:38	**3568.**	**J.J. Kelley, CT**	**3:28:53**
41.	A. Navaro, Mexico	2:20:56		**J.A. Kelley (age 80)**	**4:26:36**

Masters

1.	R. Marczak, Poland	2:17:53
2.	**B. Rodgers, MA**	**2:18:17**

Team prize

1. Italy
2. Kenya
3. Tanzania

ONE THOUSAND WOMEN

MONDAY, APRIL 18, 1988

Portugal's Mota Has No Challengers

Though 1,000 women came to run the 1988 Boston Marathon, the group included only two sub-2:30 women, Priscilla Welch and Rosa Mota. But rumor had it that Welch had injured herself. It seemed to reporters that Mota might win Boston 1988 without much fight. But in 1982 observers had expected Grete Waitz to win in a waltz, and she never finished.

Welch, age 43, had astounded the world with her 2:26 in London the year before. At the 10-mile mark in this year's Boston Marathon, Finland's Tuija Jousimaa followed Mota, followed in turn by Canada's Lizanne Bussieres with a 2:36:16 best. Welch slid comfortably into 4th place; and Canada's Odette LaPierre, with a pre-Boston personal record of 2:31:31, hung in behind Welch in 5th. The women did not race in a pack, just a string woven through the mass of men. Each woman had to rely on the crowds to learn her place.

But Welch ran for stakes much higher than money. She had decided to skip her hometown British trials and qualify for the British Olympic team by running impressively at Boston. Welch's plan, at least on the surface, looked good. None of the well-known British runners ran London particularly well the day before. Welch figured she would have to do no better than 2:35 to tie up the third post on Britain's team for Seoul.

But Welch ran with an enormous problem. According to Dave Welch, her coach and husband, "She was just running to survive. She went out for a training run 2 weeks ago and walked back home."

A calf-muscle tear had plagued Welch for several weeks, since she had run the Cherry Blossom 10-miler in Washington, DC, earlier in the spring. If she didn't run Boston as planned, she would not be chosen for the British Olympic team. The British Amateur Athletics Board didn't like that three of their very best, Welch, Geoffrey Smith, and Steve Jones, had all snubbed the London Marathon, seemingly to run for better money in Boston. From the last bastion of amateur running the Boston Marathon had become the sport's pot of gold. Whatever her reasons for choosing Boston over London, at 43 Priscilla Welch couldn't easily snub Seoul in 1988 in favor of Barcelona 1992. Her coach-husband thought when he left her at the starting line that she'd never finish the race.

Strategy for the women's race certainly seemed clear: Welch would let Mota run away with it. Welch would instead run a slower, controlled pace . . . for a reasonable finishing time . . . for survival.

Mota still lived and trained in Boulder. Her Portuguese federation really had no choice but to pick her for their Olympic team. Thus, with the Olympic qualifying-time pressure off her shoulders, Mota seemed to be in Boston strictly for the money, although a few days before the race she told the press "I always want to run in Boston because there are so many Portuguese people living here."

Mota let two nervous Finns, Sinikka Keskitalo (pre-Boston best of 2:33:18), and Jousimaa (2:32:07 pre-Boston best), who were using Boston as their Olympic team trials, lead for the first couple of miles before they inevitably slowed down. From there Mota took control. "I like to run alone, actually. . . . especially for an entire race!" She won with ease and without doubt on anyone's part. On the road behind Mota, Welch sneaked into fourth place.

With 400 meters to go, LaPierre nipped Welch, but Welch thought she easily secured her Olympic team spot by snagging fourth place with a time of 2:30:48, 5 minutes under what she thought she "needed." But the British selectors, known for their whimsy, had other ideas. After the race, Welch bubbled, "My calf was a bit tight, but I'm ready to run again!" She smiled, and so did Dave Welch. And so, of course, did LaPierre, who shaved almost a full minute off her best and earned her Canadian team vote for Seoul.

The Canadian Olympic team lined up with Lizanne Bussieres and Ellen Rochefort running. (Jackie Gareau had cramped and crashed in London, crawling in with a 2:36:04 and missing any chance to make her country's team).

The British selectors decided to keep one Olympic position open for Veronique Marot, pending her recovery and a good performance. Dave Welch was furious upon hearing that Priscilla was not selected on the basis of her Boston performance; he gave the selectors one week to decide on Priscilla or she would "not be available." Some said that the selectors frowned on British runners who lived outside their country, others felt they especially favored Marot, a French runner who adopted the United Kingdom. Others accused the selectors of being perverse by not expecting an old lady to do well when she had just shown she could. A week passed. Monologues from the Welches intersected with their own ultimatums while the selectors turned deaf ears. Priscilla Welch did not go to Seoul.

In second place, Tuija Jousimaa had bettered her best with a 2:29:26. After the race she confided, smiling wryly, "I am most happy to have beaten Sinikka [Keskitalo]. She is considered to be #1 in Finland, you know." The three top Finns made their country's team for the 1988 Olympic marathon.

Runner and playwright Israel Horovitz wrote about the 1988 Boston Marathon for *New England Runner* magazine: "But Mota's lonely run in Boston gets the imagination wandering across the waters to Seoul, South Korea. What a good shot she will have, really! Ingrid, like Grete [Waitz] may well be a bit beyond it, now. So, it is entirely possible that in South Korea, Rosa Mota will be the one to beat."

Mota won the Olympic marathon. She and the male Olympic champion, Gelindo Bordin, would return to Boston, but not for 2 years.

Checkpoint Splits

5K	Rosa Mota	16:22
5 miles	Rosa Mota	32:21
7 miles	Rosa Mota	37:48
15K	Rosa Mota	50:49
10 miles	Rosa Mota	54:42
25K	Rosa Mota	1:25:09
23 miles	Rosa Mota	2:06:54
24 miles	Rosa Mota	2:12:19
40K	Rosa Mota	2:17:02
25 miles	Rosa Mota	2:17:55

1988 Women's Results

1.	R. Mota, Portugal	2:24:30	16.	H. Darami, France	2:44:29
		(63rd overall)	17.	G. Corona, Mexico	2:45:40
2.	T. Jousimaa, Finland	2:29:26	18.	L. Bouchard, Canada	2:46:02
3.	O. LaPierre, Canada	2:30:35	19.	L. Mohanna, NE	2:46:09
4.	P. Welch, England	2:30:48	20.	C. Iwahashi, CA	2:48:57
5.	L. Bussieres, Canada	2:30:56	21.	J. Regan, MA	2:49:30
6.	E. Rochefort, Canada	2:31:36	22.	M. Hoshi, Japan	2:49:50
7.	S. Keskitalo, Finland	2:34:12	23.	K. Ginder, MA	2:50:13
8.	S. Kumpulainen, Finland	2:35:24	24.	C. Gibbons, NJ	2:52:29
9.	S. Stone, Canada	2:38:48	25.	L. Paddock, NY	2:53:52
10.	G. Beschloss, NY	2:40:08	26.	C. Soby, IL	2:54:38
11.	A. Hearn, NY	2:40:15	27.	J. Ullyot, CA	2:54:48
12.	G. Horovitz, NY	2:40:26	33.	P. Catalano, VT	2:57:35
13.	R. Lemettinen, Finland	2:41:58	40.	D. Potter, ME	3:00:03
14.	L. Marjaana, Finland	2:42:57	326.	S. Newton, MN	3:30:03
15.	K. Rauta, Finland	2:43:54	768.	E. Gillanders, VA	4:00:02

Team prize

1. Finland
2. Liberty AC
3. Forerunners TC

MORE AFRICANS

MONDAY, APRIL 17, 1989

Hussein, Ikangaa Top Field for Race

The Olympic Games burdened Ibrahim Hussein by forcing him to choose between the needs of his personal training and his duties and obligations as the standard bearer and captain of his country's team. Those duties, added to the training for a marathon, strained him. First he had to leave New Mexico, where he had developed a personal system of training and had no distractions. There he had time and place to train for the sport he loved, but he had to go back to Kenya for a month culminating in the team trials. As team captain he could not pass on that obligation. Next he had to go to Korea a month before his race. As flag bearer he could not hide in New Mexico to train on familiar trails, then fly to Seoul at the last possible moment. The opening ceremony in which Hussein would carry Kenya's flag was the first event to enter the Olympic stadium and the marathon was the last event to enter it—a month after his arrival in Korea. Still, Hussein thought about Kip Keino, the glorious Nandi disembarking in Nairobi, wearing the sombrero and drinking the drink of victorious warriors, the fermented milk from the calabash of his clan. After an Olympic victory, Hussein too could do that. If only he could feel as good as he had in the Boston Marathon when he had speed to spare.

In addition to the stress of the excessive travel was the fact that fellow team members called upon Hussein to solve their personal problems. As captain he had to respond; he had the capacity and the duty. Already on the fine edge between training and overtraining, he broke under the load and became ill. He raced and dropped out of the Olympic marathon. He went home to Kenya. He disembarked without celebration. He built a house for his family and did not run for 3 months. When he came back to Boston he was not the invincible runner of 1988.

The invincible runners of the world seemed to be fellow East Africans—Ethiopians. A day before the Boston Marathon Ethiopian Belayneh Dinsamo, a 2:06:50 marathoner, won the Rotterdam Marathon in 2:09:39. The same day Ethiopian Zeleke Metaferia won the World Cup Marathon in Milan, Italy, in 2:10:28. Abebe Mekonnen, age 25, who had run 2:08:33 in Tokyo in February of 1988 to beat Ikangaa, led the Ethiopian team in Boston. In 1988 Mekonnen ran a fourth place of 2:09:33 in April in Rotterdam and a 2:07:35 in Beijing in October. He had finished second in the World Cross-Country Championships in 1986, fourth in 1987, and fifth in 1988. He had emerged from Ethiopia in 1984, when he finished second in both the Munich Marathon and the Friendship Games in Moscow. He had finished third in Tokyo in 1986 with a 2:08:39.

Of course Ethiopians, namely Abebe Bikila and Mamo Wolde, had been to Boston before. The Kenyans may have had an Olympic hero in 1,500-meter runner Kip Keino and their gold medalists in the steeplechase and 10,000 meters, but they had never won Olympic gold in the marathon. Ethiopians had won three gold medals—two by Bikila in 1960 and 1964 and one by Wolde in 1968. A generation of Ethiopian marathoners grew up with those heroes. Bikila's early death raised him to near-deified status with young Ethiopian runners. Mekonnen said,

> I feel so deeply about him that I sometimes even cry when I see his picture. I always pray for him. It is his great inspiration that has made us as good as we are. It is because of him that we are known worldwide. To me Abebe is almost a god—he sacrificed for Ethiopia, his country and his flag. He is an unforgettable memory. It is my dream to be like him.

That hero worship may explain how a poor country of 43 million people with a per capita income of $141 could overwhelm the running world. They had the talent, the altitude, the attitude, and the legacy.

But for political reasons the Marxist Ethiopian regime would not allow their athletes to compete in Los Angeles in 1984 or in Seoul in 1988. Drought and famine, exacerbated by the Eritrean guerrilla war and other wars and uprisings aided, in part, by Sudan and Somalia, overwhelmed parts of the country in 1984. While pictures of starving children horrified the rest of the world and mobilized relief efforts, the government, allied with the Soviet Union, spent 9.6% of its wealth on the military. Most Ethiopian runners came out of the military, but Mekonnen from Shoa province held the rank of police lieutenant. That sort of military or quasi-military support of runners born to a central plateau 6,000 to 10,000 feet high combined with the inspiration of Bikila and Wolde drove Mekonnen and his teammates. They took their training with ferocity.

When a dog attacked Tesfaye Tafa, interrupting his training run, he ran home, got a gun, ran back, shot the dog, then continued to run.

But the Ethiopian team had organization in addition to inspiration and talent. The Ethiopians suggested that the Kenyan coaches were not quite up to theirs, all of whom had physical education or sport physiology degrees from Eastern Europe, notably East Germany. But the more liberal political atmosphere in Kenya allowed its runners to seek scholarships, coaching, and running experience abroad.

"People ask why we are good marathoners," said Nigussie Robe, the head coach of the Ethiopian Athletics Federation for more than 20 years, who studied physical education in Czechoslovakia. "Some people say it is because we are at a high altitude. But to be in a high altitude is not enough. You have to have a well prepared training program. My athletes are good because they have a good training program and are well disciplined. They have more discipline than in the United States or Britain." Mekonnen said, "The Ethiopian weather is very hard. Other runners who run above the 400-meter distance—if they came here they wouldn't do half as well."

Abebe Mekonnen reacted faster than any other runner at the start. At the gun he shot out like a sprinter. He wanted the lead from the first step. For winning the Boston Marathon, Mekonnen could earn over 300 times the yearly income of his countrymen. After a dozen steps he settled into the large lead pack to wait and relax behind whichever runner led the pack. He wore an adidas green shirt and red shorts. Hussein wore a black outfit with adidas in gold. Ikangaa wore a white Asics shirt. Twenty-year-old Simon Robert Naali from Moshi, Tanzania, took the early lead through the first downhill mile in 4:33. Kathrine Switzer and Frank Shorter, broadcasting for Boston's WBZ-TV, called Naali a rabbit, a runner paid to set a fast early pace but who would not finish the race. But Naali had no rabbiting intentions. He planned to win the race. Mile after mile he ran tall, square-shouldered, and muscular. Ikangaa, Hussein, and Mekonnen ran in a pack well behind him. And well behind them ran John Treacy, the Irish 1984 Olympic silver medalist. Temperatures reached 62 °F, making the black men glisten with sweat. The highlights showed Naali's perfect musculature, tiny Ikangaa's furrowed and wrinkled face, Hussein's lithe and tapered body, but on Mekonnen nothing showed. Compared to the others, Mekonnen looked unremarkable—neither wiry nor muscular, short nor tall. His striding style was, well, ordinary. He looked indistinguishable from several thousand other men in the race. The fact that the pace stressed his lungs and muscles less than it did those of his competitors did not impress itself upon anyone. Mekonnen knew, as did everyone else in the world, especially Ikangaa, that Ikangaa had no kick. Hussein had outkicked Ikangaa at the end of Boston the year before, Seko had outkicked him at Fukuoka by 3 seconds, Mekonnen had outkicked him in Tokyo. Ikangaa had run seventh in the Los Angeles Olympic marathon. To anyone who could be near him at the end of a marathon, he looked like an easy target.

Ikangaa, condemned by his lack of finishing speed, had to push the pace to escape a repeat of 1988's kick by Hussein. Mekonnen had only to wait and watch the Tanzanian dismantle the Kenyan so he, the Ethiopian, could take over.

When Ikangaa's pressure brought the pack of three up to Naali, Naali surprised everyone by sticking to the pack. The four of them ran together, often abreast in the middle of the sun-filled road, sharing water and sponges. At each water stop Mekonnen burst ahead, snatched a cup and drank, poured some on his head, then drifted back to the pack to offer water to any of the other men who didn't get any. Perhaps he seemed more like a host supplying his guests with drinks than a runner. At times Hussein would drift a step ahead to look back at the faces of the other men and assess their fatigue. He saw none on Mekonnen. They passed the half-marathon point in 1:02:23.

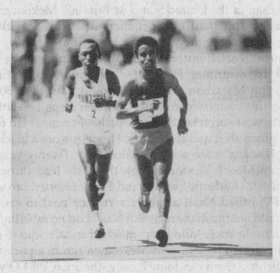

Now only two are left—Tanzanian Juma Ikangaa (#2) and Ethiopian Abebe Mekonnen (#4). © Victah/Agence Shot.

Over the hills Treacy pulled closer. He ran white and lonely with a low back-kick, a stride that served him well winning the World Cross-Country Championships over muddy, hilly ground in 1978 and 1979. He had been running alone since the 3-mile mark. The sun burned his shoulders. A bad cold had forced him to drop out of the 1988 Olympic marathon. If he could only catch the Africans and tuck in with the pack, as he had the year before. He knew he could kick with the best of them—he could certainly outkick Ikangaa—if only he could catch them.

On the hill over Route 128 Naali dropped back. Up the first of the Newton hills Hussein dropped back. Naali passed him. Treacy passed Hussein. Hussein suggested to Treacy that they work together to catch up, but soon Hussein could not stay with Treacy on the hills. Treacy had been running the hills well and had learned how to roll like Bill Rodgers on the downhills so his quadriceps muscles would not stiffen from an unnatural use as brakes. By the top of the hills Treacy passed Naali. Treacy surged to within 7 seconds of the lead, but as he surged Mekonnen took control and Ikangaa would not give up. Ikangaa stuck to Mekonnen until 2 hours and 1 minute into the race. There Mekonnen surged. Then, for the first time, contortion appeared on his face, showing that the strain of the race had at last touched him. With a snarl and a grimace he looked back, pleased that his 4:50 mile had at last produced a gap. The grimace turned to a grin as Ikangaa conceded defeat. Treacy realized with dismay that not enough race remained to close the gap on Ikangaa. Third again. Treacy would train harder and smarter and come back to try to win the marathon he regarded as the best in the world. As Mekonnen won, the growing Ethiopian community of Boston danced in the streets.

Money Talks

A close comparison of the 1989 results to results of races before prize money was awarded at Boston reveals a startling difference. The very good but not world-class local runner seems to be all but gone. The first woman ran 26th in 1989 with 2:24:33, but in 1983 Joan Benoit ran 121st with the course record of 2:22:43. The 1989 women's winner ran slower but finished better among the men because hordes of men had disappeared. In this race only two men ran times in 2:20-something, three in 2:21-something, three in 2:22, four in 2:23, and six in 2:24, for a total of 18 between 2:20 and 2:25. In 1983 80 men had finished between 2:20 and 2:25. Where did 62 men go? What could account for this curious gap? It seems that as the decade closed, the numbers of speedy collegians taking up the marathon declined. American men who may have run 4:10 to 4:15 miles in college seemed no longer to move up to the marathon. And it may be that runners of national-level ability (2:15–2:25) found it more worth their while to race in smaller races where they had a chance to win prize money. Prize money and sponsorship had definitely changed the composition of the Boston Marathon's top finishers, making the race a major international event but a minor regional championship.

Checkpoint Splits

5K	Simon Naali	14:12
5 miles	Simon Naali	23:08
10K	Juma Ikangaa	29:01
15K	Juma Ikangaa	43:57
10 miles	Juma Ikangaa	47:21
20K	Juma Ikangaa	59:03
Half marathon	Simon Naali	1:02:23
15 miles	Juma Ikangaa	1:11:54
25K	Juma Ikangaa	1:14:35
30K	Juma Ikangaa	1:30:20
40K	Abebe Mekonnen	2:03:10
One-to-go	Abebe Mekonnen	2:04:13
Last mile	Abebe Mekonnen	4:53

1989 Men's Results

1.	A. Mekonnen, Ethiopia	2:09:06	13.	G. Karagiannis, Greece	2:20:50
2.	J. Ikangaa, Tanzania	2:09:56	14.	I. Rodrigues, Brazil	2:21:00
3.	J. Treacy, Ireland	2:10:24	15.	M. Vera, Mexico	2:21:44
4.	I. Hussein, Kenya	2:12:41	16.	I. Ramirez, Colombia	2:21:57
5.	J. Campbell, New Zealand	2:14:19	17.	D. Dunham, MA	2:22:03
6.	S. Naali, Tanzania	2:14:59	18.	A. Aregha, Ethiopia	2:22:20
7.	G. Alcala, Mexico	2:15:51	19.	V. Mora, Colombia	2:22:49
8.	K. Ito, Japan	2:16:19	20.	M. Taif, France	2:23:01
9.	C. Wuresa, Ethiopia	2:17:31	21.	O. Aguilar, Chile	2:23:03
10.	H. Wills, FL	2:17:40	22.	T. Jones, CO	2:23:23
11.	R. Marczak, Poland	2:17:43	23.	B. Allen, MA	2:23:28
12.	D. Harrison, New Zealand	2:20:40	24.	T. Mimura, Japan	2:24:04

25. L. Lopez, Costa Rica	2:24:14	41. K. Kato, Japan	2:27:49
26. J. Molloy, MA	2:24:50	42. L. Denning, CO	2:28:09
27. J. Kreutz, VT	2:24:57	43. H. Chavez, Mexico	2:28:17
28. A. Romero, Canada	2:24:57	44. K. Doll, West Germany	2:28:47
29. S. Otsu, Japan	2:25:05	45. P. Masaras, Greece	2:28:51
30. J. Machalek, Sweden	2:25:25	46. D. Allen, WI	2:28:55
31. E. Lee, United Kingdom	2:25:33	47. S. Cranford, GA	2:29:23
32. N. Bergeron, Canada	2:25:35	48. R. Bieber, PA	2:29:27
33. H. Clavijo, Colombia	2:25:41	49. J. Mello, MA	2:29:40
34. M. Brochu, Canada	2:25:42	50. V. Miranda, Panama	2:30:13
35. B. Schwelm, PA	2:26:46	963. B. Menard, FL	3:00:00
36. T. McGraw, ME	2:26:56	2763. C. Glickman, NY	3:30:02
37. R. Ferguson, VA	2:27:19	**3428. J.J. Kelley, CT**	**3:46:50**
38. S. Branch, MA	2:27:31	3795. R. Flynn, MA	4:00:53
39. A. Oman, NY	2:27:40	J.A. Kelley (age 81)	5:05:00
40. M. Meyers, WI	2:27:46		

5,285 starters, 4,239 finishers.

40-49

		60-69	
1. J. Campbell, New Zealand	2:14:19	1. M. Jones, United Kingdom	3:04:46
2. R. Marczak, Poland	2:17:43	2. J. Johncock, MI	3:12:13
3. V. Mora, Colombia	2:22:49	3. B. Hoffman, AR	3:12:36
4. B. Allen, MA	2:23:28	4. R. Lussier, MA	3:12:42
5. J. Machalek, Sweden	2:25:25	5. B. Early, Ireland	3:13:19
6. E. Lee, United Kingdom	2:25:33		
7. N. Bergeron, Canada	2:25:35		
8. H. Chavez, Mexico	2:28:17		
10. R. Reimer, CO	2:31:41		

50-59

1. M. Williams, VA	2:39:40
2. F. Bradley, Washington, DC	2:42:39
3. J. Burgasser, FL	2:42:51
4. J. Fordor, OH	2:45:02
5. D. Smith, LA	2:45:47
6. R. Jamborsky, VA	2:49:23

I'LL BE BACK

MONDAY, APRIL 17, 1989

Kristiansen Wants World Record

Ingrid Kristiansen, now 33, looked to most like the woman who would win the 1989 Boston Marathon. But like so many runners before her, winning alone no longer challenged her. She wanted the world record. She had won the Boston Marathon 3 years earlier. She knew how hard it would be. She wore white cotton gloves to wipe the sweat off her face on this warm day.

She had already run a 2:21:06 marathon for the world best in 1985, and only 2 weeks before the Boston Marathon she had won the Boston Milk Run 10K in 30:59. Larry Newman, the BAA press liaison, said that based on Kristiansen's matchup with Joan Benoit Samuelson and her past few races, including a world best in the half marathon in March, there was good reason to believe that she was ready to become the first woman in history to run under 2:20. She had tried it 3 years before at Boston, but it had been too hot. She planned to go for it again. She stated the obvious: If you don't try, you'll never do it. Kristiansen was the only woman to hold the 5,000-meter, 10,000-meter, and marathon records simultaneously. She had run 19 marathons and won 11. If anyone could do it, she could. But the race against Benoit Samuelson would not happen. Benoit Samuelson had not been able to train as much as in previous years. This race came 10 years and one child after Benoit's first win in Boston, so although she would run, she would be no match for Kristiansen.

Kristiansen ran exactly the same time at 5 miles as she had in her attempt to break 2:20 in her victory in 1986. Benoit Samuelson gamely ran in second

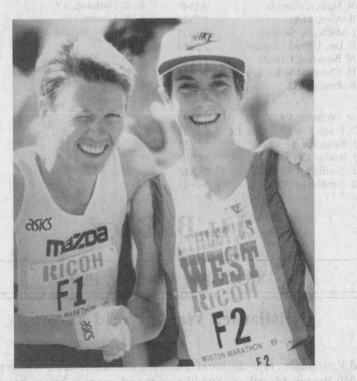

Good friends at the starting line, Ingrid Kristiansen (#F1) and Joan Benoit Samuelson (#F2) soon commit themselves to the course. © Victah/Agence Shot.

place at halfway, but her hip troubled her. After halfway Lisa Weidenbach moved into second place.

From way back in the pack a New Zealand dentist, Marguerite Buist, began her drive through the pack. She wore a one-piece bright orange suit that would have looked stylish on a beach. That it simultaneously revealed athleticism and femininity would have pleased Kathrine Switzer. Buist passed Weidenbach after 20 miles. By this time temperatures reached toward 70 °F. Kristiansen again gave up her goal of breaking 2:20. Her coach, Johan Kaggestad, said she would have to wait for an overcast, drizzling day. She ran within her abilities to insure her win.

Weidenbach dropped behind Kim Jones from Spokane, Washington, and Eriko Asai of Japan. Benoit Samuelson's hip prevented her from taking a full stride. An hour of great weight fell upon her as first one runner then another passed her, pushing her down to ninth place. Once she was the unbeatable best in the world, now she could only hobble. Fans cheered. Friends and family cheered. Nothing helped. Willpower could not stretch a stride out of her constricted hip. Still, she would not drop out. Stubbornly she staggered over the finish line. But at the postrace press conference, almost in tears, she said that people expected her to announce her retirement:

> A lot of people are expecting me to say, "This is it." They have been expecting me to say that before, but this is not it. I've been spending as much time in physical therapy as in training. I just can't go on doing that, I just can't go on with my responsibilities as a wife and mother and spend as much time in physical therapy. . . . I've run some good races and I think I have some very good races left in me and I want everyone to know that it's still there. . . . I will run again.

As Benoit Samuelson left the press conference the purportedly professionally disinterested press had apparently become fans: They applauded. I have been duly humbled, she thought. But I will be back. It is not the end of Joan Benoit Samuelson's career.

Checkpoint Splits

5 miles	Ingrid Kristiansen	26:00
10 miles	Ingrid Kristiansen	52:50
13.1 miles	Ingrid Kristiansen	1:09:31
15 miles	Ingrid Kristiansen	1:20:08
20 miles	Ingrid Kristiansen	1:48:17
25 miles	Ingrid Kristiansen	2:18:10

1989 Women's Results

1.	**I. Kristiansen, Norway**	**2:24:33**	20.	C. Iwahashi, CA	2:51:23
		(26th overall)	21.	P. Donovan, NH	2:51:27
2.	M. Buist, New Zealand	2:29:04	22.	S. Meltzer, OK	2:51:53
3.	K. Jones, WA	2:29:34	23.	T. Martland, RI	2:53:29
4.	E. Asai, Japan	2:33:04	24.	S. Kessler, NY	2:54:30
5.	**L. Weidenbach, WA**	**2:33:18**	25.	L. Hruby, PA	2:54:43
6.	L. Welch-Brady, MA	2:34:16	26.	A. Lilburn, FL	2:55:07
7.	P. Welch, United Kingdom	2:35:00	27.	C. Venture-Merkel, VA	2:56:18
8.	O. LaPierre, Canada	2:35:51	28.	J. Hutchinson, MO	2:56:29
9.	**J. Benoit Samuelson, ME**	**2:37:52**	29.	K. Haulenbeek, NJ	2:56:43
10.	L. Binder, CA	2:39:21	30.	B. Larson, WA	2:56:55
11.	C. Mentlewicz, Poland	2:40:25	31.	C. Virga, FL	2:57:13
12.	N. Corsaro, MA	2:41:13	32.	K. Beebee, MA	2:58:28
13.	A. Hearn, United Kingdom	2:41:39	33.	L. Scofea, VA	2:59:05
14.	L. Kindelan, OR	2:42:41	34.	V. Johnson, TN	3:01:10
15.	C. New, Canada	2:42:56	35.	N. Wadden, Canada	3:01:38
16.	M. Yli-Ilkka, Finland	2:45:51	98.	K. Airoldi, MA	3:15:08
17.	M. Tanigawa, Japan	2:46:11	282.	B. Capasso, WI	3:30:00
18.	A. Wehner, DE	2:47:32	695.	J. Osborne, Washington, DC	4:00:10
19.	M. Wood, CO	2:49:05			

1,133 starters, 864 finishers under 4:30.

40-49

1.	P. Welch, United Kingdom	2:35:00
2.	L. Binder, CA	2:39:21
3.	A. Hearn, United Kingdom	2:41:39
4.	M. Wood, CO	2:49:05
5.	J. Hutchinson, MO	2:56:29
6.	K. Beebee, MA	2:58:28
7.	V. Johnson, TN	3:01:10

50-59

1.	W. Yu, NY	3:23:19
2.	E. Quinn, NJ	3:26:42
3.	M. Betz, NY	3:26:52

Chapter 10

1990-1995
New World Order?

Presidents: *George Bush, William Clinton*

Massachusetts Governors: *Michael Dukakis, William Weld*

Boston Mayors: *Raymond Flynn, Thomas Menino*

1990 Populations: *United States, 248,709,873; Massachusetts, 5,876,000; Boston, 574,283*

After the Gulf War victory of the United States–led coalition against the Iraqi regime of Saddam Hussein, U.S. President George Bush rode a 91% approval rating with the American public. Bush proclaimed that the victory ushered in a "New World Order." In the next year's election, the same American public voted Bush out of office in a world of growing unpredictability, which led the wise guys to speak of a "New World Disorder."

Because the last decade of the millennium has only half passed, we cannot revisit it as we have the earlier decades. But we can note that the rate of change of nearly everything is accelerating. We talk of global warming and global recession while nearly every village on the planet is hooked on Coca-Cola, CNN, and the Internet. The Boston Marathon can be watched via video on every continent. With every top marathoner in the world eventually finding her or his way to Boston, it is clearly a global sporting event. Yet the trend to globalization faces a countervailing and not necessarily contradictory force—ethnic sovereignty. Each ethnic group seems to want its own country.

While worldwide popular culture becomes more homogeneous, personal loyalties seem to get devoted to smaller units. With the breakup of the Soviet Union and Yugoslavia and the creation of the Czech Republic and Slovakia as well as Namibia, there are more countries in the world than in 1989. Yet as top runners differentiate themselves with national uniforms, they come together under the sponsorship of global corporations like Nike, Reebok, and John Hancock. Former Soviet citizens play an important role in the Boston Marathon as they come to run for Russia, Ukraine, Kyrgyzstan, or Belarus. Most former Soviets, as private entrepreneurs, have sponsorship contracts with Reebok. Curiously, most runners and observers were not concerned in the 1950s whether Emil Zatopek was a Czech or a Slovak, nor did we wonder in 1958 if Franjo Mihalic was Serb, Croat, or Bosnian.

531

Beginning with the close of World War II the long-distance running sub-culture erased national differences, adopting successful training strategies regardless of their origin.

The 1990s emphasize the international breadth of the Boston Marathon fields. Fewer and fewer Americans fill the ranks of the elite runners; they have been joined by all-star teams of Ethiopians, Portuguese, Italians, Germans, Kenyans, Tanzanians, Mexicans, Colombians, Brazilians, and Spanish as well as the traditional groups of Finnish, Swedes, Irish, Japanese, English, Scottish, French, and Canadian runners. The long-banned South Africans have joined Moroccans and Algerians as well as Chinese and returning Koreans.

The role of the John Hancock Financial Services and their quiet international operatives like Patrick Lynch in assembling crack fields becomes apparent in the 1990s. Some wonder whose race it is since 1986, the BAA's or Hancock's. In fact every winner, man and woman from 1986 until 1995, was a Hancock-sponsored athlete. A week before the 1989 race Hancock replaced their 10-year, $10-million sponsorship with a 15-year pact worth $18 million. They maintained in a press release that their sponsorship agreement with the BAA would maintain stability well into the 21st century if they exercise their 5-year sponsorship option. Critics feel the arrangement makes the race too dependent on a single major sponsor. (In this decade the BAA gets minor sponsors such as Adidas and Citgo.) But the relationship with Hancock has worked to bring together the top marathoners from all over the world.

Yet many countries of the world had war rather than athletics on their minds early in the 1990s. On October 2, 1990, Iraq invaded Kuwait. On September 30, 1991, the Yugoslav (Serbian) army moved on Croatia. By 1995, the United Nations was still powerless to quell the conflict. On December 13, 1991, the Soviet Union broke up, ending years of Cold War. The American economy continued its relative decline, leading some pundits to say that the Cold War had two losers. In 1992 Americans elected Bill Clinton president on a platform pledging change.

Clinton, who runs 3 miles at 8:00 minutes per mile daily, invited the 1993 Boston winners to run with him in Washington a few days later. The Road Runners Club of America reported that membership applications increased because of President Clinton's avid jogging. Could this presidential attention to running precipitate another boom as Kennedy's interest in fitness did in the 1960s?

During the Boston Marathon of 1993, images of flaming buildings interrupted television coverage of the race. Agents of the Federal Bureau of Alcohol, Tobacco, and Firearms stormed the enclave of the Branch Davidians in Waco, Texas. The resulting fire in the enclave killed 72 Davidians. On April 19, 2 years later, a bomb, later said to be planted in revenge for the Waco deaths, exploded in front of the federal building in Oklahoma City, Oklahoma, killing 169 people.

In American midterm elections, the nation's citizens elected virtually a new Congress, creating a new Republican majority in opposition to the Democratic president. Amid this apparent confusion the country's economy continued robust demonstrations of the profitability of American business with record prices in the stock market.

Things look very good for the Boston Marathon in this seemingly disorderly world as up to 50,000 runners—10 times the usual field—prepare to celebrate the 100th running of the race in April of 1996. The Boston Athletic Association intends to find and invite every living winner to join the party.

THE JINX AND THE MAD AFRICANS

MONDAY, APRIL 16, 1990

Can Olympic Gold Medalist Win at Boston?

In the months before the 1990 Boston Marathon another apparently scandalous incident riled Boston Marathon runners and fans. The consequence of seeming bureaucratic bungling set off attacks and counterattacks in the Boston and national media. Boston people got as passionate about a change in rules as they had about Rosie Ruiz and Marshall Medoff.

At first no one saw a problem in a simple rule change. But some past winners got angry at The Athletics Congress (TAC) (now USA Track and Field). Bill Rodgers said that TAC was taking things too far:

> Traditionally, TAC has been anti-athlete and Stalinistic. They're going to wipe out history? It's like the secret police in an Eastern bloc country. . . . My question is do they know anything about marathoning? They're up in their ivory tower and they don't understand the effect of the Boston hills when you push hard or what happens when the race is warm.

"[The people who made this rule are] obscure statisticians in back rooms who couldn't even run half a marathon. I believe it has come down to a matter of ego with these guys," said Alberto Salazar.

At TAC's 1989 convention in Washington, DC, in early December, the technical people on the rules committee passed a new rule:

> For all road records: The course must not have a net decrease in elevation exceeding one part per thousand (i.e., 1 meter per km).
> The start and the finish of the race must lie closer than 30% of the race distance apart, as measured along the straight line between

them, except that when it can be shown that the average component
of the wind direction for the duration of the race did not to any
extent whatsoever constitute a tail wind. The method of determin-
ing wind direction shall be as specified by the Road Running Technical Committee.

Guy Morse, director of the Boston Marathon, emerged from the meeting
and announced, "We lost, I can't believe it; we lost."

The Boston Marathon course from point to point is basically a straight
line, west to east, that drops from 490 feet above sea level in Hopkinton to
10 feet at the finish. In New England the prevailing winds come from the
west. The Boston Marathon course fell outside the rule. So it appeared that
future world record times set on the Boston Marathon course would not
count. Under the new rule Yun Bok Suh's 1947 world record of 2:25:39,
Liane Winter's 1975 world record of 2:42:24, and Joan Benoit's 1983 world
record of 2:22:43 would not have counted. In fact, the rule was seen as
retroactive. Those world marks, as well as Rodgers's, Salazar's, and Benoit's
American records set on the Boston course, would be stricken from the books.

That revelation unleashed a volley of media exchanges that ignited normally introverted runners to threaten to burn their TAC cards. TAC membership cards are the ID—the road runner's drivers license—of members of the
Congress-appointed governing body of amateur athletics in the U.S. This is
the organization that replaced the Amateur Athletic Union. The technical
people who enacted the change were not usually movers and shakers but
measurers and counters. They carried calculators. One of them, Alan Jones,
had even invented a counting device to precisely measure the distances of
road race courses. These men and women had done good, important, careful
work in bringing state-of-the-art technology to the sport of road racing.
Their pens, maps, charts, calculators, and Jones-counters had brought added
respect. The proliferation of TAC-certified courses allowed runners to be
certain at last of their road racing personal records. But the new rule slipped
into being without public relations response from the TAC leadership or
the directors and sponsors of the big marathons, New York and Boston.
Suddenly the biggest and most prestigious races appeared banned from
world record consideration. The threat that world records, American records,
and personal records would be confiscated by a bunch of bureaucrats lingered in the air.

The BAA vs. TAC controversy broke in the *Boston Globe* in mid-January
of 1990. The *Globe* said that TAC had discredited the Boston Marathon course.

But, had the Boston Marathon ever been credited? If so, by whom? What
was the real Boston Marathon record? As we have seen in the past, the exact
distance of the Boston Marathon was not set in stone, asphalt, or dirt, so
there were many records for the various course lengths over the years. But
the 2:07:51 run by Rob de Castella in 1986 remains the undisputed best
time ever on the Boston Marathon course. There is a slight but important

distinction between *best* times and *record* times. From the beginning of the sport of marathoning there had not been recognized world records for the marathon or any other road race, because all courses were too different; there were *world bests*. The term *world record* applied only to track races, run in controllable arenas built for the sport. Road races, on the other hand, had virtually no rules. Engineers had designed the roads for automobiles, not runners. Yet the technologies had developed to such a precision that marathon courses could now be measured exactly and compared with one another.

Past distances for road races have been only approximate. Up until the 1970s New England was the most active region in the country and perhaps the world for road races. But a "10"-miler could actually be 8 or 12 miles long. A course measured to the nearest tenth of a mile was a rarity. Runners could not compare one race to another. They could not be sure of their own personal records, let alone regional, national, or world records set on the roads. Journalists could not compare one runner to another to judge who might really be the favorite for an upcoming race unless they could refer to a track race. Race directors and sponsors could not defensibly say that a best time for their particular race distance was set on their course, although they could be fairly accurate about a course record. As the sport of road racing grew throughout the 1970s and '80s, accuracy became more important to more people.

The movement toward greater accuracy started in the 1970s with Ken Young of Arizona, the self-appointed head of the self-financed, self-operated National Running Data Center. (Young had to be self-appointed because in those days governing bodies—the AAU—had no funds for his efforts.) His data bank was the first of its kind. But he often did not know if a submitted time had been really run over the entire distance that the runner and race director maintained. Fast times were automatically suspect. Standards of acceptance for entry into the data bank became essential. The time had arrived to establish precise techniques for measuring courses. No longer was it enough to drive the course and note the odometer reading—automobile odometers differed wildly. Young needed more precision to compare courses across the nation. During the late 1980s people with technical abilities and inclinations joined TAC and formed the Road Running Technical Committee. Race courses became more accurate. Yet in the months before the Boston Marathon of 1990, the controversy raged.

Negotiating a way out of this mess fell to Boston Marathon Race Director Guy Morse. The view out of Morse's 8th-floor window underlooked the slender 62-story John Hancock tower. The race's million-dollar sponsors were up there somewhere. Morse hefted a file of news clippings. He was not happy.

> I went to the [TAC] convention because I knew this rule would come
> up. At other conventions we and friends of the Boston Marathon

were able to keep it shelved. This year I talked to each of the sports committees in the meetings, the men's and women's long distance running committees, the rules committee, the technical committee, the records committee, the masters committee. I went to each to argue that the rule should not exclude Boston from record status.

"I think the press, sponsors, and public don't care about wind or hills unless they are extreme," said Morse. Weather, Morse contended, was an act of God and should not be standardized, but a course itself was an act of race directors, so courses could of course be designed merely to allow records to be set. "But such races," Morse continued, "are short sighted." Morse said that if race directors and sponsors set out to design ever-faster, downhill, wind-tunnel courses they would quickly run out of locations. But Boston and New York would not be moved to get faster times or slower times, said Morse. "We won't adjust the course one inch." Would TAC adjust? Who would budge or blink, Boston or TAC?

In their search for increasing degrees of precision, The Athletics Congress Road Racing Technical Committee forgot the reason for sport in society. They forgot that road racing is a reprieve from the confines of the track and that the marathon is as much a celebration as a race against time. Technology need not be applied to a problem simply because the technology is available.

In the past course measurement had been sloppy. Most embarrassing had been the disappearance of about 1,200 yards due to road reconstruction in the mid-1950s. It took years for anyone to notice that the course was about 5 minutes shorter.

Precision does take vigilance. But sometimes marathoners, sponsors, administrators all begin to wonder what marathoning is for. For most participants sport is supposed to be for fun and celebration; it is what makes life worth living between bouts of work. There is a sweetness to being able to spend effort in nonessential activity. The Boston Marathon was born out of celebration, not precision.

TAC and the big marathons reached a compromise: All performances would be listed, and race conditions such as slope and wind would be noted against those apparently "aided" times.

The Jinx

From Johnny Hayes and Bill Sherring in the early years of the century on to Albin Stenroos, Delfo Cabrera, and favorite Abebe Bikila in 1963—no Olympic gold medalist had won the Boston Marathon. The jinx seemed to be a disease that struck every Olympic gold medalist who ventured to Boston.

Many had tried, but all had failed: Thomas Hicks, who won Olympic gold in 1904, ran in Boston many times but never won; nor did Johnny Hayes, gold in 1908. The 1948 Olympic champion Cabrera finished 6th in Boston in 1954; 1924 Olympic champion Stenroos came to Boston, but Johnny Miles beat him. Between Olympic victories Abebe Bikila came to Boston in 1963 and lost; Frank Shorter, gold in 1972, later finished 23rd and 75th in Boston. The Boston media portrayed the possibility of an Olympic gold medalist's winning the Boston Marathon as an organically impossible achievement.

Two women, Joan Benoit and Rosa Mota, had won the Boston Marathon and then went on to win Olympic gold medals, but as holders of Olympic gold, neither had won at Boston. So it seemed that if you had the gold you couldn't have Boston. But Mota and Gelindo Bordin thought they could be different.

Four brothers born in the small town of Lumignano, near Venice in northern Italy, had preceded Gelindo Bordin's entrance into his world on the second of April in 1959. These sons of a farmer lived in a big house in the country with four other families. The children all lived in one big room set up like a barracks; 22 of them slept and played like crazy cousins. Gelindo worked hard on the farm in the summer. Until age 14 he defended his team's goal against soccer balls. His older brother Nerino had run 5K in 15 minutes and a marathon in 2:22. He brought Gelindo to a race for the first time. Nerino won.

Within 2 months Gelindo won his regional cross-country championship. It was running, not soccer, that captured him—it would be his sport for life. Bordin spent a year as a runner in the military at age 18. He grew to be tall, strong, and gregarious. He usually wore a short beard, giving his strong-featured face a biblical force, yet he could play the clown. During a training run with Bill Rodgers and Greg Meyer, Bordin dropped a step behind as they passed a stop sign. Bordin reached up and whacked the sign with his palm and fell to the ground, holding his head. The loud sound horrified Rodgers, sure that Bordin was seriously injured. As Rodgers bent over Bordin to attend to his injuries or administer last rites, Bordin burst into crazy laughter.

He committed another of his jokes on Italian national television. Several months after he won the Olympic gold medal in 1988, he announced with a sad face his retirement from sport. The next day's headlines read "Bordin Annuncia Il Suo Retiro." By noon he revealed his joke to the world.

But racing Bordin took seriously. By 1978 he ran 19th in the International Junior Cross-Country Championships in Glasgow, Scotland. But it all nearly ended on an ordinary training run in 1981.

Bordin had no idea what had happened to him when he suddenly awoke in a hospital after a 6-hour coma. He didn't know where he was or how he had gotten there. His skull was broken, shards of glass imbedded in the bone. Seven vertebrae were broken, and ligaments were torn in his left knee. For the next 4 months Bordin saw double. He had been hit by a car, found by the roadside, and taken to a hospital, but the impact of his skull against the pavement had destroyed all memory of the collision.

The doctors told Bordin not to run for 6 months, but in 3 weeks he ran, bent painfully over. Breathing came with difficulty. Days passed as he gradually recovered. Fortunately the accident left only an eerie memory of waking up in a hospital. By 1986 Bordin won the European Championships. He finished third in the World Championships in 1987. For 1988 he focused on the Olympic marathon; he ran Boston that year only because it offered the most competitive field in the world and would best prepare him for the Olympics. He decided he would have to come back another year to win.

Once Bordin won the Olympic marathon in Seoul he had to return to win Boston, because in 1988 it had reclaimed its position as the world's most competitive marathon. He wanted to show that he, the Olympic champion, could win in spite of "The Jinx"—that recurring bad luck that struck Olympic gold medalists, preventing them from winning in Boston. Jinx or no, Bordin liked Boston; lots of Italians lived in its North End, a place that would become almost a second home to Gelindo.

Gelindo Bordin liked a lot of things. He liked to eat. He liked to cook. With glee, gusto, and garlic he cooked big meals for his friends. He made a savory meal for Joan Benoit Samuelson and her family on a visit to their Maine seaside home. Bordin liked clothing; he even designed athletic clothes. His girlfriend—tall, blond Patrizia Cassard, a half-French 2:06 half-miler and architecture student from Turin—wore his creations well. His designs courageously combined colors and shapes not ordinarily found in nature. They pressed against the fine edge of fashion violation. Bordin had studied design and he held a degree in "Geometra"—something less than an engineer or architect but between them in function in the construction industry. As an employee of the Bottacini construction company from 1979 to 1986, he specialized in home design, selecting and coordinating materials and re-working specifications.

Bordin worked hard at his job, and he worked hard at running. He lived in Verona, Italy. For 5 years he committed to a daily routine: 13 miles in the morning, work until noon, 13 miles, work until late. He experimented by running over 200 miles in a single week. He had no time to clown, party, or relax. He got a skin rash. It itched. He could not sleep. No medicine helped. He could not work full-time and train his best for racing. By that point in his life Bordin had run a 2:11 marathon and placed in the top 10 in the World Cross-Country Championships. He faced a choice, realizing that he had to understand what he did to train his body. In a strong sense, for Bordin training his body offered a full-time engineering and design project. The job at Bottacini stood in the way of his improvement as a runner. Bordin began to think of training for running as his profession. He would take the risk—a turned ankle or another car accident might leave him with no livelihood. But he had to quit Bottacini. He needed the time to design and engineer his body to become a perfect running machine. He had to see how good he could get.

Bordin took on a coach, Luciano Gigliotti, to help him understand what worked and what did not work in his training and to act as his agent. With Gigliotti, a masseur, and himself, Bordin had the team to extract everything possible from his body. He went to Tenerife Island in the Canary Islands to train at altitude, because the island raised hills in the shadow of Pico de Teide at 3,718 meters—and it offered no distractions from running up them and growing stronger. Bordin came to Boston with Patrizia Cassard and Coach Gigliotti.

When Gigliotti saw how the Africans ran the first miles of the Boston course, he said that they were funny guys, crazy guys; it was just not possible to run like that. He called their pace ludicrous. But the Africans could not save themselves from the sway of competition.

In 1990 the biggest field yet for the Boston Marathon—9,362 people—packed together behind the starting line. These were official entrants who qualified for the race, not the total volume of people waiting to run out of Hopkinton. The official qualifying times were relaxed by 10 minutes each to 3:10 for open men and 3:40 for open women. Behind the official runners waited uncountable thousands, maybe three, of unofficial, numberless runners. Race officials affectionately called them *bandits*. In other races without qualifying times, like the New York City Marathon, fields reached 20,000. From a distance these races looked like mass migrations, calling to mind caribou, wildebeest, or lemmings.

The masses of pressed-together racers generated astonishing heat on a warm spring day. At the gun they gave way like a loosed cliff that fell, thinning as it tumbled, down the slipface to Boston. At the crest ran exuberant, incorrigible Kenyans, Ethiopians, and Tanzanians. Provoked by the 1988 winner, Ibrahim Hussein, they surged, fell back, surged again, and passed the first mile in 4:26, the next in 4:32, and the next in 4:37. In 1985 observers had called Geoff Smith's pace crazy, but he had run only 4:40 miles. Smith himself watched from a place behind the pack of mad Africans. He ran those same 4:40 miles as in 1985 and could not believe all those guys were running ahead of him. Smith ran with Greg Meyer, who pointed ahead and said that those guys had to be totally crazy—they couldn't possibly be that good. The two former winners reassured themselves that their own pace was right. Both were in good shape. Meyer had trained at high altitude in Alamosa, Colorado, for 2 months. Smith had run a 1:03:32 half marathon a month earlier. Smith and Meyer each planned to be factors in the race, if not outright repeat winners. But for now they could not catch up to get into the race, let alone dominate; they ran behind without influence, watching the receding pack, hoping that all the Africans had blundered and would slam into the proverbial wall en masse. Meyer and Smith kept wondering who all those lunatics were up there anyway.

Rob de Castella, the 1986 winner and course record holder, likewise watched in amazement. He thought that the Africans actually raced each other, egging each other on in a private competition, oblivious to the rest of the world. Did they think they were 800-meter track runners who could run a fast first lap and hang on for the next? De Castella thought the Africans had a very short memory of previous marathons or didn't respect the race.

But it was not only Africans who ran ahead of de Castella, Smith, and Meyer. Alone in the turbulence, but well behind the lead pack, ran a man at a merely crazy pace. Bordin ran telling himself that he ran a crazy pace but that all those raucous ebony men who ran ahead of him would come back to him. In the 1988 Boston Bordin had run 2:09:27 for fourth place behind two of them. At this rate it looked to him as if he might run 2:05 and place seventh. But he kept telling himself that ahead raced a mob of insanity. He ran *pazzo*, but they ran *pazzissimo*. The Africans seemed spooked, like a herd of gemsbok leaping and bounding away from a hungry lion. Bordin saw panic on the Serengeti Plain. If he could stay cool and control his emotions he might have a chance. But his incorrigibly Italian upbringing had produced a man of emotion and passion, art tempered with science. Science said slow down, yet he had to stay close regardless of the danger. Like the sons of the wind ahead of him, Bordin ran at the mercy of his origins.

The Tanzanians, Juma Ikangaa and Simon Robert Naali; two Ethiopians, Zeleke Metafaria and Tesfaye Tafa; and two Kenyans, Ibrahim Hussein and Kipkemboi Kimeli, did not look like the funny guys Gigliotti saw. They ran through 5 furious miles in 23:05. Yet Ikangaa did not feel he ran too fast at all. He had finished second to Hussein in 1988 and second to Mekonnen in 1989. He did not want to again finish second to another African. De Castella once explained Ikangaa's motivation from his own experience.

Eight years after de Castella beat Ikangaa by a few seconds to win the 1982 Commonwealth Games Marathon, the two of them found themselves together again in that race, but this time both were fading out of the top 10 and just running to finish. With 5K to go de Castella turned to Ikangaa to offer to run together. Ikangaa agreed, saying it would be a nice thing to do; so de Castella thought Ikangaa had agreed to finish with him and not sprint. But another African runner gained on them. De Castella turned to Ikangaa to say that maybe they ought to pick up the pace to stay ahead of him, but de Castella began to think that he really did not care if he finished 11th or 12th. With 50 meters to go the other African caught them. Ikangaa detonated a sprint and beat the other African. De Castella watched them go. After the finish he asked Ikangaa what had happened to their agreement. As if it explained everything, Ikangaa said, "Ah, yes, but he was from Zimbabwe."

This year Ikangaa and Hussein set a scorching pace to burn off the newcomers. But the newcomers had enormous talent. Kimeli, 24, was the 10,000-meter Olympic bronze medalist with a 27:25.16; Metafaria, 21, had won the World Cup Marathon in Milan a year earlier; and Tafa, 25, had just run a course record of 1:03:24 in the hilly, hot San Blas Half Marathon in Puerto Rico. Naali led the 1989 Boston Marathon for half the race before finishing sixth. Since then he had won the Honolulu Marathon. Some of these men might have newly come to Boston, but none were neophyte runners. They did not burn off easily.

Ikangaa himself had trained to his physical and philosophical limit. He often said, "The will to win means nothing without the will to prepare." The Africans ran at course record and world record pace, but because of a recent ruling by The Athletics Congress, any such supposed record might not be official. The problems caused by the ruling—problems of measurement, wind, and slope—ripped up the Boston Marathon running community almost as much as had the Marshall Medoff affair. But road racing is at heart a matter of running wild through the streets, which was exactly what this pack of Africans did, much to the distress of one tall, bearded Italian.

At 10K Bordin thought that the Africans could not finish the race at that pace, but he did not chase them. He ran alone. He took his mind off racing and waited to push himself later. But he worried, not about the runners ahead, but about a runner behind, one running a sane pace—maybe Smith, maybe Meyer, maybe de Castella. Bordin passed the half marathon 45 seconds behind Ikangaa's 1:02:01 checkpoint record. De Castella followed him.

Bordin thought of the course as "free for the mind, but hard on the body." He knew the Boston course would not allow him to run at a specific, mechanical pace, as is most efficient on a flat course. Because each section of the course is different, he could not click off even split times like a machine; instead he had to release his mind and emotions to run as his body felt best over all the little hills in Natick and Wellesley. And he knew that the downhills would rend his quadriceps muscles with microtears.

But the fact that he ran alone may have helped him, because unlike the surging Africans, he had no obligation to respond to someone else's pace just to stay with the pack. The men in the lead pack ran to avoid the conspicuous disgrace of falling off the group. They had to drive their bodies into oxygen debt, perhaps just at the moment when they needed to cruise, relax, and recuperate. Bordin had no such pressures. He pushed, cruised, relaxed, and recuperated at the rate his body required.

Bordin saw Naali coming back after 25 kilometers. He could finally see the digital clock on the lead vehicle. He focused on that. Up the hills he passed the Ethiopians and Hussein. Hussein would soon drop out of the race with what he feared was a career-ending injury to his Achilles tendon.

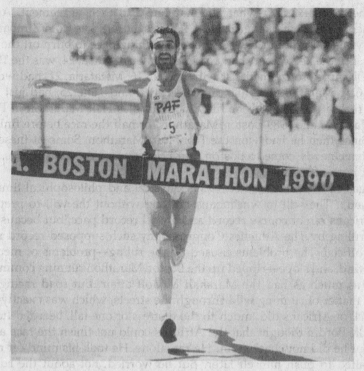

Were it not for the fact that Gelindo Bordin was in seventh place at the half marathon point in 1:02:46, his pace would have been deemed crazy. © Victah/Agence Shot.

At last only Ikangaa ran between Bordin and the lead. At the crest of the hills Bordin carefully passed Ikangaa. By scrupulously keeping to the opposite side of the road Bordin hoped he would not inspire Ikangaa to run away on the downhill. But Ikangaa had problems.

At halfway Ikangaa expected to run 2:08 and win, but his calf muscle tightened. A cramp took control. He thought that if he tried to follow Bordin in order to win, the calf muscle would not permit it and he would risk losing second place. For the first time in the race Ikangaa adopted a defensive tactic. He let Bordin pass. Would he have let another African pass, or would he have ignored the protesting muscle and run full speed ahead?

Ikangaa survived to take second place for the third straight year. Again he had run a fast and aggressive pace, leading from the start, just as he had in his other two Boston Marathons and his Olympic marathon. But again it did not produce victory. He said he was very disappointed but that some things were beyond his control. He said he felt unlucky to finish second so many times but that he would keep coming back and keep trying.

Bordin broke the jinx. He became the first Olympic gold medalist to win the Boston Marathon. He had to chase down a pack of pace-crazy Africans, but he succeeded where so many Olympic champions had failed. Bordin's exuberance, intelligence, and friendliness made him a great hit with the Boston crowds.

Rolando Vera of Ecuador ran an even pace to finish third. John Campbell of New Zealand ran an even pace to finish fourth. He was 41 years old. His time of 2:11:04 broke countryman Jack Foster's 16-year-old world masters record. Campbell had an odd running history; he kept quitting and returning. At age 19 he had made the New Zealand team for the World Junior Cross-Country Championships, but he had placed a dismal 69th. He decided he did not like running, quit running, got married, had two kids, and became a trawler fisherman. In 1974 Campbell returned to running and ran 5,000 meters in 14:01, only to fail to qualify for the Commonwealth Games by one second. So he quit running again. In 1983 his marriage ended, so he began running again. This time he made the Commonwealth team and by 1986 ran a 2:15:55 for 14th place in the New York City Marathon. In 1987 the New Zealand selectors left him off the national team. Again he got angry and quit running. This time he bought a new fishing trawler and went to sea.

A year later Campbell returned yet again to running. He had read Jack Foster's *The Tale of the Ancient Marathoner* two or three times. The book inspired him to go after the author's world record. He quit fishing. At times he ran as much as 180 miles in a week. He married again, had a son, and opened a dairy store. In 1988 he had placed 12th in the Olympic marathon; in the 1988 Boston, 6th with a 2:11:08 at age 39; and now, 4th at age 41, he had run his best race and fastest time. But he had to live with the disquieting notion that a masters athlete really has no future.

Checkpoint Splits

5K	Simon Naali	14:04	
5 miles	Juma Ikangaa	23:05	
10K	Simon Naali	28:44	(Gelindo Bordin, 7th, 29:31)
15K	Simon Naali	43:29	
10 miles	Juma Ikangaa	46:53	(Gelindo Bordin, 7th, 47:32)
20K	Juma Ikangaa	58:41	
1/2 marathon	Juma Ikangaa	1:02:01	(Gelindo Bordin, 7th, 1:02:46)
15 miles	Juma Ikangaa	1:11:15	
25K	Juma Ikangaa	1:13:51	(Gelindo Bordin, 6th, 1:14:47)
30K	Juma Ikangaa	1:29:40	(Gelindo Bordin, 3rd, 1:30:29)
20 miles	Juma Ikangaa	1:36:53	(Gelindo Bordin, 2nd, 1:37:09)
35K	Gelindo Bordin	1:45:58	
40K	Gelindo Bordin	2:01:24	
25 miles	Gelindo Bordin	2:02:12	
One-mile-to-go	Gelindo Bordin	2:03:18	
Finish	Gelindo Bordin	2:08:19	
Last mile	Gelindo Bordin	5:01	

1990 Men's Results

1.	**G. Bordin, Italy**	**2:08:19**	43. L. Lopez, Costa Rica	2:25:30
2.	J. Ikangaa, Tanzania	2:09:52	44. F. Rivas Paz, Guatemala	2:26:22
3.	R. Vera, Ecuador	2:10:46	45. P. Massaras, Greece	2:26:41
4.	J. Campbell, New Zealand	2:11:04	46. H. Clavijo, Colombia	2:26:47
		(master)	47. T. Coffin, ME	2:27:04
5.	**R. de Castella, Australia**	**2:11:28**	48. W. Muenzel, West Germany	2:27:15
6.	I. Rico, Mexico	2:13:02	49. G. Tomlinson, Canada	2:27:26
7.	**G. Smith, England**	**2:13:38**	50. M. Keohane, NJ	2:27:40
8.	S. Qocqaiche, Morocco	2:13:53	51. J. Da Silva, Brazil	2:27:44
9.	F. Shinohara, Japan	2:14:10	52. A. Duzzu, Cuba	2:27:51
10.	P. O'Brien, Great Britain	2:14:21	53. C. Bloor, FL	2:28:02
11.	T. Tafa, Ethiopia	2:14:29	54. M. Slavin, MA	2:28:28
12.	G. Curtis, Ireland	2:14:37	55. M. Bressi, PA	2:28:29
13.	P. Maher, Canada	2:15:25	56. T. Jones, CO	2:29:00
14.	D. General, MD	2:15:28	57. S. White, DE	2:29:07
15.	T. Eickmann, West Germany	2:15:51	58. D. Banville, Canada	2:29:15
16.	O. Monoe, Japan	2:16:02	59. S. Kendall, VA	2:29:32
17.	K. Stahl, Sweden	2:16:19	60. A. Riscado, Portugal	2:29:50
18.	A. Boileau, Canada	2:16:26	61. R. Roybal, CO	2:30:11
19.	S. Spence, PA	2:16:40	62. G. Horner, CA	2:30:16
20.	D. Dos Santos, Brazil	2:16:44	63. Z. Gassmann, TX	2:30:23
21.	R. Marczak, Poland	2:16:44	64. C. Hummel, NJ	2:30:31
22.	R. McCandless, Hayward, CA	2:16:56	65. M. Fitzgerald, Ireland	2:30:43
23.	J. Leuchtmann, St. Louis, MO	2:17:25	66. J. Molloy, MA	2:30:44
24.	M. Cuevas, Mexico	2:17:30	67. J. Stein, GA	2:30:50
25.	V. Ruguga, Uganda	2:17:46	68. K. McGovern, MA	2:30:55
26.	I. Rodriguez, Colombia	2:18:13	69. P. Riley, MA	2:30:56
27.	G. Genicco, Italy	2:18:40	70. G. Corbett, MA	2:31:01
28.	P. Herlihy, New Zealand	2:18:45	71. R. Marion, MA	2:31:21
29.	J. Alves-Desouza, Brazil	2:18:53	72. T. Bernard, RI	2:31:27
30.	M. Kawagoe, Japan	2:19:54	73. K. Stumpf, CA	2:31:31
31.	**B. Rodgers, MA**	**2:20:46**	74. P. Millard, ME	2:31:35
32.	A. Aregha, Ethiopia	2:21:16	75. J. Langworthy, MN	2:31:44
33.	E. Beatriz, Mexico	2:21:31	**298. R. Hill, England (age 51)**	**2:45:22**
34.	L. Zajcz, Hungary	2:21:31	824. E. O'Reilly	2:57:43
35.	D. Long, United Kingdom	2:21:36	994. D. Sargent, MA	3:00:00
36.	A. Navaro, Mexico	2:23:07	3490. R. Orgovan, CT	3:29:08
37.	H. Wills, FL	2:23:30	5666. W. Collamore, MA	4:00:00
38.	Y. Yoneyama, Japan	2:23:59	5786. R. Flynn, MA	4:03:52
39.	T. Smoot, GA	2:24:13	6517. D. Dimond, NH	4:59:21
40.	K. Lasecki, Poland	2:24:29	**J.A. Kelley**	**5:05:00**
41.	R. Foley, Australia	2:24:52	G. Meyer, I. Hussein, DNF	
42.	P. Vhah-Vahe, Finland	2:25:23		

Team prize

Central Mass Striders

A ROAD TO FREEDOM

MONDAY, APRIL 16, 1990

Can Gold Medal Woman Defy Jinx?

The year 1990 will be remembered as the one when the Berlin Wall crumbled. The crumbling touched the world—pictures were published and broadcast around the globe showing citizens selling as souvenirs the pieces of what had been a barrier against free markets.The falling touched the Boston Marathon with the appearance of women who would not otherwise have been allowed to come to Boston. The Cold War had held most Eastern European athletes, men and women, behind a political wall and away from Boston until this year—45 years after the war

An East German woman came, a Polish woman, a French woman, a Portuguese woman, a Mexican woman, and an American woman—each saw the race from Hopkinton to Boston as a road to freedom.

the world began its final phase of recovery. Franjo Mihalic, the Yugoslavian winner in 1958, had been an exception. This year an East German woman came, a Polish woman, a French woman, a Portuguese woman, a Mexican woman, and an American woman—each for her own reasons saw the race from Hopkinton to Boston as a road to freedom. Russians themselves would come.

Those in the 1990 elite women's field milled around in the basement of the Congregational church across from the common in Hopkinton before the 94th running of the Boston Marathon. Officials allowed in only runners with orange stickers. Runners with other colors had to wait and warm up outside. The elite stretched, stood in line for the restroom, or relaxed however they could.

A number of these women had survived great political as well as athletic difficulties to get to this elite basement. Some had much more in common than the pure desire to race fast. Survival for Jane Welzel, who had been born in Hopkinton and now trained in Ft. Collins, Colorado, had been more than political. Several years earlier, when she and her husband were driving on winding roads in New Zealand, their car had swerved, pitched down an embankment, and rolled onto its roof. The accident left Welzel in a body cast for months. Some people thought she would never run again. Once freed from the body cast she slowly recovered, first her health and then her road racing fitness. She went home to explore new territory.

The first running race in Jane Welzel's life had been the Boston Marathon of 1975. Nineteen then and a sophomore at the University of Massachusetts, she struggled along in 3-1/2 hours. Fifteen years and more than as many marathons later she came back to Hopkinton. She wanted a 2:31 and a top 10 finish. She says that in her mind she never left New England and will be back to live there eventually.

Near to Welzel, German Uta Pippig from East Berlin relaxed by listening to a tape by singer Kenny Rogers. Ten years younger than Welzel, with what one Boston newspaper described her "movie-star good-looks," she had short blond hair and a perfect orthodontal symmetry that she displayed with quick smiles. Pippig had left Communist East Germany for a permanent stay in the West on January 6, 1990. She spoke through an interpreter but laughed at a reporter's joke before it was translated—her English was better than she let on.

Pippig lived a restricted life in East Berlin before she realized that she could make money with athletics; she studied medicine and planned to specialize in pediatrics. The official bureaucratic apparatus of the East German athletic federation told her when and where to race. But after the Berlin Wall was dismantled, Pippig and her marathon coach, Dieter Hogen, walked over the rubble to West Germany, where they took up residence and began an unrestricted life together in a small town outside of Stuttgart. At last Pippig could do with her life what she wished.

Welzel's father had been born in Berlin, where he lived until he escaped during World War II to come to live and raise a family in Hopkinton, Massachusetts. Jane, her father, and her family planned to travel to Berlin in the fall of 1990 for the Berlin Marathon. Her father hoped to point out the houses and streets of his youth.

In West Germany Pippig transferred to the school of medicine at the University of Tübingen. At last she could select her own races. In the Boston Marathon she could make her first international expression of that new freedom. Before coming to Boston Pippig selected and won a 15K in 49:37 and placed second in the Boston Milk Run 10K a week before the marathon with 31:39, en route setting her 5K PR of 15:31. She had run 10 prior marathons with two wins in Leipzig: a 2:36 in 1985, and a PR of 2:30:56 in 1987. She had placed third in the World Cup in 2:35 and before the Milk Run held a track 10K PR of 32:40. As Pippig relaxed to her tunes, Olympic gold medalist Rosa Mota of Portugal waited in line.

Mota could not relax. She worried. Her best time of 2:23:29 had been back in Chicago in 1985. She did not feel ready to break that time. She knew she

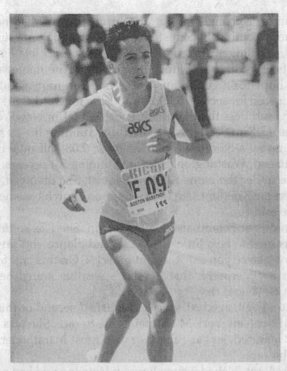

Rosa Mota had more trouble with her Portuguese federation than with the field in the 1990 marathon. © Victah/Agence Shot.

faced a stronger field of women than she had seen in 1987 and 1988, the years when she had won Boston. Now she was the Olympic champion—could she keep it up? Eventually something would go wrong in one of these races, and there was that jinx on Olympic champions. She knew that Pippig could run a full minute faster than she could over 10K. Zoya Ivanova, the quiet Russian who had arrived in Boston only a day earlier, had beaten Mota in Los Angeles.

The American hope, big and blond Kim Jones, at the top of her game, liked to come from behind, and Mota liked to run from the front. It would be a race of nerves—the ninety pound, dark-haired, nervous Mota pursued by a relatively large, confident All-American girl and a rookie East German refugee medical student. Mota's training had been interrupted by vicious public disputes with her Portuguese national athletic federation, who wanted to dictate her races. She said, "They said things about me in the newspaper that made me sad. I think they were jealous of the publicity I had been getting. In my country and outside of it, people like me, but they were jealous."

Mota was nervous. Her preparations could not have been complete without scheduled competitions. She and her coach could not plan under a federation that might not let her race where she wanted. "I would train, but then I'd say to myself, 'What am I training for?' because I didn't know if I'd get to come to Boston." She had wanted to race in the London Marathon before Boston for a change and for a fast time. But she had not been ready for a fast time at London. "I come to try to win (Boston), not run a fast time."

Jones, the marathoner ranked #1 in the U.S. by *Track and Field News*, said, "I've never been fitter than I am right now. . . . The homework is there. I just have to hope for a good day." Jones had run four marathons in 1989: 2:32:31 in Houston for second, 2:29:34 in Boston for third, 2:31:42 in the Twin Cities to win, and, less than a month later, 2:27:54 in New York City for a second. Jones, as Kim Seelye, had started her running life as a quarter- and half-miler running a 55-second quarter and a 2:08 half mile in high school at Port Townsend, Washington. She quit running for 5 years, married, and began to race under the name Kim Rosenquist. She divorced, then married again and became Kim Jones. In the Hopkinton church basement she waited to go outside and run.

Kamila Gradus of Poland also waited to run. She was so tiny that at first glance she seemed to be a little girl. At second glance you saw a gymnast's body. At third glance you saw the taut muscles. Gradus laughed easily. She said through an interpreter that the day's weather suited her—somewhat warm, about 60 °F and dry.

Italian Laura Fogli, aged 30, who had finished second or third each of the last 6 years at the New York Marathon, came to race. She was raven-haired, with a softer featured, less angular face than most marathoners. She did not talk before the race.

Veronique Marot, 34, had beaten Jones in Houston and had come to Boston with a marathon best of 2:25:56. *Track and Field News* ranked her #2 in the world. She had come in 1976 from the north of France to study in the north of England and became a British citizen in 1983. Her accent when she spoke English melted into a delicious mix of the French and that almost-a-Scot-brogue that they speak up near Newcastle. Before the Boston Marathon she complained of shin splints. To avoid further injury she had been training exclusively on grass and trails, avoiding track work and fartlek, taping and icing her shin, and taking ibuprofen.

Mexican-American Maria Trujillo, a very frequent road racer, had never broken 2:30 but wanted to. When her father lost the family farm to a gambling debt, Trujillo accepted a track scholarship to Arizona State University and began to train seriously. She represented Mexico in the 1984 Los Angeles Olympic marathon but by 1988 had become an American citizen.

Russian Zoya Ivanova, age 38, didn't speak to the press. Ranked #3 in the world, in her long career she had won the World Cup Marathon in 2:30:39 and placed second to Mota in the World Championships. She had finished third in Tokyo with a personal record of 2:27:57. In the 1989 Los Angeles Marathon she had defeated Rosa Mota with a 2:34:42 to 2:35:27, but Mota had run poorly rather than Ivanova running well.

Dimitra Papaspirou, aged 26, from Athens had run only 2:34:24, a time similar to Finnish, Ritva Lemettinen, aged 29, who had won the Helsinki Marathons in 1988 and 1989.

Anne Roden, aged 43, the old lady from Surrey, England, came to race. She could boast only a 2:38:24. But the experts picked Christa Vahlensieck, aged 40, of Wuppertall, West Germany, to win the women's masters race. She had placed second at Boston in 1974 and came with a 2:33:22 PR.

When the time came to start, the orange-stickered runners filed through a snow-fence chute to a human-chain chute to the starting line. Pippig and Welzel filed. Had history been a bit different might they have been running as teammates? Contained by officials to keep the nervous elite from starting too soon and more behind to keep back the eager green-stickered pretty-good runners, the racers all waited for the start.

At the noon gun, gold medalist Rosa Mota bolted. She liked the lead. She had won the Boston Marathon twice before—why not again? She seized the lead with a 5:09 first mile and defended it with an average of 5:22 through 5 miles. At 5 miles the women's lineup was Mota, Trujillo, Jones, Pippig, Paivi Tikkanen, Ivanova, Odette LaPierre, Welzel, Fogli, and Gradus. Mota's 26:48 did not match Ingrid Kristiansen's 1986 record of 26:00—that was no surprise. The surprise was Maria Trujillo; very few people picked her for a top five finish.

Trujillo thought that the only way she could win would be if Mota broke down. Both runners fought to hold their positions. It became a double defensive battle. In fact all positions changed little until after 20 miles. Trujillo closed at one point to within 100 yards of Mota. "I was mentally prepared," said Trujillo. "I pushed myself from the start, but I was a little afraid. I beat her before when she had cramps or something. I think that because she is human, something like that can happen, but I wasn't hoping for that. But she pulled away at 10 miles. I lost sight of her at 12 miles." In that pursuit Trujillo ran a personal record for 10 miles, breaking 55 for the first time with a 54:24.

Mota said, "I felt nervous before the start because maybe I was not in shape, but once the race started I was able to concentrate and forget my nervousness." She was even more able to forget her nervousness when partway through the race her coach, José Pedrosa, shouted, "No one is close. . . . Enjoy. . . . Don't kill yourself." But still there was that jinx that everyone talked about, that Bostonians seemed to be proud of. Olympic gold medalists aren't supposed to win the Boston Marathon. But Rosa Mota had no respect for jinxes.

Marot passed 10K in a very fast 33:10, which worried her because a week earlier she had run the Milk Run in only 34:02. Regardless, by 10 miles Marot moved up to seventh place past Gradus, Fogli, LaPierre, and Welzel. She passed the favorite Finn, Tikkanen, by the half marathon. She didn't feel bad, so she continued with her fast early pace.

Mota passed 10 miles in 54:03, the half marathon in 1:11:16, and 15 miles in 1:21:51.

Marot's shins began to hurt at 17, but there she passed Ivanova. Because of her shin injury Marot had rarely run on asphalt; now the paved downhills aggravated her sore shins. She knew they had compromised her training but she thought, "Better to be 90% fit than 100% injured, but better yet not to finish, as the French say, in the cabbages."

Welzel passed the half in 1:15:30. But by 18 miles her plan to run 2:30 slowly fell to pieces. By 22 miles she could not find even the pieces. Her thighs hurt. Her calves hurt. Her footsteps, now tiny and taken at an 8:00-mile pace, each hurt. "There was nothing I could do." But this was the Boston Marathon, not some road race through desolation. Welzel was known in Boston, and people cheered for her by name. "I've never died in a race that was so enjoyable to finish. The crowd, I knew, would get me to the finish."

The crowd knew Mota, too, and helped her as well. She liked Boston. She liked the support she received from the Portuguese community. She liked to see the Portuguese flags. She passed 20 miles in 1:50:03.

Pippig moved on Trujillo at Heartbreak Hill. She heard the crowds count down that she had 90 meters, 20 meters, then 10 meters to catch up. By the top of the hill the German passed the Mexican-American. A year earlier the East German Pippig could not imagine herself in Boston. She could not have imagined herself working for herself. Now she would be able to keep the prize money and use it to start her new home in Stuttgart. She had not gone out too quickly—34-something for 10 kilometers. She had early thoughts about catching Mota, but she felt wilted from the heat and, hearing that Mota ran 2 to 3 minutes ahead, she got rid of those thoughts. Second place at Boston earned $24,000, a sum impossible for an East German to earn before the collapse of the Berlin Wall.

The French-born Englishwoman Marot worried about a cramp and the figurative wall. She had long since resolved in which country she would live, but she had yet to resolve her race. Would it get worse? "From 20 on I wanted a hill. My quads hurt. I liked the Citgo hill" (the small turnpike overpass just before Kenmore Square where a huge sign advertising the Citgo gasoline company dominates). Marot wondered how fast she could run the last 10 kilometers. Forty-two minutes? Ivanova, the Russian, pursued, still close. Marot's cramp relaxed its grip. Through the crowd of male runners who were contending for 75th place or so as the racers all snaked between rows of screaming spectators, at 25 miles Marot caught sight of Jones and sprinted. "She looked so far away. I thought I might catch her if I tried. . . . But if I really believed it, I might have done it."

Gradus sneaked up on Trujillo, who said, "I didn't know she was near me. I didn't want to know."

Rosa Mota didn't need to sprint. Her nearly 3-minute cushion made that unnecessary. She won the race, and the money and prestige that winning brought her freed her from her stodgy federation. At last she could race when and where she wanted.

Before the race Mota had said she wasn't fully prepared. Perhaps she was more fit than she thought. Perhaps her standards of training perfection were higher than everyone else's. Perhaps her statement was a trick, but more likely she had a depth of fitness far greater than anyone else who came to Boston.

Uta Pippig went back to Germany and back to school with her boodle of cash and promised to come back to Boston to run faster in the next 2 years. Her medical interests changed from pediatrics to sports medicine. She would be back.

Maria Trujillo got her sub-2:30 and managed a 3-second margin on Kamila Gradus, who ran a personal best by 9 minutes. That meant $16,000 for Trujillo—perhaps more than the cost of a Mexican farm. And Gradus won $13,000 to take back to Poland, where a pair of running shoes could cost nearly a month's salary in *zloty*, a currency that could not buy bananas or oranges. But dollars could buy anything. She too would come back.

Kim Jones, suffering from blisters, Veronique Marot, and Zoya Ivanova finished within 14 seconds of each other. Ivanova won $7,500—that would buy more than rubles. Jones ran slower than she had in 1989. She vowed she would improve on that. Jones would be back.

1990 Women's Results

1.	R. Mota, Portugal	2:25:24	23.	C. Gibbons, NJ	2:50:09
		(43rd overall)	24.	M. Griffith, Canada	2:50:40
2.	U. Pippig, West Germany	2:28:03	25.	M. Wood, CO	2:51:09
3.	M. Trujillo, Phoenix, AZ	2:28:53	26.	S. Silsby, MA	2:51:46
4.	K. Gradus, Poland	2:28:56	35.	M. Dickerson, MA	2:55:14
5.	K. Jones, Spokane, WA	2:31:01	36.	G. Clewes, Australia	2:57:48
6.	V. Marot, England	2:31:09	37.	K. Haulenbeek, NJ	2:58:02
7.	Z. Ivanova, USSR	2:31:15	38.	C. Iwahashi, CA	2:58:41
8.	R. Lemettinen, Finland	2:38:44	39.	T. McCourt, CA	2:58:57
9.	D. Papaspirou, Greece	2:38:45	40.	L. Senatore, MA	2:59:04
10.	A. Roden, England	2:39:36	41.	T. Busby, NV	2:59:07
11.	J. Welzel, CO	2:42:04	42.	S. Lovejoy, MA	2:59:12
12.	C. Matsuda, Japan	2:42:14	43.	J. Reicher, NJ	2:59:29
13.	C. Vahlensieck, W. Germany	2:42:18	44.	S. Barfoot, New Zealand	3:00:07
14.	C. New, PQ	2:44:08	45.	J. McKeown, CT	3:00:32
15.	G. Horovitz, NY	2:45:00	46.	J. Dehaye, GA	3:01:45
16.	J. Aiello, CA	2:45:02	47.	K. Hurley, IL	3:01:54
17.	C. Taroni, Italy	2:46:32	48.	K. Beebee, MA	3:03:34
18.	C. Saito, Japan	2:47:28	49.	S. Marshall, CA	3:03:44
19.	J. Hutchison, MO	2:47:55	50.	S. Gillis, MA	3:03:45
20.	K. Norling, MN	2:49:13	269.	D. Bain, NY	3:30:02
21.	J. Hine, New Zealand	2:49:30	962.	L. Bartnicki, CT	4:00:00
22.	J. Kawakami, Japan	2:50:04	1433.	C. Bellinger, MA	4:59:53

1,743 entrants.

Team prize

Warren Street Social and Athletic
Club (New York City)

INSHA'ALLAH

MONDAY, APRIL 15, 1991

Japanese-Trained African Leads Marathon Field

Ibrahim Hussein had not raced since his dropout in 1990. For a whole year he had not pinned on a number and tested himself. No one had seen him run publicly. No one but him considered him to have a chance to win this year's race. In 1990 his Achilles tendon had forced him to drop out, making him think that his career had ended. No one from the press had bothered to ask him why he dropped out—they simply assumed that he could no longer handle the fast pace. Only Hussein knew why he could not finish. The press just forgot about him. He went back to Kenya, then to Flagstaff, Arizona, to run and recover his fitness. He loved to train on trails in the thin, dry, cool air. He thought he would win the Boston Marathon again as he had in 1988, but everyone else thought another Kenyan, Douglas Wakiihuri from Mombasa, would win. But Hussein held the Muslim attitude toward his fate: *Insha'allah*—if it is God's will. It is God's will if you win or if you drop out, if your tendon heals or it does not.

Wakiihuri appeared to American runners and the American press as an invincible hybrid. In him the mysteries of Africa and the Orient combined. Tom Fleming called him the Kenyan-Japanese Zen master of running. Born on September 26, 1963, Douglas Wakiihuri grew up on the coast of Kenya in Mombasa, not at altitude. His mother worked as a civil servant. He never knew his father. He was a Kikuyu, not a Nandi like Ibrahim Hussein. In high school he ran in track events but did not excel. He saw the marathon as his only Olympic hope, but he would have to dedicate himself totally, mind and body, to its pursuit to fulfill his dream, the dream of nearly every Kenyan schoolboy—running in the Olympic Games. Wakiihuri had heard of Seko and his win in Boston in 1981 and of his coach, Kiyoshi Nakamura. In 1983, at age 19, Wakiihuri went to New Zealand, where Nakamura conducted a training camp. Wakiihuri came to believe Nakamura's teaching that the fusion of body and mind negates the ego. Nakamura became the father Wakiihuri never knew.

After Nakamura died in May of 1985, Shinetsu Murao, a former Nakamura runner, became Wakiihuri's coach. They prepared scientifically and spiritually. When asked by reporters how many miles he trained each week, Wakiihuri answered with a Zen mystery, "Sometimes I run farther than the day before, other times I run less."

Michoko Nakamura, the coach's widow, told Kenny Moore of *Sports Illustrated*, "When my husband first met Douglas, he told him, 'From today, I

am your father. If you are ever lonely or in pain, come and we will talk.'
Douglas had a pure heart. They made a good son and father."

In 1990 Wakiihuri trained in Japan under Murao, who had coached and
managed Toshihiko Seko. Wakiihuri often trained in New Zealand and lived
in Sweden. He spoke fluent English, Japanese, and Swahili. Unlike Hussein,
Wakiihuri remained distant from his fellow runners. They seemed to believe
he possessed an arcane invulnerability, and they planned to follow him
closely during the race. John Treacy, twice third in Boston and 1984 Olympic
silver medalist, said, "He's got the legs of a Kenyan and the mind of a
Japanese." Nearly all the journalists polled before the race thought Wakiihuri
would win. They seemed to think that the blending of East African talent
with Japanese discipline would prove invincible.

Wakiihuri's record alone seemed to predict his victory. In 1987 he had
won the World Championship Marathon in Rome in 2:11:48; in 1988 the
silver medal in the Seoul Olympic marathon in 2:10:47; in 1989 the London
Marathon in 2:09:03, the Commonwealth Games Marathon in 2:10:27 in
Auckland, New Zealand, and the New York City Marathon in 2:12:39. Why
not Boston? But that's what Juma Ikangaa thought too.

Ikangaa, now a major in the Tanzanian army, came to Boston to improve
on his three straight second-place finishes in the previous 3 years at Boston,
but his leg bothered him. He trained in Alamosa, Colorado, at 7,500 feet,
running 170 to 180 miles a week. He usually spoke quietly and often referred
to himself in the third person. He could speak any of five languages. Yet
he frequently seemed to speak in parables preceded by the phrase, "Let me
explain something . . ." Back in Arusha, Tanzania, Ikangaa was an important
public figure, so he carefully weighed his responses to questions. Usually
he answered them with grace and dignity in addition to vagueness, but he
always answered politely.

But when asked about the health of his leg before the race, Ikangaa grew
uncharacteristically testy and abrupt. This time the reporter had struck a
nerve. Ikangaa would not talk about his leg injury—how it occurred or if it
had healed. Grace had vanished. Ikangaa wanted to win the Boston Marathon, and like Tom Fleming and both of the Kelleys, he felt that he had
finished second too many times. Ikangaa had run six sub-2:09 marathons—no
other marathoner had done that. He had won marathons in New York,
Cairo, Melbourne, Tokyo, Fukuoka, and Beijing—why not Boston? And why
not with a world record? He had said that as long as he was an active athlete
in the marathon he was always thinking of the world record. And he was
thinking about his leg.

Ethiopian Abebe Mekonnen thought about Wakiihuri. Mekonnen decided
to run in Wakiihuri's shadow and, if he could stay with him, to outkick
him. Mekonnen knew he had more speed than Wakiihuri. Treacy, Geoff
Smith, Ed Eyestone (the American hope), Alejandro Cruz, Rolando Vera,
Salvador Garcia, and 20 other top men decided to stay with whatever pace

Wakiihuri set. The weather did not suggest the necessity of a slow early pace. In fact a temperature of 51 °F and 45% humidity predicted the opposite.

Following the example of the impulsive Africans of the year before, Florence Wangechi of Kenya took the lead for the first half mile. Never before had a woman led the Boston Marathon. (She finished in 1081th place in 2:56:52, the 45th woman.) The men followed her in a gigantic clump and then passed, reaching the mile mark in 4:57. Hussein ran in the lead but no faster than necessary. He felt no pressure from behind. Sensitive to the men behind him, Hussein essentially followed from the front. It is a delicate and subtle technique, but a runner can lead a race subject to the pace of the runners behind and still be able to relax as much as in their slipstream, provided she or he is fit and fast enough. Hussein in his white gloves looked the picture of relaxation and confidence.

The other men looked around. They scanned the crowd of 25 runners to see who ran with them and especially to judge the location of Wakiihuri. Mekonnen, much shorter than Wakiihuri, tucked in behind and occasionally peered out from behind Wakiihuri's elbows.

At the 6-mile mark all the men ran together, surrounding Wakiihuri. Only Hussein and Ikangaa paid no attention to him. At a water stop Ikangaa missed the cup. He looked angry and annoyed. Various men took their turns leading—Naali, Treacy, Cruz, Smith, Eyestone, and young Andy Ronan. Ronan, an Irishman, followed the same route to the United States through Providence College as had Smith and Treacy. He hoped to run 2:12 that day in only his third marathon and impress the Irish Olympic selectors for the 1992 Barcelona Games. Ronan ran with his shirt untucked, making him look brash.

At 11 miles a pack of 10 broke away, stimulated by Naali. Wakiihuri elected not to respond. His delegates, including Treacy and Mekonnen, stayed with him. Hussein chased Naali into Wellesley. Hussein knew all the others would not take him and Naali seriously after what they had done the year before, going out at a crazy pace only to have the more reasonably paced Bordin catch them and win the race. Hussein kept looking back in amazement that Wakiihuri, Treacy, and Mekonnen stayed back. Hussein and Naali did not run a crazy pace.

In Wellesley Naali stopped for water, ceding the lead to Hussein as they passed the college. Hussein laughed and mockingly put his white-gloved fingers in his ears to acknowledge the loud cheers of the students. Hussein ran in a very good mood.

Still in Wellesley, Garcia of Mexico chased Hussein and Naali, passing Naali and dragging him up to reestablish contact with Hussein. Cruz and Eyestone joined this breakaway and, like bicycle racers, tried to steal away. Treacy loomed up from behind.

Ikangaa's leg problem forced him to drop out of the race just past Wellesley. But he would be back the next year.

On the hills Ronan and Hussein dropped Cruz, Eyestone, and Naali. Only Treacy ran within sight. Hussein tossed off his white gloves. He worried that Ronan looked so strong going up the hills and wondered how much speed work he had done because he thought he would need a kick to the finish. But Treacy had other plans.

He felt excellent. Ronan and Hussein had only 20 yards on him. Treacy felt the strength, power, and speed that he had often felt before. Whenever he had had that feeling before, he won his race. Now he had that feeling in the Boston Marathon. His victory seemed a certainty. The feeling had never lied to him before. Five miles remained.

At 21 miles, as Treacy readied himself for the kill, a cramp seized his hamstring. Every time he lifted his leg the hamstring muscles contracted and would not release. He could not run. Every other part of his body and mind felt ready to sprint to the finish. He sat on the curb as Wakiihuri and the bunch of them slowly caught up. Treacy had to wait for the dropouts' bus, where he sat shivering for 3 hours. The officials could not give him as much as a dry T-shirt. The bus left him off to hobble three quarters of a mile to his hotel. When he arrived shivering at the door, BAA officials would not let him in because the lobby was too crowded. They would not let him pass because he could not produce a room key. Treacy was frustrated and furious. A reporter asked him a question. Had he had the strength, Treacy might have hit him. He expected triumph and victory, but this abject rejection crushed him. (The next year Treacy went on to win the Los Angeles Marathon.)

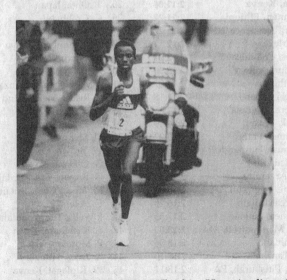

While everyone watched Douglas Wakiihuri, Ibrahim Hussein slipped away for the win in 1991. © Victah/Agence Shot.

Meanwhile Mekonnen woke up to the realization that Wakiihuri had no intention or ability to catch Hussein and Ronan. Mekonnen pulled out of Wakiihuri's shadow in a panic over his foolishness and flew down Beacon Street in pursuit of Ronan. Mekonnen clearly held the greatest fitness and speed of anyone in the race. Hussein ran on in the relaxed, carefree stride that had left Ronan hanging on to second place. In the last mile Mekonnen charged past Ronan, but like so many runners in the Boston Marathon, like Tom Laris in 1967 and Victor Mora in 1972, his valiant stretch run brought him only close enough to watch Hussein, smiling and relaxed, break the victor's tape.

Checkpoint Splits

5 miles	Ibrahim Hussein and 30 others	24:59
10 miles	Ibrahim Hussein and 25 others	50:22
1/2 marathon	Ibrahim Hussein and 20 others	1:05:28
15 miles	Andy Ronan, Ed Eyestone, and Ibrahim Hussein	1:15:22
20 miles	Andy Ronan and Ibrahim Hussein	1:40:01
25 miles	Ibrahim Hussein	2:04:53

1991 Men's Results

1.	I. Hussein, Kenya	2:11:06	
2.	A. Mekonnen, Ethiopia	2:11:22	
3.	A. Ronan, Providence, RI	2:11:27	
4.	A. Cruz, Mexico	2:12:11	
5.	C. Grisales, Colombia	2:12:33	
6.	D. Wakiihuri, Kenya	2:13:30	
7.	T. Tafa, Ethiopia	2:14:07	
8.	A. Sakauchi, Japan	2:14:18	
9.	L. Chengere, Ethiopia	2:14:28	
10.	A. Witczak, Poland	2:14:49	
11.	J. Charbonnel, France	2:15:22	
12.	P. Zimmerman, Pittsburgh, PA	2:15:32	
13.	R. Vera, Ecuador	2:15:46	
14.	J. Juarez, Argentina	2:15:55	
15.	E. Eyestone, Bountiful, UT	2:15:58	
16.	I. Ellis, Great Britain	2:16:20	
17.	J. Kortelainen, Finland	2:17:55	
18.	G. Smith, Mattapoisett, MA	2:18:00	
19.	P. Roto, Finland	2:18:04	
20.	T. Naali, Tanzania	2:18:10	
21.	K. Judson, Pittsburgh, PA	2:18:11	
22.	M. Kawagoe, Japan	2:18:22	
23.	M. Amway, PA	2:18:26	
24.	S. Naali, Tanzania	2:19:19	
25.	T. Ohta, Japan	2:19:46	
26.	C. Crabb, NJ	2:19:51	
27.	A. Navaro, Mexico	2:20:23	
28.	M. Ngumbao, Kenya	2:20:52	
29.	M. Slavin, MA	2:21:13	
30.	M. Cuevas, Mexico	2:21:22	
31.	J. Mashishanga, Tanzania	2:21:43	
32.	P. Rischl, Switzerland	2:21:47	
33.	L. Barthlow, MA	2:23:01	
34.	R. Tbahi, Morocco	2:23:15	
35.	H. Shiraiwa, Japan	2:23:27	
36.	W. Brown, OK	2:23:34	
37.	G. O'Hara, NY	2:23:37	
38.	D. Brown, Great Britain	2:23:40	
39.	M. Hoey, Great Britain	2:24:22	
40.	G. Peters, FL	2:24:45	
41.	J. Wells, The Woodlands, TX	2:24:49	
42.	T. Kashihara, Japan	2:24:59	
43.	P. Moreton, MA	2:25:00	
44.	L. Zajcz, Hungary	2:25:09	
45.	W. Kiplagat, Kenya	2:25:18	
46.	A. Sorrell, NH	2:25:41	
47.	S. Warren, MA	2:25:43	
48.	G. Wersinger, NJ	2:26:00	

49.	V. Kriyoy, USSR	2:26:13
50.	D. Nelson, IL	2:26:21
51.	J. Pelarske, MN	2:26:33
52.	R. Bieber, PA	2:26:52
53.	G. Guillemette, RI	2:26:54
54.	C. Simons, CA	2:27:01
55.	F. Sula, Guatemala	2:27:21
56.	K. McGovern, MA	2:27:32
57.	D. Petersen, OR	2:27:57
58.	C. Norman, OH	2:28:01
59.	R. McOmber, OH	2:28:04
60.	J. Straub, NY	2:28:30
61.	R. Ferguson, VA	2:28:37
62.	J. Dowling, NH	2:28:37
63.	J. Rasch, FL	2:28:38
64.	M. Soto, Mexico	2:28:40
65.	B. Robinson, NJ	2:28:43

7,124 entrants.

66.	J. Alexander, FL	2:28:44
67.	N. Galasso, NY	2:28:59
68.	C. DelCastillo, Venezuela	2:29:02
69.	C. Moore, WA	2:29:24
70.	E. Bruni, NY	2:29:26
71.	M. Whittlesey, CT	2:29:26
72.	N. Wheaton, MA	2:29:43
73.	M. Meyers, WI	2:29:47
74.	K. Wu, VA	2:29:48
75.	J. Garcia, Leominster, MA	2:29:53
250.	T. Mather, MA	2:40:10
631.	T. Hartge, OR	2:50:26
1368.	E. Ellisen, CA	3:00:03
4299.	J. Bates, MI	3:30:00
5549.	R. Flynn, MA	3:53:30
5550.	P. Barrett, MA	3:53:31
	J.A. Kelley (age 83)	**5:42:54**

40-49

1.	K. Judson, Pittsburgh, PA	2:18:11
2.	A. Navaro, Mexico	2:20:23
3.	M. Cuevas, Mexico	2:21:22
4.	V. Kriyoy, USSR	2:26:13
5.	J. Pelarske, St. Cloud, MN	2:26:33

50-59

1.	F. Bradley, Washington, DC	2:40:24
2.	J. Linnell, MA	2:43:40
3.	P. Teachout, VT	2:46:26

60-69

| 1. | J. Wood, Middlesex, England | 2:47:23 |

NOT FADE AWAY

MONDAY, APRIL 15, 1991

Fastest Women's Field Ever

In January of 1990 a friend drove down a narrow Maine road looking for the home of Joan Benoit Samuelson to go for a run with her. It was bitter cold. He was late and on the wrong road. She lived in a big old house on a coastal point. Suddenly the friend saw a runner wearing the green of the Maine Track Club up ahead. He didn't recognize the stride or form. As his car pulled closer he recognized the face of Joan Benoit Samuelson on top of a body expanded to accommodate 8 months of pregnancy. She had started the run without him. He rolled down the window. "You're on the wrong road," she said. He jumped out of the car to run the last bit with her. After a mile she asked, "Is the pace too fast for you?"

Back at her house Benoit Samuelson built a fire against the winter cold and looked out at the ice on Casco Bay as the tide came in underneath. She talked about the last decade.

When Joan had entered the dark tunnel under the Olympic stadium all alone and certain to win the 1984 Olympic gold medal in the marathon—the first one ever offered to women—a curious notion crossed her mind. She didn't have to do it. She knew her life would be forever different once she emerged into that light. People would expect things of her, things she had never bargained for. She could have sat down in that coolness, leaned back against the concrete, and waited for the rest of the field to pass by. But she knew she would run full-tilt into the stadium where friends, family, and fiancé waited. But running there in the coolness, she thought about what it all would mean. In years past she used to recite an Emily Dickinson poem about fame and adulation: "I'm Nobody! Who are you? Are you—Nobody—Too?" ending with the lines "How dreary—to be—Somebody! How public—like a Frog—To tell one's name—the livelong June—To an admiring Bog!" Benoit Samuelson said to herself, Once you leave this tunnel your life will be changed forever. She looked at her shoes and kept running. Her mother said later that Joan looked like a little gray mouse skittering out of a hole. Benoit Samuelson was right, after the Olympic victory people did expect things from her. They expected her to act and talk like a perfect Olympic champion. They expected her to retire and spend her evenings giving inspirational talks to civic groups. But she hadn't finished her running.

In the fall of 1984 Joan Benoit married Scott Samuelson in a pleasant ceremony, full of runners without any racing to do. The guests stood on the shore down from the tent where they had eaten the chocolate-zucchini wedding cake and threw birdseed as Joan and Scott left in a boat Scott had built. Married life and requests for public appearances presented new challenges for Benoit Samuelson, but the driving passion to run a truly fast marathon remained unchanged.

Ingrid Kristiansen ran a 2:21:06 marathon in April in London in 1985. Benoit Samuelson met her at the Chicago Marathon in the fall. The two of them ran together until Benoit Samuelson, tired of Kristiansen's sitting on her pace, threw in a 5:30 mile between miles 20 and 21. Ingrid fell back and Joan won in 2:21:21.

Benoit Samuelson had a second operation on her heels in early 1986. She didn't run a marathon that year. In 1987 she was pregnant with daughter Abby.

In 1988 at the New York City Marathon Benoit Samuelson had to endure the indignities of a "pit stop" during which Kathrine Switzer, working for a TV station, tried to interview her on camera and then a collision with a spectator that sent her slamming onto the mean streets of Central Park to earn her third place in 2:32:40. It was less than satisfying to struggle behind runners she had so easily run away from in 1984. But she pulled together and planned for the 1989 Boston Marathon, where she placed ninth.

In the winter of 1990 Benoit Samuelson waited for the birth of her second child, due in February. A fire roared in the big fieldstone fireplace, ice on the bay cracked and fell as the tide receded. Benoit Samuelson was content, but still drumming in the back of her mind beat the number 2:20, 2:20. She was only 32, and sometime in the 1990s she would want to try to run faster than she had ever run before. Reality, responsibilities, joints, bones, muscles, and connective tissue spoke against a comeback to world record, gold-medal standards.

> My running? she said. I've been happy with my role as mother, but as far as my running is concerned I've been totally frustrated since Abby's birth. Biomechanically I am not the same runner as I was before. My biomechanics have always been the key to my success, my efficiency. I am hoping that #2 will knock everything into place that Abby knocked out. I certainly will make one more effort to come back to high-level competitiveness. I think I'm going to have to concentrate on the shorter distances and forget about the marathon until I can race without my leg and hip and back giving out on me. By no means do I close the door on my career. I'd like to come back as quickly as possible, but if it doesn't seem to be working I could become a recreational runner for 4 or 5 years until the kids are in school. Then I could make a real legitimate attempt to come back. But the first thing I've got to do is get to the bottom of this biomechanical fault. That's going to mean a couple of different things. I've seen physical therapists, massage therapists, osteopaths, chiropractors, orthopedic surgeons. I've seen them all, but the one person I haven't seen is a neurologist. I have to race shorter than 12 miles for a while.
>
> I remember Priscilla Welch [at age 44] going past me at Boston, and I said, Hey, I could take 10 years off and still come back.
>
> Life has been good to me. My career has been good to me. My focus has changed. My priorities have shifted. I have run through this pregnancy because running has become such a part of my life that I can't get going if I don't run. It's been more of a maintenance thing than anything else. I truly think that I can run personal records at any distance from 10K to the marathon. If I didn't think that then I'd throw in the towel.

In 1991 Benoit Samuelson came back to Boston, but only a few of the experts picked her to place third or fourth. Those were sentimental picks. She publicly said she would be happy with a top 10 and a sub-2:30.

But at the start Benoit Samuelson looked highly nervous. Her friend Gillian Horovitz said it was because she probably had already decided to go out fast. She went out with a 15:38 for the first 3 miles. Benoit Samuelson said later that she had to loosen up, to shake out some biomechanical kinks. It seemed suicidal. She seemed to be in a time warp, and observers feared she had split with reality and blasted away like in 1983, when she set the course record. She had run only a mediocre 52-minute 15K in Cincinnati going into the marathon. She had probably trained through that race, but at Boston she went through 15K in 49:55—way too fast. It seemed that disaster loomed. Why wouldn't she just run an even pace and try to slip into the prize money? Why try to win the whole thing—after all those years? Why crash and burn? Why risk it?

But Benoit Samuelson had committed herself. She ran mile after mile as smoothly as ever, and the biomechanical kinks melted away. Except for the new color of her Nike uniform, she looked like the runner she was in 1983. But there was something different in this women's Boston race. For the first time the top women ran in a tight pack. Ingrid Kristiansen and Wanda Panfil joined Benoit

> *It was a beautiful sight to see— three fit, flying women headed for a low-2:20 marathon.*

Samuelson, and the three formed a wedge flying through the field of men. It was a beautiful sight to see—three fit, flying women headed for a low-2:20 marathon.

Wanda Panfil, born in Poland but living in Mexico, in 1990 had won the New York City Marathon in 2:30:45, the Goodwill Games 10,000 in 32:01, and the London Marathon in 2:26:31. Running with a potent stride, her face hawkish, Panfil moved at the peak of preparation for her fierce vocation. She had rearranged her life to run, changing continents, cuisines, and languages.

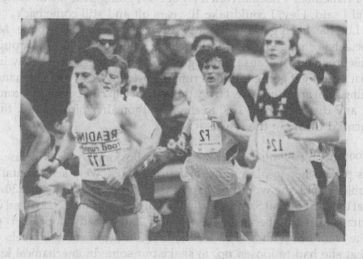

Wanda Panfil (#F2) runs in a crowd including the partly visible Ingrid Kristiansen (behind #177) and Joan Benoit Samuelson (behind #124). © Victah/Agence Shot.

Just behind the leaders ran three more voracious women. Uta Pippig, Kim Jones, and Kamila Gradus did not wait on a conservative pace, but ran in hot pursuit.

Pippig, aged 25, of Germany had a 2:28:03 personal record from her second place Boston of 1990. More wealthy, more western, and more famous than she had been a year earlier, Pippig had run a recent 1:10:35 half marathon. Jones, aged 31, of Spokane, Washington, had run fifth the year before and wanted to at least catch Pippig and Benoit Samuelson.

Just outside Wellesley, Panfil ran away from Benoit Samuelson and Kristiansen. Kristiansen dropped back. Her feet and lower legs suffered from the pounding. She had trained through the winter on skis so had not hardened herself to the asphalt. Kristiansen drifted back to sixth place, and her appearance in the sights of the younger runners no doubt encouraged them. Pippig and Gradus followed in the wake of Jones as she prowled up to Benoit Samuelson. Jones wore sunglasses that made her look like a predatory wasp. She worried that if she pushed herself too hard too soon, cramps might grip her. She had been slowing through the hills, fearing a cramp in her calf. She noticed too that the women's field, except Panfil who ran invulnerably far ahead, had dangerously begun to bunch up. But with a mile to go at Kenmore Square, Jones pounced and drove by Benoit Samuelson. Jones said later that she wanted to warn Benoit Samuelson that Pippig and Gradus approached, but she passed in such a rush that she overshot any window for conversation. She did not want to give encouragement to Benoit Samuelson by a timid encounter, yet she did not want the other runners to jump Benoit Samuelson. Jones said Joan Benoit Samuelson had inspired her to begin racing marathons. Benoit's courageous run at the Olympic trials in Olympia, Washington, and her subsequent Olympic victory in Los Angeles motivated Jones from a Spokane homemaker and mother of two who ran 30 miles a week in preparation for the local road race to an international level competitor. But inspiration or not, this was a race! Jones pumped her arms, stared straight ahead, and stomped past Benoit Samuelson into second place.

Meanwhile Pippig closed; Gradus closed on her. The field that had been strewn about the course coalesced. Down Boylston Street Panfil ran alone to cheers of the crowd; no one could catch her, but the others strained in fear and hope. Panfil crossed the finish line wearing a relaxed, satisfied smile.

Benoit Samuelson feared that she might fall apart. She knew she was running faster than she had hoped and that third place exceeded her plan. But she held her pace. Pippig knew she herself was quick—quicker than most marathoners. She stretched every meter per second of speed out of her Colorado-tanned legs. Her cover girl good looks yielded to a gnarled, gnashed mug shot as she strained to catch Benoit Samuelson.

Little Kamila Gradus turned over her pale Poland-wintered legs and balanced above them with the poise of a ballerina. She churned down Boylston Street so quickly that expert television commentators positioned above the finish line did not see her. They missed the tightest, most exciting finish in women's marathoning history. Like Pippig, Gradus flickered in and out between the male runners. It was entirely possible for her to catch both Benoit Samuelson and Pippig. These sprinting women had to find a plumbline through the tangle of racing men. A man could, in his fatigue, inadvertently influence the fortunes of a female marathoner by thousands of dollars. Fortunately every woman maneuvered through these dodge'ems with skill and grace. No man interfered with a woman or tripped her in an attempt to get to the right finishing chute. Pippig passed Benoit Samuelson at the line by two seconds. Gradus failed to catch Benoit Samuelson by one second. The three women finished within a four-second span—Pippig, Benoit Samuelson, and Gradus. Never before had five women run under 2:27 in the same marathon. It looked like the finish of a 1,500-meter race rather than a marathon.

Her fourth place in 2:26:54 so delighted Benoit Samuelson and exceeded her expectations that she did not mind Jones's passing her in the last mile, nor was her happiness tempered by Pippig's cutting ahead just before the finish to beat her by two seconds. She was so happy to be running well that she was oblivious to Gradus, bearing down 1 second behind her. Joan lost $12,000 in the last mile and nearly another $3,000, but she still cried tears of joy. For runners time is not money—time is better than money. In 1989 when Benoit Samuelson promised not to quit she had shed tears of frustration. Now they were tears of joy.

Wanda Panfil of Poland won the 1991 Boston Marathon in her personal record of 2:24:18. She lived in Mexico City with her husband, Olympian Mauricio Gonzales. When it was time to go, Panfil went, and no woman finished within 2:22 of her. She ran away from the world record holder, Ingrid Kristiansen of Norway (2:21:06), and the course record holder, Joan Benoit Samuelson of Freeport, Maine (2:22:43).

1991 Women's Results

1.	W. Panfil, Poland	2:24:18	17.	L. Binder, San Diego, CA	2:43:25
		(39th overall)	18.	J. Hine, New Zealand	2:44:25
2.	K. Jones, Spokane, WA	2:26:40	19.	L. Bullen, Ireland	2:44:31
3.	U. Pippig, Germany	2:26:52	20.	J. Moss, CA	2:47:19
4.	J. Benoit Samuelson, ME	2:26:54	21.	S. Silsby, Yarmouthport, MA	2:47:25
5.	K. Gradus, Poland	2:26:55	22.	A. Nielsen, Argentina	2:47:45
6.	I. Kristiansen, Norway	2:29:51	23.	C. Iwahashi, Sacramento, CA	2:47:49
7.	M. Ferreira, Portugal	2:30:18	24.	L. Senatore, Medford, MA	2:48:18
8.	M. Birbach, Poland	2:32:13	25.	M. Kon, Japan	2:49:16
9.	O. LaPierre, PQ	2:32:55	26.	C. Tudoce, France	2:50:00
10.	M. Machado, Portugal	2:33:08	27.	M. Pastizzo, CT	2:50:01
11.	R. Bonney, Great Britain	2:35:35	28.	C. Skarvelis, PA	2:50:13
12.	C. McNamara, Venice, CA	2:36:21	29.	C. New, PQ	2:50:29
13.	G. Striuli, Italy	2:37:10	30.	Y. Ishikawa, Japan	2:51:01
14.	K. Rauta, Finland	2:37:35	31.	A. Kattwinkel, NC	2:51:32
15.	R. Lemettinen, Finland	2:38:19	32.	K. Amato, NJ	2:52:53
16.	G. Horovitz, Gloucester, MA	2:40:46	33.	B. Reinhold, KY	2:53:41

34. J. Moreton, MA	2:53:46	43. M. Rutter, KS	2:56:10
35. C. Snow-Reaser, NC	2:54:02	44. A. Wehner, DE	2:56:27
36. R. Malloy, MD	2:54:13	45. F. Wangechi, Kenya	2:56:52
37. S. Gillis, MA	2:54:45	46. H. Fetherston, CA	2:57:10
38. B. Frick, GA	2:55:16	47. D. Beck, CT	2:57:27
39. C. Dodge, CA	2:55:31	48. A. Lutz, MO	2:57:32
40. B. Powell, NY	2:55:53	49. D. Kee, NY	2:57:37
41. S. Nicholson, MD	2:55:58	50. J. Rood, NH	2:57:44
42. A. Bagneres, France	2:56:02		

1,562 entrants.

40-49

1. G. Striuli, Italy   2:37:10
2. L. Binder, San Diego, CA   2:43:25
3. J. Hine, New Zealand   2:44:25

COACH HUSSEIN

MONDAY, APRIL 20, 1992

Africans Expected to Dominate Race

The 1989 Boston Marathon winner, Abebe Mekonnen, promised himself and his Ethiopian teammates that it would not happen again. He would not be caught unawares behind the wrong runner at the wrong pace, as he had been in 1991 in the shadow of Kenyan Douglas Wakiihuri. Mekonnen had learned his lesson; he would not have to learn it twice. Ibrahim Hussein, the apparent beneficiary the year before of Mekonnen's poor judgment and of a benign neglect when the press threw all its expectations at Wakiihuri, this year felt the press heat—at least half of the press corps picked him to win. The other half picked Mekonnen. The 1992 start proved to be much faster than the year before, establishing that this race would develop an entirely different character from 1991's wait-and-see-what-Douglas-does race. It appeared more like the 1990 race of the mad Africans.

The lead line looked like a team training run in East Africa, with Kenyans and Tanzanians stretched across the road. Kenyan Simon Karori, a big and lumbering runner, ran yards ahead, like a drum major clearing the way for his teammates and their neighbors. He ran at reckless, near-record pace, but it seemed easy, festive. He had finished third in the World

The lead line looked like a team training run in East Africa.

Cross-Country Championships, but he had never run a marathon. He did not know yet how bad it could get. Curiously Abebe Mekonnen, the 1989 winner and 1991 runner-up to Hussein, could not be seen with the leaders. Mekonnen thought he should have won the 1991 race. He swore he would not make his mistake again. But he appeared to be doing just that, unless he had guessed correctly that the leaders' pace, initiated by a first mile of 4:36, would destroy the entire bunch. Mekonnen gambled.

While Mekonnen with his calculated guess hid in the security of the gigantic second pack, Hussein ran far ahead of them in a light and playful manner, wearing white gloves and his adidas uniform in the 53 °F air under a cloudy sky. A slight breeze followed from the southwest. Hussein's teammates wore new powder-blue uniforms recently supplied by Reebok. Before the race Hussein said he wanted a fast pace—a pace like 1990 but with a 1988 result. As he ran along he felt like he would win. Without arrogance or effort, he simply felt superior to everyone around him. He imagined the course stretching in front of him and saw himself in total control of the time and distance. He seemingly had the power to reach out and pull the finish line to him. While bounding to Boston, Hussein thought about also wanting a fast time. He already had the third fastest time on the course with his 2:08:43 from 1988. But he wanted a personal record. It had been 4 years since he had run under 2:09. He needed to prove to himself and everyone else that he could run fast, kick, and win. Hussein's master plan would have revealed a Boston win in record time, then Olympic gold in Barcelona. Mekonnen assumed that the fast pace of Hussein and his cohorts would leave no one in the lead pack standing. So he waited.

Hussein's immediate plan involved his teammates. He wanted to pose a dilemma for the rest of the field. If he and his teammates went out fast would the others follow, or would they regard the leaders as a pack of crazy Africans and run a conservative pace, expecting Hussein and his phalanx to die from their fast pace? Surely some of them would die, but would they all?

Hussein ran flanked by younger Kenyan runners Godfrey Kiprotich, Sam Ngatia, Boniface Merende, and Sammy Nyangincha. They deferred to Hussein's pace. He frequently spoke with the other Kenyans, encouraging them and dispensing advice about how to pace in anticipation of approaching elements of the course. (The Kenyans communicated in various languages—a tribal language if they didn't want the Tanzanians to understand them, Swahili if they did want other East Africans to understand, and English if they wanted the world to know.) Hussein wanted his teammates to stay with him as long as possible. At 14 kilometers one said in Kisi, "Ikangaa looks tired." Then all the Kenyans picked up the pace just a trifle. But Hussein knew that none would stay with him all the way.

After 10 miles the sun broke through the overcast.

Karori cracked first. He ran his first half marathon in 1:02 and his second in 1:51, a 3:42 marathon pace. As Hussein and his group caught Karori, Hussein did an odd thing. He moved from the extreme left of the line behind all the other runners to come up alongside Karori. He thanked him for his fast pace and suggested he drink some water and try to stay with the group. Karori tried . . . for a while. Still Mekonnen and the Ethiopians waited.

Juma Ikangaa pushed the pace out of Wellesley.

Hussein won the gamble against the conservative pack. Ikangaa and Merende would fare well from the fast starting tactic. Karori, Sammy Nyangincha, Kiprotich, Ngatia, Simon Robert Naali, and Juma Mnyampanda would not. As Hussein, his friends, and Ikangaa passed over the long Route 128 uphill overpass, Hussein looked at complete ease. Ikangaa pumped his arms vigorously, but Hussein seemed to run without having to use his arms. He casually pulled off his gloves and gently tossed them to the side of the road.

Hussein knew that Ikangaa fiercely wanted to win this race. He had placed second too many times. Ikangaa tried to break away on the hills, but Merende and Hussein would not yield. Hussein liked to float ahead of the pack by a step or two so he could look back at the faces of the other runners to see how they were doing. At 18 miles the habitually front-running Ikangaa gave up trying to push the pace and uncharacteristically tucked himself in behind the two Kenyan runners. Before the 19th mile on the second hill Ikangaa dropped off Merende and Hussein's pace.

When Merende started to drop off, Hussein motioned for him to keep up. Merende tried but could not.

Only when Hussein found himself running alone did he begin to run hard. He started at Cleveland Circle. There his arm carriage lifted and he began to forge his way. No longer did he run playfully, acknowledging loud

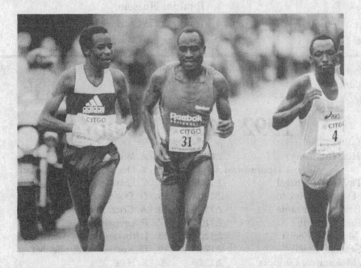

As Ibrahim Hussein fiddles with his gloves, he thanks Simon Karori (#31) for his fast early pace. Juma Ikangaa is #4. © Victah/Agence Shot.

applause by putting his fingers in his ears. His lip quivered from his effort. No longer was he coaching others; he drove himself to run his best time. He gave no thought to anyone following him, because he ran so fast that he knew no runner in the world could catch him. He drove himself hard, but in complete control, to set a personal record and chase the course record.

Now Hussein's year of training on the trails in the thin air of New Mexico paid off. He had not raced often; he would descend from the hills to do track work with young fast runners, but otherwise he had not tested himself. After a pent-up year of solitary training he had risked everything on winning the Boston Marathon for the third time; he burst forth to victory by more than 2 minutes. There could be little doubt that Hussein had reached his physical and emotional peak.

For the first time in his racing career Ibrahim Hussein broke into tears at a finish line. He pushed his face into his hands and cried. Two years ago he had feared that his racing career was ended, but now he had run faster than he had ever run, faster than Bordin had run. He knew as he broke the Boston tape that the next one he might break could well be the one for Olympic gold in Barcelona a few months later.

Checkpoint Splits

5 miles	Simon Karori	23:07
10 miles	Simon Karori	46:54
Half marathon	Simon Karori	1:02:41
15 miles	Ibrahim Hussein	1:12:14
20 miles	Ibrahim Hussein	1:37:35
25 miles	Ibrahim Hussein	2:02:17

(In 1986 de Castella took 6 minutes to run 1 mile, 385 yards; Hussein took 5:57 for the same distance.)

1992 Men's Results

1. **I. Hussein, Kenya**	**2:08:14**	
	(second fastest yet)	
2. J. Pinheiro, Portugal	2:10:39	
3. A. Espinosa, Mexico	2:10:44	
4. J. Ikangaa, Tanzania	2:11:44	
5. J. Rocha, Brazil	2:11:53	
6. B. Merende, Kenya	2:12:23	
7. J. Santana, Brazil	2:12:25	
8. **A. Mekonnen, Ethiopia**	**2:13:09**	
9. I. Miranda, Mexico	2:13:14	
10. T. Tafa, Ethiopia	2:13:36	
11. S. Jones, Great Britain	2:13:55	
12. A. Witczak, Poland	2:14:06	
13. Y. Osuda, Hino City, Japan	2:14:54	
14. C. Grisales, Colombia	2:15:09	
15. D. Dos Santos, Brazil	2:16:21	
16. A. Cruz, Mexico	2:16:31	
17. P. Levisse, France	2:16:46	
18. J. Mnyampanda, Tanzania	2:16:49	
19. D. Kurtis, Northville, MI	2:17:03	
20. R. Haas, PA	2:17:36	
21. A. Navaro, Mexico	2:17:48	
22. M. Erixon, Sweden	2:18:06	
23. P. Roto, Finland	2:18:29	

24.	I. Saito, Kawasaki-Shi, Japan	2:18:49	55.	F. Mayiek, Kenya	2:26:23
25.	D. Simonaitis, Tewksbury, MA	2:18:59	56.	D. Brown, Great Britain	2:26:23
26.	I. Vaananen, Finland	2:19:39	57.	J. Barnard, Great Britain	2:26:31
27.	B. Walshe, Ethiopia	2:19:50	58.	C. Mercado, Puerto Rico	2:26:38
28.	G. Sloane, Great Britain	2:20:27	59.	G. O'Hara, NY	2:26:50
29.	T. Mimura, Japan	2:20:31	60.	Y. Sakurada, Japan	2:26:59
30.	S. Nyangincha, Kenya	2:21:06	61.	R. Couture, Canada	2:27:10
31.	Y. Morita, Japan	2:21:38	62.	P. Farrell, IN	2:27:16
32.	S. Andriopoulos, Greece	2:21:42	63.	M. Bunsey, NC	2:28:01
33.	K. Manyisa, Kenya	2:21:45	64.	M. Hoey, Great Britain	2:28:19
34.	I. Salum, Tanzania	2:21:58	65.	M. Henschel, NY	2:28:22
35.	J. Corro, Venezuela	2:22:03	66.	R. Adkins, KY	2:28:25
36.	A. Aregha, Ethiopia	2:22:07	67.	T. Orlando, PA	2:28:32
37.	T. Kazuno, Japan	2:22:17	68.	W. Krivoy, Commonwealth of Independent States	2:28:34
38.	M. Vera, Mexico	2:22:20			
39.	Y. Nakato, Japan	2:22:28	69.	J. Garcia, MA	2:28:46
40.	S. Ngatia, Kenya	2:22:34	70.	P. Fey, Great Britain	2:28:52
41.	S. Poulton, Australia	2:22:38	71.	D. Mullan, LA	2:28:55
42.	K. Hurst, Switzerland	2:22:46	72.	P. Madar, Czechoslovakia	2:29:02
43.	G. Mthembu, Swaziland	2:23:22	73.	J. Madelon, France	2:29:09
44.	B. Schwelm, PA	2:23:37	74.	J. Nolan, PA	2:29:46
45.	G. Guillemette, RI	2:23:40	75.	D. Keenan, NY	2:29:47
46.	Z. Siemaszko, Poland	2:24:12	76.	W. Kessenich, HI	2:29:48
47.	H. Yokota, Japan	2:24:26	77.	G. Gillson, Canada	2:29:49
48.	V. Miranda, Panama	2:24:48	78.	L. Mutai, Kenya	2:29:54
49.	S. Naali, Tanzania	2:24:53	79.	L. Floyd, GA	2:29:57
50.	M. Harrison, VA	2:25:39	80.	G. Kaplan, Washington, DC	2:30:18
51.	J. Reyes, Mexico	2:25:53	308.	E. O'Reilly, MA	2:45:19
52.	F. Rivas, Guatemala	2:25:59	601.	S. Karori, Kenya	2:53:56
53.	A. Masai, Kenya	2:26:20	5863.	J.J. Kelley, CT	4:07:32
54.	D. Verrington, MA	2:26:21			

9,625 entrants.

WINNING IS NOT ENOUGH

MONDAY, APRIL 20, 1992

Polish Star Seeks Record Run

For some people winning is not enough. Such was the case for Wanda Panfil, born of Poland and nurtured by Mexico. She trained in the thin air outside of Mexico City with some very fast runners under the direction of her husband, 10,000-meter Olympian Mauricio Gonzales. Her mother-in-law prepared Mexican food for them—she did not eat Polish food and she spoke Spanish—yet she retained Polish citizenship and represented Poland, not Mexico, in international competition. Panfil dedicated herself completely to running. She had won the Boston Marathon in 1991; this year she wanted to set a personal record (2:24:18), break the course record (2:22:43), and break the world record (2:21:06). No small ambitions, these. She could simply run a cagey race to pocket the $60,000, but she considered herself the fittest woman marathon runner on the earth, duty-bound to her gender to chase records rather than money. (Although there *were* bonuses of $25,000 for the course record and $50,000 for the world record, so a decision to risk a run for the records was not without financial incentives.) Whatever her motivation, it propelled her to within 2 seconds of the course record at 5 miles with a 26:02.

Joan Benoit Samuelson, the only woman who had ever set out to break the course and world records at Boston and succeeded, worked for Channel 5 television providing expert commentary. She knew how a runner in pursuit of a record had to fling herself at the course and run irrationally in each step, not thinking about the future 3 miles down the road. This Olympic year Benoit Samuelson planned to qualify for the trials in the 10,000 meters. She threw herself at the track, but she missed the track trials qualifying time by 1.6 seconds. It is not a rational thing to run against a clock.

Grete Waitz of Norway had felt that same lack of reason in 1982 when she set a record pace out of Hopkinton, only to crash, burn, and drop out in the hills of Newton. Waitz was in town in 1992 for the marathon but wouldn't touch this unkind course again. Her compatriot, Ingrid Kristiansen, felt the urge for going for a record not once but twice, in 1986 and 1989. She failed both times to break a record, but she did gather herself to finish and win. Panfil's rush for the record this year held all the trappings of irrationality her predecessors had experienced. But no woman ever had behind her the kind of howling pack that pursued Panfil.

First Uta Pippig, her face flushed pink with effort, pulled up behind Panfil. By 3 miles (15:21) Pippig tried to settle in behind Panfil and relax. She could almost do it, but Panfil's speed proved to be just a bit too fast. Pippig's coach/boyfriend, Dieter Hogen, chased her along the course in the *New England Runner* magazine van driven by John McGrath, pursuit driver and publisher. Hogen said at the first stop, "It's a crazy, crazy pace." At 6 miles he gave up worrying. There was nothing he could do to help. His girlfriend ran beyond his reach. He said, "Maybe it's too fast or maybe she makes her own tactic now—I have no idea. She looks not too bad." Pippig teetered on the aerobic–anaerobic edge as they passed mile after mile up to 8 miles in 42:14 (5:17 per mile). By 10 miles Pippig voluntarily dropped off the chase as Panfil passed 10 miles in 53:23 and the half marathon in 1:10:33 (equivalent to the world record pace). Pippig cleverly remained 30 seconds back and that retreat into the safety of the aerobic zone allowed her to recover.

During that recovery young Yoshiko Yamamoto of Japan, Manuela Machado of Portugal, and Olga Markova of Russia charged past, but Pippig's recovery allowed her to stay close to them. Dieter Hogen, in the van speeding from checkpoint to checkpoint, said, "She looked not to be afraid of the other girls coming." But once they had paraded past her his helplessness became evident. Although Hogen watched and encouraged Pippig from eight different checkpoints along the way, he boiled with frustration because he could not see her except as she flashed past checkpoints. "I cannot watch it on TV, I must be at the race. I must have the feeling to be with her, to touch her." On the steep downhill into Newton Lower Falls, Yamamoto gained on Panfil. On the long uphill over Route 128 Panfil could no longer hold her pace. She dropped her arms and tried to relax. She knew the hills waited for her. Dieter Hogen said—about Pippig, but it applied to Panfil as well—"She went too fast in the beginning and now you pay, that's the trouble."

Markova gave steady chase, running with precise pixie steps. She flittered along; she did not look powerful like Panfil, but she picked off the women ahead of her one by one as she ran up the hills. Markova had spent the previous months preparing for the Boston race in Gainesville, Florida, along with six other Russian women, all sponsored by John Hancock. Perhaps training in the warm, humid Florida air helped Markova, while conversely the thin, dry air of Mexico City provided Panfil no preview of the thick air of Boston. On the last hill Markova could see Panfil ahead of her. Both women wore classic Reebok shorts with the red, white, and blue stripes on the sides (but done up for this season on a magenta base). Markova caught Panfil at 18 miles, but her long-sought moment in the race proved anticlimactic. Panfil had no race left in her, and Markova had too much. Panfil gave Markova a glance, but for more than a minute she did not try to contest the lead. She knew she had no response left. All she could do was finish on legs that had become painful posts. Panfil plodded on as five more women ran past her. Her courage impressed Benoit Samuelson, who commended her for her performance on the air.

After the hills Pippig moved from fifth to third by the finish. Being young yet, with medical studies that had restricted her training, she might be able in another year to sustain the kind of early rhythm she could not quite hang on to. She would be back to Boston, about which she said, "I have this marathon a little bit in my heart." She ran the last 50 yards blowing kisses to the crowd—some of them may have left with a little bit of Uta in their hearts.

Jane Welzel, age 36, had this marathon a lot in her heart, too. She had watched her first Boston Marathon at age 11 months. Her family lived in Hopkinton, where her mother rolled baby Jane to the start in her stroller. She had run an unsatisfying 2:35:55 for ninth place in the 1992 Olympic marathon trials in January. She had had the flu then and didn't feel 100%, so she decided to try the Boston Marathon. She wanted a sub-2:30 personal record, but before the race she said she would be satisfied with a top 10 finish and a mid-2:30s time. Other than her initial Boston Marathon in 1975 Welzel had run Boston twice before, with a best of 2:42:04 for 11th in 1990

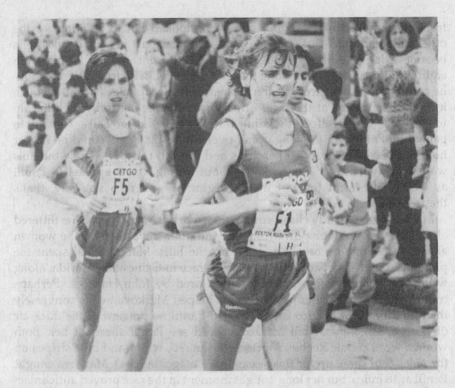

Olga Markova of Russia is about to catch Wanda Panfil of Poland, but both have contracts with the same shoe company. © Jack McManus/Agence Shot.

and a 2:48:26 for 22nd in 1981. At 10 miles this year she ran in 8th place at 57 minutes, a half marathon in 1:14:30. Her second 10 miles took 59 minutes, but her last 10K took 39:20. Odette LaPierre and Ritva Lemettinen ran by, pushing Welzel down to 10th place. With a mile to go her clock read 2:30. "If only I can summon up a sub-6:00 mile . . . ," she thought. But all she could manage was another 6:20. She left Boston with sore thighs. "The course has never been kind to me." She had trained 90 to 100 miles a week, making a point of running loops with long downhill finishes, but still the Boston downhills ruined her quadriceps. Back at her temporary home in Fort Collins, Colorado, she would continue to train, because she still felt she had that sub-2:30 in her. "Maybe next year."

The $60,000 in prize money would make Markova a wealthy woman in her Russian hometown of St. Petersburg. That and a personal services contract with John Hancock and a promotional contract with Reebok made her a wealthy woman in America. Her coach, Viktor Smirnov, and her translator,

Gregory Viniar, traveled with her. Markova said Smirnov had become father, brother, and friend to her in the years since he began coaching her in 1980. (Her father died of cancer in 1987.) Initially Markova had to ask Smirnov for permission to join the sports club where he coached. In her school she had won many races, but no one thought she really would be a great runner, probably because of her dainty stride. So no one had invited her to join a sports club, as was the custom. She had to ask for herself.

But Markova felt that after this Boston performance she would not have to ask for a place on the Russian Olympic team. As the year wore on, no woman in the world ran a faster marathon, but the Russian selectors, like frowning politbureaucrats, ignored Markova's Boston victory and chose three other runners. One of them, Valentina Yegorova, won the gold medal, but with only a time of 2:32:41. Many people (perhaps Markova herself, but she was too polite to say so), thought that medal should have been Markova's.

1992 Women's Results

1.	O. Markova, Russia	2:23:43*	26.	V. Sukhova, Russia	2:48:44
		(47th overall)	27.	K. Goff, RI	2:50:22
2.	Y. Yamamoto, Japan	2:26:26	28.	J. Blanca, Mexico	2:51:18
3.	U. Pippig, Germany	2:27:12	29.	C. Poenisch, MI	2:51:25
4.	M. Machado, Portugal	2:27:42	30.	B. Walz, NY	2:51:32
5.	M. Birbach, Poland	2:28:11	31.	F. Levasseur, Canada	2:51:58
6.	W. Panfil, Poland	2:29:29	32.	J. Foster, CT	2:52:37
7.	I. Bogacheva, Russia	2:32:45	33.	L. Senatore, MA	2:53:08
8.	O. LaPierre, Beauport, PQ	2:34:19	34.	J. Wanklyn, Australia	2:53:34
9.	R. Lemettinen, Finland	2:34:30	35.	J. Hine, New Zealand	2:53:52
10.	J. Welzel, CO	2:36:21	36.	E. Willis, MI	2:54:12
11.	S. Minegishi, Japan	2:37:13	37.	C. Lifschultz, MA	2:54:53
12.	A. Roden, Surrey, England	2:37:37	38.	M. Button, CA	2:54:57
13.	J. Nagy, Budapest, Hungary	2:38:33	39.	T. Schmidt, NV	2:57:14
14.	L. Dewald, Arlington, VA	2:39:22	40.	D. Hanson, UT	2:58:30
15.	G. O'Rourke, New Zealand	2:39:36	41.	C. Bengston, CA	2:58:47
16.	B. Portenski, New Zealand	2:39:56	42.	E. Coyne, NY	2:59:29
17.	G. Horovitz, New York, NY	2:40:52	43.	C. Iwahashi, CA	2:59:34
18.	P. Guevara, Mexico	2:41:04	44.	K. Guderyon-Goetz, WI	3:00:13
19.	E. Gueuara-Weinst, FL	2:41:48	45.	P. Degnan, MA	3:00:53
20.	N. Kawaguchi, Japan	2:43:11	46.	L. Roman, CT	3:00:59
21.	R. Smekhnova, Russia	2:43:46	47.	M. Rutter, KS	3:01:12
22.	A. De Jesus, Mexico	2:43:46	48.	B. Powell, NY	3:01:17
23.	C. Matsuda, Toride-Shi, Japan	2:45:41	49.	A. Iglehart, CA	3:01:32
24.	B. Adkins, Overland Park, KS	2:48:21	50.	M. Gilluly, Washington, DC	3:01:40
25.	J. Mercon, Clearwater, FL	2:48:24			

1,893 entrants.

*Fastest time yet at the Boston Public Library finish line (used since 1986).

THE WAY AND THE LIGHT

MONDAY, APRIL 19, 1993

Kenyan Runner Set to Win Again

Two neatly dressed, trim, and fit-looking gentlemen accompanied Kim Jae-Ryong to Boston. They comported themselves with dignity and obvious pleasure. BAA officials treated them like royalty. After absences of 46 and 43 years, former Boston Marathon winners Yun Bok Suh, 1947, and Kee Yong Ham, 1950, had returned. Both carried business cards identifying them as vice presidents of the Korean Amateur Athletic Federation. Yun Bok Suh had taught high school, coached the national team, and still ran regularly, but Kee Yong Ham, now a retired bank manager, no longer ran, yet he looked as if he did, and he held a keen interest in the sport. Both held expectations that they had come to Boston in the company of the next Korean winner—Kim Jae-Ryong. Kim's training partner, Hwang Young-Jo, had won the gold medal in Barcelona. Now came Kim Jae-Ryong's turn to win a big marathon.

Kim came to Boston as the first elite Korean runner since the all-Korean top three sweep in 1950. The Koreans had been the best marathoners in the world that year, and with their 1992 Olympic gold they wanted to regain preeminence. Kim had the credentials: He had finished 10th in the Olympic marathon, had won the Seoul Marathon in 1992 in 2:09:30, and had won a silver medal in the Asian Games 10,000 in 1990. He had the speed, the background, and the backing. A win by Kim in Boston would signal that not only had Korea survived its civil war of the early 1950s—along with its emergence as a world industrial power challenging Japan as a source of high-quality, inexpensive automobiles—but that the country had returned as an athletic force as well. The Barcelona Games were the first time since 1936 that a Korean, Ki Chung Sohn (Kitei Son representing Japan in some record books) had won the Olympic gold medal.

While the Koreans had their eyes on victory, everyone else had theirs on Ibrahim Hussein. But he carried burdens to Boston. He had not won Olympic gold in Barcelona; he struggled instead to finish 37th. He carried the weight of three Boston victories and two Olympic losses. Many expected him to win Boston again, but Hussein knew the difficulties in becoming a four-time Boston Marathon winner—a feat accomplished only by Clarence De-Mar, Gerard Cote, and Bill Rodgers. If he won, it would not happen by luck alone, but for Hussein the training itself had become difficult.

In Kenya Hussein had become famous. Celebrity, wealth, and power can for Africans bring as many obligations as they do freedoms. In Western countries people have traded extended family and community obligations for options that celebrity, wealth, and power allow them to execute. They are free and expected to make personal use of earnings and windfalls. But in Africa expectations differ; wealth must be shared with the family and the community, if not literally, then symbolically. These symbolic expectations hampered Hussein, who tried to excel in a sport that is by nature selfish and individualistic. He could not train in Africa. Before the Boston race in 1993 he said,

> There are some runners who can train in Kenya, but I cannot. When I am in Kenya, the people invite me to drink tea with them, or to share food with them . . . And in my country, it is considered a great insult to refuse such an invitation. If I go, and I do not drink tea, or I do not eat a lot of food, then they think: "What is with Ibrahim? Why won't he drink tea with me? Why won't he eat more food?" And, of course, you are expected to invite them to your home to share food, as well. So you see, I always gain weight when I visit Kenya, and it's difficult to stay in top condition. But in the U.S., I can concentrate on my training—and people must call me before they can come to visit.

Hussein brought some members of his family out of Africa. In the U.S. his younger brother Mbarak Hussein had run 1:46 for 800 meters and 3:40 for 1,500 meters. But so many runners from Kenya are plying the opportune roads of the U.S. (and nearly all have upstart younger brothers or friends who can also run fast) that one wonders what effect road-race earnings like the $65,000 for first place in Boston might have on the Kenyan economy, with its per capita gross domestic product of $380.

With ridiculous ease Kenyans took the top five places in the 1993 World Cross-Country Championships. Ten Kenyans, all with astounding running achievements, came to Hopkinton. Benson Masya of Machakos had once run the first mile of a 10,000-meter race in 4:06. He had run a half marathon in 1:00:24. He had won the Honolulu Marathon in 1991 and 1992, most recently with a 2:14:19. His boyhood friend, Cosmas Ndeti, had placed second by a mere 9 seconds. Other fast Kenyans, like Boniface Merende, who had finished sixth in 1992 with a 2:12:23, Sammy Lelei, and Sammy Nyangincha, hoped to seize their moments.

But in the week before the race some Kenyans visited a Massachusetts school in part of a Hancock-sponsored cultural awareness project called "adopt a marathoner." Hussein, Merende, Lelei, Nyangincha, Godfrey Kiprotich, and Lemeck Aguta visited the Elmwood Middle School in Hopkinton with Fred Treseler, Boston Running Club coach and Hancock and Reebok representative. The runners themselves took to explaining their lives, the similarities and differences, to the schoolchildren—that the U.S. and Kenya were both once British colonies, that running is a way of life for Kenyan schoolchildren. Lelei told how as a boy he had the responsibility for taking the family's cattle out to graze 5 kilometers away. He told how he would join the elders to hunt antelope, a source of good lean meat. He ran for hours, carrying a stick, with a dog at his side to drive the antelope into a trap. The stick kept the dog moving and the dog kept the antelope moving.

Merende, a military officer in Kenya, used the blackboard to explain Kenyan houses. He drew the houses of different tribes—round, square, thatched roof, tin roof, mud-and-sticks construction, Nairobi suburban. Hancock gave the children Kenyan flags and red-and-black hats to wave and wear at roadside on race day. During the race the Kenyan runners would weave to the side of the road to touch the children's hands.

Never before had so many fast marathoners crowded the same starting line. Hussein proclaimed it better than the Olympics—at the Olympics there were only three Kenyans.

Not only East Africans but *South* Africans came to run. Banned from international competition for 32 years because of their country's apartheid policy of racial separation, South Africans came back into international athletics in 1991. South Sotho tribesman David Tsebe, holder of the fastest marathon time in the world for 1992, a 2:08:07 in Berlin in September, came to Boston. He worked in a clerical position in the Bafoking North Platinum mine in the high veldt of the northern Transvaal. Tsebe came with Lawrence Peu, 2:10:39; Michael Scout, 2:10:47; and Xolile Yawa, a 1:01:41 half marathoner, all of whom had also endured the frustration and guilt created by the ban that intended to help black South Africans but ironically prevented specific athletes from openly pursuing international competition. Before the lifting of the ban Tsebe had to enter marathons under assumed names and travel with a false passport. In the Honolulu Marathon he entered as Brandt Nava, a Peruvian. After he ran well in the race Alberto Salazar attempted to interview him in Spanish. Tsebe, aka Nava, of course did not speak Spanish; thus his nationality was revealed.

In 1971 John Halverstadt, a white South African and student at Oklahoma State, ran Boston and placed third to Mejia and McMahon. He had been allowed to run that year because of his student status but had been banned in other years or forced to run as a bandit. As an outspoken opponent of apartheid, Halverstadt was branded by South Africans as an "athletic terrorist." But all South Africans were banned from Boston. Halverstadt and other South African runners of the 1970s, including Bernie Rose, felt that it may have been fun and a youthful and defiant thing to sneak into marathons claiming that sport should be kept separate from politics, in a sort of ideological apartheid, but that ultimately it was a selfish thing to do. Halverstadt later said that such banditry was a big mistake because it was a surrender of integrity. He came to regret selling out on his principles in order to run;

looking back, he said he would never do it again because it made no state-ment. Halverstadt said that sport is in fact at the leading edge of society and that sports and politics do and should mix. So as a matter of world public policy the 1993 Boston Marathon celebrated the arrival of the South African marathoner.

Mark Plaatjes, a "coloured" South African, had become an American citizen residing in Colorado. He had entered the Boston Marathon in 1985. The BAA gave him entry and paid his expenses—no one told him he couldn't run. In those years many South Africans raced in America, but they did so undercover. The Athletics Congress was sloppy in its enforcement of the ban, and the BAA was careless in processing entrants. Plaatjes had to read in the *Boston Globe* that he was banned. He returned to South Africa and, to serve notice that he might in fact be the best marathon runner in the world, on May 4 ran a 2:08:58 in Port Elizabeth. It is a fair bet that Plaatjes would have given Geoff Smith a run in 1985. In 1993 the BAA paid his way to Boston. He wanted to qualify for the United States team for the World Championships in Stuttgart, Germany—a race he would end up winning.

An astounding Japanese runner also came to Boston in 1993. Hiromi Taniguchi had run about a minute behind first place in the Olympic marathon after having fallen and lost nearly a minute. Many experts said he would have won otherwise. The fall did not diminish his good humor and love of running. He had won the World Championships in 1991, and *Track and Field News* ranked him #1 in the world the next year. Taniguchi had a marathon best of 2:07:40 from Beijing in 1988, where he finished 5 seconds behind Abebe Mekonnen. Mekonnen also would run this year's Boston. Taniguchi would be careful not to fall down on Boston's streets.

Hussein said he wanted a fast first mile of 4:35, but the bright sun and slight following wind produced a gigantic but cautious lead pack, who bumbled through the first 2 miles in 4:55 each. The entire pack watched Hussein and paced off his every nuance. He wore white gloves. He didn't need them. It was 67 °F at the start and would reach 77 °F.

The lead pack presented the greatest assembly of long-distance runners ever packed into 8 square meters. Bronze medalist Stephan Freigang of Germany, like Juma Ikangaa, Steve Jones, Mekonnen, and Joaquim Pinheiro (the 1992 second-place Boston runner), had every reason to believe that victory would be his. The group passed 5 miles in a cautious 24:46, nowhere near Ikangaa's record of 23:05 from 1990. In all about 20 runners pressed together, including Kenyans Merende, Nyangincha, Lemeck Aguta, and Lelei; South Africans Tsebe, Scout, and Peu; Irishman Andy Ronan; Japanese masters runner Takeshi Soh (who had run 2:08:55 in Tokyo in 1983); Ethio-pian Tena Negere (who had run 2:09:04 in Fukuoka the previous December); and a newcomer, Lucketz Swartbooi, of the new African country of Namibia.

American Paul Pilkington, a teacher from Roy, Utah, ran in that multicul-tural conglomerate, as did Risto Ulmala of Finland, Severino Bernadini of Italy, and Andres Espinosa of Mexico. They all seemed to watch Hussein,

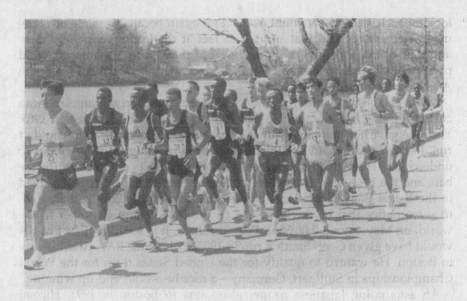

Two dozen in Natick: Cosmas Ndeti is barely visible at the very end of this pack running next to Benson Masya. Kim Jae-Ryong (#25), Boniface Merende (#32), Ibrahim Hussein (#1), Lucketz Swartbooi (#30), Stephan Freigang behind (wearing glasses), Sammy Nyangincha (#39), Steve Jones behind Juma Ikangaa (#4), Hiromi Taniguchi (#12), Mark Plaatjes behind, Paul Pilkington (#9), master runner Takeshi Soh behind. © Victah/Agence Shot.

who with his white gloves ran in the center of the mass as if he were the conductor of a choir. He took one of the gloves off and tossed it aside. He used the other to wipe the copious sweat from his forehead. He did not look comfortable. The mass passed 10 miles in 49:35, 2:42 slower than Ikangaa's 1990 checkpoint record.

The race strategy seemed like a poker game, with everyone calling everyone else's bluff. Kim Jae-Ryong had come to follow gloriously in the tradition of Yun Bok Suh, Kee Yong Ham, and Hwang Young-Jo, yet the pace piddled along. Knowing he could kick with the best of them, he felt eager to break away, but he did not try. Instead he floated to the front of the pack and periodically tested their resolve with little surges that were promptly and eagerly matched by Taniguchi and the others. In all, these little flurries served to gradually quicken the pace.

Taniguchi, a runner with irrepressible humor, ran with an odd upper body carriage. His head would tilt to the right or list to starboard while he held his arms as if gripping an invisible helm. The effect proved quite comical as he scooted ahead of the pack, looking left and right, maneuvering himself to each aid station. Each runner had arranged for his special drink to be placed on the table, and many runners identified their bottles with some kind of unique mark. Taniguchi marked his with a pink parasol—the kind served with tropical drinks to lounging poolside vacationers. He snatched his silly drink as he scooted into the lead and sipped it, seemingly oblivious to the world's most talented marathon field looming inches behind him.

By Wellesley Hussein had removed his remaining glove. He did not look as smooth and playful as in 1992. He did not react to the screaming Wellesley crowd as he had in 1991 by sticking his fingers in his ears and smiling. In fact Hussein grimaced and ran with more motion in his arms and shoulders than in previous years. He had taken too much water at the start of the race, and the bulk of it sloshing in his belly had given him painful cramps. He had been waiting for over an hour for the cramps to go away. They did not, so he dropped back and eventually out.

The slightly dwindling pack passed the half marathon in 1:05:12, 3:11 behind Ikangaa's 1990 record run. The pace was quickening. Then it slowed. By 15 miles they ran 3:23 behind Ikangaa's 1990 record of 1:11:15 with a 1:14:38.

With the momentum of the downhill into Newton Lower Falls, the least experienced runner in the pack, 27-year-old Swartbooi, took the lead with a swooping surge. It fractured the pack as his 4:39 mile left them like debris in his wake. It looked as if a new marathon star had been born. Swartbooi looked utterly different from the East Africans and South Africans. His burnt orange furrowed skin evoked the colors of a Kalahari sunset. He did not gleam black with sweat. He seemed to sweat hardly at all. With a minimal musculature he floated lean and efficient on spindle limbs. Compared to the lush equatorial climate of East Africa, Swartbooi's Namibian homeland granted little mercy to living things. As a desert dweller from a long line of desert dwellers, he felt no distress from the dry sun on his shoulder. The day seemed a cool one by standards of his town of Windhoek in the Namibian desert. Two years earlier in his first marathon ever, with his only running practice gathered from soccer, he ran 2:30; a year later he ran a 2:11:23 marathon to qualify for the Barcelona Olympics, which he led halfway before dropping out. He had come to Boston looking for a good finishing position, not to win the race, but opportunity presented itself and away he went. He ran smoothly and silently and he never heard the runners coming from behind.

Kim Jae-Ryong joined Swartbooi but would not pass. After several miles of the Newton hills with Kim in dogged pursuit, Swartbooi grew annoyed. At 30 kilometers he gestured that Kim should take his turn leading, but Kim refused. Kim, sweating profusely, looked far more tired than Swartbooi. Swartbooi looked calm, in control and unbeatable. With Tsebe and Lelei dropping back, no one else seemed in contention.

But 22-year-old Kamba tribesman Cosmas Ndeti had run the early parts of the race with his boyhood friend Benson Masya. The two had grown up together in mile-high Machakos, where their parents farmed coffee, maize, and beans. They had trained together in the hills of Kenya and the streets of Liverpool, England, where they had spent time with their agent, Jerry Helm. Now they lurked just behind the sweltering pack at 15 kilometers. They enjoyed their whirlwind good fortune to be skilled runners, able to travel to England, Japan and other countries. It had been a lark when they finished within 9 seconds of each other in the Honolulu Marathon. And it had been a party when a John Hancock representative invited both of them to run in Boston, and the ease continued when Alberto Salazar, representing Nike, offered Ndeti a few hundred dollars to wear a Nike shirt for the race. In the early miles of the Boston Marathon Ndeti wanted to run up with the leaders, but Masya cautioned him, "No, no, stay back, stay back." They planned to later uncork a big move together. But the fun stopped when Masya developed back problems and could not keep the pace with Ndeti. It saddened Ndeti to have to go on alone without his friend, but his newfound Christian faith buoyed him. On his shoe he had written Christ's message: "I am the way and the light," and he added the words "Jesus Saves."

Ndeti passed runner after runner. He passed Tsebe to move into fourth. When Ndeti passed Lelei they spoke briefly. Then Ndeti flew away. He ran his miles under 4:50, gaining 10 or 15 seconds a mile on the leader. Later he would say he "felt nice" because he had been in Kenya climbing high mountains. He said that only with 4 miles to go did he feel he would win. Kim had fallen off Swartbooi's pace. Ndeti caught him. Kim surged. Ndeti swept past regardless. When he caught Swartbooi, Ndeti paused. He matched strides and listened, performing a silent medical exam on Swartbooi: breathing, reflexes, hydration, attitude. To detect attitude Ndeti had to look at Swartbooi's face. Ndeti turned to look hard into Swartbooi's eyes. Swartbooi did not turn his head to return the glare. Ndeti glanced at the course ahead, then turned back to Swartbooi to look again for a spark. If the eye is the window to the soul, these windows were closed. One mile remained in the race. Ndeti diagnosed that Swartbooi could not resist, so he shrugged and took off.

Swartbooi in fact could not follow. Ndeti had run the second half of the race in 1:04:10, and the last 10K in 29—both faster than anyone had ever run. He coasted the last half mile in case anyone wanted to sprint. He had plenty of energy left, but no one could catch him. Kim caught Swartbooi as all three broke 2:10.

After the race Ndeti said he has four brothers and five younger sisters back in Machakos, that 20-year-old Josphat Alaia Ndeti is faster than Cosmas and that already he (Cosmas) is training his 7- and 8-year-old sisters. Cosmas's wife gave birth to a son, Gideon, 2 days before the race. More Africans will be coming to Boston.

1993 Men's Results

1.	C. Ndeti, Machakos, Kenya	2:09:33
2.	K. Jae-Ryong, Seoul, Korea	2:09:43
3.	L. Swartbooi, Namibia	2:09:57
4.	H. Taniguchi, Japan	2:11:02
5.	S. Lelei, Eldoret, Kenya	2:12:12
6.	M. Plaatjes, Boulder, CO	2:12:39
7.	B. Merende, Kisii, Kenya	2:12:50
8.	S. Bernadini, Italy	2:12:56
9.	K. Brantly, Ormond Beach, FL	2:12:58
10.	C. Tarazona, Venezuela	2:13:37
11.	S. Nyangincha, Nairobi, Kenya	2:14:23
12.	A. Ronan, Ireland	2:14:58
13.	A. Espinosa, Mexico	2:15:12
14.	X. Yawa, South Africa	2:15:28
15.	S. Jones, Great Britain	2:15:30
16.	J. Romera, Spain	2:15:48
17.	D. Mungai, Kenya	2:17:12
18.	T. Shibutani, Funabaski, Japan	2:17:37
19.	J. Charbonnel, Antony, France	2:17:44
20.	B. Turbe, Ethiopia	2:17:56
21.	L. Aguta, Nairobi, Kenya	2:18:05
22.	J. Ikangaa, Tanzania	2:18:06
23.	D. Tsebe, South Africa	2:18:15
24.	J. Nzau, Kenya	2:20:33
25.	M. Scout, South Africa	2:20:57
26.	J. Montero, Pamplona, Spain	2:21:13
27.	L. Lopez, San Jose, Costa Rica	2:21:33
28.	C. Bloor, Lorgo, FL	2:21:43
29.	S. Lopez, Coyoacan, Mexico	2:22:51
30.	D. Kurtis, Northville, MI	2:22:57
31.	T. Soh, Miyazaki, Japan	2:23:08
32.	I. Bloomfield, Great Britain	2:23:14
33.	B. Masya, Kenya	2:23:25
34.	R. Guerrero, Tampa, FL	2:23:28
35.	P. Gschwend, Switzerland	2:23:38
36.	M. Ochoa, Anaheim, CA	2:23:56
37.	J. Corro, Venezuela	2:24:02
38.	R. Haas, Pottsville, PA	2:24:27
39.	N. Richardson, Ireland	2:25:22
40.	J. Leuchtmann, Ballwin, MO	2:25:24
41.	G. Sloane, Clinton, NJ	2:25:26
42.	D. Verrington, Bradford, MA	2:25:40
43.	G. Mutisya, Kenya	2:25:42
44.	H. Araki, Hanamatsu, Japan	2:25:52
45.	G. Devison, Australia	2:26:12
46.	L. Zajcz, MA	2:26:32
47.	V. Krivoy, Ukraine	2:26:57
48.	Y. Hashimoto, Japan	2:27:24
49.	O. Kitahara, Japan	2:27:36
50.	M. Gozzano, Italy	2:27:36
51.	S. Warren, Stoughton, MA	2:27:53
52.	G. Romesser, Indianapolis, IN	2:28:12
53.	A. Filho, Brazil	2:28:42
54.	B. Schwelm, PA	2:29:00
55.	F. Rivas, MA	2:29:12
56.	R. Denesik, CO	2:29:36
57.	L. Teran, Ecuador	2:29:39
58.	W. King, PA	2:29:59
59.	C. Bennion, UT	2:30:14
60.	L. Zubrod, Milwaukee, WI	2:30:43
61.	J. Garcia, Leominster, MA	2:30:56
62.	C. Del Castillo, Venezuela	2:30:58
63.	M. Bunsey, NC	2:31:20
64.	C. Demet, Great Britain	2:31:21
65.	F. Rivera, Mexico	2:31:26
66.	J. Conforti, Boston, MA	2:31:51
67.	S. Jayson, TX	2:32:01
68.	A. Ceruti, MA	2:32:01
69.	T. Orlando, Erie, PA	2:32:15
70.	B. Crane, Lowell, MA	2:32:39
71.	R. Ulmala, Finland	2:32:55
72.	R. Marino, Annapolis, MD	2:32:59
73.	M. Harrison, VA	2:33:24
74.	T. McCluskey, OH	2:33:25
75.	L. Peu, South Africa	2:33:39
76.	A. Diantonio, NJ	2:33:43
77.	F. Klevan, PA	2:33:47
78.	L. Moseev, Russia	2:34:01
79.	D. Lampasi, Merrick, NY	2:34:05
80.	J. Muldowney, Pottsville, PA	2:34:09
81.	B. Miller, Decatur, GA	2:34:15
82.	J. Nolan, Schwenksvil, PA	2:34:29
83.	J. Mello, Jamaica Plain, MA	2:34:36
84.	L. Briggs, West Hartford, CT	2:34:40
85.	L. Floyd, Albany, GA	2:34:55
86.	L. Olsen, Millis, MA	2:35:08
87.	C. Norman, Medford, NJ	2:35:23
88.	R. Sica, Indianapolis, IN	2:35:33
89.	J. Stromann, Germany	2:35:35
90.	M. Gonsalves, Canton, MA	2:36:04
91.	K. Lauenstein, Greensboro, NC	2:36:12
92.	K. Gartner, Falmouth, MA	2:36:19
93.	M. Warner, AL	2:36:45
94.	W. Sieg, FL	2:36:51
95.	G. Norton, ME	2:36:56
96.	P. Riley, Concord, MA	2:36:59
97.	K. Shilling, Washington, DC	2:37:18
98.	B. Topalian, Hollywood, CA	2:37:28
99.	Y. Castrillo, Costa Rica	2:37:32
100.	S. Marsalese, NY	2:37:36

Olga With the Chip on Her Shoulder

MONDAY, APRIL 19, 1993

Russian Women Come to Battle in Boston

Olga Markova came to Boston the clear favorite. The Olympic gold medalist, Valentina Yergrova, came to Boston too. They trained together in Florida but rarely spoke. They were not friends.

The year before Olga Markova had not followed the rules. She had won the Boston Marathon in what would remain the fastest marathon time for any woman in the world in 1992—but she did not follow the rules of the Russian Olympic team selectors. They had specified that all Russian contenders for their Olympic team must have run in the Los Angeles Marathon, in March. But Markova waited for Boston. Valentina Yegorova had followed the rules, and she ran 2:29:41 for fourth place at Los Angeles in 1992. The selectors selected her and two teammates. Then maverick Markova came to Boston and ran 2:23:43. She thought that if she beat Madina Biktagirova's winning Los Angeles time of 2:26:23, surely the selectors would notice. She expected her dominating time to guarantee her a place on the Olympic team. But with politbureau inertia, the selectors waited until the last moment to tell Markova that they would not send her to Barcelona.

Markova had been training and dreaming until she learned she would not go to the Olympics. The thought nearly extinguished her. She was indeed the fastest woman marathoner in the world. That thought made Markova angry. But it is difficult to imagine her angry. At 100 pounds, with an artistic child's face, Baltic blue eyes, a sweet and sensitive manner, limbs unmuscled except for calves like twisted cables, she was not the picture of a raging athlete. The anger and effrontery had to bubble within. Having been raised in a society where communism, conformity, and state control of wealth insisted that one follow the rules, Markova had had to gather tremendous will to break the rules. She had mustered entrepreneurial audacity to win lucrative endorsement contracts with Reebok and John Hancock. But because she broke the rules, the best woman marathoner in the world did not go to the Olympic Games.

Instead Valentina Yegorova, who followed the rules, won the Olympic gold medal with a slow 2:32:41, and was named to the *Track and Field News* #1 world ranking. Markova stayed under control, made her resolutions privately, and publicly said, "It's okay. I'm only a little bit angry."

Markova had spent June in a secluded forest camp training for the Olympic Games, but she used her Olympic fitness for the next biggest marathon in the world. Markova placed second in New York with a 2:26:38, but still *Track and Field News*, the bible of the sport, placed her only third in the world in 1992. If you didn't have the gold . . .

But if you don't have the gold the next best thing to do is to meet the woman who has the gold and beat her—to symbolically take it. Here in Boston Markova had that opportunity. If she could beat Yegorova, run a fast time, and win the race, then who could say she would not have been the gold medalist? With that chip on her slender shoulder, Markova came to Boston.

In the early miles of the 1993 Boston Marathon, a pack of women formed— Markova, Tatiana Titova, Irina Bogacheva, Wanda Panfil, Joan Benoit Samuelson, Manuela Machado, Olga Appell, and Valentina Yegorova.

By 2 miles Benoit Samuelson—hoping for a repeat of the thrilling day of 10 years before when she had won the race in a world record of 2:22:43, remembering the chilling days of the previous week and all the last winter, feeling the heat beating down on the pavement as well as the back of her neck—took a tactical retreat. She said to herself, "This is crazy. These guys

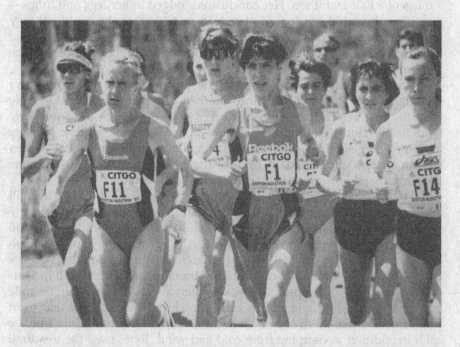

From left, Olga Appell (with headband), Irina Bogacheva (#F11), Wanda Panfil (with sunglasses), Olga Markova (#F1), Manuela Machado (behind Markova), Valentina Yegorova, and Tatiana Titova (#F14). © Victah/Agence Shot.

are going to beat up on each other." Benoit Samuelson knew herself and the course too well to let irrational hope overtake experience.

By 5 miles only Yegorova, Panfil, Titova, and Markova remained. Soon Titova dropped off. Panfil ran with laboring effort. By 9 miles she could no longer stay with the Russians. Past 10 miles the Markova–Yegorova duel began.

Markova and Yegorova contrasted in running styles as much as they clashed over the Olympic selection process. Yegorova ran thick and sweating, her straight dark hair plastered to her head. Markova moved mechanically, with metered steps, her skinny arms—skinnier than the year before— locked at the elbows, her eyes nailed on the road ahead.

At Markova's side Yegorova wrestled with her own inadequacies. Two women from the same country, now on the opposite side of the globe, raced each other, but each ran apart from the other, each within her own inner world of effort. When Yegorova dug deep inside she confronted her own lack of preparation. She had run well in hot weather such as this in winning the Olympic marathon—this day in the mid-70s °F was not as hot as that—but 6 weeks earlier in Japan she had been hospitalized for 3 days with influenza. She had been invited to Japan to run a race. Optimism lifted her from her hospital bed to the starting line, but the illness reduced her to a walk after 3 miles of a half marathon. Her conclusions lodged in her legs and lungs— then, that she could not fool Mother Nature; now, that she could not stay with Markova after only 6 weeks of tentative training. Yegorova watched Markova's pixie steps disappear ahead of her. She dropped out of the race at 22 miles.

Meanwhile Kim Jones appeared to be dropping into the race. Many thought her day had gone by since she had dropped out of the Olympic trials the year before. She had been ranked #1 in the U.S. by *Track and Field News* in 1989 and 1991, but now 2 weeks shy of her 35th birthday, perhaps her time had passed. Her best marathon had been at Boston in 1991, when she ran a 2:26:40 for second. In 1989 she had placed third in 2:29:34. But few people realized how well she had prepared for this race.

In late winter Jones had migrated from Spokane, Washington, to a small and solitary apartment in Boulder, Colorado, where she could train for 7 weeks without distractions. To be close to her coach/advisor, Benji Durden (who ran third in Boston in 1983 in 2:09:57), she left her family and the harsh Spokane winter. Yet the high altitude March weather in Boulder was not balmy either. She did her highest quality training on the treadmill in Durden's house. She did repeat 1,000-yard intervals on it at a 5-minute mile pace. But it was her long run in early March on the treadmill that most impressed Durden as she ran 22 miles in 2:20. The treadmill didn't lie, he said. In addition to escaping from cold and wind, Jones used the treadmill to escape the trigger of her pollen-induced and exercise-induced asthma.

Her allergic reaction was so strong that on days when pollen was flying she could not breathe. On many training runs and in some important races she had had to stop because she could not get enough air. At other times she had found that running too fast in the early stages of a race could induce an asthma attack, so she had to control her early pace so she did not, as she said, "get anaerobic." But on a treadmill either at home or in Boulder she could turn on an air-purifying device and run alone in a room with two machines to completely control her environment. Indoors and out, her training mileage averaged 100 miles a week. The concentration and seclusion paid off.

From 6th place in Natick, Jones moved into 2nd place by Newton. Carmen De Oliviera of Brazil rose from 10th place at 10 miles to pass Machado in the hills.

No one challenged Markova. She ran on, looking thinner and frailer than she had in 1992, yet unrelenting in her pace. She won by 4:33 over Jones, or about a mile, and placed 42nd overall. At the postrace press conference, Yegorova said, "I am very pleased with Olga Markova's result because, as myself, she trained hard for this race. It is a good result and I am happy for her."

As if to recognize that the 1993 Boston Marathon was only one battle in what would be an ongoing war, Markova said, "Valentina Yegorova was not prepared well enough to compete with me today." Perhaps Yegorova had rushed herself in trying to run in Boston.

1993 Women's Results

1.	O. Markova, Russia	2:25:27	20.	S. LaChance, Lunenburgh, MA	2:53:05
		(42nd overall)	21.	K. Pier, Seattle, WA	2:53:15
2.	K. Jones, Spokane, WA	2:30:00	22.	C. Dodge, CA	2:53:26
3.	C. De Oliviera, Brazil	2:31:18	23.	M. Hurta, Freeport, TX	2:53:30
4.	M. Machado, Braga, Portugal	2:32:20	24.	J. Moreton, Cambridge, MA	2:53:40
5.	A. Galliamova, Russia	2:35:12	25.	G. Beschloss, Great Britain	2:54:15
6.	J. Benoit Samuelson, ME	2:35:43	26.	C. Allen, VA	2:55:41
7.	N. Prasad, France	2:37:11	27.	K. Ise, Yuzawa-Shi, Japan	2:56:06
8.	T. Titova, Russia	2:37:42	28.	L. Clayton, CA	2:56:19
9.	J. Smith, Houston, TX	2:38:35	29.	J. Strait, NC	2:56:38
10.	G. O'Rourke, New Zealand	2:39:09	30.	M. Rutter, KS	2:58:24
11.	J. Welzel, Ft. Collins, CO	2:39:38	31.	T. Yamada, Ibaraki, Japan	2:58:34
12.	I. Bogacheva, Kirghizia	2:41:09	32.	M. Button, Los Angeles, CA	2:59:26
13.	B. Portenski, New Zealand	2:41:18	33.	K. Driscoll, Pennsville, NJ	3:00:02
14.	L. Belaeva, Moscow, Russia	2:43:06	34.	H. Tolford, Tillamook, OR	3:00:36
15.	I. Bondarchuk, Russia	2:43:15	35.	E. Oberli-Schuh, Germany	3:01:19
16.	A. Roden, Great Britain	2:44:10	36.	B. McReynolds, Colchester, VT	3:01:59
17.	M. Kitajima, Miyagi, Japan	2:48:49	37.	P. Kolakowski, Arlington, VA	3:02:37
18.	J. Hine, New Zealand	2:52:20	38.	C. Virga, Boca Raton, FL	3:03:05
19.	A. Adams, Canada	2:52:32	39.	J. Willette, Greenwich, CT	3:05:19

40. L. Lielke, Lynnwood, WA	3:05:37	46. G. Sly, Grand Blanc, MI	3:07:35
41. A. Wehner, Hockessin, DE	3:06:10	47. E. Wilmoth, Hurricane, WV	3:09:01
42. B. Powell, NY	3:06:35	48. E. Phillips, Canada	3:09:02
43. C. Christensen, San Jose, CA	3:06:36	49. L. Dodson, Macungie, PA	3:09:19
44. M. Astrop, Richmond, VA	3:07:09	50. D. Smyers, Wethersfield, CT	3:09:49
45. R. Smekhnova, Belorussia	3:07:14	51. J. Wightman, Rochester, NY	3:09:55

Valentina Yegorova, **Lisa Weidenbach, Wanda Panfil,** DNF

40-49

1. B. Portenski, Wellington, NZ	2:41:18
2. I. Bondarchuk, Russia	2:43:15
3. A. Roden, Great Britain	2:44:10
4. J. Hine, New Zealand	2:52:20
5. C. Dodge, CA	2:53:26

MY GOD IS ABLE

MONDAY, APRIL 18, 1994

Can a Kenyan Win Again?

When Cosmas Kitavi Ndeti of Machakos, Kenya, came to Boston in 1994 to defend his title, he had written a new message on his shoe. Ndeti had trained long and hard on mile-high hills outside his hometown. Unlike the many Kenyan runners who trained three times daily, Ndeti trained only once a day. But he ran very fast for 25 to 40 kilometers. Ndeti coached himself because he felt that adhering to a coach's schedule would force him to run when he felt tired and needed to rest. When he needed rest, he rested. When he needed to run hard, he ran so hard he could not speak. Ndeti listened to his body to find his training, and he listened to his God to find his inspiration. On his shoe this year Ndeti had written "My God Is Able."

Called bumptious by one journalist and written off by most pundits as a one-shot winner, Ndeti bumbled around press conferences displaying his year-old son—named Gideon *Boston* Ndeti—to commemorate the boy's birth, which coincided with his father's victory in 1993. In his dual boosterism of his religion and himself, Ndeti alternated preaching his born-again Christianity and promoting his running prowess. Whenever Ndeti mentioned God and Jesus, the reporters stopped writing, but they resumed when with divine logic Ndeti asked, "If God let me win last year's race, if He allows me to wear number 1 on my jersey, then why not again be number 1 this year?" Such self-promoting is unusual in an African, but in America such behavior is accepted, as long as the promoter wins. But a repeat victory was not guaranteed for Ndeti.

In fact, recent races pointed against Ndeti's running well in Boston. In August's World Championships marathon in Stuttgart, he had dropped out at 23 kilometers. In December he placed second to South Korea's Lee Bong-Ju in the Honolulu Marathon. After those travels Ndeti went back to Kenya to train. When he came to the United States, he spent three days with 1982 Boston Marathon winner Alberto Salazar in Portland, Oregon. Salazar told Ndeti not to try the same come-from-behind tactic he had used the year before but to stay with the lead pack. Salazar also helped sign Ndeti to a lucrative product endorsement contract with Nike. But the Boston newspapers picked someone else as their favorite—Mexican Andres Espinosa.

Hard-bitten, mustachioed Espinosa, age 31, who won the New York City Marathon in 1993 with a 2:10:04 over Bob Kempainen, came to Boston to run his best-ever marathon. The press expected it. A former steelworker in Montclova, Mexico, the third of nine children, Espinosa said he had an obsession to win in New York after twice finishing second there. To win Boston and New York would be a special treat and would bolster Mexico's challenge to Kenya for the birthplace of the world's best marathon runners. Espinosa ran third in Boston in 1992 in 2:10:44, but in 1993 he had finished only 13th, with a 2:15:12.

Another Mexican (but now a U.S. citizen), Arturo Barrios, had finished a disappointed third in New York with a 2:12:21. Barrios had once held the world record for 10,000 meters, 27:09.23, set on August 18, 1989, in Berlin. Many important events in Barrios's life happened in Boston. On a whim he first came there to race in 1986. He boldly pursued Rob de Castella in that runner's course record 2:07:51 before fading to fifth. "At the time," Barrios said, "I was running a 2:08 pace, and all of a sudden, with about five kilometers to go, that's when I died. I mean I was dead. But I don't think that's going to happen [this year]. In New York I slowed down. I didn't die. There's a big difference between slowing down and dying." Barrios thought of himself as a 2:08 marathoner. He desperately wanted to legitimize himself with a 2:08 in Boston. Barrios had married Joy Rochester in Boston in 1987, just a few blocks from the finish line. He still held the world record for 20 kilometers in 56:55.6, set May 30, 1991, in La Fleche, France. Barrios felt he was too old at age 31 for world-record track racing. He wanted to prove himself in the marathon. But so did Espinosa.

Espinosa said, "Of the more prestigious marathons we [Mexicans] only have to win Boston and London. There is a possibility that some of the guys from our club who are going to London Sunday have a chance to win there, and I'll try to do the same in Boston." (Mexican Dionicio Ceron won at the London Marathon in 2:08:51.) Salvador García paid his own way to Boston and entered at the last minute to join the Mexican group. Barrios added, "Obviously, it would be great for our country. I guess it would be very gratifying in terms of a Mexican runner winning the race. But it would be even more gratifying if that Mexican runner were me." Both Mexicans had prepared themselves for this race better than for any other in their lives. Espinosa said, "I mean, just imagine, winning both New York and Boston."

But imagine also winning the Olympic marathon and the Boston Marathon. That's what Hwang Young-Jo of Seoul, Korea, could easily envision. But after winning the gold medal in the 1992 Barcelona Olympics, he hurt his foot, and after surgery missed an entire year of competition. On a hot day in Barcelona Hwang ran 2:13:23 to win. His best ever is a Korean record of 2:08:47. No Korean had won at Boston since Yun Bok Suh in 1947 and Kee Yong Ham in 1950. Both victors had come to Boston in 1993 to watch Kim Jae-Ryong win but left disappointed that he placed only second. His teammate, Lee Bong-Ju, the man who not only had beaten Ndeti in Honolulu in 1992 but also had won the 1992 Korean marathon championship in 2:10:27, of course thought that he should be the runner to win for Korea.

The race started mildly as Brazilian Aniello Montuori Filho led the first mile in 4:53. Shortly thereafter an American, Floridian Keith Brantly of Ormond Beach, at age 31 holding a marathon best of 2:12:49 in New York in 1993 and ninth the same year in Boston, found himself in an easy lead. He looked the part of the golden beach boy—muscular, wearing white gloves and a New Balance shirt, blond hair blowing ahead of him in the wind. Perhaps his 3:57 mile speed made the pace feel easy, but in fact the pace was easy for everyone. Brantly's time of 9:51 for a downhill two miles was mild for the extremely fit group of men who followed him. No one felt any discomfort.

Brantly's pace for 5 and 10 miles looked reckless because the pack allowed him to run so far ahead, but his times of 24:40 and 49:30 were within the range of hundreds of runners. His pace was nowhere near as crazy as Juma Ikangaa's mad dash in 1990. None of the runners could feel the wind; the most experienced knew they ran with a big tailwind. The official Boston wind readings, taken by the National Weather Service at Logan Airport, 5 miles east of the finish, showed a western tailwind of a constant 19 mph. The hills, buildings, and trees along the race course made the actual wind speeds for the runners unmeasurable, but Brantly's times were clearly measurable. He ran alone and ahead of the field, but by only 25 seconds. The field seemed to have no interest in catching Brantly, nor did he seem to have any interest in either running away from them or settling back into the comfort of the pack. No one seemed interested in racing at all. As Brantly ran, stuck ahead of the pack but at the same speed, everyone else waited. To observers the tactics seemed quite strange.

Perhaps they all had visions of negative splits running through their heads. That tactic, running the second half faster than the first, had worked for Ndeti the previous year, but no other winner had ever used it. Until the pack decided what to do, they created a constant, recursive feedback loop of watching each other, waiting, and running. Hwang watched Espinosa, who watched Barrios, who watched Lucketz Swartbooi, who watched Steve Jones, who watched Moses Tanui, who watched Kempainen, who watched Benson Masya, who could not see Ndeti. Ndeti dallied at the back of the pack and watched the watchers, none of whom showed the slightest interest in chasing Brantly. Ndeti's younger brother, Josphat, ran a little ways back in the second pack, watching Cosmas. Cosmas paid special attention to the whereabouts of Masya, his childhood friend. As kids in Machakos they had shaved their heads to become known about town as the two coconuts. Masya very much wanted to win the Boston Marathon, as had his friend Cosmas, and he thought since he had faster times in shorter races, his day in the marathon would come. It deeply bothered Masya that his marathon break-through had not yet arrived.

Randomly, various of the runners floated to the front of the pack to tease and test the rest. Still, no one wanted to chase after Brantly. Brantly himself was not trying to run away; neither did he want to break into a jog to wait for them. He knew the pack would be along soon enough.

At 10 miles the pack still waited 17 seconds behind Brantly. At 12 miles Brantly removed a glove to drink water, then replaced it. Had it been a warm day he would have left the glove off. Yet, if it was such a good day for running, cool with a tailwind, why was the 10-mile time nearly 3 minutes slower than the course record? Soon someone was going to get impatient.

At 14 miles, Swartbooi initiated the charge to catch Brantly. As Cosmas Ndeti stayed in the now 14-man pack watching the Mexicans, the Koreans quickly joined the chase. Like hounds recruited for the kill, Tanzanian Lorry Boay Akonay and Kenyan Jackson Kipngok of Nairobi joined as well. The rest of the pack had to follow. Within a mile they had swallowed Brantly. Later Brantly would say, "They were being way too tactical. These are guys who can run a world record, and I definitely believe the world record should have fallen today."

Suddenly at 16 miles a pack of eight runners surged away. They smelled blood in the water. Salvador García led the charge with a 4:41 mile against a pace

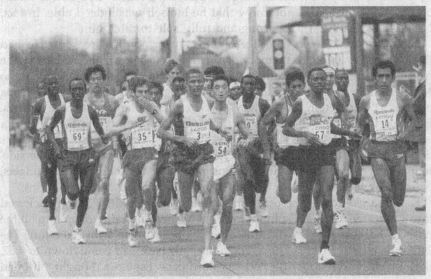

While Brantly ran bravely ahead, at 9 miles the pack waited with visions of "negative splits" running through their heads. Lucketz Swartbooi (#3), Arturo Barrios (#14), Cosmas Ndeti (#1), and the rest all bided their time. © Victah/Photo Run.

that had been averaging 4:56. Bong-Ju, Hwang, Espinosa, Swartbooi, Kipngok, Akonay, and black South African Gert Thys followed García. While not officially part of the surge, Barrios and Ndeti followed a respectful 5 yards back.

At 17 miles five runners surged: Swartbooi, Espinosa, Akonay, Kipngok, and Hwang. García fell off. At 19 miles Swartbooi and Akonay surged, with Espinosa, Hwang, and Kipngok following. This mile passed in 4:38. It seemed like the moment of breakup. Each surge had sharply increased the pace, but after each surge the pace did not settle back to the original. It seemed as if the pack had strung out for the final struggle to the finish. But behind these surging men ran Ndeti, still calmly watching it all. He had not initiated a surge yet. Carefully he observed the men ahead as he tailed them. He needed to understand their weaknesses. He needed the psychological advantage of knowing how they felt while they did not know the same about him. An observer might say that he ran defensively. Ndeti saw many weaknesses, but he also saw that Espinosa had none.

Before 21 miles Swartbooi began to fall off Akonay's pace. Akonay, who has run only a 2:16 marathon and has never won a major race, sensed that Swartbooi was tired. But Akonay made a mistake. He relaxed. Perhaps the relaxing was inevitable because of fatigue, but at that moment the ever-vigilant Ndeti prepared his one and only big surge. Like a resting reptile sensing prey, Ndeti mobilized his attack. Quickly he zipped up to Akonay and lingered next to him. As he had with Swartbooi in 1993, Ndeti took a long and lingering look deep into his rival's eyes. No response. Akonay had been drained. Ndeti accelerated again because he knew Espinosa would not be fooled long by his sudden surge. Ndeti had written "My God is Able" on his shoe, but he did not know that he himself was indeed able. In fact, Ndeti knew Espinosa was strong and fully able to catch him.

Espinosa knew it too. He, like Ndeti, ran for spiritual reasons. He had dedicated this race to the memory of a man he had known and respected: the recently assassinated Mexican presidential candidate Luis Donaldo Colosio Murrieta. Colosio had been killed after delivering a campaign speech in Tijuana on March 23. Something larger than sports or prize money drove these runners. Espinosa wanted to win at Boston to be invited to the White House to run with President Clinton. Espinosa chased after Ndeti. Espinosa could see Ndeti's tired, flat-footed stride and circling right arm as it whipped out to the side, reminiscent of the form of four-time Boston winner Bill Rodgers. Like Rodgers, Ndeti did not want the race to come down to a man-against-man sprint.

Espinosa closed to 4 seconds on Hereford Street. Ndeti looked back and saw a monster coming. Espinosa lowered his head and dug deep into all the push he harbored. Ndeti did the same, his head tilting with the effort. The 24th mile passed in 4:35. The average per-mile pace had come down to 4:52. Each man ran well under the course record pace. Espinosa thought, "If I had started chasing Ndeti a mile sooner, I might be able to catch up." But anything can happen, so Espinosa did not relent or relax. The 3 miles from 22 to 25 passed in 13:48. Ndeti and Espinosa turned for the long last straightaway down Boylston Street to the finish in front of the public library. The TV cameras with their super-zoom lenses magnified the men, distorting their images and making them look like rippling figures against a foreshortened background. Both men fought all their demons and fatigue on that last run in. As they flashed past the screaming spectators, no one could be sure who would win. To the very last step the gap—4 seconds—remained unchanged. Both runners had broken the course record. For all their contorted straining, neither looked especially tired. It had been a good day to run fast.

A step after the finish, Ndeti warmly gripped Espinosa's hand. A few steps later, Ndeti held son Gideon Boston in his arms. Father and son charmed the city of Boston.

Ndeti won $70,000, plus a $25,000 bonus for breaking Rob de Castella's course record (the bonus was also awarded to Espinosa). The winnings would buy Ndeti much in Machakos. Now there would be no end to Kenyans coming to Boston.

Split Times Compared to 1990 Record Times

	Record	1994
5 miles	23:05	24:40
10 miles	46:53	49:30
Half marathon	1:02:01	1:04:52
15 miles	1:11:15	1:14:13
20 miles	1:36:53	1:37:56

Leader's Time for Each Mile

1.	Aniello Filho	4:53	14. Keith Brantly	4:56
2.	Aniello Filho	4:58	15. Keith Brantly	4:57
3.	Keith Brantly	5:00	16. Salvador García	4:41
4.	Keith Brantly	4:49	17. Lucketz Swartbooi	4:54
5.	Keith Brantly	4:59	18. Lucketz Swartbooi, Andres Epinosa	4:50
6.	Keith Brantly	4:55	19. Lorry Boay Akonay, Lucketz Swartbooi	4:38
7.	Keith Brantly	5:00	20. Lorry Boay Akonay, Lucketz Swartbooi	4:43
8.	Keith Brantly	4:57	21. Lorry Boay Akonay	4:58
9.	Keith Brantly	4:56	22. Cosmas Ndeti	4:34
10.	Keith Brantly	5:03	23. Cosmas Ndeti	4:39
11.	Keith Brantly	4:58	24. Cosmas Ndeti	4:35
12.	Keith Brantly	4:53	25. Cosmas Ndeti	4:45
13.	Keith Brantly	4:58	Last mile + 385 yards, Cosmas Ndeti	5:49

1994 Men's Results

1.	C. Ndeti, Kenya[CR]	2:07:15*	51.	D. Rathbone, Great Britain	2:21:43
2.	A. Espinosa, Mexico	2:07:19*	52.	H. Welten, Canada	2:21:45
3.	J. Kipngok, Kenya	2:08:08	53.	N. Horio, Japan	2:22:19
4.	Y. Hwang, Korea	2:08:09	54.	A. Limo, NV	2:23:26
5.	A. Barrios, Mexico	2:08:28	55.	J. Michailov, Russia	2:23:26
6.	L.B. Akonay, Tanzania	2:08:35	56.	L. Mosejev, TX	2:23:36
7.	B. Kempainen, MN	2:08:47	57.	G. Sloane, NJ	2:23:45
8.	L. Swartbooi, Namibia	2:09:08	58.	R. Verney, CA	2:23:51
9.	S. Nyangincha, Kenya	2:09:15	59.	R. Denesik, CO	2:24:02
10.	M. Tanui, Kenya	2:09:40	60.	D. Tsebe, South Africa	2:24:05
11.	B. Lee, Korea	2:09:57	61.	V. Krivoy, MA	2:24:09
12.	M. Fiz, Spain	2:10:21	62.	D. Beauley, NH	2:24:16
13.	L.A. Dos Santos, Brazil	2:10:39	63.	A. Filho, Brazil	2:24:34
14.	L. Aguta, Kenya	2:11:19	64.	Y. Oosuda, Japan	2:25:01
15.	T. Moghali, Lesotho	2:11:40	65.	P. Anderman, Sweden	2:25:17
16.	J. Kagwe, Kenya	2:11:52	66.	T. Birnie, New Zealand	2:25:39
17.	B. Masya, Kenya	2:12:35	67.	J. García, MA	2:25:46
18.	E. Bitok, Kenya	2:12:45	68.	M. Henschel, NY	2:26:19
19.	C. Tarazona, Venezuela	2:12:49	69.	L. Baker, MI	2:26:39
20.	K. Brantly, FL	2:13:00	70.	G. Rose, MA	2:27:15
21.	J. Pinheiro, Portugal	2:13:12	71.	C. Prior, CO	2:27:20
22.	M. Coogan, MA	2:13:24	72.	K. Loeffler, Germany	2:27:37
23.	S. Lelei, Kenya	2:13:40	73.	D. Audet, NH	2:27:42
24.	D. Held, WI	2:13:50	74.	J.D. Blodgett, MA	2:27:42
25.	Z. Miano, Kenya	2:14:16	75.	M. Groom, CT	2:27:47
26.	J. Ndeti, Kenya	2:14:26	76.	K. McGovern, MA	2:27:49
27.	D. García, Spain	2:14:35	77.	C. Del Castillo, Venezuela	2:27:52
28.	A. Cruz, Mexico	2:15:32	78.	F. Mullen, MA	2:28:35
29.	D. Kurtis, MI	2:15:48	79.	J. Nolan, PA	2:28:48
30.	P. Levisse, France	2:17:13	80.	D. Lampasi, NY	2:29:25
31.	D. Steffens, WA	2:17:34	81.	J. Wilde, Holland	2:29:32
32.	S. Jones, Great Britain	2:17:40	82.	R. Chisolm, KS	2:29:34
33.	I. Bloomfield, Great Britain	2:17:42	83.	J. Trettin, CA	2:29:40
34.	J. Hill, WA	2:17:44	84.	M. Condori, IL	2:29:40
35.	Y. Iwasa, Japan	2:18:28	85.	M. Harrison, VA	2:30:10
36.	P. Piper, NC	2:18:33	86.	A. Polania, NY	2:30:22
37.	R. Pierce, CO	2:18:53	87.	W. Kessenich, HI	2:30:35
38.	M. Mondragon, Mexico	2:19:17	88.	A. Ruben, NY	2:30:42
39.	J. McVeigh, GA	2:19:23	89.	D. Black, MI	2:30:45
40.	J. Barbour, MA	2:20:26	90.	G. Norton, ME	2:30:48
41.	S. Karasyev, TX	2:20:34	91.	D. Blachnio, Poland	2:30:52
42.	A. Khellil, Algeria	2:20:38	92.	P. Kodama, WA	2:31:06
43.	K. Hurst, Switzerland	2:20:52	93.	P. Gillooly, MA	2:31:09
44.	R. Sayre, OR	2:20:52	94.	G. Towne, CA	2:31:15
45.	R. Wilder, SC	2:21:14	95.	D. Cobine, OR	2:31:31
46.	B. Schwelm, PA	2:21:22	96.	P. Allen, NJ	2:31:37
47.	H. Shimazu, Japan	2:21:26	97.	J. Mulligan, MA	2:31:38
48.	T. Harding, CT	2:21:26	98.	J. Schoenberg, CO	2:31:40
49.	E. Roesner, Germany	2:21:36	99.	H. Aoya, Japan	2:31:43
50.	J. Corro, Venezuela	2:21:36	100.	J. Waldron, MA	2:31:45

*The top two broke the old course record.

LOVE AND MUSCLE

MONDAY, APRIL 18, 1994

Olympic Gold Medalist Favored

Valentina Yegorova came to Boston in the best shape of her life. She had trained herself to be stronger and faster than ever before. She wanted to take no chances against Olga Markova and the rest of the field. Some people considered Yegorova's Olympic victory in Barcelona a fluke, that in the heat she had not run well but rather everyone else had run poorly. Her time, 2:32:41, was much slower than Markova's Boston runs in both 1993 and 1992. There was, rightly or wrongly, a taint of illegitimacy about Yegorova's Olympic medal—a suggestion that she was strong like a bull, tough and impervious to heat, but not swift like a deer and not quick enough to run away from fast runners. Some thought Markova should have been selected to represent Russia and would have won.

This year Yegorova, with a new marathon PR of 2:26:40 from Tokyo in 1993 and a 1:09:35 half marathon in St. Petersburg, Russia, came to crush Markova. For 2 years she had wanted to prove she was indeed the best female marathon runner in the world. She came to Boston fit enough to prove her point. Yegorova remembered dropping out of the 1993 Boston Marathon and how she eventually found her way back to the Copley Plaza Hotel, sweat-plastered and shivering. She swore such a thing would not happen again. She seethed with intent to beat Markova. Markova herself expressed faint doubts about her own fitness in prerace conversation. She had finished only third in a 10-miler in Washington a week earlier. She alluded to her worry, mentioning "a lot of good girls coming up."

One of the up-and-coming good "girls," Elana Meyer, the 10,000-meter Olympic silver medalist, arrived in Boston for her first marathon. She held the fastest 10K credentials—31:11—and a knack for show*woman*ship. In the Olympic 10,000 meters, Meyer, a white Afrikaner, and black Ethiopian Derartu Tulu ran a happy victory lap together, symbolizing the world's hopes for Africa's future. Bright-eyed and effervescent Meyer beamed through the entire 400 meters.

Uta Pippig, however, was not beaming on the days before the Boston race. She remained in her room, nursing a bad cold. She had every reason to believe she would not start or, if she did start, would not finish. Why did she have to get a cold now? She and her coach–companion, Dieter Hogen, hid out in their hotel room and waited.

As the race began, Veronica Kanga of Kenya, a dark, muscular young woman, took the lead with a 5:07 first mile. Barbara Moore of New Zealand took the next mile until the German Pippig took the lead at 3 miles. Either Pippig's cold had evaporated or she had decided to go out in a blaze of glory, echoing the sentiments of marathon gold medalist Frank Shorter, who had said about racing that if he were going to die he'd prefer to die from the front.

At that point Pippig, Meyer, Albertina Dias of Portugal, Markova, Yegorova, Colleen de Reuck, Maria Luisa Muñoz of Spain, and Alena Peterkova of the Czech Republic ran together. Monica Pont of Spain, Sachiyo Seiyama of Japan, and Carmen De Oliveira of Brazil ran nearby. De Reuck, in a blue crop top, moved with the powerful bounding strides of a runner full of speed and impatient to use it. Peterkova, blond hair bouncing in a ponytail, had run well in the Boston Alamo Five Miler a week earlier with a 25:54. Dias, in an orange top and pants, had finished second to Lynn Jennings in the world cross-country championships at Franklin Park in Boston in 1992, and had placed 1 second ahead of Meyer in the world cross-country championships in Budapest, Hungary, 2 years earlier. She also had run a 2:26:49 debut marathon and held a 10K best of 31:33. Meyer had run a 1:07:22 half marathon in Tokyo in 1993, so each had recently proved her fitness.

Pippig came to race Boston in 1994 having run second in 1990 with a 2:28:03, third in 1991 with a 2:26:52, and third in 1992 with a 2:27:12, plus a first place 2:26:24 several months earlier in the New York City Marathon. She had won the Peachtree 10K in Atlanta, Georgia, in 32:17 in the heat and the Bolder Boulder 10K at altitude in 33:39. She won the Berlin Marathon twice, in 1990 (2:28:37) and 1992 (2:30:22), and had placed seventh in the Barcelona Olympic Marathon. Pippig had showed strength and versatility.

De Reuck led through the 6-mile checkpoint with the pack close behind in 32:20, averaging 5:24 per mile. As the group churned through the next several miles, various runners technically held the lead at the specific checkpoints. Pippig led at 7 and 8, de Rueck at 9 and 10. Ten miles passed in 53:56, an average 5:24 per mile. Joan Benoit's course record split was 51:38. Pippig ran 2:18, nearly a half mile behind what Benoit had run. Pippig yearned to set a course record, but she felt she was not yet strong enough to get it.

In the next miles, as Pippig put in a tiny surge, Yegorova matched it, and Meyer tagged merrily along with the track runner's kicking confidence. Meyer seemed to be having no trouble with the pace. She seemed to run on a spree. The next miles passed in 5:30, 5:25, and 5:23, with the half marathon passing in 1:10:48, a bounding de Rueck leading the pack by 8 yards through 13 miles. Benoit had run 1:08:22 for the half marathon. One could imagine the pack of '94 chasing the memory of Benoit's solo run of '83 from 2:26 behind.

By 14 miles Pippig and the pack had come back to join de Rueck. At 15 miles Yegorova took a 5-yard lead with her efficient shuffling stride. At 15 miles (1:21:20) the group ran 2:24 behind Benoit's record pace. Then Pippig stretched out and took a big swoop down the hill into Newton Lower Falls with a 5:12 mile. She picked up 15 yards on Yegorova and Meyer, but she took long looks back as if to say she didn't believe that she had broken away so easily. The surge killed off de Rueck. It should have done the same for Yegorova and Meyer, but Meyer set off in pursuit and took back the lead by 18 miles. Pippig was right—she could not break away so easily. The pack came back. Pippig in the pack of three set off in dead earnest with a 10-second increase in pace, for a 5:20 next mile. Meyer looked to be floating along. She seemed to be smiling and later would say she loved every minute of it. Pippig kept looking back and spitting. They all gained on the record pace.

Meyer and Pippig ran together, with Meyer usually lurking behind. At times Pippig would gesture to Meyer to come up and share the lead. Because of her inexperience, Meyer declined. Meyer reached for cups of water but frequently missed or spilled them. Pippig neatly snatched the cups from the spectators and dumped the contents on her head. Meyer showed no such skill as they romped through the Newton hills. Pippig kept looking back to check on Yegorova.

At 19 miles Pippig opened a gap, but this time Meyer could not respond. The quick little steps that had allowed her to close all the previous gaps would not come. Instead her thighs felt heavy, wooden,

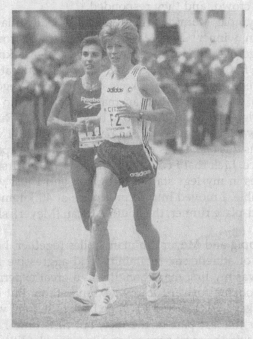

Smiling and shadowing Uta Pippig (#F2), Elana Meyer showed that the marathon may be her best event. © Victah/Photo Run.

unresponsive. She poured water on them as if to prime them. It did not work; they would not pump. She slowed dramatically. Yegorova passed as Meyer slowed to almost a walk. Pippig passed 20 miles in 1:48:22. In 1983 Benoit had gotten to 20 miles 1:38 earlier. Clearly Pippig was rapidly gaining on the record. Now released of the shadow of the kicker, Pippig flew away after the course record. In her head she calculated how she gained on the record time, and she just as easily calculated the bonus money. She cranked out miles of 5:12, 5:18, and 5:10, chasing Benoit's ghost. She said to herself, Just win, in 2 or 3 years you can get the record.

Those 140-mile weeks paid off. The tailwind pushed Pippig along. She went for the record and in the process risked her win. At any moment a sudden cramp could seize her leg muscles. Such a thing has happened to many runners before. Perhaps Pippig agreed with Joan Benoit's preference: "I'd rather burn out than rust." Instead of exercising caution, she chased the ghost of Joan Benoit. Somewhere along Beacon Street Pippig caught the ghost. Benoit (now Joan Samuelson), working as color commentator on Boston's Channel 5, saluted the attempt.

Three miles later Pippig ran along Boylston Street in sight of the finish line, a minute under the course record, blowing two-handed kisses to the crowd, pumping her clenched fist in the air and pointing to her biceps. There it was, a sublime exposition of muscles and love. She demonstrated that love to the crowd, and they responded.

The 1992 Olympic Marathon gold medalist Valentina Yegorova and two-time Boston winner Olga Markova traded fates from the previous year, when Yegorova had dropped out. This year Markova stayed with the lead pack for about 9 miles and dropped out at 20. This year Yegorova crushed Markova as Markova dropped out. Yegorova said, "All I wanted to do was set the Russian marathon record to prove that I'm stronger than Olga Markova." Yegorova beat Markova's Russian record by 10 seconds. "I wasn't surprised by the pace," she said. "I was very happy that the pace was this fast. I was prepared for it and felt capable that I could run at a 2:22 pace. I felt that I could win the race for the first half marathon; then the muscles in my legs started to tighten and I just wanted to finish as high as possible. I moved into second place at 40 kilometers. Then was when the second-place runner, the South African [Meyer], slowed to almost a walk."

In Boston, Pippig and Meyer ran many miles together, both exhibiting a perfect balance of athleticism, femininity, and aggressive running. Meyer gushed, "This was my first marathon. It was a great experience. I loved it, and I am now looking forward to my next marathon. But I am not giving up the track. I also love that, and I will go back to it. I am very happy with my time. I blew the last part of the race, but next time I will improve. I thought I could win the race, even when Uta opened a little gap. But in the last couple of miles, I did not feel very good. My legs were very sore. And

I just wanted to finish the race. But for most of the race, I felt in control. Heartbreak Hill was the easiest part of the race. The last 3-1/2 miles seemed very far. I just couldn't go any faster. When [Pippig] made a little surge, I couldn't keep up. Over the last part of the race I really backed off. The next time, I'll be better prepared for the last part of the race. When I prepare on the track, I know what shape I'm in. It was just amazing for me to be a part of the Boston Marathon."

Pippig said about Meyer, "I was not so surprised with how well Elana ran. Also, I was surprised she couldn't stay with me at the end. I thought about the record with about 3 to 4 miles left. But I was really tired at miles 25 and 26, and I just wanted to finish. I said, C'mon, just win. I trained for a 2:22, so this was a good run. I need maybe 1 or 2 more years to break the record. It is harder and harder to find ways to improve. I've made my easy days hard. A hard day is 30 to 35K. But it's always on the hills. I never run on the track. I have more time to train. I study [for medical school] only 2 to 3 hours a day."

With her welcoming good looks and charismatic German accent, Uta Pippig found herself running with the president of the United States and invited onto the David Letterman show on national television. She knocked Letterman over with her description of 5:30 miles in the early part of the race and descending to 5:17, then 5:10 in the latter miles. He asked about her training, and she reported having trained 140 miles a week for 10 weeks. The comedian was aghast. He had to sit down.

Pippig and her coach–companion, Dieter Hogen, are eminently likable. Hogen, by force of personality and a voracious appetite for coaching information, forms half of the partnership that is undoubtedly the source of Pippig's success. Hogen had been coaching her since her start in athletics. But it is Pippig, the medical student who will eventually be Dr. Pippig, who understands and applies the science Hogen unearths. Hogen may have been the catalyst, but together they are a team. Pippig, for all her outgoing, funny, pleasing manner, is celebrated both as a great athlete and an example of grace, good looks, and personality.

There is certainly a shrewdness under the clear skin. As the cover-girl spokeswoman she never misses the chance to sweet-talk a cameraman or TV reporter to get the right angle to show her sponsor's logo. And over the negotiating table Pippig could drive a hard bargain. She is not the sullen, serious, kill-joy fitness fanatic that makes the public cringe with guilt. She doesn't make the public see exercise as punishment for excess eating or drinking. She makes no talk of sacrifice and pain, but viewers could feel her exuberance in having performed so well; and more importantly, they could see her exultation during the race. Exercise and training itself is the excess, the self-indulgence in which Uta Pippig revelled. Uta Pippig was joy in victory.

Uta Pippig won $70,000 for first place, plus $25,000 for her course record. She placed 52nd overall. Pippig and Hogen will be back to Boston.

Leader's Time for Each Mile

1. Veronica Kanga	5:07	13. Colleen de Reuck 5:30
2. Barbara Moore	5:27	14. Uta Pippig 5:28
3. Uta Pippig	4:55	15. Valentina Yegorova 5:38
4. Olga Markova	5:37	16. Uta Pippig 5:12
5. Maria Luisa Muñoz	5:37	17. Uta Pippig 5:32
6. Colleen de Reuck	5:37	18. Elana Meyer 5:30
7. Uta Pippig	5:20	19. Uta Pippig 5:20
8. Uta Pippig, Valentina Yegorova, Albertina Dias, Elana Meyer, Colleen de Reuck	5:23	20. Uta Pippig 5:28
		21. Uta Pippig 5:39
9. Colleen de Reuck		22. Uta Pippig 5:12
10. Colleen de Reuck, Uta Pippig	5:23	23. Uta Pippig 5:18
11. Uta Pippig, Valentina Yegorova	5:30	24. Uta Pippig 5:10
12. Uta Pippig, Colleen de Reuck, Elana Meyer, Valentina Yegorova, Olga Markova	5:25 5:23	25. Uta Pippig 5:30

1994 Women's Results

1. U. Pippig, Germany	2:21:45[CR]	
	(52nd overall)	
2. V. Yegorova, Russia	2:23:33	
3. E. Meyer, South Africa	2:25:15	
4. A. Peterkova, Czech Republic	2:25:19	
5. C. De Oliveira, Brazil	2:27:41	
6. M. Pont, Spain	2:29:36	
7. M. Tenorio, Ecuador	2:30:12	
8. K. Jones, WA	2:31:46	
9. C. de Reuck, CO	2:31:53	
10. A. Dias, Portugal	2:33:21	
11. E. Scaunich, Italy	2:33:36	
12. S. Seiyama, Japan	2:35:46	
13. G. O'Rourke, New Zealand	2:36:30	
14. I. Bondarchouk, Russia	2:36:53	
15. M.-L. Currier, CT	2:37:01	
16. A. Ivanova, Russia	2:37:15	
17. V. Kanga, Kenya	2:38:46	
18. L. Edmark, OR	2:39:38	
19. N. Galouchka, Belarus	2:40:09	
20. S. Betancourt, Mexico	2:40:55	
21. M.L. Muñoz, Spain	2:41:18	
22. K. Webb, Canada	2:41:22	
23. S. Ciric, Germany	2:41:46	
24. B. Acosta, CA	2:43:36	
25. S. Gilbert, CA	2:43:46	
26. M. Daigo, Japan	2:44:02	
27. B. Portenski, New Zealand	2:45:37	
28. L. Norwood, TX	2:45:47	
29. M. Button, CA	2:46:50	
30. D. Tracy, CA	2:46:56	
31. M. Jones, CA	2:48:06	
32. J. Hine, New Zealand	2:49:46	
33. D. Hanson, UT	2:51:15	
34. S. Stubler, MN	2:51:46	
35. M. Rutter, KS	2:52:35	
36. C. Dowling, NE	2:52:51	
37. F. Levasseur, Canada	2:52:59	
38. C. Christensen, CA	2:55:05	
39. C. Dube, MA	2:55:22	
40. Z. Wieciorkowska, CT	2:56:37	
41. L. Nelson, MD	2:56:59	
42. R. Balder, MN	2:57:17	
43. M. Whitlock, FL	2:57:17	
44. M. Shapiro, GA	2:57:24	
45. T. Martland, RI	2:57:39	
46. K. Perini, MA	2:57:41	
47. J. Gaskill, KY	2:58:14	
48. A. Kawano, Japan	2:58:14	
49. M. Schoeler, Canada	2:58:29	
50. M. Stewart, TX	2:58:41	
51. S. Vos, CT	2:58:48	

New World Order? 597

SECRETS AND AGENTS

MONDAY, APRIL 17, 1995

Kenyan Faces Monstrous Field

"The 'Mzee' race starts at 1 o'clock," Cosmas Ndeti said laughingly to a tall, thin, gray-headed American man. Ndeti gestured for the old man to take his suit and shoes off and approach the starting line in Nairobi at the Kenyan cross-country championships in mid-February. The American man had come to learn the secrets of Kenyan running. Here the outside world would get its first look at what will be the planet's dominant long-distance running talent. From this group will emerge the top marathon runners in the world.

Many barefoot young men had come down from the hills to test themselves against other young runners, to begin their running careers and perhaps follow the success of great Kenyan runners like Kip Keino, Henry Rono, and Ibrahim Hussein. These runners became world famous and nearly as well known as Kenyan president Mzee Jomo Kenyatta, the first president of the country after the colonial English left. Mzee is the Swahili title denoting respect. It is usually applied to gray-haired men in suits. As the best cross-country runners in Kenya assembled, a few important gray-haired men in suits watched. In the mid-1990s Kenyan runners have been the best in the world. With half of the country's population of 26 million under the age of 15 and fewer than 5% over the age of 60, a demographic figure that accounts for the rarity of "Mzees," they are likely to continue to be the best in the world.

The Mzee that Cosmas Ndeti cajoled to race was an old Boston Marathon runner, Larry Barthlow from Boston. Barthlow had last run Boston in 1991, finishing 33rd in 2:23:01. At his best he had run 10 minutes faster, so he knew running talent when he saw it. Barthlow had come to Africa because he and his new firm, Global Athletics, had become Ndeti's agent, and they wanted to sign the next generation of African running talent. These young, talented, and unknown runners were the secrets the gray-haired men in suits—the agents—sought. They observed the awesome display of running skill as hundreds of earnest young men warmed up; Cosmas, joking, urged the older men to race. The agents would have loved to; they were young men at heart and members of the same worldwide tribe of people who loved to run. To Cosmas, to his younger brother Josphat, to his childhood friend Benson Masya, steeped in the culture of fast young men in a rapidly changing youthful country, the idea of gray-haired men running races was funny. But actually it is the young men who are really funny. Josphat is more than funny—he is zany, the clown of the group. Josphat has a plan to find a wife for Barthlow's partner, Mark Wetmore. Josphat, Cosmas, and their friends have arranged for many young women to send photos and descriptions to Wetmore's office in Boston. The letters keep coming and coming.

The young men also make fun of one another. They call one fine runner Twiga, the Swahili word for giraffe. Eighteen-year-old Jackson Kabiga from Kianyaga is Twiga. Twiga was living in Cosmas Ndeti's house along with Ndeti's wife, Jane, and the couple's children, Gideon Boston and newborn Serafina. Twiga trains with Cosmas, or tries to, but as Josphat says, "Nobody can train with Cosmas." Josphat might actually be a faster runner than Cosmas, but the older brother's personality dominates. Cosmas takes care of the people around him. He is training his sisters. He has two cars. He is a Kenyan *mensch*, but he still joins in the fun at Twiga's expense.

When chased by hunters on foot, a giraffe will run for days. It does not slow down no matter how tired it gets. But when the animal has fully depleted its energy sources, it suddenly goes from full speed to full stop. Jackson Kabiga raced and trained like a hunted giraffe. Twiga tried to keep up with Cosmas. But frequently out in the bush he stopped running far from home. Cosmas left him for dead, and Twiga walked home. Kabiga raced like prey. He had only two speeds: full and stop. He had run a half marathon in 1:01:00, 28:44 for 10,000 meters. The older Kenyan runners had faith in Kabiga but teased him unmercifully—"Twiga! Twiga!" Cosmas brought Twiga with him to Boston to race his first marathon.

But in Kenya in February the watchword is cross-country: the Kenyan national championships. The Kenyans dominate cross-country running in the 1990s like the Japanese dominated marathon running in the early 1960s, when they fielded more sub-2:20 marathon runners than the rest of the world combined. It can be argued that the Kenyan national cross-country championships is a better race than the actual world event because an unlimited number of Kenyans can compete. Runners of renown like Tergat, Kirui, Songok, Sigei, Ondieki, and Ngugi drive young men to race each other for the coveted positions on the Kenyan National team.

Moses Tanui watched Cosmas clowning with the "Mzees." Tanui could not figure out the older Ndeti. Tanui was a serious man, not one of the jocular boys. He had finished 10th in Boston in 1994 and had run a half marathon faster than anyone (59:47), but he could not understand why Ndeti started the cross-country race so lackadaisically. After the first 100-meter sprint Ndeti, wearing training shoes, ran in dead last place by 20 yards. Gradually he picked off 100 runners and finished 140th, and he immediately began to joke around, as if his poor performance had not touched his pride. Tanui could not fathom that Ndeti's performance held no meaning for him. All Ndeti cared about was Boston. But Tanui planned to beat Ndeti there.

In his large western-style house, with an adjacent shamba—a garden full of cabbage, onions, and corn—Ndeti lived unfazed by impending competition. His driver had a room in the house, as did Twiga. The driver used the red Toyota wagon named *Boston, Massachusetts*, but Cosmas alone drove the white Japanese sports car he called *The Airplane*. One must understand that Kenya is a country filled with young men who like to drive at top speed on roads with few rules and little enforcement. Anything goes in Kenya as drivers speed recklessly along narrow red-dirt roads, honking at pedestrians, animals, and lurching lorries overloaded with passengers clinging to every handhold. On such roads and under such duress, Cosmas, Josphat, Twiga, the agents Barthlow and Wetmore, and the driver traveled 4 hours north along the east escarpment of the Great Rift Valley to the training camp at Embu. Josphat drove *Boston, Massachusetts* at maximum speed. His hands twitched oddly as he lightly held the steering wheel, and could have signaled his nervousness. One of the white-knuckled "Mzees" asked Josphat if he had ever driven before. "Oh, yes, twice."

Cosmas trained at Embu, in the shadow of Mt. Kenya. He proclaimed his training methods secret, and mockingly refused to divulge them. His agents would not reveal them either. The idea of training secrets was, of course, a young man's joke on those who wanted to believe in such things.

For Cosmas Ndeti and his family and friends in Machakos, life formed a pleasant daily cycle: training, a lot of socializing, and eating. In a country where the economy is stagnant and where the dictatorship government is without tradition and operates to maintain its power to the exclusion of all else, what counts is kin and community. The importance of the tribe and centuries-old loyalties to traditions shuffle aside individual accomplishments and expressions. Kenyans are not usually braggarts or self-promoters or even accurate about their accomplishments. Rarely do they make predictions about race outcomes. They might say something vague, like "I will do my best," or "God will decide." A Muhammad Ali–type, saying "I am the greatest!" would not emerge from Africa. Too much attention paid to the self usually works against the cohesion of community. Ndeti is unusual in Africa. He has his new-born Christian religion, and through it he is a rare African practitioner of individualism. But at the same time, he is also a man of his community. He has become a famous individual in his town. Daily Ndeti lunches at the T.Tot Hotel in Machakos, usually eating rice with a mild meat sauce, and always with company. Everyone in town recognizes and greets him. And always he carries with him the message of his god, which he readily shares.

Once in Boston for the marathon, the Kenyans congregated at Mark Wetmore's South End home. There Ndeti took special pains to make Kenyan food for the Kenyan contingent, especially Tegla Loroupe. Hearing that she felt ill from the American food, he made a meal from home—comfort food. Loroupe had won the New York City Marathon in a surprise come-from-behind surge over the final 5 miles. But in Boston her stomach felt upset, so Ndeti made ugaalli—a thick cornmeal mash with a sauce of cabbage and onions. The Kenyans lined up to wash their hands before eating and laughed at the agents who did not bother. The Kenyans scooped up the cornmeal with three fingers and dipped it into the sauce. The agents used forks.

Perhaps Ndeti had a special respect for Loroupe because in March she had almost beaten him in the Lisbon Portugal half marathon. He had run only 68:18 and she 68:32. After that race his confidence seemed to vanish. He was sullen. His agents couldn't get a laugh out of him.

But in Boston all had changed; the confidence had returned. Ndeti said, "I know my body, and I know I can win more times. I can win five or six times." Then he began to sing the praises of the Kenyan training system: "There are a lot of Kenyans here and they're a good example. They encourage me. It's not a problem. It's our training. Kenyan training is harder than [that of] the other guys. You find in our country many people are good runners, and you have to work hard to beat your friend. There are about 40 guys who can qualify for the World Cross-Country, so everyone has to work hard to qualify."

But not only Kenyans came to Boston. Benson Masya said, "The Koreans will be the biggest threats to the Kenyans, I believe." Of the four Koreans three were named Kim: Kim Jae-Ryong, second in Boston in 1993, Kim Wan-Ki, 2:08:34 in the Dong-A marathon in 1994, and Kim Min-Woo. The fourth Korean was Sohn Moon-Kyu.

Old Johnny Kelley led the race in a convertible. He sat on the back of the rear seat and waved to the crowd. He was named the new grand marshal because he had run the race more times than anyone. Kelley wanted to run the race again, but at age 88 he didn't want to make people wait that long at the finish line. Barnabas Rotich started the race so quickly he seemed to be trying to catch Kelley and jump in the car with him. Rotich ran the first mile in 4:34, all alone.

A pack of 25 caught him in Ashland, Ndeti leading. But then Ndeti drifted to the back of the pack and seemed to adopt the role of mobile spectator. He seemed content with the pace. Rotich took off again to resume his solo leadership. No one in the big pack cared to close the gap. Just as Brantly had run alone the previous year, so did Rotich. For amusement Rotich could look ahead to the truck-mounted pace clock to see the elasped time, the current pace per mile, and the projected time. It read 2:07:15.

At 13 miles Kim Jae-Ryong led the charge to catch Rotich. Perhaps the pack felt the urge to gather momentum to finish the second half faster than the first. Lucketz Swartbooi dropped out at 14. The term "negative splits" had become popular, following a new fashion to run the second half of the marathon faster than the first. Ndeti had run negative splits in the 1993 and 1994 Boston Marathons. It seemed the pack wanted to be in fashion all together. They caught Rotich at 15 miles, but he stayed with them and forged back into the lead at 16. Kenyans Paul Yego, Lemeck Aguta, Moses Tanui (2:09:40 at Boston in 1994), Sammy Nyangincha (2:09:15 at Boston in 1994),

Gilbert Rutto, and Charles Tangus; Koreans Kim Wan-Ki and Kim Jae-Ryong; and Spaniard Alberto Juzdado composed the lead pack. Juzdado, age 28, of Madrid, had run 2:11:39 at San Sebastian, Spain, in 1992. Ndeti took over with a 5:02 mile to push the pace over the long Rt. 128 uphill overpass so no one would be able to rest before the turn up into the Newton Hills. The pack became 12, then 8, including Kim Jae-Ryong; Aguta, Nyangincha, Yego, Tanui, and Rutto. The day seemed warm, and there was a headwind.

Kim Jae-Ryong took the pace. The pack shrank to five runners by 19 miles. One of the casualties was Twiga, Jackson Kabiga. He suddenly stopped. He could not run another step. He waited by the side of the road for the lions to eat him.

At 20 miles Ndeti and Aguta ran side by side, leading a pack of five. Nyangincha and Rutto disappeared. At 22 miles the fight in the pack of five grew vicious. Ndeti floated ahead of the pack and turned to look back. His look carried a threat. Ndeti followed through on the threat as he tossed in a 4:39 mile. TV color commentator Bill Rodgers watched Ndeti and saw something of his own fierce self. "This is where the race begins. Cosmas is a strategic genius. He knows how to exert pressure. He is just squeezing these guys. You can see them drop one by one—they are just collapsing. You can see it in their faces. He loves this race."

At last Ndeti ran with Moses. Only Moses Tanui, the rapid 10,000-meter runner, remained. He did not look distressed. Ndeti started to panic. He had to get rid of Tanui. He turned the screws with a 4:47 mile. To Ndeti, Tanui was a real threat. He was not just one of the guys. The last 2 miles had passed in 9:26. The 23rd mile killed Tanui. Ndeti ran on alone.

Ndeti ran through the finish with his arms extended, one finger pointing up as if to say "I am number 1." Then he waved three fingers jauntily: "I have won three times in a row." Then he pushed three fingers of each hand in the air. Did he mean that he intended to win six times in a row? A couple of minutes later Ndeti said "I would like to be like Johnny Kelley and run here as often as possible." On the sidelines the "Mzees" stood nodding their gray heads and smiling. They knew the secrets—they had been to Africa.

Checkpoint Splits

5 miles	Barnabas Rotich	24:16
10 miles	Barnabas Rotich	49:13
Half marathon	Barnabas Rotich	1:04:52
15 miles	Large pack	1:14:19
20 miles	Cosmas Ndeti, Lameck Aguta	1:38:48
Last mile + 385 yards	Cosmas Ndeti	6:10

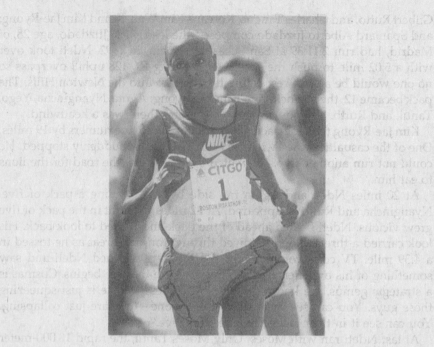

Cosmas Ndeti has his eyes fixed on the finish line, and the future. © Victah/
Photo Run.

Leader's Time for Each Mile

1. Barnabas Rotich	4:34		15. Large pack		4:59
2. Barnabas Rotich	4:45		16. Barnabas Rotich		4:44
3. Barnabas Rotich	4:57		17. Cosmas Ndeti		5:02
4. Pack of 20	5:00		18. Kim Jae-Ryong		4:56
5. Barnabas Rotich	5:00		19. Cosmas Ndeti, Kim Jae-Ryong, Sammy Nyangincha, Paul Yego, Lameck Aguta		4:51
6. Barnabas Rotich	4:50				
7. Barnabas Rotich	4:52				
8. Barnabas Rotich	4:57		20. Cosmas Ndeti, Lameck Aguta		4:56
9. Barnabas Rotich	5:03		21. Cosmas Ndeti, Moses Tanui		5:17
10. Barnabas Rotich	5:15		22. Cosmas Ndeti, Moses Tanui		4:39
11. Barnabas Rotich	5:03		23. Cosmas Ndeti		4:47
12. Barnabas Rotich	4:55		24. Cosmas Ndeti		4:46
13. Barnabas Rotich	5:08		25. Cosmas Ndeti		4:55
14. Barnabas Rotich	5:01				

1995 Men's Results

1.	**C. Ndeti, Kenya**	**2:09:22**	51.	K. McGovern, MA	2:28:47
2.	M. Tanui, Kenya	2:10:22	52.	K. Kelly, PA	2:29:54
3.	L.A. Dos Santos, Brazil	2:11:02	53.	D. Kurtis, MI	2:30:05
4.	L. Aguta, Kenya	2:11:03	54.	J. Stein, GA	2:30:16
5.	P. Yego, Kenya	2:11:13	55.	M. Prinzel, TX	2:30:22
6.	A. Juzdado, Spain	2:12:04	56.	A. Breidbach, MA	2:30:27
7.	J. Kim, Korea	2:12:15	57.	R. McGarry, PA	2:30:36
8.	S. Nyangincha, Kenya	2:12:16	58.	R. Bieber, PA	2:30:47
9.	G. Rutto, Kenya	2:12:25	59.	T. Murdock, MA	2:30:59
10.	T. Moqhali, Lesotho	2:12:56	60.	D. Lampasi, NY	2:31:05
11.	I. Rico, Mexico	2:13:10	61.	P. Leonard, PA	2:31:09
12.	W. Kim, Korea	2:13:32	62.	J. Courcelle, VT	2:31:10
13.	C.K. Tangus, Kenya	2:14:08	63.	N. Shertzer, PA	2:31:13
14.	B. Rotich, Kenya	2:14:25	64.	S. Warren, MA	2:31:23
15.	P. Maher, Canada	2:14:33	65.	J.D. Blodgett, MA	2:31:25
16.	M. Kim, Korea	2:15:08	66.	M. Henschel, NY	2:31:27
17.	M. Mondragon, Mexico	2:16:29	67.	C. Koehler, VA	2:31:34
18.	J. Marquez, Mexico	2:16:50	68.	G. Neysmith, Canada	2:31:37
19.	C. Wathier, Brazil	2:17:49	69.	A. Castle, TX	2:31:52
20.	H. De Jesus, Mexico	2:18:45	70.	D. Ciaverella, FL	2:31:55
21.	J. Lopez, Colombia	2:19:09	71.	B. Crane, MA	2:31:55
22.	B. Katui, Kenya	2:19:31	72.	T. Jones, CO	2:31:58
23.	Y. Mikhailov, Russia	2:19:37	73.	H. Kitame, Japan	2:32:00
24.	R. Verney, Australia	2:19:41	74.	A. Samarron, NM	2:32:11
25.	A. Navarro, Mexico	2:20:31	75.	D. Bebinger, TX	2:32:21
26.	K. Koskei, Kenya	2:20:46	76.	J. Schoenberg, CO	2:32:26
27.	H. Steffny, Germany	2:21:38	77.	H. Haava, KY	2:32:29
28.	T. Buckner, Great Britain	2:21:40	78.	G. Towne, CA	2:32:36
29.	M. Whittlesey, CT	2:22:48	79.	D. Newman, PA	2:32:42
30.	S. Karasyev, Russia	2:22:53	80.	J. Trettin, CA	2:32:44
31.	C. Fram, NH	2:22:58	81.	J. Montgomery, NJ	2:32:53
32.	J. Corro, Venezuela	2:22:59	82.	B. Burns, OH	2:33:00
33.	C. Del Castillo, Venezuela	2:23:13	83.	G. Svendsen, NJ	2:33:08
34.	J. Correa, Colombia	2:23:48	84.	T. McGrath, LA	2:33:09
35.	T. Redding, FL	2:23:55	85.	F. Mullen, MA	2:33:31
36.	M. Sohn, Korea	2:24:09	86.	T. McCluskey, OH	2:33:32
37.	G. Guillemette, RI	2:24:18	87.	S. Clark, NH	2:33:32
38.	S. Fader, OH	2:24:46	88.	P. Peterson, MD	2:33:32
39.	A. Montuori Filho, Brazil	2:24:51	89.	M. Cooney, MA	2:33:33
40.	V. Krivoy, MA	2:25:12	90.	P. Allen, NJ	2:33:33
41.	M. Carpenter, CO	2:25:57	91.	J. Swift, CT	2:34:11
42.	T. Covington, VA	2:26:02	92.	A. Kuramata, Japan	2:34:45
43.	J. Brunswick, RI	2:26:34	93.	K. Wilson, NM	2:35:03
44.	T. Harding, CT	2:26:38	94.	K. Amundson, NJ	2:35:06
45.	J. Conforti, MA	2:26:41	95.	R. Stefanovic, WI	2:35:07
46.	N. Kiguchi, Japan	2:26:53	96.	A.J. Bruder, NY	2:35:15
47.	R. Meyer, NE	2:27:32	97.	V. Connelly, MA	2:35:23
48.	B. Simmons, MN	2:28:02	98.	L. Moseev, Russia	2:35:25
49.	W. Rabbitskin, Canada	2:28:25	99.	J. Knap, OH	2:35:33
50.	J. Nolan, PA	2:28:37	100.	S. Greenspan, AZ	2:35:34

A Kiss Is *Not* Just a Kiss

MONDAY, APRIL 17, 1995

German Medical Student Returns to Defend

Outside the church in Hopkinton, shortly before the start of the 99th Boston Marathon, Dieter kissed Uta. The kiss was not the good luck kiss of a coach to an athlete, nor was it the passionate kiss of new lovers. It was an "airport kiss" of the long-married, who know that the traveling or the staying could change their lives. As coach Dieter Hogen kissed runner Uta Pippig outside the church in the sunshine, both knew they parted at the start of a journey similar to many others. But like couples separating at airports, neither dared feel that the parting was routine. Lives change during separations, even brief ones. Nothing is taken for granted.

For 8 years Hogen had coached now 29-year-old Pippig, the defending Boston champion, course record holder (2:21:45), and race favorite, who the previous year had worried that a cold would hurt her race but who this year held no such worries. The two refer to each other as companions. They have a house together in Berlin, Germany, and another in Boulder, Colorado. They share 10 secrets of training and diet that they would not reveal before the race. So why did Coach Hogen have a gnawing feeling in his stomach as he watched Pippig walk from the church through the shade of the nearby graveyard with the other elite runners to their starting position ahead of 2,175 qualified female entries? Because things do go wrong. One of the graves they passed was that of 12-year-old Jeduthun Perry, who died in 1817. The words Pippig could not stop to read on his tombstone: "Death is a debt to Nature due. As I have paid it, so must you."

Hogen wanted to be with Pippig as she ran, to watch and advise her if anything went wrong, but the Boston Marathon course has some logistical problems. How could nervous Hogen get out on the course while thousands of police officers, uniformed militia, and a million spectators blocked the course?

The exact way Hogen followed Pippig must remain a trade secret, but John McGrath, publisher of *New England Runner* magazine, had painstakingly worked out the procedure, including times of departure and lengths of stay at each checkpoint. Zipping in a van from checkpoint to checkpoint, the members of Team Hogen could listen to the radio or watch an onboard TV monitor. Each person in the entourage received printed instructions as precise and complex as the plot in a cinematic spy-and-counterspy thriller.

A German television crew followed in another vehicle. No margin for error remained. Everyone wore black-and-white Boston Marathon press jackets and carried either a notebook or a camera. Except Dieter Hogen. He dressed in black sweatpants and wore a black Nike baseball cap backwards. Everyone followed Hogen and watched Hogen. The entire operation was conducted in German, except for Hogen's nervousness, which he communicated in universally understood gestures.

The players in the operation had to leave Hopkinton immediately after the kiss. Amby Burfoot, Boston Marathon winner of 1968 and now executive editor for *Runner's World* magazine, was one of only two non-German speakers in the operation. In the van, Burfoot watched Hogen display his anxiety. He twitched. He yawned. He stroked his forehead, removed his hat, replaced it. Again and again he drew his index finger and thumb from the corners of his mouth to the tip of his chin. Asked how he felt, he poked his fingers deep into his abdomen and shook his head. Something was eating him.

Hogen and company arrived at 5K without incident. The crew filed out of the van in close order and ran after Hogen to the course. The lead men powered past, then Hogen waited in the gap until he could see the women's lead vehicle. He caught sight of Pippig. She led with no one in sight. Her time was about 16:45. Hogen ran alongside her, shouting in German and clapping his hands. The camera crew followed as best they could.

Pippig had been running 5:20 miles and looked good. She seemed to be running for the course record and a sub-2:20. Hogen seemed relieved that no other runners were around, but he remarked that it was early yet. Then he rubbed his stomach. He had done his job as coach. He had thought intensely about his athlete, had done endless research about diet and exercise physiology. He knew the East German training methods. He knew their strengths and weaknesses. He had devoured nearly everything written on nutrition and the training of long-distance runners and had applied it to Pippig and the other athletes he coached. Now all he could do was rub his stomach.

At the 10K Valentina Yegorova, Elana Meyer, and Franziska Moser arrived to worry Hogen. A headwind had destroyed any attempt at record pace. The three hung behing Pippig. Yegorova's fluorescent orange outfit clashed with Pippig's mustard-yellow Nike suit. The other two wore sensible blue. Yegorova, age 31, of Cheboksari, Russia, was the current Olympic champion. She placed second in 1994 in Boston with a 2:23:33 personal record. Meyer, age 28, from Stellenbosch, Republic of South Africa, had placed third the previous year in her debut Boston Marathon with a 2:25:15. She was the current Olympic silver medalist in 10,000 meters. Meyer had won the World Cup 10,000 meters in 30:52:51 and the Tufts 10K in 31:39. Moser, age 28, of Spiegel, Switzerland, had won the Frankfurt Marathon in 2:27:44 the previous year. As the runners passed, Hogen ran alongside, shouting in German. Pippig looked at him and nodded. He had told her to give up running for time and go instead for place, but she had already decided that. Hogen turned and ran back for the van.

Leading the file out of the van at the 10-mile checkpoint, Hogen saw that diminutive Tegla Loroupe of Kenya had passed Moser and approached Pippig. New York City Marathon champion Loroupe, age 21, looked quite at ease and dangerous. The stomach problems that had troubled her in the preceding days did not seem to be slowing her now. Perhaps the ugaalli Cosmas Ndeti had made for her had settled her innards. Loroupe, although as far from threatening as a person could appear, looked like a threat to run away with the race. Hogen again matched strides with Pippig and her entourage of Yegorova and Meyer.

In her first marathon in New York, Loroupe had come from behind to win in 2:27:37. Many observers of marathon racing expected a great surge of women marathoners to follow the men out of Kenya, and they saw young Loroupe as the crest of the wave. Here on the course in Boston, she had already run 31:29 for 10K. The day, warm and sunny, seemed suited to one born on the equator. Hogen seemed to be shouting specific instructions at Pippig.

After the sprint back to the van, Hogen was asked if he had told Pippig that Loroupe approached. He said no. He had told her to run a tactical race because the sun, heat, and headwind made conditions bad for a record attempt. Eagerly the vanful headed off to the half-marathon point to see whether the Kenyan would join the other African, the Russian, and the German. Hogen jumped out of the van and ran along to see that indeed a pack of women seemed to be forming but had not quite coalesced. Pippig passed in 1:11:23. Back in the van on the way to 30K Hogen could see on the TV monitor that the women's pack formed and tightened at miles 16 and 17. Now it looked like a track 10,000-meter race.

Pippig, Yegorova, Meyer, and Loroupe ran together toward the 30K mark, where Hogen and the vanload waited. Never before had that many women been so tightly bunched so late in the Boston Marathon. They raced each other up the hills but generally followed Pippig, forcing her to lead into the brunt of the headwind. Pippig had been training on steep mountains in Colorado, so the Newton Hills did not faze her. To Pippig Heartbreak Hill felt "like a little bunny hill." To this point she felt that her training served her well. At a checkpoint table she grabbed her special water bottle filled with chamomile tea and ran on, gradually trying to wear down her followers. She had been leading and pace-setting since the start, but what appeared to observers as Meyer and the others settling in behind Pippig in a tactical wait for a kick, as in a track race, was really a recognition of her physical superiority.

None of the others had been willing or able to train three times a day and log in over 150 miles a week. Pippig knew that few other women would dare train so hard. She took massages regularly and strictly monitored her diet. She trained like a Kenyan man and, in fact, trained with many of them, who also worked under Hogen's instruction. Pippig ran her tactical race and essentially followed from the front. Hogen thought Pippig was in control, but he could not be sure. She let her feelings of how the other runners were faring dictate her pace, wanting to keep full pressure on them so they could not relent.

Yegorova relented first. She had been running with quick, choppy strides that suddenly slowed to a shuffle. Soon she dropped out, as she had in 1993 at about the same place. She was taken to Brigham and Women's hospital, where she was rehydrated and released. At 19 miles Pippig approached the elite athletes' water table. Deftly she snatched her waiting bottle of chamomile tea. Meyer casually reached to the table to pluck her bottle from the lineup but instead knocked it and several other bottles to the ground. In a year she still had not learned how to neatly grab a drink. Loroupe's bottle fell, and the two runners stumbled around each other, grabbing for the bottles as Pippig sped away. Inexperience often shows itself in the small things; later Loroupe nearly tripped Meyer. Pippig glanced back when she felt no one on her shoulder.

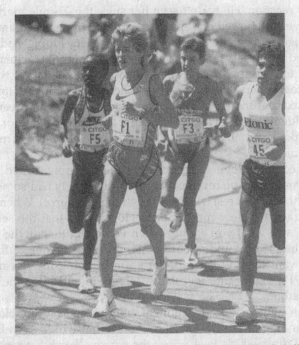

Tegla Loroupe (#F5), once a shy schoolgirl from the remote, high hills of western Kenya, ran more than 33,000 miles before the age of 20. She is running just behind Uta Pippig (#F1) and ahead of Elana Meyer (#F3). © Victah/Photo Run.

Soon the two Africans would catch back up to the German, but at a cost that would be fatal to Loroupe's chances. Almost immediately upon returning to Pippig's shoulder, Loroupe, looking even smaller and younger than usual, began to drop back. She faded to ninth place by the finish, then collapsed into a medical wheelchair. She closed her eyes and curled up, her comfort gone, her stomach pains returned.

Still Meyer followed. Pippig felt confident of her fitness and her present feelings. She also felt a growing blister on her foot. She said later, "This is sport and anything can happen. It would be no good if you had absolutely no problems. It would be too easy." The blister became the spice of her race on the downhills after Boston College. Every time Pippig looked back she said, "I could see a little person with blue clothes."

But Meyer, the little person with blue clothes, had problems of sport too. Her quadriceps muscles began to cramp. So cramps followed blister as both women slowed to performances considerably slower than the previous year's. But Pippig's high mileage and consequent extra strength kept her from slowing too much. Gradually her lead stretched to over a minute. The blister did not inhibit her exuberance on the Boylston Street finish promenade. She glanced back, saw her lead, and blew kisses to the crowd.

Meanwhile Hogen waited beyond the finish chutes. Unable to see Pippig, he could only infer her approach from the public address announcer and the crowd's reaction. He hadn't seen her since the 22-mile mark. He didn't know if Meyer still lurked on Pippig's shoulder with a coiled and poisonous kick. As Hogen heard the announcement that Uta Pippig had won, a big smile flashed across his face, and he began hopping in excitement. But he had to wait to see Pippig. First she had to receive the laurel wreath, smile for the photographers, and blow kisses. She worked her way toward where Hogen waited, parting the mass of photographers like an ocean liner parts the sea. Suddenly seeing Hogen, she burst through the wall of admirers to give him a powerful hug and a real kiss, the kiss of the returning traveler safe and home.

When asked about their 10 secrets of training, Pippig turned to Hogen to ask if they could now be revealed. He said the secrets had something to do with diet, training, and rest (as does everything, of course). When a persistent reporter begged to know more, Coach Hogen said that the secrets had to do not only with what you eat but when you eat it, that all the information is there in the medical and scientific literature for anyone to find. He said he did not want to spoil the reporter's fun in doing the research but that Hogen and Pippig would reveal the secrets in full after the next year's Boston Marathon.

In 1996, an estimated 50,000 runners will descend on tiny Hopkinton for the 100th running of the Boston Marathon. What would Tom Burke—who back in 1897 dragged his heel across the narrow, hard-dirt road in front of Metcalf's Mill in Ashland to start 15 men on the way to Boston—think of his race a century later?

Leader's Time for Each Mile

1. Uta Pippig	5:26	15. Uta Pippig, Valentina	5:37
2. Uta Pippig	5:22	Yegorova, Elana Meyer	
3. Uta Pippig	5:23	16. Uta Pippig	5:20
4. Uta Pippig	5:21	17. Elana Meyer, Uta Pippig,	5:51
5. — —	— —	Valentina Yegorova,	
6. Uta Pippig	11:03	Tegla Loroupe	
7. Uta Pippig, Valentina Yegorova,	5:24	18. Uta Pippig, Tegla Loroupe,	5:38
and 3 others		Elana Meyer	
8. Uta Pippig, Valentina Yegorova	5:22	19. Uta Pippig	5:33
9. Uta Pippig, Valentina Yegorova	5:28	20. Tegla Loroupe,	5:45
10. Uta Pippig, Valentina Yegorova	5:32	Elana Meyer, Uta Pippig	
11. Uta Pippig	5:33	21. Uta Pippig	5:49
12. Uta Pippig, Valentina Yegorova,	5:21	22. Uta Pippig	5:22
Elana Meyer		23. Uta Pippig	5:29
13. Uta Pippig, Valentina Yegorova,	5:32	24. Uta Pippig	5:35
Elana Meyer		25. Uta Pippig	5:51
14. Uta Pippig, Valentina Yegorova,	5:31		
Elana Meyer			

1995 Women's Results

1.	U. Pippig, Germany	2:25:11	26.	M. Shapiro, GA	2:49:57
		(40th overall)	27.	S. Christoff, CT	2:50:39
2.	E. Meyer, South Africa	2:26:51	28.	M. Rhoden, KS	2:50:48
3.	M. Biktagirova, Belarus	2:29:00	29.	M. Perkins, CT	2:51:36
4.	F. Moser, Switzerland	2:29:35	30.	S. Reedy, PA	2:51:47
5.	Y. Danson, Great Britain	2:30:53	31.	J. Briggs, CA	2:52:42
6.	Y. Yamamoto, Japan	2:31:39	32.	L. Mendoza, CA	2:53:18
7.	M. Tanigawa, Japan	2:31:48	33.	K. Kent, CO	2:53:27
8.	S. Mahony, Australia	2:33:07	34.	C. Dube, MA	2:53:58
9.	T. Loroupe, Kenya	2:33:10	35.	L. Ruptash, Canada	2:55:11
10.	M. Tenorio, Ecuador	2:33:34	36.	Z. Wieciorkowska, CT	2:55:33
11.	L. Somers, CA	2:34:30	37.	L. Kelp, PA	2:55:38
12.	C. Metzner, Germany	2:36:22	38.	A. Durham, DC	2:55:48
13.	A. Sugihara, Japan	2:37:07	39.	D. Snowberger, FL	2:55:57
14.	M. Kosaka, Japan	2:37:59	40.	L. Fitzsimmons, WI	2:56:12
15.	V. Yenaki, Moldova	2:38:15	41.	P. Leisher, NJ	2:56:19
16.	G. Loma, Mexico	2:39:31	42.	A. Morse, FL	2:56:42
17.	T. Pozdniakova, Ukraine	2:40:26	43.	L. Fitzpatrick, FL	2:56:55
18.	I. Bondarchouk, Russia	2:43:42	44.	J. Rood, NH	2:56:55
19.	A. Suzuki, Japan	2:44:18	45.	R. Bonilla, Mexico	2:57:07
20.	I. Gonzalez, Colombia	2:44:45	46.	D. Grossert, Germany	2:57:11
21.	K. Yoshida, Japan	2:45:26	47.	E. Krznarich, WI	2:57:16
22.	M. O'Connor, New Zealand	2:47:03	48.	K. Stopyra, NY	2:57:18
23.	M. Schoeler, Canada	2:47:58	49.	M. Hynes-Johanson, MA	2:57:39
24.	C. Keeler, FL	2:48:02	50.	B. Addis, NJ	2:58:08
25.	L. Holda, GA	2:49:40	51.	N. Schubring, MI	2:58:17

A Short History of Wheelchair Racing in the Boston Marathon

1970: Almost an hour before the noontime start of the 1970 Boston Marathon, Eugene Roberts of Baltimore, who had lost his legs to a landmine in Vietnam, left Hopkinton for Boston propelling himself in his wheelchair. Because he had been a 10:04 two-miler at Forest Park High School in Baltimore the marathon came as an obvious challenge to him. He would finish just after six o'clock. Roberts was the first racer to complete the Boston Marathon course in a wheelchair.

1975: Five years later, 24-year-old Bob Hall of Belmont, Massachusetts, set his chair down at the start. Hall had already been participating in shorter road races and had designed and built racing chairs for himself. He took half as long as Roberts to finish (2:58).

1977: No wheelchair racers came to Boston in 1976, but in 1977 the race became the National Wheelchair Marathon Championship. Sharon Rahn of Champaign, Illinois, ran the course in 3:48:51 to become the first woman to complete the course in a wheelchair. Hall smashed his course record to win again with a 2:40:10 over a field of six men.

1978: The wheelchair field expanded to 18 men and 2 women. George Murray of Florida bested Hall's record by over 13 minutes to post a 2:26:57 victory. Curt Brinkman of Utah finished second as he had in 1977. Ken Archer of Ohio finished fourth. Susan Schapiro of California won the women's race with a 3:52:53.

1979: Over wet slippery roads, Murray pushed hard to escape Archer. He drove himself over the Newton hills to lose Archer. But Archer would not get lost. He upset Murray by 1:14 to win with a 2:38:59. Sheryl Bair of Sacramento, California, easily won the women's race with a 3:27:56 world record.

1980: Murray came back to Boston prepared to win. He had trained harder than ever and had improved his equipment and technique. By the top of Heartbreak Hill he had a mile on second place. It was all downhill from there, and Murray flew past Boston College with his four wheels spinning in the sunlight. But as Murray crossed the trolley tracks at Cleveland Circle his left front wheel caught in the track. He tried to free it but it sheared off in his hand. Brinkman made up his 1-mile deficit as Murray desperately tried to fix his wheel. But by the time he repaired it and finished eighth, Brinkman had won in a world record of 1:55:00. Jim Martinson of Puyallup, Washington, finished second. Sharon Limpert of Minneapolis, Minnesota, set a course and American record of 2:49:04 in beating Karen Jacobs by 10 seconds.

1981: Martinson won in 2:00:41 and Candace Cable-Brookes won in 2:38:41, an American and course record.

1982: Perhaps no one could have had a more perfect preparation for wheelchair racing than Jim Knaub. He had been an excellent pole vaulter. Vaulting, like wheelchair racing, is a technical event that requires courage, speed, shoulder and arm strength, and a willingness to practice subtleties. A vaulter as good as Knaub pays great attention to details like the placement of hands. A wheelchair racer likewise must attend to the placement of hands against the driving rings of the chair. Without that attention to details of technique, the speed and big shoulders are useless. If the ring is not engaged perfectly, energy from the athlete's muscles is not efficiently transferred to the road to make the chair go its fastest. Wheelchair racing is as much a sport of finesse as of endurance.

In the 1982 Boston Marathon, Murray raced Knaub until the final moments, when Knaub won by a mere 2 seconds in a world record 1:51:31. Cable-Brookes finished 12th overall among wheelchair racers, lowering her world record to 2:12:43.

1983: This year speeds exceeded many racers' ambitions. Knaub arrived with a chair and a body trimmed to perfection. He commanded the race from the start to earn a new world record of 1:47:10. Sherry Ramsey of Colorado ran 2:27:07 to Californian Jennifer Smith's 2:46:08.

1984: Wheelchair entrants became official at last. Just as the BAA was slow to recognize an official women's division in the running race, it was 9 years after Hall's sub-3:00 run and 14 years after Roberts's pioneering nearly 7-hour trek before the board of governors allowed the inclusion of an official BAA wheelchair division. Previously the wheelchair race had been supported by the National Spinal Cord Injury Foundation. Now the BAA presented awards to all division winners. Pushing into a headwind and a cold drizzle, Andre Viger of Sherbrooke, Quebec, won in a slow 2:05:20 while Ramsey won again in 2:26:51.

1985: Murray hadn't won since 1978, but he had placed second twice since and had suffered that frustration of losing his wheel while leading with 3 miles to go in 1980. Nothing makes endurance athletes redouble their efforts more than placing second. In preparation for the 1985 race, Murray trained as he never had before, and he was pushed by Viger and Knaub to set a new world record (1:45:34). Cable-Brookes won her race with a new world record of 2:05:26.

1986: John Hancock provided prize money for the foot-racers and the chairracers in 1986. The winner of the chair-race, Viger, reversed the 1985 order and beat Murray with yet another world record (1:43:25) and received $10,000 ($2,500 for first place, $7,500 for the record). Cable-Brookes received equal prize money for her 2:09:28. Angela Ieriti of Canada finished second.

1987: Wheelchair racers had gotten faster and more aggressive every year. They were men and women who liked the idea of going fast. Like bike racers, surfers, and sky divers, they had no hesitation about taking risks. They loved speed, thrill, and danger, and the first mile of the Boston Marathon course offers plenty of all three. The course immediately descends from 463 feet, so chairs can reach speeds of 36 miles an hour.

In the 1987 race something happened on the early downhill; no one could sort out the exact chain of events, but suddenly chairs flew in all directions. Some tangled with each other, others tipped and slid on their sides. The public watching in person and on television was horrified by the sight of people with disabilities crashing. Collisions and wipeouts by other athletes in other sports had become commonplace, but calls for safety procedures in wheelchair racing rang out.

Viger wound up on his side. The crash did not bother him much, nor did it bother most of the other racers. Some thought it quite interesting. Viger righted himself, and by Wellesley he had gotten back into the race. By the finish Viger ran 7 minutes ahead of his nearest rival, winning with a 1:55:42. Cable-Brookes suffered a flat tire in the crash. She quickly threw on a new tire, caught up to Ramsey, and passed her to move into the lead and win the race in 2:19:55.

The public viewed wheelchair marathon racers differently from the way they looked at other racers. They were seen as unfortunates, who with exemplary courage and fortitude had overcome their disabilities to complete a marathon in a wheelchair. They were held up as public examples of courage and virtue. The public seemed to believe that the wheelchair racers' disabilities caused their courage. But the fact is that wheelchair racers were by and large courageous people who liked the thrill of speed and the idea of racing long before they acquired a disability.

Although wheelchair racing is not nearly as dangerous as bicycle racing—the rider in a chair is close to the ground, strapped in and surrounded by a metal frame—the sponsor, an insurance company, decided it could not be associated with accidents happening to people with disabilities.

1988: The public outcry for safety forced the BAA to control the wheelchair start in 1988. A lead vehicle enforced a maximum speed limit of 15 mph on the downhill out of Hopkinton. Viger raced France's Mustapha Badid into Ashland, where Viger blew a tire. Badid defeated a record field of 56 to win in yet another world record of 1:43:19. Phillippe Couprie, his training partner and neighbor in Meton, a suburb of Paris, finished a distant second while Viger faded to seventh.

Former winners Archer and Hall finished 12th and 23rd. Cable-Brookes finished 18th overall and ahead of all other women with a 2:10:44.

1989: Badid brought his training partner Couprie, a public relations executive, to Boston. Couprie and Viger raced together for 19 miles as part of their prerace pact to go all-out for a world record. Couprie beat Viger by 41 seconds in the fastest mass wheelchair race yet, where the first eight broke Badid's year-old course and world record with Couprie's 1:36:04. (Badid finished eighth because he had stomach flu.)

Connie Hansen, a physical therapist from Denmark, smashed the previous women's course record by 15 minutes and the world record by 8 minutes to win with a 1:50:06. Cable-Brookes set a new American record of 1:52:34, and Ramsey finished fifth.

1990: Early in the race Couprie and Knaub collided slightly, damaging Couprie's chair. Badid and Switzerland's Franz Nietlispach raced through 18 miles before Badid pulled away. He won in another record smashing time, 1:29:53, while eight men followed under Couprie's record. Viger finished seventh. Couprie himself limped into third, braking with one hand and accelerating with the other. Jean Driscoll of Illinois won the women race, defeating her training partner, Ann Cody-Morris, who ran 1:44:09, and Connie Hansen (1:44:32) with a new world record of 1:43:17. Only

3 years earlier Driscoll's time would have been a men's world record.

1991: This year more racers than ever appeared for the wheelchair division. Knaub won, setting an American record of 1:30:44 and beating the fearsome Craig Blanchette of Springfield, Oregon, by about 4 minutes. Blanchette, who appears at races with pierced ears, a pierced nose, and dreadlocks, had won all eight of his spring road races. Couprie finished sixth.

Driscoll won the women's race again, setting a world record of 1:42:42. She also won $26,000. Cody-Morris took second and Hansen third.

1992: Knaub set the course and world record with a 1:26:28. Couprie finished 2nd. Badid finished 15th and Viger 23rd. Driscoll matched Knaub with a 1:36:52 world record for women. Hansen finished 2nd by about 4 minutes.

1993: Knaub and Driscoll broke their own world records again.

1994: Jim Knaub returned to Boston ready to win again: Under the ideal racing conditions and thanks to his excellent conditioning, it appeared Knaub would indeed win again. It looked like he would do so until 10K. But the push rim attached to the wheel suddenly came detached, and all the power of Knaub's massive shoulders could not reach the wheels. He stopped for repairs twice and was never again a factor. Better luck befell Heinz Frei, a 36-year-old cartographer from the town of Etziken in mountainous Switzerland. Frei loves the hills and pulled away from Tom Sellers, who had trained on the flat land of Florida. He said, "Where the biggest hill, I guess, is a bridge."

No one thought that the dominant Jean Driscoll could be beaten on the Boston Marathon course. Ideal conditions producing a record speed assured the race's competitiveness. Louise Sauvage of Perth, Australia, took the lead from Driscoll several times. At 17 miles Driscoll took the lead, but Sauvage stayed close. Driscoll finished only 23 seconds ahead, as both women broke Driscoll's world-record and course times. Driscoll won for the fifth time. "I'm not that dominant," Driscoll said, "I'm just blessed on this course."

1995: Early in the race Heinz Frei, the 1994 winner, felt he was having a normal day, not the excellent day he had had the year before. Frei also felt that his countryman Franz Nietlispach was having a very good day. In fact, the race never had another leader; Nietlispach took an early lead and never relinquished it.

Jean Driscoll won for the 6th straight year, though the headwind slowed her from her 1994 record. She dominates this race perhaps like no one has ever dominated any athletic event.

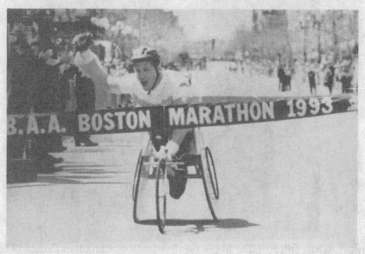

Jim Knaub wins the 1993 wheelchair division. © Victah/Agence Shot.

1995 Men's Results

1. F. Nietlispach, Switzerland	**1:25:59**	
2. H. Frei, Switzerland	1:27:49	
3. P. Couprie, France	**1:27:56**	
4. P. Wiggins, Australia	1:31:38	
5. M. Badid, France	**1:33:11**	
6. C. Issorat, France	1:33:12	
7. G. Mueller, Switzerland	1:33:13	
8. K. Tatsumi, Japan	1:33:13	
9. G. Van Damme, Belgium	1:33:14	
10. A. Viger, PQ	**1:33:14**	
11. K. Schabort, South Africa	1:33:15	
21. C. Blanchette, WA	1:41:13	
22. J. Knaub, CA	**1:41:14**	
29. T. Sellers, FL	1:45:18	
33. B. Hall, MA	**1:47:41**	

1995 Women's Results

1. J. Driscoll, IL	**1:40:42**
2. D. Sodoma, CA	1:47:43
3. R. Winand, MA	1:48:35
4. L. Sauvage, Australia	1:52:01
5. K. Hatanaka, Japan	1:52:42
6. T. Grey, Great Britain	1:56:13
7. L. Anggreny, Germany	1:56:13

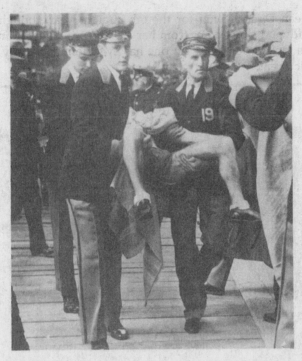

At 23 miles, while still running in the top five in 1938, Canadian Duncan McCallum collapsed and had to be carried from the course. Later he had no recollection of the incident. Courtesy of the Boston Public Library, Print Department.

Chapter 11

1996–1999
Boston Marathon History
Preface to Third Edition

I tell the stories of the contenders. Others see something of themselves in these stories. In the results I list a scattering of other names to give the reader an idea of how many finished under certain standards, and I include names of interesting or notable runners. My wife, Cynthia Hastings, ran 3304th place in 2000 but insists that I use her start line to finish line time, or chip time, of 3:53:30. I did that only for her. Yes, runners are particular about such things, but other than for reasons of domestic tranquility, I go with gun or official times and not chip or mat or elapsed times, because those times would not match the order of finish which we have to hold as cardinal.

I put the stories in the context of their years because the Boston Marathon reflects the general history of Boston, the U.S., and the world.

In reporting results I list the top runners and then skip to 3:00, 3:30, 4:00, and the last listed finisher to give the reader an idea of the overall quality and size of the race, as may have been caused by weather conditions or allowed entries.

Feel free to pencil in any additional results. Everyone's results count, they just all won't fit.

I want to tell the stories of the races and not fill the book with results of all the teams, all the age groups, and all the finishers. I have to stop somewhere or you would hold a 2,000-page book in your hands and the narrative that all runners share with the top contenders would be lost to a tome of data. The same limit applies to photos. Every competitor in the Boston Marathon has a story, and my hope is that you can see all the possible stories reflected in the few I am able to tell about the contenders. Every entrant is a contender at the gun. Everyone's story is special.

I hope someone writes a book about the "Masters of Boston" and about the wheelchairs, maybe the "Wheels of the Hub."

The names in the results in **Boldface** are those of current, previous, or future winners. In the case of future winners I do not tell you in which year they will win. You have to read forward to find out. With only a few exceptions I tell the stories in ruthless chronological order. So the reader, just like the contestants in a particular year, do not know the future. One exception is that I will tell something of the future of someone who will not return to the narrative after that year. I may from time to time mention something pertinent to that year's race that happens later in that year but does influence the next year's story.

I hope runners will use this book to prepare for a marathon by starting 120 days before their race and reading one year's story each day before your daily Boston Marathon training run. Bill Rodgers told me that he kept a copy of the first edition in the smallest room of the house so he could read a daily story as he readied himself for his run.

*Mambo Baddu**

MONDAY, APRIL 15, 1996

Kenyan Looking for Fourth Win in Biggest Marathon Ever

* Swahili for "The best is yet to come."

In his State of the Union Speech, President Bill Clinton declared, "We have the lowest combined rates of unemployment and inflation in 27 years." He said "The era of big government is over. But we cannot go back to the time when our citizens were left to fend for themselves." In April, the Whitewater trial was under way with Special Prosecutor Kenneth Starr calling witnesses.

The United States had the largest economy in the world. China was 7th, just ahead of Brazil.

Al-Qaeda, formed in 1988 by Osama bin Laden and other fighters who had been allied with the U.S. in the war against the Soviet Union invasion of Afghanistan, had not yet conducted terrorist acts against the U.S.

The big news in Boston was that this, the 100th running of the Boston Marathon, would be the biggest Boston Marathon ever and prove to be the biggest marathon anywhere in the world, ever. The U.S. Postal Service issued a special 32-cent stamp commemorating the marathon. The starting field of 38,708 was bigger than the population of three towns on the course: Hopkinton, Ashland, and Natick. The $600,000 in prizes made the 100th running of the Boston Marathon the richest marathon ever. Winners would make a special mark in marathon history. Three-time-winner Kenyan Comas Ndeti came back to make his mark and go back to Kenyan a very wealthy man.

At the BAA bib presentation ceremony, Ndeti accepted the traditional returning winner's bib with the #1. Like prize fighters he admires, Ndeti waved the bib in the air proclaiming, "This is my number! Don't forget! This is my number! Number one (will) still remain #1!" He wrote a special message on the front of his white Fila racing shirt, "The Blood of Jesus on." He wanted to make a statement by winning the 100th Boston Marathon, setting a course record, and thanking his God for helping him do that. God had not revealed his plans.

Where and how did all this Kenyan running start? The place is Toyko in 1964 and the person is Kip Keino. He finished fifth in the 5000m. Four years later he came to Mexico City for the Olympics. He brought other Africans. Keino won silver at 5000m and gold at 1500m beating American Jim Ryun. Kenyan Neftali Temu won the 10,000m, beating Ethiopian Mamo Wolde. Wolde had raced in Boston in 1963 along with double gold Olympic Gold medalist Abebe Bikila. Thus you have the spark of the connection. Ibrahim Hussein, who as a child revered Keino, brought Kenyans attention to Boston by winning in 1988 and again in 1991 and 1992. The 1996 Boston was the Kenyan men's Olympic trials, and Cosmas Ndeti, Sammy Lelei, and Boston runner-up Moses Tanui are a formidable trio. Lelei ran history's second-fastest time (2:07:02) in Berlin Sept. 24, 1995.

Cosmas Ndeti came to Boston to win again. He had won each of the previous three years. He planned to do it again in a new, big, and glorious way. Announcer Larry Rawson likened Ndeti to the boxer Mohamed Ali because of his showmanship and big-shoulder, prize-fighter display of immodest confidence. That is not the way the typical Kenyan child is raised. Before the race Ndeti said, "You should not tell me good luck, but tell me congratulations because I have already won." With $100,000 on the line for the 100th running and with three wins in the previous three years, he thought, *why not win running away*? Win big and go home a very rich man.

Ndeti lived in a house in Machakos, Kenya, at the end of a twisting road with his daughter Serafina, his wife, and his son, born two days before his father's victory in 1993. Yet he wasn't always such a family man.

He used to be a break dancer in city discos. Dancing, the night life, and bars became too much a part of his life. A boyhood friend, Richard Kombo, took him aside and talked to him about changing his lifestyle. Nedeti told *Boston Globe* reporter Joe Concannon, "He told me to commit my life to Jesus and see what can happen to my life. From that time I've seen God bring great things to my life." Ndeti wanted to bring great things to Boston: a fourth win, to match Bill Rodgers.

Ndeti trained in isolated Embu, Kenya, at 7,000 feet above sea level. There is a steep hill on red clay soil where he ran with his training partner Alfornce Muindi. They ran it 20 times. They call it Funia Kifua, Heart Killer hill. Ndeti said, "I get to Heartbreak Hill, and I think nothing of it after this hill."

"Training is good," said Ndeti. "It's almost like 1994. I have won Boston three times. I have the record. I think on this course I can break the world record."

There is no pressure, he maintains, even though he is the favorite.

When asked about the weather, "It doesn't make any difference," Ndeti told Concannon and his agent Mark Wetmore, "because God does not change His

mind. I want to run my own race and not run against anybody. I'll be happier to run my own race. I can run the first half fast. Or the second fast. Or run
both fast. So to me it doesn't matter if there's anybody or if it's a strong field. It
doesn't matter. I know the course like the back of my hand. They can go out fast
and I know where to make my move."

Ndeti has a ministry in his homeland and says he wants to be preaching
when he's not training, says he is "over-confident." Concannon said this was a
blunt way of stating he was ready.

"God has all the power in this world," Ndeti said. "If He says I'll win, I'll
win. It doesn't matter who will be in Boston or how the weather will be in Boston. The God who created me is the God who created the weather."

God created Moses too, and gave him a mission and a burden to bear. The
BAA gave Moses Tanui #2 because he had placed second the last year. He had
trained hard for the entire year, but not to run second to Ndeti. Moses Tanui
came to Boston with the burden, the fear, the revenge, and a host of other emotions that have been common to any runner in any race who came back to try to
win after having finished second. The propinquity of victory can inspire or paralyze a runner. It is easy to try too hard, and hard to try to hold back. Control in
a marathon can sometimes be more important than talent. Tanui certainly had
the talent. Did he have the control? He was the first man to run a half marathon
in under an hour with a 59:47 in Milan, Italy, on April 3, 1993.

Tanui said, "I started running as a very young boy. In Kenya we normally
look after cattle and sheep. We are walking and running all the time. We don't
have cars so we normally run to school in the morning, at lunch time, and again
in the evening."

He lives in Eldoret, Kenya, with his wife and three children. He works as
a farmer and does the height of his training in Brescia, Italy, with Dr. Gabriel
Rosa. Rosa himself writes passionately about Africa and his experiences there.
Rosa wrote a book, published in 2014, *Correre la Vita*, or "Running Life," in
which he wrote about Africa and explains his passion for African runners and
their passion for running:

> Africa is a land of emotion. Where you plunge into your past,
> often not understanding it and sometimes even despising it.
> However, if you look at that world with pure eyes, you can
> only be moved by the pride of the people's faces, the ten-
> derness of the children's smiles. Africa is youth despite her
> age . . . Looking at the world through Africa, you perceive a
> sense of unity. It emerges from the depths of the eyes of Af-
> rican children, who miraculously harbor surprise, awe, and
> confident hope from the tough and brutal reality of adult life.
>
> Africa fills me with deep emotion. No country or continent
> on Earth can grab and press my heart like the villages in that
> part of the world. Like the schools in the Great Rift Valley
> where the children, poor in everything but dignity, wearing

> nothing but worn out colored uniforms, show great respect
> and admiration for their teachers, and for whomever with
> age, has crumbs of wisdom to give them.

This Boston Marathon would serve as the Kenyan Olympic Marathon Trials. Ndeti had already won three world-class Bostons; Tanui had not.

Race director Guy Morse ventured into new territory because more people were coming to run his marathon than had ever come to run a marathon before. He tried to anticipate everything in a campaign that took on military overtones. Military analogies came easily to all involved in organizing the biggest marathon in world marathon history. The potential for a race disaster loomed huge.

There was a problem of crowd control from two sides, unlike sporting events in stadiums where a small number of players perform on a field and tens of thousands watch from numbered seats. In the marathon, a city's worth of people would be on the playing field and anyone could march to any part of the course on either side. So the marathon had a stadium 52 miles long and no seats. Where should crowd control be concentrated? What if crowds pressed in from each side of the road and pinched off the stream of humanity hell bent on getting to Boston? Guy Morse stayed awake worrying about these and any other nightmarish, insomnia-generated possible scenarios. But he did have some help finding solutions.

Morse and company tried to avoid a logistical nightmare. "[It was] Desert Storm in Hopkinton," said Dave McGillivray, nine-year technical adviser to the race and a long-time Greater Boston runner and race organizer. The marathon needed 840 buses to shuttle the runners to athletes' village.

"We're trying to think of everything," said McGillivray. "We're busing approximately 90 percent of the people and dropping them off at the village." First, the BAA had to feed its guests. Just as an army marches on its stomach, marathoners run on theirs. On the day before, the pasta company Ronzoni invited the entire race field to dinner. Ronzoni advertised that the runners would be "burning" their pasta. Guy Morse, Boston Mayor, Tom Menino, and Bill Rodgers, among many others, dished out pasta and tomato sauce to their "army." The city sat in high party mode.

Food may fuel marathoners, but money fueled the entire eastern Massachusetts venture. An estimated 136 to 140 million dollars poured into the economies of all the towns and cities, airports, restaurants, and hotels. These were tourists with friends, family, money, and a mission.

This was not the first time Boston Marathon runners ate well the day before racing, but it would be the first time they ran with computer chips to separate their actual time from crossing the starting line to crossing the finish line instead of only time from when the starting gun fired to the finish. Because of the large crowd, some runners would be far down the road to Boston when others had not reached the starting line. The post-race question would then arise for the first time, "What was your chip time compared to your gun time?"

Mixing metaphors, some people compared the Hopkinton athlete's village to Woodstock. Maybe even more so with John A. Kelley moving runners to tears with his singing of "America" and "Young at Heart." Kelley would ride in the open lead vehicle and wave to the crowd to herald the approach of the runners. The final entrant would cross the starting line 28 minutes and 32 seconds after the start of the gun. Senator John Kerry who would run for president of the U.S. in 2004 and eventually become Secretary of State, would fire the starting gun for the wheelchair race.

Bright sun, 48°F. No early headwind. The day could not be sweeter. But there was a hard race to run and hard runners came to run it.

At the gun Ndeti took the lead, dragging along a pack of 17 through 10k in 29:27 and ten miles in 47:50 and the half in 1:03:22. Thirteen Kenyans ran in the back, two Ethiopians, one Korean, and one Moroccan. The Kenyans wanted to make their Olympic Team. Ndeti wanted to make history. Ndedti ran with an easy loping style, oblivious to the string of runners following him. Tanui rested in the pack. Yet Ndeti ran much faster than in his previous victories. It was a confident move—one in keeping with his prediction of certain victory. He showed no trace of fatigue in the early miles. The 1989 winner, Ethiopian Abebe Mekonnen, also ran in that pack to the amazement of many. He would be picked to represent Ethiopia in the Olympics. He wore a high number, indicating that he was a late entry.

Paul Yego, Tanui, Ezequiel Bitok, Lameck Aguta, Charles Tangus, and Sammy Lelei ran in the 15-man pack following Ndeti's loping lead. Occasionally Ethiopian Turbo Tumo ran nervously alongside. The old pro Andres Espinosa monitored the pack from the middle. Australian great hope Stephen Moneghetti

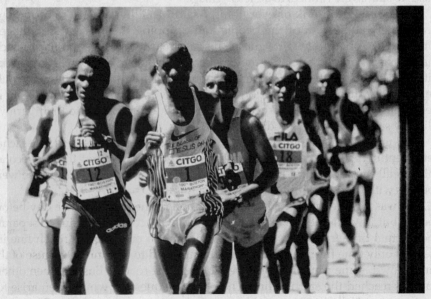

Comas Ndeti (#1), with "The Blood of Jesus on" written on his shirt, leads, with Mekonnen a step behind and Tanui buried in the pack. Photo by Victah Sailer.

lingered well back, playing the predator to pick off the inevitable causalities, but from the press truck no one could be seen racing on the road behind the lead pack.

The pace and hills ground off all but 9 men. Lameck Auguta, looking bright and alert, snatched his turn at the lead running side by side with Ndeti. The only non-Kenyan who remained in the pack was Mekonnen in all red with ETHIO-PIA across his chest. The Kenyans wore all white with the name of their team sponsor, FILA, an Italian shoe and sports apparel maker, or their other sponsor Nike's Swoosh. A headwind came up in the second half of the race. The Kenyan "coach," Dr. Gabriel Rosa, closely monitored the race. By Lake Street at the bottom of the hills near Boston College, Tanui at last made his presence known. He burst into the lead with a Blitzkrieg surge, ripping the pack to pieces by swooping around the turn down Chestnut Hill Ave to Beacon Street at Cleveland Circle and leaving all but two men drifting behind like a trail of spent shavings. Lameck Aguta and Ezikiel Bitok stuck to Tanui. Ndeti ran behind and out of the picture as Tanui's assault put 20 meters on the rest. Soon the pace discarded Aguta as Tanui continued alone. Ndeti had closed in other years with a surge. He settled back into the chase pack to rest. Bitok, who had looked to have given up the chase, suddenly surged up to join Tanui. Aguta remained the third Kenyan. Ndeti would have to dig deep to at least make the Kenyan Olympic team.

With a mile to go, the crowds in Kenmore Square dangerously thickened with the release of Boston Red Sox baseball fans from Fenway Park. They instantly became screaming marathon fans. Winning the race would not be possible for Ndeti without an unlikely collapse of Tanui and Bitok, but a top three among Kenyans would still be possible. That would mean finishing third. Aguta threatened to keep his third place. Only by 40 kilometers did Tanui pull away from Bitok for a small victory margin. Ndeti might have wished that he had held back from his early boasting pace. Ndeti used all of his speed and endurance to charge back past Aguta to his place on the Kenyan Olympic team. Tanui crossed the finish line with his index finger in the air: #1. Bitok used his index finger to stop his wrist watch.

Agent Mark Wetmore had this to say about his client's performance: "I think the headwind was more significant than he thought. His idea was to go out there and make them beat him. And he did. I thought he ran very bravely. Everyone is going to say he lost the race but that's not giving Moses the respect he deserves."

After the race Ndeti said, "I thought the pace was alright. I was taking the lead and to me the pace was OK. I'm not disappointed. Losing was not a shock. I am the third guy to win this race three times in a row and I still hold the course record." Ndeti planned to come back to win a fourth time. And so passed the biggest marathon the world had seen. The planning and execution of the race passed almost free of flaws.

Race director Guy Morse, a man of detail, generosity, and precision, said, "I'm unbelievably pleased with the overall way the event unfolded. The challenges were considerable and the complexities enormous. The organizing bodies and the town of Hopkinton really rose to the occasion."

Marathon fans and organizers immediately wondered what could possibly improve on this 100th running. The racers, however, did not wonder. Within a week they began preparations to come back.

1996 Men's Results

1. Moses Tanui, KEN	2:09:15	
2. Ezequiel Bitok, KEN	2:09:26	
3. Cosmas Ndeti, KEN	2:09:51	
4. Lameck Aguta, KEN	2:10:03	
5. Sammy Lelei, KEN	2:10:09	
6. Abebe Mekonnen, ETH	2:10:21	
7. Charles Tangus, KEN	2:10:28	
8. Paul Yego, KEN	2:10:49	
9. Carlos Grisales, COL	2:11:17	
10. Stephen Moneghetti, AUS	2:11:17	
11. Luis Dos Santos, BRA	2:11:48	
12. Gilbert Rutto, KEN	2:12:28	
13. Andres Espinosa, MEX	2:13:04	
14. Sammy Maritim, KEN	2:13:13	
15. Jan Huruk, POL	2:13:13	
16. Joao Lopes, POR	2:13:15	
17. Simon Lopuyet, KEN	2:14:33	
18. Eric Kimaiyo, KEN	2:14:37	
19. Andre Luis Ramos, BRA	2:14:50	
20. Turbo Tumo, ETH	2:14:59	
21. Salvatore Bettiol, ITA	2:14:59	
22. Shin Nakashima, JPN	2:15:28	
23. Jacinto Lopez, COL	2:16:54	
24. Simon Peter, TAN	2:16:56	
25. Patrick Muturi, KEN	2:17:43	
26. Asaf Bimron, ISL	2:17:58	
27. Abderazzak Haki, MAR	2:18:15	
28. Dov Kremer, ISR	2:18:31	
29. Joseph Kamau, KEN	2:18:46	

30. Kevin Collins, NY	2:18:54	
31. Herbert Steffny, GER	2:19:33, First 40+	
32. Juriy Mikhaliov, RUS	2:19:50	
33. Romas Sausaitis, LIT	2:20:11	
34. Naasi Gwagwe, TAN	2:20:22	
35. Osmiro, Silva, BRA	2:20:35	
36. Artemio Navarro, MEX	2:20:39	
37. Heiko Schinkitz, GER	2:20:50	
38. Alfredo Norvello, ITA	2:20:54	
39. Risto Ulmala, FIN	2:20:56	
40. El Hadi Moumou, FRA	2:21:07	
56. Glen Guillemette, USA	2:25:13	
58. Rachid Tbahi, MAR	2:25:18	
87. Masahiro Sato, JPN	2:30:00	
183. Paul Gompers, USA	2:35:43	
243. Eamon Coghlan, IRL	2:37:47	
1155. Jack Fultz, USA	2:52:50	
1207. Bill Rodgers, USA	2:53:23	
1866. Neil Cusack, IRL	2:58:28	
2124. Bruce McLaren, USA	3:00:00	
2859. Keizo Yamada, JPN	3:05:27	
4283. Ron Hill, GBR	3:13:13	
7991. Steve Flanagan, MA	3:29:19	
8362. Scott Samuelson, ME	3:30:43	
9453. Darrin Messina, USA	3:30:25	
15664. Joseph Franco, USA	4:00:00	
21613. Amby Burfoot, USA	4:38:31	
27371. Robert Crowther, USA	7:37:51	
last recorded finisher		

Men's Winning Teams

1.   Central Park Track Club, NY, 7:45:15
2.   West Side Runners, 7:47:12
3.   Greater Lowell, MA, 7:47:44
4.   Chico TC, CA, 7:48:33
5.   Boston Athletic Association, 7:48:37
6.   New York Harriers, 7:52:48
7.   Whirlaway Racing Team, MA, 7:53:45

"I had some problems . . ."

First Lady Pippig Is a Prohibitive
Favorite to Win Third Straight

For the past six months, what she'd been avoiding were finish lines. Pippig hadn't raced since her victory in the Berlin Marathon the previous fall. Despite her fine performance, she had a sore foot. For a month she had rested and run little. She underwent lots of physical therapy. Without the required travel and interruption of races, she could concentrate on her training and nutrition. She said she had had some difficulties with digestion but had not shared that information with the press on race weekend. In January, she settled into Boulder to train for her third Boston win. At last the foot felt fine.

Last year Uta Pippig and her boyfriend/coach Dieter Hogen left Boston hinting at secrets of preparation, diet, and training that might be revealed in the future. But nothing reveals secrets like performance. Running is a sport with few secrets. Hogen had concluded that she might be her own worst enemy by training too hard and ignoring the signs that normal people hear that tell them to back off, to rest, to recover. "I fear that she will run to death," said Hogen. Pippig had been pressured by herself and by expectations to repeat her three victories—two in Berlin, one in New York—and now with the press and public looking for a fourth win in the biggest of all marathons, Boston.

Her agent, Tom Ratcliffe, also served as a comforting and congenial host for her, Hogen, and other runner/friends who were Ratcliffe's clients. She had no real cause for nervousness, something was wrong . . . To compound the compounded, it was an Olympic year and she wanted to run, and win for Germany. Yes, it's stress, but stress that was not making her body stronger. Fame may be counter to the solitude an endurance athlete needs to prepare.

After her 1995 victory President Bill Clinton had invited Pippig to Washington for a run along the Potomac. She ran on one side of the president, and men's Boston winner Cosmas Ndeti ran on the other. The president wore a big, white T-shirt. She greeted him playfully, "Good morning, Mr. President." He replied while running, "Good morning, Uta, and if you are not going to sweat could you at least breath."

This year seeking some solitude, Pippig sequestered herself. She did not meet and greet the public and friendly reporters. She took her meals in her room. She stayed out of sight of the press and the pre-race ceremonies. She did not attend the traditional press event to accept her competitor's racing bib #1. She did not wave her index finger in the air promising victory.

She told *Boston Globe* reporter Barbara Huebner, "Maybe it's also how long can you stay on this level, how many more years," said Pippig. "It's more a question to yourself. I don't see an end. The training is good and I feel focused. The nice thing is you don't know what will happen in one year. Other people maybe don't like it, but I like it very much. I try to run even faster in the next year. We have some ideas in training. My body I think, in the end, is a good machine."

But during the race this good machine felt gut pains or cramps. Something was wrong. This was too early for the pain of fatigue. This was the pain of disease.

Madina Biktagirova of Belarus felt no disease. She had placed third last year and wanted to win. Biktagirova competed in the Barcelona Olympics in 1992 competing for the Unified Olympic team. She placed 4th, but after the race, she tested positive for norephedrine and became the first Olympic marathoner disqualified for failing a drug test. The drug is common in over-the-counter cough and cold preparations. To Pippig, Biktagirova posed serious competition. But there were others. Thirty-one-year-old Nobuko Fujimura of Japan had run a marathon in 2:26:09, Alla Jiliaeva of Russia had run 2:27:38. Of course Franziska Moser of Switzerland had finished 4th last year in 2:29:35 when she raced the leaders and wanted to be the winner of the 100th Boston Marathon. They passed 10k in 33:22 with front-running American Kim Jones wearing a peloton yellow Nike outfit in charge. No one seemed to notice tiny Tegla Loroupe a brief 12 seconds back until Pippig took a quick glance back and held it for a few strides to be sure that she had identified Loroupe in the running crowd. She had been dangling furtively at the back of the pack. Pippig saw a danger running there.

Tegla Loroupe was a 22-year-old postal office auditor from Kenya.

In her Boston Marathon debut a year ago, Loroupe fought off a stomach virus that left her dehydrated. She staggered across the finish line in 2 hours, 33 minutes, 10 seconds. Last November, in defending her New York City Marathon win, she overcame her grief at the death of her 33-year-old sister, Albina, from unknown causes a few days before the race. She won the NYC Marathon for the second time but in 2:28:06. Her personal best was 2:27:37 in NYC in 1994.

After the NYC win Loroupe said about her sister, "She was an inspiration to me, she gave me a lot of advice. It gave me a lot of courage to go through the pain. The situation I had last year was terrible."

Loroupe grew up in Kenya to the far west of the Rift Valley in the isolated, rural West Pokot district. It is not an area rich in runners like Kikuyu, Kamba, Kisii, Kalenjin, or Nandi. The dialect is not easily understood by Nandi so has led to some unease between the tribes. But unease was greatest within Loroupe's family when her father had initial doubts about her running. She started running in school and the usual paternal questions rose about a career as a runner. She ran to school and home and ran races. Her mother and sister supported her running ambitions. She got a job at age 18 in the post office. Her first invitation to race in Europe came via her post office job connections. She advanced rapidly in Europe as she learned more about racing and training. Painfully polite, quiet, and small, belied her stern intention to find her own way to excellence. She learned from her past Boston Race. She came prepared.

Michael Vega wrote in the *Boston Globe*, "But that was last year. And none may ever be as turbulent for Loroupe. Tomorrow, when the No. 5-ranked women's marathoner by *Track and Field News* toes the line in Hopkinton for the 100th running of the Boston Marathon, Loroupe will pose a threat to end Uta Pippig's reign as champion."

Allia Jiliaeva of Kursk, Russia, led early running next to Kim Jones. Pippig and several other women contenders hid behind them and the many men running at the same pace. (The separate women's start would be some years in the future, but now men and women started together.)

Pippig had serious competitors all around her, but the biggest threat chewed at her from inside her own digestive tract. Sharp pains jabbed her with every striding jostle. She felt gurgling and feared the need to stop or have an unsightly accident while under the lens of press cameras. By 20k in 1:08:20 not much had changed internally nor externally. She did not know at the time that she suffered from ischemic colitis, where a lack of blood to parts of the colon causes rupture and bleeding. No one had any inkling that she had ischemic colitis. The condition can lead to tissue death and perforation of the colon and peritonitis when the contents of the colon leak into the abdominal cavity, initiating rampant infection, and can be life-threatening.

Kim Jones had her own health issues. She has asthma so cannot start quickly but must build into the race. She had a point to prove in this race, since it was an Olympic year and she was forced to drop out of the U.S. Olympic Trials. This was her Olympic marathon. Nobuko Fujimura ran in that bunch but with her short stature was hard to see in the big scrum of running men. At around 8 miles she took the lead as if to test the competition to see who was willing to go with her.

In Natick, Pippig reached back, apparently to her hamstring, feeling for something. She was checking to see if she was having an unsightly accident. She seemed to be trying not to push the pace or encourage anyone of the other six nearby women to do so.

Biktagirova, Fujimura, and Kenyan Salina Chirchir ran together, with Pippig 25 meters behind. By the half marathon in 1:11:58, Loroupe and Pippig had joined Biktagirova and Fujimura in the lead. Then on the downhill into Newton Lower Falls Pippig took the lead and looked to be storming alone to another victory, pushing up over Route 128 in advance of the hills. No one could see what she felt inside. She kept hoping the feelings would just go away. But Tegla Loroupe responded. Loroupe took the lead going up the Newton Hills. But at an aid station she missed her designated water bottle and went back a step for it. Pippig caught up. The invited marathoners send their own specially marked bottles to each of the aid stations. These bottles are kept in a chain of custody so an athlete cannot receive unexpected aid or performance-decreasing substances from strangers along the road. An athlete could inadvertently receive a substance that would cause a positive post-race drugs test. Or be sabotaged. Loroupe returned to stretching out her lead.

The 22-year-old Loroupe, slight and seeming impervious to gravity, leaped up the Newton Hills on her own apparent parade to victory. Pippig faded back to stew in her own intestinal turmoil. Loroupe had 30 seconds at the crest of the hill. Pippig thought she could not catch Loroupe. "They told me that I was not too far behind and to 'go' because I could catch her," Pippig said later. "I thought I could not catch Tegla. She was too far away." Oddly, the Kenyan lives and trains in Germany and the German lives and trains in the States.

At a water station Loroupe looked unbeatable, but she again overran the spot where her designated drink sat. She twisted around awkwardly to reach for it. She missed. The stretch wrenched her hip, slowing her pace by a minute per mile.

Pippig ran from 30 to 35 kilometers in 18:30 while Loroupe ran only 18:43. Only then Pippig saw the possibility.

Loroupe began to limp. Pippig began to push. In her mind Pippig had to separate the discomfort of athletic effort from the non-athletic demons eating away at her innards. Loroupe held a big lead but kept looking over her shoulder. She knew how she slowed and knew that the race might be up to whomever ran in second. She could not at first see.

Observers saw that Pippig would catch Loroupe in Kenmore Square at mile 25 after Loroupe seemed barely able to overcome the slight hill on the bridge over the Mass Pike before Kenmore Square. She reached for needed water and got it this time and slowed to drink it. It would not help. Pippig, now energized, came on. Pippig too reached for her water bottle and drank it but without slowing and threw it hard away and bore down on Loroup. It was an aggressive move. Loroup took a long and hopeless look at closing Pippig. Pippig sprinted past. She dumped a cup of water on her head. She pushed hard, not wanting to relax and assume Loroupe was in fact as bad off as she looked. Pippig ran her final mile in 5:40 while Loroupe had left everything on her gravity-defying sprint up the Newton Hills and had energy left for only a 6:50 stagger to the finish. Pippig faced another dichotomy.

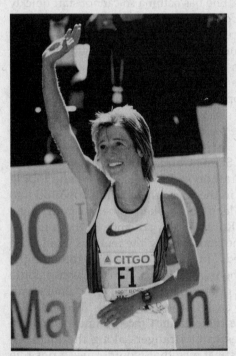

Uta Pippig, wrapped safely in a blanket, waves with the relief of victory. Photo by Victah Sailer.

She felt the joy of victory, the pain in her belly, and the dribble of diarrhea and blood down her leg before spectators and cameras in the biggest marathon in history. Only in the last minutes had she dared to think she had the race won. She replaced her grimace with a brief incredulous toothy smile, then returned to the grimace and the final thrust to get the race done and the pain to stop.

Photos of her approach to the finish would appear on the internet under the title of most disgusting running photos. She beamed a big smile as she broke the finish banner. At the line she received a blanket that she wrapped around her waist to conceal her embarrassing leakage. She accepted the laurel wreath and medal but kept a hand on the blanket as the German national anthem played.

"I had some problems with my period. I didn't expect it would become this worse. After 4 miles, I was thinking several times to drop out because it hurt so much. But in the end, I won."

After winning Pippig wanted to party, but the little problems were big problems. Medical officials confined her to the hospital for observation and treatment for exhaustion and dehydration. She spent three days in the hospital. No party.

The race, the 100th running party, the celebration of the towns and cities along the way, and the relief that all went well when so much could have gone wrong told everyone that the best was yet to come. Immediately the winners and near winners, those who set personal bests, and those who had setbacks, began to plot their returns to Boston.

1996 Women's Results:

1. Uta Pippig, GER	2:27:12	19. Eiko Yamazaki, JPN — 2:38:52
2. Tegla Loroupe, KEN	2:28:37	20. Ingrid Kristiansen, NOR — 2:39:00
3. Nobuko Fujimura, JAP	2:29:24	21. Emma Scaunich, ITA — 2:39:14
4. Sonja Krolik, GER	2:29:24	22. Taeko Terauchi, JPN — 2:40:33
5. Larisa Zouzko, RUS	2:31:06	23. Lorraine Hochella, USA — 2:41:38
6. Franziska Rochat-Moser, SUE	2:31:33	24. Mieke Hombergen, NE — 2:41:55
7. Madina Biktagirova, BLS	3:31:38	25. Sharon Stubler, USA — 2:42:35
8. Lorraine Moller, NZL	2:32:02,	26. Terumi Hatazawa, JPN — 2:43:20
	First 40+	27. Honor Fetherston, USA — 2:44:36
9. Alla Jiliaeva, RUS	2:32:32	33. Christa Vahlensiech, GER — 2:48:20
10. Valentina Enaki, MOL	2:33:58	76. Akiko Kawano, JPN — 3:00:06
11. Marcia Barloch, BRA	2:34:27	106. Jacqueline Gareau, CAN — 3:04:46
12. Salina Chirchir, KEN	2:34:33	?? Charlotte Teske, GER — 3:17:01
13. Solange Cordeiro, BRA	2:34:51	463. Margaret Beardslee, AUS — 3:30:07
14. Stefanija Statkuviene, LIT	2:36:42	1129. Gayle Barron, USA — 3:46:35
15. Lizanne Bussieres, CAN	2:36:55	2310. Elda Caraco, USA — 4:00:01
16. Sissel Grottenberg, NOR	2:37:28	7801. Nina Kuscsik, USA — 5:35:47
17. Stella Castro, COL	2:38:00	8172. Roberta Gibb, USA — 6:02:24
18. Ai Sugihara, JPN	2:38:50	8497. Alison Burleigh, USA — 8:01:05

Women's Winning Teams

1. Forerunners, FL, 8:54:55
2. Northwest Club Runners, 8:59:58
3. Boston Athletic Association, 9:28:11
4. Cambridge Sports Union, MA, 9:44:35
5. Impala Racing Team, CA, 9:47:05
6. Cape Cod AC, MA, 9:56:47

Cosmas vs. Moses?

MONDAY, APRIL 21, 1997

Kenyan Is Favorite

The most widely observed comet of the 20th century, the Comet Hale-Bopp, looped closest to Earth on March 22. Ezequiel Bitok, who "suffered" to place second to Tanui last year, came back to Boston to make everyone else suffer so he could take over. Before the race, Moses Tanui told about training for two weeks in the rain at home in Kenya and that he chose to try to race 10,000m in the Olympics instead of the marathon, but he did not make it through the Kenyan Olympic Trials to make the team to go to Atlanta. Later in the year he had dropped out of the NYC Marathon. He did not talk boastfully about defending his title as had Cosmas Ndeti the previous year. But Tanui is quiet by nature and had by no means given up on winning the Boston Marathon. Setbacks may be the thing that define a champion competitor. When asked about his race plan he said, "I don't want to say. I have to wait for that day. I know there will be plenty of people pushing."

At pre-race press events our colleagues of the fourth estate tried to provoke a verbal fight between Tanui and Ndeti. Tanui smiles often but says little. When he saw training partner Eric Kimaiyo run 2:08:08 in London and finish 4th he told Boston Globe reporter Joe Concannon, "It gives me more motivation, because I know how we were trained together, and this gives me the feeling I am ready to run. In training sometimes you cannot tell, but I feel I also can run well after training very hard with him. Where we train are a lot of hills, the same course as Boston." Tanui and Kimaiyo spent the last several months running hard, hilly weekly 38k runs in Kenya. Tanui had prepared well, maybe too well, but did not want to announce a race strategy. "It's very important to run the best time—to win, but to run the best time," said Tanui. "Winning is also good, but the best thing is to run the best time. The only problem I have now is I have a little bronchitis."

All the reporters wanted to hear Tanui's plan. They wanted to hear him say that he came to Boston to beat Ndeti again.

They asked him again: your game plan?

"I don't want to say. I learned what I need to do in the race. Now if I'm in that situation, I know what I want to do. But in athletics there is no way you have a favorite. Everybody runs on the course. I will try my best."

Reporters wanted Ndeti to thump his chest and supply them with braggadocio copy. But Ndeti was oddly reticent.

Kenyan Joseph Kamau had won the Bobby Crim 10 Miler in a course-record 45:43 which is the sort of thing Greg Meyer did before he won at Boston in

1983. A couple of Mexicans, Dionicio Ceron and German Silva, came to Boston with their own ideas. Marathon watchers thought Sammy Lelei, who had run 2:07:02, was the one to watch. A couple of Americans came to do more than watch. Mark Plaatjes and Keith Brantly also planned to upset the Kenyan apple (mango) cart.

True to his ambition and talent, Plaatjes led a pack of 50 men through 5k in 15:41 along with Mexican Isidro Rico. The first downhill mile had gone in a gentile 5:01. Under clear skies and a start temperature of 47°F that would reach upper 50s by race end, and with a constant headwind of 5–10 mph, fast times did not seem likely. Everyone still bunched together at 10k in 31:23. They seemed to all be trying to hide behind each other. Through the half marathon in 1:06:11, Ndeti and Tanui seemed to have eyes only for each other. Joseph Kamau and Ceron sometimes braved the wind to lead the gang.

Lameck Aguta seemed merely another pack filler. But he came with a prophecy. When a youthful Lameck Aguta first met the 1988 and 1991 Boston Marathon winner, Ibrahim Hussein, he heard the prophecy from the prophet. Aguta said, "We ran together with him one day in Boston and he told me, 'You look like you'll be a very good runner.' And he told me, 'One day you'll win.'" Aguta placed 21st in 1993 and 14th in 1995 and had finished 4th in his two previous Bostons, so he came armed with the necessary experience and persistence. Most importantly, perhaps more so than prophecy, he had the necessary recent training. It began to appear that Ndeti and Tanui did not.

"The pace was too slow," said Aguta, a Kisii raised on a farm in the wild west of Kenya. "It helped me a lot. I didn't want to push. I pushed with Ndeti last year from the beginning, and I paid the price. I knew if I was going to push I would push from behind and then push at the end. I knew there would be a push because all the guys were very strong at that point." Aguta spoke clearly and intelligently.

The Mexicans came determined to win Boston for the first time, and they raced to unseat the Kenyans. "The plan was to stay together in a group," said Ceron. "I never like to look at the clock, but the race was slow. I don't know why. I only tried to win this race. I was thinking all the time of a victory, but the pace was slow and you could not do too much after a slow half. All the time, I push to the end of the race."

Silva, who gained fame at the 1994 NYC Marathon for winning the race after making a wrong turn off the course near the finish, fell in Ashland after a water-stop tangle with Joshua Kimaiyo. But both sprung up and raced on.

"Nobody knew who was working," said Silva. "It was one of the strongest and most competitive races I have been in. I wasn't tired, but the course was tough and my legs are gone." Lameck Aguta looked the best of all.

Ten kilometers passed in 31:23 bunched together. So slow they were that master's runner Martin Modragon from Mexico led the bunch.

Kamau and Ceron led through the half marathon in 1:06:11.

The rest of the pack eyed Tanui and Ndeti as they eyed each other. By 25k, only 5 remained. Ndeti was not one of them.

Ndeti later said he had contracted malaria in February and missed training, "I've run this course four times under 2:10," said Ndeti. "My training didn't go well the last two months. I tried my best the last six weeks. I said, 'I must finish and see what position I finish.'"

Brantly stopped at 15k and and Plaatjes at halfway.

Ceron and Kamau pushed, and Aguta, Tanui, and Silva followed. Aguta still looked good and was waiting.

Agent Kim McDonald first saw Lameck Aguta in 1993 when he showed up a 5k time trial in Nairobi, Kenya. Lots of young eager runners show up for these trials. They hear via the bush telegraph and somehow, all before everyone in Africa acquired cellphones, these hopeful young men show up. Aguta had blasted out in 4:26 for the first mile and of course died, figuratively. McDonald told him to train for two months and come back. He did and this time ran a little slower at the start and didn't die and ran about 14 minutes flat. Now he trains with the best of partners and coaching.

In 1997, Aguta trained with the world's top 3000m and 5000m runner, Daniel Komen, and elite steeplechaser Moses Kiptanui under Dieter Hogen's coaching. He looked to be well on the way to a successful professional running career.

"I've been training hard to come here to win," said Aguta.

Coach Hogen said to wait until 40k and make one big push. That mark is where Beacon Street rises over the Mass Pike. Aguta threw down his big one. No one could respond. Aguta ran on alone with Kamau pushing as hard as he could, but on the Hereford Street and Bolyston, Aguta stayed ahead to win. He expected his life to change.

His wife, Regina, was expecting their third child in July. They already had twin sons (Aguta himself was a twin), so he had good reason to train hard to win and provide for his family. First place would win $75,000. "I've been training for the last 5k. I needed more strength. Today, when I reached 5k [to go], I was feeling strong. I knew I had the speed from [Komen and Kiptanui]. We'd been training together, and at the end I was catching them. I was waiting for anything to happen in the last mile, but I knew in the last 5k I could go with them with my speed."

Aguta continued his story:

"I saw all of us together with 7k to go. I tried to see who was looking better. When I was watching the videos of the times I've been coming to Boston, my coach told me, 'There's no way they can go with you with your speed.' He told me, 'There's nobody who can catch you.' I give the credit to my coach. He told me, 'Don't push from the 5k because all the guys are ready for you.'"

The coach and Hussein's prophecy proved to be right. Again Dieter Hogen had coached a Boston Marathon winner. Aguta left Boston with his $75,000 in first place prize money. That is an enormously life-changing amount of money for rural Kisii where he grew up with his twin brother, Shem. But the good life that such large winnings promised would not stay.

Things looked very good in July 1997 as Aguta rode from Nairobi to the Western Highlands with Shem. They carried a briefcase with $10,000 in cash because the Kenyan banking system did not work well. The young driver didn't know the road and missed a turn. The car ran off the road and stuck. The accident did not hurt him, his brother, or the driver seriously, but it had been observed. Often in Kenya victims of automobile accidents become opportunities for thieves.

When the opportunists realized they had a famous, rich person in their control, they wanted money. Aguta did not hand it over readily. The robbers hit him in the head. "They beat me so I almost died." Aguta had to be airlifted to Nairobi Hospital.

After that attack, he said that he "talked nonsense" due to his injuries. His agent/manager Kim McDonald arranged for him to be transferred to a London hospital that specialized in the re-education of the motor functions damaged in the attack. Aguta wanted to race again. He wanted to come back to Boston. He wanted back his life as an athlete.

1997 Men's Results:

1. Lameck Aguta, KEN	2:10:34	
2. Joseph Kamau, KEN	2:10:46	
3. Dionicio Ceron, MEX	2:10:59	
4. German Silva, MEX	2:11:21	
5. Moses Tanui, KEN	2:11:38	
6. Gilbert Rutto, KEN	2:12:30	
7. Jimmy Mundi, KEN	2:12:49	
8. Andre Ramos, BRA	2:13:10	
9. Jose Luis Molina, CRC	2:13:34	
10. Tesfaye Bekele, ETH	2:14:02	
11. Nelson Ndareva, KEN	2:14:12	
12. Charles Tangus, KEN	2:14:34	
13. Ezequiel Bitok, KEN	2:14:57	
14. Joshua Kimaiya, KEN	2:15:29	
15. Andres Espinosa, MEX	2:16:19	
16. Thabiso Moqhali, LES	2:16:32	
17. Sammy Lelei, KEN	2:17:20	
18. Belay Wolashe, ETH	2:18:13	
19. Daniel Gonzales, CA	2:18:30	
20. Dominique Chauvelier, FRA	2:19:10, First 40+	
21. Paul Yego, KEN	2:19:16	
22. Antoni Niemczak, POL	2:21:43	
23. Johann Hopfner, GER	2:21:48	
24. Joseph McVeigh, NJ	2:22:01	
25. Sergei Karasyev, RUS	2:22:16	
26. Martin Mondragon, MEX	2:22:19	
27. Cosmas Ndeti, KEN	2:22:56	
28. Doug Kurtis, MI	2:23:10	
29. Sammy Bitok, KEN	2:23:45	
30. Bedaso Turbe, ETH	2:24:04	
31. Romas Sausaitis, LIT	2:24:56	
32. Dick Hooper, IRL	2:25:03	
43. Budd Coates, PA	2:30:03	
746. George Holland, MA	3:00:00	
3196. Bruce Sparfuen, RI	3:30:00	
3450. Keizo Yamada, JPN	3:33:14	
5056. Gerald Lee, CO	4:00:01	
6416. Eddie Schmidt, LA	5:08:00	

Men's Team Winners:

1. Boston Athletic Association, 'D,' 7:46:36
2. Berlin Oldies, 2:51:06
3. Atlanta Track Club, 8:02:38
4. Central Park Track Club, 8:06:37
5. Tri-Athletics, 'A,' 8:06:40
6. Berwick Ramblers, 8:11:01
7. Central Florida, 8:13:21
8. St. Louis Track Club, 8:15:09
9. Summitt AC, 8:19:30
10. Greater Boston Track Club, 8:23:42

Uta Four in a Row?

Formidable Field Faces Three-Time Champ

Uta Pippig had had a tough year. First she had to deal with her stomach problems. But then she had to train. People expected her to perform. She expected herself to perform. She simply had to represent Germany in the Olympics in Atlanta. She developed lower back problems. She got a pelvic stress fracture. She failed to finish the Olympic Marathon. But Boston kept pulling her back.

Considering the bad last year she had had and the ever-present possibility that a marathon can be full of surprises, she and her coach, Dieter Hogen, decided on a conservative strategy—linger at the back of the herd like a hungry wolf and wait to pick off the stragglers, one by one. She had come from behind last year to win. Stranger things have happened. The logic is impeccable: if you don't show up you can't run a bad race . . . but you can't win either. Of course appearance money might have had something to do with the decision too. She will get paid, as a previous winner, by just showing up and making a serious shot at competing. Who knows? It might work. She would not be able to continue running well forever. But maybe, maybe this year would be okay.

American women may be factors this year. Kim Jones, a 38-year-old veteran of the course, this year brings speed along with experience. She recently placed third in the 15k River Run in Jacksonville, Florida, in 50:36, only 23 seconds behind winner Lynn Jennings. Olga Appell, a 10,000m Olympian last summer, reportedly was in top shape; Kristy Johnston, native of Coos Bay, Oregon, who won Chicago in 1994 with a 2:31:34; and Debbie Kilpatrick who had finished 6th in the 1996 Olympic Trials.

Elana Meyer, South African silver medalist at 10,000m in the 1992 Olympic Games, was coming off a world-record half marathon performance. She had raced the Boston course twice, finishing 3rd in 1994 and 2nd in 1995. She expected that the combination of her 10,000m speed and experience would carry her to the win.

Olympic gold medalist Fatuma Roba was the foremost marathoner in the world. She beat a loaded field to win Olympic gold for Ethiopia in Atlanta. She beat Pippig. But Roba had not raced at Boston before. She said, "I am ready enough to win the race, and I am sure I will win." She was 26 years old. Joan Benoit Samuelson said, "They're eyeing Uta's record, and I think they're going to go for it." She called this the strongest group of women assembled since the Chicago Marathon in 1985, when Portugal's Rosa Mota and Norway's Ingrid Kristiansen helped push Samuelson to a 2:21:21 win. That time was still the American record, and second-fastest women's marathon ever. But first the weather and tactics had to cooperate.

Derartu Tulu, running her first marathon anywhere, had beaten Meyer to win 10,000m gold in Barcelona and took second at the World Cross-Country Championships. Tulu, too, is from Ethiopia. Kenyan Tegla Loroupe decided to skip Boston in favor of Rotterdam's flat, fast course, which she won the day before Boston in 2:22:07, setting a mark to provoke the Boston field.

Toss in Japan's Junko Asari, with a personal best of 2:26:10; Delilah Asiago, a Kenyan 10k road racer making her wild card debut at 26.2 miles; and Colleen De Reuck, a South African looking for vengeance after a disappointing race here in 1994.

Boston weather is fickle: the sea breeze kicked in at the gun.

Roba did not preview the course, despite its hills and its complexity owing to deceptive early downhills.

"I begged her," said her agent Troy James, "I said, 'I don't want this to come down to whoops, I didn't know that turn was there.'"

The women went out slower than in the past, hunkered together against the wind. Ten kilometers passed in 34:29. They reached the halfway point in a large association: Roba, Meyer, and Junko Asari in 1:12:51. No course record seemed possible, nor did a time to match Rotterdam.

Roba led a slowly shrinking pack of up to 8 women—including Meyer, Asari, De Reuck, Pippig, Ethiopia's Derartu Tulu, Asiago, and Mexico's Maria Carmen Diaz—through 12 miles when she threw in a surge to drop anyone uncertain of her fitness. Meyer and Asari quickly made up the gap, with De Reuck and Pippig giving chase just behind, but none remained in view of the lead vehicle.

Pippig did what she could. She ran to the limit of her fitness. If those ahead of her ran out past the limit of their fitness, they would come back to her. If they did not, they would not come back to her. Winning the race moved out of Pippig's grasp.

But it was Roba who had a handle on things. "I think she was in charge a big part of the race," said Meyer.

By the 15-mile mark, De Reuck and Pippig were about 50 yards behind the leaders, but by mile 16, De Reuck had caught the lead pack, while Asari began to slip back. At the firehouse turn onto Commonwealth Avenue in Newton, it was Roba, Meyer, and De Reuck, with Pippig and Asari 80 yards behind. Three women raced through the Newton hills. Roba, who had been a stride or two ahead for most of the race, relinquished the lead for the second time to rest—the first had been heading up the hill over Route 128 toward Newton-Wellesley Hospital—and joked later that she was merely being polite.

"Up to that point I was leading all the while," she said, "but at that point I said, 'Let them have the chance.'"

In Newton, Ethiopian flags propagated. Several times jubilant fans ran along, waving them as if joining a conquering army massing to invade Boston proper.

"We thought that was going to be a factor," said Troy James. "There's a large Ethiopian community here, just like there was in Atlanta."

Nonetheless, the race unfolded as Roba had planned with James. Knowing of Meyer's superb speed at 10k, Roba did not want this to come down to a sprint from Kenmore Square.

"I just wanted her to break her [Meyer] beforehand," said James as he explained via translation his client's intention and execution to the press after the race.

Meyer planned to train harder and be back fitter so she would not be dropped and could kick to victory. Roba, of course, did not want that to happen.

1997 Women's Results:

1. Fatuma Roba, ETH	2:26:23	18. Josette Columb-Janin, FRA	2:40:53
2. Elana Meyer, RSA	2:27:09	19. Sissel Grotenberg, NOR	2:42:07
3. Colleen De Reuck, RSA	2:28:03	20. Lynn Clayton, AUS	2:43:31
4. Uta Pippig, GER	2:28:51	21. Shoko Sakaguchi, JPN	2:44:32
5. Derartu Tulu, ETH	2:30:28	22. Yoshiko Yamamoto, JPN	2:45:33
6. Junko Asari, JPN	2:31:12	23. Gillian Horovitz, GBR	2:46:32
7. Alla Jiliaeva, RUS	2:31:55	24. Mary Alico, FLA	2:47:44
8. Sonia Maccioni, ITA	2:31:59	25. Reiko Kawamorita, JPN	2:48:38
9. Kim Jones, WA	2:32:52	26. Delilah Asiago, KEN	2:48:57
10. Debbie Kilpatrick, OH	2:36:04	27. Mary-Ellen Kelley, SC	2:49:27
11. Maria Carmen Diaz, MEX	2:37:16	28. Mary Button, CA	2:49:47
12. Tamara Karlioukova, RUS	2:37:33	29. Cindy Glass, OH	2:49:54
13. Yukari Komatsu, JPN	2:37:44	30. Florinda Camayo Lapa, PER	2:54:12
14. Ida Mitten, CAN	2:39:27	49. Cathi Campbell, MA	3:00:33
15. Svetlana Vasileva, RUS	2:39:59	360. Maryclair Premo, VA	3:30:01
16. Maria Trujillo, CA	2:40:49	1454. Kim O'Callaghan, MA	4:00:00
17. Ludmila Petrova, RUS	2:40:52	2477. Margaret Long, NY	5:07:57

Women's Winning Teams:

1. Boston Athletic Association, 9:05:15
2. Forerunners, 9:22:18
3. DC Road Runners 'A,' 9:40:27
4. Boston Running Club 'A,' 9:56:32
5. Greater Lowell, RR, 9:59:13

Kenyan Invasion

MONDAY, APRIL 20, 1998

Tanui Back, but is He in Shape?

Pre-race stories in the Boston papers retold Aguta's story: "A year ago, Lameck Aguta was thanking God for finally, gloriously granting his wish to be first across the finish line of the hallowed Boston Marathon."

Aguta remembers nothing of the accident. If the large amount of cash—commonly carried for business in a country not known for checking accounts—was ever found, it has not been returned.

"It's a totally different culture," said Aguta's agent Kim McDonald. "Obviously it's a lot easier to go to a police station here and look at the documentation as to what happened."

What is known is that Aguta was in a coma for two weeks, unable to move, sustaining brain damage that left him with impaired coordination and no memory.

"I am OK," he said last week. "I hope one day I can run in a race."

Physically healed from his head wounds, Aguta was discharged at the end of July to a life he barely recognized. He had forgotten about the new baby, and insisted it was not his child. He would chat in the afternoon with fellow runner Godfrey Kiprotich about coming to his house that morning when they hadn't seen each other in weeks. He would go into town and forget the way home.

"The mind he had was just telling him to go, but not to come back," his wife explained.

"I was getting lost," Aguta said bluntly. For his family and friends, worry grew.

"His speech was slurred, he was very confused," said Tom Ratcliffe in Boston who worked with McDonald. Something had to be done.

In November, McDonald had Aguta flown to England for neurological tests. When he arrived in London, his balance was so impaired that he couldn't stand on one leg without falling over. It was quickly decided that he should remain for therapy to help him regain both his motor skills and his memory, so he moved in with Kenyans who regularly train in nearby Teddington.

Aguta stayed for six weeks, after his therapists, concerned about his apparent depression, thought his recovery would be speeded if he resumed training.

"We would try our best to keep him occupied, training with the other Kenyans, so he wouldn't have too much time to spend thinking about the past," said McDonald. "In his mind, he had everything and all of a sudden he thinks, *Am I ever going to run again?*" He had thoughts of Boston within a week of his first run in England. He was making great strides. After a Christmas reunion with his family, he spent another six weeks in England before returning to Kenya for good.

The Boston newspapers covered Aguta's story with sympathy and hope. The people of Boston always want their heroes to return. He tried to run again, managing a marathon in 2:34:04 in the White Rock Marathon in Texas in 2004, but he never again approached world-class fitness. Reports years later had him working as a janitor somewhere in the American South.

"To me, Boston is the best marathon in the world," said Dr. Gabrielle Rosa of Italy, whose clients include Boston favorite and centennial champion Moses Tanui of Kenya. "The winner is No. 1 in the world outside of the Olympic Games and the World Championships."

"Without a men's defending champion, I think it's wide open," said Toni Reavis, who planned to do color commentary on Boston's Channel 7 TV said. "You have the Ndetis, the Tanuis, the Cerons, the Silvas, who are proven warhorses. They all have something to prove again. They all want to show it's not over for them, and they can reconstruct themselves. Somebody is going to be able to come out of that group."

Reavis continued, "You have all these young studs on the other side of it, all on the rise. You have Chebet. Kagwe, Gomez, and others like Philip Taurus who have run high-quality races this year. They're free and wild, who have never been humbled by the distance, and absolutely free to go nuts. Then you have Kagwe, who wants to prove New York wasn't a fluke. Kamau was second in Boston last year. There's no one in between. You have all these people who are old and have something to prove or who are young and ready to roll."

USA Track & Field CEO Craig Masback said in the pre-race press room that he wants stipends and performance bonuses for American male and female runners who develop into world-class stars. Those runners would, in return, agree to compete in American races and engage in promotional activities and clinics. He has talked about a team concept in road racing where various countries can compete and score as units. To oversee all of this, Masback said he wants to hire a national long-distance administrator.

Kenyan runners on the roads of this country caused some race directors from Boulder to Jacksonville to Red Bank, New Jersey, to cut back prize money when the Kenyans enter the race in large numbers. They dominate, sponsors become irritated, and there are some races that present the prize money to only Americans.

David D'Alessandro, the president and COO of John Hancock, said he wasn't concerned. It's the federation's problem that it hasn't been stepping forth since the days of Bill Rodgers, Frank Shorter, Joan Benoit Samuelson, and Alberto Salazar. John Hancock hands over upward of $2 million a year to back the Boston Athletic Association's running of the Boston Marathon.

"The Americans are always complaining," said D'Alessandro to Boston reporters in comments before the race. "I've never heard a high-quality athlete say, 'I don't want to compete because there's no chance I can win.' I find it fascinating . . . There are a lot of American runners who want to compete. . . I think with the new head (Craig Masback) we're going to see the potential of a resurgence in this country. The colleges are the feeders. Let's say we put up $3 million, $5 million, $10 million for the resurgence of track and field . . . the problem is corporations can't do what a Federation can do in the middle. They can bring in the feeders, the colleges. You're talking about marketing the sport to sponsors and television."

The federation struck back. "I, as someone involved in leading the sport, need to be at the Boston Marathon and other events like that," said Masback. "It's going to take a lot of hard work to get where we want, where we need to be."

Such questions about Americans versus foreigners are not new to the Boston Marathon. One hundred years ago marathon fans complained of Canadians, then Native Americans, (okay, not really foreigners); then in the 1950s, the Finns and the Japanese. Now, it's the Africans. But the consideration of money and the business of marathon presentation is different. There is much more at stake than national pride.

Of course Tanui wanted to win again—so did Cosmas Ndeti, but it may be some law of nature that the more you have won, the less likely it is that you will win again. Eventually returns diminish. But Tanui had entangled himself in several new business ventures like publishing Kenya's first running magazine, *The Athlete*. With that inaugural issue he said, "…we can assure you we are here to stay. "That may be said for the Kenyans as a whole regarding the Boston Marathon. Tanui and a lot of fast Kenyans came to race—some of whom may likely challenge him. But he appeared sharp, having won the Toyko half marathon in January with a 1:00:24 and won again in Kyoto in March. He said he had had bronchitis last year and that is why he placed fourth. This year he had no such malady. At 10k, Joseph Chebet and Philip Tarus seemed to be setting the pace for Tanui, and Mexicans Gabino Apolanio, Margarito Xamora, and Jorge Marquez seemed to be servicing their compatriot, German Silva, to win. Twelve disciples of the marathon clumped together at the half in 1:02:44. Ndeti would drop out at 16 miles. This put an end to his top racing at Boston.

Thys, Ceron, Ramos, Gomez, Nderva, Ndirangu, Kimani, Tumo, and Kagwe ran fast. No gaps of mercy opened among them. Not a scrap of mercy for Tarus for setting the pace for 30k in 1:29:55. The service used him up. His name would not appear in the results.

Chebet took over pushing the pace. Kagwe pushed ahead at 35k, going 15:21 for the 5k. Still Gert Thys, from South Africa, and Chebet hung on as the savage pace ripped the pack apart. They ran close to Ndeti's course record.

Tanui had been hanging back sometimes as much as 14 seconds behind the leaders. He had not participated in pushing the pace. He seemed to gain ground on the uphills and flats only to lose it on the downhills. He said, "I can run on the flat and I can run uphill, but on the downhill they pulled away. I cannot run down hills." Four together raced through Cleveland Circle, including clever Tanui. After the race Tanui would say, "I was very confident during the first half of the race because I thought the pace was a little too fast, and I didn't think the leaders would last, but at 35k I was worried, and I thought, 'These people can run.'"

Chebet may have heard the thought and decided it was his time to break away. He took off wearing the same Fila-sponsored shirt as Tanui. Tanui responded with his own breakaway. But it did not work. Both were trained by Dr.

Gabriele Rosa in Italy with money from their sponsor—Fila, an Italian brand of sportswear founded in 1911. The support helps them benefit from the best training technology. They knew each other. Thys and Brazilian Andre Ramos went with Tanui. Mercy and relief were nowhere. They ran abreast down Beacon Street, no man yielding to another. Yet all felt the bone-crumbling fatigue of pushing and catching up. They ran miles 23, 24, 25, in 4:52, 4:53, and 5:05.

One block from the finish line Tanui gave Chebet a look. The look penetrated. Then Tanui kicked away. No mercy with even a block to go. Tanui said after the race, "By good luck, I still had some energy when I caught the pack, but I waited until 200 meters to test Chebet and see if he had the energy to run with me. But when I sprinted he could not respond . . ."

"I knew the winner would come from behind, because it hurt, " said Thys, who was provoked because perhaps he hadn't completed the race in his previous visit four years ago. "I tried to hold back, but I couldn't. If I did, I would run alone. I had to stick with the group. I feel Moses could win the race, because he came from behind and didn't use up too much. He didn't go too fast in the first half."

Chebet said, "I lost it with about 100 meters to go."

The race was worth $80,000 in prize money to Tanui; Kenyans have won the last eight Bostons, and since 1994, they have placed an astonishing number of runners in the top places.

Tanui, who is the unofficial mayor of his home city, Eldoret, met the official mayor of Boston when Thomas Menino placed the laurel wreath on his head at the finish line.

As the Swahili goes, "Mambu Baddu, meaning the best is yet to come."

1998 Men's Results:

1. **Moses Tanui, KEN**	**2:07:34**	
2. **Joseph Chebet, KEN**	**2:07:37**	
3. Gert Thys, RSA	2:07:52	
4. Andre Ramos, BRA	2:08:26	
5. John Kagwe, KEN	2:08:51	
6. German Silva, MEX	2:08:56	
7. Alejandro Gomez, ESP	2:12:34	
8. Turbo Tumo, ETH	2:13:06	
9. Jose Ramon-Rey, ESP	2:13:12	
10. Takayuki Inubushi, JPN	2:13:15	
11. Akinori Kuramata, JPN	2:13:53	
12. Margarito Zamora, MEX	2:14:05	
13. Peter Ndirangu, KEN	2:14:20	
14. David Buzza, GBR	2:14:59	
15. Andrey Kuznetsov, RUS	2:15:27, First 40+	
16. Belay Wolashe, ETH	2:16:42	
17. Joseph McVeigh, NJ	2:16:48	
18. Keith Anderson, GBR	2:17:08	
19. Kenichi Suzuki, JPN	2:17:16	
20. Nelson Ndereva, KEN	2:17:43	
21. Peter Koech, KEN	2:18:02	
22. Dominique Chauvelier, FRA	2:20:49	
23. Shun Yamanaka, JPN	2:20:59	
24. Budd Coates, PA	2:21:35	
25. Ruben Hinojosa, MEX	2:22:01	
26. Jim Hage, MD	2:22:44	
27. Joseph Himani, KEN	2:25:32	
28. Robert Morrison, NY	2:25:41	
29. Timothy Root, MA	2:26:47	
30. Naofumi Sasaki, JPN	2:26:55	
42. Jesse Darley, MA	2:29:50	
140. William Cockerell, GBR	2:39:52	
986. Jeff Garber, TX	2:59:59	
4177. **Amby Burfoot, PA**	**3:35:32**	
4419. **Keizo Yamada, JPN**	**3:38:50**	
5572. Stephen Spohn, MA	3:59:59	
7146. Kafina Martin, MA	6:09:04	

Men's Team Winners

1. New York Harriers, 7:40:45
2. London Ontario Flying Force, 2:45:35
3. Boston Running Club, 2:47:18
4. Whirlaway Running Club, MA, 7:48:00
5. Central Park Track Club, NY, 7:48:27
6. Boston Athletic Association, 7:50:10
7. Greater Boston Track Club, 7:57:21
8. Cumberland Valley, MD, 7:57:59
9. Gate City Striders, NH, 7:59:22
10. Warren Street, NY, 8:01:02

The Flags of Victory

MONDAY, APRIL 20, 1998

Roba Wants Win, Meyer Out

News of the Bill Clinton–Monica Lewinsky affair broke in January 1998. The scandal filled the news for months. Uta Pippig had an operation on her foot in October 1997. She had gone to New Zealand to recuperate. She could not race, but she came back to Boston to work with the fundraising arm of Dana-Farber cancer institute and to provide color commentary for the race with WBZ's Channel 4 TV sports announcers Bob Lobel, Frank Shorter, and Kathrine Switzer. "This is 'no excuse' weather," Channel 4's Frank Shorter said. Fatuma Roba, the Olympic gold medalist and last year's winner, came back to defend her title. She seemed to come with unfinished business. She knew that the world best was 2:20:47, set in Rotterdam on Sunday before this year's Boston by Tegla Loroupe of Kenya. Wouldn't it be sweet for Roba to break that record the day after it was set?

South African Elana Meyer came to Boston with a blue, burning intention sparked by having placed second, as she did in 1995 and '97. That steady flame aimed at Boston would not die. She had run a world-best half marathon on March 8 in Toyko with a 1:07:29. She had trained hard. Desire might burn, but reality is cruel. Lower back pain snuffed the fire. She said she ran a 30-minute trial in Boston to test the injury, then decided that the best decision was to withdraw.

"I had troubles in the back and trouble walking," said Meyer. "It's an extremely big disappointment, but there is always a chance of being injured in sport. I've been through a couple of bad injuries. I'll be back, and I'll be tougher."

The job looked easy for Roba to win again—no Meyer, no Pippig—but the fickle demon of endurance training, injury, haunted her too. For three weeks she said, "I felt a terrible pain in the right leg." She rested and did not feel the pain so she decided to start the race. Desire is a dangerous thing. Shortly after the start of the race she felt the pain again. Business may remain unfinished.

Many pre-race prognosticators picked South African Colleen De Reuck, who had finished third last year, as the one with the experience to capitalize on Roba's right leg pain. De Reuck came to Boston hot off a 52:16 run in the Cherry Blossom 10 Miler earlier in April.

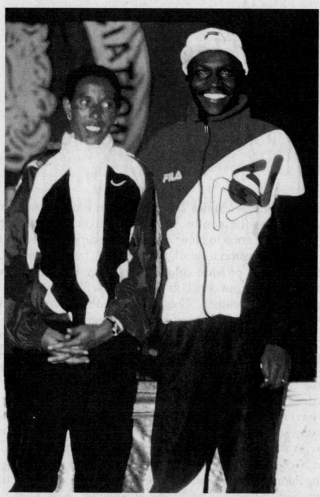

Fatuma Roba and Moses Tanui. Photo by Victah Sailer.

Through 5k in 16:48 the lead group consisted of Roba and De Reuck and Manuela Machado of Portugal, (2:27:42 PR) raced with the support of three-time Boston winner, her compatriot Rosa Mota, and palindromic Romanian Anuta Catuna (who had won the NYC marathon in 1996), and Irina Kazakova of France.

By 15k Kazakova and Catuna had dropped off and slowly Machado dropped back, leaving the two Africans alone to share water past 25k. Roba took the lead. "Actually, Fatuma didn't surge," said De Reuck. "I was just out of gas and started to fall back." De Reuck moved to a defensive strategy. "Once I realized that I couldn't win, I was thinking, *just protect second, second is still good*." Then passing out of Brookline Renata Paradowska, who had held back from the early racing, marched on past. "Oh, well, finishing in the top three is okay," revised De Reuck. But the marathon is oblivious to rationals. Catuna eased past. De Reuck re-revised, "All I was thinking after that was, *Just get home. Just finish the race*."

Roba ran past men who struggled, as throngs of spectators chanted her name. Ethiopians darted into the street, flags unfurled, to cheer the re-crowning of their gold medal marathon queen. The Ethiopian flag blossomed along the course. All 7,000 Ethiopians living in the Boston area seemed to have come with fluttering flags.

By mile 16, the only opponent Fatuma Roba hadn't left behind was the terrible pain in her right leg. She said she would have run three minutes faster but for the pain in her leg. She had set her sights on the world record that Tegla Loroupe had set the day before in Rotterdam.

1998 Women's Results:

1. **Fatuma Roba, ETH**	**2:23:21**	
	(27th overall)	
2. Renata Paradowska, POL	2:27:17	
3. Anuta Catuna, ROU	2:27:34	
4. Manuela Machado, POR	2:29:13	
5. Colleen De Reuck, RSA	2:29:43	
6. Irina Kazakova, FRA	2:30:44	
7. Jane Salumae, EST	2:31:20	
8. Hiroko Nomura, JPN	2:31:58	
9. Irina Timofeyeva, RUS	2:32:32	
10. Arica Buia, JPN	2:34:17	
11. Mary-Lynn Currier, MA	2:35:18	
12. Libbie Hickman, CO	2:35:37	
13. Fusai Okamoto, JPN	2:37:06	
14. Cindy Barber-Keeler, FL	2:39:49	
15. Yumiko Furuya, JPN	2:40:40	
16. Gillian Horovitz, GBR	2:41:15	
17. Alice Thurau, PA	2:41:58	
18. Marie Boyd, NM	2:42:26	
19. Irina Bondarchuk, RUS	2:42:44	
20. Maria Polyzou, GRE	2:42:53	
21. Alina Karwowski, BRA	2:44:59	
22. Jane Welzel, CO	2:45:44	
23. Shauna Whitmer, OR	2:45:50	
24. Mary Burns-Prine, CA	2:47:24	
25. Lynn Deninno, MA	2:49:20	
26. Mary Sweeney, GA	2:50:43	
27. Mary Button, CA,	2:51:25	
28. Cheryl Harper, UT	2:51:40	
29. Inglandini Gonzalez, FL	2:51:53	
30. Teresa Dejesus, FL	2:53:01	
49. Cheryl Simoni-Schultze, CT	3:00:10	
481. Adrienne Brooks, IL	3:30:03	
1819. Sandi Ludwa, NY	4:00:00	
3143. Lynn Buttoph, MA	6:13:14	

Women's Team Winners

1. Boston Athletic Association, 8:59:10
2. Sojourners, UT, 8:59:38
3. Greater Lowell Road Runners, 9:19:56
4. Forerunners, FL, 9:26:52
5. Tidewater Striders, VA, 9:29:51
6. Atlanta Track Club, GA, 9:39:43

The Last Race
of the 20th Century

MONDAY, APRIL 19, 1999

Patriots Day on Patriots Day

On April 19, in Kosovo, Serbian paramilitaries killed 20 Albanian men. They shot 11 in a vacant lot and killed 9 more in their homes. NATO forces moved into Kosovo. In Belgrade, black smoke filled the sky after NATO warplanes hit several plants. NATO officials said they had struck oil facilities and had devastated Yugoslavia's ability to refine crude oil.

The Battle in Boston would cause damage to egos and expectations—things that runners and reporters hold dear. When you finish 2nd in a marathon, does it make you crazy? The taste is there. Joseph Chebet could see Moses Tanui three seconds ahead last year. Was this year Chebet's turn after making pace for Tanui for all but the last 200 meters of the race last year? He felt he was due for victory. But would Tanui do the same thing to him again—a burst a half minute from the finish line? Or would some Boston debutante spoil the obvious succession?

Chebet finished 2nd too many times to maintain sanity. His 2nd-place finishes at both Boston and New York a year ago could plunge him into road-racing psychosis. Chebet did win his first two marathons, in Amsterdam in 1996 (2:10:58) and Turin in '97 (2:08:23), but was runner-up in his last three (he was also second to Kagwe in the 1997 NYC Marathon). Chebet won in Luxembourg's Route du Vin Half Marathon in 1997 in 1:00:53. His 2:07:37 in Boston last year might make him the pick this year. That time stands as the fourth-fastest time over the course. Almost winning may have pushed Chebet into a motivation crescendo. The reports came that he started his training for Boston two months ahead of schedule. Chebet sought a secret weapon. He consulted Bill Rodger's Greater Boston Track Club coach, Bill Squires. Billy Squires said with full confidence that he knew who would win and it would be Chebet. He picked up a piece of paper and wrote down the name "Joseph Chebet." He underlined it. "Chebet came to me on Saturday. He sought me out. He said, `I want the American coach to take me out on the course.'"

"I showed Joseph the 'move' spots and the 'pull' spots," Squires said, referring to the Newton Hills.

"He knew that the hill at Newton City Hall was the place to start and that after that he was going to own the real estate," declared Squires. "He knew he'd be in command by the 22-mile mark." *Boston Globe* reporter Bob Ryan listened to Squires's predictions and mentoring. How did Squires know? Or did he?

John Kagwe, from Kenya, ran 5th last year in 2:08:51, with recent performances similar to Tanui's, threatened Chebet and Tanui. He won the last two New York City Marathons. Last year he waited to kick until in sight of the finish line by the Tavern on the Green in Central Park before outkicking Chebet. This bad dream of being outkicked in the last minutes of a marathon haunted Chebet and drove him to train more than ever. Kagwe won New York by 3 seconds. He won by a more comfortable margin of 1:15 over Chebet in 1997. Kagwe had to stop on three occasions to tie his shoelaces, and he still beat Chebet. So if Chebet looks back and sees no one running, Kagwe could be hunkered down tying his shoes. Not seeing is not necessarily believing. Racing against ghosts taunts a runner's sanity. Two weeks prior to Boston last year, Kagwe was fifth at the Cherry Blossom 10-miler in Washington, D.C. Chebet is from Miharati, Kenya, where he owns a farm, but he does a lot of his training on the trails of the Valley Forge Reservation near Norristown, Pennsylvania. He probably didn't really believe in ghosts.

So here is the problem for Chebet, Tanui, and Kagwe: What tactic to use? Traditionally when off to the hunt, one follows the old man. He knows the game. That is Tanui at age 33, compared to age 28 for Chebet and 30 for Kagwe. They clearly decided that they would take their cues from Tanui. Watch the old man. Copy his moves. Then, in the last moments, turn the tables and succeed to the throne.

The day granted ordinary temperatures of 51°F and a light SW wind, warming to 73°F by mid race and cooling to 68°F by the finish. But at the first mile Chebet found himself running stride for stride with Sun Yingjie, the straight-armed young woman from China running her first and exuberant Boston Marathon. Such company was not ordinary for Kenyan men in a marathon. Chebet looked to be wondering that this was not the hunt of his ancestors. But by 10k, in 31:27, he had worked his way up to the lead pack next to Kenneth Cheruiyot, the designated pacesetter. Kagwe surged at 7 miles and opened up a 6-second gap. Perhaps he planned to launch his coup d'état early? The designated pacemaker hustled to get back on the job, but a mile later Tanui and the pack with Korir, the Mexican Isaac Garcia, the Ecuadoran Silvio Guerra, South Africans Frank Pooe and Abner Chiopu, and more Kenyans: Julius Ondieki,

Peter Gituka, and Luka Kibet. They passed the half marathon in 1:05:29. The 14-runner pack looked content, but that would not last.

First Lima fell off, then Ondieki, then Garcia. The pack swooped down the hill into Newton Lower Falls, shedding runners like broncos bucking off bad cowboys. They could hear the Charles River water rushing over the falls on its own tortuous trip to Boston. Like the Marathon, the Charles River starts at Echo Lake in Hopkinton, but the river is 80 miles long and the water takes weeks to get to Boston. But as the river surprises at every turn, so does the marathon, as an unknown took command over RT 128 on the firehouse turn.

Silvio Guerra had trained hard in the thin air of Ecuador—thin as the air in the Kenyan highlands. He felt good and comfortable running with the Africans, so went with the feeling. He said, "It was just a little move, but when no one went with me, I made it a big move. "The Kenyans waited on Tanui," said Guerra after the race. "When you are feeling good, you can take a risk. At the time I didn't know if I could win, but I was ready to try for it." But Tanui was not feeling good. Chebet waited for Tanui's signal.

Thirty-four kilometers into the race, Moses Tanui felt pain in his stomach. The urge to vomit overwhelmed him. He stopped. He walked. He sipped water. He attempted to run again. Tanui was out of the hunt and off the race course.

"I'm not happy because everybody cried when I stopped, but I had no other way," said Tanui. "It was very sad. Everyone was waiting, and all of a sudden this problem came."

Tanui said his training this year was much better than in 1998, when he won the race in 2:07:34. But over the last three weeks, according to his coach Dr. Gabriele Rosa, Tanui said he did not feel well and had symptoms similar to a chest cold. Rosa suggested Tanui get a checkup, but the Tanui declined, telling Rosa not to worry.

But it was Chebet's time to worry. An Ecuadoran was leading and two South Africans were pushing. Who were these guys? Abner Chiopu and Frank Pooe. Chipu was a good cross-country runner, having placed 57th at 12k in Belfast, Ireland, in the IAAF World Cross Country Championships. That is considered the toughest running race in the world, but that is not a performance that would have earned him a reputation for Kenyans to fear. Pooe had run a 1:01:17 half marathon the year before, but that was in Durban, South Africa, on the other end of a big continent so Kenyans were not aware.

The three led the race up to Boston College. But Chebet, having no Tanui or teammates to follow, remembered the advice of the original Greater Boston Track Club coach, Bill Squires. He said to move on this downhill. So Chebet moved.

Chebet said after the race, "I tried my best since last year. I very much wanted to get the title at Boston. Last year I tried my best for Boston also, but I got tired at the end. This year I changed something in my training so that would not happen again."

He had been 27 seconds behind at 30k and then began to push alone. He caught the South Africans. Down through Cleveland Circle he caught the Guerra. Chebet did not pass quickly but lingered at Geurra's side, perhaps gathering strength or assessing the opposition and measuring his relative strength. Satisfied with his evaluation, Chebet ran away with the 24th mile in 4:49. He ran the next in 4:57. He stopped after the finish line, passing it with no celebration, and looked back to see Guerra cross. Perhaps it was a gesture of respect, of communion with a runner who ran 2nd in palpable proximity to victory, not to celebrate in his face. Guerra himself did not seem crushed.

"The race was great," said Guerra. "The first half was not so fast, so that is why I decided to go after it at 25k. I was feeling great and strong. But I am very new to the marathon. This is only my fourth, and I'm just learning how to run it. I tried to run the race. You never know in the marathon. Anything can happen."

It seemed as if he had some to Boston in reconnaissance and quite pleased with the future he saw for himself. He planned that his turn would come.

Guerra said, "I'm used to being around just Kenyans; I'm the only one half-white in that group." He is half-black, half-Incan. "I'm really prepared to run with the Africans. They are the best in the world. I am very happy to be here with these guys."

At the post-race press conference reporters asked Guerra if he would have done anything differently. "Yes," he said. "I would have won the race."

1999 Men's Results:

1. **Joseph Chebet, KEN**	**2:09:52**	
2. Silvio Guerra, ECU	2:10:19	
3. Frank Pooe, RSA	2:11:36	
4. Abner Chipu, RSA	2:12:46	
5. John Kagwe, KEN	2:13:58	
6. Peter Githuka, KEN	2:14:04	
7. Andrey Kuznetsov, RUS	2:14:20,	
First Master, age 41		
8. Jose Luis Molina, CRC	2:14:27	
9. Ruben Maza, VEN	2:41:41	
10. Julius Ondieki, KEN	2:15:28	
11. Masaki Oya, JPN	2:15:45	
12. Joshua Kipkemboi, KEN	2:25:56	
13. Joseph LeMay, CT	2:16:11	
14. Franklin Tenorio, ECU	2:16:32	
15. Luka Kibet, KEN	2:17:50	
16. Isaac Garcia, MEX	2:18:14	
17. Andres Espinosa, MEX	2:18:47	
18. Rod DeHaven, WI	2:19:23	
19. Joseph McVeigh, NY	2:20:21	
20. Tesfaye Bekele, ETH	2:21:20	
21. William Ramirez, COL	2:22:03	
22. Toshiaki Kurabayashi, JPN	2:22:30	
23. Budd Coates, PA	2:22:52	
24. Bob Schwelm, PA	2:23:42	
25. Heiko Schinktz, GER	2:24:22	

26. Peter Hammer, MA	2:24:33	
27. Jan Myrda, POL	2:25:20	
28. Glen Guillemette, RI	2:25:25	
29. Ruben Hinojosa, MEX	2:26:01	
30. John Barbour, MA	2:26:02	
43. Todd Lipin, NY	2:30:15	
48. Jesse Darley, MA	2:31:04	
62. Christopher Lawrence, RI	2:33:20	
65. James Garcia, MA	2:33:44	
66. Mel Gonsalves, MA	2:33:50	
75. Mark Reeder, MA	2:35:16	
97. Arnold Seto, MA	2:38:23	
720. Jack O'Conner, RI	3:00:01	
785. Stephen Peckiconis, MA	3:01:23	
3205. Tom Varns, IN	3:30:00	
3710. Don Kardong, WA	3:36:05	
3741. Keizo Yamada, JPN	**3:36:26,**	
	First 70+	
5393. Richard Rockwood, RI	4:00:00	
7511. Cameron Hugh, MA	6:00:15	
Bill Rodgers DNF		

Winning Men's Teams

1. Boston Athletic Association, 7:30:17
2. West Side Runners, NY, 7:38:10
3. Greater Boston Track Club, 7:41:57
4. BAA, B Team, 7:43:40
5. Boston Running Club, A Team, 7:47:08
6. Whirlaway Running Club, 7:57:30
7. Central Park Track Club, NY, 7:57:57

Charming Champion Suspended

MONDAY, APRIL 19, 1999

Roba Back to Defend

In April 1998 Uta Pippig visited her parents in Berlin, Germany, when there came a knock on the door. It was the Deutscher Leichtathletik Verband (DLV) at the door to give her a surprise out-of-competition drug test. The DLV is the country's athletic federation, its official governing body. Pippig had no reason to suspect she would be compelled to take a test, since she had not been competing for about a year. *Why now*, she wondered?

It is routine, the German officials said. They did not appreciate that she had been inactive because of injuries. In August 1998, Dieter Hogen, her coach and partner, received a phone call that there was a drug test abnormality. When he told her the news, she said she went ballistic. Her agent, Kim McDonald, told her to calm down because it might be a mistake. But the DLV suspended her in October 1998. No mistake, the officials said, but was the test accurate, fair, or revenge? The test showed an abnormal ratio of testosterone to epitestosterone in her urine. The accepted ratio of testosterone, the male sex hormone, to epitestosterone, an inactive metabolite that is used as a marker, is 6 to 1; anything above that is considered to indicate the possible use of testosterone as a performance-enhancing anabolic steroid.

The test cannot distinguish naturally produced (endogenous) testosterone from injected or otherwise taken testosterone, even a high ratio is no guarantee an athlete has taken testosterone.

A ratio of 10:1 is considered by many to be in a gray area. Pippig says her ratio of 9.2:1 was not due to high testosterone but rather to low epitestosterone, perhaps resulting from a number of conditions specific to gender and health issues that she has been battling since her epic run in 1996. There is little evidence that the bowel condition she calls ischemic colitis causes a decrease in epitestosterone.

A great deal of doubt and innuendo follow her. Rumors circulate inside the running community about Pippig's high training mileage and rapid recovery after races. Many runners can't believe her training routine. She trains in Boulder. But runners there called her excessively private. They cite her East German background. Many East German athletes found to have used performance-enhancing drugs have been banned. But until last fall, Pippig never had failed any of the dozens of drug tests in her career.

She said that while still living in East Germany in 1984, she briefly took "some kind of drug" that her trainer told her was vitamins, but she stopped within a few weeks, saying her parents told her to stop.

Others have said that the prize money she won in races was obtained fraudulently and should be theirs. Still others have said that in private conversations she has admitted drug use from the very start. But of course such things are rumors and hearsay. She has been accused by the failed test, but there are experts who question the tests.

"I'm skeptical about the validity of the test, especially in women," said Dr. Robert Barbieri, chief of obstetrics and gynecology at Brigham and Women's Hospital, who had sent a letter to the German federation on Pippig's behalf. "This test has been most widely used in male athletes, and then it's been applied to females kind of by analogy. In my mind, when we finally work out the details, we will abandon it as a test for women."

Especially in question, Barbieri believes, are the effects on the t/e ratio of oral contraceptives—which Pippig was taking at the time—and medical conditions involving the bowel, through which the hormones are cycled. Pippig was hospitalized for tests after the episode during the 1996 Marathon, and said that intestinal problems, including diarrhea, and a severe hormone imbalance persisted even up to the time of the drug test last April.

"I think it's kind of a sad thing," Pippig said of the accusations. "But I feel sorry for them. People who say this can be jealous." She said about medical complexities, "It's obvious I had a lot of problems with my intestinal tract during the last years," she said.

Pippig's contract with Nike expired and Nike did not offer to renew. She had to pay her own legal fees, and lost perhaps hundreds of thousands of dollars in appearance fees and potential prize money.

"I don't wish any person on Earth this," said Pippig. I know I didn't do anything. It's hard. It's just not fair." The suspension and the extensions to a ban of some length is the subject awaited under appeal. "I am very often asking my people what is going on," said German Federation president Helmut Digel. "It is very important the period of suspension shouldn't last too long." At the point of this year's Boston Marathon, the suspension had been going on six months, but the commission in Germany had not set a hearing date. Pippig was unable to compete while the case was pending.

The threat of a lawsuit against the DLV followed. Was the DLV taking revenge against Pippig for living in the U.S. instead of Germany? Were they making an example of her? Could she be the only German athlete accused of using performance-enhancing drugs? Certainly not, since others had been found out and banned. As Uta Pippig came to Boston to defend her reputation, Fatuma Roba came back to Boston to defend her title. The marathon had made her rich, famous, and comfortable as well as a gracious host. She built herself a new house in Arsi.

When Roba first came to Boston she came as the Olympic Marathon Gold medalist, the same as in 1963 when Abebe Bikila came to Boston. But he did not run well. In fact, no Olympic Gold medalist had won at Boston and when Bikila, the barefoot winner of the Rome Olympics who opened the door to African long-distance running, failed to win, Boston became known as the graveyard of Olympic gold medalists. Reporters said that he was cut down by the cold east wind and ran only 2:24:43. Roba had run over a minute faster last year. Asked at the Saturday press conference if she was aware that her time here last year was faster than Bikila's in '63, Roba looked puzzled. *What is your question?* she wanted to know. He must have had a bad race, she insisted, quick to defend the legend of Bikila. "My dream is to win again the Olympics, like my countryman," she said this week through a translator, a day after arriving from Addis Ababa, Ethiopia. "To match the same story. I am not a hero like him, but a lot of people know me because I make the same history at the Olympics," said the first black African woman to win marathon gold. "Especially children. Now they want to be like me."

In the 1964 Olympics in Toyko, Bikila won Gold again, this time in 2:12:12, a world record.

"He opened the door not only for all Ethiopians, but for all Africans," said Roba, who was born in 1973 before Bikila died of a brain hemorrhage long after being left paralyzed from a car crash in 1969. He received a state funeral in Addis Ababa. He was indeed the perfect runner, with grace and fluidity, just as Roba runs with an enviable smoothness. But then she added: "I'm hoping to make my race even faster this year." *Boston Globe* writer Huebner wrote about her: "Roba's style, fluid and seemingly without idiosyncrasy. Her carriage, one of grace and subtle authority."

Roba has won Boston twice. But, oddly, she has not run well elsewhere. At the World Championships in Athens in 1997, she dropped out midway with a leg injury. At Tokyo in 1997 she ran 4th, in 2:30:39; last year she could manage no better than 8th there in 2:36:22, running with a cold. Roba said racing well has a lot to do with chance.

"Not entirely," said her agent, Mark Wetmore of Global Athletics & Marketing. "I don't think she's as good on a flat course," he said. "She's very much faster on a difficult course. She thinks if she can break the world record, she can do it here."

Colleen De Reuck from South Africa had spent the last year training at altitude in Colorado under the catalyst of having almost won the Boston Marathon. Might this be her year? Last year's 2nd place came back, Renata Paradowska of Poland. She won the San Jose Mercury News 10K in March in 33:49. Franziska

Rochat-Moser returned—besides being an elite runner, she was a lawyer and owner of the gourmet restaurant Girardet in her hometown of Crissier, Switzerland. She earned notice in the United States with her win at New York in 1997 (2:28:42), but she's no stranger to Boston, either, with a 4th in 1995 (2:29:35) and a 6th in 1996 (2:31:33). She was 18th in the Atlanta Games in 1996 and set her personal best (and a Swiss record) by winning at Hamburg in 1994 (2:27:44). Rochat-Moser was a popular and charming athlete among her competitors and fans.

But Roba, Olympic gold medalist, has never lost on the Boston course. She has dominated it, her 2:23:21 last year the third-fastest time in Boston's history. But Joan Benoit Samuelson said the race could come down to either the experienced Roba or two newcomers to the distance—Catherine Ndereba and Lynn Jennings. "I think we'll either have a three-peat champion or a duel between the debut queens," said Samuelson, hedging her bets.

Jennings was a Liberty AC teammate of Benoit Samuelson, and many-time world cross-country champion. Ndereba, the 26-year-old Kenyan who has twice been ranked the No. 1, took a year off for the birth of her daughter, Jane, in May 1997. In 1998, she won 16 of the 21 races she entered, including the Falmouth Road Race and Samuelson's own Beach to Beacon 10K in Cape Elizabeth, Maine. At a clam bake after that Maine race, a server placed a freshly boiled whole lobster on her plate. Ndereba's eyes got very big. Someone asked her if she liked lobster. She answered, "I like to look at them."

"She's relaxed," said Samuelson. "She's just going to go out and have fun. That's a great way to approach this race."

Another unknown was Japan's Yuko Arimori, running Boston for the first time. The two-time Olympic medalist—silver in 1992, bronze in 1996—living in Boulder has not raced a marathon since Atlanta. She said she needed a rest, and lost several weeks when she banged herself up in a fall on the ice while training a month ago. But Arimori is known for running well when it counts. Franca Fiacco was prolific, having run more than a dozen marathons since 1994 and winning three, including New York (in a 2:25:17 personal best), last year.

"All I want from my marathon is a good race," said De Reuck (2:26:35 lifetime best), "one that when I get to the finish I feel every step of the way I've given what I've got to it."

"She's been so close so many times," said Samuelson.

For this year's race most eyes will be on Jennings. No American woman has won here since Lisa Weidenbach in 1985, but if the 1992 Olympic bronze medalist at 10,000m from Newmarket, New Hampshire, is anywhere in contention coming out of the hills. Said Samuelson, "I wouldn't bet against her. Lynn has a lot of speed."

Jennings had been modest about her chances. She said her only goal was to run 2:42 or under to earn a qualifying time for the Olympic Trials, which would give her the option of trying to make the U.S. team at either 5000m, which she did in 1996; 10,000m, which she did in 1988 and 1992; or the marathon. She was not exactly brand new to the marathon. When she was 17 in 1978 she finished

3rd at Boston in 2:45, but she was one year too young to officially register. Sam-uelson, however, predicted she would run under 2:30 this time, and that if she was near the leader in Brookline, she would get the energy boost of her life. "The crowd will be going nuts."

Twenty-year-old Sun Yingjie from Liaoning, China, came to Boston to run her fifth marathon, but her first outside her country. She seemed excited. She ran only 13 seconds behind the men at 5k in 15:58 and ahead of the nearest woman by 51 seconds. She continued to lead the women by 65 seconds by 10k in 32:30. She ran with an odd carriage to her arms as if reluctant to bend her elbows. The pack of women did not know Yingjie ran so far ahead. Since the men and wom-en started together, the (mostly) taller men blocked the view of the field. Only by 15k did Ndereba and Roba realize Yingjie led the race. They ran in a pack with Arimori, Catuna, Ndereba, Rochat-Moser, and Russia's Ludmila Petrova.

"I think no one was taking her seriously," said Rochat-Moser. "I think all the girls looked at [each] other but not at the Chinese girls."

"At first I didn't know (that someone else was in the lead)," Roba said. "Later I noticed, and just decided I had to change my pace. I wasn't scared of the Chi-nese runner." But regardless she took off running the next 5k in 16:27—faster than any 5k she had run in all of her Bostons. Those were run in a relentlessly steady pace free of surges, but now she surged. Only Ndereba dared to follow. Sun's eagerness took her through the half in 1:10:20, a pace to break the world record. Roba and Ndereba caught her just after 25 kilometers. After that Sun would fade. The race was down to Roba and Ndereba. For 3 miles, Ndereba ran right on Roba's shoulder, matching her stride for stride, with both still on a pace to run the fastest women's marathon in history as they made the turn by the firehouse on Commonwealth Avenue. The previous year Roba had broken Colleen DeRueck long before that on the downhill to Newton Lower Falls.

Beyond the fire house, the hills played to Roba's strength. At 18 miles, she ran 20 yards ahead of Ndereba. Again, as last year Ethiopian Bostonians invaded the course waving flags and shouting. By 20 miles, on Heartbreak Hill, Roba had another 160 yards, and soon the press in the lead vehicle could no longer see Ndereba. On the final hill Roba accepted and donned a headband of Ethi-opian colors. At 21 miles she ran faster than Pippig's record, but blisters had formed on her feet. She slowed to 5k split of 17:25. It disappointed her not to break the course record, but she finished overjoyed to have won three in a row. "Winning three in a row here makes it very special for me." Roba won another $80,000. She could go home to finish her house.

8 March 2002: Franziska Rochat-Moser, Lausanne, Switzerland, died after an accident in the Swiss Alps. Rochat-Moser climbed on a snow ledge near the 2,340-meter (7,670-foot) La Para peak. The ledge suddenly collapsed. She fell 2,300 feet. She was found alive, but died the next day. Rochat-Moser was trained to be a lawyer but gave up the practice of law when she married Chef Philippe Rochat in order to to help him run Girardet, a gourmet restaurant in the L'Hotel de Ville in her hometown of Crissier. She was 35.

1999 Women's Results

1. Fatuma Roba, ETH	**2:23:25**	**18.** Melanie Ellis, GBT	2:46:55
	(24th place overall)	**19.** Ai Dongmei, CHN	2:47:11
2. Franziska Rochat-Moser, SUI	2:25:51	**20.** Michelle Lafleur, GA	2:49:19
3. Yuko Arimori, JPN	2:26:39	**21.** Maribel Burgos, PR	2:49:47
4. Colleen De Reuck, RSA	2:27:54	**22.** Lisa Goldsmith, CO	2:50:17
5. Martha Tenorio, ECU	2:27:58	**23.** Cheryl Harper, UT	2:50:33
6. Catherine Ndereba, KEN	**2:28:27**	**24.** Yumiko Otsuka, JPN	2:50:51
7. Ludmila Petrova, RUS	2:29:13	25. Lisa Valentine, FL	2:51:40
8. Mitsuko Sugihara, JPN	2:30:34	26. Lee Dipietro, MD	2:51:51
9. Renata Paradowska, POL	2:31:41	27. Janice Posey, AZ	2:53:39
10. Anuta Catuna, ROU	2:33:49	28. Chiyomi Munakata, JPN	2:54:03
11. Sun Yingjie, CHN	2:37:11	29. Kimberly Harrity, PA	2:54:15
12. Lynn Jennings, NH	2:38:37	30. Laurel Kjorlien, CAN	2:55:08
13. Julia Kirtland, ME	2:39:45	38. Lane Tracey, FL	3:00:00
14. Josette Colomb-Janin, FRA	2:40:36	409. Carrie Okay, NJ	3:30:00
15. Danuta Bartoszek, CAN	2:43:18	1974. Dona Brown, CA	4:00:00
16. Maki Nakagawa, JPN	2:43:28	3763. Annmarie Bonapane, MA	5:57:24
17. Gillian Horovitz, GBR	2:46:31	**DNF Ingrid Kristiansen at 18 miles**	

Winning Women's Teams

1.   Forerunners Track Club, FL, 8:49:26
2.   Sojourners, UT, 9:14:05
3.   Hi-Tek Racing, CT, 9:04:07
4.   Boston Athletic Association, 9:18:49
5.   Atlanta Track Club, GA, 9:21:40
6.   North Medford Club, MA, 9:28:00
7.   Tidewater Striders, VA, 9:32:21
8.   Central Park Track Club, NY, 9:45:33
9.   Knoxville Track Club, TN, 9:48:30

Chapter 12

2000–2009
Y2K?

Presidents: *William Jefferson Clinton, George W. Bush, Barack Obama*

Massachusetts Governors: *Arego Paul Cellucci, Jane Maria Swift, Mitt Romney, Deval Patrick*

Boston Mayors: *Thomas M. Menino*

2000 Populations: *U.S. 282.2 million, Massachusetts 6.361 million, Boston 590,433*

The touted end-of-the-world year 2000 shutdown of computers worldwide, or a second coming or any calendar-generated apocalypse, never happened. But terrorism and economic depression did. The Boston Marathon in contrast flourished, providing a yearly anchor to the city of Boston and the Marathon world. The decade started with America looking unstoppable and ended with American frailties exposed.

It seemed to the United States' political, business, and military leaders that theirs was the strongest country in the world. With the collapse of the Soviet Union and with populous China and India having much weaker militaries, what was once a bi-polar world was now a unipolar world—one with a single superpower. American politicians felt that no country posed a threat to the U.S. The expectation was that a Pax Americana would by sheer strength and goodness impose peace on the world. Few people saw any challenge to American Power. George W. Bush was elected president and took the oath of office with Dick Cheney on January 20, 2001. The U.S. seemed so powerful that it could make its own reality.

All that would change on September 11, 2001, with the terrorist attack on the World Trade Center and other places. The lives of all Americans and people worldwide changed in a way that the Cold War, with the possibility of mutually assured nuclear destruction, had not changed them. Either there would have been world-wide nuclear holocaust or not. But all terrorism is local. If war is politics by another means then so is terrorism. But with whom could leaders demand an armistice or negotiate surrender?

The UN passed a resolution on Iraq in 2002 in a search for weapons of mass destruction. They found none. In 2003 Bush declared the mission accomplished, but by decade's end Iraq would have no peace. On August 29, 2005, Hurricane Katrina struck the Gulf Coast and the second Bush administration did not have the power, money, organization, nor will to respond quickly. On September 16, 2008, big financial institutions in the United States failed, due primarily to the vulnerability of securities composed of packaged subprime lending and credit default swaps. On October 11, 2008, the head of the International Monetary

Fund (IMF) warned that the world financial system was teetering on the "brink of systemic meltdown." U.S. investment markets lost half their value. Later in 2008 Obama/Biden defeated McCain/Palin.

The world talked about global climate change but did little about it. Kenyans dominated the Boston Marathon, and marathons worldwide in this decade—although their neighboring Ethiopians tried to dispute that. The reasons were mostly economic. The prize money alone would instantly make a runner wildly wealthy at home and likely the wealthiest person in the village or town. That was good reason to train hard and often.

For the Boston Marathon, everything improved in this decade, from prize money to sponsorships to worldwide affirmation that the Boston Marathon was the premiere running event in the world. The Boston Athletic Association increased its staff and involvement in the community by most obviously hosting more events, starting with the BAA half marathon run in the fall. Guy Morse and the BAA board of governors led the organization through this upgrade. Race director Dave McGillivray sought every logistical and technical way to make the race more accommodating to more runners and less intrusive to the cities and towns on the course. Marketing and communications manager Jack Fleming tried reach everyone in the world with the message of the Boston Marathon.

A New Century for the Marathon

MONDAY, APRIL 17, 2000

Into the Teeth of the Wind

1955 Boston Marathon winner Hideo Hamamura died on May 7 in Yamaguchi, Japan, of cancer at age 71. Joe Concannon, who for years was the *Boston Globe*'s lead Marathon writer, died. Seats in the press room and on the press vehicle that lead the race were reserved in the name of Concannon, who had retired the previous fall. Around 10,000 to 15,000 protesters demonstrated at the International Monetary Fund and World Bank meeting. On April 16 and 17 the number of those arrested grew to 1,300 people. The essence of the protest was that the movement of capital across international borders undermined local political control. Forces pushed countries to isolate themselves, and other forces such as the Boston Marathon pushed countries and athletes together.

The Kenyan Federation decided that it would use the Boston Marathon to pick two of its three Olympians for the Sydney Olympics. That put more pressure on the favorite, Moses Tanui. The pressure of the Kenyan trials looked like an opportunity for Ecuadorian Silvio Guerra, "It is good because I have a bunch of Africans who will be pushing the race, so I don't have to worry about that, and they will have the pressure to qualify for the Olympics. I have already qualified, so I don't have the pressure to get on the team. I just can go for the win."

On the eve of the Boston Marathon, David D'Alessandro, president of Marathon sponsor John Hancock Financial Services Inc., talked to Boston Globe reporter Michael Madden about U.S. Track & Field's reluctance to use Boston for the United States Olympic Trials.

"USATF is afraid," said D'Alessandro. "They can only make money by going to Pittsburgh [for the men's qualifier] and South Carolina [women's]."

The Boston Marathon never has been used as the U.S. Olympic qualifier "because they have this ridiculous rule that the course is too hilly," said D'Alessandro. "They have this rule about how much grade you can have in the course.

"But my point is that if [the United States] is supposed to post up its best three runners who can run against international competition, then why do we insist on this incestuous race with just Americans?"

Many of the world's best marathoners are in Boston today, he said. "This is the only event in America where enough of the international players come in in the time frame to qualify for the Olympics. What better race to qualify for the Olympics than one of the world's more competitive marathons?" said D'Alessandro. The only sure thing about the U.S. Olympic Trials "is that an American is going to win," he said. "Since when do American athletes run—or compete—out of safety? It's not the American mentality and, supposedly, not our heritage. We're supposed to be risk-takers and out front in everything we do."

The temperature was 50°F. A sea breeze would drop it to 47°F by the finish. Japanese runner Makoto Sasaki took an early lead into the 5-minute-a-mile headwind. The rest of the field let him have it. So did the wind. He would pay dearly and finish far behind the leaders.

Simon Mpholo of South Africa and Kenyan David Busienei led through the half marathon in 1:05:41, followed by a second pack with another South African, Lavan Nkete, and a couple of Ethiopians, Abraham Assefa, Gezahene Abera, Hideyuki Obinata, and Ryoji Maeda of Japan, Alejandro Cruz of Mexico and also a herd of Kenyans, Philip Tarus who had pushed the pace in 1998, Isaak Kipronon, Jackson Kabiga, Joseph Chebet, Ondoro Osoro, John Kagwe, the Nandi, Elijah Lagat, and of course, Moses Tanui. Ecuadorian Silvio Guerra, with his hunger from having placed 2nd the year before, watched the Kenyans watching each other while keeping a third eye on the Ethiopians. Each Kenyan wanted his position on the Olympic team, but none of them wanted an Ethiopian to beat them. They raced with a mixture of pride and caution. By 25k it was Kabiga who decided he would toss caution to the wind to break things up with a surge. He took 7 seconds from the pack. When Kibiga was 18 he lived in Cosmas Ndeti's house and tried to keep up with him in training. But like a hunted giraffe he would run full speed until exhausted, then not slow down, but suddenly stop.

The guys in his training group teased him and nicknamed him "giraffe," in Swa-hili it is Twiga. "Twiga," now 23, was stronger and wiser, but also in the company of other strong, wise runners. He had come to Boston with Ndeti in 1995, but his name does not appear in the results. He pushed but the only thing he broke was himself as he faded back. But he would not stop. Not this time.

Elijah Lagat ran in the pack waiting and watching. Sometimes it was hard to see Tanui in the pack so cleverly he ran tucked inside and protected, waiting to use the kick that had given him victory. In the pack runners jostled each other, hiding from the wind and testing each other. "At 25 kilometers, I was going to pull out," Abera said after the race. Abera claimed Tanui and Lagat were jos-tling and tripping him.

"I was in between them and it was very difficult," he said. "They were push-ing me and kicking me. I can't say if it was intentional or not." But the Kenyans later said that if Abera wanted to lead he was welcome to do so.

To explain how Kenyan runners instinctively use team tactics, Sammy Lelei told agent Tom Ratcliffe about how 11-year-old Kenyan farm boys hunt togeth-er in the pastures when they see wild antelopes pass through. They cut short sticks called *rungu* from hardwood with a dense knot at the end. They chase the antelope toward their friends, confuse the animals, tire them, and whack them with the *rungu* to bring home meat to fortify the family's *ugali*. Tanui may have wished he carried a *rungu*.

At 22 miles Tanui decided that he would stop trying to play the invisible man when all sly eyes watched him. He surged to the lead. Lagat thought that was the end. The boss had taken over, so Lagat set himself to race the other guys for 2nd place. That point at Cleveland Circle had a special significance for Tanui. That is where he had dropped out a year earlier. So he made his defiant statement.

But Abera was not ready to yield; nor was Lagat, who wanted to defend his position for the Kenyan Olympic team. Abera went with Tanui. Lagat followed. The three men continued their jostling and testing. After the race Abera said, ". . . one was in front and the other came from behind and kicked me so that I got a strain on my muscles, that is what created a problem for me." But Lagat said, "I had the same problems. Those who were watching might say that it was Abera who was kicking me, but I did not think of it as being intentional. I know that when somebody's concentrating on following, these things can happen."

Tanui, however, still held a grudge against Halie Gerbresellassie from the 1993 world track 10,000m when the Ethiopian appeared to deliberately and repeatedly step on Tanui's shoe to remove it. The tactic worked and Tanui had to try to sprint wearing only one shoe. Now he suspected Abera of using the same tactic. Tanui said after the race, "He kicked me two or three times when I was in front. And this is not correct that he is accusing Kenyans. He is the one who was doing it, and that is his problem." The three of them took the final turn off Hereford Street on to Boylston. They had about a minute and half to run. They suddenly came abreast of each other. They lined up like sprinters for the shot down Boylston Street. At exactly 26 miles with only the appended 385 yards remaining, Tanui lifted his knees into full sprint posture. He opened a gap. Abera closed it. Lagat watched. But the two leading men had started kicking too soon. With less than 200 meters to go, as oxygen debt seized Tanui and Abera, Lagat began his kick. Lagat had a step on Abera by the finish.

At the Olympics later in the year Abera won and Silvio Guerra placed 14th. The first American was 69th. Elijah Lagat did not finish.

Many runners had problems at the finish. Many were cold and shaking. They filled the medical tents. In the past, reporters could freely course the tents interviewing runners. But the tent had become more sophisticated with much more medical equipment such as intravenous needles, tubes, bottles of saline solution for dehydration, and defibrillators to save the life of a runner in cardiac arrest. In an effort to protect patient privacy, journalists were allowed only to stand at the entrance. "[Our legal team] told us because we were doing invasive procedures, they believed that we crossed the threshold into being more like a hospital," said Marathon spokesman Jack Fleming. "So we had to follow hospital-like protocol."

2000 Men's Results

1. **Elijah Lagat, KEN**	**2:09:47**	
2. Gezahegne Abera, ETH	2:09:47	
3. **Moses Tanui, KEN**	**2:09:50**	
4. Ondoro Osoro, KEN	2:10:29	
5. David Kiptum Busienei, KEN	2:11:26	
6. John Kagwe, KEN	2:12:26	
7. Laban Nkete, KEN	2:12:30	
8. **Joseph Chebet, KEN**	**2:12:39**	
9. Julius Ruto, KEN	2:13:26	
10. Silvio Guerra, ECU	2:14:18	
11. Alejandro Cruz, MEX	2:2:15:09	
12. Michal Bartoszak, POL	2:15:24	
13. Jackson Kibaga, KEN	2:16:13	
14. Makhosonke Fika, RSA	2:16:27	
15. Ryoji Maeda, JPN	2:17:04	
16. Philip Tarus, KEN	2:17:09	
17. Joshua Kipkemboi, KEN	2:17:11, First Master	
18. Hideyuki Obinata, JPN	2:17:24	
19. Fedor Ryjov, RUS	2:17:38	
20. Abraham Assefa, ETH	2:18:22	
21. Sadayuki Kigure, JPN	2:19:13	
22. Jose Luis Molina, CRC	2:19:40	
23. Arsenio Ortiz, MEX	2:21:54	
24. Jamie Hibell, PA	2:22:09	
25. Chris Verbeek, BEL	2:22:52	
26. Maximo Oliveras, PR	2:23:06	
27. Budd Coates, PA	2:25:10	
28. Christopher Ashfield, CA	2:25:14	
29. Bob Schwelm, PA	2:26:59	
30. Johnny Loria Solano, CRC	2:27:08	
36. Francisco Tomas, IL	2:30:05	
80. Mokoto Sasaki, JPN	2:37:24	
1204. Andrew Young, NY	3:00:00	
4721. **Keizo Yamada, JPN**	**3:27:31**	
7887. Toshiyasu Miyazaki, JPN	4:00:00	
10199. Ludovic Kabran, MA	6:00:58	
Jack Fultz, DNF		

Winning Men's Teams

1. Leigh Valley Road Runners Club, PA, 7:28:33
2. Hoy's Excelsior RC, CA, 7:38:55
3. Greater Boston Track Club, 7:42:31
4. Whirlaway Running Club, MA, 7:44:06
5. Bryn Mawr RC, PA, 7:44:34
6. Boston Athletic Association, 7:47:13
7. Greater Lowell Road Runners, MA, 7:47:16

Roba Back for #4 Win?

Eyes toward Sydney Olympics

Fatuma Roba decided to come back to Boston. She said before the race that she knows that no one has won four Boston Marathons in a row and that she had been training intensely to make history.

Although the spotlight in the women's race of the Boston Marathon has focused sharply on how Fatuma Roba's opponents, of course, will try to shove her off the stage. "You don't win the Olympics and three Bostons without being a class athlete," Elana Meyer. "Hopefully, she can't do it for a fourth."

"She's [Elana Meyer] been the bridesmaid so many times. She keeps coming back because she really wants this," said Joan Benoit Samuelson.

Catherine Ndereba, who ran with Roba through 17 miles last year, came back as well. "I just wanted to be challenged, and that's exactly what happened," said Ndereba, who had finished 2nd in the New York City Marathon the previous fall.

Lornah Kiplagat ran a fast 1:06:54 half marathon, and has gone 2:25:30 in the marathon.

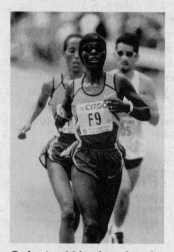

Catherine Ndereba takes the lead from Fatima Roba. Photo by Victah Sailer.

Sun Yingjie of China, with a 2:25:45 personal best, was now 21 years old and ready to risk it all for a win.

The cool temperatures and headwind predicted slow times and a hide-and-seek tactical race. Catherine Ndereba said, "Last year I tried to stay with the leaders, but the pace was too fast for me and I faded over the last 6 miles. This year, I want to run my own race." But that is not what happened. Everyone ran, not her own race, but the race allowed by the weather. The raw headwind forced the field to bunch up behind their own bulwark, trading little peeks into the wind from the safety of the pack as if checking to see if the wind still blew and it was safe to go outside. Roba, Meyer, Yingjie, Catuna, and Bogacheva stuck together in a mutual defense pact. But Ndereba and Lornah Kiplagat ran together a little off the leaders;

they seemed to be losing contact with the leaders running behind by 10 seconds, then 39, then 51 at the 10k, 15k, and halfway. Those who thought they were contenders hung with Roba. By 25k Ndereba and Kiplagat made up 20 seconds. The leaders didn't know they were coming.

Roba sensed their approach, and by the firehouse at the Commonwealth Ave turn she tried to flee into the hills. Her move strung out the pack as the Ethiopian flags rushed out of the side streets. Roba looked effortless and seemed to be about to run away to another victory. Sun Yingjie ran in 2nd place, her arms resolutely pointing straight down by her sides. Ndereba passed Romanian Anuta Catuna and Sun Yingjie then pulled even with Roba at the top of the hill. Roba glanced over to Ndereba, acknowledging her arrival, but Ndereba stared stoically forward. Roba was not as fit as she had been. So Ndereba ran on alone. Bogacheva pushed desperately in pursuit of Roba to the finish. She caught Roba at the line to take 2nd place by a judge's decision. Boston had its first Kenyan woman winner.

Roba said, "I personally did not have any problems. The only obstacle that I face was the kind of weather that we do not experience back in Ethiopia." In the Sydney Olympic Marathon Roba finished 9th, Loroupe 13th, and Bogocheva 14th, but Ndereba did not run: the Kenyan selectors did not select her, however she said about Loroupe, "I want to see whether I could be one like her," said Ndereba, referring to Kenyan Tegla Loroupe, the world record–holder. "Even if I am not exactly, I am in the process to be like her." Loroupe has the world record of 2:20:43 set in Berlin in 1999.

2000 Women's Results

1. **Catherine Ndereba, KEN**	**2:26:11**	18. Maria Trujillo de Rios, CZA	2:42:24
2. Irina Bogacheva, KGZ	2:26:27	19. Melissa Moon, NZL	2:452:41
3. **Fatuma Roba, ETH**	**2:26:27**	20. Kristin Schwartz, CO	2:44:44
4. Anuta Catuna, ROU	2:29:46	21. Jacquine Merritt, PA	2:45:07
5. Lornah Kiplagat, KEN	2:30:12	22. Marie Boyd, NM	2:45:58
6. Ai Dongmei, CHN	2:30:18	23. Sandra Branney, GBR	2:46:32
7. Ornella Ferrara, ITA	2:30:20	24. Lee DiPietro, MD	2:47:00
8. Sun Yingjie, CHN	2:31:22	25. Gillian Horovitz, GBR	2:47:49
9. Marta Tenorio, ECU	2:31:49	26. Dorian Meyer, NJ	2:47:54
10. Elana Meyer, RSA	2:32:09	27. Christine Stief, GER	2:49:29
11. Firiya Sultanova-Zhdanova, RUS	2:32:21	28. Katherine Koski, MN	2:50:17
12. Renata Paradowska, POL	2:33:45	29. Maribel Burgos, PR	2:50:57
13. Gite Karshoj, DEN	2:35:11, First Master	30. Laurie Corbin, NJ	2:51:41
		58. Joan Hunter, PA	3:00:10
14. Annemari Sandell, FIN	2:35:12	651. Sheila Foley, CAN	3:29:58
15. Tatyana Pozdnyakova, UKR	2:35:43	3304. Cynthia Hastings, MA	3:53:30
16. Gabrielle O'Rourke, NZL	2:39:37	5469. Alice Mansfield, MI	5:59:44
17. Danutas Marczyk-Teschner, POL	2:41:57		

Winning Women's Teams

1. Forerunners Track Club, FL, 8:42:35
2. Valley Forge Striders, PA, 8:57:21
3. Utah Sojourners, A Team, 8:57:44
4. Utah Sojourners, B Team, 9:26:48
5. Bryn Mawr RC, PA, 9:31:13
6. Boston Athletic Association, 9:35:32
7. Hi-Tek, CT, 9:37:00
8. North Medford Club, MA, 9:37:27

In Memory of the Father

MONDAY, APRIL 16, 2001

Ecuador, Korea, vs. Kenya

Commenting on the race, American middle distance Olympian Marty Liquori said, "When you lose the Olympics by 3 seconds, it tends to stay with you for a while—like every day for the rest of your life (so) when you're in that situation again, you try not to get 2nd again." It was in Atlanta in 1996 that Lee Bong-Ju placed 2nd by a mere 3 seconds. In Sydney he placed a humble 24th. He did not want to be humble in Boston. Other Koreans had run well in Boston. In 1947 Yun Bok Suh ran 2:25:39 to win and set a world record, and Kee Yong Ham led a Korean sweep in 1950. Now Koreans were back.

Lee Bong-Ju had his doubts after Sydney and considered quitting the sport. "I was disappointed and it undermined my confidence a lot," he said. "I felt if I didn't pull myself together it could be the end of my career."

He regrouped two months later to be runner-up at Fukuoka in 2:09:04. It restored his confidence and fed his appetite. But winning would be good.

With sunny skies and a temperature of 56 degrees, conditions were near ideal at the start, and South Africans Makhosonke Fika and Simon Mpholo ran to an early lead. By 2 miles they had almost 200 meters on a pack of 30, and soon were slapping hands with spectators as they cruised along. By 9 miles the pack had closed the gap, catching up during a fluid-stop fiasco in which Fika stopped to sort through several bottles until he found his own. The hand slapping stopped.

The pack read 10 miles in 49:45 on the clock; the field featured 8 runners with personal bests under 2:10 and they watched each other within that massive pack. Still in the hunt were a number of Americans, including Rod DeHaven,

Mark Coogan, and Josh Cox—bold and blond, who briefly took the lead just before the midway point. Coming into Wellesley Center, the pack began to spread out, and at the halfway point (1:05:19) the South Africans briefly retook the lead.

Just past 14 miles, Josh Cox fell off the pack with a side stitch "that felt like someone was stabbing me with a knife."

By the Newton firehouse turn onto Commonwealth Avenue, the pack slimmed to 13, and on the downside of the first of the Newton hills it shrunk as Guerra extracted more effort from anyone who wanted to stay with him. The real race had begun, with Guerra deciding to push the pace. When no one responded, he settled back into a somewhat smaller pack. Lee Bong-Ju still ran in that pack. He wore a white headband with the traditional Korean red and blue Taeguk symbolizing balance, and a professionally acquired SAMSUNG shirt tucked into Asics shorts.

Going up Heartbreak Hill, just after the 20-mile mark, Ethiopian Gezahegne Abera—one of the three runners in last year's closing sprint down Boylston Street and the Olympic Gold medalist—began to look distressed and fell back. Soon the pack was down to 3, and at mile 22 Lee took a slim lead over Guerra and Chelang'a. Lee slowly fattened his lead. With 2 miles left, he ran alone. Lee pumped his fist as he crossed the line. Koreans were back to Boston after fifty years, when Kee Yong Ham led a 1-2-3 finish of his countrymen in 1950. And yes, of course winning is good.

"Fifty years is a long time," said Lee through a translator, "and a long time makes this honor much bigger."

Lee Bong-Ju felt haunted by having missed his father's death. He won the race to honor his father. Bong-Ju wasn't there for his father Lee Hae Ku. He told Boston Globe reporter Michael Holley the day after the race that his mother, his sister, and his brother-in-law were in the tiny house, but no one actually witnessed the death. For some Koreans, it is important for children to watch as their parents breathe for the last time. It is a way to honor them. "I felt that my father was with me today," said Bong-Ju. "I felt him when I needed encouragement and confidence." He raised the family in a village of about 35 houses and 100 people. He smoked, he drank, worked hard, and said little. When Bong-Ju, his youngest, won the 1996 Olympic silver medal, he offered to move the family to a nicer home in a big city such as Seoul, but the father declined. "'No, son,' he said. 'We are farmers. We love the land. We belong here, where we can be close to the earth.'"

Although he managed to finish 16th in 2:17:04, Abera wound up in the emergency room at New England Baptist Hospital on race night, under observation for a suspected sinus infection and preparing to undergo an MRI.

2001 Men's Results

1. **Lee Bong-Ju, KOR**	2:09:43	4. David Kiptum Busienei, KEN	2:11:47
2. Silvio Guerra, ECU	2:10:07	5. Mbarak Hussein, KEN	2:12:01
3. Joshua Chelang'a, KEN	2:10:29	6. Rod DeHaven, WI	2:12:41

7. Laban Nkete, RSA	2:12:44	22.	Kim Je-Kyung, KOR	2:21:25
8. Fedor V. Ryzhov, RUS	2:13:54,	23.	Samuel Lopez, MEX	2:21:28
	First	24.	Sammy Ngatia, KEN	2:23:07
	Master	25.	Scott Larson, CO	2:23:43
9. Makhosonke Fika, RSA	2:14:13	26.	Paul Zimmerman, OR	2:23:46
10. Timothy Cherigat, KEN	**2:14:21**	27.	Jacob VanWyk, RSA	2:24:22
11. Joshua Kipkemboi, KEN	2:14:47	28.	Kevin Beck, NH	2:24:25
12. Moses Tanui, KEN	**2:15:05**	29.	Yukinobu Nakazaki, JPN	2:25:01
13. Joao N'Tyamba, ANG	2:16:00	30.	Jamie Hibell, PA	2:25:17
14. Josh Cox, CA	2:16:17	43.	Simon Mpholo, RSA	2:26:41
15. Shem Koria, KEN	2:17:02	43.	John Mortimer, MA	2:29:55
16. Gezahegne Abera, ETH	2:17:04	841.	David Lavalle, MA	3:00:00
17. Elijah Lagat, KEN	**2:17:59**	3701.	Robert Larosa, MA	3:29:59
18. Motsehi Moketsana, RSA	2:18:13	**4590.**	**Keizo Yamada, JPN**	**3:39:32**
19. Mark Coogan, MA	2:18:58			**First 70+**
20. Makoto Ogura, JPN	2:20:24	6029.	John MDonough, MA	4:00:00
21. David Morris, NM	2:21:10	8592.	Charles DeFillipo, MA	5:59:51

Winning Men's Teams

1.   Leigh Valley Road Runners Club, 7:25:13
2.   Central Mass Striders, 7:35:03
3.   Boston Athletic Association, 7:46:11
4.   Atlanta Track Club, GA, 7:50:35
5.   Greater Boston Track Club, 7:59:26
6.   West Side Runners, NY, 8:02:10
7.   Bryn Mawr Running Club, PA, 8:09:24

Roba vs. Ndereba

MONDAY, APRIL 16, 2001

Catherine the Great

Catherine Ndereba was third born in a family of nine in Gatung'ang'a village, Nyeri district. Ndereba started athletics early in life and started competing while at Kahiraini primary school in Gatung'ang'a. By the time she finished her running career she would have a fine house in the former expats' affluent sub-urb, Karen, outside Nairobi—named for Karen von Blixen (the Danish writer, penname Isak Dinesen, featured in the book and film *Out of Africa*). But Ndere-ba would have a long road to run before taking up retirement.

In 1990 she joined Ngorano secondary school in Nyeri, specializing in the 3000m, and reached the national secondary schools finals. By the end of her secondary school education, she had attracted attention from several teams and Kenya Prisons moved in, recruiting her in 1994. She met her future husband Anthony Maina at Kenya Prisons training college. In 1995, Ndereba won 13 of her 18 races.

Ndereba returned in 1998 after taking time off for the birth of her daughter and, in 1999, ran the world's fastest times at 5k (15:09), 15k (48:52), 12k (38:37), and 10 miles (53:07). She also represented Kenya at the World Half Marathon championships, winning an individual bronze medal and playing a part in team gold. She made her debut in the Boston Marathon in 1998 finishing 6th (2:28:27) and in November in New York she finished 2nd (2:27:35).

Ndereba came back this year to Boston as defending champion. In the words of Toni Reavis, Ndereba went through her requisite pre-race assignments with an elegance, grace, and contentment that masked a steely determination. But of course she was not the only racer with steely determination, iron will, or just plain brass.

The day gave the field a 53°F with a slight N/NE wind. At 4 miles, 6 women ran under 2:26 pace. Ludmila Petrova of Russia, the 1995 London Marathon winner Malgorzata Sobanska of Poland, Nderba's good friend Lornah Kiplagat hot off her world record half marathon at Lisbon of 1:06:34, Honolulu Marathon course record holder Luybov Morgunova of Russia, and Ndereba and Roba. The two previous Boston winners and fierce rivals from different countries wore identical uniforms from their sponsor, Nike, and wore bid numbers FI and F2. Battles between Kenyans and Ethiopians always prove to be merciless.

For miles, the pace flowed leisurely enough that any of the front-runners might have had a chance. At one point, Morgunova veered off to a water station and came back to find herself in front. So closely were they grouped that Russia's Ludmila Petrova took a tumble near the 16-mile mark when someone clipped her heel. "This was not an impressive pace," observed Sobanska, who led for most of the first 15 miles. "It was comfortable for me." In such luxury they all passed the half marathon checkpoint. It was comfortable for everybody, until Ndereba decided to make it uncomfortable for everybody.

Later Ndereba revealed, "I just wanted to maintain a pace of 5:30 to 5:33 in the first half and then push it in the second half." That first half went in 1:13:05. In 1983 Benoit had been 1:08:43 at the half. But the fashion of marathon racing had turned to negative splitting—run the second half faster than the first.

She and Roba took the lead running downhill into Newton Lower Falls. Then at 16 miles, Ndereba disappeared from sight of the lead vehicle. She had stopped to retie her shoe. But although the press noticed, it seemed the pack did not and no one surged at that moment. She caught back up and joined Roba, matching strides as well as Nike uniforms into the turn at the fire station.

"When Catherine ran, it was too fast," conceded Sobanska, who would run a personal best by 48 seconds but lose sight of Ndereba by Newton City Hall.

Roba felt that she had gone hard too soon last year and planned to wait until later in the race like 22 or 23 miles to break away. But she never got that far. Ndereba pushed up the hills. She ran her last half marathon in 1:10:48, 5 seconds faster that Pippig's record form 1994.

"Once she made that gap between myself and herself, I was not going to make it," conceded Roba, who was thwarted again in her bid to become the first woman to win Boston four times. "I was a little weak today," said Roba. "I wasn't in very good condition. It just so happened I couldn't make it."

"I was capable," said Ndereba, who ran the second half of the race in 1:10:53 and whose time was the 7th-fastest in race history. "I was feeling like my body was responding. I had the confidence I can move at the same speed until the finish."

She did not say that she felt sweet revenge toward the Kenyan bureaucrats who refused to select her for the team for Sydney last year after she'd won in Boston. She vowed (not out loud) to extract sweet revenge without fail and to prevail.

"I want something special," said Catherine, who had garnered the nickname Catherine the Great. "To hold a world record."

Something else special was Bobbi Gibb, who came to run to celebrate 35 years since her first run and to call attention to Mass General Hospital that cared for a friend who had died of cancer in the early 1990s. She vowed she would finish the race no matter what, but early reports came in that she had dropped out. Fighting a case of bronchitis, Gibb had trouble on Heartbreak Hill, according to her running partner [Ed Rice], and dropped out at a Red Cross aid station at mile 21. After the medical vehicle in which she was getting a ride made several other stops, the determined Gibb asked to be let back out where she had gotten in. She resumed running and crossed the finish line at 6:40 p.m., 40 minutes after the official clock was turned off.

2001 Women's Results

1. **Catherine Ndereba, KEN**	2:23:53	13. Gitte Karlshoj, DEN	2:36:36,
2. Malgorzata Sobanska, POL	2:26:42		First Master
3. Lyubov Morgunova, RUS	2:27:18	14. Jill Gaitenby, RI	2:36:45,
4. Lornah Kiplagat, KEN	2:27:56	15. Susannah Beck, OR	2:37:12
5. **Fatuma Roba, ETH**	**2:28:08**	16. Shireen Crumpton, NZL	2:40:25
6. Irina Timofeyeva, RUS	2:28:50	17. Rachel Hopkins-Cook, MA	2:41:00
7. Ludmila Petrova, RUS	2:29:23	18. Beth Whitney, RI	2:41:42
8. Wei Yanan, CHN	2:29:52	19. Gordon Bakoulis, NY	2:43:16
9. Bruna Genovese, ITA	2:30:39	20. Rosa Gutierrez, OR	2:43:18
10. Kaori Tanabe, JPN	2:31:31	21. Mai Tagami, JPN	2:43:37
11. Albina Galliamova, NM	2:32:45	22. Josette Colomb-Janin, FRA	2:44:39
12. Zhang Shujing, CHN	2:33:43	23. Gabrielle O'Rourke, NZL	2:44:53
		24. Meghan Arbogast, OR	2:45:52

25. Lori Stich-Zimmerman, OR	2:46:35	46. Marge Belliusle, RI	3:00:18
26. Maribel Burgos, PR	2:47:16	474. Dona Cimino, IL	3:30:01
27. Lee DiPietro, MD	2:47:40	2460. Cori Book, NM	4:00:01
28. Jeanne Hennessy, NY	2:49:50	4814. Nicole Harris, MA	5:59:49
29. Mary Sweeney, GA	2:49:53	**Bobbi Gibb, MA**	**6:40 (unofficial)**
30. Gillian Horovitz, NY	2:50:26		

Women's Winning Teams

1. Bears Running Club, NY, 8:48:22
2. Greater Boston Track Club, 8:59:47
3. Boston Athletic Association, 9:06:15
4. Atlanta Track Club, GA, 9:55:21
5. Forerunners Track Club, FL, 9:55:46
6. Central Mass Striders, 9:59:40
7. Greater New York Racing Team, 10:00:15
8. Central Park Track Club, 10:01:07

Is Their Security Enough?

MONDAY, APRIL 15, 2002

Kenya Team Comes to Fight Back

The terrorist attacks on the World Trade Center on September 11 of the previous year would not leave anyone's mind. The city of Boston symbolized freedom, as the birth of the American Revolution and the marathon celebrated that on Patriots Day. Logic led dark thinkers to expect a terrorist attack on the marathon. The original name for what we call the Boston Marathon was the American Marathon. It was founded by BAA members to be the American contribution to the sport after the first modern Olympic Marathon in 1896. The marathon always did have a political and military component to it, but generally sports, and especially the Olympic Games, promote peace. The Boston Marathon is an offspring of the Olympics, yet its origins require that authorities consider it a possible target for terrorists. They did. About 15,000 police were set to guard the competitors and fans, assisted by 415 National Guard troops, 1,500 law enforcement personnel, and a sizable contingent of emergency medical workers. Three police helicopters flew over the course.

The race had always been closely monitored—mostly to intervene in cases of rowdiness or drunken incivility—officials increased their vigilance following the September 11 terrorist attacks. "Obviously, things have changed since [Sept. 11]," said Secretary of Public Safety James Jajuga. "Public Safety has to stay vigilant and alert, more than ever."

Jajuga planned to spend race day in the Framingham bunker alongside representatives of 36 state, federal, and local agencies, including police and fire departments, MassHighway, and the MBTA. For the first time, the FBI had joined Massachusetts in protecting runners and spectators.

Many police would be undercover, said Deputy Superintendent Charles Cellucci. That includes 300 off-duty police who are running in the marathon but have been asked to react in the case of an emergency. Specialized units have been trained to respond to chemical or biological terrorism.

Yet the possibility of a terrorist attack on the marathon itself did not occupy the minds of spectators or competitors—just the dark thinkers. Most people thought it could never happen at the Marathon. The race occupied their minds.

Nothing dark occupied the mind of the defending champ Lee Bong-Ju. But perhaps Lee had a distraction. He planned to marry the following Sunday. Surely he would like to give her another Boston victory as a wedding gift . . . with the $80,000 first place prize money.

Silvio Guerra, having finished 2nd twice, wondered . . . might this be his time? He said, "If I can win the race this time, it will be . . . a big impact." He hopes to become the first South American winner here since Colombia's Alvaro Mejia in 1971. "The Kenyans are the best, but there are other people who can do it."

Venezuelan runner Luis Fonseca came to race. But the Kenyan men would yield nothing to South Americans and did not want to yield to a Korean again. Rodgers Rop said, "Our goal is to make sure we win." He finished 3rd in his marathon debut in New York last autumn. "We are now fighting back to reclaim our title." The fickle New England weather might defeat them all with a forecast scheduled to reach the 80°F. But as with the weather, things don't always follow predictions.

A little rain stopped in the morning and a 50°F foggy mist remained. The fog lifted but clouds remained for the day. The temperature would not go into the 60°F. But as predicted Kenyans formed the majority of the lead pack. An ever-game and popular 6'3" Elly Rono took the early pace. He attended the University of Southern Indiana where he was an NCAA Division II champion in cross country, the indoor 5000m, and the outdoor 10,000m. He had run a 1:06:35 half marathon in Naples, Florida, in January, so he was fit, but not favored to contend. He said later, "I wanted to get myself out there for all to see."

It took until halfway for the pack following Rono, often called a gentle giant, to decide that the weather was not going to turn warm. The giant posted a big 1:05:19.

Rodgers Rop made a push at the half, but most of the pack came back. He tried again at an aid station at 25k when his competition had split apart to identify their specially marked drinks. While the drinks distracted them, Rop scooted away. Fred Kiprop and Chelang'a went with Rop, and shortly others caught back up, Christopher Cheboiboch and Elias Chebet. It was an all-Kenyan party. But at 30k, 5 of them pulled a 4:38 mile to make the separation clean.

Mbarak Hussein, the younger brother of two-time winner Ibrahim, said, "Coming up the hills, the pack put in some really tough surges. I let them go. I thought they'd come back, but they didn't." Approaching Heartbreak Hill, Rop surged again with a 4:44 mile. Only Cheboiboch stayed with him. Rop kept surging like a prize fighter making little jabs to wear out the opponent. But after opening a gap, Cheboiboch came back again and again. He just would not lie down on the mat and take the count. Through Cleveland Circle and all along Beacon Street this "punching" continued. Not until 1 mile to go at Kenmore Square did Cheboibohe seem to drop back. But not too much. He was known for a deadly kick. Perhaps he held this knockout punch for Boylston Street. He kicked hard after Rop down the corridor of wild cheering. The gap shrunk by seconds, but the race ended with 3 to go. Cheboiboch said, "I thought I was still strong. I thought I could still catch him. But it was fine with me."

Lee Bong-Ju left Boston to go marry Kim Mi-soon in front of 20,000 people at Seoul's Olympic stadium in a ceremony that would be broadcast on national TV.

2002 Men's Race

1. **Rodgers Rop, KEN**	2:09:02	14. Fedor Ryzhov, RUS	2:13:04
2. Christopher Cheboiboch, KEN	2:09:05	15. Keith Dowling, VA	2:13:28
		16. Elly Rono, NC	2:15:17
3. Fred Kiprop, KEN	2:09:45	17. Clint Verran, MI	2:15:19
4. Mbarak Hussein, KEN	2:09:45	18. Noriaki Igarashi, JPN	2:15:55
5. **Lee Bong-Ju, KOR**	2:10:30	19. Mark Coogan, MA	2:17:35
6. Elias Chebet, KEN	2:10:40	20. Kazuaki Wakimoto, JPN	2:17:58
7. Simon Bor, KEN	2:11:39	54. Mark Cucuzzella, CO	2:30:00
8. Getachew Kebede, ETH	2:11:39	911. Dick Beardsley, MN	2:58:48
9. Luis Fonseca, VEN	2:11:49	1025. Peter Cooper, MI	3:00:00:
10. Silvio Guerra, ECU	2:12:28	4271. Patrick Dunleavy, PA	3:30:00
11. Joshua Chelang'a, KEN	2:12:40	7545. **Keizo Yamada, JPN**	**3:57:49**
12. Joshua Kipkemboi, MA	2:12:48, First Master	6673. Primo Jazbec, SLO	4:00:02
		7081. Bill Billing, CT	4:08:01
13. David Busienei Kiptum, KEN	2:13:04	9234. Michael Welsh, MA	7:58:31

Winning Men's Teams:

1.   Boston Athletic Association, 7:25:52
2.   Greater Lowell Road Runners, 7:29:22
3.   Central Mass Striders, 7:34:03

Ndereba the Great Returns

MONDAY, APRIL 15, 2002

Looking for a Little Respect

Catherine "the Great" Ndereba came back to Boston crowned by the press and pundits as the overwhelming favorite. She had run 2:18:47 to set the world record at the Chicago marathon last fall so who could possibly challenge her? Roba was not back and neither was Loroupe. Naoko Takahashi, who set a short-lived world record a month before Ndereba of 2:19:46, was not coming to Boston. There was no one else . . . or was there? To find out is why we have races, not just to coronate royalty. Predictions were that hot weather would rule the race, but it never arrived so cool conditions allowed for fast running. John Powers of the *Boston Globe* wrote before the race about Ndereba, "Should she take teammates Wanjiru and Okayo with her ahead of Ethiopia's Elfenesh Alemu and Romania's Nuta Olaru, the Kenyans will become the first country to sweep the women's medals since the Americans (Lisa Larsen-Weidenbach, Lynne Huntington, and Karen Dunn) did it in 1985, the last year before prize money was offered."

But on the world stage, economically ascendant China desperately wanted a little marathon respect. As the most populous country in the world they likely had an equally ascendant runner. They again sent Sun Yingjie to shine for them. She had the experience at Boston. She placed 8th in 2000. Now she wanted her notch in marathon history.

But Margaret Okayo had beaten Roba at the San Diego Marathon last June. Roba had beaten Ndereba. Marathons don't work like logical syllogisms, but there is a hard logic to marathon racing.

The pack at halfway at 1:10:40 contained Okaya, Ndereba, Sun Yingjie, and Ethiopian Elfenesh Alemu. Under the low clouds in the cool air, conditions were good for running fast. Paula Radcliffe had won the London Marathon in 2:18:55 only the day before. Faster would be better.

Suddenly Sun Yingjie shocked the field with a 5-minute mile down into Newton Lower Falls. Ndereba passed her back and Okayo joined her. They ran in lockstep. The two Kenyans pushed up the incline up from Newton Lower Falls over Rt 128 (I95). When Okayo's coach, Dr. Gabriele Rosa, saw this, he thought Okayo had pushed foolishly hard to stay with Ndereba.

Ndereba seemed confused by water stations earlier in the race. She was in front on the right side of the course just before the Mile 13 marker, with China's Sun Yingjie close behind, when she came to the next water station. Ndereba ran over to the station and seemed to pause, picking up her bottle. Yingjie snatched up hers and passed Ndereba. Later Ndereba and Okayo would be seen randomly switching sides of the road. After taking the lead, Okayo kept running from one side of the course to the other, with Ndereba usually following. Between Route 128 and Boston College, the two switched sides nine times.

Asked about the switching, Okayo said, "I was crossing over because I was looking for water." Boston Athletic Association official Jack Fleming said elite water stations are set according to number, odds on one side of the course, evens on the other. Okayo, who wore #6, retrieved water on the right. Ndereba, who wore #1, retrieved water on the left. He said the move is to avoid pileups at elite stations. Sometimes those little things are hard to remember when all the blood drains from the brain to the legs. Observers like Dr. Rosa waited for Ndereba to make her big move. But Okayo was not waiting. She was running.

Later Okayo said, "I knew that even if she [passes and] finishes with a 2:21, I would finish with a 2:22, so she was helping me," said Okayo. Runners do sense where other runners are by the sound of footsteps and breathing and by timing the rise of the next wave of cheering. You don't have to look. "I never looked back to see where Catherine was," said Okayo. "I was just focused on running my own race."

"The last mile, I had problems with my right hamstring," said Ndereba. "I didn't want to push anymore." Okayo ran that crucial mile in 5:12. She ran alone down Boylston Street to a 58-second course record beating the one set by Uta Pippig. Ndereba also broke the 1994 one.

Soon after finishing, Ndereba sought Okaya and gave her a warm hug. It was sisterly, not a brief, perfunctory post-race embrace. Catherine the Great looked triumphant. "I was happy that Margaret won," she said. "I'm not discouraged. I'm very happy and very proud that my fellow Kenyan athlete won. We are on the same team."

"I am very happy with my [time]. My aim was to break the course record, and I did it," she said. Commonly Kenyans, unlike runners from other countries, genuinely feel and express joy in the success of their compatriots. Envy and jealousy seem not to be a part of their cultural upbringing.

"She is my fellow Kenyan athlete," said Ndereba. She apparently held no animus toward her homeland for leaving her off the 2000 Olympic team. "I felt proud to hear the national anthem, if not for me then for Margaret. Our anthem was still being played."

"I couldn't push," Ndereba explained. "As we were going, I could see Margaret was strong, and I was just feeling OK. If Margaret won, it would have been much better."

"I'm very happy to have set the course record. I didn't expect it," said Okayo. "The course was fine, even if it was a hard course. I came to Boston looking for respect as a runner and I felt I got it," said Okayo. "I knew that I trained well for me to run well."

"There was a lot of pressure on me," Ndereba said. "Not just from the media and back home, but from the other competitors. They were all looking at me."

Many years later in 2016, Kenyan police would hold Federico Rosa, son of Dr. Gabriele, on various doping-related charges. Whether the charges had any validity or were products of common Kenyan corruption has not been decided. But cases against Sun Yingjie were brought and closed.

In October 2002, she won her 2nd straight Beijing Marathon title with terrific time of 2:21:21.

Sun Yingjie times in 2005 Helsinki improved from the 2004 summer Olympics in Athens; she placed 11th in 5000m (14:51.19) and 7th in 10,000m (30:33.53); she had previously run 15:07:23 and 30:54:37. She won her 4th Beijing Marathon in the even better time of 2:21:01. The after-competition drug test came back negative. Two days later she raced in Nanjing, finishing 2nd in 10,000m behind Xing Huina in the Chinese National Games. Following the race, she tested positive in a drug test and was banned from competing for two years and disqualified from the 10,000m. Her two-year ban was upheld despite a civil court ruling that another athlete, Yu Haijiang, had spiked her drink with androsterone.

2000 Women's Race

1.	**Margaret Okayo, KEN**	**2:20:43***	18.	Ayumi Noshita, JPN	2:44:47
2.	**Catherine Ndereba, KEN**	**2:21:12**	19.	Kelly Keeler, MN	2:45:00
3.	Elfenesh Alemu, ETH	2:26:01	20.	Cathi Campbell, MA	2:46:17
4.	Sun Yingjie, CHN	2:27:26	21.	Carol LeGate, WI	2:47:57
5.	Firaya Sultanova-		22.	Laura Hruby, PA	2:48:49
	Zhdanova, RUS	2:27:58,	23.	Kristen Till, MD	2:48:52
		First Master	24.	Heather Gardiner, CT	2:49:39
6.	Bruna Genovese, ITA	2:29:02	25.	Monique Maddy, MA	2:50:10
7.	Nuta Olaru, ROU	2:30:26	26.	Maryse LeGallo, FRA	2:50:20
8.	Mai Tagami, JPN	2:32:00	27.	Lisa Valentine, FL	2:51:04
9.	Gitte Karlshoj, DEN	2:35:01	28.	Cheri Rosenblatt, NC	2:51:31
10.	Yukari Komatsu, JPN	2:35:34	29.	Nancy Corsaro, MA	2:53:13
11.	Jackie Gallagher, AUS	2:35:46	30.	Katrina Blanch, CAN	2:53:19
12.	Irina Timofeyeva, RUS	2:36:47	35.	Gillian Horovitz, NY	2:54:29
13.	Jill Gaitenby, MA	2:38:55	47.	Nikki Kimball, NY	3:00:10
14.	Gordon Bakoulis, NY	2:42:47	554.	Jane Gillham, NY	3:00:01
15.	Norimi Sakurai, JPN	2:43:09	2707.	Anne Hope, NV	4:00:00
16.	Janelle Burgmann, AUS	2:43:46	5339.	Stephanie Woolwich-	
17.	Esther Wanjiru, KEN	2:44:32		Holzman, VT	5:59:51

Women's Winning Teams

1.   Boston Athletic Association, 8:44:43
2.   Forerunners, FL, 8:50:10
3.   Central Mass Striders, 8:50:45
4.   Cambridge Running Club, 9:01:44
5.   Baltimore Running Coalition, 9:10:42
6.   Green Bay Runnaways, MN, 9:17:09
7.   Whirlaway Running Team, 9:24:43

Weapons of Mass Destruction

MONDAY, APRIL 21, 2003

Grand Marshall, John Adelbert Kelley

The U.S. invaded Iraq on March 19. The invasion continued during the marathon. In announcing the invasion President George W. Bush said, "At this hour, American and coalition forces are in the early stages of military operations to disarm Iraq, to free its people and to defend the world from grave danger." But during this time of war, the Boston Marathon proved to be good and peaceful business for the city.

CEO of the Greater Boston Convention & Visitors Bureau, Patrick Moscaritolo said that the direct and indirect economic impact to Greater Boston is $74.2 million. Almost 1,200 media personnel form 259 media outlets covered the marathon. In terms of media credentials, the Boston Marathon ranks behind only the Super Bowl as the largest single-day sporting event in the world. Four Red Sox baseball games are included in the money figure.

Two F-15 fighter jets again flew over the start to commemorate Patriots Day. The country, as comfortable as it was, was still at war. Kenyan young men came to Boston to do battle.

A few days before the race, reporters asked Rodgers Rop, "Can anyone not from Kenya win this race?" The rest of the Kenyan invaders sat around him. "No," he concluded matter-of-factly. "I don't think. If their mission was to intimidate the competition, well, that mission was accomplished."

This time 27-year-old Rop was only the third-fastest Kenyan to arrive. Both 26-year-old Vincent Kipsos (2:06:52 in Berlin last year) and 32-year-old Benjamin Kosgei Kimutai (2:07:26 in Amsterdam last year) have faster personal bests. "Rop is one of the favorites for sure," said Guerra, who is back again. "But there are other Kenyans with the same level." Besides Rop, who ran 2:08:07 when he had won New York the previous autumn, seven Kenyans had broken 2:10, as had Italy's Giacomo Leone (2:07:52), Estonia's Pavel Loskutov (2:08:53), Tanzania's John Nada Saya (2:08:57), and Guerra (2:09:49).

At the noon time gun, the men bolted out after the women who had started ahead of them for the first time. The 29-minute lead would allow for the press to follow the women's pack without risk to the men and would isolate the women competitors from any men who incidentally ran at the same pace and allow the women to see their competition.

Vincent Kipsos took the pace out rapidly. He ran at course-record pace for the first 10 miles, and why not? His 2:06:52 was tops in the field. It was cool and maybe his obligation to take the lead and set an example for his countrymen.

His 4:49 first mile gave him a 40-yard lead. He kept leading by as much as 80 meters. He passed 10k in 30:26. Two 40-plus-year-old competitors ran in the pack. Russian Fedor V. Ryzhov and American Eddy Hellebuyck born in Deinze Oost Vlaanderen, Belgium, had run 2:11:53 on London in 1996. These "old" men were the only non-Kenyans contending. But the day turned warm and windy and Kipsos began to suffer. He was not interested in running a slow race. By halfway in at 1:05:06 the pack closed on him twice. He no longer ran sub 2:07 pace, but managed to surge a little faster than the pack was willing to match. Twice he did that. But on the third time, the pack consumed him. Shortly he bailed out. "I can see I am going to run a poor time," said Kipsos, "so I decide to leave."

Now Rop took over looking strong and confident. Timothy Cherigat, Robert Cheryiyot, Benjamin Kimutai, and Christopher Cheboiboch looked good too.

The dead air turned into a headwind and the temperature, predicted to be around 60, climbed to 70, and the race became a survival test rather than a speed test. On the hills Cheruiyot and his friend Benjamin Kosgei Kimuta led looking smooth. By the time they arrived at the Newton hills, the pack dwindled to six: Kimutai, Rop, Cheruiyot, Lel, Cherigat, and Cheboiboch. The other guys ran behind, surviving, waiting. Rop sensed he was done. "I don't know what happened." Cheruiyot, who'd won his only other marathon outing (2:08:59) last December in Milan, said later, "When I was at 25 kilometers, (I said to myself) *Okay, I will win this.*"

But the pair crested the hills together passing 20 miles in 1:39:50. Cheruiyot threw in a couple of 4:50 miles without looking back. He then ran on alone without Kimuta. He began to enjoy himself. He waved the victory V sign to the crowds. He said, "This [was] my second marathon. I enjoyed it because I like the way people give encouragement along the way. They are happy about Africans. I like that very much." But he kept looking back behind, but did not seem to be slowing. When asked why he looked back, he said, "I was looking for my friend, [Benjamin Kosgei Kimutai], I was expecting him to be behind me." As Cheruiyot ran he looked over his shoulder, waiting for Kimutai's challenge. But Kimutai could not join his friend. "I had nothing to offer," said Kimutai. When asked about how he felt with 2 miles to go, he said "I could see he was 100 meters from me. So I was thinking, *Let me keep my position.*"

With 5 miles to go, Cheruiyot pushed hard. He threw in a blazing 4:37 mile coming down the other side past Boston College, opening a 30-meter lead over Kimutai running beside the quiet cemetery before Cleveland Circle. Cheruiyot said, "If somebody goes in front of me, I am ready to defend and be with him, "

"It is very nice to win this marathon, because you make your name in your country." Cheruiyot owes a farm and supermarket in the Nandi District. He collected an $80,000 paycheck.

In 2004, when Eddie Hellebuyck was 43 and his 25-year running career was enjoying a sudden, blazing renaissance, he failed an out-of-competition drug test administered by the United States Anti-Doping Agency (USADA). He contested the results, which showed that he had used the banned substance erythropoietin (EPO), but his plea did not stand. In December 2004 he was issued a two-year suspension. After six years he admitted that he had cheated. Such offenses, suspicion of such offenses, testing, and denials will haunt the rest of this narrative. Like the politics of war, sports is sometimes not what it seems at first to be.

2003 Men's Results

1. **Robert Kipkoech**		17. Ken Pliska, MA	2:30:12
Cheruiyot, KEN	**2:10:11**	18. Robert Dickie, HI	2:30:21
2. Benjamin Kosgei Kimutai,		19. James Lander, MI	2:30:25
KEN	2:10:34	20. Daniel Feldman, CA	2:30:27
3. Martin Lel, KEN	2:11:11	21. Eric Beauchesne, MA	2:31:27
4. **Timothy Cherigat, KEN**	**2:11:28**	22. Michael Danahy, NJ	2:32:03
5. Christopher Cheboiboch,		23. Lowell Ladde, MA	2:32:34
KEN	2:12:45	24. Jeffery Day, OH	2:32:55
6. Fedor V. Ryzhov, RUS	2:15:29,	25. Jason Bodnar, FL	2:32:57
First Master		26. Todd Snyder, PA	2:33:05
7. **Rodgers Rop, KEN**	**2:16:14**	27. Matt Pelletier, RI	2:33:22
8. David Kiptum Busiene, KEN	2:16:16	28. Damien Angus, MA	2:33:34
9. Elly Rono, KEN	2:17:00	29. Nicholas Iauco, NC	2:33:46
10. Laban Kipkemboi, KEN	2:17:50	30. David Williams, WI	2:34:24
11. Silvio Guerra, ECU	2:18:31	557. Paul Miller, MI	3:00:00
12. Karl Johan Rasmussen, NOR	2:18:55	3298. Bill Greer, MI	3:30:00
13. Salvatore Bettiol, ITA	2:22:06	6555. Ruben Garcia, TX	4:00:00
14. Diego Colorado, COL	2:23:59	6886. **Amby Burfoot, PA**	**4:03:37**
15. Wieslaw Perzke, POL	2:29:00	7379. **Keizo Yamada, JPN**	**4:10:11**
16. Guennadi Temikov, TUS	2:29:59	10728. Jason Pisano, RI	7:42:55

Winning Men's Teams

1. Greater Lowell Road Runners, MA, 7:47:46
2. Westside Runners, NY, 8:00:03
3. Omaha Running Club, NE, 8:04:42
4. Boston Athletic Association, 8:12:25
5. Greater Boston Track Club, 8:20:36
6. Front Line Racing Team, MI, 8:23:01
7. Bowerman Athletic Club, OR, 8:23:45

From Russian with Love

MONDAY, APRIL 21, 2003

Record Holder Back to Defend

"Margaret has shown herself to be exceptional," acknowledged Marla Runyan, the top American hope here after running a startling 2:27:10 in her 26-mile debut at New York last year. "If she brings her A-game . . ."

Well, that was the question. Last year Okayo did bring her A-game, but a year had passed. She may have had an A+ game . . . or not. "She is the defending champion, but that was a year ago," said countrywoman Esther Kiplagat, who beat Okayo in New York. "Anybody can win this." Maybe that runner would come from Russia?

Svetlana Vladimirovna Zakharova never had an A-game. She had come to Boston in 1997 and finished 15th with a time of 2 hours, 39 minutes, 59 seconds. She was not happy with that and didn't want to ever come back to Boston where she had had such a miserable experience. She said, "It was a very difficult experience. It was a very difficult recovery after that race. I wasn't ready to run such a big race and prestigious marathon. It was difficult to make this decision to come to Boston." But here she was with her coach and without a resume including a win at a major marathon. She had won the Honolulu Marathon twice, but that is a good, but not major marathon. She ran 2:21:31 in Chicago last year for 4th place. She has been quite prolific, tough, and consistent. At London she took 2nd twice in 2:24:04 and the next year 2002, 2:22:31. But running well is one thing and winning is another.

With Ndereba missing (she was 2nd in London a week earlier), Okayo is clearly the favorite. But if cool weather descends and the Newton hills aggravate the back problems that bothered her in New York, Okayo may not be able to defend. Or Okayo's Kenyan teammate Joyce Chepchumba, the Olympic bronze medalist, may be the one.

"My goal is to improve my time and place," says Runyan, who was 4th in New York, "which means I'd like to be top three here." Runyan, who is legally blind, would have a cyclist riding alongside her.

Okayo took off at the gun. It seemed the course record holder wanted to break her own record. She zoomed through 5k in 16:45. But that was in fact slower than course record time. Zakharova ran 23 seconds behind her at 10k. Okayo again had problems with her back. Zakharova, like most competitors, is a keen observer of her competition. She had run against Okayo when she ran her best, winning NYC. "I noticed that Margaret was running a little different this year," Zakharova said. "I ran against her in New York in 2001, and I was confident that I was in better shape this time. I saw that Margaret fell back and tried catch up again, and that's probably not the way to do it. I had a lot of confidence that I would be able to overtake Margaret, especially on the hard part of the course. So I wasn't really concerned about Margaret or any of the other runners."

So Zakharova began to push at 10k. "Most of my races have been different strategy than this race," Zakharova said. "For this race, my coach and I decided to accelerate after the point and push as hard as I could through the difficult parts." Runyan and the other Russian, Lyubov Denisova, made the pack of four through 15k. Zakharova continued her experimental strategy by surging at 12 miles. That lost Runyan and Denisova. With Okayo the two passed the halfway in 1:12:39. On the insidious hill over Rt 128 up from Newton Lower Falls it was Okayo who threw in a surge. After the race Zakharova would say, "It was an interesting battle with Margaret."

As the runners picked up the pace, the wind picked up. Smaller Okayo did not hide behind the taller runner to shield from the wind. Then past the turn by the fire house, Zakharova surged again, snatching 2 seconds by 25k. But as Okayo seemed to have paid for her early pace, she said later, "I think I started a little fast," Zakharova began to pay. Denisova, who had not be playing the surge game, watched from 21 seconds back, but then found herself gaining on the tiring runners ahead. She caught them and briefly took the lead. But they would not give it up. Runyan gave up her position to Joyce Chepchumba. "I wasn't feeling so good until after the half marathon," she explained later. Zakharova pushed to the front as Okayo continued chasing up Heartbreak Hill, but that broke Okayo. She began her slide back into the pack. "I had a cramp [in her side and calf] at the 16- to 17-mile point," said Runyan. Denisova had no such problem. After passing Okayo, Denisova moved right behind Zakharova at 19 miles and made her move at the base of Heartbreak Hill. Denisova put on a major push, running a 5:40 split to take the lead.

Denisova thought, "There was a possibility that I could win the race." But Zakharova had more tricks left. She threw down a 5:37 mile on the hill. Then she ran alone. To cement the trickery, she squeezed out a 5:19 mile at mile 23. That opened a 35-second gap.

After the win, reporters asked Svetlana Zakharova if she was concerned about Denisova after she overtook her for the lead at the 21-mile mark.

Zakharova paused. She leaned into the microphone and replied: "*Chestno govorya, nyet*," meaning, "Honestly speaking, no."

When Zakharova's comments were relayed to Denisova, she said about the well-trained winner. "I didn't think I could beat Svetlana today." Zakharova trains in the mountains. "We don't train together," said Denisova, who trained near her home in Moscow. The two, however, seemed to derive little national pride from the feat. They did not gloat that they had defeated the Kenyans. They seemed most gracious in victory. "Not just the Russians," Zakharova said, "but all the women prepared equally hard for the race."

"Now I'm No. 1," said Zakharova, who also was $80,000 richer. "And I know this course is not something I cannot run. I'm very happy and just overwhelmed at this moment. It just happened here that the Russian women ran stronger," she said. "I don't really know how to explain why we did better. Maybe because it's a difficult course and the Russian women, we like to go through the difficulties. Maybe that's the reason."

2003 Women's Results:

1. Svetlana Zakharova, RUS	2:25:20		17. Lisa Valentine, FL	2:50:52
2. Lyubov Denisova, RUS	2:26:51		18. Sharon Stubler, NM	2:51:41
3. Joyce Chepchumba, KEN	2:27:20		19. Heather May, IN	2:53:33
4. Margaret Okayo, KEN	2:27:39		20. Lee DiPetro, MD	2:55:00
5. Marla Runyan, USA	2:30:28		21. Shannon Hovey, CT	2:55:57
6. Albina Ivanova, RUS	2:30:57		22. Kristin Pierce Barry, VA	2:57:36
7. Firaya Sultanova-			23. Elizabeth Seeley, PA	2:58:24
Zhdanova, RUS	2:31:30,		24. Jane Johnson, FL	2:58:47
	First Master		25. Simonetta Piergentili, MA	2:58:51
8. Milena Glusac, USA	2:37:32		26. Lynn Dempsey, CAN	2:59:30
9. Jill Gaitenby, USA	2:38:19		27. Veena Reddy, PA	3:00:02
10. Esther Kiplagat, KEN	2:38:43		28. Kyla Barbour, GA	3:00:09
11. Gitte Karlshoj, DEN	2:40:52		29. Kimberly Duclos, MA	3:00:45
12. Emily Levan, ME	2:41:37		30. Christine Reaser, ME	3:00:59
13. Alysun Deckert, WA	2:47:19		363. Lisa Drew, AL	3:30:00
14. Maribel Burgos, PR	2:48:03		2239. Lene Poulsen, NY	3:59:59
15. Cori Mooney, ID	2:48:29		6302. Megan Robb, DC	6:04:07
16. Linda Smith Somers, CA	2:49:41			

Winning Women's Teams

1. Greater Lowell Road Runners, MA, 9:16:06
2. Whirlaway Racing Team, MA, 9:18:46
3. Central Mass Striders, 9:31:53
4. Boston Athletic Association, 9:40:45
5. Team Utopia, NY, 9:51:50
6. Atlanta Track Club, GA, 9:56:04
7. Cambridge Running Club, MA, 9:59:03

Can You Beat the Heat?

MONDAY, APRIL 19, 2004

Africans Have Heat Advantage?

John Powers writing for the *Boston Globe*, in the column "With Another Run for the Hoses" (referring to the 1976 race when temperatures on parts of the course reached 100°F), predicted for the 108th Boston Marathon temperatures were expected to be in the mid-80s. The Boston Athletic Association was advising the 20,000-plus starters to "run safely and smartly." Meaning, they should pace themselves sensibly and rehydrate frequently. "It'll be the Boston Massacre," said four-time champion Bill Rodgers.

Many marathon observers criticized the traditional noon start. The Boston Marathon is blessed by a rich tradition, but that richness also makes them resistant to change. Noon worked for over 100 years. So what if fickle New England weather presents an occasional scorcher? Some runners might welcome it.

"It will be good for us," said Ethiopian Hailu Negussiee, who has won three of the six marathons he's entered (including the Xiamen Marathon in China last year), is the man most likely to challenge the usual pack of Kenyans. "It will combine both the heat and the terrain. I think we [Ethiopians] are lucky."

"This race will be a mystery," said defending champ Robert Kipoech Cheruiyot. "The heat will affect the performance of each and every one of us," said Rodgers Rop. "We will not expect better times. I think everyone will be together."

The battle would likely be among most of the previous year's contenders: Cheruiyot, runner-up Benjamin Kosgei Kimutai, Martin Lel, Timothy Cherigat, and Rop—plus Negussie, who had the third fastest time (2:08:16) in the last two years.

When asked about getting boxed in by the Kenyans, "I'm not worried about that," said Negussie. "This has happened many times. We are used to it. We are careful, because we are small in numbers." This East African rivalry between Ethiopia and Kenya would play out in Boston many times.

All pre-race worries were not about the natural weather. Many people wondered about the growing number of cases of performance-enhancing drug use. The BAA planned to maintain use of the same drug-testing system they've run for several years: a urine sample taken at random from top finishers, looking for everything from steroids to hormones that increase endurance.

"My sense, and it's only a sense, is that marathoning in particular is as clean as any sport out there in the world," said Dave McGillivray, race director of the Boston Marathon. "I feel the amount of abuse is minuscule."

In long-distance running, finding any abuse that does exist can prove a daunting, and sometimes impossible, task. The drug that most worries officials in endurance sports is erythropoietin, or EPO, a potentially dangerous hormone that boosts the supply of red blood cells that carry oxygen to muscles and quickly passes from the system.

"I'm becoming more of a doomsayer given what we're seeing in baseball," said Jack Fultz, winner of the hot 1976 Boston Marathon. In the recent past, distance runners would inject a donor's blood to boost their reservoir of oxygen-laden red cells. Later, they began storing their own blood for re-injection months afterward. Called blood doping, the practice is banned by track and field federations.

Training at high altitude, which is not banned, increases red blood cells. This is because at high altitudes, lower air pressure does not allow the lungs to jam oxygen into red blood cells, so more blood cells with a proportionally greater surface area makes up for the lower air pressure.

In the late 1980s, for patients stricken with a type of anemia that is often related to kidney failure or cancer treatments, scientists developed a synthetic version of EPO. It worked marvelously, reversing anemia in patients. Athletes quickly recognized that it could help them, too.

"And in effect, it's very analogous with what you would see with blood doping," said Roger Fielding, a specialist in exercise physiology at Boston University's Sargent College of Health and Rehabilitation Sciences in a Boston Globe article. "By improving the oxygen-carrying capacity of your blood, it essentially can improve your ability to perform endurance-type activities like the marathon."

Widespread testing for EPO began at the Sydney Olympics in 2000 and spread to other elite athletic events, such as the Boston Marathon, said Rich Wanninger, spokesman for the United States Anti-Doping Agency. Neither marathon organizers nor the Anti-Doping Agency revealed precisely how many runners would be tested at the end of today's race, although race director Dave McGillivray said a certain segment of the top 15 men and top 15 women would be sampled, as well as a group of other runners.

"It's not 100 [who will be tested]," McGillivray said, "but it's also not two." Marathon officials said that it's not realistic to expect events to test every athlete, given that each test costs several hundred dollars.

The Globe article reported, "In a perfect world, you'd want to be testing those people weeks before the marathon," said Frank Uryasz, president of the National Center for Drug Free Sport, a testing company that works extensively with the NCAA. "But we don't live in a perfect world. Sometimes, the post-event test is the best we have."

Two former winners came to face each other: Rogers Rop from 2002 and Robert Kipkoech Cheruiyot. Stephen Kiogora and Jackson Kipng'ok led early, then the pack quickly dwindled to 8: Cherigat, Cheboror, Kiogora, defending champion Robert Kipkoech Cheruiyot, previous winner Rodgers Rop, last year's runner-up Benjamin Kosgei Kimutai, New York victor Martin Lel, and Ethiopia's Hailu Negussie. They passed the halfway in 1:05:30.

"I was really surprised," said Cherigat, who'd come to ruin last year trying to answer Cheruiyot's surge atop Heartbreak and finished 4th. "I thought he was a great challenge today. But he had dropped off, and I had to take advantage."

Shortly after the firehouse turn, starting up the hills, Cherigat and Rop ran alone in front.

Timothy Cherigat ran with ease in the midst of the pack.

Cherigat, who had run Boston twice before and finished 3rd in last fall's BAA half marathon, had that advantage. He knew what was up ahead and Cheboror did not.

"I was afraid to go forward," Cheboror said, "because I didn't know the course." At 16 miles that passed in 1:19:48, Timothy Cherigat decided to assert himself. But when he reached for his water bottle as Rop led the race he missed it, knocking it to the ground. Cherigat stopped to pick it up and drink. Then instead of conserving his energy by gradually rejoining the group, he charged

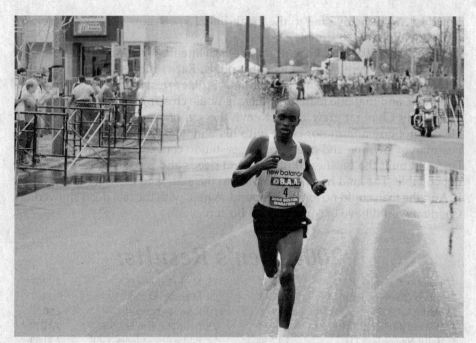

The town opened up the fire hydrants on this hot day to spray the runners. Timothy Cherigat #4.

up to the pack, through the middle of it and to the lead with Rop, and pushed the pace. That move reduced the pack to Lel, Cheboor, and Rop.

He threw in a very fast mile suddenly opening a 19-second lead cresting the hills with a 4:52 mile. Cheruiyot and Rop dropped out. Reported temperatures on the course reached 87°F.

Uta Pippig watched nervously on the monitors in the press room at the finish in the Copley Plaza Hotel.

"When I fell behind," said Cheboror, "it was too hard to catch up."

"I had to ensure that this year I came to Heartbreak Hill strong," Cherigat said, "so I could be able to race faster toward the finish. I trained for this move. I knew that if I made it, it would drive me to the finish line. I moved without much trouble."

Before Cleveland Circle, Cherigat seemed to run with ease. The sun beat down, but it did not seem to bother him. At Coolidge Corner, 2 miles from the finish, his lead was nearly a minute. By Kenmore Square, Cherigat might as well taking a victory lap.

Winning Boston is great, but the Kenyan selector would not pick Cherigat for the Kenyan Olympic team.

"You must respect the team that has been chosen," said Cherigat, who won an $80,000 prize. "Maybe I wait for my time, and it will come."

"Maybe I could have run faster," said Cherigat, "but I can't speak of that, because that's what the weather was today. I knew that the move I made, when

I made it, would drive me to the finish line. I knew how the guys were, so I moved without much trouble."

More than 1,100 entrants required medical attention during or after the race. More than 140 were taken to local hospitals. Race officials said two runners, whom they would not identify, went into cardiac arrest but were said to be out of danger, and that one man broke his leg while crossing the finish line.

Timothy Cherigat grew up in Kenya the son of an engineer, not a farmer. He did not buy a farm nor cattle with his winnings, but wanted to be a businessman by owning and operating a gas station convenience store. He bought land and built the business, but laws and deeds and records in Kenya are not dependable. The land had not belonged to the man who Cherigat had paid for it. And the man could no longer be found. A man with the real deed showed up. Cherigat would have to come back to Boston.

2004 Men's Results:

1. **Timothy Cherigat, KEN**	**2:10:37**	18. Mario Fattore, ITA	2:29:17
2. Robert Cheboror, KEN	2:11:49	19. Michael Wardian, VA	2:29:57
3. Martin Lel, KEN	2:13:38	20. John Mentzer, RI	2:30:50
4. Stephen Kiogora, KEN	2:14:34	21. Laban Kipkemboi, KEN	2:31:17
5. **Hailu Negussie, ETH**	**2:17:30**	22. Eddie Ernest-Jones, GBR	2:31:53
6. Benjamin Kosgei Kimutai, KEN	2:17:45	23. John Mirth, WI	2:32:32
7. Joshua Kipkemboi, KEN	2:18:23	24. Henry Wanyoike, KEN	2:33:20
8. Andrew Letherby, AUS	2:19:31	25. Hiroaki Taskeda, JPN	2:33:22
9. Fedor V. Ryzhov, RUS	2:21:24, First Master	26. Ryan Lindin, MI	2:33:32
		27. Brian Spangerberg, CA	2:33:57
10. Elly Rono, KEN	2:22:45	28. Minoru Isono, JPN	2:34:07
11. Alexander Prokopchuk, LAT	2:23:48	29. Jason Saitta, CO	2:34:14
12. Wilson Komen, KEN	2:24:06	30. Jesse Williams, VA	2:34:38
13. Christopher Zieman, CA	2:25:45	299. John Gleeson, HN	3:00:00
14. Salvatore Bettiol, ITA	2:26:15	1719. Doug Reimer, NJ	3:30:01
15. Kentarou Suzuki, JPN	2:27:15	4412. Gilbert Martinez, CA	4:00:00
16. Dawit Trfe, ETH	2:27:54	10496. Brendan Sullivan, MA	6:45:19
17. Eric Post, VA	2:29:13		

Winning Men's Teams

1. Pacers Racing Team, VA, 7:58:58
2. Greater Lowell Road Runners, MA, 8:07:03
3. Boston Athletic Association, 8:08:07
4. Greater Boston Track Club, 8:11:46
5. Moose Milers and Marathoners, NH, 8:19:56
6. Westside Runners, NY, 8:29:42
7. United States Air Force, AA, 8:30:19

No Top Americans

MONDAY, APRIL 19, 2004

Heat Will Be the Foe

For the first time ever in 2004, the invited women would start 29 minutes ahead of the men, so most likely a woman would break the tape before a man. What a reversal of history! This ensured that the women's race could play out before the cameras with no men obscuring the view of the competition and with no dangerous camera vehicle trying to follow them by weaving around men. "I was pushing for it as far back as 1980," said Billy Squires, Greater Boston Track Club's original coach. Olivera Jevtic was all in favor of the new format. "Yes," she said, "I prefer to run with the women." But the day loomed hot and hard. Anything could happen. But not for Americans. The women's Olympic Marathon Trials were in St. Louis to select the Athens team only two weeks earlier, using up any possible American contenders. But there were plenty of others.

Who can deny that Catherine "the Great" Ndereba, whose personal best (2:18:47) was more than 5 minutes faster than anyone else's in the field, was the favorite. "If I win, it just happens," she said. "It would mean a lot to me. This was the first marathon that I ever ran and my first victory."

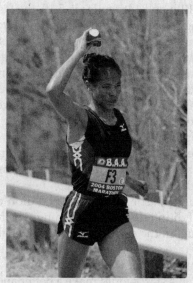

Elfenesh Alemu pouring water on her head to cool off in 2004. Photo by Victah Sailer for PhotoRun.

But challengers abounded. Maybe it would be Ethiopian Elfenesh Alemu, who shocked Olympic champion Naoko Takahashi in Tokyo the last fall. She came to race. "I'm extremely happy," said Ndereba, who hoped to become the first Kenyan of either gender to win the Olympic gold medal in Athens this summer. "We will be able to tell who is there and who is not. And now, you can know the splits, because you have that big clock ahead of you."

Joan Benoit Samuelson waved the starter pistol with its cord attached to the electronic timer connected to big clock and fired. The small women's elite field took off as everyone else waited. No wind blew. It was 83°F. Malgorzata Sobanska of Poland took the lead through 5k in a slow, slow 18:01. That was 2:32 pace. Elfenesh Alem did not like that. "The pace was slow and I made a decision to go out," said Alemu. "That's why I made my move." She bolted to the lead to ratchet up the stakes, hauling everyone through 10k in 35:15 a split that projected a 2:28:44 time. Eastern Europe followed: Serbian, Jevtic; Russian, Friya Sultanova–Zhdanova; Latvian, Nuta Olaru; and Romanian Jelena Prokopcuka. Ndereba, Leah Malot of Kenya, and Ai Yamamoto of Japan followed as well. The acceleration continued, passing 15k in 51:56 to project even faster to 2:26:05. Then there were three: Ndereba, Jevtic, and Almu. Friya Sultanova–Zhdanova and Leah Malot would drop out. Alemu pushed ahead by 8 seconds. Later Ndereba said, "I went with my own pace." So it was for the next 5 miles. It seemed that Ndereba did not want to push the pace but lingered back within sight of Almu hanging out to dry alone. When Almu picked up the pace, Ndereba kept the same gap. When Almu slowed, Ndereba slowed. So it continued being not obvious to anyone watching that they observed hunter and prey or two athletes equally suffering on a hot day. They ran apart, but together.

Alemu said, "I was aware that she was behind me. It did not make me nervous." Alemu ran the 12th and 14th miles in 5:19, the fastest of the day. Then at 25k she slowed, forcing Ndereba to run with her. Ndereba joined her, shaking her arms in a way runners commonly do to relax the shoulders after over an hour of running. She wore bug-eye sunglasses. Jevtic ran 1:24 behind. The two Africans matched strides for the next 10 miles. By 25 miles Ndereba suffered leg cramps. Alemu suffered too—her back hurt. The temperature reached 85°F. Ndereba risked a collapse if leg cramps totally took over her and stopped her running, but seized the lead and built upon it, inflicting pain upon herself. Unlike in other sports, opponents do not face each other and any pain inflicted on the opponent has to be equally endured by the inflictor. "I felt dead. That was the worst pain," she said. "I could not be standing." In 1999, she finished 6th and collapsed into a wheelchair at the finish.

"This was much tougher," she said. "In 1999, I didn't have enough training. This time, it's not like I didn't do enough training. The heat was just too tough. It was the women's duel in the sun as pivotal as the Salazar-Beardsley duel in 1982. Those two never raced as fast again. But the toughness of the competition and the toughness of the women wrote a confirmation that the idea of a separate professional women's start would make a better and more exciting competition. "Oh yes, I prefer the women-only start," said Ndereba. It was so great. We had all the room and all the road." Joan Benoit Samuelson said, "With the new start, the women were able to put on a show. That was a great race. We've proven our abilities. I think, relatively speaking, that the women's times were more impressive than the men's."

Marathon racing needed good news to offset the growing cloud of controversy over the use of performance-enhancing drugs. Two of the top 10 finishers were involved in that controversy. Lyubov Denisova in 2007 would be found guilty of using Prostanozol, testosterone according to reports, "Doping Rule Violation - Lyubov DENISOVA." (iaaf.org. IAAF. 11 May 2007. Archived from the original on 15 October 2015. Retrieved 18 October 2015.)

Olivera Jevti⊠ had received a public warning and disqualification from the 2002 New York City Marathon for use of Ephedrine according to IAAF news Feb 28, 2003. At the August Olympics in Athens, Greece, Ndereba placed 2nd; Alemu, 4th; and Jevtic 6th.

2004 Women's Results:

1. **Catherine Ndereba, KEN**	**2:24:27**	
2. Elfenesh Alemu, ETH	2:24:43	
3. Olivera Jevtic, SCG	2:27:34	
4. Jelena Prokopcuka, LAT	2:30:16	
5. Nuta Olaru, ROU	2:30:44	
6. Lyubov Denisova, RUS	2:31:17	
7. Malgorzata Sobanska, POL	2:32:23	
8. Victoria Klimina, RUS	2:33:20	
9. Ramilia Burangulova, RUS	2:34:08	
10. Ai Yamamoto, JPN	2:34:32	
11. Rika Tabashi, JPN	2:41:41	
12. Jessica Galvan Rodriquez, MEX	2:50:57	
13. Andrea Niggemeier, GER	2:50:59	
14. Greta Varchi, ITA	2:54:15	
15. Yumiko Une, JPN	2:54:15	
16. Julie Spencer, WI	2:56:39	
17. Angela Batsford, CAN	2:57:06	
18. Mary Ann Protz, FL	2:57:58,	
First Master		
19. Kim Donaldson, FL	2:58:15
20. Lee DiPietro, MD	2:58:59
21. Tracy Fischer, CA	2:59:36
22. Stephanie Hodge, CAN	3:00:00
23. Simonetta Piergentili, MA	3:01:00
24. Caroline Dobbyn, IRL	3:01:57
25. Sarah Llaguno, NC	3:02:06
26. Lisa Valentine, FL	3:02:19
27. Shannon Hovey, CT	3:03:30
28. Jane Johnson, FL	3:03:44
29. Nancy Corsaro, MA	3:04:04
30. Carrie Greenway, TN	3:04:30
31. Margaret Bradley, MA	3:04:54
41. Emily Bates, MA	3:09:59
52. Jessica Blake, MA	3:14:44
148. Tina Juillerat, IL	3:30:03
264. Laura Hayden, MA	3:38:54
1080. Allison Gillmore, TX	4:00:01
6237. Catherine McAleavey, MA	6:20:09

Winning Women's Teams:

1. Greater Boston Track Club, 9:58:32
2. Boston Athletic Association, 10:11:22
3. Somerville Road Runners, MA, 10:22:38
4. Team Utopia, NY, 10:40:01
5. Front Line Racing Team, MI, 10:40:53
6. Central Mass Striders, 10:45:28

Culpepper American Hope

MONDAY, APRIL 18, 2005

Cheruiyot and Cherigat and
Kenya Expected to Dominate

"I have the ability to win," said 32-year-old Alan Culpepper from Colorado. Ryan Shay also came to spark an American resurgence. "I didn't come here to take a back seat and be along for the ride," Shay said. Culpepper, who had won national championships at 5000m, 10,000m, and cross country, said, "I feel like my best opportunity lies with the marathon." Peter Gilmore, age 27 from San Mateo, California, came to race. He made his marathon debut in 2002 at the LaSalle Bank Chicago Marathon where he struggled home with a 2:21:48. He worked with the scientific coach Dr. Jack Daniels over the next two years, and four marathons later in 2004, had improved his personal best to 2:14:02 when he finished 2nd at the California International Marathon.

The Athens Olympics inspired hope in many American marathoners after two of them won marathon medals. The notion took hold—Americans can do this . . . they are not shut out of the marathon. Meb Keflezighi took a silver and Deena Kastor a bronze. "I think both of them [Culpepper and Shay] are going to be in the top 10," said Bill Rodgers. "I think they can duke it out with anybody in the field. They're real marathoners. Your heart has to be into the event and they're into it now. They're in the hunt." This turn of expectations may have reminded Rodgers of the old days in 1979 when Rodgers and his teammates placed, 1-3-8-10. His club, GBTC, was better than countries.

"To look at it realistically, we have two runners who are clearly world-class," said Alberto Salazar. Shay ran his first marathon soon after graduating in the top of his class in economics from Notre Dame in 2002. "I think that's the way to go for young runners," he says. "Try a marathon early and then decide if that's something they want to pursue or not." Shay found he was born for this event. It would consume his life.

Shay trained with Kastor and Keflezighi at Team Running USA's California camp, one of several long-distance incubators. These Americans would go against the favorites, Cherigat, Cheruiyot, and the rest of the Africans. Might it have put undue pressure on the Americans? "That's a good thing," Culpepper said. "I'm excited by the fact that the U.S. has a little more expectations now."

Boston Globe reported a pre-race interview with Tom Ratcliffe, who represents Cherigat. He believes Cherigat not only can win today but can compete at the highest level for years to come. "In terms of the marathon, based on his training over the last year, we think he has as much potential as any marathoner in the world," said Ratcliffe.

"Going into last year, Timothy went in fully expecting to win the race. Outside of our small group, most people didn't rate him very highly because you had a great field compared to Timothy's somewhat modest results. But now, obviously, he's gone from being one in the group to the one that is expected [to excel]."

Ratcliffe said he expected Cherigat's chief opposition to be Kenya's Robert Cheruiyot and James Koskei. "Based on the results from 2003 and based on the results of the Lisbon half marathon, I would say Robert Cheruiyot," said Ratcliffe. "I think Timothy [training under Dieter Hogen] is well-prepared and I assume Robert Cheruiyot is well-prepared, so I do think it will be a great race."

Kenya's Stephen Kiogora and Morocco's Khalid El Boumlili charged into a gentle, cooling headwind at 3 miles. The little wind cooled them, but also sucked moisture out of them by quickly evaporating sweat, giving the men a false sense of comfort. These two slowly destroyed themselves with splits of 25:12 at the net downhill 5 miles and accelerated to 50:18 by the relatively flat 10-mile mark. They led the more conservative pack by half a minute. But by 15 miles in 1:15:53 the pack swallowed them and spit them out by the roadside—dried up and done. Neither would finish the race.

Hailu Negussie nestled in the pack. He had finished an unnoticed 5th last year. He said, "Day and night I was dreaming of winning the Boston Marathon."

But others had their own dreams. Five of them were up front up into the hills with Negussie: defending champion Timothy Cherigat, Robert Kipkoech Cheruiyot, Benson Cherono, Benjamin Kipchumba, and Wilson Onsare. The American, Culpepper, who had come to Boston to win, dropped back. Perhaps this was a clever defensive move, or a necessity. He ran in 6th place. But at the top of the hills Cheruiyot appeared to be weakening. From 50 meters back, Culpepper could see his weakening. The other four looked comfortable. They passed 20 miles in 1:40:40. Negussie put in a surge. Surprisingly this seemed to revive Cheruiyot and only he responded. But the surge was massive. A 4:29 mile coming off the hill shook everybody, leaving Cheruiyot and Negussie alone. They registered a 4:47 for the next mile. But instead of hammering his competition into oblivion, oblivion stuck Cheruiyot, this time permanently leaving him like a ship taking on water and listing to starboard—out of the fight and barely underway. Culpepper set his sights on his victim. Tim Cherigat felt the same fecklessness and faltered as Culpepper clipped past.

Onsare and Cherono did not falter, but up front the man from Showa, Ethiopia, showed no distress. By the time he got to Coolidge Corner, Negussie could relax. "I knew I was going to win," he said.

He steamed ahead blissfully and buoyant. "I am so happy to win this race after so many years," said Negussie. "For Ethiopia, it is a big win." He was sure that his shocking burst enervated the Kenyans. He made the rules. He did not want to stay in a pack and play their game. "I was worried about that because it happened last year," he said.

"This is right up there with the Olympics for me," said the 32-year-old Culpepper, who was 12th in Athens last summer. "This is very special."

The fine showing by Americans lifted the spirits of all American marathoners and their fans. Ryan Shay resolved to do everything to get better, especially in preparation for the 2008 Olympics to be held in Beijing, China.

Ryan Shay set out to be a better marathoner than he had ever been. Ryan and other top athletes underwent medical testing in Flagstaff, Arizona, with Dr. Jack Daniels, where he trained last spring, and he was cleared for running, said his father Joe Shay. "He said the doctors told him that because your heart rate is so low, when you're older you may need a pacemaker to make adjustments on that," said Joe Shay, adding that his son first was diagnosed with a larger than normal heart at age 14. Ryan Shay went to the U.S. Olympic Trials in NYC in 2008 to make the team. He was running in a normal and fine way early in the race. Suddenly something went wrong, terribly wrong.

"He crossed right in front of me and stepped off the course," said runner Marc Jeuland of Chapel Hill, North Carolina, who did not see Shay collapse. "He nearly tripped me." Shay hit the ground near the Central Park boathouse. A statement from USA Track & Field said Shay immediately received CPR. He was taken to Lenox Hill Hospital, where he was pronounced dead on arrival.

"If you probably asked him if there was any way he wanted to go, it was out on the race course," said Terrence Mahon, who coached him in Mammoth and would later become the BAA coach in Boston.

SCD, or sudden cardiac death, is characterized by a thickening of the heart muscle, which means the demand for blood flow is increased. When the blood flow is restricted, the heart muscle firing becomes unstable and the fatal arrhythmia can occur. Cardiac arrhythmia due to cardiac hypertrophy with patchy fibrosis of undetermined etiology was the natural cause of Ryan Shay's death.

In more evidence that life is not fair, Johnny A. Kelley, who ran the Boston Marathon 61 times and won twice in 1935 and 1945, died on October 6, 2004, at age 97. Ryan Shay ran Boston only once.

2005 Men's Race

1. **Hailu Negussie, ETH**	**2:11:45**	16. Wilson Komen, KEN	2:19:41
2. Wilson Onsar, KEN	2:12:21	17. Redor Ryzhov, RUS	2:20:28
3. Benson Cherono, KEN	2:12:48	18. Terefe Uae, ETH	2:20:42
4. Alan Culpepper, CO	2:13:39	19. Jae-Young, Hyung, KOR	2:23:47
5. **Robert Kipkoech Cheruiyot, KEN**	**2:14:30**	20. Chris Lindstrom, CA	2:23:50
6. **Timothy Cherigat, KEN**	**2:15:19**	21. Stuart Hall, GBR	2:24:26
7. Benjamin Kipchumba, KEN	2:15:26	22. Matt Pelletiter, RI	2:24:55
8. Andrew Letherby, AUS	2:16:38	23. Carl Rundell, MI	2:24:59
9. Mohamed Quaadi, FRA	2:16:41	24. Eric Post, VA	2:25:22
10. Peter Gilmore, CA	2:17:32	25. Michael Wardian, VA	2:25:43
11. Ryan Shay, MI	2:18:17	26. Jacob Fry, MI	2:26:28
12. Benjamin Kosagi Kimutai, KEN	2:18:22	27. Gidey Amaha, ETH	2:26:56
13. Thomas Omwenga, KEN	2:18:57	28. Takehisa Okino, JPN	2:27:09
14. Pavel Loskutov, EST	2:19:04	29. Terrance Shea, MA	2:27:20
15. Joshua Kipkemboi, KEN First Master	2:19:28,	30. Piergiorgio Conti, ITA	2:27:36
		31. Sean Nesbit, CO	2:30:17

569. Doug Shaw, CAN	3:00:00	**8109. Keizo Yamada, JPN**	**4:28:05**
3032. Edward Tateosian, MA	3:30:00	10881. Paul Clerici, MA	6:00:00
6187. Robert Rickert, MI	4:00:00	10884. Jason Pisano, RI	7:25:28

Winning Men's Teams

1. Greater Boston Track Club, 7:40:28
2. Greater Lowell Road Runners, MA, 7:42:15
3. Boston Athletic Association, 7:43:27
4. Running Heritage, RI, 7:8:05:03
5. Raleigh Running Outfitters, NC, 8:09:58
6. Whirlaway Racing Team, MA, 8:10:49

My God Is Bigger

MONDAY, APRIL 18, 2005

Champion Expected to Repeat

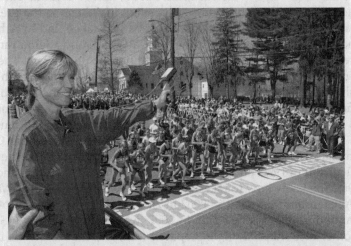

Uta Pippig fires the electronically connected starting gun. Photo used with permission from the BAA.

Paula Radcliffe had run 2:17:34 in London recently and still held the world record 2:15:25, from 2003. *Boston Globe* reporter Bob Ryan asked Ndereba what would happen if Radcliffe decided to race at Boston next year.

"If she comes, I know my God is bigger than anybody in this world."

The temperature read 68°F at the 11:31 a.m. elite women's start. Bright sun might have led the field to expect a hot day like the previous year. They started cautiously. Russia's Lyubov Morgunova led the first, easy downhill mile in 5:52. Hearing that, the pack jacked up the pace to 5:22 and 5k in 17:13.

But none of these racers were new to the course or to each other. Everyone knew every risk and reward ($100,000). At 5k, Ndereba ran in 7th place at 17:37, a time that projected to only 2:28:40.

Nuta Olaru of Romania and Elfenesh Alemu of Ethiopia led by mile 4. Observers poured their attention on Alemu because they expect the painful burn lingering from last year's 2nd place to drive her to force a confrontation with Ndereba, who seemed to be having a bad day.

Elfenesh Alemu, born in the Arsi highland not far from the town of Bekoji in Ethiopia, grew up with her sister, who was a runner. Her sister, Asnakech, did not continue running after marriage, but Elfenesh decided to continue her running career after marrying Gezahegne Abera, the Olympic marathon champion, in a nationally celebrated wedding held in a giant stadium and attended by 25,000 people. Guests included the president of the country and Haile Gebrselassie.

Almeu wanted to win an Olympic marathon medal at Athens to match the gold her husband won at Sydney. She did not want to match her husband's 2nd-place finish at Boston in 2000. That's why she led the race.

The two had run shoulder to shoulder last year with Ndereba prevailing, so where was she? She ran 23 seconds behind at 5k, and 59 seconds back at 10k. Alemu had run to the heartbreaking 4th position in Athens so the press corps expected her appetite to be voracious. Ndereba had taken 2nd in Athens but did not look in contention today. At the halfway Olaru and Alemu ran 1:12:11 and Ndereba in 4th ran 1:20 behind. She could not see the leaders. The gallery of reporters in the press truck could not see her. Alemu ran to 25k with Olaru.

Elfenesh pushed away from kind-hearted Nuta who began her drift back into the field. But meanwhile Ndereba seemed stuck in a four-woman pack with 2003 Boston winner Svetlana Zakharova, Moroccan Zhor El Kamch, who had won Rotterdam Marathon in 2:26:10 last year, and three-time Olympic distance medalist Gete Wami of Ethiopia. She had finished 3rd in the Atlanta Olympic 10,000m in 1996, and in Sydney in 2000, 3rd in the 5000m, and 2nd in the 10,000m. She knew how to race and likely knew Alemu's ability. Wami had won the Amsterdam Marathon in 2002 in 2:22:19. She would go on to win the World Marathon Majors Series Title in 2007, which she would win $500,000. About another race she said, "I've prepared well, and the results are in God's hands. If God wills it for me, nobody can take it away from me. Apart from that, it's a sport, I've trained well, and I'm just focusing on doing well. I'm not thinking too much about what will happen beyond that."

She could not be thinking about what was happening behind her. She could see the pack around her and had an idea of what was happening ahead, and saw Olaru falling back but could not see the Italian, Bruna Genovese, running her third Boston Marathon, sneaking up behind. She is from Montebelluna, Italy, and is coached by Salvatore Bettiol. He had run Boston himself in 2003 in

2:22:15 for 14th at age 42. (2:10 at his youthful peak.) So she had received experienced advice. She said she had started slowly, "Because it is hot, it is better to run slowly at the beginning." She had run 2:25:35 in Toyko in 2001.

Metaphors about strategy in the marathon abound. The voice of the marathon, Toni Reavis, says that most marathons require the strategy of checkers, but the Boston Marathon, because of the variables of weather and topography, is chess.

Ndereba did not know what moves she would make or how far behind she ran. Later she said, "I'm glad I didn't know. If you believe you can do it, you can." If you don't know then we can suppose it helps you to believe. A pack of more than half a dozen competitors followed Ndereba, confident that she had picked to right distance to play behind the leader. Too far back and the pursuit would be futile and too close would risk the same blow-up as a runner running too fast, too early under the day's conditions, giving the race to a smarter someone further back. Perhaps this tactic is possible because the faster 40 women in the race are invited to start alone about a half hour ahead of the men, so a chasing woman can see the competition ahead without a clog of obscuring men as in past years.

Russian Lyubov Morgunova, in a compromise, ran alone between the leaders and the pack. Ndereba seemed to be pulling the pack along in her wake while she had a line attached to the runners a minute ahead of her.

So chasing her belief, she took off—a flight of faith. In the 5k from miles 20 to 25, she crawled 28 seconds closer to the lead. By 30k she saw and caught Olaru and Morgunova and moved into 2nd place. She now had Alemu in sight. The target pulled her on. Alemu looked over her shoulder and saw Ndereba. Alemu said later, "I was doing the best I could to keep my pace."

But could Ndereba sustain that push? She had made up 80 seconds in 7 miles. Many runners have started their races wisely, but picked up the pace too hard, too soon. Alemu had been slowing but was not staggering in a death march. In fact she looked quite fluid and graceful. Ndereba pulled alongside. Award-winning reporter Barbara Huebner wrote of the beauty of the two running together, "The pair ran side-by-side-sometimes in perfect, elegant synchronization-for the next two miles, but their hearts were going in opposite directions."

Alemu said, "The pace was a normal pace. I wanted to run 17 minutes for 5k and so that was the right pace and that's why I went out the way I did. I was doing my best and keeping my pace."

Ndereba after the race said, "I felt like my legs were kind of heavy when we started and I didn't like to take a chance of pushing it," she said. "I kept on doing it, taking it easy, and I found myself running like normal. My body started responding towards 20 kilometers and I kept on trying to push the pace, and toward the finish, I just felt great."

From there Ndereba ran her fastest 5k of the race with in 16:46, but Alemu and Olaru had run that split from 5k to 10k, about an hour and a half earlier. Perhaps that made the difference, because Alemu fell apart in the last 5k, running over a minute slower than Nderaba. Perhaps her god was weaker, or perhaps deities should run their own races.

After the race Alemu said, "I am not disappointed because there is winning and not winning. It happens, so I'm not worried about that."

"Boston is my finest and my favorite milestone," said Ndereba. She has said she'd be an elementary school math teacher if she wasn't a professional athlete.

"I like the people and the atmosphere down there because they are very friendly. I like the location of the race itself and the fans are very welcoming. The course is very challenging and it's so prestigious. In the marathons I've done, I think Boston is the most challenging course, but it is the best for myself."

"It means a lot to me," Ndereba said. "I just run according to how my body was feeling," she said. "As I kept on pushing the pace, I could feel like my body was moving. I thought like 'Wow, I can do it.' Last year, it was kind of tough for me because it was hot and humid. Towards the finish, it was like everything was gone from my body and I was so sick. [For the final] few meters, I was battling cramps. I thank God, for this year I didn't have this problem. It is more than a thrill, I tell you. Because I can see what my God can do, and how much he has in store for me."

"It feels very good and I thank God for the history that I've made," said Ndereba. "I know it's not by my might or my power but by the power of the Holy Spirit. It's only because God was on my side. I know the power of winning comes from my God."

In the finish area Ndereba found the microphone and thanked John Hancock, the BAA, and God. Clearly, she had learned more than skillful tactics in her three previous victories. First thank those who provide the appearance money. Later with professional poise, she said about her fourth, unprecedented win, "The lord's kingdom is still flying high."

A band of guerrilla marketers accosted naive Kurt Belhumeur, 23, a simple courier from Beverly, Massachusetts. They offered him $50 if he would jump into the race wearing a sandwich board advertising their product, ManiaTV. He accepted, ran down an alley, a side street, and then onto Boylston Street to join a pack of marathon runners on the course. Officers grabbed him and dragged him off the course. They arrested Belhumeur and arraigned him in Boston Municipal Court on charges of disorderly conduct. The company could have paid for marathon sponsorship and not be a danger to public safety by jumping on to the playing field.

Guy Morse, the executive director of the Boston Athletic Association, said, "It troubles me from a public safety perspective first and foremost. Our first priority is the safety of the runner and that the runners have a safe course on which to compete."

Morse was further quoted in the *Boston Globe* saying he is not sure how the marathon can improve security for future races. He added that protecting the 26.2-mile course is "simply a police matter."

Women's Results 2005

1. **Catherine Ndereba, KEN**	2:25:13	3. Bruna Genovese, ITA	2:29:51
2. Elfenesh Alemu, ETH	2:25:03	4. **Svetlana Zakharova, RUS**	2:31:34

5. Madina Biktagirova, RUS	2:32:41,	20. Lee DePietro, MD	2:53:34
	First Master	21. Eri Matsubara, JPN	2:54:21
6. Lyubov Morgunova, RUS	2:33:24	22. Lisa Haas, PA	2:54:23
7. Shitaye Gemechu, ETH	2:33:51	23. Diona Fulton, MA	2:55:08
8. Zhor El Kamch, MAR	2:36:54	24. Nathalie Vasseur, FRA	2:55:16
9. Mina Ogawa, JPN	2:37:34	25. Edie Perkins, NY	2:55:42
10. Nuta Olaru, ROU	2:37:37	26. Caroline Kondoleon, MA	2:56:04
11. Firaya Sultanova-Shdanova, RUS	2:41:05	27. Becki Marshall, NC	2:26:27
12. Emily Levan, ME	2:43:14	28. Kimberly Fitchen-Young, CA	2:56:40
13. Caroline Annis, CA	2:43:46	29. Danyelle Phelps, NH	2:56:46
14. Carly Graytock, MI	2:44:02	30. Shannon Nobis-Scherer, UT	2:56:54
15. Yuko Sato, JPN	2:47:00	39. Shannon Hovey, CT	3:00:06
16. Christine Brough-Glockenmeier, NJ	2:29:45	320. Emily Bates, MA	3:29:58
17. Kimberly Fagen, CA	2:50:07	2011. Sarah Moberg, MO	4:00:00
18. Michelle Rorke, NY	2:50:10	6644. Kelley Lucket, GA	6:27:02
19. Simonetta Piergentilli, MA	2:51:35		

Winning Women's Teams

1. Impala Racing Team, CA, 8:50:37
2. U.S. Navy, VA, 9:03:30
3. Greater New York Racing Team, 9:24:16
4. Front Line Racing Team, MI, 9:33:07
5. Hi-Tek Racing Team, CT, 9:33:08
6. Boston Athletic Association, 9:37:41

Sweet Chariot

MONDAY, APRIL 17, 2006

Can THIS Be the America Year?

This year saw the first multi-wave start. In 1969 the first field of over 1,000 runners seemed to overwhelm officials. Those were the days of stopwatches and results written in pencil by a human hand. By 2006, technology and logistical innovations allowed almost 20,000 finishers and with a new method to prevent runners from having to wait so long to reach the starting line on the narrow street in Hopkinton.

On Wednesday before the race, officials from Greece and local boosters unveiled a bronze statue in honor of Stylianos Kyriakides. Kyriakides won the

1946 Boston Marathon to publicize the plight of Nazi-devastated Greece. The statue was called "Spirit of the Marathon" at the 1-mile mark near Weston Horticultural Nurseries. It was a gift from New Balance to the Hopkinton Athletic Association. Dimitri Kyriakides came to Hopkinton for the unveiling of his father's statue. "For me, it's like a dream come true, because ever since I was young I would hear my father talking about the Marathon, Hopkinton, Boston, Johnny Kelley."

As reported in the *Washington Post*, on the eve of the third anniversary of the Iraq invasion, President Bush promised to "finish the mission" with "complete victory," urging the American public to remain steadfast but offering no indication when the war would be over. On the other hand, American soldiers stationed in Iraq held a "Boston Marathon" there compete with a Boston Marathon start/finish banner. The BAA supported the race, making it officially unofficial. About 150 runners finished, with one under 3 hours. The race started at 6 a.m. to avoid the heat, but by the last hour the temperature reached triple digits.

Just as America seemed bogged down in Iraq, American marathoners seemed bogged down in Boston. Greg Meyer is often called the last American to win the Boston Marathon and that was back in 1983. He did not like being called the "last" American. The press decried the lack of wins for the home team. The *Boston Globe*'s John Powers wrote: "A Seoul man led the parade down Boylston Street five years ago. An Ethiopian busted five Kenyan tickers on Heartbreak Hill last April. Could this be the time when a Yankee Doodle Dandy finally wins here on Patriot's Day?"

"I definitely feel that sense of, finally, we're at a point where this could happen," said Alan Culpepper, who finished 4th last year. "You watched Meb in New York last year," said Culpepper. "He was in the hunt. And I was in the race here. I was part of the whole scene." Referring to race sponsor John Hancock, who assumes the responsibility for inviting top marathoners and paying their appearance fees, "They did a good job of bringing in a great field," said Meb Keflezighi. He came to Boston after finishing twice in the top 3 in New York. "They could have made it easier if they just wanted an American to win it, but they didn't." Speaking for the Americans, Keflezighi said, "It's going to be challenging, but that's what we want. If we win, we want to do it against the best."

These top race field in top marathons do not happen by themselves. The best do not just randomly show up on race day. But they are not just hired guns. They are products of art—some business to be sure, but ultimately fields are assembled by skill, sensitivity, and artistry. The Boston Marathon's artist for a span of 26 years was Pat Lynch. Lynch got his running start as a member of the Greater Boston Track Club during the Bill Rodgers era. He had run about a 3-hour marathon but trained with the very best and learned the needs, hopes, and fears of top marathoners. He was employed as a marathon consultant to sponsor, John Hancock. He traveled to the athletes and got to know them, their coaches, friends, agents, and family and developed a sense of how each fits into a potential race field. He wanted runners who knew each other but he also wanted a mix of strangers in the field to bring in an element of uncertainty. He never took the easy way of buying a star and filling the field with lesser lights.

Lynch wanted athletes who would come back for several years with growing prowess and reputation. He wants the athletes to spread the word that racing the Boston Marathon is good for their careers. They are individuals coming together to produce an exciting competition that none of them could do alone. Contracts include drop-out clauses in most races, but Lynch saw that it would be a travesty of the sport to put the athletes up on blocks for an auction or even for the athletes to shop around for simply the race that would pay them the most. It was a negotiation to Lynch—a long-term negotiation where everyone from the public to the racers themselves come away happy to be part of an exciting, challenging race.

Cherigat would be running Boston for the fifth time, Cheruiyot for the fourth. The Kenyans did not want an Ethiopian to win again. Politely denying the rivalry, Wilson Onsare said, "We do not feel an enmity. But most of the time Kenyans have been winning."

Fifty-five degrees at noon. Perfect for running fast. A giant, unwieldy pack of confident men swooped downhill out of Hopkinton led by Tanzanian John Yuda to a 4:57 mile, then 24:20 at 5 miles, 48:07 at 10. Culpepper, the great American hope, Keflezighi, Benjamin Maiyo, Deriba Merga, John Korir, Negussie, Cherigat, Onsare, William Kiplagan, and the Japanese runner, Jenjiro Jitsui ran happily at that rapid pace. Keflezighi and Culpepper wore white Nike uniforms with a big USA on the chest. Brian Sell, running for the Hansons' Club out of Rochester, Michigan, wore the club's red/black/yellow harlequin uniform. Maiyo pushed first into the air ahead of Yuda. Somewhere thereafter his confidence in himself vanished. Keflezighi and Merga went with Maiyo. The pack thinned, stretched, and broke apart like salt water taffy pulled beyond its tensile strength, replacing the expected sweetness of the day with bitter disappointment for those who could not stick. The greater the expectations, the harder the fall. Last year's winner Hailu Negussie dropped out of the race.

Twenty meters back, past winners Cherigat and Cheruiyot ran together with John Korir. The leaders hit halfway in 1:02:43 with the three observers back by 12 seconds. Maiyo said later, "I was feeling it was fast, but my tactic was to run the course record. Talking [the previous night] with my group, we said, 'Let's try to run a fast race. Let's not go very slow.'"

At the start of the hills, Keflezighi, Merga, and Maiyo led, but pursuit had begun. Cheruiyot said later, "Sometimes, the hills are good for me. To climb is very easy for me." He eased himself up to the leaders. Merga vanished. Korir would not finish. But Cheruiyot may have had his doubts. He had not won a major marathon since his Boston win three years earlier. Maybe a lack of confidence set him to go out more easily and less in pursuit of a record.

"A marathon is a long distance," he said. "Twenty-six miles is a big distance." "But [training partner/world record-holder] Paul Tergat told me: 'Don't run too fast, you only need to win.'"

Cheruiyot ran up behind Maiyo through the hills. Maiyo gestured for him to take the lead by turning back and waving his arm. "I was trying to tell Robert to assist me in pacing," he said, "but Robert refused." Cheruiyot declined until the crest. Then he pushed hard. But perhaps too hard. "When I was at 40k, I think maybe I can run 2:06," said Cheruiyot. He suffered over the last 2 miles. The confidence for 2:06 and a record dissipated. He leaned back to Tergat's advice. "You only need to win." Win he did, beating Ndeti's record for 1994 by a trifling, but valuable, second. That second won him the $25,000 bonus.

"I think it was very well done," said Keflezighi. "It was a tremendous effort by all of us. I really thought I had a good chance at winning this," said Keflezighi. "I came in to win it, and I positioned myself, but this course takes a lot of strategy, a lot of patience, and I don't think I was patient today. But at the same time, you know, when you're trying to win, you can't let guys have too much of a gap. "It's a delicate balance," said Culpepper, who decided to stay back and pick off stragglers, as he did last year. "Because you don't want the race to go without you. I do not follow the guys, because I know the race is too fast," said Cheruiyot. The fast pace floored Keflezighi, "Wow," he said to himself. "If we keep this up, I don't know what we are going to do on Heartbreak Hill. We both played into Cheruiyot's hands, I have experience here, I was thinking that he was going to slow down maybe," said Maiyo. "But he was very strong." Cheruiyot said, "I see that the clock is at 2:07 and I say, 'I can make it.'"

American men finished in 11 out of the top 22 places. That led Bill Rodgers to declare, "A new day for the Boston Marathon." Rodgers worked for Channel 5 TV as color commentator and commented colorfully: "I think in the U.S. there's so many other sports, and marathoning and road racing is not really on the radar screen. The Boston Marathon, yeah, okay, it's once a year. But I think for the first time Americans are starting to get some coaching and some support. Some of these programs are starting to pay off, and if we support our young people, they'll always come through, and that's what we saw today. They might not run quite as fast as the great Kenyans, but they'll run pretty darn good. To see that happen today, it was pretty powerful, especially here at Boston, which had gone through a long kind of a drought. Occasionally, runners would take fourth or fifth, like Culpepper ran great here last year, but to see the depth is nice."

Quite responsible for that depth is the Hanson Brothers' project. Kevin and Keith Hanson of Rochester, Michigan, took the model of the Greater Boston Track Club of the 1970s to bring coaching and organization to top American distance by bringing them all to the same place so they could train together and have some employment and health benefits. This system seems to be working.

The team seems to have a chant that goes like this . . . the team that trains together, competes together, lives together, and wakes up early for a day of running together is also a team that wins together.

Culpepper said, "We've seen it coming for a while and we've seen it building," he said. "This has been a work in progress for the last five or six years. For myself and Meb, this started 10 years ago and Brian [Sell] showed today that, you know, the fruits of his labor are paying off. I think it bodes very well for the future. I think three or four years ago, I don't know if there would have been as many guys to pick up the slack there when the Kenyans were fading or when some of these other guys started to really fade. In years past, they just would have maintained their placing, whereas now guys are coming up from behind and running them down."

Some people were surprised that American men ran so well. Culpepper said, "For those of us that are in it, who make our profession this way, we're probably not as surprised as some other people are, honestly." Sell said, "I just kind of let the pack go and hoped I would see them again." Sell ran 1:05:17 at the half, not 1:02:45 like Keflezighi did. Sell let the leaders go early on, as did winner Cheruiyot, then pushed the last half of the race, gaining confidence with each fading runner he passed. "I saw John Korir. It was nice to pass him."

Sell caught and passed Culpepper on the course's final left turn at the corner of Hereford and Boylston. That move earned him the ten millionth dollar paid out by John Hancock in prize money. That is a big step from 1979 when Bill Rodgers was paid nothing. Entry fee for next year's qualifiers will be $95, with a $50 late fee for entries postmarked after March 1, 2007. $150 for international qualifiers.

2006 Men's Results:

1. **Robert Kipkoech Cheruiyot, KEN 2:07:14***
2. Benjamin Maiyo, KEN 2:08:21
3. **Mebrahtom Keflezighi, CA 2:09:56**
4. Brian Sell, MI 2:10:55
5. Alan Culpepper, CO 2:11:02
6. Kenjiro Jitsu, JPN 2:11:32
7. Peter Gilmore, CA 2:12:45
8. William Kiplagat, KEN 2:13:26
9. Wilson Onsare, KEN 2:13:47
10. Clint Verran, MI 2:14:12
11. Luke Humphrey, MN 2:15:23
12. **Timothy Cherigat, KEN 2:16:09**
13. Julius Ruto, KEN 2:17:02
14. Wilson Komen, KEN 2:18:26
15. Chad Johnson, MI 2:19:29
16. Chris Lundstrom, MN 2:19:37
17. Kazuo Letani, JPN 2:19:40
18. Lyle O'Brien, MI 2:19:57
19. Trent Briney, MI 2:20:10
20. Marzuki Stevens, CA 2:20:11
21. Miguel Nuci, MEX 2:20:45
22. Martin Rosendahl, MI 2:21:12
23. Johnathan Little, MO 2:23:17
24. Peter Vail, CAN 2:25:06
25. Shinobu Minami, JPN 2:23:16
26. Jesse Williams, WA 2:26:24
27. Sammy Nyangincha, KEN 2:26:37, First Master
28. Paul Rades, MD 2:26:56
29. Tobias Van Ghenmen, GER 2:27:00
37. Michael Wardian, VA 2:29:51
1063. Robert Rene-Gael, FRA 2:59:59
5202. Jerry Flanagan, CA 3:30:00
8939. Choi Chang Oun, KOR 4:00:00
9973. **Keizo Yamada, JPN 4:16:07**
12059. Vincent Messina, TN 6:05:34

Winning Men's Teams

1. Hanson-Brooks Distance Project, MI, 6:40:30
2. United States Air Force, 7:41:55
3. West Side Runners, NY, 7:45:13
4. Whirlaway Racing Team, MA, 7:49:04
5. PR Mose Milers Racing Team, NH, 7:55:36
6. Greater New York Racing Team, 7:57:19
7. Greater Boston Track Club, 8:00:26

Passport to Victory

MONDAY, APRIL 17, 2006

Weak American Field

From the gun, a pack of about a dozen runners broke away, led by Japan's Reiko Tosa. The first mile passed in 5:24 and Tosa continued with metronomic precision. Tosa ran 5th in the Athens Olympics and has a marathon best of 2:23:57 from winning the Nagoya marathon in 2004. In 2005 she ran 10,000m in 32:07.66. Called Miss Consistency in Japan, she has rarely run a bad marathon. She has trained at altitude in Kunming, China and Boulder, Colorado.

Her father was a distance runner, her mother a javelin thrower, and her sister a sprinter.

Tosa came to general notice after joining a corporate track team, Mitsui Kaijyo. In her first year with the team, after a 40 days of high-altitude training at Boulder, Tosa finished 6th in the 1999 Sapporo half marathon with 1:10:59. With this performance Tosa was selected for the Japanese team at the 1999 World Half Marathon championships, where she finished 5th with 1:09:36. In 2001, Tosa and Lidia Simon of Romania entered the stadium together. Tosa had been trying to break the Romanian to avoid a final sprint. She could not. She finished 2nd. Tosa jokingly said, "Had my sister been dueling with Simon in Edmonton, she could have out-sprinted her!"

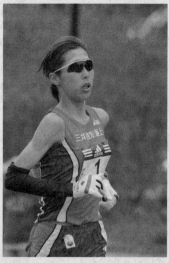

Reiko Tosa set the pace for Boston 2006.

At 10k, 9 women ran together at 34:07. The previous 5k passed a little faster than the first in 16:57. Jelena Prokopcuka of Latavia held the vanguard at the checkpoint. The next 5k matched the first but spectators counted only 8 in the pack.

The same 8 held the same pace through 20k but pursuers had dropped behind by 500 meters. Tosa led on a day of comfortable temperatures. They all continued through the half together in 1:12:19.

Tosa led the next steady 25k and lost Zivile Balciunaite of Lithuania.

At halfway in 1:12:19, 8 runners sat in position to outkick Tosa. Jelena Prokopcuka from Latvia had been to Boston before and bided her time. Experienced was Bruna Genovese of Italy, but Zivile Gaslciuante of Lithuania, another Japanese runner, Kiyoko Shimahara, and many-time Boston racer, Olivera Jevtic of Serbia and Montenegro, Alevtina Biktimirova of Russia, and the Kenyan rising star, 25-year-old Rita Jeptoo of Kenya, all relative newbies.

Jeptoo completed the bulk of her training surrounded by hills and mountains in Kapsabet, Kenya. She knew the Boston Marathon course had hills, but training on hills was ordinary in her neighborhood. She had started racing in Italy in 2000 where she had gone with Jonah Koech to train under the renowned coach Renato Canova. In the world championships in Helsinki she ran with Catherine Nderaba and Paula Radcliffe after catching them at halfway before fading to 7th in 2:24:22. But all that preparation might have had to wait in defeat by Afro-Italian bureaucratic fumbling except for the last-minute magical appearance of the essential passport. But her 6 p.m. Saturday arrival in Boston did not allow Jeptoo the final bit of preparation—a course tour. So she had to start the race blind to its vicissitudes.

By 18 miles, attrition shaved everyone off the pack but four: Tosa, Jeptoo, Prokopcuka, and Genovese. A surprise to reporters it was that Genovese took the lead and pushed. But the move sliced no one from the pack as they all matched her. All she managed to do was cut herself out of the running.

Then there were three.

Tosa and Prokopcuka wore sunglasses and often ran on each side of Jeptoo. Jeptoo with her red-tinted hair stacked on top of her head, with earrings and a necklace, looked down from the height of fashion. Tosa wore #1, Prokopcuka wore #2, and Jeptoo #5. They ran in synch. But Tosa had lost recollection of the hills and at 22 miles Jeptoo pushed the pace to the fastest mile of the day, 5:19. Jeptoo said, "I'm not feeling to go very fast, because I think [Prokopcuka] is faster than me," Jeptoo said. "But when I'm 38 kilometers, I'm feeling to go. I'm feeling to move, so I cannot wait. "The pace slowed only slightly through the hills but the effort had increased painfully. Then only four ran together: Bruna Genovese of Italy, Jeptoo, Tosa, and Prokopcuka. A 17:03 next 5k lost the Italian. Tosa began to look uncomfortable. Was it the arm warmers or the pace? Jeptoo took that moment to test the other two with a 100-meter surge. She said later, "I said my body was still strong. I saw the two ladies and sensed they were finished." Just to make sure, she danced her way to a 5:06 mile. The knot of hair colored by henna piled on top of Nandi woman, Rita Sitienei Jeptoo from Kenya looked completely undisturbed by 24 miles of racing.

No one joined her. Prokopcuka gambled that the surge would not last and a kick with bring her to victory. Prokopcuka planned that Jeptoo would fade like in Helsinki. After all, in 2000 Prokopcuka had run 14:47.71 for 5000m in Stockholm. Tantalizingly close she ran to Jeptoo—10 seconds was not too long to kick in a marathon and a final push might be safer than one too soon. She hoped for a kick. Prokopcuka felt stronger than she had two years ago. Jeptoo looked back and thought that Prokopcuka ran to catch her and was fast enough to do it. She ran in fear. Fear and hope balanced in the last miles, keeping the gap steady. Jeptoo won by the same gap she had created in the surge at 38k.

About her win at the post-race press conference, she said, "At the last minute I come here, and I feel very happy to come here and to post my fastest." Then she rambled on in fatigue, happiness, and relief that she actually solved the passport problem and made it to the race on time. "This is my fastest marathon . . . so I am happy, so much, and I won and this is my best time. I don't know. I don't have anything I can tell because I'm happy so much."

"This," Jeptoo said, "is happiness for me to win Boston."

2006 Women's Results:

1. **Rita Jeptoo, KEN**	2:23:38	
2. Jelena Prokopcuka, LAT	2:23:48	
3. Reiko Tosa, JPN	2:24:11	
4. Bruna Genovese, ITA	2:25:28	
5. Kiyoko Shimahara, JPN	2:26:52	
6. Alevtina Biktimirova, RUS	2:26:58	
7. Olivera Jevtic, SCG	2:29:38	
8. Madina Biktagirova, RUS	2:30:06, First Master	
9. Olesya Nurgalieva, RUS	2:30:16	
10. Zivile Balciunaite, LTU	2:32:16	
11. Chika Horie, JPN	2:34:40	
12. Tatiana Titova, RUS	2:36:57	
13. Emily Levan, ME	2:37:01	
14. Kutre Dulecha, ETH	2:37:08	
15. Svetlana Demidenko, RUS	2:39:53	
16. Michelle Lilienthal, PA	2:40:23	
17. Michelle Rorke, NY	2:43:08	
18. Carly Greytock, MA	2:43:19	
19. Melisa Christian, TX	2:46:30	
20. Tere Stouffler, TN	2:48:15	
21. Jenny DeWeese, NC	2:49:07	
22. Phebe Ko, NC	2:51:39	
23. Simonetta Piergentili, MA	2:52:28	
24. Helena Crossan, IRL	2:52:48	
25. Veronika Ulrich, GER	2:53:45	
26. Christina Seehan, MA	2:54:13	
27. Johanna Thomas, MA	2:54:20	
28. Leslie Gold, CAN	2:54:37	
29. Gina McGee, PA	2:55:03	
30. Denise Robinson, CAN	2:55:10	
38. Kara Haas, MA	2:58:09	
39. Mega Doshi, MA	2:58:10	
49. Gi Sook Moon, KOR	2:59:56	
968. Erin Hewitt, NY	3:30:00	
4404. Judy Mink, OH	4:00:00	
7619. Jo Dee Messina, TN	6:05:34	

Winning Women's Teams

1. Boston Athletic Association, 8:19:57
2. Impala Racing Team, CA, 9:26:39
3. Greater Boston Track Club, 9:31.01
4. Front Line Racing Team, MI, 9:39:49
5. Whirlaway Racing Team, MA, 9:41:47
6. DC Road Runners, DC, 9:45:53

Defending Champ Returns

MONDAY, APRIL 16, 2007

Northeast Storm Could Ruin Race

A northeast storm churned off the coast of New England, driving wind and rain into the coast and raising a storm surge causing flooding and shutting roads in coastal communities at high tide. A major Nor'easter was expected to dump more than 4 inches of rain and threatened severe flooding inland and on city streets. Some weathermen predicted snow, but as the storm approached it pulled some warm air north, changing the predictions to driving sheets of rain. Weather and emergency personnel advised people to stay inside and avoid the roads. The Coast Guard warned fishermen not to venture out to sea.

The second largest entry field in Boston Marathon history, at 23,869 entrants, would assemble this year starting at 10 a.m. for the first time instead of noon. Every year management of the race grew in complexity.

That year Guy Morse thought there would be no end in sight to his work improving the marathon. But a diagnosis of prostate cancer in late 2007 and subsequent treatment and complications in 2008 shocked him into a different outlook on life. The work and a daily 4-hour commute began to wear him down.

With treatment as a patient at Dana Fabre Cancer Institute, it became evident to him that he would not be able to carry on as the Executive Director. He would suggest in 2010 to divide the leadership of the BAA into two parts, the Executive Director and the Senior Director of External Affairs. The change allowed him to contribute but with relief from some day-to-day operations. He retired completely from the BAA at the end of 2012 but continued to be present at marathon events.

The one man picked to win was the man who had won twice before. Robert Kipkoech Cheruiyot had won twice and dropped out once. The Boston Marathon changed his life perhaps more that it had changed the life of anyone. John Powers writing for the *Boston Globe* recorded, "The $80,000 paycheck might as well have been a billion-dollar lottery ticket." "When I got home, I bought a big farm with a plantation and a small house with electricity," Cheruiyot told Powers. "And I brought my parents together. That was what I wanted."

Cheruiyot's life started on a doorstep where his parents had left him and his brother Stephen Biwott because the family had collapsed. His father had inherited a farm from a white settler who had left Kenya, but he sold it and wasted the money. That left the two boys on the lowest end of Kenyan society. They had no land and worse, they had no immediate family. Eventually instead of school, Cheruiyot got a job in a barber shop. "I was making 20 bob [30 cents] a day."

In a good turn of luck other relatives found him and took him in as a surrogate son and he began training again—he'd shown promise as a distance runner in school. Cheruiyot fondly recalled the exact moment that inspired him to pursue running: "The 1996 Olympics were in Atlanta and we watched on a black and white television set back in Kenya. The guy standing on the podium was my classmate!"

A driver for one of the local FILA running camps noticed him running and Cheruiyot met Moses Tanui at the camp. "Moses was very tough, like a president in those days," Cheruiyot says. "You didn't go say hello."

Cheruiyot said that when his coach, who thought he was eating more than he was running, wanted him out, Tanui decreed that he stay. Tanui saw promise in that lanky frame (6 feet, 2 inches, 140 pounds), which Paul Tergat, the future world record–holder, noticed after their first run together. Tergat gave Cheruiyot his training shoes and urged him to apply himself.

When Cheruiyot won a local 10k, he won enough Kenyan shillings to seem like a fortune for a young person who once had worn the same clothes for a year. "I used 50 shillings to feed myself," he recalls. "And then 1,000 to buy clothes."

As he continued to train and race well he received a contract from FILA, which brought him to Italy in 2001 for an advanced apprenticeship. "Robert was very simple, very nice, very poor," said his agent, Federico Rosa. "But he showed always a big heart."

"Ten years ago, we were next to beggars," said Biwott, who has since run a 2:11:16 marathon and who is also entered in this year's Boston race. John Powers further wrote, "Against all odds, the old family has become new again, with land and a house that will never vanish." One thing, though, has changed.

Cheruiyot decided to come to Boston in 2003 because he had asked Elijah Lagat, who won Boston in 2000, what it was like to run that race. "It's okay," Lagat said, so Cheruiyot came to Boston and won by 23 seconds in only his second marathon.

"I was known because I won in Milan," he said that day after becoming the youngest Boston victor in nine years. "This makes my name bigger."

But the Kenyan Federation did not select him for the Olympic team for Athens; instead, the Kenyan Federation named Tergat, Sammy Korir, and Eric Wainaina. But the Federation knew that Cheruiyot had run "only" 2:10:11 in Boston and that he'd missed three months of training because of a leg injury.

But last year he dominated Boston, sitting back because he sensed that the early pace was unwisely fast, then caught countryman Benjamin Maiyo on Heartbreak Hill who was racing to break Cosmas Ndeti's 12-year-old course by one second record with a 2:07:14. Then Maiyo slowed only to 6th place. He would be back, fitter and wiser.

In Chicago the previous fall, Cheruiyot won but in a terrifying moment that made observers think of Pheidippides' mythical "rejoice we conquer," then dying. Cheruiyot approached the last steps before the slick timing matt across the finish line. Only then sure he had outsprinted Daniel Njenga, Cheruiyot started to slow himself down, and dug his heel into into the mat that sported the sponsor's logo. But the mat was slick plastic, not rough asphalt. His heel slid in front of him and he fell backwards, slamming the back of his head, which was 6'2" above his slipping shoe, against the asphalt. He did not get up.

"It was almost finishing my career," said Cheruiyot. Cheruiyot didn't know if he'd won (his torso slid across the line). Officials peeled him off the pavement, took him off in a wheelchair, and kept him in the hospital for two nights after a CAT scan showed bleeding inside his head. "I was not sleeping for one and a half months," he said. He feared a career-ending back injury. But he had crossed the finish line officially so had won the race and his career did not end. Yet the fall haunts him. "There is pain inside my head. When I run too much I feel it. I want to be back to run well like before."

His career focus is on big races with big prize money. "He can make much more money from long races," said Rosa, "than from getting $10,000 in small races every weekend."

Cheruiyot's Boston victory last year earned him $100,000, plus a $25,000 bonus for the course record. Winning in Chicago meant another $125,000 plus 25 more points in the World Marathon Majors race. If Cheruiyot won this third world major's race in Boston, he likely would win the WMM title, which is worth an extra $500,000.

But his head hurt and a coastal storm approached. Cheruiyot said, "I may have trained well but due to the headaches, I cannot say that I am 100 percent. But I'll give it my all. One of my strongest points is that I believe in myself and I'm confident of doing well. "

The storm came early, disturbing the elite women's start more than the later starters. The rain stopped and only gusts remained by the men's start. Race officials breathed a sigh of relief as runners at the gun just breathed.

Josephat Ongeri and Jared Nyamboki seemed blown down the road by their own gusts, but actually ran into the wind. Did they not know what they were doing? They opened up a lead of 2 minutes by 10 miles. But the pace was not fast. The leading pair only ran 1:07:07 at the half. They were not the favorites. They are Kenyans but listed as coming from Fayetteville, Ga. Some thought that their leading had something to do with promoting the shoes they wore. They seemed to be delivering on their marketing mission by leading through six checkpoints. The marathon has become a marketing opportunity. So maybe they did know what they were doing. In fact, the guys in the pack that thought themselves the contenders wondered who those two guys leading in the funny shoes were. If the good guys are back here, who are those guys? But no one ran fast or seemed to want to run fast. "I was thinking maybe the race will be 2:20," said Cheruiyot. The pack trailed the leaders by 1:37. "Everyone was around. Nobody wanted to go ahead. Nobody wanted to remain behind." Sixteen guys ran in that pack wondering who or what would help them. Sometimes the wind gusted to 30 mph in their faces. Who wants to take that in the face?

Help came from gravity that dragged those two show-stealing runners back into the pack. Someone started pushing and cranked out a 5:02 mile up the hills—the hills that blocked much of the wind. The push blew away all but seven—Cheruiyot, Kwambai, Stephen Kiogora, James Koskei, Benjamin Maiyo,

Teferi Wodajo, and Philip Manyim. The Georgia boys were nowhere to be seen. "From 35 kilometers," said Cheruiyot, "that is when we start the marathon."

Cheruiyot drifted to the front of the pack. He unleashed a 4:45 mile between miles 22 and 23. The next he cranked down to the race's fastest mile, 4:37.

With a little more than 2 miles to go, the race came down to Cheruiyot, Kwambai, and Kiogora. Kiogora dropped off, then Cheruiyot and Kwambai ran shoulder to shoulder. Kwambai had to decide what to do: dash away in perhaps foolish defiance of the champion and risk cramps and a crash out of the money or settle for 2nd and a $40,000 payday?

"I was staying behind because I wanted to be careful," said the 24-year-old Kwambai, who'd won in Beijing and Brescia last year but was stepping up market. "Some other people could come and get me."

Cheruiyot did not look back. He said, "When a lion is chasing an antelope, he doesn't look back. He has to eat. "So three wins for Cheruiyot. Maybe he buys another farm with the $100,000. He did win the WMM $500,000. Maybe he will retire. No one believes a runner can win seven times like Clarence DeMar or even four times like Bill Rodgers. "I think that maybe this is the last generation—myself—to win Boston three times,' said Cheruiyot. "Boston is not so easy. It is very tough."

Would he come back? They don't always. Look at the results below. The 79-year-old 1953 winner came back in 2007. How can Cheruiyot stay away?

2007 Men's Results

1. Robert Kipkoech Cheruiyot, KEN	2:14:13	21. Nathan Wadsworth, KS	2:2:22:13
2. James Kwambai, KEN	2:14:33	22. Matt Lavassiur, CO	2:22:50
3. Stephen Kiogora, KEN	2:14:47	23. Ross Martinson, PA	2:23:51
4. James Koskei, KEN	2:15:05	24. Thomas Frazer, IN	2:24:01
5. Teferi Eodajo, ETH	2:15:06	25. Jerome Ross, AK	2:24:47
6. Benjamin Maiyo, KEN	2:16:04	26. Patrick Moulton, NH	2:24:58
7. Ruggero Pertile, ITA	2:16:08	27. Robert Krar, AZ	2:25:44
8. Peter Gilmore, USA	2:16:41	28. Matthew Byrne, PA	2:25:48
9. Samuel Ndereba, KEN	2:17:04	29. David Bronfenbrenner, CA	2:25:50
10. Robert Cheboror, KEN	2:18:07	30. Terrance Shea, MA	2:25:54
11. Stephen Biwott, KEN	2:19:04	36. John Mortimer, MA	2:26:36
12. Ulrich Steidl, WA	2:19:54	50. John Friedman, MA	2:30:33
13. Hosea Kiprop Rotich, KEN	2:20:04	63. Michael Wardian, VA	2:33:22
14. Hiroki Tanaka, JPN	2:20:10	145. Eric Narcisi, MA	2:43:02
15. Miguel Nuci, CA	2:20:18	159. Abebe Mekonnen, ETH	2:44:12
16. Cecil Franke, IN	2:20:43	899. Robert Smith, MD	3:00:00
17. Christopher Lundstrom, MN	2:21:24	4702. John Lum Young, TRI	3:30:00
18. Philip Manyim, KEN	2:21:34	8822. Glen Hann, CA	4:00:01
19. Zachary Freudenburg, MO	2:21:40	10378. Keizo Yamada, JPN	4:24:07
20. Konrad Knutsen, CA	2:22:02	12363. Eugene Kern, FL	6:29:28

Winning Men's Teams

1. Adidas Transports Racing Team, CA, 7:08:10
2. Boston Athletic Association, 7:19:54
3. Philadelphia Runner Track Club, 7:22:26

Strong Field for Patriots Day Marathon

MONDAY, APRIL 16, 2007

Kastor American Hope

A strong field of women faced a little tougher conditions with their earlier start against the fading storm. One could argue that the early, or elite, women's start faced different conditions and was thus a different race than the first wave of runners who started 28 minutes later. Thus are the perils of the fickle New England spring weather.

Also unpredictable is the assignment of USA Championships. The American governing body declared this year's Boston Marathon to be the country's championship. So a strong field of American women came led by Olympic Athens bronze medalist Deena Kastor. Also coming to impress their own country was the Hansons' women's team from Michigan. The Hansons' men's team had won the previous year so why not complete the set? They came with a formidable team and couple of talking coaches. Kevin and Keith Hanson, according to Marc Chalufour writing in the BAA post-race racer's *Record Book*, talked a big game. Last year the men won by a whopping 21 minutes, so why not repeat? They brought their big guns: Melissa White, Dot McMahan, and Desiree Davila. But the host Boston Athletic Association team did not want them to walk away without a fight.

And a fight the race promised to be. The press corps picked no overwhelming favorite. The last year's winner, Kenyan Rita Jeptoo, had not been racing well, but last year's runner up, the charming Lativian Jelena Prokopcuka, had proven herself a constant threat with her consistency, but suffered recently from the flu. They both faced the American Olympian, Deena Kastor, and the ever-lurking mysterious Russians, Lydia Grigoryeva, who had won the Los Angeles marathon in March 2006 and Paris in April 2005, and Lyubov Denisova who had finished 2nd in Boston in 2003.

The remains of the storm spat annoying bursts of rain on the elite women and buffeted the field, forcing cautious racers to try to hide behind each other for protection. Kastor folded herself into the middle of the pack and hunkered under her dark baseball cap as the pace per mile lagged to 6-plus minutes at the half marathon mark. Wind blew from the east at 30 miles per hour during the first hour, then from the southeast at 22 miles per hour for the rest of the race. No one was eager to take the lead, often leaving Prokopcuka and Jeptoo as the reluctant front-runners as the race progressed through Framingham and Natick.

Prokopcuka felt used by the pack who seemed to want to hide behind her height. But at one time or another she had defeated everyone in the pack who had run against her. They all seemed to conspire to force her to lead. She displayed her annoyance after the race, "I was a bit disappointed because it's a difficult job to run against the wind. No one wanted to help me, so I had to run alone and try to make the pace, because I don't like jogging."

Grigoryeva in her Boston debut decided to follow the favorites and not lead. "I stayed behind Deena the first few miles but realized something was different with her. She was slowing down in downhill running."

With the old pro Prokopcuka in front, the top women passed the halfway point in 1:17:10. The warm-up was over and as the wind direction changed to a less direct headwind, they began to shed clothing—arm warmers, long-sleeved T-shirts, hats, gloves. The pace intensified, dwindling the pack to six. Kastor and Giovanna Volpato dwindled. Kastor ran 5 seconds behind by the 14-mile mark, then trailed the top group by 43 seconds a mile and a half later. She felt stomach cramps. Kastor had to stop at one of the well-placed portable toilets. She said afterwards, "I HAD to stop."

That the top American at Boston with a personal best of under 2:20 could not stay with the pack even before the hills chagrinned many American marathon fans.

"I just had a really bad day out there," said Kastor. "There was a lot of toying around with fast and slow paces. The pace was very pedestrian, so I was comfortable with that but my strength is going out and making a steady tempo run out of a race."

When she stepped out into the light she found herself in 9th place. After Heartbreak Hill, Mexican Madai Perez tried to separate herself from the Eastern Europeans, Grigoryeva and Prokopcuka, but they would not let her go. "The most important part was Heartbreak Hill," said Prokopcuka, "After that part, the last 7k, I knew the wind would be very strong in face. When your legs haven't enough strength, unbelievably hard." Jeptoo dropped back at 18 miles.

Prokopcuka had come down with the flu a month before the marathon and could not train exactly as she planned. She grimaced. The three often ran side by side navigating around puddles. They clung until Grigoryeva pushed ahead just before the 25-mile mark, separating with the fastest mile of the race, a 5:10. "During my training in Russia, the weather conditions were very similar," said Grigoryeva. "I am not surprised. I did a lot of long runs during cold, windy weather. She turned around to see a gap. She looked forward and ran, then checked back later to see the same gap. That moment gave her confidence.

"The leading group of about eight people started slow, but I decided to stay behind them and go through the pace. In the last half of the race, I felt very strong and confident in my ability to win the race," said Lidiya Grigoryeva.

Neither Prokopcuka nor Perez could close the gap, and on the contrary Grigoryeva pried it wider. Grigoryeva trains at altitude in Cheboksary, and Kislovodsk counted on her 10,000m experience to sustain the push. The wind and the surge were too much for Prokopcuka. She grimaced more and had to give up the hope and settle for 2nd.

Steps from the finish line, Grigoryeva veered to her right to pluck a Russian flag from the crowd. She clasped it in her right hand then glanced skyward with a look of thanks and relief. She crossed the finish line with her flag and her damp pony tail flapping in the breeze over the still wet, puddled pavement.

"I prepared for a faster race and time," said Grigoryeva, "but with the weather conditions, I had to make changes."

But Deena Kastor won herself an extra $25,000 for winning the U.S. Women's Marathon Championships that was this year declared a subset of the Boston Marathon. For someone with a personal best of 2:19:26—10 minutes ahead of the second contender, she only squeaked through to victory. Ann Alyanak and Kristin Price took the next two places, and qualified for the 2008 Olympic Trials.

Lyubov Denisova of Russian originally placed 7th but was removed from the results for having tested positive for prostanozol testosterone in an out-of-competition test. Reported by Frank Litsky on May 10, 2007, for the *New York Times* that she failed the drug test on March 20. She received a two-year ban.

2007 Women's Results:

1. **Lidiya Grigoryeva, RUS**	**2:19:18**	20. Lori Stich Zimmerman, TX	2:46:28
2. Jelana Prokopcuka, LAT	2:29:58	21. Phebe Ko, MD	2:36:30
3. Madai Perez, MEX	2:30:16	22. Norimi Sakurai, JPN	2:46:31
4. **Rita Jeptoo, KEN**	**2:33:08**	23. Kasie Enman, VT	2:47:26
5. Deena Kastor, CA	2:35:09	24. Veena Reddy, PA	2:48:18
6. Rove Tola Guta, ETH	2:36:29	25. Lava Tamara, CA	2:49:05
7. Alice Chelangat, KEN	2:38:07	26. Sopagna Eap, OR	2:49:16
8. Ann Alyanak, USA	2:28:55	27. Caryn Haffernan, WA	2:51:33
9. Kristin Price, USA	2:38:57	28. Angela Bestwick, NV	2:51:57
10. Mary Akor, USA	2:41:01	29. Laurie Knowles, GA	2:52:54
11. Christine Lundy, CA	2:41:14	30. Diona Fulton, MA	2:53:28
12. Janelle Krause, RI	2:41:24	34. Mega Doshi, MA	2:54:49
13. Zoila Gomez, CO	2:41:36	35. Heidy Lozano, TX	2:56:03,
14. Melissa White, MI	2:42:56		First Master
15. Kelly Flathers, CA	2:43:52	36. Emily Raymond, MA	2:56:16
16. Dot McMahan, MI	2:43:56	46. Brett Ely, MA	3:00:24
17. Turena Johnson Lane, FL	2:44:23	838. Melissa Sinning, OH	3:30:01
18. Desiree Davila, USA	2:44:56	4176. Tarra Richard, IA	4:00:00
19. Jenny Crain, WI	2:45:07	7973. Kristin McGrath, MA	6:35:19

Winning Women's Teams

1. Hanson-Brooks Distance Project, MI, 8:11:48
2. Boston Athletic Association, 8:29:14
3. Greater Boston Track Club, 8:55:00

Riots and Panics

MONDAY, APRIL 21, 2008

Kenyan Goes for Fourth Win

On New Year's Day 2008 rioters killed over 50 unarmed Kikuyu women and children, some as young as a month old, by locking them in church and burning them alive in Kiambaa village near Eldoret, Kenya. These violent protests began after the disputed election in late December, but were soon taken over by targeted ethnic violence. At first it was directed mainly against Kikuyu people, the largest ethnic group in the country, living outside their traditional settlement areas, especially in the Rift Valley. Later the violence spread to the cities. The violence continued sporadically for months, particularly in the Rift Valley.

This ethnic violence profoundly endangered the Kenyan running community and embarrassed them because those who compete internationally like to think of themselves as all Kenyan brothers and not members of disunited, squabbling tribes. They were not happy to explain what happened.

"We are still here," said Robert Kipkoech Cheruiyot, who is from the Nandi District near Uganda. Cheruiyot went off to train in Brazil, returned home for a week, then left for the safety of Namibia on the other corner of Africa. Wesley Ngetich, who'd won the Grandma's Marathon in Duluth, Minn., last year, was killed by an arrow in January during the tribal fighting. "It was by mistake he was killed," said Timothy Cherigat. "But it came as a shock."

The American economy generated a different sort of shock. Irrational exuberance, low inflation, stable growth, greed, and an oblivious attitude toward risk spun together to put the American financial system on the verge of collapse. It would fall later in the year. Companies made home mortgage loans to people who could not pay them back, and then sold the right to collect those payments to other people who had no knowledge that the original loans went to borrowers who had little income to pay them back; then unconnected, uninformed other financial agents bundled those securities backed by mortgages into insurance pools that were supposed to spread the risk of default widely enough to be safe.

Everyone said it was safe. But the demand for housing pushed up prices into a bubble that would burst. Property values fell. They fell below mortgage obligations. Incomes fell. People walked away from the houses they could no longer afford. Regulators such as Fed chairman Alan Greenspan had fallen asleep at the wheel. The big investment company Lehman would go bankrupt. Jobs vanished. Markets plunged.

For the first time since he became race director in 1985, Guy Morse would not be at the starting line in Hopkinton this morning. "It was a tough decision, but I thought better of it," said Morse. His title now was Boston Athletic Association Executive Director. He was recovering from surgery after rupturing both quadricep tendons in February and had to use crutches.

The weather seemed to cooperate with a start temperature of 53°F and no wind.

To win the Boston Marathon for the fourth time would be so sweet for Robert Kipkoech Cheruiyot. It would put him in the book with Bill Rodgers, but other runners had other ideas. Kenyan Lawrence Saina set the early pace, leading at seven of the first eight checkpoints. They all clocked 30:20 at 10k. Cherigat, Kwambai, Cheboibock, Kosei—the usual suspects. But some dangerous strangers lingered—a couple of unusual suspects.

Ten miles passed in 48:11.

Cheruiyot pushed away from James Mwangi Macharia at the 13-mile mark, planning to win and break the course record. At the half marathon in 1:03:07 he pushed the pace and thinned a lead pack of six runners to four. The unusual suspects still hung on: Abderrhime Bouramdane, Kasime Adillo, and Gashaw Asfaw. Two Moroccans and an Ethiopian. No more Kenyan friends accompanied the three-time king and the tallest man in the pack.

By the firehouse turn heading up Commonwealth Avenue, the whittled pack of four—Cheruiyot, countryman James Kwambai, Morocco's Abderrahime Bouramdane and Ethiopia's Kasime Adillo—ran together. Cheruiyot knew he could beat Kwambai, because he ran away from him last year. He wasn't sure about the others.

At the 18-mile mark, Cheruiyot split 4:37 for the mile, his fastest of the day. That wrung submission from the two 30-year-old Moroccan pursuers. "Two guys and I don't know them," Cheruiyot said. "When I decide to move," he said, "I don't look back." Perhaps he did not dare look back. A backward glance could encourage the dangerous Moroccan hunters. "For me, it was better to kill them before," Cheruiyot said. "When the lion wants meat, he has to kill."

"I just wanted to go fast," said Cheruiyot. "I wanted to make this race faster and better this year, and also to achieve my goal of running a 2:07."

"This was the hardest one," Cheruiyot said after the race. "I wanted the race to be very fast and so I started from the first kilometer."

He wanted a course record, however a late sea breeze prevented that, but only slightly. He suffered in miles 20 and 21 with only a 5:17 split. The aggressive racing from the first kilometer took its toll on him, but also on everyone else. In marathon racing if you want to make your opponents suffer, you must be willing to suffer too. "It's very difficult when you're running alone here in Boston," Cheruiyot said. "You need company."

Once he broke away he lost the help of competitors' rhythms and had to concentrate alone. The chance at a new course record slipped away.

"Boston is very different from the other marathons," Cheruiyot said. "As usual, the course was very difficult and I tried to push harder this year." Cheruiyot explained, "Hills are challenging, but I enjoy running in the hills." He finished just 32 seconds short of his course record.

Cheruiyot celebrated by dropping to his knees and twice kissing the pavement. He stood and pumped his fist four times—one for each win. Turning to the crowds he displayed four fingers. Winning is good. "When I come to America, everyone will know I have won four times," Cheruiyot said. "I am in the book with Bill Rodgers."

For Bouramdane, a sock subverted his Boston debut, but his explanation at first left reporters confused. At the post-race press conference he apologized, saying his English wasn't so good. Then he said he was fluent in French and Arabic, for those in the media who would like to ask questions in those languages. No one did. The press stuck with English, so Bouramdane tried.

"The trouble started at 18 with my suck," he said. "It slipped off my foot."

Your "suck?" asked an incredulous reporter.

"Yes," Bouramdane said. "My suck."

When he took off his right shoe, reporters could see that Bouramdane referred to his "sock," that had caused an angry red blister on the inside of his big toe. "I would like to congratulate Robert Cheruiyot," said Bouramdane. "He's very, very strong. It was a strong course and a strong marathon."

Winning is good. Finishing 2nd is good too. But not everything is good. For instance, cheating is bad. Famous cyclist Lance Armstrong ran wearing bib No.100. He has since been totally discredited. He came to Boston to raise money. "Boston and New York are the two big ones," he said.

His name appears in the results below, but he was found guilty of doping and had his Tour de France titles striped from him. Armstrong denied doping for more than a decade before finally admitting it in a televised interview with Oprah Winfrey in January 2013. Armstrong has been banned from sanctioned cycling events for life. His name will no longer appear in this book. Indeed, a year of violence and fraud.

2008 Men's Results:

1. **Robert Kipkoech Cheruiyot, KEN**	**2:07:46**	
2. Abderrahime Bouramdane, MAR	2:09:04	
3. Khalid El Boumlili, MAR	2:10:35	
4. Gashaw Asfaw, ETH	2:10:47	
5. Kasime Adillo, ETH	2:12:24	
6. **Timothy Cherigat, KEN**	**2:14:13**	
7. Christopher Cheboiboch, KEN	2:14:47	
8. James Kwambai, KEN	2:15:52	
9. James Koskei, KEN	2:16:07	
10. Nicholas Arciniaga, MI	2:16:13	
11. Abdelhadi El Mouaziz, MAR	2:16:51	
12. Tesfaye Girma, ETH	2:18:40	
13. Shadrack Kiplagat, KEN	2:18:55	
14. Jason Schoener, VA	2:19:18	
15. March Heuland, NC	2:20:57	
16. Edward Kimosop, KEN	2:22:22	

17. James Lander, CA	2:22:34		29. Cecil Franke, IN	2:25:50
18. Katsuhiko Fulunaga, JPN	2:23:15		30. Mbacha Mangeh, CMR	2:25:51
19. Gino Van Geyte, BEL	2:23:36		50. Thomas Martin, CT	2:30:18
20. Bruce Deacon, CAN	2:23:56		478. ~~Lance Armstrong, TX~~	~~2:50:58~~
21. Oleg Strizhankov, RUS	2:24:16		1185. Mark Snyder, NJ	3:00:00
22. Patrick Rizzo, MI	2:24:27		5558. Steve King, NY	3:30:01
23. Eric Blake, CT	2:24:30		**8513. Amby Burfoot**	**3:51:04**
24. Dan Vassallo, MA	2:25:10		9551. Tim Wampler, KY	4:00:00
25. Alan Horton, TN	2:25:14		**12682. Kiezo Yamada, JPN**	**5:18:23**
26. Jason Bodnar, NC	2:25:22			(age 80)
27. Ben Reynolds, GBR	2:25:23		13019. Steven Witt, VA	7:35:19
28. Tariku Aboset, ETH	2:25:35			

Men's Winning Teams

1. Boston Athletic Association, 7:34:37
2. Pacers/Brooks Racing Team, VA, 7:35:26
3. Greater Boston Track Club, 7:36:55
4. Georgetown Running Company, DC, 7:39:48
5. Knoxville Track Club, TN, 7:44:40
6. Whirlaway Track Running Club, MA, 7:45:51

No American Women This Time

MONDAY, APRIL 21, 2008

Two-Marathon Weekend: Olympic Trials and Boston

No American women would play a role in the 2008 Boston Marathon. Deena Kastor may well have been a contender, and most likely would have run better than last year's race, when she was interrupted by a cramping stomach that forced a toilet stop. But this year she had run the day before, winning the Olympic Trials on a loop course along the Charles River between Boston and Cambridge.

The women's race slipped from the starting line at 9:35 a.m. Joan Samuelson, who had run the day before in the 2008 Olympic Trials Marathon, fired the starting gun in Hopkinton under cloudy skies and 50°F temperatures. They hit the easy first mile in 5:23 and the 5k in 17:09, which put them on record pace. Prokopcuka led. She had trained at altitude and in the canyon of San Luis Obispo in California before the race. She had won the NYC Marathon and the Osaka Marathon in 2:22:56.

The wind blew in their faces, weakening the next 5k to 17:41. The next 5k slowed slightly to 17:43, and grossly to 18:14. They had slowed to some miles of 5:57 reaching halfway in 1:14:45 and 25k in 1:28:37. Six women had taken turns leading. Each popped into the lead to push the pace but the wind, pushing back, undermined their confidence and made each in turn revise the plan and seek shelter in the pack. Young Dire Tune tried her pull at the front but hesitated and melted back into the pack. Tune comes from the same Arci region in Ethiopia where many of the country's great distance runners grew up, including the legendary Haile Gebrselassie.

As the miles passed the pack became increasing nervous.

The turn-taking stopped at mile 22 when Russian Alevtina Biktimirova summed up her pre-race confidence and charged with a 5:08 mile, and then followed it with a 5:12. Gradually Prokopcuka, Grigoryeva, and finally Jeptoo lost grip. But Dire Tune only held on. Brash underdogs seemed to have less fear of the wind. The two of them strained toward the ever-less-distant finish line having left the formidable Rita Jeptoo and Jelana Prokopcuka behind. Two women ran yielding nothing to each other and each dreading a race that would come down to a final sprint. Resolving a race sooner would be better. It would be nice to run down the corridor of cheers on the Bolyston Street. How wonderful it would be to look around and see the crowds and acknowledge them and maybe accept your country's flag and wave it in solo glory. But the perfect match of these two athletes would not allow such a luxury. First place would win twice as much money as 2nd, $150,000 to $75,000. And further winning would be good to impress their respective countries' Olympic selectors to go to China. Both wanted to sprint away, but neither were sprinters which of course is why they became marathoners. Biktimirova had run 1500 meters in 4:18 and Tune only 4:25. They had been trying for hours to drop each other but they stuck to each other like Tango dancers. Biktimirova displayed admirable abdominal muscles. Tune led down Beacon Street but nearly lost the race at that point because, in her fatigued state, she started to follow the press truck as it left the course to continue down Beacon off the course instead of taking the turn onto Hereford Street. Spectators and officials pointed her in the right direction and she swung back into stride with Biktimirova. Neither had been picked as favorites with the press approving Jiptoo, Prokopcuka, or the previous year's winner, the Russian Grigoryeva.

The lead switched twice as Tune and Biktimirova turned onto Boylston Street. Seemingly willing to race herself into a coma, Tune pinned herself to the lead and with all the energy she had left, she surged ahead and regained the lead with 150 yards to go. The two of them ran down Boylston Street with the slow-motion feeling exhaustion brings to running as fast as possible. At last Biktimirova could not respond.

It proved to be the closest women's finish in Boston history. Tune crossed the finish line, kneeled, and kissed the ground. Biktimirova followed two seconds later, swerving slightly to avoid the ground-kissing Tune.

"Coming to the finish, I realized that Biktimirova was very strong," said Tune through a translator. "The only thing that was going through my mind was,

'Even if I collapse at the finish line, I will get the victory.' The Boston Marathon is such a big marathon that when I go back to my country and tell people I won here, it will make a big name for me."

"In the last two years, when she started having big wins and setting new personal records, she started thinking big," said Hussein Makke, Tune's manager. "She wants to put her name with the best of the best in Ethiopia like Fatuma Roba and Derartu Tulu. "She has everything any champion needs. She just needs more time and experience. She's a very, very determined athlete and a fighter."

"When I was not able to run away from her earlier in the race, I conserved my energy to use for a final kick," said Tune. "I tried to pass, but it was a little bit windy. When I go back behind her, she protected me from the wind. I am a smart racer and know how to listen to my body."

"On Heartbreak Hill, I tried to get away," said Biktimirova, through a translator. "I was leaning forward and trying to push it. I am a good uphill runner. I tried several times to make a move on the hills. "

"Even before I came to Boston, I was confident I could win the Boston Marathon," said Tune. "From the beginning to the end of the race, my training and the way I ran helped me finish strong. Once I saw the finish line, I was certain I would finish first."

Dire Tune ran 2:31:16 for 15th in the 2008 Olympic Marathon.

2008 Women's Results

1. **Dire Tune, ETH**	**2:25:25**	18. Makie Makajima, JPN	2:50:42
2. Alevtina Biktimirova, RUS	2:25:27	19. Emily Landis, PA	2:50:50
3. **Rita Jeptoo, KEN**	**2:26:34**	20. Christa Benton, FL	2:51:03
4. Jelena Prokopcuka, LAT	2:28:12	21. Sonia O'Sullivan, IRE	2:52:10
5. Askale Tafa Magarsa, ETH	2:29:48	22. Gabrielle O'Rourke, NZL	2:53:12
6. Bruna Genovese, ITA	2:30:52	23. Elle Pishny, NC	2:54:04
7. Nuta Olaru, ROU	2:33:56	24. Jennette Seckinger, OR	2:54:48
8. Robe Tola Guta, ETH	2:34:37	25. Bean Wrenn, CO	2:55:10
9. **Lidiya Grigoryeva, RUS**	**2:35:37**	26. Becky Angeles, TX	2:55:28
10. Stephanie Hood, CAN	2:44:44	27. Sue Pierson, WI	2:55:31
11. Denise Robson, CAN	2:45:54	28. Allison Krausen, CO	2:55:45
12. Magdaline Chemjor, KEN	2:46:25	29. Rachel Rich, WI	2:56:37
13. Firaya Sultanova-Zhdanova, RUS	2:47:17, First Master	30. Corina Canitz, WI	2:56:51
14. Eliza Mayger, AUS	2:47:36	31. Megan Doshi, CA	2:57:15
15. Ashley Anklam, NM	2:48:43	54. Kristin West, IL	3:00:00
16. Kelly Jaske, OR	2:48:49	1146. Ulrike Lange, GER	3:30:00
17. Kim Duclos, MA	2:49:31	5000. Issy Nelson, RI	4:00:00
		8927. Stacy Durma, MA	6:31:01182

Winning Women's Teams

1. Central Massachusetts Striders, 8:52:02
2. Team Red Lizards, OR, 8:52:12
3. Impala Racing Team, CA, 8:55:15

God's Plan Plays Out:
The Last Lion Standing

MONDAY, APRIL 20, 2009

Ryan Hall, the New American Hope

Ryan Hall came to Boston to win. He wasn't the first person to think of that, but his faith told him that he would prevail.

"I don't try to force my faith on people, but at the same time I'm not going to hide it, especially because it's such a big part of me," said Hall. "It is who I am. It is impossible for me to talk about my running without talking about my faith because it plays into every single day, every single run and every part of who I am."

"When I think about how I am as a runner, what I worry about most is going out too fast. I love running downhills. So, I know it's going to take a lot of self-control to not just rip it the first half and go out really hard. I know I'm going to have to run with a lot of wisdom and discernment and humility out there because I've never run this course. I haven't [raced] Heartbreak Hill yet. I'm going to need to make sure I'm going to be able to make it through that tough section of the course."

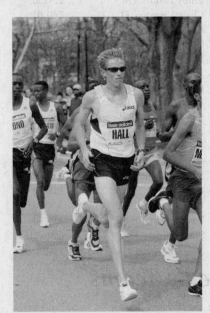

Hall won the 2008 U.S. Olympic Team Trials Marathon in a Trials-Record 2:09:02, then placed 10th in the Olympic Marathon in Beijing.

Ryan Hall may have had God on his side but all the pressure weighed on Robert Kipkoech Cheriyot to win for a fifth time. A lot of things have to go right to win a major world marathon. The runner has to be at his best. That is hard to maintain for six years, but then the experience of racing the best in the world and winning is a priceless power for continued success.

Hall bolted at the 10 a.m. gun, flying down the hill out of Hopkinton to a 4:38 first mile. The temperature was ideal at 51°F but the wind blew in their faces at 9.2 mph. Hall said, "My plan was to run my

Ryan Hall, tall, blond, Californian, "My day will come."

own race from the get-go." He was still go-getting at 5k in 14:33. A mob of 13 runners hung on to that pace, 50 seconds faster than course record speed. No one was letting Hall run away with it. Ethiopians Gashaw Asfaw, Tekeste Kebede, Solomon Molla, and Deriba Merga contested in that pack with Kenyans Daniel Rono, James Kosgei, Stephen Kiogora, and three Cheruiyots, Robert, Evans, and the other Robert [Kiprono].

All these racers clicked through 10 miles in 48:06 and slowed to a mere 1:03:39 at the half. They ran together with strength in numbers, snatching water, splashing some on their colored shirts with their sponsors' logos. There may have been Ethiopians and Kenyans but also there were Nike and Adidas and the blond, blue-eyed American in a Japanese brand, Asics. Hall ran in the middle of all these East Africans. He said, "I wanted to make it a full 26-mile race and not let it come down to the final 10k. I wanted to make it an honest race."

All together all these guys knew someone, sometime would inject a surge and spoil the party.

It was the Ethiopian lion, Merga, who threw in the spoiler. Regardless of a building headwind, he said to himself that he wanted to be the last lion standing. "There are a lot of strong athletes with us," he said. "If I didn't push, maybe I didn't have a chance to win." But Molla and Rono gamely went with him. "At 18k, he is coming from behind," Merga said. "After that, he did not come. I think this day is not for him." Hall fell back to 9th place. But Merga had created some pain in those who tried to follow even at some distance, leaving them vulnerable to Hall. Most famous among them was Robert Kipkoech Cheruiyot, who dropped out at Cleveland Circle and had to be taken to St. Elizabeth's Hospital for observation and later released—no fifth win. Hall fought back. But Merga crested the hills full of power at 20 miles in 1:37:37. No one would catch him. "I am looking behind," he said of his observation at the crest, "and there is nobody behind of me." Victory did indeed taste sweet for Merga. He had dropped out of his first Boston in 2006. "Boston is one of the biggest marathons in the world. Because of that, our people are very happy." With his $150,000 prize money so was he.

"Would I have liked to win? Yeah," said Hall. "Did I think I had a legitimate shot? Of course. But a lot of guys have legitimate shots and don't win."

Hall said, "My day will come. " Hall would be back. The Boston Marathon is a sweet lure to its champions and nearly all champions come back.

So many come back to Boston. Past winner (1953) 81-year-old Keizo Yamada returned to this year's race. It would be his last. Bill Rodgers came back, as did the old BAA runner, John DiCommandrea, who did his best racing in the 1950s, and the now 40-year-old contender Silivo Guerra from Ecuador came back. The pull of the Boston Marathon is strong.

2009 Men's Results

1. **Deriba Merga, ETH**	2:08:42	4. Tekeste Kebede, ETH	2:09:49
2. Daniel Rono, KEN	2:09:32	5. **Robert Kiprono Cheruiyot, ETH**	2:10:06
3. Ryan Hall, USA	2:09:40	6. Gashaw Asfaw, KEN	2:10:44

7. Solomon Molla, ETH	2:12:02	24. Eric Blake, CT	2:23:54
8. Evans Cheruiyot, KEN	2:12:45	25. Carl Rundell, MI	2:24:19
9. Stephen Kiogora, KEN	2:13:00	26. John Thompson, KY	2:24:23
10. Timothy Cherigat, KEN	**2:13:04**	27. Tracy Lokken, MI	2:24:39
11. James Koskei, KEN	2:14:52,	28. Kalib Wilkinson, VA	2:24:46
	First Master	29. Michael Mckeeman, CA	2:25:33
12. Grigoriy Andreev, RUS	2:16:27	30. Crosby Freeman, CA	2:25:36
13. Lee Troop, AUS	2:16:21	38. Silvio Guerra, ECU	2:27:50
14. Brian Sell, PA	2:16:3	55. Michael Wardian, VA	2:30:50
15. Patrick Rizzo, MI	2:17:05	1275. Brian Walsh, MA	3:00:01
16. Luke Humphrey, MI	2:18:48	6088. Robert Smart, IL	3:30:00
17. Sergio Reyes, CA	2:19:22	10231. Stephen Dunkley, BER	4:00:00
18. Todd Snyder, MI	2:19:55	**10722. Bill Rodgers, MA**	**4:06:49**
19. Kyle O'Brien, MI	2:20:55	13533. John Di Commandrea,	
20. Gino Van Geyte, BEL	2:22:00	MA	6:06:23
21. Stephen Drew, CAM	2:22:15	(age 81, 12th in 1955)	
22. Allen Wagner, PA	2:23:36	**13540. Keizo Yamada, JPN**	**6:16:56**
23. Katsukiko Fukunaga, JPN	2:23:51	13545. Michael McBride, CO	7:31:36

Winning Men's Teams

1. Hanson-Brooks Distance Project, MI, 6:52:24
2. Asics Aggies Running Club, 7:14:26
3. Boston Athletic Association, 7:23:09
4. Greater Boston Track Club, 7:36:12
5. Whirlaway Racing Team, 7:42:16
6. Adidas Transports, CA, 7:47:37

To the Kicker Belongs the Spoils

MONDAY, APRIL 20, 2009

Goucher Carries American Hopes

Still no signs that the nation's worst recession since the Great Depression would end. The U.S. economy had lost more than 7 million jobs since the recession began in 2007; and in 2009 the unemployment rate stretched past 10 percent, its highest rate in over 25 years. But marathoners came to Boston just as they did in the Great Depression in the 1930s, but the 1930s' unthinkable idea of women racing, as well as the sheer size of the race, uplifted spirits. An accomplished Boston Marathoner said once that it didn't matter if you are unemployed as long as your running is going well.

Kara Goucher herself charmed and lifted the city, but she came to Boston like Atlas, carrying the weight of the world on her shoulders. Expectations pressed on her like a planet: expectations from her coach, her husband, her sponsor, and most weightily of all, herself. The cover of *New England Runner Magazine*'s pre-marathon issue blared a quotation from Kara Goucher, "My goal is to win Boston."

When this author learned of a quotation from the Duluth, Minnesota, *News Tribune* that she is an avid reader of earlier editions of *Boston Marathon* history book and wants her own chapter of Boston Marathon history (!), all semblance of disinterested journalism on the part of this writer vanished. She said, "I'd love to be a chapter in the book." Here it is.

She flattered fans of American marathoning by stating boldly her intention to be the first American woman to win the Boston Marathon since 1985. Nearly every American wanted Kara Goucher to win. But the marathon is a tough and tricky business. The odds always favor the field over any individual. Partisanship cannot spin the results that occur on asphalt and hills. And odd things happen.

Ethiopian Bezunesh Bekele came to town with the fastest time, 2:23:09.

Forty-five-year-old Colleen De Reuck felt surprised to be leading. No one wanted to take the lead and block the wind for everyone else by pushing the pace. Goucher said, "Someone would go to the front and then just stop. It was so windy, nobody wanted to be in the front."

Frequently De Reuck found herself drifting to the front during the first 10 miles.

The laughably slow women's race gave Tomoe Yokoyama and Hiroko Sho some unexpected international camera exposure as they ran at the head of the elite women's pack. Yokoyama had suffered injuries since winning February's Ome Marathon 30k road race and hoped only to break 2:40, meaning that the lead pack's speed throughout the first 10k of the race suited her fine. As the pace crept glacially forward, Sho drifted away, but Yokoyama moved to the front and alternated the lead with veteran American Colleen De Reuck.

The women's elite field ran the first mile at a cold molasses pace with Colleen De Reuck leading. She said afterward, "I was a little embarrassed leading in 6:28—you get paid a lot to come to the race." But at the mile, she took control to get the field moving to a 6:01 next mile, but still the entire bunch of seventeen ran only 18:59 at 5k or a pace projecting to a 2:40 marathon. The weather was cool and the headwind real, but not very strong.

Seventeen runners ran slowly, milling around each other with various runners in the lead but no one daring to take the initiative. No miles clicked by faster than a 5:34 at mile 16.

Americans Elva Dryer, Mary Akor, De Reuck, and Goucher ran in various places in the big pack. Goucher looked vigilant, remaining in about 3rd place in the group so she could see and respond if anyone surged. At about 15 miles, while De Reuck led, the pack surged, leaving De Reuck behind, but to her amazement the pack slowed, so De Reuck caught up and then dutifully took the lead that she held until mile 20. De Reuck aimed to run 2:30 to win the master's women's race but never expected to be leading the whole thing. The race became a waiting game.

Goucher said, "I knew someone was going to flip the switch and start the racing, I just didn't think it would be me . . ." At 22 miles, Goucher seized the lead and began the push to the finish running the next 5k in 16:22, the fastest of the race by more than 90 seconds. The pace had dropped for the first time to below 5:30 per mile with a 5:21, then a 5:20, then a 5:09. Then there were only three runners left.

As she emerged from the Mass Ave. underpass, Goucher ripped off her gloves to prepare symbolically for the big kick past the two remaining runners, Dire Tune and Salina Kosgei.

But Goucher could not lift to a kick. The last mile did not accelerate but only registered 5:19. Kosgei had not studied the course, something that in a close race can be fatal. "When I was coming to the finish, I thought the first turn was the finish. So after I saw another turn (onto Boylston Street) I was like, *wow—I'm not going to finish!*"

Ahead of Goucher by 5 seconds, Tune and Kosgei exchanged leads down the final stretch. Last year, Tune kicked to victory by 2 seconds. This year she faced Kosgei, who had started her running as a 400/800-meter runner. But it was Tune who took the lead in sight of the finish line. Kosgei said, "At the end I had given up when [Tune] when in front." But she may not have studied the course, but she had studied sprinting. She said afterward, "So I know about sprinting." She lifted up on her toes and danced past Tune. Kosgei won by a second. Tune fell on the finishing mat and had to be raised by medical staff. The slow 2:32:16 won the Boston Marathon—the slowest winning time since 1985, and was Kosgei's personal worst. Imagine winning the Boston Marathon with the slowest marathon time of your life? Goucher staggered in 3rd—utterly spent, and cried into her husband's shoulder as Salazar consoled her. "I wanted to be the one who won for everybody."

"What she proved today was that she has the wheels," declared Bill Squires, the original Greater Boston Track Club Coach. "I was very impressed. She is still a marathon rookie. You need experience to run Boston, with its rolling terrain. This is the toughest course in the world, no doubt. What do Old John Kelley, Johnny Kelley, and Bill Rodgers all have in common? They were all dropouts in their first Boston Marathons."

"For her first time here, she did great. It's not like other courses. You've got 7.5 miles of treacherous hills that will really beat you up, and then you go flat. And when you talk about a kick, in road racing the kick may start with a mile to go. Here it starts with 4 miles to go."

"It was a great race, and she ran a great race," said Samuelson. "And she made the race. She really pushed it when it needed to be pushed. She got them back on pace."

"It was too slow for all of us," Goucher said.

"Very honestly," she said, "I thought I'd have that kick. My legs felt 'poppy,' and my legs had lots of control. I can tell you I did not feel 'poppy' in New York. All day long I thought I'd have that extra gear, but it wasn't there. No one expects any more out of me than I do myself," she pointed out. "For people to have high hopes for me is, I think, a good thing."

Shortly, she recovered her balance. She will be back to Boston. "My first comment to [Goucher] after she crossed the finish line," said two-time champion Joan Benoit Samuelson, "was, 'You've experienced Boston now, you'll know what to do.' When she comes back, she will bring friends."

2009 Women's Results

1. Salina Kosgei, KEN	2:32:16	19. Nathalie Vasseur, FRA	2:47:04
2. Dire Tune, ETH	2:32:17	20. Tomoe Yokoyama, JPN	2:47:57
3. Kara Goucher, USA	2:32:25	21. Denise Robson, CAN	2:48:15
4. Bezunesh Bekele, ETH	2:33:08	22. Allison Kerr, CA	2:49:34
5. Helena Kirop, KEN	2:33:24	23. Hiroko Sho, JPN	2:49:37
6. Lidiya Grigoryeva, RUS	2:34:20	24. Meghan Arbrogast, OR	2:49:46
7. Atsede Habtamu, ETH	2:35:34	25. Tamara Karrh, GA	2:49:50
8. Colleen De Reuck, USA	2:35:37	26. Jutta Merilaine, CAN	2:49:51
9. Alice Timbilili, KEN	2:36:25	27. Sheila Casey, NJ	2:50:02
10. Alina Ivanova, USA	2:36:50	28. Christa Benton, FL	2:50:05
11. Sheri Piers, ME	2:37:04	29. Andrea Pomaranski, MI	2:50:55
12. Elva Dryer, CO	2:38:50	30. Shelby Joslyn, MI	2:51:29
13. Mary Akor, CA	2:41:09	68. Michelle Kelley, UT	2:59:54
14. Heidi Westerling, NH	2:43:11	1204. Stephanie Hordequin, MA	3:30:00
15. Anzhelika Averkova, UKR	2:44:19	5468. Jill Ludwig, CA	4:00:00
16. Veena Reddy, VA	2:45:46	6880. Andrea Hatch, ME	5:12:37
17. Jennifer Feenstra, CAN	2:46:16	(25+ finishes)	
18. Adanech Zekiros, ETH	2:46:51	9298. Maryellen Loucks, MA	7:16:03

Winning Women's Teams

1. Boston Athletic Association, 8:51:34
2. Somerville Road Runners, MA, 9:07:26
3. Whitby Tigers Running Club, ON, 9:10:49
4. Greater Boston Track Club, 9:13:32
5. Reebok-Rhode Island, 9:15:27

Chapter 13

2010–2016: Terrorism Comes Back to Boston

President: *Barack Obama*

Massachusetts Governors: *Deval Patrick, Charlie Baker*

Boston Mayors: *Thomas Menino, Martin J. "Marty" Walsh*

2010 populations: *United States, 309.3 million; Massachusetts, 6.6 million; Boston, 620,451*

This decade saw the U.S. pull out of a financial recession. From a low of 6,507.04 on March 9, 2009, the Dow Jones returned to pre-recession levels. But the sting of the economic recession gave rise to authoritarian candidates supported by those who did not benefit from the economic recovery and blamed others for preventing their prosperity. The conflict between globalism and nationalism spread around the world, and the hopes in what was called the Arab Spring dissipated into local power disputes.

Hillary Clinton battled Donald Trump for the U.S. presidency in the dirtiest political campaign in over 150 years. A toxic media-defined tribalism took over the country, organized by cable networks like Fox, NPR, CNN, and CNBC, and gerrymandered districts guaranteed the election of extreme candidates.

Some other events that characterize this decade:

On April 20, 2010, a final cement seal of an oil well in the Gulf of Mexico failed, causing oil and methane gas to spew from an uncapped wellhead a mile below the surface of the ocean for 87 straight days.

On September 17, 2011, the Occupy Wall Street action received global attention and spawned the Occupy movement against social and economic inequality worldwide. The movement is said to have also spawned the candidacy of Vermont Senator Bernie Sanders for the democratic nomination for U.S. president and set battle lines between the 1 percent richest people and the 99 percent who weren't. In October 2012, Hurricane Sandy caused such destruction in NYC that officials canceled the New York City Marathon.

On March 13, 2013, Jorge Bergoglio of Argentina was elected the 266th Roman Catholic Pontiff, Pope Francis.

On March 8, 2014, Malaysia Flight 370 disappeared in the South Pacific.

In 2016, in a manifestation of the politics of resentment, a majority of Brits blamed the European Union for their failure to rise economically and forced Britain to leave the European Union.

In the fall of 2016, U.S.-Russian relationships met a new and dangerous low around the political upheaval in Syria. Russia deployed nuclear weapons in the

Mediterranean. U.S. and Russian forces came dangerously close to each other over Syrian cities such as Aleppo.

In October 2016, Ethiopia declared a state of emergency because of protests in Oromia.

In this decade, the Boston Marathon would suffer its greatest shock and trauma as terrorist bombs exploded at the finish area. The bombs killed three people and injured many more and set off a long, paralyzing manhunt. Yet in the subsequent year, the marathon would find its future in bringing its past full circle to define itself as a symbol of a people overcoming adversity. The bombing would stimulate many films and videos depicting the crime, the suffering of the victims, their courage in overcoming adversity, and described at the end of this chapter, a documentary embracing the entire history of the marathon.

More Cows and a Few Sheep

MONDAY, APRIL 19, 2010

Fast Field Assembled

On April 14 the Eyjafjallajökull volcano in Iceland entered its second phase of eruption, sending an abrasive ash cloud up 30,000 feet to hover over Europe. Airlines canceled nearly two-thirds of all European flights because of the thick cloud of volcanic ash that might damage plane engines.

The 1970 winner, Ron Hill, accepted a BAA invitation to come to Boston to be recognized 40 years after his win. But he could not get a flight out of the U.K. "Just when you think you've dealt with everything, now we add volcanoes to the mix," Guy Morse said.

On February 17, 2010, David Lelei died in a motor vehicle accident while traveling with Boston winner and friend Moses Tanui along the Nairobi-Nakuru highway (A104 road), about 200 kilometers from Nairobi. Tanui sustained serious injuries to his chest and legs, and was rushed to the nearby St. Mary's hospital before being transferred to Nairobi hospital for specialist treatment. Doctors have described his condition as "out of danger."

Ryan Hall arrived in Boston from California three weeks earlier and trained on the course. He planned to win and would leave nothing to chance. His preparation was meticulous.

At pre-race press events the runners talked about the race, the course, and their experiences in and on it. "After last year, I felt I didn't have a great understanding of the course," said Hall, who along with Meb Keflezighi was half of the great American hope to win Boston. About the last year Hall said, "The learning curve is so tough. This is the most technical course in the world. Knowing the ins and outs, knowing how to spend your energy on the hills. There's so much to glean from the course."

Particularly reckoning when and where to make your move—and when not to is essential. In his first effort here four years ago, Keflezighi succumbed to optimism by joining Ethiopia's Deriba Merga and Kenya's Benjamin Maiyo in a mad dash through Wellesley, hitting the midway point more than 2 minutes under Cosmas Ndeti's course record.

"I looked at my watch and I said, *Wow!*" recalls Keflezighi. "This is going to be a big day for a PR—or it's going to be a long day." It was long.

Robert Kipkoech Cheruiyot, who had won, knew the pace was insane, so he sat back, waited until the firehouse turn heading into the hills, then made his move and off the early fast pace set the course record of 2:07:14.

"It's become the norm that an African will win a major race," said Hall. "But Meb won in New York. It's just a matter of time." But Americans have to learn how to race Boston's diabolical contours.

Keflezighi knew that last year he could have made better tactical decisions. He finished third and wanted to go back to school on the course. He asked the BAA to send videos of the course for him to study.

It's one thing to see the course," Keflezighi said. "It's another thing to run on it."

"You learn it by getting your butt kicked," said Bill Rodgers.

"They're not making it any easier for Ryan or me," said Keflezighi. "But we want to be the best in the world."

Greg Meyer, who was in Boston to watch the race, is surprised that no other American has won it in 27 years. He didn't like being called the "last" American to win Boston, because that sounds like there will never be another. He'd rather be called the most recent American winner of the Boston Marathon.

"I thought I'd win again," he said about his 1983 victory. "We had three guys under 2:10 that day (Meyer, Ron Tabb, and Benji Durden) and a bunch of guys under 2:12. I assumed it would keep going. It's been overdue."

"The course is very tough," said Merga, who has run in London, Berlin, Beijing, Houston, Paris, and Fukuoka. "It is up-down-up-down. You cannot run constant."

The first miles are downhill, tempting runners to try to push the same fast pace when the course flattens.

"You have to keep your cool," said Bill Rodgers.

"The uniqueness of Boston is how eccentric the course is," said Terrence Mahon, who coached Hall. "It hits you hard at all the wrong times."

Hall went for a run with Rodgers to learn the master's wisdom.

"He shared a couple of his little tricks," Hall said. When asked what those tricks were, Hall did not answer precisely for the press to report to his competition.

"He'd say things like, 'This is a spot on the course where I've pushed it,'" Hall said.

The weather is a big, unpredictable factor in Boston. "It's so much different here than back home," said Hall.

Merga ran his first marathon in Boston in 2006 and dropped out. Keflezighi and Benjamihn Maiyo ran a crazy pace. "I didn't calculate the distance," Merga said. "I lost my energy and dropped out. Now, I know the course. I know which part is difficult."

Last year Merga waited as Hall pushed the pace, then made his move before the firehouse, dropped everybody on the hills, and ran alone to the finish.

"You want to be in the catbird seat, where Merga was, where you can watch the action," said Rodgers. "He ran it perfectly last year." Hall listened carefully to Rodgers, but did not broadcast the intelligence he received.

"If six guys go, two guys might survive and four might not," said Keflezighi.

It took Keflezighi five tries at New York before he finally won there last year and became the first American victor since Alberto Salazar in 1982.

"The one who wins will be the one who is the strongest and the fittest," Keflezighi said, "and the smartest."

Keflezighi learned caution, Merga learned caution, and all the runners contending to win the race knew all those things that everyone knew about how important it is to save energy for the hills. Maybe Rodgers gave Hall priceless wisdom, or maybe not.

Ryan Hall led the race to a 4:52 first mile. He had run repeat miles on the course in 4:50 so figured if he ran a pace that he could maintain, he would win. Simple. Not so. Or maybe so. "My goal was to have fun and to run free." The field would not let him run free of their company. So it seemed that everyone was having fun at 5k in 14:58. Hall—carefree, tall, with blond hair blowing in the wind, wearing contrasting dark glasses and a red USA racing singlet—looked like a beacon. Merga, Robert Kiprono Cheruiyot [not the previous winner], Meb Keflezighi, Kebede, Goumri, Cheruiyot, Moses Kigen, Gashaw Asfaw, John Komen, and David Mandago all followed the flowing beacon.

Hall pushed ahead through 10k in 30:06, making veteran observers think that he had succumbed to temptation and would soon crash like bubbled-up financial markets. The conventional wisdom followed in a tight pack. Did Rodgers tell him to do that? Keflezighi, the Olympic medalist, would never bolt to the lead ahead of such talent as surrounded him now. At 9 miles in 43:32, Merga jumped Hall and moved ahead. Hall did not go with him. This looked like the end of Hall's show. Only Merga's fellow Ethiopian Chala Dechase gave chase, with Kenyan John Kigen bolstering the pursuit. The tight pack stretched thin. So much so that it seemed the end for Hall's God-driven braggadocio. The pundits in the press truck thought they would see him no more.

Then Merga and Cheruiyot ripped off a 4:35 mile running through Natick. Hall dropped 100 yards off and bided his time. "If somebody is champion, you try to go with him," Cheruiyot figured. "So I try to come with Merga."

"I knew if I went, I might blow up," Hall said.

But Merga was not out to murder the field, not just yet, so slowly the pack reformed like a shoal of herring after an orca attack. The pause allowed Hall to rejoin the school at Wellesley College as they all passed the halfway mark at 1:03:25. Someone was going to teach a lesson to this school of 20 men. Were they all going to run double time to 2:06:50? Hills were coming. They can't all do that. No one had run faster than 2:07:14. Boston is a tough course. The press waited in their truck to record the carnage.

"I was happy with our halfway split, felt like it was plenty fast," Hall said. "When they moved, I just didn't move with them. I was going to save my energy for those hills, thinking about Bill Rodgers and what he told me. He just maintained [speed] on the hills, then tried to fly down them. I was thinking that going up the hills that I would maintain, then try to fly down the back side. I kind of did that, but I didn't fly down quite as quickly as I was hoping. "

John Komen felt the urge for going. But this time the pack ignored him and stuck together. Hall sat next to Keflezighi and Gourmi. They all looked so easy, as if sitting in an open tour bus taking in the scenery in cozy comfort.

"My hat's off to those guys," saluted Hall. "They were rolling. It was fun to be up with them for a while."

They all seemed to be waiting for the hills. Some were waiting for Heartbreak. Fourteen miles passed with a split of 4:43, with the next clicking off in 4:38. They seemed to have decided not to wait for Heartbreak but only to inflict its gravity on Hall, the new American hope, by going hard before Heartbreak. Robert Kiprono Cheruiyot instigated this surge by the Newton Fire Station, taking the right-hand turn to face the hills. A next mile of 5:09. Merga followed, as did most of the pack, but neither American. At 18 miles Cheruiyot provoked a 4:42 split. All but Merga one by one fluttered away as their physiologies could no longer find available carriers for the oxygen their muscles needed to mount the hills. Two months earlier in Kenya, Robert "the Younger" Cheruiyot had consulted Robert "The Elder" Cheruiyot (no relation) about race strategy.

"He said if you stay in a group, it is very nice," the Younger related. "When you see them going slowly, try to move. I was trying what Robert told me." By the top of the hills, only these two remained in contention. Cheruiyot pushed the ante up with a 4:36 22nd mile then a cruel follow-up 4:44. Distress wrote its name over Merga's face while Cheruiyot looked serene and boyish at age 21—six years younger than anyone in the top 10. Keflezighi, at age 34, was the senior citizen.

Hall said, "At mile 24, I saw the helicopter kind of off in the distance and I was like, *Well, I don't think* [the leaders] *are coming back*. At that point I knew I was running my own race."

Hall passed Keflezighi at the 25-mile mark. He rubbed Keflezighi's shaved head as he ran by. He'd rather have been passing the leader than a countryman.

"Yeah, I wasn't too excited about that," said Hall. "He wasn't the guy I was hoping to pass at that point in the race."

"But I see I am going to break the course record," Cheruiyot said. "So I push."

Alone now, young Cheruiyot ran another 4:36 mile. Still no stress at mile 24. And no one remaining in sight behind him by the finish.

"We ran our heart out," Keflezighi said. "I cried afterward because the vibrations were still going, 'U-S-A! U-S-A!' As long as you try your best, and Ryan and I gave our best . . . if you run your best and somebody beats you, that's the nature of the game. When they made their move, I tried to do what I did in New York, stay 3 to 5 seconds behind. I was trying to rubber-band it, keep it up for a long time, but it got really tough for me."

"That would have been my new lucky number," said Keflezighi. "I'm just delighted to be part of it. It's wonderful to be back. I hadn't been here since 2006, and [this race] reminds me how special it is. I did my best. I came to win." He would have to try again.

But what did the young man who won say when asked what he would do with his $150,000? He said he would use it to buy some more cows . . . and maybe a few sheep.

2010 Men's Results

1. **Robert Kiprono Cheruiyot, KEN**	**2:05:52***	
2. Tekeste Kebede, ETH	2:07:23	
3. **Deriba Merga, ETH**	**2:08:39**	
4. Ryan Hall, CA	2:08:41**	
5. **Mebrahtom Keflezighi, CA**	**2:09:26**	
6. Gashaw Asfaw, ETH	2:10:53	
7. John Komen, KEN	2:11:48	
8. Moses Kigen Kipkosgei, KEN	2:12:04	
9. Jason Lehmkuhle, MN	2:12:24	
10. Alejandro Suarez, MEX	2:12:33	
11. Cuthbert Nyasango, ZIM	2:12:40	
12. Antonio Vega, MN	2:13:47	
13. Elijah Keitany, KEN	2:14:48	
14. Stephen Kiogora, KEN	2:14:50	
15. Chala Dechase, ETH	2:14:57	
16. Drew Polley, MI	2:16:36	
17. Dmytro Baranovskyy, UKR	2:17:15	
18. James Koskei, KEN	2:17:28, First 40+	
19. Chad Johnson, MI	2:17:41	
20. Jason Delaney, CO	2:19:17	
21. Seth Hutchinson, VA	2:20:56	
22. Gilbert Yegon, KEN	2:21:12	
23. Reuben Chesang, KEN	2:21:15	
24. Lucan Meyer, CT	2:21:29	
25. Tomoyuki Kawakami, JPN	2:21:44	
26. Jason Fogel, IA	2:21:51	
27. Jesse Davis, IN	2:22:59	
28. Antonino Liuzzo, NY	2:23:00	
29. Jorge Eliecer Real, NY	2:23:08	
30. Marc Jeuland, NC	2:23:33	
44. Paul Ryan, MA	2:27:14	
67. Ian Nurse, OR	2:29:26	
72. Jim Johnson, NH	2:30:00	
92. Junyong Pak, MA	2:32:59	
112. Ioannis Papadopoulos, MA	2:34:54	
152. Darren DeReuck, CO	2:37:42	
1272. Julian Saboisky, MA	3:00:00	
4286. **Gelindo Bordin, ITA**	**3:21:27**	
5806. Paul Sackles, CA	3:30:00	
9902. Jim Miller, FL	4:00:01	
13117. Yong Ho Lee, CA	6:24:50	

Men's Winning Teams

1. Hanson-Brooks Distance Project, MI, 6:58:24
2. Boston Athletic Association, 7:15:59
3. Runablaze Iowa, 7:28:42
4. Whirlaway Racing Team, MA, 7:33:01
5. Greater Boston Track Club, 7:33:12

No American Women
Favored to Win

MONDAY, APRIL 19, 2010

Hope and Fear

"She runs like a boxer," coach Squires said, as he sat with the pundits and prognosticators in the BAA press room in the posh Copley Plaza Hotel. Others agreed. "She over strides," said one. "She lumbers." Ethiopian Teyba Erkesso did run brashly, like a big-shouldered rookie, blasting away from a cautious pack at 5 miles. They tripped along, having slowed to slightly under 6-minute-per-mile pace. Her 5:17, 5:18, 5:23, and 5:06 miles swooping down into Newton Lower Falls at mile 16 left the rest of the women's field out of sight. The know-it-alls of the press thought she would die, so they hovered like vultures and waited.

Previous winners had come to race: Kosgei, Grigoryeva, and Tune; but who was this brazen woman leading and looking like a rookie? Well, she is from Arsi, where many Ethiopian running stars come from. That's a clue. Maybe they didn't know that still dealing with a knee injury, Kosgei was not in top shape. Erkesso was 27 years old and had been racing in world-class competitions since she was 16, but she was only a rookie at Boston. She had won the Houston Marathon the previous two years with a 2:24 and a 2:23. She had run excellent cross-country races, a talent many runners, including Bill Rodgers, expanded upon for the marathon. She is the real deal, but the skeptical reporters did not see it. In 2007, she ran 31:13.67 for 10,000m. But why did she leave the safety of the pack? Entering Wellesley Center, Ethiopians Erkesso and Dire Tune and Korean Yal had pushed ahead of the lead pack. Running a 5:17 mile, the three opened a 150-yard gap on the rest. It remained a 3-woman trio until the runners crossed over Route 9 and dropped Tune who had slowed because of stomach pains. She would not finish. The previous two women's Boston Marathons had come down to a sprint. Did Erkesso want to make this one boring by running away and hiding from the cooperating pack?

"My intention was to run my own race. I was not really trying to make a surge or break away, just trying to stick with my own racing plan. When I pushed the pace, nobody came with me and I just kept with my plan," said Erkesso.

They passed the half marathon in 1:14:52.

On the open climb over Route 128 Erkesso pushed the pace, quickly separating herself from Yal. Her mile time dropped from 5:23 to 5:06. "I wanted to test myself and the other competitors."

As she passed Newton-Wellesley Hospital, Erkesso held a 50-meter lead over Yal. By the time Erkesso hit the 30k mark just past the Newton Fire Station, she led by almost 80 seconds. And she would maintain her sizable advantage as she tackled the Newton hills.

Despite boxer-like side-to-side arm movement, Erkesso looked strong and at ease on the toughest Heartbreak Hill. She consistently clicked off miles slightly quicker than 5:30 as she ran through Newton alone. There was no one else in sight. She had a 1:19 lead.

Pushkareva captained the chase pack and smiled and waved at the press cameras. She said, "I felt great, I am still young in the marathon. My tactic was to stay a little bit back and run faster in the second half."

It looked like there would be no contest. A knockout. "During training, I prepared very well," said Erkesso, "I just wanted to push the pace. When I go too fast, everybody is left behind. Because of that, I kept pushing because I'm in good shape." Erkesso ran and in the press truck there wasn't much to do. In the press room the reporters watching on the universal feed monitors saw one woman running alone so decided this was a good time to go for coffee.

Back with their cups in hand, the reporters smelled drama. They no longer needed their caffeine. When Erkesso had reached Cleveland Circle she felt abdominal pains. She discreetly reached down toward her left side, pushed in with her hand and pushed out to make the pain go away. She took deep breaths.

"I suffered acid reflux and I reduced my speed," said Erkesso after the race. "I tried to wait and see if I could recover. After I recovered, I tried to pick up my pace again. I knew that somebody might see me and pick up on this weakness."

Yes, indeed. The Russian was coming. Erkesso looked over her shoulder: 22 seconds behind and closing.

"I was thinking about who was coming behind me. I knew the Russian was coming. From my experience, I knew the Russians have very, very good finishes to the marathon. "

Pushkareva said, "I see only how close I am getting to her. I am hoping."

Now the ferocious Russian, Tatyana Pushkareva, sensed weakness ahead of her. She quickened her hunt. She had begun her running life as a 1500-meter runner so shared a quality of speed with last year's winner, Salina Kosgei, who had beaten Ethiopian Dire Tune in a last-second kick for the closest women's finish in Boston Marathon history. Pushkareva wanted to do that to Erkesso.

Making the turn onto Boylston Street, Pushkareva thought it was possible.

Erkesso feared a duel on city streets with Pushkareva. She felt the classic bad dream where the monster is coming and you cannot run. Erkesso had been pushing to avoid any final sprint drama. Monsters were not in her plan. "In the last [miles] when I saw her, I change my power. She doesn't pass me today, I am thinking in my mind." Victory is sweet when you can savor the last mile. By the Back Bay, Pushkareva had all the push. The gap narrowed. "I was hoping to catch her," said Pushkareva. "The only thing I was thinking was how close I was getting to her. I saw only one runner in front and how close I was to her and the finish line. That was all I was thinking." Pushkareva left Erkesso no time to savor the screaming fans. "It came into my mind," said Erkesso. "I was fighting hard to keep my chances alive." Last year Erkesso had watched the kick finish at home in Addis Ababa and decided that she would not let that happen to her this year. She took off early in a gamble that she would not die.

The contest didn't look like a contest to people who don't know the sport. These two women very much battled as if they were in contact like boxers yet at times could not see each other.

"I didn't want to lose the race like Dire," said Erkesso. Pushkareva pushed as Erkesso eked every bit of stride out of her stiffening legs. In the last miles they could see each other. The Russian ran relentlessly. Pushkareva could see Erkesso directly and Erkesso could feel the pressure wave of 2nd place cheering creeping up behind. She could steal a glance. Pushkareva never lost hope, and Erkesso never lost fear until she crossed the line 3 seconds ahead of the Russian locomotive.

"When I was coming down the last meters, I heard a lot of noise," said Erkesso through a translator. "If I didn't look behind and see her coming closer, maybe she wins the race. After I saw her, I increased my speed." But the victory came at a terrifying and distasteful cost: she out-lasted Pushkareva by 3 blessed seconds. After crossing the line, Erkesso weakly lifted both arms in celebration. Minutes later she vomited. But shortly, the stomach problems gone, Erkesso smiled and could enjoy the moment. She removed a few yellow roses from her winner's bouquet and tossed them to the crowd at the finish area.

About 2 minutes later Kosgei again outsprinted an Ethiopian, Waynishe Girma, at the line for 3rd. "I was not expecting to be in the top three this year," said Kosgei. "I tried to keep up with Tatyana. I tried to close in on her, but she was stronger than me.

"I knew that I was not going to be able to catch up. I tried my best to push in the last few seconds. I was expecting to be fourth and was very happy to finish in third."

Nailiya Yulamanova finished 9th, but because of a drugs suspension backdated to February, her name that appeared in the media immediately after the race was removed from the historical results.

The team race in a big event like the Boston Marathon is impossible to see. The BAA has made it possible to imagine it unfolding electronically on their website via Team Tracking. Like the race for 1st place among women, an invisible team drama played for the entire race.

The BAA won the team cup, a valuable set of crystal glass bowls awarded at the glittering ceremony in the Copley Plaza Grand Ballroom that looks like an academy awards gala, with all the athletes dressed in evening clothes. They look quite glamorous and of course all wear their clothes better than any supermodels. The Boston Athletic Association does a classic and elegant service in celebrating athletic achievement. An article in the *Boston Globe* on December 19, 2010, brought the BAA to task for lacking diversity in its membership.

Bob Hohler wrote the *Globe* story, "Revealing a Lack of Diversity." He examined the membership of the board and the association. The board consisted of 11 members and the Boston Athletic Association of 120 members. The BAA is different from the BAA Running Club that has membership open to a larger number of competitive athletes. Those racers, with only a few exceptions, are not members of the BAA and do not vote for the board of governors. Hohler wrote,

"Blood runs deep in the organization responsible for the Boston Marathon. Diversity? Not so much." He wrote that after 123 years, the membership resembles the gentry of an upper-crust suburban country club. The membership has only two African Americans and has no minority employee on its 15-member administrative staff. "At least 8 BAA members are descended by ancestry or marriage from George V. Brown, the organization's first athletic director." He reported that the average age is 60 and that at least 26 others have relatives or spouses in the membership. Hohler characterized the board as having "a clannish tradition that Thomas S. Grilk recently extended as board president when his 20-year-old sons, Christopher and David, joined the membership."

Grilk subsequently replaced Guy L. Morse as executive director and Joann F. Flaminio was elected to succeed Grilk as president. Flaminio is quoted in the article, "The more diverse the membership, the better." Hohler reported that Morse's total compensation reached nearly $300,000. (Morse left management at the end of 2012 and the 990 federal income tax form by 2012 reported total compensation for Grilk at $249,699. By 2016 the board had three new members, including African American runner Wayne A. Levy.)

Meanwhile, Kim Smith, born in 1981 in Papakura, New Zealand, who came to the U.S. to attend Providence College, a week later would run 2:25:21 in the London Marathon, placing 6th and beating Boston 2003 winner Svetlana Zakharova. Why not Boston next? New England runners considered her to be one of their own. She was courageous and fast, very fast. She'd run 10,000m in 30:35.54 at Stanford only two years earlier. She cast her eyes to Boston.

2010 Women's Results

1. **Teyba Erkesso, ETH**	**2:26:11**	19. Catherine Mullen, NY	2:40:16
2. Tatyana Pushkareva, RUS	2:26:14	20. Chaofeng Jia, CHN	2:40:33
3. **Salina Kosgei, KEN**	**2:28:35**	21. Sheri Piers, ME	2:40:46
4. Waynishet Girma, ETH	2:28:36	22. Michelle Frey, IA	2:42:38
5. Bruna Genovese, ITA	2:29:12	23. Denise Robson, CAN	2:43:16
6. **Lidiya Grigoryeva, RUS**	**2:30:31**	24. Melisa Christian, TX	2:44:01
7. Yurika Nakamura, JPN	2:30:40	25. Laurel Burdick, NY	2:44:16
8. Weiwei Sun, CHN	2:31:14	26. Karen Barlow, CA	2:44:19
(9. Nailiya Yulamanova, RUS	2:31:48)	27. Jeanne Cooper, CAS	2:45:20
Removed from results in 2012		28. Heidi Wolfgang Peoples, PA	2:45:51
(All move up one place)		29. Lori Kingsley, PA	2:46:45
9. Albina Mayorova-Ivanova, RUS	2:31:55	30. Kelley Fathers, CA	2:46:53
10. Agnes Kiprop, KEN	2:33:21	33. Jill Boaz, CA	2:49:15
11. Yal Koren, ETH	2:33:48	40. Sarah Bard, VA	2:53:09
12. Paige Higgins, AZ	2:36:00	79. Elizabeth Randell, NY	3:00:11
13. Madai Perez, MEX	2:36:04	1306. Christine Doherty, MA	3:30:00
14. Meseret Legese, ETH	2:37:00	3303. **Jacqueline Gareau, CAN**	**3:44:17**
15. Mary Akor, CA	2:38:12	5635. Christine Banks, CO	4:00:01
16. Jennifer Houck, NM	2:39:02	6053. **Lisa Rainsberger, CO**	**4:04:00**
17. Heidi Westover, NH	2:39:14	9550. Shannon Kohitz, MI	6:28:55
18. Loretta Kilmer, NY	2:40:07		

Winning Women's Teams

1. Boston Athletic Association, 8:48:28
2. New York Athletic Club, 8:57:52
3. Willow Street Athletic Club, 9:03:59
4. Greater Boston Track Club, 9:06:40
5. Whirlaway Racing Team, 9:15:15 (40+)
6. Cambridge Running Club, 9:35:07

Run Like the Wind

MONDAY, APRIL 18, 2011

Sweet Cheruiyot Back to Defend

John J. Kelley (Dec 24, 1930, to Aug 21, 2011), the only BAA runner to win the Boston Marathon (1957), died the previous August. He later coached and mentored Amby Burfoot, who won in 1968 and who inspired his college roommate, Bill Rodgers, who first won in 1975. There is a legacy and a lineage. Runners, friends, and family packed the very hot Union Baptist Church in Mystic, Connecticut, for Kelley's funeral.

Burfoot spoke elegantly and boldly and despite his obvious grief, held the congregation close. But later in the car, he spoke softly and loosely but, like most runners, with a holy reverence for the "loop." With his friend he toured the asphalt, ordinary asphalt, but gave it meaning. Things happened on that pavement.

He showed the flat road by the harbor where Kelley used to push the pace in anticipation of the infamous Cliff Road. Cliff Road started innocently but turned vicious as it continued undulating uphill toward Pequot Ave. Kelley liked to be tired when he started running up the hill.

Burfoot pointed out the woods behind Kelley's house on Pequot Ave where Kelley led his tribe of runners on paths before workers bulldozed through an access road to the new interstate.

Kelley changed running in the U.S., and maybe the world, and sent countless runners on hunts after the elusive perfect fitness or deeper understanding. His rebellious spirit grew in his front yard. Trees grew where other houses have lawns. While residents of residential neighborhoods mowed on weekends, Kelley ran races. Kelley started his rebellion young.

He was the first American to take track speed and ply it on the roads. All of American running owes John J. Kelley for being the first to step off the track and onto the roads without slowing down. Americans who seek to win the Boston Marathon follow Kelley's footsteps.

The Boston newspapers reported that the Kenyan prime minister came to Boston as part of his week-long visit to the U.S. to spur trade. Brand Kenya had a booth at the John Hancock Sports & Fitness Expo at the Hynes Convention Center. Kenyan marathoners had become the country's athletic ambassadors. "More than anything else they have put Kenya on the global map," said Mary Kimonye, chief executive officer of Brand Kenya, which promotes trade and tourism. Kenyan Prime Minister Raila Odinga was visiting on marathon weekend, as was Kenyan ambassador Elkanah Odembo. He attended Bowdoin with Joan Benoit, and he ran Boston in 1979—in the days when Americans Benoit and Rodgers won and Kenyans still ran cross-country, track, and steeplechase, but not marathons.

It made sense for Raila Odinga to come to Boston where Kenyans are already lucratively trading running fast for money. The marathon is business, and the term, first heard from Boston Marathon director Dave McGillivray, was the "Running Industry." The top earners are the top runners. "Being a Boston Marathon champion follows them throughout their lives," said agent Tom Ratcliffe.

The prize money is life changing. The annual per capita income in Kenya is $1,600, Cheruiyot earned $175,000 last year for a little more than two hours' work. His status took a gigantic leap upward. Back home he bought a tea plantation and land for his family and relatives. When he shows the farm, he says, "I tell the people, this is my sweat from Boston."

An invitation from Patrick Lynch, the longtime race recruiter for sponsor John Hancock, is an opportunity that can make a bigger difference for a Kenyan than for an American being accepted to a fine ivy-covered college. "After making results in smaller marathons, they want to move up to a big marathon," said Gerard van de Veen, Geoffrey Mutai's manager. "Boston is one of them."

The Kenyans, who generally are polite, modest, seldom loud, and often diplomatically humorous, get along well. They know they can win only with the cooperation of others. The marathon is business. Good business. Almost all the top marathoners are Kalenjin, yet most of them don't know each other well. "There are a thousand runners," said Moses Kigen Kipkosgei, who trained with Robert Kiprono Cheruiyot in Kapkitony. "Every year a new runner, a new runner." There has to be a race and there has to be competitors, spectators, sponsors—for which the Kenyans are grateful. A generation before had few options other than working the land. The runners explained to the Boston press that they'll share the workload during the race. "We have to do teamwork," said Kigen. "You cannot win a race on your own. You have to be assisted."

The Kenyans refer to each other as "colleagues." But in the hills of Newton, the colleagues become rivals. "They'll celebrate a Kenyan victory but they want to win themselves," said Ratcliffe. "They're not going to sacrifice themselves for anyone else. "

"Everything in Kenya now is marathon, marathon," said Kigen. But for all the Boston media expectation of a Kenyan dominance, a tall white man and a big wind made the day.

Loping lithely, lightly, lingering . . . in the air Ryan Hall spun a magic spell on this Patriots Day. Buffed by a tailwind, his deep-breathing chest filled like a spinnaker at the starting gun, pulling the field along like men on the deck of a racing yacht. Four minutes and 38 seconds later the mile mark bobbed by. About clicking off the mile at such a rapid 4:38, he later said, "I feel comfortable in the lead...I felt really comfortable at that pace, and I like to arrive ahead of schedule." Five miles clicked by in 23:18 and 10 in 47:03. He wore his billowing red, white, and blue USA racing singlet and sunglasses like a splendid America's Cup racing yacht under a bright sun on a sharp sea. Like a crew hiked out on the high side, all the favorites hung out to balance their ship as the wind hurried over the flood.

Defending champion Robert Kiprono Cheruiyot—and crew members Gebremariam, Moses Mosop, Evans Cheruiyot, Geoffrey Mutai, Bekana Daba, Robert Kipchumbas, Philip Kimutai Sanga—all seemed comfortable and blithely uncalculating that the 10-mile split projected to a 2:02:40 finish time. Impossible! Yet they sailed on, following Hall. Hall, seeming to have the time of his life, passed Wellesley College, where the gleeful students cheer in dizzy decibels; he put his hand to his ear as if they weren't loud enough. This rocking pack hit halfway in 1:01:56, slowing to a slightly less impossible projected finish of 2:03:52. Sometimes Hall would drop back into the back, then reemerge to push the pace. It was as if the pack rejuvenated him so he burst back into the lead.

At 18 miles Hall still pushed again at the prow, but a mutiny brewed behind him. Mutai took command. He ran ahead alone for a while, then Mosop joined him as first mate and Gebremariam tried but could not stay on board. Hall could not believe what he was seeing, or not seeing. "I couldn't believe it, I was running 2:04 pace and I couldn't even see the leaders." Mosop and Mutai tried to break each other, but only kept running faster. They reached a mile to go in 1:58.31 . . . Beacon Street to Hereford right and left on to the swing to Boylston and the first sight of the finish line. Not until 200 meters to go did it become clear that Mutai had a sprint left.

"The course was so nice, it reminded me of where I was training [in Kenya]," Mutai said. "I'd been training on hills. I had it in my head that this course was so tough." A new course record.

"When you're in good form and you get good weather, you can push it," Mutai said. "Everybody was so strong." The day was cool and dry and had a tailwind. It happens once every ten years.

"These guys obviously showed us what was possible," said Ryan Hall, who took 4th in 2:04:58, the fastest marathon ever run by an American. "I was just blown away by the day. For me to be out there and run a time like that, I'll remember it the rest of my life. It will go down as one of the best marathons ever run. I kept thinking the pace was going to slow. Well, it never slowed."

Mutai said, "When I'm alone, I know I'll control my pace; when I'm with someone, I don't know." Mosop said, "When I caught him, I thought I'd try my best, but I was feeling tired. I was thinking maybe 2:07 or 2:08. I was surprised to run 2:03."

Mutai said, "I'm happy for this moment. I was not coming here to break the world record, but I really enjoyed my time here. I always knew my future was here in Boston."

But immediately all the press wags started wagging about a sub–2 hour marathon. Well, the wind could have blown harder. Or there is some magic on the course or some magic in the runners. Or maybe there's magic in money.

"He helps a lot because he pushed all the time," said Mutai. "He was like a pacemaker."

"When I was coming to Boston, I was not preparing to break a world record," Mutai said. "I see it as a gift from God."

A world best, certainly, but not a world record, says the rule book. Sponsor John Hancock paid Mutai a $50,000 bonus for his world-best effort to go along with his $150,000 winner's prize, plus $25,000 for the course record.

This seems like the lucrative trade that Kenyan Minister Raila Odinga came to the U.S. to spur.

Fans delighted in seeing the fair-haired Hall in a USA uniform leading the race. American runners want to win the Boston Marathon once again. Clarence DeMar won 7 times, but in a less competitive world. Great American hopes began coming back in 2006 when Meb Keflezighi, Brian Sell, and Alan Culpepper finished 3-4-5, and now Hall placed 4th for a second time. This time Hall took the captain's chair for most of the race. They all promise that an American's time to win the Boston Marathon will come. "We're knocking on the door," proclaimed Hall. "It's going to come. It's just a matter of time."

"For some reason, whenever I break through, I'm in a race of people who are all breaking through as well," said Hall. "One of these times, I'm going to break through when everyone else is having an off day, and come away with the victory."

It was his first marathon since splitting with Coach Terrence Mahon in October, after which he went through health issues and a disappointing finish in the New York half marathon. He altered his preparation for Boston, coming down from altitude two weeks before the race.

"My plan was just to run my own rhythm," Hall said. "It felt very smooth and very comfortable and very relaxed out there. I was just having a good time. I was just enjoying the streets, enjoying running through all the neighborhoods, enjoying the crowds. I love Boston. I think I should move here. I feel like a hometown boy here."

But Boston is a peculiar town and its marathon is a peculiar race so you can't set a world record at Boston, but Mutai apparently just did. So what is the story? World records are banned in Boston. Why?

Regardless of how fast you run on the Boston Marathon course, you cannot set a world record. Ever. It is against the rules to set a world record on the Boston Marathon course. Although the Boston Marathon has been around since 1897, the BAA, which manages the Marathon, knows the rules full well, but defies them for good reason.

Here are two portions of rule 265 in the 2013 International Athletics Federation rule book:

2013 USATF Competition
Rules • 158

For all road records:

(a) The course must not have a net decrease in elevation from start to finish exceeding 1 part per thousand (i.e., 1m per km).

(b) The start and finish of the race must lay no more than 50 percent of the race distance apart as measured along the straight line between them.

(c) The course must be verified (i.e., re-measured) as late as possible before the race, on the day of the race or as soon as practical after the race, in accordance with Rule 240.3.

There are other rules about how the course must be measured to be accurate. They involve bicycles whose tires have been calibrated to a steel tape before and after they have been ridden over the course in a proscribed manner, in case a change in the temperature changes the tire circumference. The Boston course is accurate—measured by the book—but the course will not conform to an attempt to tame it by binding it to approximate a running track. Nevertheless, it is point to point and downhill. The course is almost a straight line, not anything like an oval. From the start to the finish in a perfect straight line, regardless of roads, the distance is 24 miles, so it curves very little. This means that the wind can blow at the runners' backs, aiding them for all the race. That was the case in this year's race. The course loses 495 feet from start to finish, or 3.3 meters per kilometer, clearly in violation of rule 265. The Boston Marathon course does not comply with the rules meant to standardize marathon courses throughout the world so times could be compared and records set, like on a track. The lack of potential for a recognized world record instead of a mere "world best or fastest" is a business loss. It is good marketing to be able to promote a marathon course as having the potential for a world record. Then the race can invite the world record holder or almost world record holders and provide the means to deliver great advertising value to their sponsors. That would be good business, but Boston is famous for its tradition and notorious because the course can be very hard and slow when the weather is bad.

The downhills take a toll on a runner's thighs, and all the little rolling hills through Wellesley and Natick bang bones and muscles into each other. On a day with a slow, warm, following wind, runners easily overheat because the wind can approximate their running speed, giving them little help but preventing their own sweat from evaporating in the stillness of runner and air moving together. On some days in April in Boston temperatures have reached over 100°F. On other days in April rain slightly above freezing has fallen. Northeast storms have blown off the ocean into the runners' faces, pushing their cold, wet hair back like soggy mops. A loop course would even these extremes with a change in wind direction. A loop of course would start and finish at the same elevation.

Times from year to year would not be so radically different. But standardization is not why Bostonians founded their marathon.

Boston will not change the course of the Marathon to make it more uniform. One could design a loop course that starts and ends in the city—like the women's Olympic Trials in 2008. The course could follow Paul Revere's ride, but those roads barely exist, and Paul did not post a Google map of his route. An out-and-back course would conform to the rule. Run to Wellesley and turn around. Then you would have to run the Newton Hills twice—Heartbreak Hill from each side. In Boston, the prevailing winds blow from the west, so often the race has a tailwind. Geoffrey Mutai ran 2:03:02—faster than a marathon had ever been run. The wind blew him to Boston at 15 to 20 mph. Four men broke 2:05. In other years, no one broke 2:10. That is the way the wind blows. The winds of change in the marathon world, however, brought a need to be able to sanction and certify a world record, because it is good business to have a world-record story to tell. Boston listens to a longer tradition than most marathons because it is older, cantankerous, and stubborn and has its own story to tell. And will tell it regardless of a lack of world-record certification. "All I know is that I've run a 2:04 and I have that next to my name," Hall said. "I'm very proud of that time, regardless of what everyone else thinks. I'm a 2:04 marathoner."

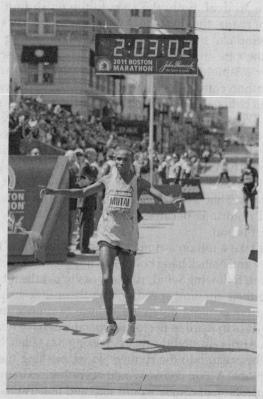

Geoffrey Mutai: the clock says it all.

2011 Men's Results

1. **Geoffrey Mutai, KEN**	**2:03:02**		19. Franklin Tenorio, CO	2:17:56
2. Moses Mosop, KEN	2:03:06		20. Chris Pannone, NJ	2:18:05
3. Gebregziabher Gebremariam, ETH	2:04:53		21. Boudalia Said, ITA	2:18:31
4. Ryan Hall, CA	2:04:58**		22. Kalib Wilkinson, VA	2:19:53
5. Abreham Cherkos, ETH	2:06:13		23. Terrance Shea, MA	2:20:48
6. **Robert Kiprono Cheruiyot, KEN**	**2:06:43**		24. Ben Payne, FL	2:21:01
7. Philip Kimutai Sanga, KEN	2:07:10		25. Jacob Bradosky, MT	2:21:11
8. Deressa Chimsa, ETH	2:07:39		26. Jason Delaney, CO	2:22:05
9. Bekana Dab, ETH	2:08:03		27. Alex Taylor, MA	2:22:19
10. Robert Kipchumba, KEN	2:08:44		28. Antonio Sousa, POR	2:22:21
11. Peter Kamais, KEN	2:09:50		29. Nathan Kra, MA	2:22:24
12. Juan Carlos Cardona, COL	2:12:17		30. Nick End, PA	2:22:30
13. Gilbert Yegon, KEN	2:13:00		76. Scott Leslie, MA	2:29:58
14. Migidio Boufiga, ITA	2:13:45,		1426. Jeremy Miller, NV	3:00:00
	First 40+		6302. Clive Bradley, CAN	3:30:01
15. Toyoyuki Abe, JPN	2:15:48		10346. Frank Fantasia, MA	4:00:00
16. Zachary Hine, MI	2:16:54		13778. Neil Weygandt, PA	5:52:14
17. Paul Petersen, UT	2:17:35		45th in a row	
18. Diego Colorado, COL	2:17:54		13839. Miguel Vasquez, IL	7:37:43

Winning Men's Teams

1.   Boston Athletic Association, 7:05:31
2.   Air Force, CA, 7:08:14
3.   New York Athletic Club, 7:15:19
4.   Melbourne Midday Milers, AUS, 7:38:29
5.   Knoxville Track Club, TN, 7:46:23
6.   Greater Boston Track Club, 7:49:54

Minus the Not Winning

MONDAY, APRIL 18, 2011

Kim Smith in the Best Shape of Her Life

Kim Smith sticks her tongue out when she runs. She doesn't mean to stick her tongue out, but there are so many other things to think about and control . . . Desiree Davila thought she could run with anyone, but at the gun Smith stuck out her tongue and took off, forcing anyone with any thoughts of winning to put them aside and wait for Smith to falter. Maybe Davila could run with anyone, but that did not mean she should, at least not in the early miles. Kara Goucher came to win. She said so. She'd given birth less than seven months earlier, but that hiatus seemed to fuel her ambition, not dampen it. Davila's coach, Kevin Hanson, said they had come to Boston to win. Goucher, Davila, and in an adopted sense Smith, wanted to end the dearth of American women winning. Smith, a native New Zealander, came to the States to attend Providence College and had stayed for a decade, becoming a local New Englander by fact rather than citizenship. Her proximity living in Rhode Island may make her more a part of the New England family than Goucher and Davila who live on other parts of the North American continent.

Smith, running at course-record pace, put herself nearly out of sight as she ran first at 30 seconds ahead at 5k and by 11 miles all alone; the reporters in the press truck could see only Smith and a distant indiscernible pack. Smith wore a pale blue top, slightly darker shorts, and with her blonde hair, blue eyes, fair skin, and a flying pace propelled by a jet-stream tail wind [21 mph at the start], she looked like the sky. Davila later said, "I felt like she was going to get reeled in."

"My plan was just to run with the pack as long as possible," said Goucher. Smith's shot to the lead left everyone with only that option or a solo chase after a woman running faster than course-record pace. To do that the chaser would have to run much faster than course-record pace—a risk no one wanted to take. "Although I had great training, felt really strong, this was kind of a big step," said Goucher." I felt like the race was very hard. Desi went by me [at mile 16] and encouraged me to keep my eyes up, and it was like I was standing still. I was like, *OK, go get 'em*."

Smith, who knew the course better than anyone on the women's field, ran past the half marathon in 1:10:52. She floated down into Newton Lower Falls and up over Route 128 toward the firehouse showing no signs of slowing, fatigue, or discomfort.

Smith charged up the hills, seeming to be full of energy until one particular step. Without warning a sharp pain sprung from the center of her calf. It was a pain unlike any she had ever experienced. Her left leg buckled. She nearly fell over. She caught her balance. Then she lurched and stumbled. An essential muscle would no longer work. She tried to make it work. The perfect charging machine would no longer charge without that component. She tried to change the way she ran—use other muscles—but she could not make the pain ease. The mind was willing but the broken cog snapped the essential chain of energy. She stopped and tried to rub away the muscle spasm like exorcising a demon. The devil remained in her details. Quickly the pack arrived. She tried to run with them. "I felt great when I stopped. It got to the point where I physically couldn't do it anymore." Smith left the race course at 18 miles. The sky had fallen. "I felt great all the way," she said afterward. Until she didn't.

The pack of 4—Sharon Cherop, Caroline Kilel, Alice Timbilili, and Dire Tune—thought only they would take over the lead from Smith, but Davila, with her eyes up, joined them. She did not linger at the tail of the pack to conserve her energy but moved right up to the front to take charge. A mile later Tune dropped back. Off the hills and past Boston College and into Cleveland Circle, Timbilili dropped off. Only Davila, Cherop, and Kilel remained. At Cleveland Circle, Davila spotted her coach, Kevin Hanson, in the crowd. She smiled and nodded in his direction, signaling that she felt good, that she would contend until the very end.

Davila followed Kilel. She is the mother of a three-year-old and had run a personal best marathon of 2:23:55 in Frankfurt the previous fall. Just past Coolidge Corner Kilel surged. Cherop answered. Davila hesitated then skipped a water station and caught up.

"I was really just trying to keep contact [because] I didn't want anyone to settle so it was a back-and-forth anytime the pace got soft." Down Beacon Street to the turn onto Hereford Street. "I'd regroup and catch up, regroup and catch up. I threw down everything I had."

Davila sensed she had to go and break these two right then and not wait for Boylston Street. She shot around the right turn and into the lead. But Kilel took it back on Boylston. The two faced the interminably long shot to the finish. The line, the banner, the photo bridge, the clock, the grand platform with the mayor, the dignitaries, and the laurel wreath seemed not to get closer. With 500 meters to go Davila came back on Kilel to thrill the crowd with the expectation of the first American woman's win since 1985. On glorious Boylston Street, Desiree Davila heard chants of "U-S-A, U-S-A." Her legs had little left. She held the lead with 250 meters remaining. "The last 800 meters, my legs were fried . . . I kept thinking, *Keep contact, keep contact.* You are kind of bargaining with yourself: 'Well, I've made it pretty far, doing OK. People will be happy.' Then you're like, 'No! I've worked too damn hard. Don't give up. Don't give up.'" Four hundred meters to go and Kilel, with perhaps the same mental self-talk, sprinted. She hit the line first and crumbled to the pavement.

"I'm happy because I won a close one," said Kilel. "I love Boston. I would love to run here many times, if they invite me. I feel very happy."

She plans to take her $150,000 prize money, buy a plot of land in Kenya, and build a house to watch her three-year-old grow up.

"It was my first time running the Boston Marathon," said Cherop. "Toward the last part, that was where my legs became tired. That's why I managed to be No. 3. It was a great achievement for me."

Goucher said after the race, "It was tough, but it was a great first step and I was really pleased to get a PR [personal record]. I want to win here; Desi wants to win here. We all want to be the one that ends that [American] drought. But it wasn't my day. I wasn't even close to being the one. I just go home and I just want to work even harder and get more time under my belt. This was my first step back. It was a good, solid performance. It wasn't good enough today. That doesn't mean that it's over. It just means this was one more step toward that goal."

Davila did everything correctly. She set a personal best by almost 4 minutes.

"I felt I could run with anyone today," said Davila. "I know that's a bold statement beforehand, especially when you look at the field. But I don't think I would have placed where I did if I didn't believe that coming in . . . As the race broke and my race plan was unfolding, it just went perfect for me, minus not winning."

Davila trains with the Rochester, Michigan–based Hanson-Brooks Distance Project. She was confident that years of training would allow her to keep pace with the Kenyans.

"[Hanson-Brooks] has taken me from being an average runner and put me here," said Davila. "The training group and training methods helped me develop. Everything's been one step at a time. And knowing that I don't have to be great tomorrow has allowed me to take the necessary steps to get here instead of just going for the fences and failing.

"Everything's been small steps, and it's working well."

At the pre-race press conference not many reporters pressed to interview Davila.

"You felt somewhat unappreciated," said Hanson. "There were lots of areas where they said, 'Yeah, but . . . Desi will run a solid race. She'll do a good job, but she doesn't have a chance to win.' I knew no matter what happened she wasn't going to get dropped," said Hanson. "She might get beaten, but she was not going to get dropped because all of a sudden the wheels fall off."

"She was in nobody's mind. From that aspect, it was good for her to have this," said Joan Benoit Samuelson, the first women's Olympic Marathon gold medalist. "Desi's put America back on the boards big-time."

2011 Women's Results

1. **Caroline Kilel, KEN**	**2:22:36**	
2. Desiree Davila, MN	2:22:38	
3. **Sharon Cherop, KEN**	**2:22:42**	
4. **Caroline Rotich, KEN**	**2:24:26**	
5. Kara Goucher, OR	2:24:52	
6. **Dire Tune, ETH**	**2:25:08**	
7. Werknesh Kidane, ETH	2:26:15	
8. Yolanda Caballero, COL	2:26:17	
9. Alice Timbilili, KEN	2:26:34	
10. Yuliya Ruban, UKR	2:27:00	
11. Trifi Tsegaye, ETH	2:27:29	
12. Woynishet Grima, ETH	2:28:48	
13. Hellen Mugo, KEN	2:29:06	
14. Silvia Skvortsova, RUS	2:29:14	
15. Tatyana Pushkareva, RUS	2:29:20	
16. Clara Grandt, WV	2:29:54	
17. Larisa Zyusko, RUS	2:34:22, First Master	
18. Jennifer Houck, MN	2:34:28	
19. **Svetlana Zakharova, RUS**	**2:35:47**	
20. Caroline White, TX	2:37:22	
21. Nan Kennard, CO	2:38:12	
22. Sheri Piers, ME	2:39:23	
23. Kasie Enman, VT	2:39:55	
24. Caitlin Smith, CA	2:41:37	
25. Louise Knudson, VA	2:42:42	
26. Sarah Bashinski-Flament, OH	2:43:37	
27. Shannon McHale, CT	2:43:46	
28. Anna Beck, PA	2:44:03	
29. Elle Pishny, MA	2:44:30	
30. Megan Grindall, NM	2:45:16	
44. **Joan Samuelson, ME**	**2:51:29, First 50+**	
78. Verity Breen, CA	2:57:51	
106. Helen Olafsdottir, IDL	3:00:43	
1400. Michelle McKenzie, GA	3:30:00	
1463. Abby Samuelson, OR	3:30:36	
5898. Deanna Medvidofsky, FL	4:00:00	
10074. Tracey Bowling, CA	6:23:41	

Winning Women's Teams

1. Boston Athletic Association, 8:10:45
2. Running Republic of Boulder, CO, 8:40:50
3. Impala Racing Team, CA, 8:52:09
4. Somerville Road Runners, 8:59:10

Hotly Contested

MONDAY, APRIL 16, 2012

Fastest Man Back to Defend:
$813,000 in Prize Money at Stake

The first Gallup poll of the 2012 election campaign showed Mitt Romney edging out President Obama.

Romney, the former Massachusetts governor, had the support of 47 percent of registered voters nationwide, while Barack Obama has the support of 45 percent. That race would take seven months to play out; but the Boston Marathon would take one day, and for some runners it will be a very long day.

Leadership change at the BAA developed internally and organically. That January Tom Grilk became Executive Director, while Guy Morse became Senior Director of External Affairs—reducing his work load for health reasons, and Dave McGillivray became race director—something that would prove to be not good for his health. McGillivray ran a marathon in 2:29:58 and, like Tom Grilk, got his start running for the Greater Boston Track Club with coach Bill Squires, Bill Rodgers, and a host of very fast runners. Grilk's wife happened to teach with Bill Rodgers's wife in Wakefield, Massachusetts, so the running idea implanted itself. Grilk worked as a corporate attorney and found, like many, that work may be intellectually satisfying, but was athletically bereft. Most of the GBTC men had been top runners in their high schools and colleges and highly competitive, but Tom Grilk was an eager late comer. He had completed a stint in the army, but had never been a competitive athlete. But once he had gotten the running bug in 1976 and joined the GBTC, he was hooked. In those days runs often started at Bill's store in Cleveland Circle (equipped with a shower) and proceeded out Beacon Street to the Hospital in Newton then back on the marathon course. The runs started slowly with social conversation. These guys knew enough to not make their runs into races. But inevitably such a bunch of competitive men would liven the pace. To delay that and stay with the party,

Grilk asked lots of questions. The longest that ever worked was halfway. Then they would talk louder and run away up the marathon hills on Commonwealth Ave and Grilk would be left to find his own way back to the store. In the group, the guys were careful not to race each other, not to throw surges into their training run, but each pretended that the pace was easy as they all ran faster and faster. As long as someone was talking, the pace was not too fast. The consequence was twofold. Bill Rodgers became a great talker as well as runner and Tom Grilk got down to a 2:49:03 marathon. He did in fact qualify for Boston in the years when the qualifying standard was 2:50. But he got injured and that year marathon announcer, GBTC member Larry Newman, wanted to race so Grilk agreed to be the finish-line announcer starting in 1979.

Dave McGillivray's idea of nutrition was that if the fire was hot enough, you could eat everything, and anything. In time he developed heart problems, but disciplined his diet and overcame them.

At the 10 a.m. start the temperature read 79.2°F. By the finish it would read 85°F.

Alberto Salazar, who won the Boston Marathon in 1982, was at the Boston Public Library on Sunday to discuss his new memoir, *14 Minutes*, which is named for the 14 minutes he was clinically dead after suffering a heart attack in 2007. Salazar, who appeared at the library with his *14 Minutes* coauthor, John Brant, was also one of two subjects in Brant's book *Duel in the Sun*, which followed Salazar and competitor Dick Beardsley through the 1982 race and its aftermath.

The marathon incumbent, Mutai, came back to race. In the intervening year, with his winnings he had built himself a beautiful house for his wife and two daughters in Eldoret, Kenya. Geoffery Mutai had arrived wealthy and relaxed. He would like to do it again. In a country where the per capita income is $1,600, a man can set himself up for life with one marathon win. "They win, and then you never see them again," is said about many Kenyan runners. Mutai, who won $225,000 in prize money and bonuses in Boston and another $200,000 in New York, came back to Boston to be seen. The Kenyans have the reputation of being more interested in money than medals. With the London Olympic Marathon coming later in that year, the question lingered: Kenyans can make money, but can they win Olympic Glory?

Glenn Randall from Mesa, Colorado, shot into the lead with a 4:51 first mile. Nick Arciniago went with him for a little while then thought the better of it and drifted back to the pack, leaving Randall out to roast. He took the first 5k in 15:05, half a minute slower than everyone last year, but the pack would have no part of it. Alone he still led at 4 miles in 19:25 with the pack 22 seconds behind. Randall was a top class cross-country ski racer with hopes of making the U.S. winter Olympic team. In skiing, he was a member of the 2007 NCAA championship skiing team and won the 2008 10k NCAA title in cross-country skiing. In cross-country running he qualified individually for the 2008 NCAA championships, where he was 61st. He beat many celebrated collegians in the process. He ran 30:00.40 for 10,000m at the 2008 Penn Relays.

Randall won the 2010 Pikes Peak Ascent in his home state of Colorado, and last fall ran his marathon debut at Chicago in 2:20:40, good for 20th place. "During every good race of my life, I've been aggressive," said Randall. "People thought I was being stupid, but I live by the sword and I die by the sword. Sometimes it doesn't work out. I'm at peace with this. It's not always going to be your day." This race did not work out for Randall and it wasn't his day so he vanished from the lead but does appear deep in the results.

Ten kilometers passed in 31:02 with the temperature in Framingham at 82°F. Temperature ruled the day and ruled more severely for slower runners, with the day's peak coming at 12:30 p.m. in Framingham of 89°F. For the lead runners the temperature would not exceed 84°F. On this day, it was cooler to be fast.

Still the leaders passed no mile in under 5:00. They hit the halfway at 1:06:11. In the pack ran Mutai, Korir, Chebet, Gebremariam, Matebo, the conspicuous Muzungu Mkubwa, in Swahili, Jason Hartman, and Matthew Kisorio. It was a pack of hot desperadoes waiting for someone to draw and take the first shot.

Kisorio took it at 14.5 miles. He kept the lead for a while. Everyone ran 4:53 in the next mile as they assembled and set up for a shoot-out on the hills. A mile in 4:50 took them to 17 miles. Matebo and Kisoro put on the pressure. Mutai hung close and Wilson Chebet—a four-time sub–one hour half marathoner—strained to close the gap, as did Laban Korir. But Wesley Korir did not join this pressure group. Just before Heartbreak Hill a spectator shouted to him that he was in 6th place.

"I thought, if I finish number 5 in Boston that would be awesome," Wesley Korir said. "After I passed number 5 I thought, let me get to 4th. I wasn't thinking about winning. I was thinking about counting one person at a time. One by one, it just happened." The pack withered to 6. Mutai, the fast man from last year, stopped with stomach cramps and left the race course. "This is the will of God," said Mutai, the 2:03:02 man from last year amid perfect conditions. "I can't blame anything or anyone. I am still happy."

By not finishing here, Mutai might have sealed his chance of earning one of the three places on Kenya's Olympic team. "It is only depending on Athletics Kenya," said Mutai. "For me, I can't say whether I will be there or not be there." Gebremariam vanished. Kisorio and Matebo pulled ahead further with an uphill mile of 4:56 to reach 18 miles. Suddenly Kisorio no longer looked sharp and powerful. He wilted. Matebo looked calm and faultless with a 150-meter lead. This looked like his day at 23 miles in 1:55:35. The gentlemen in the press truck began to relax and all but write their story leads about Matebo winning.

But the reporters could not feel the fatigue that weighed on Matebo. The sun sucked energy from him. He slowed. Wesley Korir had been charging through the faltering aspirants. He pulled even with Matebo at 24.5 miles. Korir sacrificed a few seconds while slowing for water, but quickly caught Matebo again. It seemed to be quite a confident move to stop for water so late in the race with the lead a step away. But Korir had been marshaling his resources for the entire race and water was just another one of them. Korir took off. Matebo gave no chase. Korir reached the finish alone.

After the surges, American Jason Hartman, the big white man of the pack, worked his way past the tired men, as did Korir. That is the gamble of marathon racing on a hot day. How much might you dare to sit back and wait for the runners ahead to self-destruct . . . all the time wondering, *what if they don't? Or what if I do?*

"It was just a battle," said Hartmann, who had run a poor 32nd in the U.S. Olympic trials in Houston in January. "So many times you wanted to throw in the towel but you just fought on." Last year's pace would have put the winner about 2 miles ahead of this year's winner. This is the cruel whimsy of the marathon gods of Boston.

"To see the great Kenyans running this slow shows that the heat is the biggest challenge," said Bill Rodgers. "This is classic Boston. That's what makes Boston the greatest test of all."

Winning the Boston Marathon would profoundly change Wesley Korir's life and test many of the assumptions of how he thought his life would go, and have an equally profound effect on Kenyan parliamentary politics.

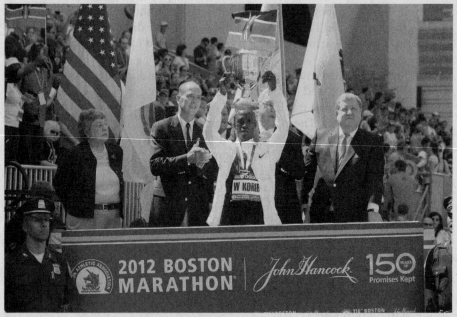

2012 Winner Wesley Korir would go on to win a seat in Kenya's Parliament. The BAA vice president, Gloria Ratti, watches carefully that the tired marathoner does not drop the trophy.

2012 Men's Results

1. Wesley Korir, KEN	2:12:40
2. Levy Matebo, KEN	2:13:06
3. Bernard Kipyego, KEN	2:13:13
4. Jason Hartman, USA	2:14:31
5. Wilson Chebet, KEN	2:14:56
6. Laban Korir, KEN	2:15:29
7. Michael Butler, NED	2:16:38
8. David Barmasai, KEN	2:17:16
9. Hideaki Tamura, JPN	2:18:15
10. Matthew Kisorio, KEN	2:18:15
11. Tim Chichester, NY	2:21:10
12. Sergio Reyes, CA	2:22:06
13. Brendan Martin, MI	2:22:32
14. Gebregziabher Gebremariam, ETH	2:22:56
15. Uli Steidl, WA	2:23:08, First Master
16. Franklin Tenorio, ECU	2:24:04
17. Kota Shinozaki, JPN	2:25:45
18. Koji Hayasaka, JPN	2:27:08
19. Scott Mindel, CT	2:27:15
20. Matt Hensley, FL	2:29:17
21. David Bedoya, MA	2:29:34
22. Kieran O'Conner, NY	2:30:09
23. Jake Krong, UT	2:30:21
24. Tracey Lokken, MI	2:31:06
25. Arron Hohn, MO	2:31:09
26. Josh Whitehead, AL	2:31:16
27. Jason Ryf, WI	2:31:50
28. Craig Coon, NY	2:32:20
29. Patrick Kuhlmann, DC	2:32:55
30. Sebastien Baret, NY	2:33:13
54. Glenn Randall, CO	2:37:13
174. Kyle Heffner, TX	2:48:36
502. Ryan Tellock, MT	3:00:02
2666. Rick Decarr, NY	3:30:01
6204. Robert Kujawski, NY	4:00:00
12594. Paul Clerci, MA	7:16:42
12621. Alfred Buccilli, MA	9:30:16
Geoffrey Mutai DNF	

Men's Winning Teams

1. Boston Athletic Association, 7:51:24
2. Greater Boston Track Club, 7:55:43
3. Willow Street Athletic Club, NY, 8:18:11
4. Dick Pond Fast Track Racing Team, IL, 8:29:13
5. Urban Athletics, NY, 8:35:38
6. Warren Street Social and Athletic Club, NY, 8:36:30
7. Central Park Track Club, NY, 8:37:13

Group Think

MONDAY, APRIL, 16, 2012

Few Americans in This Olympic Year

The front page of the *Boston Globe* on Tuesday April, 10, 2012, reported that politician Elizabeth Warren had raised twice as much money as her opponent, Scott

Brown, for a Massachusetts Senate seat. That story appeared under another one about raising charity funds for marathon entry by *Globe* staff writer Beth Teitell, titled, "Racing to find donors—as Marathon nears, pressure on charity runners builds." According to the report, the number of charity runners who promise to raise money for charity in return for a qualification time waiver increased from $500 in 1994 to $2,285 in 2011. The amount of money each raised increased from $1,547 to $6,977 each. The $4,000 minimum increased by $750 since 2011.

Caroline Cheptanui Kilel said, "Boston, I love Boston. I am happy to come back." And why not? She won last year in a delightfully fast time, holding the Boylston Street crowds in suspense to the last seconds. It was a thrilling show. Kilel happened to be in Houston to run the open marathon on the day after the U.S. Olympic Trials. Shalane Flanagan won in 2:25:38, with Desiree Davila and Kara Goucher following and clocking in well under 2:30. Kilel went out of her way to approach the Hanson brothers, who coach Davila, to tell them she would cheer for Desiree. "I like the way she runs." But Desiree would come to Boston but only to race the BAA 5k that year. Kilel expected to have the marathon to herself with the competition out of the way. But she did not anticipate that her biggest competition would be relentlessly meteorological.

Kilel has a four-year-old son in Kenya where she trains apart from any group but with her husband Vincent Kipkemoi. She is easy going until the race gets going when she becomes an aggressive competitor. She stayed on in Boston to compete at the inaugural BAA 10k, which she also won in a time of 31:58 minutes, beating Kim Smith.

Unnoticed in last year's thrilling back-and-forth duel between Davila and Kilel was Sharon Cherop in 3rd, only 6 seconds behind. In a race as long as a marathon such a small difference means the athletes are physiologically the same. What will separate them is something else, perhaps tactical—maybe Cherop could have kicked or pushed sooner. She will never know about that race. The image of the two ahead of her battling down Boylston Street repeatedly played in her head for a year. Sometimes the differences are not just tactical but psychological, as the image of being so close after coming so far simmers, cooking a year of training to perfection. For Boston Marathon racers, finishing 2nd generates a very useful psychosis. But two weeks before the race Cherop had developed a problem with her right knee. She received physical therapy right up to race time. She said, "If my knee allows me, I will run better than last year."

Danger in the beating heat and unshaded sunshine generates yet another psychosis. At 10 a.m. the temperature read 79.2°F and rising. The weather becomes everyone's competitor. In the face of danger, a group may panic and scatter, freeze in indecision, or conversely, all may glom together for protection. What a group does depends on its incentives and upbringing. In the women's race, the incentive of prize money, $150,000 for 1st compared to $75,000 for 2nd, clashed with the culture of growing up as a woman in East Africa—where it took a village. In the face of the day's heat, the lead group of women decided to stick together under the threat of burning daylight that might fry and embarrass anyone.

At the press conference the top two women repeatedly referred to each other as "my friend." Sharon Cherop and her friend and training partner Jemima Jelagat Sumgong ran together, reinforced in their knowledge of each other. By 2 miles, they had run 90 seconds slower than last year.

At 5k the entire pack ran like an episode of friends grouped around Caroline Kilel and Sharon Cherop. With them ran three Ethiopians, Firehiwot Dado, and Genet Getaneh with Kenyans, Caroline Rotich, who was 4th last year, Georgina Rono, Rita Jeptoo, who had run 3rd and 1st respectively at Boston in '08 and '06, Diana Sigei, Agnes Kiprop, Sumgong, and many others.

All wanted water at every opportunity. At the stations they grabbed for their personalized, special bottles with their own unique markings or cups of plain water. More than once their grab and go knocked other containers off the table and splashing to the pavement.

Together they all clicked off miles slower than 6 minutes. No one wanted to push the pace. Mayumi Fujita of Japan joined them briefly as the pace dipped into the 5:50s toward the half marathon mark in a mass 1:17:11—6.5 minutes slower than Kim Smith last year.

The pack withered on the blazing 128 uphill overpass. The passage burnt Caroline Rotich to a standstill and off the race course. The same happened to Diana Sigei. Spectators brought their own shade with umbrellas.

Rita Jeptoo slowed while Genet Getahah and Agnes Kiprop evaporated from the course.

The survivors continued to the bare-branch, semi-shaded climb past the fire station at the start of the hills. At 18 miles a water station loomed like an oasis. A thirst-crazed pack of five approached. A water station volunteer, perhaps heat crazed herself, stepped into the pack to distribute cups. Suddenly the road race became a line of scrimmage as runners halted and dodged. In the confusion Caroline Kilel collided with the volunteer. She collected herself, rejoined the pack, but grimaced, then faded. She would be reduced to a walk and by a mile to go, and far out of contention, removed herself from the competition. Cherop, Dado, Rono, and Sumgong sustained the pace, but followers fell a minute behind. Heartbreak Hill broke Dado. With the rival Ethiopian gone, Cherop looked to relax and fly down the hills in the fastest pace of the day. She had been practicing running downhills—a great boon to racing on the Boston Marathon course. Her coach, Gabriele Nicola, moved her training to Marakwet from Iten to use the long downhills there to simulate the Boston course. "She learned how to save energy . . . how to roll down the hills." He thought she would win the race that way.

The question of Cherop's knee remained. It was, after all, attached to flesh and bone leg, not a wheel.

In an additional 5k only three remained: Cherop, Sumgong, and Rono. Through Kenmore Square, Rono took a long look over her shoulder and, seeing the safety of the Kenyan sweep, dropped off. The two friends in the lead ran together and one or the other would look back and appear to report to the other that no one closed. The ghosts of Ethiopians could rise from anywhere. As the miles passed the incentive to win superseded friendship.

Sharon Cherop had much earlier decided that any Ethiopian runners would pose more of a short-sprint threat than any Kenyan runners, so she decided she would start her sprint at the final turn with 580 meters to go only if she arrived at that point with a Kenyan rather than an Ethiopian. This would be the only pace change or surge of the race. "This time I knew the course. I had already decided. I was going to start my sprint at the corner," said Cherop. "We work together, so I knew how [Sumgong] runs."

Cherop and Sumgong had pulled away from what had been a 5-runner lead pack by mile 23, creating separation and making it a test between friends. A test of endurance, test of strategy, test of mental and physical limits. Cherop made the decision to go first, only looking back to see if Sumgong could follow. She could not.

"I was with my friend Sharon until maybe 300 meters to go, then she broke free," Sumgong said. "It was a comfortable pace, but she was pushing hard at the end and I couldn't do it." Cherop said about her race plan, "It depended on the person I was going to be with. If it was a Kenyan I needed to speed up at 600 [meters] and again at 300 meters," Cherop said. "If it was an Ethiopian, you have to be careful because they're known for having a stronger finishing kick than Kenyans.

"This time around I was really prepared. I stuck to a plan. I'm so happy." Cherop burst away from Sumgong knowing she could not respond quickly to draft until the final meters as she feared an Ethiopian runner may have done. Sumgong did rally in the last 200 meters to close to a mere 2 seconds—Cherop

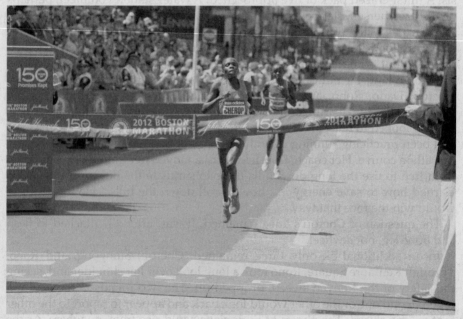

Sharon Cherop out kicked Jemima Sumgong a step before the tape. Sumgong would eventually win Olympic gold in 2016 in Rio.

turned and embraced her friend, genuflected, then crossed herself looking heavenward in thanks.

The friendship would stay but the Kenyan selectors would have to pick the women for the Olympic team and would have to compare a hot, slow, courageous, smart Boston win with a cool, fast-paced London race. The selectors sometime later picked Mary Keitany, Edna Kipolagat, and Priscah Jeptoo who had swept London instead of the Kenyan team that swept Boston. Piscah Jeptoo won silver in the London Olympics and Keitany finished 4th.

2012 Women's Race

1. **Sharon Cherop, KEN**	**2:31:50**	18. Akiko Kudo, JPN	256:20
2. Jemima Jelagat Sumgong, KEN	2:31:52	19. Jen Nicholson, CAN	2:56:01
3. Georgina Rono, KEN	2:33:09	20. Meredith Lambert, PA	2:56:42
4. Firehiwot Dado, ETH	2:34:56	21. Dalena Custer, NC	2:48:00
5. Diana Sigei, KEN	2:35:40	22. Rachel Stanton, AUS	2:58:14
6. **Rita Jeptoo, KEN**	**2:35:53**	23. Hollie Estupinian, CA	2:29:23
7. Mayumi Fujita, JPN	2:39:11	24. Denise Robson, CAN	2:59:43
8. Nadezhda Leontyeva, RUS	2:40:40	25. Suzanne Evans, CAN	2:59:50
9. Svetlana Pretot, FRA	2:40:50,	26. Elle Pishy, MA	2:59:52
	First Master	27. Lauren Philbrook, MA	2:59:56
10. Sheri Piers, ME	2:41:55	28. Megan Malgeri, VT	2:59:56
11. Genet Getaneh, ETH	2:42:11	29. Christine Kennedy, CA	3:00:42
12. Larisa Zyusko, RUS	2:47:47	30. Heather Lieberg, MT	3:01:00
13. Sheila Croft, USA	2:38:31	409. Ima Briebesca, NY	3:30:00
14. Paula Keating, CAN	2:48:58	2454. Michaela Kramper, NE	4:00:00
15. Hilary Dionne, MA	2:51:56	8995. Rebecca Holland, MA	8:02:40
16. Shannon Miller, FL	2:55:47	**Caroline Kilel, DNF**	
17. Lindsay Willard, MA	2:55:53	**Caroline Rotich, DNF**	

Winning Women's Teams

1. Boston Athletic Association, 8:47:41
2. Somerville Road Runners, MA, 9:30:26
3. Central Park Track Club, NY, 9:39:49
4. Nittany Valley Running Club, PA, 9:43:29
5. Fast Running Blog, UT, 9:46:54
6. Impala Racing Team, CA, 9:49:56
7. Greater Boston Track Club, 9:56:28

Touch and Go Tactics

MONDAY, APRIL 15, 2013

East Africans Expected to
Dominate: Kenya vs. Ethiopia

Reports of violence continued to make the world news.

An attack on the main law courts in the Somali capital of Mogadishu killed at least 20 people. According to witnesses, gunmen entered the courts, detonating explosives and opening fire. It is not clear who carried out the attacks against random members of the public.

Violence broke out at the U.S. military's Guantanamo Bay detention center after the commander there ordered prisoners moved from communal living areas into single-person cells. The violence came after at least several dozen detainees staged a hunger strike to protest their treatment and the dim prospects for release. Some of the prisoners had to be force-fed to maintain their health.

A drone attack conducted by the United States killed at least five people in Datta Khel, North Waziristan, Pakistan.

But spring came quietly to Boston.

The only approaching conflict in Boston seemed to be between two racing teams, Kenya and Ethiopia, in the Boston Marathon. What a sweet and profitable way to settle differences. Last year's winner went home a wealthy man. All the combatants face the same direction, and if they fall to the street at the finish, they soon get up free and ready to race again.

Wesley Korir came back to Boston to defend his title. Much had changed for him in the past year. He was now a Member of Parliament—something he never intended nor dreamed would happen. He had hoped only to escape destitution. When Wesley Kipchumba Korir, the son of Nehemiah Kip Korir Koros, left Kenya in 2004 for a scholarship at a U.S. college, he planned never to return to Kenya. He said, "I remember telling God, Hallelujah. I've left the poverty land. I'm going to the land of riches. In my heart and head, I never thought I would go back."

He got to college in the States with some help. Olympic 800m gold medalist Paul Ereng used his contacts with college coaches to get a place at Murray State in Kentucky for Korir. When Murray State dropped its men's track and cross-country programs Korir transferred to the University of Louisville.

In 2007, he returned to Kenya to visit his family, only to be caught up in the violence that followed the country's elections that year. For a short time, he was conscripted into a roving gang; he soon escaped across the Uganda border, spending two weeks as a refugee before he was able to return to Louisville.

Korir recalled, "As I was going across the border, I looked at my cousin, who had to go back, and told him, bye bye. I won't see you again. I'm going to America and I'm going to be in America forever. That's what my heart was saying. But let me tell you, God had a different idea. When I said that, I believe God in heaven was laughing."

In March, Bostonians learned that Wesley Korir, 2012 John Hancock Boston Marathon winner, had taken a seat in Parliament for Cherangany Constituency in Kenya. According to Kenyan political source Sylvia Chelimo, Wesley Korir won an independent seat, as many feel Korir will serve a beneficial role in providing a rebuilding for the country of Kenya. But life was not only running and politics for Korir. He had a heart and a sense of humor, and he could dance.

Korir met Canadian runner Tarah McKay on the Louisville track and field team in March 2010, they married and now they have a daughter named McKayla. He and his wife founded the Kenyan Kids Foundation to improve education and health care in his homeland, and they assisted with the construction of a new hospital in Korir's hometown of Kitale.

When Wesley was a child in Kitale, a snake bit his younger brother. His mother wanted to take him to the hospital, but it was 20 kilometers away. There was no ambulance or bus, there was only the matatu. The *matatu* is an often colorfully painted, privately owned mini-bus or truck that plies the rural roads of Kenya giving inexpensive but slow and unscheduled rides. Wesley's mother and snake-bitten little brother had to wait for the matatu to make all its stops. During the ride, Wesley's little brother died. That is why when Korir made a lot of money in the U.S., he wanted to build a hospital in Kitale.

When he told his mother that he wanted to run for a seat in Parliament, she said to wait until 2017. But he asked, "What if I die before 2017 and stand before God and he asks what I have done?"

In addition, after he became rich, he went home to pay his old school back. They said they did not want his money but wanted him to do the same for someone else. He started a foundation and has paid school fees for 300 children.

Once word reached his district of his marathon victories and that he gave his own money to help educate children, his election was assured. He does not see himself as a politician but as a leader. There is an adage: Beware of fat men in thin countries. Korir is certainly no *mufata mzee* (greasy old fat man in a spiffy suit).

Before his election to the Kenya National Assembly, the family divided its time between Louisville, Canada, and Kenya; they lived full-time in Kenya during his five-year term in office.

"The difference between being a politician and being an athlete is everything you do, you don't do it for yourself anymore," Korir said. "Everything you do, you do it for your country and you do it for your people. So I have to represent my people well."

Korir made a point by campaigning as an independent in a country that went through a wrenching civil war half a dozen years ago and still is riven by partisanship.

"I wanted to show the Kenyans that you can elect somebody for what he is, not for what party he is in," he says. "We got independence 59 years ago, but now we are colonized by party politics."

Korir explained that Nike would have tripled his sponsorship pay when he became a U.S. citizen, but now more than money drives him. Korir is a permanent U.S. resident, but he has put his pursuit of citizenship on hold. "Honestly, I haven't thought about it," he says. "I have to have full undivided attention toward serving my people."

Since becoming a member of Parliament, Korir has taken up the cause of clean water in his constituency and throughout Kenya: "Water is medicine. If you can get water, you get rid of 80 percent of our diseases. That's why water is the song I am going to sing for the next five years. I'll get money from the government. And I'll put as much money as possible in water projects. But it won't be enough. That's why I will partner with people. Every dollar people give us in our area, I'm going to match it."

To that end, he briefly returned to Louisville in August 2013 to establish partnerships with individuals, businesses, and nonprofits to assist him in his effort and to get training for Kenyans in repairing water pumps. A Swedish group had installed pumps in villages throughout his region in the early 1990s, but most of them broke down and had not been supplying water for more than 15 years.

He is also concerned with larger problems in sport. "What is happening right now is a very good step to curing the problem of doping, especially when we move away from thinking about time," Korir said. "From my honest opinion and from what I see in Kenya as an athlete and leader, the issue of time and the under-two-hour marathon—that is the problem right there. When you put that pressure on an athlete, running 2:03, running 2:02, running 2:01, it is superhuman. We have very few super humans that can run that time."

Korir believed that setting lofty aspirations such as the world record or first sub-two-hour marathon will push the youth of the sport to take whatever means, illegal or legal, to get there.

"When you have a kid that is just starting to race and their mind is telling them that for you to make it and become successful as a runner you have to run those times, you're pushing them to go overboard," Korir said. He knew that desperately poor young men will take great risks to get out of poverty and said, "You're pushing them to something that is not acceptable. We need to go back to the past. We need to go back to the sport that we all love . . . of competition and giving everyone an equal opportunity to win and become successful in this sport."

But at the gun in 2013 in Hopkinton the runners did not seem to be very desperate or aggressive. They seemed as if they had already gone back into the past to run with no aspirations of a 2-hour marathon. Not a course record. Not even a 2:05. No physical explanation presented itself. The weather provided ideal conditions at 50°F and only the slightest of winds. They arrived refreshed at the mile in 5:09. North Americans Jason Hartmann and Fernando Cabada, both from Colorado, and a Canadian, Robin Watson, led the race. Wesley Korir, as the last year's winner, presided in the caucus of the lead pack like a committee chairman. Later Korir, the political leader, acted as the spokesman and explainer of the group pace choices. "It was quite tactical. It was Ethiopia versus Kenya. A day like today is when you needed a guy like Ryan Hall, because Ryan likes to go out hard and push the pace. When you see more than five Ethiopians in a race, you have to be very careful. They run tactically, as a team." Of course the Ethiopians would say the same thing about Kenyans running tactically as a team.

Three miles split at 15:06, with the North Americans leading by 16 seconds. They reached 5 miles in 25:04.

Korir ran in good position to win again. He seemed to be the party boss of the pack…or at least the boss of the Kenyan party in the pack.

Thirty-two-year-old Deriba Merga, the 2009 winner, seemed to be the captain of the Ethiopian pack. He and Gebre Gebremariam, Raji Assefa, Lelisa Desisa, and Markos Geneti mixed, mingled, and touched elbows with 2010 winner Robert Kiprono Cheruiyot, Levy Matebo, Dickson Chumba, and Micah Kogo as well as Korir. Africa swallowed up the North Americans and jostled along to a 30:53 10k in Framingham and a Natick 10-mile of 49:21. The mile splits jostled a bit too, ranging from 4:42 to 5:07 at 11 to 12 miles. Were they all acting like cautious politicians?

Shortly after 12 miles the North American firm of Hartmann, Watson, and Cabada rejoined the lead group. That sort of thing doesn't happen often. Then they took the lead through the Scream Tunnel of Wellesley College.

By 15 miles Watson led. But the hills and a reckoning loomed. Dickson Chumba, who had run 2:05:46 in Eindhoven, Netherland, last year, took charge. But he had dropped out of Boston last year. Would that make dropping out easier for him or had he resolved in a year to make up for that failure? Sometimes failure makes a runner tougher and stronger as it strengthens the resolve, but sometimes failure just enables failure. Chumba trimmed the pack to five: Gebremariam, Desisa, Kogo, and Matebo. Korir stayed back, perhaps planning to clean up after the hills helped these guys destroy one another. Between 18 and 19 they split 4:45. At 22 miles Korir looked to execute a takeover. He closed to within 7 seconds of the leading five. A half mile later he joined them. That's when he threw down his gambit. He said later, "When I caught up with them, I had the momentum. I had to take the chance." Sometimes runners cannot change gears to match the speed of an overtaking runner. But Kogo, Gebremariam, and Desisa responded as if they were waiting and counterattacked. Gebremariam had the fastest track times and had won the New York City Marathon, but that did not necessarily apply to this marathon on this day. Kogo ran in his first marathon. Desisa had run 2:04:45 in Dubai. There would be no political compromise. No give and take, only take.

One mile to go.

Kogo, Gebremariam, and Desisa turned right onto Hereford Street and quickly in unison left onto Boylston Street. Gebremariam tried to make a break, but Desisa saw the finish line and then flickered into a kick that propelled him to victory as the other two reached the finish line, straining and leaning in a nearly perfect match. (Road times are rounded to the nearest second, not tenths and hundredths as in track races, so they finished much less than a second apart.)

The top runners and the press corps proceeded to the interview area in the Fairmont Copley Plaza hotel Grand Ballroom. For them, the race was over. Time for the top runners to get drug tested, showered, and dressed for the early evening awards ceremony, to be held in the same ballroom. The reporters on deadline would file their stories then socialize. The nearest place was the hotel bar. But thousands of others still ran on the course while friends and loved ones waited for them. Soon all their lives would change.

Amby Burfoot, the 1968 Boston Marathon winner, had come to Boston to race the course yet another time. No longer did he come to defend his championship. Those days had passed. But for Burfoot and so many others, this marathon race lingered in them perhaps like the bits of ferrous material some scientists say are in the brains of pigeons that magnetically bring them home. The Boston Marathon draws runners like the visceral pull that sparks the migration of monarch butterflies, wildebeests across the Serengeti Plain, or birds that cross continents or equators. It is an irresistible urge. Nobody really knows why. At age 66, Burfoot still wanted to be nowhere else in the world on Patriots Day but on course for Boston. The race had fascinated him the first time he ran, as a teenager, with its pageantry and importance. Now the pilgrimage that had become his custom had seeped into a deep animal homing instinct. In the tradition of seven-time winner Clarence DeMar, two-time winner John A. Kelley, Burfoot's coach and mentor John J. Kelley, and Burfoot's college roommate, Bill Rodgers, Burfoot wanted to come back again and again, long after any hope of winning had passed.

They all kept coming back. The Boston Marathon is more than a footrace. It is a celebration of springtime in a pagan sense and is held on Patriots Day; it is a recurring celebration—the birth and rebirth of freedom.

It had been 45 years since Burfoot's victory, which had come at a great expense of training and trepidation. Burfoot was a 21-year-old college student at the time and confident that with his training he would take the lead in the marathon and push the pace up the Newton Hills. He had spent a two-week spring break in March running a marathon a day, 175 miles a week. He felt power and confidence on that hot day 45 years earlier, but with the lead he also felt a sudden terror that all his competition could see him, but he could not see them. The hidden enemy lurked behind him and could come up and sprint past at any time. Glory and fear drove him.

In contrast, on a pleasant day for running in 2013, Burfoot and friends trotted along in celebration. He paused at Wellesley College to collect kisses from coeds. In 1968, as much as he may have wanted to kiss and be kissed by Wellesley College girls, he sped by at 5 minutes a mile, but this year in celebration, he paused to gather congratulatory smooches he missed for 45 years. No hurry. No fear of competitors, most of whom were hours ahead. This was his homecoming, his party. Enjoy a runner's retirement.

He and his friends expected to finish in about four and half hours out of the third wave. The contenders had finished racing two hours earlier, as Burfoot and company triumphantly entered Kenmore Square with a mile to go. It was 2:50 p.m., and 4:09:43 since the start of the race.

Lining the finish area, people waited to see friends and family members finish. They wanted to celebrate too. The top runners had finished their press conference in the Fairmont Copley Plaza ballroom and wandered with reporters in the corridors, looking for food and drink. Police and officials who had been diligent about crowd control had relaxed as the crowds thinned. A couple of blocks away, first one explosion near the finish line and then another scattered spectators. Some lay injured on the sidewalk. Others thought the explosions and smoke had been planned as part of the festivities. Those who had military experience knew the explosions came from bombs. They rushed toward them. They found carnage. The bombs, fashioned out of kitchen pressure cookers and left in backpacks on the sidewalk, killed three spectators—eight-year-old Martin Richards; Lu Lingzi, a 23-year-old Boston University student from China; and 29-year-old restaurant manager Krystle Campbell. The bombs injured 264 people. A medical tent full of doctors and emergency medical technicians waited in the epicenter of the most medically equipped city in the world. Just a few months earlier emergency responders and medical professionals had practiced scrambling to respond to mass injuries. Doctors and police, bystanders, and a few knowledgeable runners rushed to the wounded and applied their expertise to stop bleeding and save lives within minutes. Seventeen people would require amputations. Ambulances whisked the injured to 27 hospitals. Boston had been exquisitely prepared. Police and political leaders shut down the city.

Officials shut down the marathon. Runners intent on finishing—their singular objective for the past four hours, suddenly heard shouts of "Stop!" instead of cheers of "Go!" Burfoot and friends saw crowds of people on the route ahead of them. Burfoot remembered the poor crowd control of the race back in the '60s and '70s when crowds leaned in to see the runners, leaving only a single path, then parted only slightly, like reeds in a marsh to allow narrow boats to pass. Burfoot grew angry and annoyed that some drunken college students were blocking the road, ruining his race with their revelry. But as he ran closer, he saw they were runners, not drunks. Then his phone rang. It was his wife. "There's been an explosion at the finish line. The race is over. Don't try to keep running. Get back to the hotel." He obeyed. His race and that of thousands behind him had ended. But the race had only started for law enforcement and medical responders. In a great arc around the spot that would be called Ground Zero, trained medical personnel rushed to help the wounded and protect everyone from any possible additional attacks. Emergency vehicles filled the streets as police evacuated everyone else. Information became rare and often wrong. In this fog of war, responders worked with incomplete information. Were they bombs? Gas explosions? Fireworks? Reports came in that a bomb had exploded at the Kennedy Library five miles away. No such thing had happened.

At the Fairmont Copley Plaza, security guards shoved the reporters and athletes back into the building shouting, "Lockdown!" with no explanation. The city, the subway, shut down, block by block. All transportation shut down. Security controllers shut down cell towers to prevent cell phones from detonating any more bombs. The emergency departments of the hospitals filled up. The finish line had become a crime scene. The hotel stayed in lockdown for four hours.

Some doctors who were running in the marathon, such as Dr. Natalie Stavas, sprinted to the wounded. Stavas managed to save a woman whose leg had been ripped open by the blast. Stavas used a belt as a tourniquet to stop the bleeding but wished she could have done more. Many responders who ran toward the area where the bombs had exploded wished they could have done more but saw their duty to do everything they could, regardless of the possibility that yet other bombs would explode, adding them to the dead and injured. Any of the hundreds of abandoned bags could have bombs in them ready to explode. They all had to be checked. But people do what they are intent on doing, which is not so much heroic as human and automatic: if you can help, if you are there to help, if you know how to help, you do. And if you have come to Boston to finish a marathon, that is what you want to do too.

Burfoot and others who were stopped a mile from their long-awaited and hard-earned finish line grew annoyed that something or someone had ruined what they had trained to accomplish. Most did not have phones and wifely messages. They had to rely on what they heard from crowds and other runners.

Only later would come the pain, the attempt to assuage it with charities such as the One Fund, which would collect $70 million for the injured and families of the dead. Tales of bravery and duty would fill the newspapers for the next year as the city and the nation tried to put the bombing into perspective.

But, as Burfoot said about his thoughts at 4:09:43, although he did not know exactly what had happened, he knew the marathon would never be the same. All of Boston knew the marathon would never be the same. But all longed to be the same—unchanged, unmoved, strong. Denial would slowly turn to defiance.

As the story unfolded, the city became a ghost town and armed camp. Police hunted the suspects as they made a murderous escape, killing a police officer and carjacking a civilian. Transportation and business stopped. Police shot one alleged bomber in a military-style firefight. As the other hid, wounded, citizens rallied. The term Boston Strong began to appear everywhere, and runners in the nationwide tribe of runners surged to qualify to race in the Boston Marathon of 2014.

Six months later, the Boston Red Sox baseball team would win the World Series in a marathon bombing tribute with the words B. Strong mowed into the outfield. The New York City Marathon, traditionally marked with a blue line along its entire length, in solidarity painted a yellow line beside it all the way to their finish, to match the traditional Boston Athletic Association colors.

The Boston Athletic Association, which manages the race, opened it up to more qualifiers to satisfy the urge to defy and to pronounce Boston Strong and to support and honor the victims and the courage of the first responders.

The urge seemed to be one of defiance: "They can't stop me. They cannot stop Boston." These runners structure their lives to train, and in a metaphorical sense, run through the "wall," referring to the pain and depletion of the latter stages of a marathon race. They are used to suffering but also used to succeeding and overcoming difficulty. They are endurance athletes. They come back to try and try again. But the bombing brought a new trepidation, not of the difficulty of distance and pace but of the haunting question of what other act of horror could be pushed on the race. Will runners and spectators look with fear at every young man with a backpack? Will runners glance fearfully at rooftops and high windows, fearing snipers? The two sides of a 26.2-mile road offer plenty of hiding places. There are only guesses about why someone may be driven to kill. What rationale cooks in the mind of someone who can kill uninvolved people for some political or religious cause? How can law enforcement, citizens, or runners themselves predict what may happen? The simplest explanation may be that people like those who planted the bombs first want to kill and only later want to justify the killing with some "cause." Might something similar happen again, or never again? Runners will run, some in fear and defiance and others in hope and in celebration. The marathon will remain a soft target run by very hard people.

The marathon could be a target for terrorists or demented people, but regardless, Boston is physically and spiritually home. For residents, it is our Boston, our town, and for marathon runners worldwide, the Boston Marathon is the premier marathon on the planet. Boston is the hometown of marathon racing. Other city marathons may be bigger or faster. Other marathons may offer Olympic gold medals in their ever-changing host cities, but Boston will always be home. It is home for Burfoot, for Pippig, and for so many others. Boston is the cradle of liberty. People fight for their homes, and after wars, hurricanes, earthquakes, tsunamis, or tornados, people want to go home. Seldom have cities under siege warfare surrendered. The citizens of cities bombed to rubble redouble their resistance. They go underground. People emerge to rebuild. People in a human response do not want to quit their homes, just as marathon runners do not want to quit their race.

Amby Burfoot and tens of thousands of others want to come back. It is a homing instinct. It will be spring; it will be time to get to Boston; it will be time for runners to make a statement.

2013 Men's Results

1. Lelisa Desisa, ETH	2:10:22	13. Tomohiro Tanigawa, JPN	2:16:57
2. Micah Kogo, KEN	2:10:27	14. Carlos Carballo, CA	2:17:05
3. Gebregziabher Gebremariam, ETH	2:10:28	15. Lee Troop, CO	2:17:52, First 40+
4. Jason Hartman, USA	2:12:12	16. Fernando Cabada, CO	2:18:23
5. Wesley Korir, KEN	2:12:30	17. Joseph Gray, WA	2:18:45
6. Markos Geneti, ETH	2:12:44	18. Kevin Pool, CA	2:18:59
7. Dickson Chumba, KEN	2:14:08	19. Carlos Trujillo, ID	2:19:24
8. Jeffrey Hunt, AUS	2:14:28	20. Matt Dewald, CO	2:19:35
9. Daniel Tapia, US	2:14:30	21. Christopher Estwanik, BER	2:19:55
10. Craig Leon, USA	2:14:38	22. Adam MacDowell, LA	2:20:38
11. Robin Watson, CAN	2:15:33	23. Glenn Randall, CO	2:20:56
12. Levy Matebo, KEN	2:15:42	24. Vyacheslav Shabunin, RUS	2:21:23

25. Tim Ritchie, USA	2:21:31	1964. Ken Little, NY	3:00:00
26. Alexander Varner, CA	2:21:40	6595. Rolf Friis, CAN	3:30:00
27. **Deriba Merga, ETH**	**2:21:40**	9996. Mark O'Brien, MA	4:00:01
28. Jeremy Criscione, FL	2:21:45	10648. David Pollard, IL	4:42:12
29. Ulrich Steidl, WA	2:22:05	**Amby Burfoot, halted, projected**	**4:25:13**
30. Scott Mindel, NY	2:22:25	**Robert Kipruno Cheruiyot, DNF**	

Men's Winning Teams

1. Boston Athletic Association, 7:12:19
2. Varsity Running, LA, 7:20:38
3. Dirigo, ME, 7:30:02
4. Williow Street Athletic Club, NY, 7:31:31
5. Greater Boston Track Club, 7:40:04

Jeptoo's Great Leap Forward

MONDAY, APRIL 15, 2013

Marblehead Native: American Hope

Race day started with 26 seconds of silence in honor of the victims of the Sandy Hook shooting on December 14, 2012. The women's invited field lined up at their early start time. Blue sky lighted a great day for racing. The press paid attention to more than the simple footrace ahead.

Writing for the *Boston Globe*, John Powers reported about a new history book: "While the Boston Marathon has been amply chronicled in any number of books, not so the founding Boston Athletic Association, which was established in 1887. Now comes *The B.A.A. at 125*, the organization's official history, written by John Hanc with a preface by actor Matt Damon. The book includes more than 100 rare photos from the association's archives . . . ."

The marathon and the hosting BAA have had a rich history that has mirrored world history. By the end of race day everyone would understand how the Boston Marathon reflects the world around it; in the book Hanc describes how the Great Depression pushed the BAA into bankruptcy and almost stopped the Boston Marathon. National and world events reach the Boston Marathon. It is not isolated. Powers wrote about the pre-race organization that anticipated care of injured runners at the finish.

"What do race organizers have in place to minister to the walking wounded in Copley Square? Forty defibrillators, 26 oxygen tanks, 25 EKG machines, 150 blood pressure cuffs and stethoscopes, 80 thermometers, 20 ice immersion tubs, 900 intravenous bags, 500 emesis basins, 380 cots, 500 sick bags, 4,000 Band-Aids, 2,000 tubes of antibiotic ointment, 2,000 pairs of medical gloves, 1,500 blankets, 2,000 adhesive bandages, 1,500 gauze pads, 500 tongue depressors, 250 rolls of moleskin, 175 Ace bandages, 200 bottles of antiseptic hand wash, 500 bags of ice, 500 tubes of petroleum jelly, and 400 towels." He had no idea that his hyperbole about the walking wounded would prove to be no exaggeration, as the troubles of the world would seep deeply into Boston by the end of the day. But first there was a race to write about.

John Powers took a reporter's impossible assignment of predicting the future—what would happen in the next day's race: "If recent history is any guide the women's race will come down to a dash and there'll be a new champion. The last five finishes have been the closest ever—one second in 2009 (Salina Kosgei and Dire Tune), two seconds in 2012 (Sharon Cherop and Jemima Jelagat Sumgong), 2011 (Caroline Kilel and Desiree Davila), and 2008 (Tune and Alevtina Biktimirova), and three seconds in 2010 (Teyba Erkesso and Tatyana Pushkareva). No titlist has repeated since Kenya's Catherine Ndereba won her fourth crown in 2005 . . ." If Cherop won she would move to the top of the World Marathon Majors standings for the year. A lot rode on this race. A lot of money. The top Americans, Kara Goucher and Shalane Flanagan, each wanted to be the first American woman to win Boston since Lisa Larsen Weidenbach (Rainsberger) won in 1985.

The coach/athlete relationship can be fraught with emotional and technical complexities. So it was between Kara Goucher and Alberto Salazar. For Kara's first race at Boston, in 2009, she arrived with her coach, Alberto Salazar, who had won Boston in 1982. By 2013, her third time in Boston, she had parted from Salazar and the two remained estranged.

Different technical training programs work well for some athletes and not for others. Running is much individualized—the attempt is to change a human body so it can do things that it could never do before. So the running coach/athlete relationship is not mitigated by a team, plays, and game strategies. Every runner is an experiment of one.

The temptation to second guess training is very great. Kara's husband, Adam, a world-class runner himself, was part of Salazar's Nike Oregon Project. He disagreed with Salazar. At this point Adam had passed his career peak as an athlete and no longer raced for the NOP. Kara Goucher quit being coached by Alberto Salazar because of that conflict between Salazar and her husband about how Kara should train. Salazar could not accept the interference, so the two parted company. Kara Goucher's new coach was Jerry Schumacher, and her training partner was her fellow Olympian, Shalane Flanagan. This would be Flanagan's first Boston Marathon.

"You know what would be so cool?" Flanagan asked. "You know what would be such a badass move? If I were to win the Boston Marathon and retire the next day."

She paused for dramatic effect. She laughed. The joke reveals how much the Boston Marathon means to her. The Boston Marathon took hold of her imagination when she was a child. It became a lifelong dream.

"In my heart, I would feel complete winning Boston," Flanagan said. "I would feel very fulfilled with my career. I would have exceeded all expectations. I have an Olympic medal. I'm a three-time Olympian. I have all these track records. Then, to win Boston, what's better than that? Retiring wouldn't happen, because I love running so much. I want to continue and see what I can do. But if someone said, 'If you win Boston, you have to retire tomorrow,' I'd say, 'OK, I'll take that deal.'"

Flanagan grew up in Marblehead, Massachusetts, on the shore north of Boston, and watched the Marathon. When she was in middle school, she watched from Boylston Street and cheered her father, Steve. The spectacle captivated her. She imagined racing down the historic homestretch.

This would be her Boston Marathon debut as a racer as one of 18 elite women. She was the 2008 Olympic bronze medalist in the 10,000 meters and American record-holder (30:22:22). She was 5'5" and weighed 113 pounds.

Joking with *Boston Globe* reporter Shira Springer, Flanagan said, "It would be mind-blowing, winning and ending the American drought. It would be a life-changing moment. That's why I have to remind myself to not let it get the best of me and not let the moment overwhelm me."

Flanagan's father ran a personal best of 2:18:36 at the Arizona Fiesta Bowl Marathon in the late 1970s and 2:20:42 on the Boston course in 1980 for 23rd place. Steve Flanagan reminded Shalane to "stay above the hype."

She had run three marathons and learned from nearly four years of marathon-focused training under Jerry Schumacher. She said she'd waited 17 years since her middle school days to race in the Boston Marathon.

"Hopefully, it's delayed gratification," said Flanagan. "I'm not a veteran by any means, but I definitely have learned a lot about myself and how to approach the marathon. Hopefully, I can knock it out of the park."

Schumacher said, "I'm confident that Shalane can run the marathon in any way that it's presented and be a factor. Whether or not it's her day, we'll find out. Whether or not she wins, nobody has that answer. But we work really hard to be in the game. So, when the time comes, we hope it's our day. If it is, I have a feeling the city of Boston will be pretty excited."

The life of a professional runner takes her away from husband and home. Flanagan lives in Portland, Oregon, but to compete with the Africans she must go to where the air is thin, to the Santa Fe Trail in Colorado that starts 7,250 feet above sea level. Flanagan and Goucher chose the route because it simulated the Boston Marathon. Flanagan said, "I've been kind of nervous about the course, even though I feel like I've prepared very well and I'm fit." She trained on the Boston route in December. "Whoever has their legs with 10k to go, that's the key. That last 10k is pretty brutal and you really need to have your mental game and physical aspects in line then if you want to win it."

Before the London Olympics, Flanagan and Goucher ran 120- to 130-mile weeks with three speed or quality workouts per week. Perhaps they pushed too hard. Schumacher said, "Because it was the Olympics everyone made more out of it than we needed to and may have pushed a little too hard."

Flanagan placed 10th and Goucher 11th in the Marathon at the London Olympics. Flanagan said she "almost didn't finish," that she was "too aggressive too soon," and then "tried to push through the wall and made things even worse." She lost 5 places in her final few miles. She learned that a runner can train too intensely. She learned the value of being "cautiously aggressive" in marathons.

In preparation for Boston, Schumacher decreased Flanagan and Goucher's mileage to around 115 per week with two quality sessions. "I feel if Shalane goes out there and wins the Boston Marathon, I'm a big part of it, and vice versa," said Goucher. "At the Olympics, we were saying that if one of us won a medal we would have to cut it in half because we helped each other get there. Shalane wouldn't be as good as she is and I wouldn't be as good as I am, if we didn't train with each other."

Flanagan described her training as 95 percent for the last few months.

At the Rock 'N' Roll New Orleans Half Marathon Feb. 24, Flanagan finished 2nd in a personal best 1:08:31. She followed that performance with a 10,000-meter Stanford Invitational win in 31:04.85. "I kept telling Jerry, 'Whatever you're doing, it's working,'" said Flanagan. "It's nice to be thriving off of the work instead of feeling like you're on the defense and just surviving. Right now, I could probably safely say I'm in PR shape and probably the best marathon shape I've ever been in."

Flanagan's birth mother, Cheryl Treworgy, set the women's marathon world record of 2:49:40 in 1971. It is nice to have fast parents.

Steve Flanagan was constantly asked about Shalane and the race. He joked with the *Boston Globe* reporters. "Everybody in town owns a piece of her success because she's the ultimate hometown kid," he said. "I've told people that the party is to celebrate her sister Maggie's Boston Marathon debut and that the other daughter, Shalane, will also be there," said Steve.

Maggie Flanagan, who was living in Fort Collins, Colorado, would make her Boston debut that year. She ran very well in high school, but took her life in other serious directions, such as working for the Peace Corps in Madagascar.

She told Shira Springer, "Visiting Shalane, the day-to-day lifestyle of a professional runner doesn't look that fun, she lives like a monk. She sees the payoff, but I see the tradeoffs. I'm always in awe of her focus . . . But Shalane and I never talk about running. There's a lot more to her and I think I'm part of reminding her of that."

Running at the top of the world of fantastically talented athletes is serious and risky business. There are no guarantees that hard work will pay off. A slight injury, a common cold, and half a year's pay is gone. A marathon racer can't call in sick.

Steve Flanagan said, "At 31, Shalane's been on enough starting lines where she doesn't let nervousness be negative. She never has. If you put too much emphasis on it, there's too much to lose. She'll give every ounce of whatever's in there. All Shalane has to be is Shalane."

Kara Goucher knew the Boston course and had read about its history (in this writer's book, 2nd edition), but the stress and risk of training made her question the Boston race plan.

In January, a left heel injury and a slow recovery from the physical and emotional grind of the London Olympics made her Boston buildup difficult. She asked Schumacher, "Should I be racing this?" Schumacher said, "You absolutely should. If you were going to go out there and make a fool of yourself, I would tell you." From that point, Goucher fought through less than perfect preparation.

She told reporters, "I love the race so much that I would never want to disrespect the Boston Marathon by going in when I'm not really, truly ready to run a good marathon. I'm OK with things not going necessarily perfect. But I'm still going to go for it. I know I'm ready for a solid race. Everything is headed in the right direction now. It just hasn't been a storybook training block."

Goucher ran 1:11:49 at the Rock 'N' Roll New Orleans Half Marathon on February 24, and 31:46.64 in the Stanford Invitational 10K on March 29.

"Part of the problem is I compare myself to Shalane, who's had absolutely perfect preparation," said Goucher. "I run with her every day and I can't always do what she's doing on some of the speed sessions. Really, the part that's lacking is my speed component. My coach and my husband keep reminding me that if I wanted to run track right now that would be a problem. But I'm not training for the track. So, I can handle not having a little bit of speed because it's the strength that's going to carry me those last 6 miles."

"Kara came together a little bit later in the game," said Schumacher. "I don't quite have as much information to make a really accurate assessment. I think she's going to run very well. I don't know exactly what that means because we haven't had enough time to play at that really high level."

But it's clear that even with a less than perfect buildup, Goucher and Flanagan benefit from their unique training partnership. Having the top American female marathoners work out together daily is unheard of in today's competitive distance-running world, with its training groups and high-altitude camps scattered throughout the country. In fact, neither Flanagan nor Goucher could think of a situation similar to theirs.

"It's like a marriage when you train with someone," said Goucher. "You can't just pair any two women together. You're with each other all the time. You see each other at your most vulnerable place. I feel like I've had some of my deepest conversations on runs because you're too tired to put up any walls or barriers. You become really open. You have to take that into consideration. But I think we could be doing more in this country with more women training together."

Flanagan said, "We're both hugely competitive, so that's not really a good enough reason to say you can't train with someone. We've learned how to really bring that out when we race. There's no point in using that competitiveness in training because it defeats the purpose of what we're doing. I always look at it as the fitter I am and the best athlete I can be, that makes Kara better, and vice versa."

Flanagan and running partner Goucher felt strong and ready, guided by Schumacher. The usual talented, competitive, international field of women runners also felt strong and ready to race.

Partly sunny skies and 48°F held potential for very fast times. The first mile sauntered out in a gentle 6:04. The field did not seem in the mood for a fast time. Manami Kamitanida led and soon Yuka Yano, also of Japan, joined her, as did Colombian Yolanda Caballero. They ran through 5k in 18:22, a split that projected to a 2:34:55 finish. A big mob of contenders ran 17 seconds behind. All felt the leaders remained easily in their grasp if not their reach. Sabrina Mockenhaup of Germany and then Ana Felix of Portugal seemed to be gently breaking away. At around 8 miles Kenyan Diana Sigei joined them. But the pack didn't seem to mind.

Ten miles passed in 53:04 with Sigei and Caballero leading. Observers began to conclude that the followers followed Jeptoo. They sensed she had some magic about her.

But Caballero it was who blasted off. Surprisingly, Felix alone chased her. Caballero alone passed the halfway in 1:14:02. In the next 2.5 miles Felix cut down 26 seconds to be only 6 seconds behind at 25k. At the water table Felix grabbed her drink and took off into the lead. Flanagan and Goucher, in the pack like eager puppies, wanted to chase her, but the queen of the pack, Jeptoo, did not. "It's really hard as a competitor to watch two women pull away from the field and have that faith," said Flanagan. But Schumacher had advised her not to make any first moves, so she waited. "I was really antsy. I did not like not having a full group together."

Felix led looking strong but not at ease; with miles to go, she frequently turned to look back. She kept seeing no one. She led by a minute. Could this be true? Swooping down into Cleveland Circle she took another look. They were coming. Sharon Cherop had told Jeptoo that it was time to move. "Let us move forward or this lady will end up winning."

Jeptoo led the charge. Later she said, "Last year I was not ready." Clearly something had changed within her. She reeked of power.

"It hurt, a lot," said Flanagan. "My legs felt like Jell-O, and when she went, I just said, 'Keep it close, don't give them too much room,' but I was suffering and we still had quite a bit to go. So I just said, 'I have to have one more gear, just in case.'"

"I really suffered when they pulled away on the downhills. The downhills, again, were really hard. They made some really strong moves on downhills. I thought I was going to be able to keep it close and really not let them take too much room from me. But those downhills, that's where they sealed the deal, right there."

Just before mile 25, Jeptoo caught and passed Felix with a 5:10 mile split. It was over. Felix struggled and staggered to the finish in 9th place. When Flanagan crossed the finish line, the emotions took over and she tried unsuccessfully to fight back tears.

Once she had composed herself and wiped away tears she said to the press in the converted opulent and overly gilded Copley Plaza ballroom, "I'm very grateful for today. I've been thinking about this moment and running in this race for a really long time. So I'm extremely happy I fulfilled a lifelong goal of mine, but I dreamt of winning today. I dreamt of a laurel wreath on my head, and it didn't happen. But that's the reason why dreams and goals are big and they're hard." She wavered between heavy, crushing personal loss and her intellectual understanding that she had engaged in an athletic competition, the loss of which allowed some sadness but could not descend to self-indulgent grief. "I have full faith that Kara and I and our coach will break this race down, but he already told me he's really proud of me. All we can ask of ourselves is to put ourselves in position to capitalize on the day." Although tired, distraught, disappointed, and feeling defeated, she made an effort to talk with reporters. "It made for a great race with great drama. I just wish I had more in me, more in my legs to be able to compete all the way to the finish. I genuinely felt like they wanted the win as much as I did today, and that's inspiring as an athlete," said Flanagan.

"We'll go back and assess, but I'm genuinely proud of my buildup and I'm proud of my race."

She left the press conference, passed through drug testing, and went upstairs to her room to shower and change before she would meet her husband, father, mother, and sister. Reporters congratulated race officials. BAA executive director Tom Grilk accepted those congratulations with a smile and look of pleasant relief that the prize-winning runners had been interviewed and no competitive controversy had emerged. It seemed that a good day's work had been done.

In the lobby of the Fairmont Copley Plaza a reporter asked Jack Fleming, the BAA director of communications, for a statement about the race. He was at a loss to single out anything as more newsworthy than anything else, so he bailed out with a compliment to the weather. "It was a beautiful day." Why not? When you have nothing else to talk about, talk about the weather. He heard a distant thud, but thought nothing of it since big buildings have background noises of doors slamming, machinery, loading docks, etc. But then a representative of the marathon's top sponsor came bursting through the doors, running up to Fleming in a distraught and near hysterical state shouting, "There are people on the ground . . . people on the ground." The marathon would shut down. The city would shut down. The luxury Westin Hotel across the street would become a rough command center. A sporting event would become a crime scene.

Flanagan's disappointment in not winning a road race would vanish into a world defined by high-velocity shrapnel. Grilk would be stressed to tears. Fleming would have more than the weather to talk about.

Uniformed security officers pushed reporters coming out of the press room in the Fairmont Copley Plaza back into the room, shouting "lockdown." No one knew why. The best explanation came that there had been an explosion. People thought, "Gas leak? Electrical transformer?" No one in the middle of the building heard anything. They pushed retired race director Guy Morse back into the hotel. He looked worried, stunned, and confused. Why all this security for an accident? Morse tried to guess what had happened. Then came word of a second explosion. He knew it was no accident. The horror sunk into Morse. His marathon had been attacked. He felt sick to his stomach with fear. But fear stiffened him and made him fear, not for himself—he had already dealt with cancer—but that his work would be broken. This was an attack on his life's work. The marathon to Morse was a contest against sun and wind but always brought people closer to each other, not split by suspicion and fear. The marathon to him was a celebration of good things, of a symbolic struggle of people together against benign distance and hills. He grew angry at this destruction of his work and the work of so many others. He would remain in Boston for the rest of the week hoping somehow to mend the damage.

Jack Fleming could say very little to all the urgent jangling of his phone. Something big and terrible was happening, but he had no facts. He was the spokesperson for the Marathon, a footrace, not the police or emergency medical responders, so in his professional triage for the sake of the race, he had to assemble a small group of BAA officials, Michael Pieroni and T. K. Skenderian, to determine what they could and should do and to stay out of the way of FBI swat teams, Homeland Security, Boston and State police, as well as the ambulances and doctors, but still take care of their runners. First, reroute the race around the crime scene and try to navigate the runners to retrieve their bags and get into warm clothes and stay safe from whatever else might happen. Fleming had to fend off the deluge of misinformation and be sure not to contribute to it or spread it. Reporters wanted to know what was going on, and the go-to person, Fleming, did not know.

As the bombs exploded, Frank Shorter walked to a meeting for the Marathon's wrap-up television show from the press viewing and TV anchor platform. Soon police would usher him into the safety of the hotel. As a marathon Olympic Gold Medalist, he had been a TV color commentator. He heard and felt the explosions like close lightning strikes. But he knew they were bombs. He had been in this place before. At the 1972 Olympics in Munich he had been sleeping on the balcony when terrorists started shooting and killing. The sound of the bombs seemed to trigger a PTSD reaction in Shorter. He looked more strained than during any final race sprint. Effort is more controllable than fear and rage. "I was there," he said, "I was right there." He calmed down. The building was secured.

Tom Grilk, executive director and the man nominally in charge, had just accepted congratulations for a well-run race. He accepted handshakes and back pats graciously and intended to wrap up a few details and relax in his hotel room upstairs with his family. But that room that was supposed to be for rest and comfort became a tense command center. He snapped back to his military training. He remembered a card he had been issued with instructions to platoon leaders: What do you know? What can you do? How much time? So Grilk set up a command and control area in his second-floor room 233 in Fairmont Copley Plaza with a view out toward the finish area, and gathered all the BAA officials in the building.

First they limited what they might do. They were not the police, and they were not emergency medical responders. Grilk had to limit what he could do and what he had to do and push deeply down what he really wanted to do. The BAA had an obligation to the runners still out on the course—all of whom wanted to finish and get their finishers medals and their bags of warm, dry clothes. But they could not. Their bags and medals were impounded in a crime scene. Race Director McGillivray had to be located. He had thought his day was over and he could get in a long run. By phone they arranged a route for the runners around the crime scenes and arranged to get the runners' bags out of the police cordon to the old Armory—a castle-like building on Arlington Street. Some runners took days to retrieve their bags. Grilk and company stayed at work until nothing more could be done. That was more than 12 hours after the race had started. Emergencies postpone personal indulgence, so emotional release for Grilk would only come later. Downstairs in the bar, the lockdown continued for hours. Cellphone coverage had stopped. The bar had a TV, a land line, and an oblique view of the finish area by flashing emergency lights reflected from the windows of Copley Square buildings. The TV kept running the same video of the finish area from moments after the blasts, because their cameras had been ordered away from the bombing and rescue site, that same scene played over and over on the TV screen above the bar. Something was happening, but the screen only showed what had happened, and that over and over. It seemed like a dream with no escape. Gradually the bartender got updates on the land line and conveyed them to his patrons, the reporters. Usually information goes the other way. Athletes, coaches, and managers sat at the bar or the tables eating and drinking and chatting. They could not leave the building, make phone calls, or do anything but wait. Flanagan sat with her family and friends as everyone gradually learned what had happened and resolved how it would change each of them. "We sat in such comfort while we knew that not far away people were suffering and there was nothing we could do about it right then," said Flanagan.

Only later in the week could runners get their bags and finishers medals, even if they had not been allowed to actually finish. The bags were moved to the second floor of 40 Trinity Place and runners had to go there to get their belongings.

Once there, they lingered, reluctant to leave the moment. They had come to Boston to finish the marathon—to cross the finish line and receive their medals. So Grilk, Fleming, and other officials placed a promotional poster of the finish line on the floor, creating a mock finish line. There on the second floor, amid the runners' bags, the runners prevented from crossing the real finish line on Monday crossed the symbolic finish one by one. As they crossed it, officials draped a race medal around each runner's neck, and they lingered and talked to each other. Some shed tears. The time proved cathartic and therapeutic. Emotions flowed that had been bottled up for these days. Emotions in Boston among runners and the public bubbled and festered for the rest of the year and would only find their expression a year later on the streets of Boston.

2013 Women's Race

1. Rita Jeptoo, KEN	**2:26:25**	19. Manami Kamitanida, JPN	2:38:21
2. Meseret Hailu, ETH	2:26:58	20. Sheri Piers, USA	2:39:25
3. Sharon Cherop, KEN	**2:27:01**	21. Hilary Dionne, USA	2:39:34
4. Shalane Flanagan, OR	2:27:08	22. Ariana Hilborn, MI	2:42:00
5. Tirfi Tsegaye, ETH	2:28:09	23. Nuta Olaru, CO	2:42:57
6. Kara Goucher, OR	2:28:11	24. Lauren Philbrook, USA	2:43:09
7. Madai Perez, MEX	2:28:59	25. Gina Salby, VA	2:43:23
8. Diane Nukuri-Johnson, BDI	2:29:54	26. Erica Jesseman, USA	2:44:35
9. Ana Dulce Felix, POR	2:30:05	27. Alissa McKaig, IN	2:45:02
10. Sabrina Mockenhaupt, GER	2:30:09	28. Sarah Bard, USA	2:45:26
11. Diana Sigei, KEN	2:33:02	29. Kimberlie Fowler, NC	2:46:37
12. Mamitu Daska, ETH	2:33:31	30. Maria Rivera, CA	2:46:39
13. Alemitu Abera, ETH	2:33:46	**47. Joan Samuelson, ME**	**2:50:29**
14. Yolanda Caballero, COL	2:35:10	134. Chelsea Young, GA	3:00:00
15. Stephanie Rothstein-Bruce, AZ	2:35:31	1859. Genevieve Story, PA	3:30:01
16. Yuka Yano, JPN	2:35:46	2979. Maggie Flanagan, CO	3:37:38
17. Rene Kalmer, RSA	2:37:15	6090. Belina Osborn, UT	4:00:00
18. Svetlana Pretot, FRA	2:38:19,	6951. Kristine Biagiotti, MA	5:32:55
	First Master		

Winning Women's Teams

1. Dirigo, ME, 8:12:42
2. Boston Athletic Association, 8:14:45
3. Varsity Running, LA, 8:44:49
4. Greater Boston Track Club, 9:04:23
5. Falls Road Running, MD, 9:10:11
6. Western Mass Distance Project, 9:13:07
7. Ashville Track Club, NC, 9:134:33
8. Somerville Road Runners, MA, 9:16:51
9. Central Park Track Club, NY, 9:21:24

Boston Strong

MONDAY, APRIL 21, 2014

Security at All-Time High

No one knew if other terrorists would strike this year's Boston Marathon. Would it be dangerous to run? In a great upwelling of defiance, marathon runners and citizens of Greater Boston and beyond vowed to run, or line the streets and not be afraid. Boston has been called the "Cradle of Liberty" because the American Revolution started there. Now the Marathon became an actual, physical expression of liberty and freedom.

This race, run in defiance of the bombing, in affirmation of Boston Strong, brought the fastest field, ever, to race. But the young men had no respect for the old man who took the early lead. After all, he had won his Olympic Silver medal in the marathon ten years earlier. That made him ten years older than most of the men in the field. Surely they reasonably thought that at age 38 he had gone to seed and ran out front to get a little publicity for his sponsor, Sketchers shoes. Keflezighi said he lost his running-shoe deal with Nike three years ago because of his age. He signed a new shoe deal three years ago with Sketchers, a footwear company known more for casual lifestyle shoes than hard-core . . . so, the young men thought he was now a lifestyle runner and not a threat. But the fire had not left the old man.

The editor and publisher of *New England Runner Magazine*, Bob Fitzgerald, listed the quality of the field:

Lelisa Desisa, defending champ
Moses Mosop, 2:03:06
Gebre Gebremariam, 2:04:53
Micah Kogo, who lost to Desisa by 5 seconds last year
Dennis Kimetto, 2:03:45

He concluded his pre-race analysis with the caveat that there is always young talent on the rise. There always is.

In Kenya and Ethiopia enough runners have gone through the system in the last 20 years that lore of training is passed down to young runners, who now learn a great deal about training from runners only slightly older. The young ones all have some connections to someone who has been on the global running circuit and can advise them. East African running is no longer naive. The kids are coming. Droves of them.

But it is easy to overlook the old man. Meb Keflezighi had won the Olympic silver medal at Athens in 2004. Further, Keflezighi was American—born in Africa to be accurate, but raised in the States and thus no longer of the same caliber as the Ethiopians and Kenyans who had come again race each other.

The weather developed to almost perfect—cool, sunny, 61°F with little wind. That was a good, a very good thing for the 120 people employed by the *Boston Marathon Documentary* film crew stationed along the course with 54 cameras to capture the most deeply filmed marathon ever.

But regardless of the glorious day, the lead men decided to doddle out at slower than 5 minutes per mile. What were they thinking? Were they thinking at all? Conditions were near-perfect.

But they hit 5k in 15:09. Defending champion Lelisa Desisa, sitting in the happy pack along with Kenyan Dennis Kimetto, who had won the Chicago Marathon, and fellow Kenyans Wilson Chebet and Frankline Chepkwony; Ethiopians Markos Geneti, Tilahun Regassa, and Gebre Gebremariamm; and hopeful Americans Ryan Hall, a two-time four placer, Jason Hartmann, Meb

Keflezighi, and Abdi Adbirahman. All the Americans knew that an American had not won this race since Greg Meyer in 1983, and that it was high time an American did so. The Kenyans and Ethiopians knew that too.

Maybe they waited for Hall to again bolt boldly where no man had bolted before. But he didn't. The pack would have followed him. As the pack passed 7 miles, it was Keflezighi who moved ever so gently to the front. Only Regassa joined him. A mile later they had 10 seconds on the unfazed pack. Then Regassa dropped back. Then having come from behind the pack with Nicholas Arcinaga of Arizona, American Josphat Boit moved up to join Keflezighi. Arciniaga stayed with the pack. It was early and it seemed wise to stick with the pack, relax, conserve energy, and wait. They all knew that marathons are not won at 9 miles. Maybe they relaxed too much. Maybe they thought that Keflezighi ran at the front only to promote his sponsor's product.

Keflezighi and Boit looked relaxed too, but by 10 miles in 49:08 had gained 30 seconds. Wilson Chebet seemed to be the man of the pack around whom, perhaps because of his 2:05:27 PR from Rotterdam in 2011, the young men had coalesced.

Keflezighi led and Boit followed through Wellesley and halfway in 1:04:20. So it remained, the complacent pack and two guys, one old, up ahead. But at 15 miles Keflezighi pulled ahead ever so slightly. The pack may have been looking only at Boit's back and not seen Keflezighi slip away. By 25k Boit continued his backsliding, but not obvious to the pack was that Keflezighi accelerated. The spilt at 25k of 1:15:59 showed the pack now back 45 seconds. By the turn at the firehouse at the foot of the windy hills, the pack could no longer see Keflezighi leading. Sometimes a runner in the lead is empowered by that glory and it energizes him. The so-called chase pack muddled along unsure about who should or could start the chase. It is hard to chase a ghost. "I knew the course, I knew what was coming," later Keflezighi said. "I'm not sure if he [Chebet] knew that." The ghost pushed on the hills, but the pack would have to push harder on the hills to have any chance of catching the alleged old man. The hills have killed off younger, faster runners but this man, assumed to be a decade off his prime, thundered up to the crest of the hills where a gaggle of delighted spectators chanted, "USA, USA!" While looking straight ahead and keeping his form perfect, Keflezighi raised his energized arm and gave a clenched fist pump sending the crest gang to a pinnacle of delight and maximum volume. This seemed to be the moment of Boston Strong symbolism, joy on the top of Heartbreak a year after.

But the race was not over. Now Wilson Chebet, 28, woke up. Like an aroused predator he cranked out 4:30 miles from the crest. His speed credentials trumped those of the one-decade-older man. When he caught sight of Keflezighi he riveted his eyes on the back of his quarry's head. Frankline Chepkwony, 29, rolled along for back up. Two against one.

Keflezighi chanted to himself his Heartbreak Hills mantra, "Boston Strong, Meb Strong."

Chebet ran from a maximum of 90 seconds behind the leaders at 8 miles to close to 12 seconds behind by 24 miles. No one had any reason to be con-

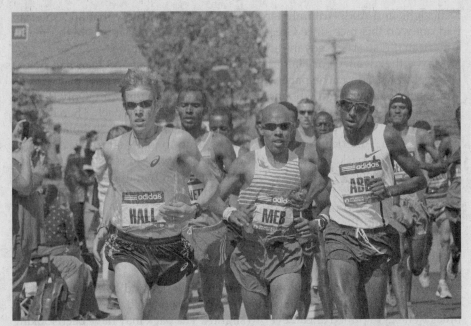

Keflezighi in the pack has not made his gentle move yet. Photo by Victah Sailer.

fident of an American victory. Keflezighi looked back. "Looking back is not a bad thing," he said. "It can save you a win." Desisa, Gebremariam, and Kimetto had dropped out. Hall's blond head could not be seen. It would be a Hollywood ending to a long and painful drama, but to Wilson Chebet, 1st-place prize money and his own country's glory rode along with him. In neat order each ran onto Hereford Street in a line simultaneously visible. Onto Boylston Street, Chebet threatened. A USA victory was not assured. Chebet was much faster than Keflezighi, but he had done a lot of catching up. He had run his last miles faster.

Later Keflezighi would say, "As soon as I got to Boylston Street, I knew I had it."

That is easy to say after the race, but with 600 meters to go in a marathon he likely could not say anything. He wanted to celebrate, take an American flag and wave it, but he did not dare. "This is it," Keflezighi told himself. "Your dream is going to come true." Marathons have been won or lost in the last meters. The crowd screamed at the prospect of an American win and the affirmation of Boston Strong. Celebrating at the point on the course where the pressure-cooker bombs exploded a year before would have been delightful visual justice. But Keflezighi had to run through the line to win. Only in the last second could he push his sun glasses over his head and stretch his arms in victory parallel to the finish line and scream in joy. Then he kissed the pavement. In congratulations, 1983 winner Greg Meyer hugged him. Americans were back.

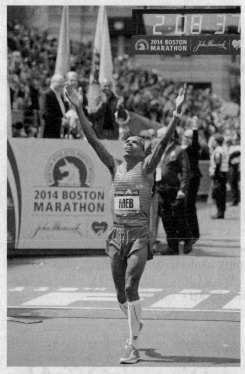

"Thank you Boston." Photo by Victah Sailer.

Keflezighi said, "My career was fulfilled 99.9 percent [and] today makes it 110 percent. This was the missing link. To have this trophy is beyond my dreams." Boston Strong indeed.

2014 Men's Race

1. **Meb Keflezighi, US**	**2:08:37**		16. Abdi Abdirahman, AZ	2:16:06
2. Wilson Chebet, KEN	2:08:48		17. Micah Kogo, KEN	2:17:12
3. Frankline Chepkwony, KEN	2:08:50		18. Brett Gotcher, CA	2:17:16
4. Vitaliy Shafar, UKR	2:09:37		19. Scott MacPherson, MO	2:17:46
5. Markos Geneti, ETH	2:09:50		20. Ryan Hall, CA	2:17:50
6. Joel Kimurer, KEN	2:11:03		21. Ruben Sanca, MA	2:19:05
7. Nicholas Arciniaga, US	2:11:47		22. Ulrich Steidl, WA	2:19:48
8. Jeffrey Eggleston, US	2:11:57			First 40+
9. Paul Lonyangata, KEN	2:12:34		23. Matt Hensley, CO	2:19:51
10. Adil Annani, MAR	2:12:43		24. Brian Harvey, MA	2:20:31
11. Josphat Boit, KEN	2:12:52		25. Vyacheslav Shabunin, RUS	2:20:43
12. Craig Leon, OR	2:14:28		26. Segundo Jami, CO	2:20:52
13. Mike Morgan, MI	2:14:40		27. Kevin Havel, IL	2:20:31
14. Koichi Sakai, JPN	2:14:56		28. Matt Flaherty, IN	2:21:20
15. Lusapho April, RSA	2:14:59		29. Tyler Andrews, MA	2:21:33

30. Eric Ashe, MA	2:21:41	**14372. Amby Burfoot, CT**	**4:42:48**
82. Michael Knutson, OR	2:30:03	16385. Bennett Beach, MD	5:26:58
2240. Vicente Jonguitud, MEX	3:00:00	47th consecutive finish	
7234. Daniel Lieberman, MA	3:29:52	17582. Kevin Counihan, MA	8:58:53
11187. Douglas Cale, MI	4:00:00	**Lelisa Desisa, DNF**	
12067. Gelindo Bordin, ITA	**4:10:37**		

Men's Winning Teams

1. Boston Athletic Association, 7:05:33
2. Western Mass Distance Project, 7:20:52
3. Wasatch Runners, UT, 7:36:40
4. Syracuse Track Club, NY, 7:27:13
5. Second Sole of Toledo, OH, 7:32:24
6. West Valley Track Club, CA, 7:32:25
7. Whirlaway Racing Team, MA, 7:34:32
8. Asheville Running Collective, NC, 7:36:37
9. Greater Boston Track Club, 7:38:37
10. Falls Road Running, MD, 7:39:39

Wicked Pissed Off About the Bombings

MONDAY, APRIL 21, 2014

Mass Native Set to Go for Victory

Did Rita Jeptoo, Buzunesh Deba, Mare Dibaba, Belaynesh Olijira, Sharon Cherop, Jemima Jelagat Sumgong, and Meselech Melkamu all watch the *60 Minutes* TV show and hear Shalane Flanagan say she was "pissed" about the bombings and "all in" for the 2014 Boston Marathon? Did they feel her rage and determination? If they did, they believed her. They would not let her run into a lead, as much as she tried to break away constantly during the race. The women would not let Flanagan go ahead alone, no matter what. One way or another, they had heard her or seen her and believed her. She wanted to bolt away at the gun and run her own race, as Joan Benoit Samuelson advised her to do. It had worked for Joan in 1983 when she ran away to win in the midst of men, but she had not broadcast her intentions to the world. She had not told the world that she was "pissed and all in." How could anyone believe that a person who said that was not a serious threat to win the race?

Flanagan ripped out the first mile in 5:11. Rita Jeptoo felt her body on fire, not ready to run that fast, that soon. Flanagan had traveled six times from her home in Portland, Oregon, to study the course. She had memorized the geometry and sliced each tangent like a surveyor to run the shortest distance.

Flanagan took the lead, passing 5k in 16:12, but she did not rip away to Joan's record time of 15:49 (there had been a big tailwind in 1983). Flanagan had expected the gang of Africans to let her go—to hang her out to dry and expect to burst past her when or if she she slowed. They had let Kim Smith go in 2011. Cherop was in the pack that had let Smith go. It worked that year, so why did they not let Flanagan go this year? It must be that they took her seriously as a runner prepared to run the best race of her life. Professional competitors do their research via television or race results. They are the biggest observers of each other.

Flanagan had run a brilliant 15k in Jacksonville, FL, a month earlier, setting an American record of 47:03. Perhaps performance says more than words.

At water stops Flanagan dropped back to keep clear of traffic. Runners don't body check other runners at water stops as if they were hockey players, but they have both a singleness of mind and a 50 percent reduction in IQ, as do all runners who are racing all-out and sending blood to their muscles instead of their brains. So accidental tangles and falls are quite likely and could instantly ruin all race preparation. But regardless of that water stop caution, Flanagan had stuck in her mind the idea of pushing the pace, so she hit 1:09:27 at halfway, with the gathered Africans behind her in a patient, calm, and poised wedge.

On the open gradual hill over the route 128 (I95) overpass, after the easy downhill to Newton Lower Falls, Flanagan pushed hard to try to shake the field. She strung them out. Whenever anyone tried to challenge her for the lead she fought them off. She did not want the race to come down to a group kick finish. On the hills Flanagan ran the shortest line through the curves. She said she wanted to know this course like a best friend. But Africans hung behind her. Cherop dropped off the group first. The others waited.

They waited past 30k in 1:39:20 to strike and then pushed past Flanagan. At 35k, Sumgong, Jeptoo, Dibaba, Melkamu, and Deba ran together. They all looked totally relaxed and virtually no different than they had looked earlier in the race. With grace and ease they flashed past the aid station and deftly snatched their special fluid bottles from the table. Through Cleveland Circle they quickened the pace off the already fast pace that Flanagan had set. Suddenly Jeptoo felt very, very good. Unease that she had felt earlier in the race vanished. Flanagan had disappeared from the view of the lead vehicle. Jeptoo stretched out the pace with a cruel ease. The other four showed distress for the first time. Deba dropped first. Jeptoo popped out a 4:47 for the 24th mile. *How could she do that?* Flanagan wondered. Jeptoo's next mile clicked off in 5:01. No one could match her as Jeptoo ran the last 3 miles nearly as fast as Keflezighi did in winning the men's race. Jeptoo ran from 35k to 40k in 15:44. It was her fastest 5k of the entire race by nearly a minute. Jeptoo ran the final 3.2 miles in 15 minutes, 56 seconds, including a 4:48 split for Mile 24. Meb Keflezighi ran 15:49.

These things don't usually happen in marathon races. It was unprecedented. That 5000m split time alone would itself have won many 5000m track races. She ran her personal best and set a new course record of 2:18:57 as the first woman under 2:20. Deba followed her under 2:20 by a second.

Jeptoo's coach, Claudio Berardelli, said, "Shalane Flanagan was the key factor in the race. She was brave." Jemima Jelagat Sumgong would go on to win gold at the Olympics in Rio in 2016. Jeptoo would not be there.

Flanagan placed back in 7th place. She ran the best marathon of her life, with a big personal best of 2:22:02. She had prepared to run a PR and did. She said after the race, "I don't wish it were easier, but I just wish I were better." Had she run a little more conservatively, she might have finished 5th, about 30 seconds faster. However, the top 4 were simply beyond the reach of any other tactic. Had Flanagan been content to sit back in the pack and let the pace lag, it is likely that no woman would have broken 2:20. Flanagan clearly had prepared herself to her lifetime peak of fitness. She made the race. She did not fail nor run foolishly. She arrived fit enough to win, but so did everyone else. That's why we have races, which are a test of preparation and bravery. But perhaps the race was a test of something else.

Jeptoo won $150,000 for 1st place and $25,000 for the course record and additional undisclosed appearance money.

At a press conference the day after the race, Jeptoo said, "The woman from the USA was pushing the race and I thought, *wow*. The way I saw everyone running yesterday was not the same Boston."

Shalane Flanagan was devastated and humiliated by her loss. She had led the race and pushed as hard as her perfect preparation allowed, yet deep into the race Jeptoo ran away with a mile, which she ran as if she had been racing a single-mile race: 4:47! How could that be?

At the press conference Flanagan had to stop several times and fight back tears. It was not the same Boston as when Jeptoo won a year earlier in 2:26 or placed 6th in 2:35 a year before that—or when she won in 2006. Jeptoo had improved tremendously. What was her magic? Such a dramatic improvement and the demonstration of virtually no fatigue at 30 kilometers into a marathon can suggest the use of a performance-enhancing substance.

Jeptoo failed a drug test conducted in September 2014 for erythropoietin, EPO. After a hearing held on January 15, 2015, by Athletics Kenya in Nairobi the authorities decided to issue a two-year ban against her. But neither AK nor the BAA could determine retroactively that Jeptoo's performance at Boston was enhanced by drugs. There was drug testing in Boston, but Jeptoo was not disqualified. The BAA would not confirm that Jeptoo was tested nor what tests were given. The ban is under appeal, but the ban is not from Boston. A press report on July 13, 2016, from Nairobi states: "Italian athletics coach Claudio Berardelli, who is facing charges of doping Kenyan athletes, was on Tuesday released on a 200,000 shillings ($1,978) cash bail. Berardelli, who has been in Kenyan police custody since July 5, becomes the second Italian to appear in court after his former boss, Federico Rosa, facing similar charges, was also released on a 300,000 ($2,960) cash bail."

If the resolution of the failed drug test rules that Jeptoo's ban extends to the date of this year's race, her name would be expunged from the record books and the BAA would seek legal action to recoup prize money paid to Jeptoo.

The revelation that Jeptoo failed a drug test came as no shock to the running community, but did bring indignation and sadness. She acquired the nickname Rita the Cheetah. Of course to Flanagan the failed test brought a shaking rage almost as great as her anger about the bombing, but this time she felt rage not about a senseless and murderous crime, but about a possible personal and professional loss of income due to fraud as well as the dismay at being beaten by a cheater. But there is no proof and little on which to base a lawsuit to recover lost income or lost potential income from opportunities for sponsorship, bonus, or appearance fees at other races.

Racing culture has made finish time, not place, the ultimate measure of a marathon. Top marathons boast flat, fast courses and hire waves of pacers to ensure a fast time. Boston has not gone full bore on the pursuit of time, perhaps mainly because it is not a world record certifiable course, but most often the goal is fast times and individual wins. We award money for fast times, so therein may lie the cause of cheating. Fast times equal big money. Cheating pays.

Money is the temptation to change the human body into something it is not— an unnatural running beastie. Soon enough, we may have the medical/technical/genetic know-how to morph runners into sublime genetically modified organisms. As we may recoil against the ethics of making money by cheating, there is ample precedent that it is all too human to do just that. Performance-enhancing drug use may be a sensible business decision. She won many hundreds of thousands of dollars, and once she was caught had to pay nothing but a two-year suspension—a vacation, putting her no worse off than had she not been a runner. The benefit is far greater than the penalty. Imagine if people who worked at a banks were to steal hundreds of thousands of dollars and receive only the penalty that they could not work in banks for the next two years? So the gamble has paid off and it was a smart gamble in the first place. The keepers of the sport have left the bank vault open and continue to do so. Run right in and help yourself. You haven't much to lose. Cheating is the best business decision.

Yes, when you put people in front of such temptations, you have to expect that a logical decision is to take the risk because that is where the money is. Corporations do that all the time. Bend the rules and break them from time to time, then pay the fine because the fine is less than the profit gained. Of course it is not ethical. Most companies follow the rules and are good citizens. Most people do not cheat. But what to do with the cheetahs?

(In October 2016, the Court of Arbitration for Sport extended Jeptoo's ban until October 2018 and stripped her of her 2014 win in Boston, plus results, prize and appearance money dating back to April 17, 2014.)

2014 Women's Race

1. Rita Jeptoo, KEN Disqualified course record	2:18:57	19. Wendy Thomas, CO	2:32:49
		20. Esther Erb, NJ	2:33:15
2. Buzunesh Deba, ETH official course record	2:19:59	21. Noriko Higuchi, JPN	2:33:39
		22. Sarah Cummings, NY	2:34:57
3. Mare Dibaba, ETH	2:20:35	23. Hilary Dionne, MA	2:35:08
4. Jemima Jelagat Sumgong, KEN	2:20:41	24. Lidia Simon, ROU First Master	2:36:47,
5. Meselech Melkamu, ETH	2:20:35		
6. Aleksandra Duliba, BLR	2:21:29	25. Andrea Walkonen, NH	2:37:06
7. Shalane Flanagan, US	2:22:02	26. Nuta Olaru, CO	2:37:29
8. Sharon Cherop, KEN	2:23:00	27. Laura Portis, MI	2:38:48
9. Philes Ongori, KEN	2:23:22	28. Magdalena Boulet, CA	2:41:36
10. Desiree Linden, US (nee Davila)	2:23:54,	29. Erica Jesseman, ME	2:42:32
		30. Bria Wetsch, CA	2:42:33
11. Belaynesh Olijira, ETH	2:24:21	31. Sheri Piers, ME	2:42:40
12. Yeshi Esayias, ETH	2:27:40	58. Joan Samuelson, ME	2:52:10, First 50+
13. Tatyana Petrova Arkhipova, RUS	2:30:29		
14. Lanni Marchant, CAN	2:30:34	131. Anne Paredes, MA	3:00:00
15. Adriana Nelson, CO	2:31:15	2099. Megan Kretz, NY	3:30:00
16. Adriana Aparecida da Silva, BRA	2:31:18	2124. Zika Rea, NC	3:30:11
17. Caroline Kilel, KEN	2:32:04	6917. Alexandra Schmidt, MA	4:00:00
18. Serena Burla, VA	2:32:27	14344. Cheryl Flynn, MA	7:52:34

Winning Women's Teams

1. New York Athletic Club, 8:00:36
2. Boston Athletic Association, 8:26:10
3. Greater Boston Track Club, 8:41:58
4. Wasatch Runners, UT, 8:43:05
5. Georgetown Running Club, DC, 8:53:26
6. Somerville Runners, MA, 8:53:50
7. Dirigo, ME, 8:55:20
8. Charlotte Running Club, NC, 9:09:10
9. Central Park Track Club, NY, 9:09:45
10. SRA Elite, CA, 9:12:43

The First Normal Race

MONDAY, APRIL 20, 2015

Ethiopian Wants to Win Again

Still the worry of the bombing lingered. No one wanted to think about it, but the more you tried not to think about it . . . Could this race put the bombing behind it? Could Lelisa Desia put all the other runners behind himself?

Lelisa Desia came back to Boston to win again. He had won in the year of the bombing, but that crime had overwhelmed everything. He had tried to win in 2014, but had to drop out. He had "died" in the race-hyperbolic way, and had to leave the course. Now in a normal year he wanted to win a normal marathon. As a show of solidarity, Desisa had returned his 2013 winner's medal to the city of Boston at the Boston Athletic Association 10K on Boston Common, two months after the bombings. Desisa told reporters he wanted the people of Boston to know he felt the pain of the attack. It went on display at the Boston Marathon RunBase store on Boylston Street. This time he intended to win and to keep the medal. Although he might have to run through some pain to do so. But the marathon footrace originated to symbolize pain and would never be free of its association with sacrifice. In more than a century the marathon championed many more symbols but always came back to stare down death in one way or another.

The Marathon served to symbolize that privilege of sacrifice for a concept larger than oneself or one's family, farm, or village. Desia's respect for Boston's suffering reflected that long history.

Keflezghi and Desia recognized that their victories meant more than their own winning for a sporting event. The winning comes in the name of some larger group than one person. The bombings have changed all that. Me, me, me had become "we."

Desia showed that the unity is not just a Boston thing, or an American thing, but a world-wide strength. The marathon has come back to its origins as a symbol to unite people in a struggle for their identity. It may no longer be the emerging nation state powered by industrial corporations but perhaps memorialized in the words of eight-year-old Boston Marathon bombing victim Martin Richard: "No more hurting people."

Do we really want to constantly call attention to the crimes that occurred during Marathon 2013? We want to wish away the bombings and all the ways they made us feel. We don't want to feel angry, afraid, vengeful, violated, or depressed. Do we have a choice? The Boston Marathon always will have a different element and deeper meaning to it because of what happened in 2013. But winning a plain, simple sporting event would be nice.

At the 10 a.m. start, the weather forecast changed by the minute. Rain and a cold wind would be coming sometime. Patrick Makau came to Boston for the first time. He had set a world record and approached marathon racing as a money maker. He is married with two children. He is motivated by using running to provide more life choices for his family and community. He has created jobs for 70 people in Manyanzwani and Nairobi, and was instrumental in providing water and electricity to his village.

Ethiopia's Tadesse Tola shot from the start, perhaps to ensure that no old man Keflezighi would be able to run away to a big lead, or perhaps because he wanted to beat the coming storm. Everyone followed through a first mile of 4:40—and the next with Gebre Gebremariam taking over at nearly the same pace. He pushed through 5k in 14:42, showing that this would not be a "tactical" race. New Boston runner Yemane Tsegay from Ethiopia took a pull at the front and Tola later returned to do the same.

After 10k, midway through Framingham, the pack thundered along at 29:43, on pace for 2:05:21. Coming through Natick there still were a dozen contenders hanging together so Desisa decided to throw in a reality check. "I try to test all the athletes to see who has more than me," he said. He pushed. Everyone else pushed back.

They passed 10 miles in 48:10. Americans Nick Arciniaga and Keflezighi ran in the pack. Matt Tegankamp and Ritzenhein seemed to have disappeared.

None had more and none less energy than Desisa. His countrymen Tsegay, Tadese Tola, and Gebre Gebremariam ran with him, as did former champion Wesley Korir and Kenyan compatriots Frankline Chepkwony, Bernard Kipyego, and Chebet. "It was four Ethiopians and four Kenyans," said Keflezighi, who was the lone American in the bunch. "I said, c'mon, Dathan."

They passed halfway in 1:04.

Dathan Ritzenhein, who was making his Boston debut at 32, ran 9th at the Beijing Olympics and has top-10 finishes in New York and Chicago. But he seemed to be cautious. Coming into Wellesley, he was 15 seconds behind the leaders. So Ritzenhein let gravity and enthusiasm swoop him downhill where he found himself 2 seconds ahead at Newton Lower Falls. It looked to spectators that an American could win this race again.

Keflezighi wore a red shirt with the Sketchers logo on the left and T-Mobile on the right, Adidas on the race bib which displayed MEB. Ritzenhein also wore red, but the Nike logo and a big USA across the chest with a little American flag.

It is not clear that the pack knew that actual world record–holder Patrick Makau, at 2:03:38 (Berlin in 2011), had stepped off the course at 5k.

At the firehouse turn it still was anybody's race, with all 10 men within a second of one another. Kenyan Bernare Kipyego had joined the race along with Abel Kirui of Kenya, and four-time World Half Marathon champion Ethiopian Zersenay Tadese, Wilson Chebet, who had nearly run down old man Keflezighi last year, and 2012 champion Wesley Korir.

Ritzenhein looked like the rabbit leading the way, running with great ease past 16 miles pushing sub-5-minute miles.

That changed after Heartbreak, where the Ethiopians began asserting themselves. But as the hills started, Ritzenhein drifted to the back of the 11-man pack. Desisa, Tsegay, and Chepkwony took turns attacking as if in a bicycle race. The pack strung out. As it did, so the headwinds continued to increase.

At the crest of the hill an odd thing happened. The pack recongealed. Perhaps the wind stood them up. A couple of miles passed in 5:24 and 5:25. Ritzenhein retook the lead looking as fresh as ever. He pushed past 20 miles in 1:39:01. After the race, Ritzenhein said, "Of course you always think maybe today is the day. But as I stepped over the hill, I decided not to go with them." Well, maybe *he* decided, but others were making decisions too.

"After 35k, knowing who was around me, I knew I was going to win because my speed was greater than theirs," said Desisa. But it was Tsegay who decided to surge and immediately powered away from Ritzenhein, but 6 runners followed the surge.

Keflezighi led briefly at 20 miles, but he couldn't go with the Ethiopians. The drink he'd gulped at the last water table rebelled on him and he stopped to vomit. "I just wanted to get to the finish line," said Keflezighi. "Took a long time."

The six men—Tsegay, Desisa, Korir, Chebet, Korir, Kipyego, and Chepkwony—solidified. Miles 22 and 23 flashed by in 4:47 and 4:42. Then observers could see that it was Desisa who controlled the pace and the others hung on for the ride of their lives. Tsegay hung most tenaciously. The sufferers dropped off like overripe fruit. Only two remained, Desisa in a ripening yellow shirt and Tsegay in green with yellow. They looked quite stylish together straining in lock step. At 23 miles, Desisa opened 20 meters, but Tsegay closed it by 24 and put his head down and charged in an aggressive move to break Desisa. It did not work. Tsegay broke himself. "I tried to push, but in the end it was impossible for me to catch up with Lelisa Desisa," said Tsegay. "That is why he won."

Desisa waved to spectators on his way to the finish line, turning Boylston Street into his victory parade.

"I started waving my hand because I love the people of Boston," said Desisa.

"I heard a lot of repeat-repeat," said Keflezighi, who would be the first American to do it since Bill Rodgers won his third straight in 1980. "I was definitely thinking of that. I thought I had a shot at it." But that stomach upset took him out of the running and he had drifted back. But racing was not over for him.

Meb Keflezighi would amazingly make the U.S. Olympic Team for Rio, where with similar stomach problems, he'd run 2:16 for 33th place. Desia would be back, too. Korir went back to Parliament. Boston would remain strong.

2015 Men's Race

1. Lelisa Desia, ETH	2:09:17	6. Frankline Chepkwony, KEN	2:10:52
2. Yemane Adhane Tsegay, ETH	2:09:48	7. Dathan Ritzenhein, US	2:11:20
3. Wilson Chebet, KEN	2:10:22	8. Meb Keflezighi, US	2:12:42
4. Bernard Kipyego, KEN	2:10:47	9. Tadese Tola, ETH	2:13:35
5. Wesley Korir, KEN	2:10:49	10. Vitaliy Shafar, UKR	2:13:52

11. Matt Tegenkamp, US	2:13:52	27. Cole Atkins, NC	2:23:21
12. Jeffrey Eggleston, US	2:14:17	28. Christian Mercier, CAN	2:24:37
14. Nicholas Arciniaga, US	2:18:02	29. Daniel Glaz, IL	2:24:44
15. Danilo Goffi, ITA	2:18:44	30. Said Boudalia, ITA	2:24:49
16. Sage Canaday, CO	2:19:12	31. Matt Lenehan, US	2:25:08
17. Sergey Zyryanov, RUS	2:19:17	32. Maxime Leboeuf, CAN	2:25:10
18. Chris Chavez, US	2:20:04	33. Takaya Sakamoto, JPN	2:25:10
19. Scott McPherson, MO	2:20:25	34. Jason Ayr, MA	2:25:14
20. Christopher Zablocki, CT	2:20:35	74. Neil Pearson, AUS	2:30:03
21. Kiyokatsu Hasegawa, JPN	2:20:42	131. Jason Butler, US	2:35:00
22. Benjamin Zywicki, CO	2:21:10	2496. Nicholas Prudhomme, CAN	3:00:00
23. Philippe Viau-Dupuis, CAN	2:21:16	7735. Randy Osbourn, OH	3:30:00
24. Ruben Sanca, MA/CPV	2:21:58	11326. Robert Wong, CA	4:00:00
25. Fernando Cabada, CA	2:22:05	**12399. Amby Burfoot, CT**	**4:18:09**
26. Malcolm Richards, CA	2:22:30	14580. William Reilly, NY	8:06:01

Men's Winning Teams

1. New York Athletic Club, 7:22:14
2. Fleet Feet Nike Racing Team, IL, 7:29:58
3. Strava Track Club, CA, 7:32:07
4. West Valley Track Club, CA, 7:33:00
5. Whirlaway Racing Team, MA, 7:34:41
6. Boston Athletic Association, 7:39:02
7. Greater Boston Track Club, 7:40:14
8. Atlanta Track Club, GA, 7:41:42
9. Bull City Track Club, NC, 7:49:03
10. Ragged Mt Racing, VA, 7:49:58

Racing Is Not Logical

MONDAY, APRIL 20, 2015

American Women Amass to Challenge Africans
Rotich Defies Logic

People cheat to win races. There is a long history to cheating in sports. The Boston Press reported richly on drugs in the marathon.

Thomas Hicks, a Cambridge, Massachusetts, brass worker, doped in 1904 when he won the Olympic Marathon in St. Louis. Hicks, who had finished

2nd in Boston that year, swallowed a combination of strychnine (rat poison), brandy, and egg whites. That may not have helped, but it goes to show that competitors have been looking for an edge since sport began. Sports do have their origins in warfare where all is fair. Many believe that East Germany's Waldemar Cierpinski used steroids to enhance recovery and thus performance before he won at the 1976 and 1980 Olympic Games. So the recent drug scandals involving Kenya's Rita Jeptoo and Russia's Liliya Shobukhova are not new.

But what do race directors, managers, and sponsors do? "Our sport should be the purest, and unfortunately that hasn't been the case," said 2014 Boston winner Meb Keflezighi, who came back to the Boston Marathon to try to win again. Last year's women's winner, Jeptoo, will not be allowed to race.

Penalties for first-time doping offenders have been doubled to four years by the World Anti-Doping Agency, also races in the Abbott World Marathon Majors will pay for out-of-competition testing for an athletes' pool that will include approximately the top 150 professional runners.

"I am ecstatic that they took such a stance," said Shalane Flanagan. "It's just mandatory. At this level you can't let anyone come in and compete when other people are doing it the right way."

The program, which is being administered by the international track and field federation and funded by the AWMM, will include testing at a first-ever laboratory in Kenya, where multiple positives have created a cloud of doubt above the planet's most dominant marathoning country.

"That will be a game-changer, as well," says London Marathon chief executive Nick Bitel, who also is the AWMM's general counsel. "It has been difficult and expensive to get samples from there to Switzerland."

The enhanced testing regimen is the only way, race directors say, to convince both clean athletes and a suspicious public that the sport is on the level. "People are watching magic when they're watching these races," said NYC Marathon race director Mary Wittenberg. "Once someone's duped and what they're watching isn't real, it erodes the authenticity of what they're watching." About Jeptoo, Wittenberg said, "We all feel burned."

Since Jeptoo's suspension is being appealed to the Court of Arbitration for Sport, her victories still stand. "We put an asterisk by them," said one official. After Jeptoo tested positive for blood-boosting EPO, and she was denied her $500,000 bonus from Chicago pending resolution of her case.

"I have and will have a high degree of confidence that we'll have athletes who've been tested in a program that's most rigorous," said Boston Athletic Association executive director Tom Grilk. "I think it leads the way."

"It's very good," says Kenya's Wesley Korir, who won the 2012 Boston Marathon. "As an athlete and as a champion of a clean sport I really encourage that. I have proposed before that they really need to make sure that the people who come here are clean athletes because what is happening is the dirty athletes are killing the sport. I think what the Majors are doing is just very commendable."

"I didn't believe they could benefit from drugs like EPO," said Bill Rodgers. "I figured altitude was enough. They're winning everything already."

"You think everybody's doing it clean, that there's no other way," said Keflezighi. "It's frustrating. In a 26.2 journey, there's no shortcut. You don't skip miles. Unfortunately, some people have skipped those things to make it happen."

Athletics Kenya, shaken to the core by the global perception that many of its distance runners are dirty, has banned Jeptoo for two years. It also suspended Rosa Associati of Italy (which represents Jeptoo) and Volare Sports of the Netherlands, two of the most prominent management organizations, from representing Kenyan marathoners for six months.

"There have been a lot of reports relating to doping in Kenya, a lot of fingers pointed at people, agents, doctors, and pharmacists," federation chief Isaiah Kiplagat, who called the doping issue "just as bad as AIDS," said at a Nairobi news conference. "We know it's an intricate issue and critical matter and we want to deal with it."

The drug testing at the Boston Marathon is paid for under contract to WADA following a protocol that the Marathon is required to keep secret so potential cheaters cannot learn how to circumvent the detection process.

"Looking back, I feel very naive now," said Amy Hastings Cragg. "One of her last miles was 4:48, something insane. At the time, I was like, *Whoa, my mind is blown. That's so crazy. Amazing.* Looking back, I'm like, *I was an idiot. That's impossible.* That's actually not possible for a woman to do at the end of a marathon. So, that's very frustrating."

Many of her competitors believe Jeptoo's two-year suspension from competition doesn't go far enough, because a positive test for the blood-booster EPO in September 2014 cannot void the Boston course record set five months earlier.

Shalane Flanagan would like lifetime bans for Jeptoo and others caught doping. She sees Buzunesh Deba (2:19:59) as the true Boston Marathon women's course record-holder. Desiree Davila Linden said she has "put an asterisk" on the Jeptoo mark. She knows it's a tricky situation because there are no positive tests to back up strong suspicions that Jeptoo cheated her way to the Boston record or earlier Boston titles.

"You've got to go by the rule book and understand how the process works," said Linden. "But the improvements she makes from cheating stick around for a long time. I guess you hope that someone can come in soon and do it the right way and erase that record for good." (In October 2016 the BAA disqualified Jeptoo and instated Deba as the rightful course record holder.)

Flanagan sometimes reviews how she raced and finished the Boston Marathon in 2013 and 2014 and imagines how it would have been different without Jeptoo in the field. If Jeptoo doped before the 2013 race, then Flanagan should move up from 4th to 3rd place in the official results. More than that, Flanagan saw Jeptoo's strong closing speed for the first time in 2013 and planned accordingly for 2014. Flanagan sped through the early miles of last year's race, rocking a 1:09:27 half marathon, because of Jeptoo.

Speaking to *Boston Globe* reporter Shira Springer, Flanagan said, "I thought, *There's no way I can let it come down to a really fast finish. I can't have Jeptoo near me in the last 5 miles. When I come off Heartbreak, I've got to have a lead. I've got to try to get her before we get there because I can't compete with that finish.* So, that's why I prepared the way I did last year."

Flanagan isn't the only elite female marathon runner who trained and strategized to beat Jeptoo. Given the way Jeptoo dominated the sport in 2013 and 2014 with wins at Boston and Chicago, her cheating created a massive ripple effect. Cragg seemed to speak for all clean elite female marathoners when she said, "You get very bitter when you start thinking about it too much . . . You can't beat these people who are on drugs."

But the testing system did catch Jeptoo, so that led some to see some hope.

"It's not a culture where you can get away with that," said Linden. "It's not a sport where the only way you can compete is if you're cheating or you're doping. It's frustrating when somebody gets caught. You're also happy and excited because it's keeping the sport clean and you see the outrage and you think, *I'm not alone in feeling like this.*"

Linden said, "You want to have that awe and shock at what the human body can do. But now it's become, 'That's unbelievable,' and it automatically raises a question mark. It's nice when those [fast finishes by runners who test positive for doping] get flushed out, but it does take away from the genuine excitement of the moment. And those moments should be special when done right."

Before races, you'd rather hear the question, *Who is going to win?* rather than speculation on who is using what chemicals. The logical thing to do is to list the competitors in order of their personal bests. But logic is not how things play out. With Jeptoo out of this year's race on a drugs ban, the logic pointed to last year's 2nd-place finisher, at 2:19:59, Buzunesh Deba, to finish 2nd again behind Mare Dibaba, who ran 2:19:52 on January 3, 2016, at Xiamen International Marathon in China. Or perhaps another Boston Marathon winner in the race, 2012 Boston winner Sharon Cherop, but she had run only 2:31:50. But logic does not always rule.

If you don't use logic to make your picks, you resort to the opposite of logic, emotion, and you pick your favorites. For Americans that would be a solid domestic sweep of Flanagan, (Hastings) Cragg, and Linden in that or any other order.

But if you are really smart, you pick nothing and sit back and watch the race play out and wonder why it plays out the way it does. This race played out like a game of chess on a board filled with queens—the most powerful piece on the board. Queen after queen would vanish from the board until only two remained. It started with an easy, downhill mile of 5:38.

At 10k, on wet roads with slight rain in the air and the fear of predicted headwinds in mind, a pack of everyone formed at 34:23. The three Americans, Amy (Hastings) Cragg who lives in Providence, Rhode Island, and recently married Irish runner Alistair Cragg; Michigan runner Desiree Linden, who as Desiree Davila placed 2nd by a whisper in 2011; and Shalane Flanagan. The pace was nothing like the fast start ignited by Flanagan the previous year in her feckless attempt to outrun Jeptoo.

The pack stuck together through the half in 1:12:45, with Linden frequently drifting to the front to push the pace, then floating through the pack to the back only to come up on one side or the other to repeat the process. Her intention seemed to be to keep pressure on the pack to lessen the chances of a mass kick in the last stage. By 30k, Flanagan began to show signs of strain by falling off the pack then struggling to reattach herself. By 35k Cragg had fallen far off and would leave the course. Flanagan could no longer rejoin the pack after Linden's relentless mild surges. Linden said, "I wanted to grind it out in a war of attrition."

Dibaba and Linden seemed to be the bosses of the pack, dictating the surge-and-respond pace. At the crest of the hill, only nine women remained in the lead pack. But by the finish Flanagan would catch one of them.

The real racing, however, started 2 hours and 3 minutes into the race, with Deba throwing down a serious surge to break away. Dibaba followed. By 2:05, Linden came back, with Caroline Rotich seeming to make her first appearance in the race. She had not been heralded prior to the race, regarded only as a field filler, with her best of 2:23:22 and a top place in a world major of only 4th and with a DNF at Boston in 2012. Although from Nyahururu, Kenya, she learned Japanese while on scholarship at Sendai Ikuei Gakuen School in Japan. She told writer Gary Cohen in a later interview, "When I got to Japan I was thinking that I wanted to go back. It was different—the food, the running—everything was different. I was homesick from the time I got to Japan so it was hard. When you get to Japan it isn't like everyone speaks English so that was hard for a while. In time I got used to it and loved it. By then I liked being in Japan and running there."

After graduation she did not get picked up by one of the Japanese corporate teams. She lived in Santa Fe, New Mexico, and trained with the Ryan Bolton group. Kenyan Joseph Mutinda was a part of that group but flunked an in-competition drug test last year for EPO, according to the USADA. He had admitted to the drug use and faces a three-year ban.

Rotich ran at 20 miles waiting to see what would happen. She focused on the race and what the other runners were doing.

Rotich tried to squeeze in between Ethiopians Deba and Dibaba but had to wait behind them. They ran a 5:07 mile at 24 miles. Linden could not respond. The race had come down to three. After the race, Rotich said that on Hereford Street she thought she would place 2nd. At the turn onto Boylston, Rotich took the lead for the first time. But when she could see the finish line, she knew she could kick. Dibaba would not let her go. Rotich told Cohen in an interview later, "It was a long way, but I was trying to go. Then I realized the finish line was so far away that I couldn't even see it. It was still far away so I thought, *Whoops, I think I made a mistake a little bit.* I didn't think I could sprint from there to the finish so I let it go for a while. Then she came so hard and I thought then that I was getting close to the finish line. So I was going to let it all out again and I knew that I had to push all of the way to the finish." Deba fell back. Rotich and Dibaba sprinted. Dibaba retook the lead. Rotich responded with very little distance left in the long race. Rotich rose up on her toes and uncorked an unanswerable kick to win by 4 seconds. She said, "But when I turned to the last part of the race, and she got the lead, I was like, *It is not over*."

"When I crossed the finish line, for about a minute it was like—whoa—this just happened. At the same time I couldn't even process what had happened."

Rotich won $150,000 and when asked after the race what she planned to do with the money, she said she had no plan. When asked if she had thought during the race about Jeptoo and her suspension, Rotich said she had not thought about her. But we are now all thinking about the logic of money, racing, sport, and the temptations.

2015 Women's Race

1. Caroline Rotich, KEN	**2:24:55**	22. Elizabeth Ryan, US	2:47:15
2. Mare Dibaba, ETH	2:24:69	23. Mayumi Uchiyama, JPN	2:47:17
3. Buzunesh Deba, ETH	**2:25:09**	24. Ji Li, CHN	2:48:07
4. Desiree Linden, US	2:25:39	25. Amber Green, UT	2:48:07
5. Sharon Cherop, KEN	**2:26:05**	26. Emily D'Addario, MA	2:48:10
6. Caroline Kilel, KEN	**2:26:40**	27. Nuta Plaru, CO	2:48:28
7. Aberu Kebede, ETH	2:26:52	28. Denise Sandahl, NH	2:48:32
8. Shure Demise, ETH	2:27:14	29. Andrea Rediger, MN	2:48:41
9. Shalane Flanagan, US	2:27:47	30. Dorota Gruca, NM/POL	2:48:49
10. Joyce Chepkirui, KEN	2:29:07	31. Hiruni Wijayaratne, JNP	2:49:05
11. Aleksandre Duliba, BLR	2:29:23	32. Marie Davenport, CT	2:49:06
12. Lisa Nemec, CRO	2:35:18	33. Kristin Barry, ME	2:49:32
13. Adriana Nelson, US	2:38:47	34. Kerri Leonhardt, MA	2:49:39
14. Megumi Amako, JPN	2:39:08	**67. Joan Benoit Samuelson, US**	**2:54:03**
15. Hilary Dionne, US	2:40:42		**1st 55–59**
16. Lauren Philbrook, US	2:41:17	149. Jordan Parker, IL	2:59:59
17. Caitlin Phillips, NY	2:44:28	2409. Stephanie Burnham, HN	3:30:00
18. Lissa Zimmer, CAN	2:44:56	7574. Cynthia Tanner, FL	4:00:00
19. Katie Misuraca, MA	2:46:22	12018. Nona Cerveny, AZ	7:59:33
20. Madeline Duhon, MA	2:46:34	Amy Cragg, DNF	
21. Liza Hunter-Galvan, TX/NZL	2:46:44		

Winning Women's Teams

1. Boston Athletic Association, 8:15:14
2. Greater Boston Track Club, 8:30:21
3. Team American Race Pacers, UT, 8:40:30
4. Dashing Whippets Running Team, NY, 9:02:27
5. Muskoka Algonquin Runners, CAN, 9:05:04
6. Impala Racing Team, CA, 9:05:05
7. Fleet Feet Nike Racing Team, IL, 9:07:57
8. Varsity Sports, LA, 9:13:59
9. Life Time Run MN, 9:14:07
10. Crow Athletics, ME, 9:20:58

Many National "Olympic Trials"

MONDAY, APRIL, 18, 2016

Weak American Field in Olympic Year

Leisa Desisa of Ethiopia again came back to Boston to win. Runners always come back to win. It is like a homing instinct. Also having won the race puts a runner's agent in a good negotiating position for appearance money. Winning is good, but ultimately hard. Others wanted to win too; the 27,491 runners who lined up in Hopkinton for the 120th running of the Boston Marathon mostly dreamed of winning, but a lean and taut handful had reason to think they may be on the line on their day. The temperatures hit 71°F under a bright sun; no humidity; a gentle sea breeze would cool them in the last miles. But the runners felt hot on the starting line as the sun beat on them. Some thought only of winning, not running fast. Lemi Berhaunu Hayle of Ethiopia came to win. He goes by Berhaunu. To do that he thought he had to beat Desisa and needed to beat him by only a little bit, so why take chances trying for a fast time? Hayle was scared of Desisa so planned to follow and not challenge, but if he lasted to the end, then challenge. But would he or might someone else?

For the New England runners, the sun had not beat on them with that intensity since last September. Of course back then such a day would be refreshingly cool, but today it shocked their pasty winter-weary skin. We presume that those raised in the tropics had no such ambiguity. As the sun beat on the runners, the ones with the serious dreams drew a bead on last year's winner.

Top Americans had peaked for and raced the Olympic Trials in Los Angeles in February, so were not strong at Boston in this Olympic year.

Japan's Shingo Igarashi zipped through the opening miles alone on a pace faster than his 2:13:14 personal best. But with the heat, the field of contenders sat back and let him go, paying homage to last year's winner, Desisa. It seems like a pack of predators played with prey, but they really watched each other knowing someone was going to do something soon, but who? By 4 miles (20:07), Igarashi still held his lead but by 5 miles (25:19), the lumbering lead pack rolled over him and, though he tried to nail himself to the bulky pack, fatigue pried him off.

Everyone who was anyone sauntered through 5k in 15:46 and 10k in 31:21. No need to list all 17 guys. Desisa, in addition to having won the Boston Marathon twice, had run 2:04:45 to win the Standard Chartered Dubai Marathon in 2013. He was 26. But the 21-year-old other Ethiopian, Lemi Berhaunu Hayle, had run 2:04:33 in January of 2016. He had, however, not won, but placed 2nd on the flat course aided by a squad of pacers. So the man of the race remained the proven winner, Desisa.

Desisa became the target. He had won twice so must know the secret. It seemed like the lead pack all decided they would follow the lead of last year's leader. Would he, could he, control the race or merely be the patsy pace maker? It is a great honor to be the man to beat and a great burden.

Lemi Berhaunu Hayle learned that he had a talent for running when he won the Assela High School Championships in the 1500m in 2005. He, like all young runners, wanted to be selected to represent his country in the Olympics. Hayle, Desisa, 2012 champion Wesley Korir of Kenya, and the previous year's runner-up Yemane Adhane Tsegay of Ethiopia swirled around in the pack. Korir also knew how to win things as diverse as marathons and political elections.

They all moseyed with their best friends through 15k in 47:06 and 20k in 1:03:13, projecting to a 2:14 finish.

Hayle watched Desisa, as did everyone else. Korir watched for another opportunity. If Desisa stayed in the group, so did Hayle.

If anyone could have been deemed to be the aggressor in the early miles, it would have been Deribe Robi from Ethiopia. Others would drift up and back, occasionally injecting an increase in tempo. But it would quickly dissipate, leaving Robi, a 2:05:58 performer from Eindhoven last year, back in the lead and controlling the charge.

The pack passed halfway 1:06:44, and everybody watched Desisa, who was watching everybody else in the 17-man pack.

When the first significant move came, it was from Desisa himself. "I am testing Yemane and also Lemi, and I decide to go. I try to go, and I try to win." He would explain later at the press conference. The gang had run through 15 miles in 1:16:43 (an average of 5:07 per mile). They passed 25K when Desisa injected a 4:34 to mile 16 to slice open the pack. The race at last had begun. But this was his sixth marathon in the last 17 months. Would he hold together?

Hayle followed, as did Tsegay. They swooped down the open road towards Newton Lower Falls, Desisa maintained his pace up over the exposed hill that does not look like a hill over Route 128/ I 95. He pushed past the fire station and up the hills of Newton. Desisa pushed, Hayle hung. They raced each other, however moreover they raced the hills. They shared water at one point. They had 24 seconds on the field by 35k.

They covered the mile between 23 and 24 in 4:56, hitting 40k (2:05:58). They had almost a minute on Korir and Yemane Adhane Tsegay.

Two Eithiopians leading, followed by another, raced slightly ahead of four Kenyans.

Hayle injected a surge just as Desisa slowed for a water table. Sharing time was over. It was common tactic to move while the other guy slows to look for water then will look up and see his pacer gone. Desisa tried to catch up but felt his left leg did not work as well as the other. Hayle gained 2, then 10, then 20 meters. Desisa snatched worried glances over his shoulder hoping to see no one. Hayle powered forward, reaching 25 miles in 2:06:39 with an 8-second margin.

"I didn't believe it until the finish line," asserted Hayle, who'd break the finish tape in 2:12:45 after celebrating on Boylston Street. Then he leaped in to the air, landed and danced a bit. "I thought that somebody would still take over. I'm so very happy. I've won some races before this one, but today feels like my birthday."

"The Boston Marathon is different to any other race," stated Desisa. "The pace was very slow, but there was a wind if you went in front. There are no pacemakers, so if an athlete goes to the front, it's hard to know how it will go."

If you were to score the race like a cross-country race between only Ethiopia and Kenya, Ethiopia would have the winning score this day.

The first American to finish was 28-year-old Zachary Hine, originally from Holyoke, Massachusetts, but now living in Dallas, Texas.

"My goal was to run conservative and have a strong last 10k," he explained. "I was hoping for top 20. I'm excited to finish tenth." Cramps had forced Hine to DNF at the Olympic Marathon Trials in February. "It was nice to bounce back," he said.

Hayle would go on to race the Olympic Marathon finishing in 13th. Keflezighi would finish 33rd, Wesley Korir would not finish at all.

2016 Men's Results:

#	Name	Time		#	Name	Time
1.	**Lemi Berhanu Hayle, ETH**	**2:12:45**		22.	Said Boudalia, ITA	2:27:41
2.	**Lelisa Desisa, ETH**	**2:13:32**		23.	Joseph Carpenter, MA	2:27:48
3.	Yemane Adhane Tsegay, ETH	2:14:02		24.	Tyler Eustance, NY	2:27:53
4.	**Wesley Korir, KEN**	**2:14:05**		25.	Alvaro Sanabria, NE	2:28:14
5.	Paul Lonyangata, KEN	2:15:45		26.	Jorge Maravilla, CA	2:28:26
6.	Sammy Kitwara, KEN	2:16:43		27.	Maharo Ikeda, JPN	2:28:53
7.	Stephen Chebogut, KEN	2:16:52		28.	Dylan Wilescas, NM	2:29:09
8.	Abdi Nageeye, NDED	2:18:05		29.	Zachary Ornelas, MI	2:29:23
9.	Getu Feleke, ETH	2:18:46		30.	Peter Bromka, OR	2:29:32
10.	Zachary Hine, USA	2:21:37		31.	Craig Coon, NY	2:29:51
11.	Cuthbert Nyasango, ZIM	2:22:02		32.	Brandon Wolfe, CA	2:30:22
12.	Tsegaye Mekonnen, ETH	2:22:21		33.	Rob Bond, GBTC	2:30:27
13.	Ian Burrell, USA	2:22:22		34.	Martin Fiz, ESP	2:30:57
14.	Jackson Kiprop, UGA	2:24:44				(age 53)
15.	Harbert Okuti, USA/UGA	2:24:46		1366.	Robert Lee, MI	3:00:00
16.	Solonie DeSilvia, BRA	2:24:54		6064.	Francois Battle, FRA	3:30:00
17.	Clint Wells, CO	2:24:55,		10248.	Robert Astrop, VA	4:00:00
		First Master		20145.	**Amby Burfoot, CT**	**4:17:48**
18.	Norio Kamijo, JPN	2:25:31		23979.	**Kenji Kimihara, JPN**	**4:53:14**
19.	Shingo Igarashi, JPN	2:26:24		14120.	Bennett Beach, MD	5:31:21
20.	Michael Kipyego, KEN	2:27:02		14463.	Daryl Farler, TN	8:25:09
21.	Andy Williams, IN	2:27:07				

Winning Men's Teams

1. Greater Boston Track Club, 7:38:02
2. Boulder Track Club, CO, 7:47:00
3. Plano Pacers Running Club, TX, 7:51:23
4. Boston Athletic Association, 7:56:57
5. Bowerman Track Club, OR, 7:57:59
6. Seattle Running Club, WA, 7:59:18
7. Central Park Track Club, NY, 8:03:05
8. Fleet Feet Nike Racing Team, IL, 8:03:39
9. Western Massachusetts Distance Project, 8:04:53
10. Adidas Garden State Track Club, NJ, 8:15:52

It's Not Over Until . . .

MONDAY, APRIL, 18, 2016

First Woman Is Grand Marshall

Bobbi Gibb, the first woman to run the Boston Marathon, rode in the honorable and celebratory lead vehicle announcing to the spectators that the women runners approached. Maybe it is symbolic, coincidental, or causal that this year a woman led the polls in the competition for the U.S. presidency. Pioneers everywhere inspire pioneers. But reality does have a way of nurtruring or crushing dreams.

Bright sun and 69°F illuminated and warmed the women's field. Like a group warm-up run, too many to list arrived all together at 5k in 18:22 after miles of 6:05, 5:47, and 5:53. Then someone pushed to a 5:38, then they all slowed to 5:54. This was weird. Many runners change their paces in fartlek or speed-play training, but this was a race, wasn't it? For one of the favorites, it soon wasn't.

Defending champion Caroline Rotich told *Boston Globe* reporter Shira Springer what she had learned from last year's close finish: "The thing I learned from last year is that it's not over until it's over. So, no matter what happens in the race, you have to keep going." But she felt a pain in her ankle at 4.5 miles. She stopped, walked, and left the course. It was over. She would seek an MRI to explain the pain. Her departure left the pack unsure of a runner to follow. Jelena Prokopcuka, the Latvian record holder with a 2:22 best from 2005, took charge reluctantly. She had been hit by a bicycle on the streets of Boston just days before the race and did not know how that would affect her.

The pack bumbled along at just barely under 6-minute-mile pace. The two Americans, Neeley Spence Gracey and Sarah Crouch, found themselves drifting into the lead. Gracey had said she wanted to have a positive experience so planned to run conservatively. Drifting into the lead was not what she expected. This was to be her first marathon. She had qualified for the Olympic Trials with a half marathon. She passed up the trials for the magic of Boston. Her father had run at Boston in 2:16:40 for 19th place on the day that Neely was born in 1990. Steve Spence later won the U.S. Olympic Trials and placed 12th in the Barcelona Olympics. But running at an easy pace, she suddenly found herself amazingly in the lead with Sarah Crouch. Crouch was born Sarah Porter of rural Hockinson in the southwest prairie of Washington state. The family didn't exactly have a farm but a few animals including a fearsome rooster named Dude. Dude had claws and did not like Sarah. One day when feeding clover to the animals in the barn she heard a rustling in the hay. Out charged the vicious bird. Sarah took off at a run. Dude chased her around the house twice, but could not catch her. Her father watched from the window. He later said, "I think I'm going to sign you up for track." So thanks to Dude the rooster, she led the Boston Marathon with Gracey with whom she had raced in college. They talked. Later, Gracey said, "We were commenting back and forth saying, 'Wow, we are leading the Boston Marathon, we need to really take this in and relish the moment.' We knew the race would get going at some point." The 5-mile mark put them front and center on the course and on the world-wide television feed. They ran with their sensible pace and with their plan. It was the rest of the pack that seemed to have no plan.

The big pack ran about 18 minutes for the next 5k, delivering the mass to 10k in 36:20.

The pace picked up a little and the 15-member pack moved ahead of the Americans. But not too much. Then next 5k passed in 17:39. The party stayed together. Then a 17:45. Maybe they all just like to party. They passed the half in 1:15:32.

The pace degenerated to as slow as a 6:12 mile at mile 14. Then someone of them, maybe Kenyans Joyce Chepkirui and Valentine Kipketer, blasted a downhill 5-minute mile. Was this a fartlek workout? Ethiopian Atsede Baysa felt a tight hamstring and did not go with them, but Trifi Tsegaye did. The move produced the fastest 5k yet of the day, a 17:28. By 30k in 1:46:32 it looked like a race with Kenyans Joyce Chepkirui and Valentine Kipketer, Flomena Cheyech Daniel against the lone Ethiopian. Daniel fell off the pace first at mile 19. That left one against two. Up over Heartbreak Hill and down into Cleveland Circle, Kipketer had dropped back. Now the race ran with only two women from two adjoining countries half a world away, and it looked like the winner would be either Chepkirui or Tsegaye because no other woman could be seen. But Tsegaye knew Baysa was fit and experienced, as the earlier exuberance allowed the hills to wear her down. She had the Godzilla complex—the dream that the monster is coming for you but you can't see it nor wake up. Tsegaye kept looking back. The monster was coming. The reporters covering the race did not know; no other runner could be seen. Baysa lingered 37 seconds behind. She had elected not to go with the 5-minute downhill mile because of worry about troubles she had had with a hamstring. She did not want to test it nor express tactical dominance that early. She ran out of sight, but not out of the Tsegaye's worry. Up the hills in stealth mode. Why was Tsegaye looking back? Again and again Tsegaye looked back. She knew something that the reporters on the press truck did not know. A yellow dot. No one could be seen. Around a bend in a twinkle Baysa appeared beside Tsegaye with a mile to go. She tried to stay with the apparition at her side, but could not. After the race she said, "I tried, but I knew she was stronger." Baysa ran the last mile alone. After the race she said, "I was going on my own pace and confident because of my good training that I was going to catch up to them." Baysa, with the confidence of an experienced stage performer, took the cue and took center stage. "Once I got to catch up with the third one, I was confident that I was going to do it," said Baysa to reporters after the race. "I knew I had the power." She had run from 30k to 35k in 16:43, but Tsegaye had run only 17:27. The she added another 42 seconds. Tsegaye finished 2nd which, as reporter Barbara Hueber put it, "isn't bad at all, when you consider that 50 years ago there was no such thing as second place."

In a gesture to history Baysa gave her trophy to Bobbi Gibb who, 50 years earlier as the only woman in the race, finished unacknowledged.

In June at the BAA 10k in Boston, Baysa finished 14th among women in 33:59. Bobbie Gibb met her there and returned the gifted trophy to Baysa at Awards Ceremony. On the awards stand in the middle of Boston Common poignant minutes unfolded. Gibb, with amazingly little gray in her long curling hair, became overwhelmed by the moment. Baysa—a well-known and accomplished Ethiopian singer—sang a song to honor both Gibb and the welcoming people of Boston. Baysa's song translated into English is "Black Winter," which is a New Year's song that looks forward to the beginning of summer.

"Boston is special for me, because I won the Boston Marathon and am able to sing in Boston," said Baysa. "To have Bobbi here, I knew that she was going to be here standing next to me, and it gave me more confidence to be up here."

A June 29 press release from Monaco states: Former Boston Marathon winner Lidiya Grigoryeva has been banned for 2.5 years for doping.

The IAAF says the 42-year-old Grigoryeva, who won the Boston Marathon in 2007 and the Chicago Marathon in 2008, was banned under the biological passport program, which tracks suspicious blood measurements over a long period.

We hope these rulings do not force us to go back and rewrite history. For the vast number of Boston Marathon racers, their battles are a fair fight to overcome adversity as complex as debilitating disease or injury or age or simply time and distance run. That competition against internal or external demons will be what lifts us all forevermore.

Women's Results 2016

1. Atsede Baysa, ETH	**2:29:19**	21. Mary Tabal, PHI	2:49:01
2. Tirfi Tsegaye, ETH	2:30:03	22. Ailsa MacDonald, CAN	2:49:59
3. Joyce Chepkirui, KEN	2:30:50	23. Hilary Dionne, MA	2:50:56
4. Jelena Prokopcuka, LAT	2:32:28	24. Elizabeth Ryan, MA	2:51:04
5. Valentine Kipketer, KEN	2:33:13	25. Kate Gustafson, CAN	2:51:13
6. Flomena Cheyech Daniel, KEN	2:33:40	26. Kirsten Allen, CO	2:51:14
7. Buzunesh Deba, ETH	**2:33:56**	27. Corina Canitz, WI	2:51:33
8. Fate Tola, ETH	2:34:38	28. Rachel Glasson, AUS	2:51:51
9. Neely Spence Gracey, USA	2:35:00	29. Sheri Piers, ME	2:52:25
10. Mamitu Daska, ETH	2:37:31,	30. Laura Hagley, NH	2:52:45
11. Sarah Crouch, USA	2:37:36,	39. Holley Rees, MA	2:54:57
12. Miharu Shimokado, JPN	2:39:21	86. Laine E. DiNoto, NY	3:00:00
13. Amane Beriso, ETH	2:39:38	661. Abby Samuelson, OR	3:19:20
14. Tiki Gelana, ETH	2:42:38	1685. Brittany Haas, WI	3:30:00
15. Tadelech Bekele, ETH	2:44:20	**2939. Uta Pippig, USA**	**3:38:40**
16. Sado Fatuma, ETH	2:45:17	6558. Carole Singelais, NY	4:00:00
17. Laurie Knowles, NC	2:45:19	11393. Patrica Huang, CA	5:17:44
18. Yuka Mikami, JPN	2:48:17	(running her 30th Boston in a row)	
19. Kana Kurosawa, JPN	2:48:47	12166. Adrianne Haslet, MA	10:30:23
20. Hilary Corno, CA	2:48:49,	**Caroline Rotich, DNF**	
First Master			

Winning Women's Teams

1. Boston Athletic Association, 8:48:59
2. Fleet Feet Nike Racing Team, IL, 8:57:40
3. Greater Boston Track Club, 9:05:50
4. Crow Athletics, ME, 9:06:02
5. Breakaway Racing Team, PA, 9:20:32
6. Dashing Whippets Racing Team, NY, 9:24:07
7. Club Northwest, WA, 9:24:13
8. Plano Pacers Running Club, TX, 9:25:18
9. Henwoods Hounds Racing Team, NY, 9:28:31
10. Western Massachusetts Distance Project, 9:30:26

The Boston Marathon and Commitment to Film

More than any other Olympic running event, the marathon is an event of memory. It lasts a long time. It creates a memory of the course itself with unique geology, geography, and culture. Each road, and each street, is unlike any other.

On April 15, 2013, however, the bombings suddenly sparked the memory of the marathon as a militant act of defiance and jarred it back to its origins. More people than ever wanted to run the marathon in 2014 to remember the sacrifice of the people killed and injured in the bombing and to honor and thank the first responders. Memory flashes back and marches forward. We can tell Clarence DeMar and Pheidippides that we still run the marathon to remember those who have gone before and have given so much. The concept of duty seems to have returned alongside, if not replacing, the concepts of fitness, self-realization, and self-congratulation. Again runners remember with reverence the symbolism of duty, of giving, of life and death, of the events of April 15th, 2013, and the exact place.

Several years ago Southern California native Jon Dunham, who would direct BOSTON, the documentary film, stood watching the water of the Sudbury River flow over the ancient dam at the site where once stood Metcalf's Mill, in Ashland, Massachusetts. He looked into the moving water for inspiration for the film he intended to make. Bits of floating leaves and sticks slowly approached the lip of the little dam and flickered over the falls to vanish in the jumble below. So many ideas, sounds, and images had to float by, offering themselves to a filmmaker who had to choose. Now the site is called Marathon Park, to commemorate the first start of the Boston Marathon, on April 19th, 1897, when Tom Burke dragged his heel across the dirt road to mark the starting line.

The film about the Boston Marathon spans more than a century. Each of the towns along the course is a character with its own history and motivation. The host, BAA, is a character in the movie too. It has a long, wrinkled, and sometimes curmudgeonly personality.

Director Jon Dunham began making films at age 13. Dunham said, "I grew up around photography. My father lived in the Yosemite Valley when Ansel Adams had a studio there, so as far back as I can remember there were these remarkable black and white landscapes of monuments like Half Dome, El Capitan, Yosemite Falls, all around the house." He graduated in 2000 from the University of Southern California's School of Cinematic Arts. Top Value Television (TVTV) pioneer Megan Williams chose him as the cinematographer for *Tell Me Cuba*, a documentary about the difficult and complex relations between the United States and Cuba. The collaboration continued with Dunham's directorial debut, *No Distance Too Far*, a documentary featuring four individuals whose lives had been touched by AIDS.

As a teenager in Los Angeles, Dunham saw L.A. Marathon entry blanks on the counter of a Subway sandwich shop. *How hard could it be?* he thought with his very young man confidence. "I run a mile every day in physical education class." On race day, he made it to his jammed corral in time for the gun. For the first mile he thought the pace was easy. "No problem. I can run forever like this," he thought. But by the halfway turn-around in Hollywood, the future filmmaker found himself walking. He didn't know how he would get back to the start. It is funny to think of the future filmmaker stuck in Hollywood. He reached the finish in 5:06:59. But the day transformed him.

He improved his marathon time to 3:22:39 in Chicago in 2001. His first marathon film, *Spirit of the Marathon*, is about the Chicago Marathon. Megan Williams is the producer of BOSTON. She is the recipient of numerous awards, including an Academy Award Nomination and the Alfred I. duPont-Columbia University School of Journalism Award. This author is Executive Producer of BOSTON. One scene shot in California was especially pleasant: "Did you see something?" Steve Edwards asked his Olympian wife Shalane Flanagan. She had been running along desolate Beartrap road in the California wilderness. "Yes, I think it was a mountain lion." The Executive Producer of the forthcoming film standing nearby [this author] said, "I saw it too." The mountain lion skulked through the live oaks on a hillside above the filming location on Tejon Ranch an hour's drive north of Los Angeles. The mountain lion eluded the camera. The director needed a beautiful road with no traffic to show the beauty and tranquility of training compared to racing in city streets. He hadn't counted on the mountain lion, but it soon wandered out of sight, perhaps figuring that Olympian marathoner Shalane was too skinny to be worth the hunt. Her husband and the producer offered more meat but they huddled close to the vehicle.

The vehicle itself was something spectacular. It is one of those movie magic things that will never be seen on screen. It is called the Ultimate Arm and is the sort of apparatus used in Hollywood action movies such as *Mad Max*. The arm is a robotically controlled appendage protruding from an SUV like a foraging dinosaur's neck, dipping and swooping above the running subject, in this case the ever-game Shalane, collecting action shots from every angle. The gyroscopic controls isolated any vibration from the vehicle or the wind to capture a crystal-clear shot of Shalane peacefully running amid the open, rolling, oak hills and broad valleys of the Tejon ranch. It is a dream place for running, looking just like it did when staked out in 1843 with quiet unspoiled hills and enticing trails. If runners can, and professionals can, they go to high and lonely places to train.

Other scenes for the film show Shalane training in Portland, Oregon, cooking at home, and interviewed in the studio. Many dozen marathon winners, historical figures, and ordinary competitors will appear within the context of the race in sit-down interviews years after their victories or in archival footage.

The film documents the 2014 race—the year after the bombing—the year of Boston Strong, and flashes back through a century of change. The planning for BOSTON started in 2007 when director Dunham interviewed me for his documentary about the Chicago Marathon. When I heard that Dunham wanted to interview me for a film about the Chicago Marathon, not Boston, I began a long rant about how Chicago at best was the second city and that a documentary film about Boston must be made. Dunham did not disagree with the ranting historian, but these things take time and money. Yes, a Boston film, maybe after 2012. Dunham made a film about the Rome Marathon, then began planning for Boston. But after the bombing Dunham questioned the propriety of making a film so soon after the crime. Dunham had started his filmmaking passion a long time ago. Dunham and producer Megan Williams knew that filmmaking takes time, money, and art, all of which are hard to compress into a single crystal.

Dunham, crew and producers traveled around the world to document the world status of the Boston Marathon. In modern Greece, he filmed a harvest of olive branches and leaves that would be plated with gold to make the Boston Marathon winner's wreath and he interviewed three-time Boston winner Rosa Mota in the beautiful marble Olympic Stadium that was built for the first modern Olympics in 1896. They interviewed Boston Marathon 1986 winner Rob De-Castella in the desert in the middle of Australia. But most of the film documents the 2014 marathon. The film crew covered that race day more closely than any marathon had ever been covered. One hundred and twenty people—camera operators, gaffers, sound ops, and deployed assorted assistants who carried equipment, managed crowds for sight lines along the course, and identified subjects for the cinematographers to shoot. Fifty-six Sony, Arri, and Panasonic cameras caught the action in full HD and 4k (8,294,400 pixels), including one on a Techocrane high over the starting line and another camera in the belfry of the South Church looking down Boylston Street. The film's agreement with the BAA included access to all the broadcast clean feeds. All the raw footage, archival and TV coverage would take about 1,000 hours, or a month's watch. Good thing that the director is an endurance athlete so he can survive the editing process. Music is composed by Jeff Beal, four-time Emmy award–winning composer who is one of the most prolific and respected composers working in film and television today. Beal's score will be performed by the Boston Symphony Orchestra and the story narrated by a Hollywood actor. All of this costs money; for instance, the Techocrane cost $12,000 to rent for the day.

The film is financed by sponsors, starting with presenting sponsor John Hancock, and BostonLog.com, RunSignUp, Clif, and small donations on https://www.crowdrise.com/BostonMarathonFilm. Private equity investors who all have a deep passion for the Boston Marathon are footing most of the costs. Executive producers are Frank Marshall and me, the author. Marshall ran 2:45 at Boston in 1980. Editor Leonard Feinstein and co-producers Eleanor Bingham Miller and Ryan Suffern round out the core filmmaking team.

BOSTON will be shown nationally as a Fathom Event. Currently, Fathom Events has access to more than 17,000 screens for promotion and more than 750 live broadcast theaters in the top 50 markets in the United States. Fathom Events will turn movie theaters into event venues. Unlike regular movies, Fathom Events films are in first-run cinemas for only one night or for limited-run encores. They can be fund raisers for running clubs or they can be adjunct events at Boston Qualifier marathons. The producers expect this film to become a cult classic viewed by runners year after year to get psyched out of their minds for their upcoming marathon. The beauty of this film, Dunham says, will shine on the big screen. The premiere was scheduled for April 15, 2017 at the Wang Theater in the Boch Center in Boston with the Boston Pops playing live.

Acknowledgments

Thanks of course to the BAA, Tom Grilk, Guy Morse, Jack Fleming, Marc Davis, T. K. Skenderian, Michael Pieroni, and Gloria Ratti. I attended the pre-race and post-race press events every year and heard all the athlete statements that were later used by me and my fellow journalists. I spoke to all the top runners who contended for victory in these races. A good source of all the statistics were each year's results book. They have more information than I could include here, such as all the age group individual and team results. Boston newspapers memorialized results, splits, and quotations. Running magazines helped with background information, as did the BAA press packets. I appreciate time spent with agent Tom Ratcliffe and with John Hancock's Pat Lynch. I benefited from insights from my broadcast friends Larry Rawson and Toni Revis. I watched every minute of all the videos of all the races live and years later. I attended all the pre and post-race press conferences with other reporters.

Some of the writing I include came from my work as senior writer in *New England Runner* magazine and I am grateful to editor Bob Fitzgerald and publisher Michelle LeBrun.

I certainly stole lots of observations and descriptions, wit and wisdom, from whoever I was near at the press events. I spoke with dozens of people every year for twenty years before, during, and after each race and all made an impression on me which are all subliminally in this book. I hope I have assimilated the essence of the Boston Marathon as expired by all observers. I apologize for the stories I have left out. The original manuscript submitted to this publisher would have produced a 1,000-plus-page book! Thanks to everyone I interviewed formally or casually. Thank you to Skyhorse Publishing, especially editorial director Jay Cassell, and editorial assistant Veronica Alvarado. Except for my mistakes, everything in this book came from somewhere.

Thanks to Bill Rodgers, Joan Benoit Samuelson, Amby Burfoot, and Shalane Flanagan for their kind forewords.

I thank Victah Sailer for his photos. It was certainly a joy working with the director of the Boston Marathon Documentary, Jon Dunham, and producer Megan Williams.

Appendix of Men's and Women's Winners

YEAR	CHAMPION	AGE	HOME	TIME
2016	Hayle Lemi Berhanu	21	Ethiopia	2:12:45
2015	Lesisa Desisa	25	Ethiopia	2:09:17
2014	Mebrahtom (Meb) Keflezighi	38	California	2:08:37
2013	Lelisa Desisa	23	Ethiopia	2:10:22
2012	Wesley Korir	29	Kenya	2:12:40
2011	Geoffrey Mutai	29	Kenya	2:03:02*
2010	Robert Kiprono Cheruiyot	21	Kenya	2:05:52
2009	Deriba Merga	28	Ethiopia	2:08:42
2008	Robert Kipkoech Cheruiyot	29	Kenya	2:07:46
2007	Robert Kipkoech Cheruiyot	28	Kenya	2:14:13
2006	Robert Kipkoech Cheruiyot	27	Kenya	2:07:14
2005	Hailu Negussie	25	Ethiopia	2:11:45
2004	Timothy Cherigat	27	Kenya	2:10:37
2003	Robert Kipkoech Cheruiyot	24	Kenya	2:10:11
2002	Rodgers Rop	26	Kenya	2:09:02
2001	Lee Bong-Ju	30	South Korea	2:09:43
2000	Elijah Lagat	33	Kenya	2:09:47
1999	Joseph Chebet	28	Kenya	2:09:52
1998	Moses Tanui	32	Kenya	2:07:34
1997	Lameck Aguta	25	Kenya	2:10:34
1996	Moses Tanui	30	Kenya	2:09:15
1995	Cosmas Ndeti	25	Kenya	2:09:22
1994	Cosmas Ndeti	24	Kenya	2:07:15
1993	Cosmas Ndeti	23	Kenya	2:09:33
1992	Ibrahim Hussein	33	Kenya	2:08:14
1991	Ibrahim Hussein	32	Kenya	2:11:06
1990	Gelindo Bordin	31	Italy	2:08:19
1989	Abebe Mekonnen	25	Ethiopia	2:09:06
1988	Ibrahim Hussein	29	Kenya	2:08:43
1987	Toshihiko Seko	30	Japan	2:11:50
1986	Robert de Castella	29	Australia	2:07:51
1985	Geoff Smith	31	England	2:14:05
1984	Geoff Smith	30	England	2:10:34
1983	Greg A. Meyer	27	Massachusetts	2:09:00
1982	Alberto Salazar	23	Massachusetts	2:08:52
1981	Toshihiko Seko	24	Japan	2:09:26
1980	Bill Rodgers	32	Massachusetts	2:12:11
1979	Bill Rodgers	31	Massachusetts	2:09:27

1978	Bill Rodgers	30	Massachusetts	2:10:13
1977	Jerome Drayton	31	Canada	2:14:46
1976	Jack Fultz	27	Virginia	2:20:19
1975	Bill Rodgers	27	Massachusetts	2:09:55
1974	Neil Cusack	22	Ireland	2:13:39
1973	Jon Anderson	23	Oregon	2:16:03
1972	Olavi Suomalainen	25	Finland	2:15:39
1971	Alvaro Mejia	30	Colombia	2:18:45
1970	Ron Hill	31	England	2:10:30
1969	Yoshiaki Unetani	24	Japan	2:13:49
1968	Amby Burfoot	21	Connecticut	2:22:17
1967	David C. McKenzie	24	New Zealand	2:15:45
1966	Kenji Kimihara	25	Japan	2:17:11
1965	Morio Shigematsu	24	Japan	2:16:33
1964	Aurele Vandendriessche	29	Belgium	2:19:59
1963	Aurele Vandendriessche	28	Belgium	2:18:58
1962	Eino Oksanen	30	Finland	2:23:48
1961	Eino Oksanen	29	Finland	2:23:39
1960	Paavo Kotila	32	Finland	2:20:54
1959	Eino Oksanen	27	Finland	2:22:42
1958	Franjo Mihalic	36	Yugoslavia	2:25:54
1957	John J. Kelley	26	Connecticut	2:20:05
1956	Antti Viskari	27	Finland	2:14:14
1955	Hideo Hamamura	25	Japan	2:18:22
1954	Veikko Karvonen	28	Finland	2:20:39
1953	Keizo Yamada	24	Japan	2:18:51
1952	Doroteo Flores	30	Guatemala	2:31:53
1951	Shigeki Tanaka	19	Japan	2:27:45
1950	Ki-Yong Ham	19	Korea	2:32:39
1949	Karl Gosta Leandersson	31	Sweden	2:31:50
1948	Gerard Cote	34	Canada	2:31:02
1947	Yun Bok Suh	24	Korea	2:25:39
1946	Stylianos Kyriakides	36	Greece	2:29:27
1945	John A. Kelley	37	Massachusetts	2:30:40
1944	Gerard Cote	30	Canada	2:31:50
1943	Gerard Cote	29	Canada	2:28:25
1942	Bernard Joseph (Joe) Smith	27	Massachusetts	2:26:51
1941	Leslie S. Pawson	37	Rhode Island	2:30:38
1940	Gerard Cote	26	Canada	2:28:28
1939	Ellison M. (Tarzan) Brown	23	Rhode Island	2:28:51
1938	Leslie S. Pawson	34	Rhode Island	2:35:34
1937	Walter Young	24	Canada	2:33:20
1936	Ellison M. (Tarzan) Brown	20	Rhode Island	2:33:40
1935	John A. Kelley	27	Massachusetts	2:32:07
1934	Dave Komonen	35	Canada	2:32:53
1933	Leslie S. Pawson	29	Rhode Island	2:31:01

1932	Paul de Bruyn	24	Germany	2:33:36
1931	James P. Henigan	38	Massachusetts	2:46:45
1930	Clarence H. DeMar	41	Massachusetts	2:34:48
1929	John C. Miles	23	Canada	2:33:08
1928	Clarence H. DeMar	39	Massachusetts	2:37:07
1927	Clarence H. DeMar	38	Massachusetts	2:40:22
1926	John C. Miles	20	Canada	2:25:40
1925	Charles L. (Chuck) Mellor	31	Illinois	2:33:00
1924	Clarence H. DeMar	35	Massachusetts	2:29:40
1923	Clarence H. DeMar	34	Massachusetts	2:23:47
1922	Clarence H. DeMar	33	Massachusetts	2:18:10
1921	Frank T. Zuna	28	New York	2:18:57
1920	Peter Trivoulidas	39	Greece	2:29:31
1919	Carl W. A. Linder	29	Massachusetts	2:29:13
1918	Camp Devens Divisional Team –		Massachusetts	2:24:53
1917	William J. (Bill) Kennedy	35	New York	2:28:37
1916	Arthur V. Roth	23	Massachusetts	2:27:16
1915	Edouard Fabre	29	Canada	2:31:41
1914	James Duffy	23	Canada	2:25:01
1913	Fritz Carlson	29	Minnesota	2:25:14
1912	Michael J. Ryan	23	New York	2:21:18
1911	Clarence H. DeMar	22	Massachusetts	2:21:39
1910	Fred L. Cameron	23	Canada	2:28:52
1909	Henri Renaud	19	New Hampshire	2:53:36
1908	Thomas P. Morrissey	19	New York	2:25:43
1907	Thomas Longboat	19	Canada	2:24:24
1906	Timothy Ford	18	Massachusetts	2:45:45
1905	Frederick Lorz	26	New York	2:38:25
1904	Michael Spring	21	New York	2:38:04
1903	John C. Lorden	28	Massachusetts	2:41:29
1902	Sammy A. Mellor	23	New York	2:43:12
1901	John P. Caffery	21	Canada	2:29:23
1900	John P. Caffery	20	Canada	2:39:44
1899	Lawrence Brignolia	23	Massachusetts	2:54:38
1898	Ronald J. MacDonald	22	Canada	2:42:00
1897	John J. McDermott	22	New York	2:55:10

YEAR	CHAMPION	AGE	HOME	TIME
2016	Atsede Baysa	29	Ethiopia	2:29:19
2015	Caroline Rotich	30	Kenya	2:24:55
2014	Rita Jeptoo	33	Kenya	2:18:57†
2013	Rita Jeptoo	32	Kenya	2:26:25
2012	Sharon Cherop	28	Kenya	2:31:50
2011	Caroline Kilel	30	Kenya	2:22:36
2010	Teyba Erkesso	27	Ethiopia	2:26:11

2009	Salina Kosgei	32	Kenya	2:32:16
2008	Dire Tune	22	Ethiopia	2:25:25
2007	Lidiya Grigoryeva	33	Russia	2:29:18
2006	Rita Jeptoo	25	Kenya	2:23:38
2005	Catherine Ndereba	32	Kenya	2:25:13
2004	Catherine Ndereba	31	Kenya	2:24:27
2003	Svetlana Zakharova	32	Russia	2:25:20
2002	Margaret Okayo	25	Kenya	2:20:43†
2001	Catherine Ndereba	28	Kenya	2:23:53
2000	Catherine Ndereba	27	Kenya	2:26:11
1999	Fatuma Roba	25	Ethiopia	2:23:25
1998	Fatuma Roba	24	Ethiopia	2:23:21
1997	Fatuma Roba	23	Ethiopia	2:26:23
1996	Uta Pippig	30	Germany	2:27:12
1995	Uta Pippig	29	Germany	2:25:11
1994	Uta Pippig	28	Germany	2:21:45
1993	Olga Markova	24	Russia	2:25:27
1992	Olga Markova	23	Comm. Ind. States	2:23:43
1991	Wanda Panfil	32	Poland	2:24:18
1990	Rosa Mota	31	Portugal	2:25:24
1989	Ingrid Kristiansen	33	Norway	2:24:33
1988	Rosa Mota	29	Portugal	2:24:30
1987	Rosa Mota	28	Portugal	2:25:21
1986	Ingrid Kristiansen	30	Norway	2:24:55
1985	Lisa Larsen-Weidenbach	23	Michigan	2:34:06
1984	Lorraine Moller	25	New Zealand	2:29:28
1983	Joan Benoit	25	Massachusetts	2:22:43
1982	Charlotte Teske	32	Germany	2:29:33
1981	Allison Roe	24	New Zealand	2:26:46
1980	Jacqueline Gareau	27	Canada	2:34:28
1979	Joan Benoit	21	Maine	2:35:15
1978	Gayle S. Barron	30	Georgia	2:44:52
1977	Michiko (Miki) Gorman	42	California	2:48:33
1976	Kim Merritt	20	Wisconsin	2:47:10
1975	Liane Winter	31	Germany	2:42:24
1974	Michiko (Miki) Gorman	39	California	2:47:11
1973	Jacqueline A. Hansen	24	California	3:05:59
1972	Nina Kuscsik	33	New York	3:10:26

Unofficial Era

YEAR	CHAMPION	AGE	HOME	TIME
1966	Roberta (Bobbi) Gibb	23	Massachusetts	3:21:40
1967	Roberta (Bobbi) Gibb	24	California	3:27:17
1968	Roberta (Bobbi) Gibb	25	California	3:30:00
1969	Sara Mae Berman	33	Massachusetts	3:22:46
1970	Sara Mae Berman	34	Massachusetts	3:05:07
1971	Sara Mae Berman	35	Massachusetts	3:08:30

Why They Will Always
Come Back to Boston

I believe that runners will always come back to do the Boston Marathon, as surely as spring follows winter. I believe that the children will be there with outstretched hands. I believe that generations to come will run at Boston as hopefully as the crocuses poke their heads from the just-thawed ground. And I do believe that the marathon is bigger than its sponsors and bigger than its creator, the Boston Athletic Association—so much so that if no one put up the money and the BAA could not manage the race, runners would still gather at the Hopkinton town green to run to Boston on Patriots' Day. If the towns refused to issue permits to allow the race to pass, I believe runners would risk arrest to run.

Yet the world has changed irreversibly since the beginning of the Boston story in 1897. Then fewer than 1.6 billion people inhabited Earth. Now 5.3 billion live here, and in another 30 years there will be more than 8 billion. By 2090—as far into the future as 1897 is in the past—the world may be unrecognizable. The next hundred years may be hell.

In this narrative we have seen that the Boston Marathon is not isolated from politics in the extreme. War contracts the marathon; the number of participants dropped during both world wars. We have seen with the cancellations of Olympic contests in 1916, 1940, and 1944 and the U.S. Olympic boycott in 1980 that politics and sport are not divorced. The ubiquitous presence of mayors and governors at the Boston Marathon reminds us that sport is an extension of politics.

Sport is also an extension of economics. When business is good, the marathon booms, as it has in the first decade of the century, the 1920s, the 1970s, and the 1980s. But numbers were down during the depression.

We have also seen a transition from the early 1980s—as the marathon whimpered along as the last bastion of amateurs, then revived in 1986 with the injection of John Hancock cash to be again the world's most important marathon. (Only athletes on the John Hancock payroll have won the marathon since 1986.) But in the next hundred years environmental collapse could do more damage than wars or the vagaries of the business cycle.

Even the purity of wilderness has ended as industrialization's legacy—global-warming carbon dioxide—permeates the air in even the most remote regions of the world, which now have 350 parts per million CO_2—10% more than when Clarence DeMar ran his best times in the 1920s. An ozone hole in Earth's atmosphere may be allowing cancer-causing ultraviolet light to pummel runners, and acid rain falls in the shadow of every industrial belt. (Perhaps today's runners should adopt the protective handkerchief headgear of DeMar and his teammates.) Perhaps the Boston Marathon of the future will be held at night, or the runners will carry parasols to avoid exposure to UV rays.

Burgeoning populations and dwindling resources may produce additional global instability in the form of chronic and festering wars. There may be no marathon-stopping world wars but rather nagging little ones feeding a growing population of world refugees. Will Americans tighten their immigration laws in a xenophobic net to keep out foreigners? Perhaps sponsors will no longer invite foreign runners, and the Boston Marathon will again become a North American event.

When people recognize problems, they are on the way to solving them. "Bricklayer" Bill Kennedy said that marathoners tend to be dreamers; they are not practical people, but dedicate themselves to attacking time and distance in the most primitive way. Like artists and scientists, they explore what has no apparent immediate benefit. Yet such are the pursuits that separate humans from all other living things. We have seen how politics—in the form of the space program, cold war rivalries, and presidential interest in physical fitness—has stimulated the sport of marathon running. After the 1993 marathon, U.S. President Bill Clinton invited the Boston Marathon winners, Kenyan Kamba Cosmas Ndeti and Communist-educated Olga Markova, to run with him around the White House. What could be more symbolic of a coming global multicultural economy than a black African, a white ex-communist, and an American president out for a run together? Such events catalyze broad public interest and show that sport offers a global forum for political, economic, and environmental consensus, just as was hoped by the original founders of the Olympic movement and their followers who established the Boston Marathon in 1897.

Perhaps technical solutions to environmental and economic problems will be found and the next generations of marathoners will live in a clean, green solar- and cold-fusion powered world where the standards of living in Africa and Asia match those in Japan and Switzerland. Perhaps runners will each wear a cellular broadcasting computer chip on their racing numbers so race splits and results can be printed instantly. Perhaps a male runner will break 2 hours for the marathon, and a woman will run 2:10.

Where will the future's performers come from? As in the 1993 race, they will continue to come from Korea, Japan, and Africa. Bill Rodgers was recently invited to Vietnam, where he tried to avoid going as a soldier in the 1960s, to run a marathon. Japan and Korea are exporting everything they can to the rest of East Asia, and along with their products will go their enthusiasm for the marathon. Japanese women are emerging as a force. One of them will soon win Boston, unless an African like Kenyan Florence Wangechi, who led the entire race for the first half mile in 1991, decides to go all the way. South Africa and the southern African countries like Namibia and Zimbabwe will be a growing source of runners.

There is a formula of sorts to predict which countries will generate marathoners. Three things are needed: a large, young population; new economic or political stability such as that emerging from the ending of a period of war; and a coaching and competitive structure complete with a national hero—like Paavo Nurmi in Finland, Abebe Bikila in Ethiopia, Kip Keino in Kenya, Jim Peters in England, Ki Chung Sohn in Korea, or Frank Shorter in the U.S.

If China or India with their huge populations could find national marathon heroes, sub-2:10 men and sub-2:25 women would pour out of their countries. Perhaps one of them will run 2:06 or sub-2:20 on the Boston course.

The future of anything is difficult to predict, but it is important and fascinating to try. The forces of change that shape the Boston Marathon of the next 100 years will be the same ones that shape the rest of our global society. I believe that we have recognized the economic, environmental, and social problems that will face us in the 21st century and that we will muster the technical means to solve them. And so every spring runners will continue to gather at the Hopkinton town green to begin their migration to Boston—all because of the undying human need to pursue something that cannot be caught.

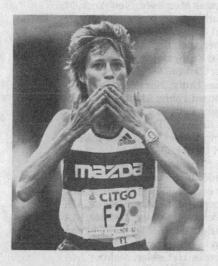

"I have this marathon a little bit in my heart," said Uta Pippig of Germany on finishing the 1992 Boston Marathon. © Victah/Agence Shot.

Appendix A

Boston Marathon Winners
Men's Open, 1897-1995

YEAR	NAME/RESIDENCE	TIME
1897	John J. McDermott, New York, NY	2:55:10
1898	Ronald J. MacDonald, Cambridge, MA	2:42:00
1899	Lawrence J. Brignolia, Cambridge, MA	2:54:38
1900	John P. Caffery, Hamilton, Ontario	2:39:44
1901	John P. Caffery, Hamilton, Ontario	2:29:23
1902	Sammy Mellor, Yonkers, NY	2:43:12
1903	John C. Lorden, Cambridge, MA	2:41:29
1904	Michael Spring, New York, NY	2:38:04
1905	Fred Lorz, New York, NY	2:38:25
1906	Timothy Ford, Cambridge, MA	2:45:45
1907	Tom Longboat, Hamilton, Ontario	2:24:24
1908	Thomas Morrissey, New York, NY	2:25:43
1909	Henri Renaud, Nashua, NH	2:53:36
1910	Fred Cameron, Amherst, Nova Scotia	2:28:52
1911	Clarence H. DeMar, Melrose, MA	2:21:39
1912	Mike Ryan, New York, NY	2:21:18
1913	Fritz Carlson, Minneapolis, MN	2:25:14
1914	James Duffy, Hamilton, Ontario	2:25:01
1915	Edouard Fabre, Montreal, Quebec	2:31:41
1916	Arthur Roth, Roxbury, MA	2:27:16
1917	Bill Kennedy, Port Chester, NY	2:28:37
1918	Camp Devens Divisional Team	2:24:53
1919	Carl Linder, Quincy, MA	2:29:13
1920	Peter Trivoulidas, Greece (NY)	2:29:31
1921	Frank Zuna, Newark, NJ	2:18:57
1922	Clarence H. DeMar, Melrose, MA	2:18:10
1923	Clarence H. DeMar, Melrose, MA	2:23:47
1924	Clarence H. DeMar, Melrose, MA	2:29:40
1925	Charles "Chuck" Mellor, Chicago, IL	2:33:00
1926	John C. Miles, Sydney Mines, Nova Scotia	2:25:40
1927	Clarence H. DeMar, Melrose, MA	2:40:22
1928	Clarence H. DeMar, Melrose, MA	2:37:07
1929	John C. Miles, Hamilton, Ontario	2:33:08
1930	Clarence H. DeMar, Melrose, MA	2:34:48
1931	James Henigan, Medford, MA	2:46:45
1932	Paul deBruyn, Germany	2:33:36
1933	Leslie S. Pawson, Pawtucket, RI	2:31:01
1934	Dave Komonen, Sudbury, Ontario	2:32:53
1935	John A. Kelley, Arlington, MA	2:32:07
1936	Ellison M. Brown, Alton, RI	2:33:40
1937	Walter Young, Verdun, Quebec	2:33:20
1938	Leslie S. Pawson, Pawtucket, RI	2:35:34
1939	Ellison M. Brown, Alton, RI	2:28:51
1940	Gerard Cote, St. Hyacinthe, Quebec	2:28:28
1941	Leslie S. Pawson, Pawtucket, RI	2:30:38

1942	Bernard Joseph Smith, Medford, MA	2:26:51
1943	Gerard Cote, St. Hyacinthe, Quebec	2:28:25
1944	Gerard Cote, St. Hyacinthe, Quebec	2:31:50
1945	John A. Kelley, West Acton, MA	2:30:40
1946	Stylianos Kyriakides, Greece	2:29:27
1947	Yun Bok Suh, Korea	2:25:39
1948	Gerard Cote, St. Hyacinthe, Quebec	2:31:02
1949	Karl Gosta Leandersson, Sweden	2:31:50
1950	Kee Yong Ham, Korea	2:32:39
1951	Shigeki Tanaka, Hiroshima, Japan	2:27:45
1952	Doroteo Flores, Guatemala	2:31:53
1953	Keizo Yamada, Japan	2:18:51
1954	Veikko Karvonen, Finland	2:20:39
1955	Hideo Hamamura, Japan	2:18:22
1956	Antti Viskari, Finland	2:14:14
1957	John J. Kelley, Groton, CT	2:20:05
1958	Franjo Mihalic, Yugoslavia	2:25:54
1959	Eino Oksanen, Helsinki, Finland	2:22:42
1960	Paavo Kotila, Finland	2:20:54
1961	Eino Oksanen, Helsinki, Finland	2:23:29
1962	Eino Oksanen, Helsinki, Finland	2:23:48
1963	Aurele Vandendriessche, Belgium	2:18:58
1964	Aurele Vandendriessche, Belgium	2:19:59
1965	Morio Shigematsu, Japan	2:16:33
1966	Kenji Kimihara, Japan	2:17:11
1967	David McKenzie, New Zealand	2:15:45
1968	Ambrose (Amby) Burfoot, Groton, CT	2:22:17
1969	Yoshiaki Unetani, Japan	2:13:49
1970	Ron Hill, Cheshire, England	2:10:30
1971	Alvaro Mejia, Colombia	2:18:45
1972	Olavi Suomalainen, Otaniemi, Finland	2:15:39
1973	Jon Anderson, Eugene, Oregon	2:16:03
1974	Neil Cusack, Ireland	2:13:39
1975	Bill Rodgers, Jamaica Plain, MA	2:09:55
1976	Jack Fultz, Arlington, VA	2:20:19
1977	Jerome Drayton, Toronto, Ontario	2:14:46
1978	Bill Rodgers, Melrose, MA	2:10:13
1979	Bill Rodgers, Melrose, MA	2:09:27
1980	Bill Rodgers, Melrose, MA	2:12:11
1981	Toshihiko Seko, Japan	2:09:26
1982	Alberto Salazar, Wayland, MA	2:08:52
1983	Gregory A. Meyer, Wellesley, MA	2:09:00
1984	Geoff Smith, Liverpool, England	2:10:34
1985	Geoff Smith, Liverpool, England	2:14:05
1986	Rob de Castella, Canberra, Australia	2:07:51
1987	Toshihiko Seko, Japan	2:11:50
1988	Ibrahim Hussein, Kenya	2:08:43
1989	Abebe Mekonnen, Ethiopia	2:09:06
1990	Gelindo Bordin, Milan, Italy	2:08:19
1991	Ibrahim Hussein, Kenya	2:11:06
1992	Ibrahim Hussein, Kenya	2:08:14
1993	Cosmas Ndeti, Kenya	2:09:33
1994	Cosmas Ndeti, Kenya	2:07:15
1995	Cosmas Ndeti, Kenya	2:09:22

Women's Open, 1966-1995

YEAR	NAME/RESIDENCE	TIME
1966	Roberta Gibb Bingay, Winchester, MA—Unofficial	3:21:40
1967	Roberta Gibb, San Diego, CA—Unofficial	3:27:17
1968	Roberta Gibb, San Diego, CA—Unofficial	3:30:00
1969	Sara Mae Berman, Cambridge, MA—Unofficial	3:22:46
1970	Sara Mae Berman, Cambridge, MA—Unofficial	3:05:07
1971	Sara Mae Berman, Cambridge, MA—Unofficial	3:08:30
1972	Nina Kuscsik, South Huntington, NY	3:10:26
1973	Jacqueline A. Hansen, Granada Hills, CA	3:05:59
1974	Michiko Gorman, Los Angeles, CA	2:47:11
1975	Liane Winter, Wolfsburg, West Germany	2:42:24
1976	Kim Merritt, Kenosha, WI	2:47:10
1977	Michiko Gorman, Los Angeles, CA	2:48:33
1978	Gayle Barron, Atlanta, GA	2:44:52
1979	Joan Benoit, Cape Elizabeth, ME	2:35:15
1980	Jacqueline Gareau, Montreal, Quebec	2:34:28
1981	Allison Roe, Takapuna, New Zealand	2:26:46
1982	Charlotte Teske, Darmstadt, West Germany	2:29:33
1983	Joan Benoit, Watertown, MA	2:22:43
1984	Lorraine Moller, Putaruru, New Zealand	2:29:28
1985	Lisa Larsen Weidenbach, Battle Creek, MI	2:34:06
1986	Ingrid Kristiansen, Oslo, Norway	2:24:55
1987	Rosa Mota, Porto, Portugal	2:25:21
1988	Rosa Mota, Porto, Portugal	2:24:30
1989	Ingrid Kristiansen, Oslo, Norway	2:24:33
1990	Rosa Mota, Porto, Portugal	2:25:24
1991	Wanda Panfil, Poland	2:24:18
1992	Olga Markova, Russia	2:23:43
1993	Olga Markova, Russia	2:25:27
1994	Uta Pippig, Germany	2:21:45
1995	Uta Pippig, Germany	2:25:11

Appendix B
Runners' Affiliations

Key: **AA** = Athletic Association; **AC** = Athletic Club; **OC** = Olympic Club; **RC** = Running Club;
RR = Road Runners; **TC** = Track Club

AAA Alpine AA
AAC Amscam AC
AC Aloysius Club
AcAA Acme AA
AirC Aircraft Club
ANC Army and Navy Club
ARC Austin RC
ARR Akron RR
ATC Atlanta TC
AthAC Athens AC
AZAA Arizona AA

BAA Boston AA
BAC Bricklayers' Club
BAFB Beal Air Force Base
BaltAA Baltimore AA
BBC Bradford Boat Club
BC Boston College
BCH Bronx Church House
BClub Boys' Club
BEEC Boston Edison
  Employees' Club
BH Bolton Harriers
BHS Brighton High School
BOC Baltimore OC
BS Boston State
BT Boston Typos
BU Boston University
BucAA Buccaneers AA
BunAA Bunting AA

CAC Cygnet AC
CALP14 Cumberland
  American Legion Post 14
CanAC Canadian AC
CAN Army Canadian Army
CapTC Capital TC
CbYMCA Cambridge YMCA
CCAC Culver City AC
CConnAA Central Connecti-
  cut AA
CG Cambridgeport Gym
CharTC Charlottesville TC
CHP Clark Haddard Post
CI Carroll Institute
CIS Carlisle Indian School
CJTC Central Jersey TC
CkG Cook's Gym
CNJTC Central New Jersey TC
ColTC Columbia TC
ConnCAA Connecticut CAA
CPTC Central Park TC

CRC Century Club
CSU Cambridge Sports Union
CTC Chicago TC
CVAC Cumberland Valley AC
CVC City View Club
CYMCA Central YMCA

DAAA Dartmouth AAA
DBC Duncan Boys Club
DC Dorchester Club
DCRRC D.C. Road Runners
  Club
DTC Dunes TC
DTF Delaware Track & Field
DVAA Delaware Valley AA

EBAC Electric Boat AC
EH Empire Harriers
EOC Edmonton OC
ETS East Tennessee State
EYTC East York TC

FAAC Finnish-American AC
FAC Fairlawn AC
FMAA Frood Mine AA
FOC Frisco OC
FS Fairfield Striders
FTC Florida TC
FurTC Furman TC

GAAA Greek-American AA
GAAC Greek-American AC
GAC Glencoe AC
GaelAAC Gaelic-American AC
GBTC Greater Boston TC
GCA Greenwood Commu-
  nity Association
GEAA General Electric AA
GermAAC German-American
  AC
GladAC Gladstone AC
GoodAC Goodwill AC
GSU Georgia State University
GU Georgetown University

HAA Harvard AA
HAC Hurja AC
HamAA Hampshire AA
HamAC Hamilton AC
HartTC Hartford TC
HC Highland Club
HCL Holy Cross Lyceum
HdC Hillsdale College
HETC Human Energy TC

HIAC Hollywood Inn AC
HOC Hamilton OC
HRR Hawaii RR
HTC Hocking TC
HU Harvard University

IAAC Irish-American AC
IAC Illinois AC
ImpAC Imperoyal AC
ISC Interstate Sports Club
ItAC Italian AC

JAC Johnstown AC

KAC Kaleva AC
KAFB Keesler Air Force Base
KC Knights of Columbus
KNS Keene Normal School
KTC Kegonsa TC

LAAC Los Angeles AC
LAC Liberty AC
LBSC Long Beach State
  College
LSAC Logan Square AC
LU Lincoln University
LUTC Laurentian University
  TC
LYMCA Lawrence YMCA

MAA Mercury AA
MAAA Montreal AAA
MAC Mohawk AC
MacAC Maccabi AC
MAFB McGuire Air Force Base
MALP45 Medford American
  Legion Post 45
MALP90 Melrose American
  Legion Post 90
MarAC Marathon AC
MC Marymount College
MCS Motor City Striders
MdC Meadowbrook Club
MedAA Medford AA
MerC Mercury Club
MercAC Mercury AC
MetAC Metropolitan AC
MFA Mount Francis Amis
MHAC Mott Haven AC
MillAA Millrose AA
MillAC Millrose AC
MinnAC Minneapolis AC
MonAC Monarch AC
MornAC Morningside AC

MPAA Mt. Park AA
MS Mohegan Striders
MSN Michigan State Normal
MT Michigan Tech
MtAC Mitch AC

NAA National AA
NAC National AC
NarrAC Narragansett AC
NBC Northwest Boys Club
NBYMCA North Branch
    YMCA
NCAS National Capitol AS
NCS Northern California
    Striders
NCTC North Carolina TC
NDAA North Dorchester AA
NEAC North End AC
NewYMCA Newton YMCA
NHAC New Haven AC
NHC Noel Hants Company
NHTC New Haven TC
NJAC New Jersey AC
NJM New Jersey Masters
NJS New Jersey Striders
NMC North Medford Club
NoAC Noel AC
NOTC Nike Oregon TC
NYAA New York AA
NYAC New York AC
NYC New York Club
NYCP New York City Police
NYMA Norfolk YMA
NYPC New York Pioneer Club

OAA Oakdale AA
OAC Olympic AC
OC Olympic Club
OccC Occidental College
OH Owairaka Harriers
OS Oklahoma State
OstAA Osterville AA
OTC Oregon TC
OU Ohio University
OWU Ohio Wesleyan
    University
OzAC Ozanam AC

PAA Peterboro AA
PAC Pastime AC
PatAC Paterson AC
PaulAC Paulist AC
PC Providence College
PennAC Pennsylvania AC
PP Philadelphia Pioneers
PYMC Polish YMC

RAA Roxbury AA
RAC Rambler AC
RBC Rambler Boys Club
RDAC Red Diamond AC

RichAC Richmond AC
RNAC Royal Navy AC
RpAC Reipas AC
RRAC Royal Rovers AC
RTC Rochester TC

SAA Svithoid AA
SAAA St. Alphonsus AA
SAAC Swedish-American AC
SABC St. Anthony's Boys Club
SAC Star AC
SAGC Swedish A & G Club
SATC San Antonio TC
SBAC St. Bartholomew AC
SBC St. Bartholomew Club
SBG South Boston Gym
SC Swarthmore College
SCAC St. Christopher AC
SCC Shanahan Catholic Club
SCS Southern California
    Striders
SDC Stonewall Democratic
    Club
SFernTC San Fernando TC
SFOC San Francisco OC
SGAC St. George AC
SH Syracuse Harriers
ShamAA Shamrock AA
ShanAC Shanahan AC
ShoreAC Shore AC
SilAC Silverthorne AC
SJC St. John's College
SJTC South Jersey TC
SLTC St. Louis TC
SMAC St. Mary's AC
SMtAC Sugarloaf Mountain
    AC
SMTC Santa Monica TC
SNTS Sampson Naval
    Training Station
SOC Seattle OC
SouthBAC South Boston AC
SPA Sportsmen's PA
SPAA St. Phillip's AA
SPAC St. Phillip's AC
SpAC Spartan AC
SSC Sacramento State College
STAC St. Anselm AC
STC Seniors TC
STCC St. Christopher's Club
SuffAC Suffolk AC
SummAC Summit AC
SWH South Waterloo
    Harriers
SWMC St. Willibrord's
    Men's Club
SyMAC Sydney Mines AC

TAC Trinity AC
TC Third Centenary

TCTC Twin Cities TC
TecAC Tecumseh AC
TFC Track & Field Club
TOC Toronto OC
TP Tappen Post
TS Tidewater Striders
TSdr Tobias Striders
TU Tufts University
TWWC Trinity WWC
TYC Ten Year Club

UC University of Chicago
UCTC University of Chicago
    TC
UG University of Georgia
UK University of Kentucky
UMass University of
    Massachusetts
US University of
    Saskatchewan
USCG United States Coast
    Guard
USMAA United Shoe
    Machinery AA
UV University of Vermont
UWO University of Western
    Ontario

VAC Vermont AC
VOC Vancouver OC
VOS Vancouver Optimist
    Striders

WAA Windsor AA
WAC Worcester AC
WashRC Washington RC
WEAC West End AC
WEYMCA West End YMCA
WHC White Horse Club
WidAC Widlon AC
WinAC Winona AC
WLAC Wolverine AC
WPAL Whitney Post
    American Legion
WPC William Paterson
    College
WRR Williams RR
WRU Western Reserve
    University
WSC Washington Sports Club
WSY West Side Y
WU Wesleyan University
WVirTC West Virginia TC
WVTC West Valley TC

YAC York AC
YMCA Young Men's
    Christian Association

Bibliography

Generally I consulted every Boston newspaper published the day before a given year's marathon, the day of the race, and the day after for race entries, accounts, and results. Usually the stories and quotations were the same and appeared in most of the papers. I list the names of the papers from which I gleaned quotations in particular years, but the same or similar quotes often appeared in other papers. I gathered the quotations and information during days of hibernation in the ancient microtext room of the Boston Public Library, located opposite the Boston Marathon finish line. I took notes with a #2 pencil into a reporter's notebook—a reverse of the process that got the information into the paper in the first place. Where a page number is given, a direct quote was taken from that page—but the source was generally used for additional information.

Introduction

Krout, John Allen. *Annals of American Sport*, The Pageant of America Series, 15 Vol (NY). Cited by Redmond.

Mandell, Richard D. *Sport: A Cultural History*, xiii. New York: Columbia University Press, 1984. This source used to debunk the Pheidippides legend.

Redmond, Gerald. *The Caledonian Games in 19th Century America*, 15. Associated University Press, 1971.

Squires, Bill, & Raymond Krise. *Fast Tracks: The History of Distance Running*, 6, 7. Brattleboro, VT: Stephen Greene Press, 1982.

Stuller, Jay. "Cleanliness Has Only Recently Become a Virtue," *Smithsonian*, February 1991, 126, 127.

Treadwell, Sandy. *The World of Marathons*, 13, 14. New York: Stewart, Tabori & Chang, 1987. Good account of the first Olympic marathon in 1896.

Whitman, Walt. *Leaves of Grass*, 1855, in a *Complete Poetry and Selected Prose*, Boston: Houghton Mifflin, 1959, 192, 199.

Chapter 1—1897-1909

Allen, Frederick Lewis. *The Big Change: America Transforms Itself 1900-1950*, 10. New York: Harper and Row, 1952.

Blaikie, David. *Boston: The Canadian Story*, 38, 39, 40, 49. Ottawa, ON: Seneca House, 1984. Excellent biographies of Caffery and Longboat.

Boston Daily Globe, 20 April 1897, 20 April 1898, 20 April 1899, 20 April 1900, 20 April 1901, 21 April 1901, 20 April 1905, 18 April 1906.

Boston Herald, 20 April 1901, 20 April 1905, 20 April 1906.

Boston Post, 20 April 1897, 20 April 1901, 21 April 1901, 21 April 1903, 19 April 1905, 20 April 1905, 20 April 1906, 20 April 1907.

Kidd, Bruce. *Tom Longboat*, 60-61. Don Mills, ON: Fitzhenry and Whiteside, 1980.

Martin, David E., & Roger W.H. Gynn. *The Marathon Footrace*, 35. Springfield, IL: Charles C Thomas, 1979. A history of all marathons up to 1978, with a list of all sub-2:20 marathons to that year.

Squires, Bill, & Raymond Krise. *Fast Tracks*.

Chapter 2—1910-1919

Blaikie, David. *Boston*, 79, 80, 91.

Boston Evening Transcript, 16 April 1912, 21 April 1914, 20 April 1920.

Boston Globe, 20 April 1917.

Boston Post, 20 April 1910, 20 April 1911, 20 April 1913, 21 April 1914, 20 April 1920.

Marshall, S.L.A. *World War I*, 7. Boston: Houghton Mifflin, 1964.

Urquhart, H.M. *History of the 16th Battalion*, 58. Macmillan of Canada, 1922. Cited by Blaikie.

Chapter 3—1920-1929

Allen, Frederick Lewis. *Only Yesterday*. New York: Harper and Row, 1931.

Blaikie, David. *Boston*, 96, 106.

Boston Globe, 15 April 1926, 20 April 1926.

Boston Herald, 20 April 1923.

Boston Post, 6 April 1923, 20 April 1927.
DeMar, Clarence H. *Marathon*, 14, 82. Shelburne, VT: New England Press, 1981.
Garraty, John A. *The American Nation: A History of the United States*, 698. New York: Harper and Row, 1966.
Kales, David, & Emily Kales. *Boston Harbor Islands*. Millis, MA: Captain George's.
Martin, David E., & Roger W.H. Gynn. *The Marathon Footrace*, 96-98.
Squires, Bill, & Raymond Krise. *Fast Tracks*, 96.
Sweetser, M.F. *King's Handbook of Boston*. Boston: Friends of Boston Harbor, (originally published in 1882).
Williston, Floyd. *Johnny Miles: Nova Scotia's Marathon King*. Halifax, NS: Nimbus Publishing, 1990. A complete biography of Johnny Miles.

Chapter 4—1930-1939

Boston Daily Globe, 19 April 1930.
Boston Post, 19 April 1931, 20 April 1931.
Burroughs, Edgar Rice. *Tarzan of the Apes*, 122. New York: New American Library, 1990 (originally published in 1914).
Lewis, Frederick. *That Golden Distance* [Video]. Boston, 1985.
Semple, John D., Tom Murphy, & John J. Kelley. *Just Call Me Jock*, 51, 55, 56, 133. Waterford, CT: Waterford Publishing, 1981. Jock Semple's own story, told in part by Boston Marathon winner Kelley, for whom Semple became a "father confessor."

Chapter 5—1940-1949

Beagan, Gerry, ed. *Charley Robbins Scrapbook: Running with the Best Since 1936*. Transcribed and edited scrapbook/training log.
Blaikie, David. *Boston*, 135-149.
Boston Globe, 17 April 1940, 19 April 1943, 20 April 1943, 20 April 1945, 20 April 1946.
Boston Herald, 20 April 1942.
Boston Post, 20 April 1948.
I.F. Stone's Weekly, 26 April 1941.
Keegan, John. *The Second World War*, 488, 588. New York: Viking Penguin, 1989.
Semple, John D., Tom Murphy, & John J. Kelley. *Just Call Me Jock*, 125.

Chapter 6—1950-1959

Beagan, Gerry, ed. *Charley Robbins Scrapbook*, 68, 138, 139.
Boston Globe, 20 April 1950, 20 April 1951, 20 April 1952, 21 April 1953, 19 April 1957.
Boston Post, 14 April 1950, 15 April 1951, 12 April 1952.
Boston Traveler, 12 April 1951, 20 April 1951.
Kelley, John J. "Kelley on Kelley." In Frederick Lewis and Dick Johnson, *Young at Heart—The story of Johnny Kelley, Boston's Marathon Man*, 131. Waco, TX: WRS Press, 1992.
Peters, Jim. *In the Long Run*, Chapter 15. London: Cassell, 1955.
Semple, John D., Tom Murphy, & John J. Kelley. *Just Call Me Jock*, 93, 133-137.

Chapter 7—1960-1969

Boston Globe, 20 April 1960.
Boston Sunday Globe, 19 April 1964.
Daws, Ron. *Running Your Best*. Lexington, MA: Stephen Greene Press, 1985.
Daws, Ron. *The Self-Made Olympian*. Mountain View, CA: World Publications, 1977.
Higdon, Hal. *On the Run from Dogs and People*. Chicago: Chicago Review Press, 1979.
Martin, David E., & Roger W.H. Gynn. *The Marathon Footrace*, 233.
Strasser, J.B., & Lori Becklund. *The Story of Nike and the Men Who Played There*, 149. New York: Harcourt, Brace, Jovanovich, 1991.
Wallechinsky, David. *The Complete Book of the Olympics*. New York: Viking Press, 1984.

Chapter 8—1970-1979

Barron, Gayle, with Kim Chapin. *The Beauty of Running*. New York: Harcourt, Brace, Jovanovich, 1980.
Benoit, Joan, with Sally Baker. *Running Tide*, 18. New York: Alfred Knopf, 1987. The complete Joan Benoit story.
Blaikie, David. *Boston*, 157-158, 170-171.

Burton, Sandra. Interview in *Time* quoted by Dave Prokop in *Runner's World*, June 1973.

Hill, Ron. *The Long Hard Road. Part Two: The Peak and Beyond*, 82-100. Hyde, England: Ron Hill Sports, 1982.

Karlgaard, Rich. An interview with Will Cloney, *Runner's World*, June 1977.

Prokop, Dave. *Runner's World*, June 1973.

Prokop, Dave. *Runner's World*, June 1977.

Prokop, Dave. *Runner's World* interview with Jerome Drayton, June 1977.

Rodgers, Bill. *Training Diary*, 1975, unpublished.

Rodgers, Bill, with Joe Concannon. *Marathoning*. New York: Simon and Schuster, 1980.

Rodgers, Bill. *Runner's World*, June 1977.

Tymn, Mike. "A Kick Too Late to Matter," *Runner's World*, June 1978, p. 58.

From 1970 on, much of the source material is my own recollections, observations, and conversations with contemporaries, as well as the usual journalistic interview in person or by telephone. For example, after running the 1970 race I showered in a stall after Ron Hill, and we chatted. One does pick up an attitude if not information after sharing similar experiences. Listing all those personal communications, even if I could, would be tedious and incomplete and have little meaning to subsequent researchers.

Chapter 9—1980-1989, Chapter 10—1990-1995

Benoit, Joan, with Sally Baker. *Running Tide.*

Boston Globe, 16 April 1985.

Goleman, Daniel. *Vital Lies, Simple Truths: The Psychology of Self-Deception*, 107. New York: Simon and Schuster, 1985.

Kahn, Joseph P. "An Image Emerges Clearly," *Running*, September/October 1980.

Maier, Hans. "Seko" *Runner's World*, June 1981.

McDonough, Will. "Marshall and the Marathon," *Boston Globe*, 17 April 1982.

Merrill, Sam. *The Runner*, July 1980.

Perlez, Jan. "Ethiopian Runners Regain Olympic Purpose," *New York Times*, 17 March 1992.

Runner's World, November 1984.

SJC No. M-2895 I.A. Consolidated Appendix, pp. 189-90.

Suffolk Superior Court No. 57376, 60861, on appeal from Superior Court.

Supreme Judicial Court, SJC-3401, SJC-3403.

Supreme Judicial Court: Words in quotations in the Marshall Medoff story come from the transcripts of the Supreme Judicial Court of the Commonwealth of Massachusetts No. M-2895 Vol. I-VI of testimony given over several days in October of 1982.

Temple, Cliff, "Triple Threat," *The Runner*, October 1985.

Wischnia, Bob. "The Pride of Portugal," *Runner's World*, November 1984, p. 60.

Wischnia, Bob, *Runner's World*, April 1984.

From 1983 to 1989, I consulted articles in *New England Runner*, *Runner's World*, *Running Times*, the *Boston Globe*, and the *Boston Herald*. After 1986 I was assisted by press material prepared by John Hancock and the BAA.

After 1980 a rich new source of information was videotapes of (nearly) the entire race broadcast by several Boston stations that covered the full length of the race. Of course, after 1988 the richest source of information was personal interviews done expressly for this book near the time of the race. Some of these interviews were graciously arranged by Pat Lynch of John Hancock.

Epilogue

Ehrlich, Paul, & Ann Ehrlich. *The Population Explosion*. New York: Simon and Schuster, 1990.

Harden, Blaine. *Africa*. Boston: Houghton Mifflin, 1990.

Hobhouse, Henry. *Forces of Change*. New York: Little, Brown, 1989. An unorthodox view of history.

Kennedy, Paul. *Preparing for the Twenty-First Century*. New York: Random House, 1993.

McKibben, Bill. *The End of Nature*. New York: Random House, 1989.

Weiner, Jonathan. *The Next One Hundred Years*. New York: Bantam Books, 1990.

Index

Note: Page numbers in italics refer to photos.

About the Author

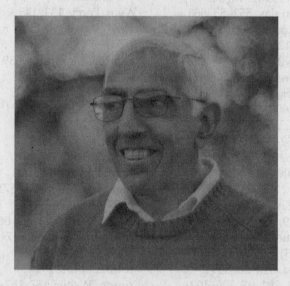

Tom Derderian ran the Boston Marathon for the first time while a senior in high school in Milford, MA, the town next to the marathon start in Hopkinton. He ran track and cross-country at the University of Massachusetts, graduating with a degree in journalism and English literature. He ran in the US Olympic Trials marathons in 1972 and 1976. His fastest Boston was 2:19:04 for 18th place in 1975.

Tom worked in design and development at Nike in Oregon for most of the 1980s. He has several US patents in his name. He has coached high school, college, and post-collegiate teams.

Tom was elected President of USATF-New England for two terms and currently serves on the board as past president.

He is executive producer of the documentary film *BOSTON*.

Today Tom serves as head coach for the Greater Boston Track Club and competes regularly in Masters races. He is a senior writer for New England Runner magazine and has written for many other running publications. Tom's book, *Boston Marathon*, the definitive history of the race, was written in collaboration with the Boston Athletic Association and first published in 1995.

Tom and his wife, Cynthia Hastings, live on the shore in Winthrop, MA, slightly east of Boston. They have two daughters, Jane and Hattie.